CURRENT PEDIATRIC THERAPY

11

SYDNEY S. GELLIS, M.D.

Professor and Emeritus Chairman, Department of Pediatrics,
Tufts University School of Medicine;
Pediatrician-in-Chief Emeritus, Boston Floating Hospital
for Infants and Children,
New England Medical Center, Inc., Boston

BENJAMIN M. KAGAN, M.D.

Director and Chairman, Department of Pediatrics,
Cedars-Sinai Medical Center, Los Angeles;
Professor and Vice Chairman,
Department of Pediatrics,
University of California at Los Angeles

W. B. SAUNDERS COMPANY

Philadelphia   London   Toronto   Mexico City   Rio de Janeiro   Sydney   Tokyo

W. B. Saunders Company: West Washington Square
Philadelphia, PA 19105

1 St. Anne's Road
Eastbourne, East Sussex BN21 3UN, England

1 Goldthorne Avenue
Toronto, Ontario M8Z 5T9, Canada

Apartado 26370—Cedro 512
Mexico 4, D.F., Mexico

Rua Coronel Cabrita, 8
Sao Cristovao Caixa Postal 21176
Rio de Janeiro, Brazil

9 Waltham Street
Artarmon, N.S.W. 2064, Australia

Ichibancho, Central Bldg., 22-1 Ichibancho
Chiyoda-Ku, Tokyo 102, Japan

**The Library of Congress Cataloged the
First Issue of This Serial As Follows:**

RJ52   Current pediatric therapy.   1964–
C8   Philadelphia, Saunders.

    v. 28 cm. biennial.

Editors: 1964–   S. S. Gellis and B. M. Kagan.

1. Pediatrics—Collected works.   2.Therapeutics—
Collected works.   I. Gellis, Sydney S., ed.
II. Kagan, Benjamin M., ed.

RJ52.C8   618.9/2006   64–10484 rev

Library of Congress   [r66i3]

Current Pediatric Therapy 11

ISBN 0–7216–1114–1

Last digit is the print number: 9   8   7   6   5   4   3   2   1

Contributors

James M. Adams, M.D.

Assistant Professor, Department of Pediatrics, Baylor College of Medicine, Houston; Director of Neonatal Intensive Care Unit and Transport Team, Texas Children's Hospital, Houston, Texas.

Tetanus Neonatorum.

Joseph C. Alper, M.D.

Assistant Professor of Medicine, Brown University School of Medicine; Staff Dermatologist and Medical Geneticist, Brown University, Roger Williams General Hospital, Providence, Rhode Island.

The Genodermatoses.

R. Peter Altman, M.D.

Professor of Surgery and Pediatrics, College of Physicians and Surgeons, Columbia University, New York; Director, Pediatric Surgery, Babies Hospital, Columbia-Presbyterian Medical Center, New York, New York.

Tumors of the Liver.

Mary G. Ampola, M.D.

Associate Professor of Pediatrics, Tufts University School of Medicine; Assistant Pediatrician, New England Medical Center, Inc., Boston, Massachusetts.

Amino Acid Disorders (Table).

John A. Anderson, M.D.

Clinical Associate Professor, Department of Pediatrics and Communicable Diseases, University of Michigan School of Medicine, Ann Arbor; Chairman, Department of Pediatrics, and Head, Division of Allergy and Clinical Immunology, Henry Ford Hospital, Detroit, Michigan.

Physical Allergy.

Philip C. Anderson, M.D.

Professor of Medicine, Chairman of Der-matology, University of Missouri School of Medicine; Attending Dermatologist, University of Missouri, Health Sciences Center, Columbia, Missouri.

Insect Stings and Arthropod Bites and Stings.

Joel M. Andres, M.D.

Associate Professor of Pediatrics, University of Florida School of Medicine; Pediatric Gastroenterologist, University of Florida Shands Teaching Hospital, Gainesville, Florida.

Cirrhosis.

Kenneth A. Arndt, M.D.

Associate Professor of Dermatology, Harvard Medical School; Chief of Dermatology, Beth Israel Hospital, Boston, Massachusetts.

Topical Therapy: A Dermatologic Formulary for Pediatric Practice.

Stephen S. Arnon, M.D.

Senior Investigator, Infant Botulism Research Project, California Department of Health Services, Berkeley, California.

Infant Botulism.

Keith W. Ashcraft, M.D.

Clinical Professor, University of Missouri at Kansas City School of Medicine; Chief, Section of Urology, The Children's Mercy Hospital, Kansas City, Missouri.

Pneumothorax and Pneumomediastinum. Chylothorax. Intrathoracic Cysts. Tumors of the Chest. Pulmonary Sequestration. Middle Lobe Syndrome.

Edward Austin, M.D.

Attending Surgeon, Cedars-Sinai Medical Center, Los Angeles, California.

Neonatal Pneumomediastinum and Pneumothorax. Preoperative and Postoperative Care of Patients Undergoing Gastrointestinal Surgery.

Felicia B. Axelrod, M.D.

Associate Professor of Pediatrics, New York University School of Medicine; Associate Attending Pediatrician, New York University-Bellevue Medical Center, New York, New York.

Familial Dysautonomia.

David W. Bailey, M.D.

Associate Professor of Pediatrics, Wayne State University School of Medicine; Associate Chief of Pediatrics, Children's Hospital of Michigan; Medical Director, Detroit Institute for Children, Detroit, Michigan.

Myelodysplasia. Spinal Diseases.

Irving W. Bailit, M.D.

Clinical Instructor in Pediatrics, Harvard University Medical School; Senior Associate in Medicine, Associate in Allergy, Children's Hospital Medical Center, Boston, Massachusetts.

Anaphylaxis.

Roberta A. Ballard, M.D.

Adjunct Assistant Clinical Professor of Pediatrics, University of California at San Francisco Medical Center; Chief of Pediatrics and Director of Newborn Services, Mt. Zion Hospital and Medical Center, San Francisco, California.

Neonatal Resuscitation.

Lewis A. Barness, M.D.

Professor and Chairman, Department of Pediatrics, University of South Florida College of Medicine; Active Staff, Tampa General Hospital; Consulting Staff, All Children's Hospital, St. Joseph's Hospital, Tampa, Florida.

Breast Feeding. Fluid and Electrolyte Therapy.

John G. Bartlett, M.D.

Professor of Medicine, Johns Hopkins University School of Medicine, Chief of Infectious Disease Division, Johns Hopkins Hospital, Baltimore, Maryland.

Infections due to Anaerobic Cocci and Gram-Negative Bacilli.

James W. Bass, M.D.

Professor of Pediatrics, Uniformed Services University of the Health Sciences, Bethesda, Maryland (Tripler Army Medical Center Affiliate); Clinical Professor of Pediatrics, University of Hawaii School of Medicine; Chairman, Department of Pediatrics, Tripler Army Medical Center, Honolulu, Hawaii.

Pertussis.

Mark L. Batshaw, M.D.

Associate Professor of Pediatrics, Johns Hopkins University School of Medicine; Developmental Pediatrician, John F. Kennedy Institute, Baltimore, Maryland.

Mental Retardation.

Arthur L. Beaudet, M.D.

Professor of Pediatrics, Baylor University College of Medicine; Chief, Genetics Service, Texas Children's Hospital, Houston, Texas.

Lysosomal Storage Diseases.

Marc O. Beem, M.D.

Professor of Pediatrics, University of Chicago; Staff Pediatrician, Wyler Children's Hospital, Chicago, Illinois.

Chlamydia.

John W. Benton, M.D.

Professor and Chairman of Pediatrics, University of Alabama in Birmingham School of Medicine; Professor, Department of Neurology (Pediatric Neurologist), Pediatrician-in-Chief, University of Alabama Hospitals; Physician-in-Chief, The Children's Hospital, Birmingham, Alabama.

Guillain-Barré Disease.

Bruce O. Berg, M.D.

Professor of Neurology and Pediatrics, Director, Child Neurology, University of California Medical Center, San Francisco, California.

Acute Ataxia. Neurocutaneous Syndromes.

William H. Bergstrom, M.D.

Professor of Pediatrics Emeritus and Assistant Professor of Biochemistry (Adjunct), State University of New York Upstate Medical Center at Syracuse; Attending Pediatrician, University Hospital and Crouse-Irving Memorial Hospital, Syracuse, New York.

Rickets. Tetany. Idiopathic Hypercalcemia.

Bernard A. Berman, M.D.

Associate Clinical Professor of Pediatrics, Tufts University School of Medicine; Chief, Department of Pediatric Allergy, St. Elizabeth's Hospital, Boston, Massachusetts.

Allergic Rhinitis.

Kenneth W. Bernard, M.D.

Medical Epidemiologist, Division of Viral Diseases, Center for Infectious Diseases, Centers for Disease Control, Atlanta, Georgia.

Rabies.

Shelly C. Bernstein, M.D., Ph.D.

Research Fellow in Pediatrics, Harvard Medical School; Fellow in Medicine (Hematology/Oncology), Children's Hospital Medical Center; Clinical Fellow, Division of Pediatrics, Dana-Farber Cancer Institute, Boston, Massachusetts.
Polycythemia.

Harry C. Bishop, M.D.

Professor of Pediatric Surgery, University of Pennsylvania School of Medicine; Senior Surgeon, Children's Hospital; Consulting Surgeon, University of Pennsylvania, and Jeanes Hospitals, Philadelphia, Pennsylvania.
Intussusception.

Iain F. S. Black, M.D.

Professor of Pediatrics, Temple University School of Medicine; Chief, Section of Cardiology, St. Christopher's Hospital for Children, Philadelphia, Pennsylvania.
Cardiomyopathies and Pericardial Diseases.

Virginia D. Black, M.D.

Assistant Professor of Pediatrics, Wayne State University School of Medicine; Associate Neonatologist, Hutzel Hospital and Children's Hospital of Michigan, Detroit, Michigan.
Hyperviscosity Syndromes.

Richard D. Bland, M.D.

Associate Professor of Pediatrics; Senior Staff, Cardiovascular Research Institute; Attending Staff, Newborn Intensive Care Unit, University of California at San Francisco, California.
Pulmonary Edema.

Bruce D. Blumberg, M.D.

Assistant Clinical Professor of Pediatrics, University of California at San Francisco; Staff Geneticist, Kaiser-Permanente Medical Center, San Francisco, California.
Genetic Diseases.

S. Allan Bock, M.D.

Associate Clinical Professor of Pediatrics, University of Colorado School of Medicine; Senior Staff Physician, National Jewish Hospital/National Asthma Center, Denver, Colorado.
Allergic Gastrointestinal Disorders.

E. Thomas Boles, Jr., M.D.

Professor of Surgery, Ohio State University School of Medicine; Chief, Department of Pediatric Surgery, Children's Hospital, Columbus; Chairman, Division of Pediatric Surgery, Ohio State University; Attending Staff, Children's Hos-

pital and University Hospital, Columbus, Ohio.
Malformations of the Intestine. Foreign Bodies of the Gastrointestinal Tract.

Bonny H. Bowser, M.H.S.A.

Burn Clinical Coordinator, Arkansas Children's Hospital Burn Unit; Research Assistant, University of Arkansas Medical Center, Department of Surgery, Little Rock, Arkansas.
Burns.

Quellin T. Box, M.D.

Associate Professor of Pediatrics and Microbiology, University of Texas Medical Branch, Galveston; Director, Infectious Disease Division, Attending Pediatrician, Child Health Center, Galveston, Texas.
Diphtheria.

William A. Brock, M.D., F.A.A.P.

Assistant Clinical Professor of Surgery/Urology, University of California at San Diego School of Medicine; Senior Staff, Children's Hospital; Attending Staff, University Hospital, San Diego, California.
Renal Hypoplasia and Dysplasia. Urolithiasis.

Itzhak Brook, M.D., M.Sc.

Associate Professor of Pediatrics, Associate Professor of Surgery, Uniformed Services University for the Health Sciences; Attending Staff, Pediatric Infectious Diseases, National Naval Medical Center, Bethesda, Maryland.
Listeria Monocytogenes.

Daniel D. Broughton, M.D.

Assistant Professor of Pediatrics, Mayo Medical School, Rochester, Minnesota.
Epistaxis and Foreign Bodies in the Nose and Pharynx.

Audrey K. Brown, M.D.

Professor and Vice-Chairman, Director of Pediatric Hematology-Oncology, Department of Pediatrics, State University of New York Downstate; Attending Physician, Director of Pediatric Hematology/Oncology, State University Hospital and Kings County Hospital, Brooklyn, New York.
Hyperbilirubinemias due to Metabolic Disturbances.

Nathaniel Brown, M.D.

Assistant Professor, Department of Pediatrics, University of California at Los Angeles School of

Medicine; Staff Physician, University of California at Los Angeles Medical Center, Los Angeles, California.
Burkitt Lymphoma. Infectious Mononucleosis.

Steven D. Budnick, D.D.S.

Associate Professor, Emory University School of Dentistry. Atlanta, Georgia.
Dental Caries. Congenital Epulis of the Neonate.

Kevin A. Burbige, M.D.

Instructor in Clinical Urology, College of Physicians and Surgeons, Columbia University; Attending Urologist, Babies Hospital, Columbia-Presbyterian Medical Center, New York, New York.
Neurogenic Bladder. Vesicoureteral Reflux.

Victor E. Calcaterra, M.D.

Assistant Professor of Otolaryngology, Tufts University School of Medicine; Senior Surgeon, Department of Otolaryngology, New England Medical Center, Boston, Massachusetts.
Disorders of the Larynx.

Fred T. Caldwell, Jr., M.D.

Professor of Surgery, University of Arkansas School of Medicine; Director of Burn Center, Arkansas Children's Hospital; Consultant, Veterans Administration Hospital, Little Rock, Arkansas.
Burns.

William A. Campbell III, M.D.

Clinical Professor of Surgery/Urology, University of Colorado School of Medicine; Chief, Urology Service and Chairman, Department of Pediatric Surgical Specialties, The Children's Hospital, Denver, Colorado.
Malignant Tumors of the Kidney.

Dennis P. Cantwell, M.D.

Joseph Campbell Professor of Child Psychiatry, University of California at Los Angeles School of Medicine; Director of Residency Training in Child Psychiatry, University of California at Los Angeles Neuropsychiatric Institute, Los Angeles, California.
Psychiatric Disorders.

Robert R. Chilcote, M.D.

Assistant Professor, University of Chicago Pritzker School of Medicine; Attending Physician, Wyler Children's Hospital, Chicago, Illinois.
Hemolytic Diseases of the Neonate.

Robert-Gray Choto, M.D.

Chairman, Department of Pediatrics and Child Health, University of Zimbabwe School of Medicine; Attending Staff, Parirenyatwa National Medical Center and Harare Central Hospital, Harare, Zimbabwe; Consultant, Ministry of Health, Republic of Zimbabwe—District and Rural Hospitals and Clinics.
Brucellosis.

Raymond W. M. Chun, M.D.

Professor, Department of Pediatrics and Neurology, University of Wisconsin School of Medicine; Attending Staff, University of Wisconsin Center for Health Sciences, Madison, Wisconsin.
Head Injury. Epidural Hematoma and Subdural Hematoma. Intracranial Hemorrhage.

Abe M. Chutorian, M.D.

Professor of Clinical Neurology and of Clinical Pediatrics, Columbia University College of Physicians and Surgeons; Attending Neurologist, Columbia-Presbyterian Medical Center, New York, New York; Consultant in Neurology, Blythedale Children's Hospital, Valhalla, New York; Director of Pediatric Neurology, Lennox Hill Hospital, New York, New York.
Benign Intracranial Hypertension (Pseudotumor Cerebri).

Richard J. Cleveland, M.D.

Professor and Chairman, Department of Surgery, Tufts University School of Medicine; Director of Surgical Services, New England Medical Center, Boston, Massachusetts.
Pediatric Cardiac Tumors.

Donald J. Cohen, M.D.

Professor of Pediatrics, Psychiatry and Psychology, and Director, Child Study Center, Yale University School of Medicine; Attending Physician, Yale–New Haven Hospital, New Haven, Connecticut.
Attention Deficit Disorder.

Arnold H. Colodny, M.D.

Associate Clinical Professor of Surgery, Harvard Medical School; Senior Surgeon, Associate Director, Division of Urology, Children's Hospital, Boston, Massachusetts.
Circumcision and Disorders of the Penis and Testis.

Harvey R. Colten, M.D.

Professor of Pediatrics, Harvard Medical School; Director of Cystic Fibrosis Program, Chief, Division of Cell Biology, Children's Hospital, Boston, Massachusetts.
Angioneurotic Edema.

James D. Connor, M.D.

Professor of Pediatrics, University of California at San Diego School of Medicine; Consultant, University of California at San Diego Medical Center, Mercy Hospital, and Children's Hospital and Health Center, La Jolla, California.

Plague.

Marvin Cornblath, M.D.

Professor of Pediatrics, University of Maryland; Lecturer, Johns Hopkins University School of Medicine, Baltimore, Maryland.

Inborn Errors of Carbohydrate Metabolism.

Kenneth L. Cox, M.D.

Assistant Professor, Department of Pediatrics, University of California at Davis School of Medicine; Chief, Pediatric Gastroenterology and Codirector of Cystic Fibrosis Center, University of California at Davis Medical Center, Sacramento, California.

Pancreatic Diseases.

Alvin H. Crawford, M.D.

Professor of Orthopedics and Pediatrics, University of Cincinnati College of Medicine; Director of Pediatric Orthopaedics, Children's Hospital Medical Center, Cincinnati, Ohio.

Orthopaedic Disorders of the Extremities.

John F. Crigler, Jr., M.D.

Associate Professor of Pediatrics, Harvard Medical School; Chief, Division of Endocrinology and Senior Associate in Medicine, Department of Medicine, The Children's Hospital, Boston, Massachusetts.

Diabetes Insipidus.

M. Douglas Cunningham, M.D.

Associate Professor of Pediatrics (Neonatology), Department of Pediatrics, College of Medicine, University of Kentucky, Lexington, Kentucky.

Intrauterine Growth Disturbances. Bronchopulmonary Dysplasia. Neonatal Atelectasis. Lobar Emphysema.

C. W. Daeschner, M.D.

Professor and Chairman, Department of Pediatrics, University of Texas Medical Branch at Galveston; Chief, Pediatrics, Child Health Center, University of Texas Medical Branch Hospitals, Galveston, Texas.

Perinephritis and Perirenal Abscess.

Murray Davidson, M.D.

Professor of Pediatrics, Health Sciences Center, State University of New York at Stony Brook;

Director of Pediatrics, Queens Hospital Center; Chief, Pediatric Gastroenterology, Long Island Jewish-Hillside Medical Center, New Hyde Park, New York.

Irritable Colon Syndrome.

Richard D. Diamond, M.D.

Associate Professor of Medicine and Microbiology, Boston University School of Medicine; Associate Visiting Physician and Associate Staff Member, Evans Memorial Hospital, University Hospital, Boston, Massachusetts.

Cryptococcosis.

Marvin L. Dixon, M.D.

Instructor in Pediatrics, Harvard Medical School; Clinical and Research Fellow, Pediatrics GI/Nutritional Unit, Massachusetts General Hospital, Boston, Massachusetts.

Ulcerative Colitis and Crohn's Disease.

Alan K. Done, M.D.

President, Association of Consulting Toxicologists; Attending Pediatrician, Children's Hospital of Michigan, Detroit, Michigan.

Salicylate Poisoning.

George N. Donnell, M.D.

Winzer Professor of Pediatrics, University of Southern California School of Medicine; Pediatrician-in-Chief, Children's Hospital of Los Angeles, California.

The Galactosemias.

Paul R. Dyken, M.D.

Professor and Chief of Pediatric Neurology, Medical College of Georgia, Augusta, Georgia.

Epidural Hematoma and Subdural Hematoma.

Heinz F. Eichenwald, M.D.

William Buchanan Professor of Pediatrics, University of Texas Health Sciences Center, Dallas; Attending Physician, Children's Medical Center, Parkland Memorial Hospital, Dallas; Consulting Physician, St. Paul Hospital, Irving Community Hospital, and Presbyterian Hospital, Dallas, Texas.

Shigellosis.

Mary Allen Engle, M.D.

Stavros S. Niarchos Professor of Pediatric Cardiology, Professor of Pediatrics, Cornell University Medical College; Director, Pediatric Cardiology, New York Hospital, New York, New York.

Congestive Heart Failure.

Moshe A. Ephros, M.D.

Research Fellow and Lecturer in Medicine, Division of Tropical Medicine, Harvard Medical School, Boston, Massachusetts; Staff, Department of Clinical Microbiology, Hadassah Hospital, Jerusalem, Israel.

Malaria. Babesiosis.

Nancy B. Esterly, M.D.

Professor of Pediatrics and Dermatology, Northwestern University Medical School, Chicago; Head, Division of Dermatology, The Children's Memorial Hospital, Chicago, Illinois.

Skin Diseases in the Neonate.

Martin Farber, M.D.

Professor and Deputy Chairman, Department of Obstetrics and Gynecology, Temple University School of Medicine; Chairman, Department of Obstetrics and Gynecology, Albert Einstein Medical Center, Northern Division, Philadelphia, Pennsylvania.

Disorders of the Uterus, Tubes, and Ovaries. Tumors of the Uterus, Tubes and Ovaries. Disorders of the Vulva and Vagina.

Ralph D. Feigin, M.D.

J. S. Abercrombie Professor of Pediatrics and Chairman, Department of Pediatrics, Baylor College of Medicine, Houston; Physician-in-Chief, Texas Children's Hospital, Houston; Physician-in-Chief, Pediatric Services, Harris County Hospital District (Ben Taub General and Jefferson Davis Hospitals); Chief, Pediatric Service, Methodist Hospital, Houston, Texas.

Bacterial Meningitis and Septicemia Beyond the Neonatal Period. Leptospirosis. Meningococcal Disease.

Sandor Feldman, M.D.

Associate Professor, Department of Pediatrics, University of Tennessee Center for the Health Sciences; Associate Member, Division of Infectious Diseases, Director of General Pediatrics, St. Jude Children's Research Hospital, Memphis, Tennessee.

Typhoid Fever. Salmonellosis.

Robert Festa, M.D., F.A.A.P.

Assistant Professor of Pediatrics, State University of New York at Stony Brook School of Medicine, Health Sciences Center; Staff Pediatric Hematologist-Oncologist, Department of Pediatrics of the Children's Hospital of Long Island Jewish-Hillside Medical Center, New Hyde Park, New York.

Aplastic Anemia.

Jo David Fine, M.D.

Assistant Professor and Director of Research, Department of Dermatology, University of Alabama in Birmingham School of Medicine; Dermatologist, University Hospital, Veterans Administration Hospital, Children's Hospital, Cooper Green Hospital, Birmingham, Alabama.

Topical Therapy: A Dermatologic Formulary for Pediatric Practice.

Richard N. Fine, M.D.

Professor of Pediatrics, University of California at Los Angeles Center for the Health Sciences; Head, Division of Pediatric Nephrology, University of California at Los Angeles Hospitals and Clinics; Consultant, Cedars-Sinai Medical Center, Olive View Medical Center, Kern County Medical Center.

Chronic Renal Failure. Hemodialysis. Renal Transplantation.

Delbert A. Fisher, M.D.

Professor of Pediatrics and Medicine, University of California at Los Angeles School of Medicine; Staff Physician, Los Angeles County Harbor-UCLA Medical Center, Los Angeles, California.

Thyroid Disease.

Abe R. Fosson, M.D.

Professor, Department of Pediatrics, Department of Behavioral Science, College of Medicine, University of Kentucky; Attending Pediatrician, University Hospital; Consulting Pediatrician, Cardinal Hill Hospital, Shriners Hospital, and St. Joseph Hospital, Lexington, Kentucky.

Histoplasmosis.

Ralph C. Frates, Jr., M.D.

Assistant Professor of Pediatrics and Rehabilitation, Baylor College of Medicine, Houston; Attending Physician, Texas Children's Hospital, The Institution for Rehabilitation and Research, and Ben Taub General Hospital, Houston, Texas.

Near-Drowning: An Update.

Ellen Mae Friedman, M.D.

Instructor, Harvard Medical School; Assistant, Children's Hospital Medical Center, Boston, Massachusetts.

Retropharyngeal and Lateral Pharyngeal Abscesses.

William F. Friedman, M.D.

J. H. Nicholson Professor of Pediatrics, University of California at Los Angeles; Chairman, Department of Pediatrics, Attending Pediatric

Cardiologist, University of California at Los Angeles Medical Center, Los Angeles, California.
Congenital Heart Disease.

Stephen L. Gans, M.D., F.A.C.S., F.A.A.P.
Clinical Professor of Surgery, University of California at Los Angeles School of Medicine; Attending Surgeon, Children's Hospital of Los Angeles and Cedars-Sinai Medical Center, Los Angeles, California.
Preoperative and Postoperative Care of Patients Undergoing Gastrointestinal Surgery.

Lawrence M. Gartner, M.D.
Professor and Chairman, Department of Pediatrics, University of Chicago Pritzker School of Medicine; Director, Wyler Children's Hospital, Chicago, Illinois.
Hemolytic Diseases of the Neonate.

Henry Gelband, M.D.
Professor of Pediatrics (Cardiology) and Pharmacology, Department of Pediatrics, University of Miami School of Medicine; Director, Pediatric Cardiology, University of Miami/Jackson Memorial Medical Center, Miami, Florida.
Cardiac Arrhythmias.

Stephen E. Gellis, M.D.
Assistant Professor of Dermatology and Pediatrics, Tufts University Medical School, Boston; Dermatologist, New England Medical Center, Boston, Massachusetts.
Warts and Molluscum Contagiosum. Miscellaneous Dermatoses.

Barbara L. George, M.D.
Assistant Professor of Pediatrics, University of California at Los Angeles: Attending Pediatrician, Attending Pediatric Cardiologist, University of California at Los Angeles Medical Center, Los Angeles, California.
Congenital Heart Disease.

Anne A. Gershon, M.D.
Professor of Pediatrics, New York University School of Medicine; Attending Physician, University Hospital and Bellevue Hospital, New York, New York.
Immunization Practice.

Hubert L. Gerstman, D.Ed., F.A.S.H.A.
Associate Professor of Otolaryngology and Head and Neck Surgery, Rehabilitation Department, Tufts University School of Medicine; Chief,

Speech, Hearing, and Language Center, New England Medical Center, Boston, Massachusetts.
Hearing Loss.

Barbara A. Gilchrest, M.D.
Associate Professor, School of Dermatology, Tufts University School of Medicine; Dermatologist, New England Medical Center Hospital, Boston, Massachusetts.
Photodermatoses.

Gerald S. Gilchrist, M.B., B.Ch.
Professor and Vice-Chairman, Department of Pediatrics, Mayo Medical School; Consultant in Pediatric Hematology and Oncology; Director, Comprehensive Hemophilia Center, Mayo Clinic and Mayo Foundation, Rochester, Minnesota.
Hemorrhagic Disorders.

Charles N. Glassman, M.D.
Fellow in Section of Pediatric Urology, Mayo Clinic and Mayo Foundation, Rochester, Minnesota; Private Practice, White Plains, New York.
Patent Urachus and Urachal Cysts. Exstrophy of the Bladder.

Bess G. Gold, M.D.
Assistant Professor of Child Health and Development, George Washington University School of Medicine and the Health Sciences; Attending Physician, Infectious Diseases, Children's Hospital National Medical Center, Washington, D.C.
Rhinitis and Sinusitis

Richard B. Goldbloom, M.D.
Professor and Head, Department of Pediatrics, Dalhousie University, Halifax; Physician-in-Chief, the Izaak Walton Killam Hospital for Children, Halifax, Nova Scotia, Canada.
General Malnutrition. Vitamin Deficiencies and Excesses. Idiopathic Cortical Hyperostoses. The Croup Syndrome. Nasopharyngitis.

Gerald S. Golden, M.D.
Professor of Pediatrics and Neurology, University of Texas Medical Branch, Galveston, Texas.
Degenerative Diseases of the Nervous System.

Dennis Goldfinger, M.D.
Associate Pathologist, Section of Blood Banking, Cedars-Sinai Medical Center, Los Angeles, California.
Adverse Reactions to Blood Transfusion.

David Goldring, M.D.
Professor of Pediatrics, Washington University

Medical School, St. Louis; Staff Physician, St. Louis Children's Hospital; Attending Physician, Barnes Hospital, St. Louis, Missouri.
Systemic Hypertension.

Gary Gorlick, M.D., M.P.H.

Assistant Clinical Professor of Pediatrics, University of California at Los Angeles School of Medicine; Attending Pediatrician, Pediatric Dermatology Clinic, Cedars-Sinai Medical Center, Los Angeles, California.
Eruptions in the Diaper Region.

Samuel P. Gotoff, M.D.

Professor and Associate Chairman, Department of Pediatrics, University of Chicago Pritzker School of Medicine; Chairman, Department of Pediatrics, Michael Reese Hospital and Medical Center, Chicago, Illinois.
Group B Streptococcal Infections.

Jeffrey B. Gould, M.D., M.P.H.

Deputy Director of Maternal and Child Health, School of Public Health, University of California at Berkeley; Neonatologist, Children's Hospital of San Francisco; Pediatric Consultant, Health Department, Contra Costa County, California.
Preparation of the Neonate for Transfer.

Alexander A. Green, M.D.

Associate Professor, Department of Pediatrics, University of Tennessee Center for the Health Sciences; Member, Division of Hematology-Oncology, St. Jude Children's Research Hospital, Memphis, Tennessee.
Neuroblastoma.

Richard Green, M.D.

Professor, Department of Psychiatry, State University of New York at Stony Brook, New York.
Homosexual Behavior.

Nahman H. Greenberg, M.D.

Professor of Psychiatry, University of Illinois School of Medicine; Attending Psychiatrist, University of Illinois Hospital, Illinois Masonic Medical Center, Chicago, Illinois.
Child Abuse.

Donald E. Greydanus, M.D.

Director, Adolescent Medicine Program, Raymond Blank Memorial Hospital, Iowa Methodist Medical Center, Des Moines, Iowa.
Adolescent Sexuality, Contraception, Abortion, and Pregnancy.

Robert C. Griggs, M.D.

Professor of Neurology, Medicine, and Pediatrics, University of Rochester School of Medicine and Dentistry; Director of Neuromuscular Disease Clinic and Neurologist, Strong Memorial Hospital, Rochester, New York.
Periodic Paralysis.

Charles Grose, M.D.

Associate Professor, Department of Pediatrics, University of Texas Health Science Center, San Antonio, Texas.
Acute Infectious Lymphocytosis.

Moses Grossman, M.D.

Professor and Vice-Chairman, Department of Pediatrics, University of California at San Francisco; Chief of Pediatrics, San Francisco General Hospital, San Francisco, California.
Neonatal Septicemia, Meningitis, and Pneumonia.

Peter C. Gruenberg, M.D.

Fellow in Pediatric Ophthalmology, Jules Stein Eye Institute, Los Angeles, California.
The Eye.

Warren E. Grupe, M.D.

Associate Professor of Pediatrics, Harvard Medical School; Director, Pediatric Nephrology, The Children's Hospital, Boston, Massachusetts.
Hemolytic-Uremic Syndrome.

Joyce D. Gryboski, M.D.

Professor of Pediatrics, Yale University School of Medicine; Attending Staff, Yale-New Haven Medical Center, New Haven, Connecticut.
Disorders of the Hepatobiliary Tree.

Jerome S. Haller, M.D.

Associate Professor of Pediatrics (Neurology), Tufts University School of Medicine; Pediatric Neurologist, Boston Floating Hospital, New England Medical Center, Inc., Boston, Massachusetts.
Cerebral Edema. Reye Syndrome.

Chrystie C. Halsted, M.D.

Clinical Associate Professor of Pediatrics, University of California at Davis School of Medicine, Davis, California.
Tularemia.

K. Michael Hambidge, M.D., F.R.C.P. (Edin.)

Professor of Pediatrics, University of Colorado

Health Sciences Center; Attending Pediatrician, University Hospital, Denver, Colorado.
Zinc Deficiency.

Ronald C. Hansen, M.D.

Assistant Professor of Internal Medicine (Dermatology) and Pediatrics, University of Arizona School of Medicine; Staff Dermatologist, Arizona Health Sciences Center; Consulting Dermatologist, Tucson Veterans Administration Medical Center, Kino Community Hospital, and Maricopa Medical Center, Tucson, Arizona.
Papulosquamous Disorders. Discoid Lupus Erythematosus.

Herbert S. Harned, Jr., M.D.

Professor of Pediatrics, University of North Carolina School of Medicine; Attending Physician, North Carolina Memorial Hospital, Chapel Hill, North Carolina.
Hypotension.

Burton H. Harris, M.D.

Professor of Surgery, Tufts University School of Medicine; Senior Pediatric Surgeon, Boston Floating Hospital/New England Medical Center, Boston, Massachusetts.
Pulmonary Embolism. Branchial Arch Cysts and Sinuses. Thyroglossal Duct Cysts.

William E. Hathaway, M.D.

Professor of Pediatrics, University of Colorado School of Medicine; Attending Staff, University Hospital and Denver General Hospital, Denver, Colorado.
Disseminated Intravascular Coagulation and Purpura Fulminans.

Michael Hattwick, M.D.

Clinical Assistant Professor, Georgetown University School of Medicine; Consultant in Medicine and Community Medicine, Georgetown University; Attending Physician, Fairfax Hospital, Washington, D.C.
Rickettsial Disease.

F. Ann Hayes, M.D.

Associate Professor, Department of Pediatrics, University of Tennessee Center for the Health Sciences; Associate Member, Division of Hematology-Oncology, St. Jude Children's Research Hospital, Memphis, Tennessee.
Neuroblastoma.

Karen Hein, M.D.

Assistant Professor of Pediatrics, Columbia University College of Physicians and Surgeons; Director, Division of Adolescent Medicine, Babies Hospital (Presbyterian Hospital), New York, New York.
Menstrual Disorders.

Douglas C. Heiner, M.D.

Professor of Pediatrics and Chief, Department of Immunology and Allergy, Los Angeles County Harbor-University of California at Los Angeles Medical Center.
Primary Pulmonary Hemosiderosis.

William C. Heird, M.D.

Associate Professor of Pediatrics, Columbia University College of Physicians and Surgeons; Associate Attending Pediatrician, Babies Hospital (Presbyterian Hospital), New York, New York.
Feeding the Low Birth Weight Infant.

Fred W. Henderson, M.D.

Assistant Professor of Pediatrics, University of North Carolina School of Medicine; Attending Pediatrician, North Carolina Memorial Hospital, Chapel Hill, North Carolina.
Bronchitis and Bronchiolitis.

Terry W. Hensle, M.D.

Associate Professor of Urology, Columbia University College of Physicians and Surgeons; Director, Pediatric Urology, Babies Hospital, Columbia-Presbyterian Medical Center, New York, New York.
Vesicoureteral Reflux.

John J. Herbst, M.D.

Professor of Pediatrics, University of Utah School of Medicine; Attending Physician, University of Utah Medical Center and Primary Children's Medical Center, Salt Lake City, Utah.
Cystic Fibrosis.

Melvin B. Heyman, M.D.

Assistant Professor of Pediatrics, University of California at San Francisco.
Resurrent Abdominal Pain.

J. Roger Hollister, M.D.

Associate Professor of Pediatrics, University of Colorado Health Sciences Center; Senior Staff Physician, National Jewish Hospital/National Asthma Center, Denver, Colorado.
Collagen Vascular Disease.

Neil A. Holtzman, M.D.

Associate Professor of Pediatrics, Johns Hopkins University School of Medicine; Attending Pedia-

trician, Johns Hopkins Hospital, Baltimore, Maryland.
Hyperphenylalaninemias.

Walter T. Hughes, M.D.
Professor of Pediatrics, University of Tennessee Center for the Health Sciences; Chairman, Division of Infectious Diseases, St. Jude Children's Research Hospital.
Pneumocystis Carinii Pneumonitis.

Sidney Hurwitz, M.D.
Clinical Professor of Pediatrics and Dermatology, Yale University School of Medicine; Attending Physician in Pediatrics and Dermatology, Yale-New Haven Medical Center and Hospital of St. Raphael, New Haven, Connecticut.
Vesiculobullous Disorders of Childhood.

Peter R. Huttenlocher, M.D.
Professor of Pediatrics and Neurology, University of Chicago School of Medicine; Attending Physician, Wyler Children's Hospital, Chicago, Illinois.
Headache.

Carol B. Hyman, M.D.
Attending Pediatric Hematologist-Oncologist, Cedars-Sinai Medical Center and Children's Hospital of Los Angeles, Los Angeles, California.
Thalassemia. Iron Poisoning.

Susan T. Iannaccone, M.D., F.A.A.N.
Assistant Professor of Pediatrics and Neurology, University of Cincinnati Medical Center; Attending Physician, Children's Hospital Medical Center and University Hospital, Cincinnati, Ohio.
Myasthenia Gravis.

David Ingall, M.D.
Professor of Pediatrics and Obstetrics and Gynecology, Northwestern University Medical School; Chairman, Department of Pediatrics, Evanston Hospital; Active Attending Pediatrician, Children's Memorial Hospital, Chicago, Illinois.
Syphilis.

J. T. Jabbour, M.D.
Director, Pediatric Neurology, Clinical Professor, Pediatric Neurology, University of Tennessee College of Medicine; Attending Staff, Le Bonheur Children's Medical Center, Memphis, Tennessee.
Hydrocephalus.

Alvin H. Jacobs, M.D.
Emeritus Professor of Dermatology and Pediatrics (Active), Department of Dermatology, Stanford University School of Medicine, Stanford, California.
Atopic Dermatitis.

Robert R. Jacobson, M.D., Ph.D.
Clinical Instructor, Medicine, Louisiana State University School of Medicine; Chief, Clinical Branch, National Hansen's Disease Center, Carville, Louisiana.
Leprosy.

D. Geraint James, M.A., M.D., F.R.C.P.
Dean and Senior Physician, Royal Northern Hospital, London, England.
Sarcoidosis.

Guinter Kahn, M.D.
Director, Pediatric Dermatology Seminars, Miami, Florida.
Skin Tumors.

Barton A. Kamen, M.D., Ph.D.
Associate Professor, Pediatrics and Pharmacology/Toxicology, Medical College of Wisconsin; Attending Physician, Milwaukee Children's Hospital, Milwaukee, Wisconsin.
Megaloblastic and Macrocytic Anemias.

George W. Kaplan, M.D., F.A.A.P., F.A.C.S.
Clinical Professor of Surgery and Pediatrics, University of California at San Diego School of Medicine; Chief of Pediatric Urology, University Hospital; Attending Urologist, Children's Hospital, San Diego, California.
Urolithiasis. Renal Hypoplasia and Dysplasia.

Collin S. Karmody, M.D.
Professor of Otolaryngology, Tufts University School of Medicine; Senior Surgeon, Boston Floating Hospital, New England Medical Center, Inc.; Consultant, U.S. Public Health Service Hospital, Boston, Massachusetts.
Malformations of the Nose. Tumors and Polyps of the Nose. Nasal Injuries. Injuries of the Middle Ear.

Arnold E. Katz, M.D., M.S.
Associate Professor of Otolaryngology, Tufts University School of Medicine; Surgeon, New England Medical Center Hospital, Boston; Acting Chief of Otolaryngology, U.S. Public Health Service Hospital, Brighton, Massachusetts.
Hearing Loss.

Henry K. Kawamoto, Jr., M.D., D.D.S.

Associate Clinical Professor, University of California at Los Angeles School of Medicine, Division of Plastic Surgery; Attending Staff, St. John Hospital, Santa Monica, Santa Monica Hospital, Sepulveda Veterans Administration Hospital, and University of California at Los Angeles Center for the Health Sciences, Los Angeles, California.
Craniofacial Malformations.

Panayotis P. Kelalis, M.D.

Professor of Urology, Mayo Medical School; Chairman, Department of Urology, Mayo Clinic and Mayo Foundation, Rochester, Minnesota.
Patent Urachus and Urachal Cysts.
Exstrophy of the Bladder.

Margaret A. Keller, M.D.

Assistant Professor of Pediatrics, University of California at Los Angeles School of Medicine; Director, Children's Ward, Los Angeles County Harbor-UCLA Medical Center.
Systemic Mycoses.

Doris Sanders Kelsey, M.D.

Associate Professor, Department of Pediatrics, Wake Forest University Bowman Gray School of Medicine, Winston-Salem, North Carolina.
Encephalitis Infections—Postinfectious and Postvaccinial.

Edwin L. Kendig, Jr., M.D.

Professor of Pediatrics, The Medical College of Virginia Health Sciences Division, Virginia Commonwealth University, Richmond; Director of Pediatrics, St. Mary's Hospital, Richmond, Virginia.
Tuberculosis.

Joseph L. Kennedy, Jr., M.D.

Associate Professor of Pediatrics, Tufts University School of Medicine; Director of Nurseries, St. Margaret's Hospital for Women, Boston, Massachusetts.
Birth Injuries.

Thomas L. Kennedy, M.D.

Assistant Professor of Pediatrics, University of Connecticut School of Medicine, Farmington; Attending Pediatrician, Pediatric Nephrologist, University of Connecticut Health Center, John Dempsey Hospital, Farmington, Connecticut.
Renal Venous Thrombosis.

Thomas P. Keon, M.D.

Assistant Professor of Anesthesia, University of Pennsylvania School of Medicine, Philadelphia; Senior Anesthesiologist, The Children's Hospital of Philadelphia, Pennsylvania.
Malignant Hyperthermia.

Maurice A. Kibel, D.C.H., F.R.C.P. (Edin.)

Stella and Paul Loewenstein Professor of Child Health, University of Cape Town; Principal Pediatrician, Children's Hospital, Cape Town, Republic of South Africa.
Infantile Colic.

George T. Klauber, M.D.

Professor of Urology and Pediatrics, Tufts University School of Medicine; Chief, Division of Pediatric Urology, Boston Floating Hospital for Infants and Children and New England Medical Center, Boston, Massachusetts.
Circumcision and Disorders of the Penis and Testis.

Jerome O. Klein, M.D.

Professor of Pediatrics, Boston University School of Medicine; Acting Director, Department of Pediatrics, Boston City Hospital, Boston, Massachusetts.
Bacterial Pneumonia.

Peter K. Kottmeier, M.D.

Professor and Director of Pediatric Surgery, State University of New York College of Medicine, Downstate Medical Center, Brooklyn, New York.
Peptic Ulcers. Gastritis.

Saul Krugman, M.D.

Professor of Pediatrics, New York University School of Medicine; Attending Pediatrician, University Hospital and Bellevue Hospital, New York, New York.
Viral Hepatitis.

John W. Kulig, M.D.

Assistant Professor of Pediatrics, Tufts University School of Medicine; Director, Adolescent Medicine, New England Medical Center, Boston, Massachusetts.
Sexually Transmitted Diseases.

Philip Lanzkowsky, M.D., F.R.C.P., D.C.H., F.A.A.P.

Professor of Pediatrics, Department of Pediatrics, State University of New York at Stony Brook School of Medicine, Health Sciences Center;

Chief of Pediatric Hematology-Oncology, Chairman of Pediatrics, and Chief-of-Staff, Children's Hospital of Long Island Jewish-Hillside Medical Center, New Hyde Park, New York.

Aplastic Anemia.

Allan Lavetter, M.D.

Clinical Associate Professor of Pediatrics and Medicine, Stanford University School of Medicine; Staff Pediatrician and Infectious Disease Consultant, Kaiser Santa Clara Medical Center; Attending Pediatrician and Infectious Disease Consultant, Santa Clara Valley Medical Center, Santa Clara, California.

Coccidioidomycosis.

Emanuel Lebenthal, M.D.

Professor of Pediatrics, State University of New York at Buffalo School of Medicine; Chief, Division of Pediatric Gastroenterology and Nutrition, Children's Hospital of Buffalo, New York.

Malabsorption Syndromes and Chronic Diarrhea.

Martha L. Lepow, M.D.

Professor of Pediatrics, Albany Medical College, Attending Pediatrician, Albany Medical Center; Consultant Pediatrician, St. Peter's Hospital, Albany, New York.

Hemophilus Influenzae Infections.

Brigid G. Leventhal, M.D.

Associate Professor, Oncology and Pediatrics, Johns Hopkins University School of Medicine; Director, Pediatric Oncology, Johns Hopkins Hospital, Baltimore, Maryland.

Lymphedema.

Lenore S. Levine, M.D.

Professor of Pediatrics, Cornell University Medical College; Attending Pediatrician, The New York Hospital, New York, New York.

Disorders of the Adrenal Gland.

Melvin D. Levine, M.D.

Associate Professor of Pediatrics, Harvard Medical School; Chief, Division of Ambulatory Pediatrics, The Children's Hospital, Boston, Massachusetts.

Constipation and Encopresis.
Disorders of Learning and Attention.

Myron M. Levine, M.D.

Professor, Division of Infectious Diseases, University of Maryland School of Medicine; Professor and Director, Center for Vaccine Develop-

opment, University of Maryland School of Medicine, Baltimore, Maryland.

Cholera.

Selwyn B. Levitt, M.D.

Adjunct Clinical Professor of Urology, New York Medical College, Valhalla; Visiting Clinical Professor of Pediatric Urology, Albert Einstein College of Medicine, New York; Codirector, Section of Pediatric Urology, Westchester Medical Center, Attending Pediatric Urologist, Albert Einstein College Hospital, Montefiore Hospital and Medical Center, and Bronx Municipal Hospital Center, New York, New York.

Hydronephrosis and Disorders of the Ureter.

Michael B. Lewis, M.D.

Associate Professor of Surgery, Tufts University School of Medicine; Chief, Division of Plastic Surgery, New England Medical Center, Inc., Boston, Massachusetts.

Diseases and Injuries of the Oral Region.

James J. Leyden, M.D.

Professor of Dermatology, University of Pennsylvania School of Medicine; Chief, Dermatology Clinic, Hospital of the University of Pennsylvania, Philadelphia, Pennsylvania.

Pyodermas.

Barbara M. Lippe, M.D.

Professor of Pediatrics, University of California at Los Angeles School of Medicine, Los Angeles, California.

Ambiguous Genitalia.

Jeffrey M. Lipton, M.D., Ph.D.

Assistant Professor of Pediatrics, Harvard Medical School; Associate in Medicine, Children's Hospital Medical Center; Assistant Physician, Dana-Farber Cancer Institute, Boston, Massachusetts.

The Histiocytosis Syndromes.

Chien Liu, M.D.

Professor of Medicine and of Pediatrics, University of Kansas College of Health Sciences; Attending Physician and Director, Division of Infectious Diseases, University of Kansas Medical Center, Kansas City, Kansas.

Psittacosis.

David A. Lloyd, M.D.

Associate Professor of Pediatric Surgery, University of Pittsburgh; Pediatric Surgeon, Children's Hospital of Pittsburgh, Pennsylvania.

Hirschsprung's Disease. Disorders of the Anus and Rectum. Chest Wall Deformities.

Anne W. Lucky, M.D.

Associate Professor of Dermatology and Pediatrics, University of Cincinnati College of Medicine; Head, Division of Pediatric Dermatology, Children's Hospital Medical Center, Cincinnati; Attending Staff, Dermatology Department, University Hospital, and Division of Pediatric Dermatology, Children's Hospital Medical Center, Cincinnati, Ohio.

Disorders of the Hair and Scalp. Disorders of Sebaceous Glands and Sweat Glands.

John N. Lukens, M.D.

Professor of Pediatrics, Vanderbilt University School of Medicine; Director, Pediatric Hematology-Oncology, Vanderbilt University Children's Hospital, Nashville, Tennessee.

Anemia of Iron Deficiency, Blood Loss, Renal Disease, and Chronic Infection.

Elizabeth R. McAnarney, M.D.

George Washington Goler Associate Professor of Pediatrics, University of Rochester Medical Center, Strong Memorial Hospital; Senior Associate Pediatrician, Strong Memorial Hospital, Rochester, New York.

Adolescent Sexuality, Contraception, Abortion, and Pregnancy. Premarital Counseling.

Wallace W. McCrory, M.D.

Professor of pediatrics, Cornell University Medical College; Director, Division of Pediatric Nephrology, New York Hospital, New York, New York.

Glomerulonephritis.

Trevor J. I. McGill, M.D.

Associate Professor of Otolaryngology, Harvard Medical School; Associate Otolaryngologist-in-Chief, Children's Hospital Medical Center, Boston, Massachusetts.

The Tonsil and Adenoid Problem.

Guy M. McKhann, M.D.

Kennedy Professor and Chairman of Neurology, Johns Hopkins University School of Medicine; Neurologist-in-Chief, The Johns Hopkins Hospital, Baltimore, Maryland.

Chronic Relapsing Polyneuropathy.

Robert H. McLean, M.D.

Associate Professor of Pediatrics, Johns Hopkins University School of Medicine; Director, Division of Pediatric Nephrology, The Johns Hopkins Hospital, Baltimore, Maryland.

Renal Venous Thrombosis.

Noel K. Maclaren, M.D.

Professor, Pathology and Pediatrics, University of Florida College of Medicine; Director, Clinical Chemistry, Shands Hospital, Gainesville; Associate, Division of Endocrinology and Metabolism, Department of Pediatrics, Shands Hospital, Gainesville, Florida.

Gynecomastia. Hyperlipoproteinemias. Inborn Errors of Carbohydrate Metabolism.

Amos E. Madanes, M.D.

Assistant Professor of Gynecology, Loyola University Stritch School of Medicine; Division of Reproductive Endocrinology, Department of Obstetrics and Gynecology, Loyola University Medical Center, Maywood, Illinois.

Disorders of the Vulva and Vagina. Disorders of the Uterus, Tubes, and Ovaries. Tumors of the Uterus, Tubes and Ovaries.

Mohammad H. Malekzadeh, M.D.

Associate Professor of Pediatrics, University of Southern California School of Medicine; Attending Pediatric Nephrologist, Children's Hospital of Los Angeles, Los Angeles, California.

Tumors of the Bladder and Prostate. Disorders of the Lower Urinary Tract.

Herbert C. Mansmann, Jr., M.D.

Professor of Pediatrics, Associate Professor of Medicine, Director, Division of Allergy and Clinical Immunology, Jefferson Medical College, Thomas Jefferson University; Director, Asthma and Pulmonary Program, Children's Heart Hospital, Philadelphia, Pennsylvania.

Bronchial Asthma.

Leonard C. Marcus, V.M.D., M.D.

Associate Professor of Comparative Medicine, Tufts University School of Veterinary Medicine; Associate Staff, New England Medical Center, Boston, Massachusetts.

Visceral Larva Migrans.

Andrew M. Margileth, M.D.

Professor and Vice Chairman, Department of Pediatrics, Uniformed Services University of the Health Sciences; Senior Attending Pediatrician, Naval Hospital, Bethesda, Maryland, Walter Reed Army Medical Center, Children's Hospital National Medical Center, Washington, D.C.

Nontuberculous (Atypical) Mycobacterial Infections.

Alan N. Marks, M.D.

Associate Clinical Professor of Psychiatry, Assistant Professor of Pediatrics, Tufts University School of Medicine; Director, Inpatient

Child Psychiatry Service, Inc., Boston, Massachusetts.

Autism.

Melvin I. Marks, M.D.

Professor of Pediatrics, Adjunct Professor of Microbiology/Immunology, University of Oklahoma Health Sciences Center; Director, Infectious Disease Service, Oklahoma Children's Memorial Hospital; Medical Director, Microbiology Laboratory, Virology/Serology Laboratories, Oklahoma Children's Memorial Hospital, Oklahoma City, Oklahoma.

Yersinia Enterocolitica Infections. Peritonitis.

Alvin M. Mauer, M.D.

Professor, Department of Pediatrics, University of Tennessee Center for the Health Sciences; Director, St. Jude Children's Research Hospital, Memphis, Tennessee.

Neuroblastoma.

Jack K. Mayfield, M.D.

Attending Surgeon and Consultant in Pediatric Orthopaedics, Phoenix Pediatric Residency Program, Phoenix Children's Hospital, Phoenix, Arizona.

Disorders of the Spine and Shoulder Girdle.

H. Cody Meissner, M.D.

Assistant Professor of Pediatrics, Tufts University School of Medicine; Attending Physician in Infectious Diseases, Boston Floating Hospital, New England Medical Center, Inc., Boston, Massachusetts.

Lyme Disease. Acute Aseptic Meningitis. Measles.

Marian E. Melish, M.D.

Associate Professor of Pediatrics, Tropical Medicine, and Medical Microbiology, John A. Burns School of Medicine, University of Hawaii; Infectious Disease Consultant, Kapiolani Children's Medical Center, Honolulu, Hawaii.

Kawasaki Syndrome.

John H. Menkes, M.D.

Clinical Professor of Pediatrics and Neurology, University of California at Los Angeles School of Medicine; Attending Staff, University of California at Los Angeles Center for the Health Sciences, Cedars-Sinai Medical Center, Los Angeles, California.

Seizure Disorders.

Harold Meyer, M.D.

Associate Executive Secretary, American Board

of Pediatrics; Clinical Professor of Pediatrics, University of North Carolina School of Medicine; Attending Pediatrician, North Carolina Memorial Hospital, Chapel Hill, North Carolina.

Pylorospasm.

Richard D. Meyer, M.D.

Associate Professor of Medicine, University of California at Los Angeles School of Medicine; Director, Division of Infectious Diseases, Attending Staff, Department of Medicine, Cedars-Sinai Medical Center, Los Angeles, California.

Legionella Species Infection.

Alfred F. Michael, M.D.

Professor, Department of Pediatrics, University of Minnesota, Minneapolis, Minnesota.

Nephrotic Syndrome.

George Miller, M.D.

John F. Enders Professor of Pediatric Infectious Diseases and Professor of Epidemiology, Yale University School of Medicine, New Haven, Connecticut.

Burkitt Lymphoma. Infectious Mononucleosis.

John F. Modlin, M.D.

Assistant Professor of Pediatrics, Harvard Medical School; Associate in Medicine (Infectious Diseases), Children's Hospital Medical Center, Boston, Massachusetts.

Enteroviruses.

Paul G. Moe, M.D.

Associate Professor of Pediatric Neurology, University of Colorado Medical Center; Chief, Neurology and EEG, the Children's Hospital, Denver, Colorado.

Intracranial Hemorrhage.

Beverly C. Morgan, M.D.

Professor and Chair, Department of Pediatrics, University of California at Irvine College of Medicine; Attending Staff, University of California at Irvine Medical Center, Children's Hospital of Orange County, and Miller Children's Hospital, Memorial Medical Center, Orange, California.

Peripheral Vascular Disease.

Andrea Morrison, M.D.

Assistant Clinical Professor of Pediatrics, University of California at Los Angeles School of Medicine; Attending Pediatrician, Cedars Sinai Medical Center, Los Angeles, California.

Congenital Hypotonia.

Thomas S. Morse, M.D.

Professor of Surgery, University of Massachusetts Medical School, Pediatric Surgeon, Berkshire Medical Center, Pittsfield, Massachusetts.
Neonatal Intestinal Obstruction.

David B. Mosher, M.D.

Instructor in Dermatology, Harvard University; Clinical Associate, Massachusetts General Hospital, Boston, Massachusetts.
Disorders of Pigmentation.

Denis M. Murphy, M.B., B.Ch., F.R.C.S.I.

Senior Registrar, Department of Urology, Meath Hospital, Dublin, Ireland.
Neonatal Ascites.

Alexander S. Nadas, M.D.

Professor of Pediatrics, Harvard Medical School; Chief Emeritus, Department of Cardiology, Senior Associate in Cardiology, Children's Hospital Medical Center, Boston, Massachusetts.
Infective Endocarditis.

David G. Nathan, M.D.

Robert A. Stranahan Professor of Pediatrics, Harvard Medical School; Chief, Division of Hematology and Oncology, Children's Hospital Medical Center and Dana-Farber Cancer Institute, Boston, Massachusetts.
Polycythemia.

Herbert L. Needleman, M.D.

Associate Professor of Child Psychiatry and Pediatrics, University of Pittsburgh; Director, Behavioral Science Division, Children's Hospital of Pittsburgh; Psychiatrist, Western Psychiatric Institute and Clinic, Pittsburgh, Pennsylvania.
Increased Lead Absorption and Acute Lead Poisoning.

Joseph P. Neglia, M.D.

Chief Resident, Department of Pediatrics, Baylor College of Medicine, Jefferson Davis Hospital, Houston, Texas.
Bacterial Meningitis and Septicemia Beyond the Neonatal Period.

John D. Nelson, M.D.

Professor of Pediatrics, University of Texas Health Science Center, Dallas; Active Attending, Children's Hospital Medical Center and Parkland Memorial Hospital, Dallas; Consulting Physician, John Peter Smith Hospital, Fort Worth, Texas.
Osteomyelitis and Suppurative Arthritis.

Mark E. Nesbitt, Jr., M.D.

Professor of Pediatrics, Therapeutic Radiology, and Nursing, University of Minnesota School of Medicine; Attending Staff, University of Minnesota Hospitals, Minneapolis, Minnesota.
Malignant Bone Tumors.

Naomi D. Neufeld, M.D.

Assistant Professor in Residence, Department of Pediatrics, University of California at Los Angeles School of Medicine; Head, Section of Endocrinology, Department of Pediatrics, Cedars-Sinai Medical Center; Attending Physician, Pediatrics, UCLA Center for the Health Sciences, Los Angeles, California.
Infants Born to Diabetic Mothers.

Thomas E. Nevins, M.D.

Assistant Professor, Department of Pediatrics, University of Minnesota School of Medicine, Minneapolis, Minnesota.
Nephrotic Syndrome.

Maria I. New, M.D.

Professor and Chairman, Department of Pediatrics, Cornell University Medical College; Physician-in-Chief, The New York Hospital, New York, New York.
Disorders of the Adrenal Gland.

Jane W. Newberger, M.D., M.P.H.

Instructor in Pediatrics, Harvard Medical School; Associate in Cardiology, Children's Hospital, Boston, Massachusetts.
Infective Endocarditis.

Victor D. Newcomer, M.D.

Clinical Professor of Medicine/Dermatology, University of California at Los Angeles School of Medicine, Los Angeles, California.
Urticaria.

James J. Nora, M.D.

Professor of Pediatrics, Genetics, and Preventive Medicine, University of Colorado School of Medicine; Director of Preventive Cardiology, University Hospital; Director of Genetics, Rose Medical Center, Denver, Colorado.
The Child at Risk of Coronary Disease as an Adult.

Edward J. O'Connell, M.D.

Associate Professor of Pediatrics, Mayo Medical School; Consultant, Pediatrics, Pediatric Allergy and Immunology, Department of Pediatrics,

Mayo Clinic and Mayo Foundation, Rochester, Minnesota.
Recurrent Acute Parotitis.

Pearay L. Ogra, M.D.
Professor of Pediatrics and Microbiology, State University of New York at Buffalo; Attending Physician, Children's Hospital, Buffalo, New York.
Acute and Chronic Nonspecific Diarrhea Syndromes.

William Oh, M.D.
Professor of Medical Sciences in Pediatrics and Obstetrics, Brown University School of Medicine; Pediatrician-in-Chief, Women and Infants Hospital, Providence, Rhode Island.
Respiratory Distress Syndrome. Disorders of the Umbilicus.

Donald P. Orr, M.D.
Associate Professor of Pediatrics, Indiana University School of Medicine; Director, Adolescent Health Section, the James Whitcomb Riley Hospital for Children, Indianapolis, Indiana.
Children Whose Parents are Divorcing.

Gary D. Overturf, M.D.
Professor of Pediatrics, University of Southern California School of Medicine; Director, Communicable Disease Service, Los Angeles County-University of Southern California Medical Center, Los Angeles, California.
Rat Bite Fever.

John W. Paisley, M.D.
Assistant Professor of Pediatrics, University of Colorado School of Medicine; Director of Inpatient Services, Denver General Hospital; Consultant, Pediatric Infectious Diseases, University of Colorado Medical Center, Denver, Colorado.
Viral Pneumonia.

Hermine M. Pashayan, M.D.
Professor of Pediatrics, Tufts University School of Medicine; Pediatrician, New England Medical Center, Inc., Boston, Massachusetts.
Diseases and Injuries of the Oral Region.

Robert F. Pass, M.D.
Associate Professor of Pediatrics, University of Alabama in Birmingham; House Staff, Children's Hospital and University Hospital.
Cytomegalovirus Infections.

Jay A. Perman, M.D.
Associate Professor of Pediatrics, University of California at San Francisco, California.
Recurrent Abdominal Pain.

Arthur S. Pickoff, M.D.
Assistant Professor of Pediatrics, University of Miami School of Medicine; Attending Pediatric Cardiologist, University of Miami/Jackson Memorial Medical Center, Miami, Florida.
Cardiac Arrhythmias.

Rosita S. Pildes, M.D.
Professor of Pediatrics, University of Illinois College of Medicine; Chairman, Division of Neonatology, Cook County Hospital, Chicago, Illinois.
Infants of Drug-Dependent Mothers.

Stephanie H. Pincus, M.D.
Associate Professor, Department of Dermatology, Tufts University School of Medicine; Dermatologist, New England Medical Center, Boston, Massachusetts.
Contact Dermatitis.

Irving M. Polayes, M.D., D.D.S.
Associate Clinical Professor of Plastic and Reconstructive Surgery, Yale University School of Medicine; Attending Plastic Surgeon and Associate Section Chief, Plastic and Reconstructive Surgery, Yale-New Haven Hospital; Attending Plastic and Reconstructive Surgeon, St. Raphael's Hospital, New Haven; Attending Consultant, Veterans Administration Hospital, West Haven; Consultant, Gaylord Hospital, Wallingford and Griffen Hospital, Derby, Connecticut.
Salivary Gland Tumors.

Donald E. Potter, M.D.
Associate Clinical Professor of Pediatrics, University of California at San Francisco; Attending Pediatrician, University of California at San Francisco Medical Center, San Francisco, California.
Peritoneal Dialysis.

Kevin C. Pringle, M.B., Ch.B., F.R.A.C.S.
Associate Professor of Surgery, University of Iowa College of Medicine; Attending Staff, University of Iowa Hospitals and Clinics, Iowa City, Iowa.
Pyloric Stenosis. Disorders of the Esophagus.

Edward F. Rabe, M.D.
Professor of Pediatrics and Neurology, Tufts

University School of Medicine; Head, Section of Pediatric Neurology, Boston Floating Hospital, New England Medical Center, Boston, Massachusetts.

Cerebrovascular Disorders. Febrile Convulsions.

Max L. Ramenofsky, M.D.

Professor of Surgery and Pediatrics, University of South Alabama, Chief, Division of Pediatric Surgery, University of South Alabama Medical Center, Mobile, Alabama.

Lymphangitis. Lymph Node Infections. Congenital Diaphragmatic Hernia.

James E. Rasmussen, M.D.

Professor, Department of Dermatology and Pediatrics, University of Michigan Medical School, Ann Arbor, Michigan.

Erythema Multiforme.

Jack S. Remington, M.D.

Professor of Medicine, Stanford University School of Medicine; Chairman, Department of Immunology and Infectious Disease Research Institute, Palo Alto Medical Foundation, Palo Alto, California.

Toxoplasmosis.

Owen M. Rennert, M.D.

Professor and Head, Department of Pediatrics, University of Oklahoma Health Sciences Center; Head, Section of Genetics, Endocrinology, and Metabolism and Chief, Pediatric Service, Oklahoma Children's Memorial Hospital, University of Oklahoma College of Medicine; Consultant, Veterans Administration Hospital, Oklahoma City, Oklahoma.

Hepatolenticular Degeneration.

Thomas S. Renshaw, M.D.

Associate Professor of Orthopedic Surgery, University of Connecticut; Assistant Clinical Professor of Orthopedic Surgery, Yale University; Director of Orthopedic Surgery, Newington Children's Hospital, Newington, Connecticut.

Congenital Muscular Defects. Torticollis.

Sylvia Onesti Richardson, M.D.

Professor of Communicology and Clinical Professor of Pediatrics, University of South Florida, Tampa, Florida.

Voice, Speech, and Language Disorders.

Harris D. Riley, Jr., M.D.

Regents' Distinguished Professor of Pediatrics, University of Oklahoma College of Medicine; Attending Physician, Children's Memorial Hospital, University of Oklahoma Health Sciences Center, Oklahoma City, Oklahoma.

Infections due to Escherichia coli, Proteus, Klebsiella-Enterobacter-Serratia, Pseudomonas *and other Gram-Negative Bacilli.*

William J. Riley, M.D.

Assistant Professor of Pediatrics and Clinical Pathology, University of Florida School of Medicine; Associate Director of Clinical Chemistry and Endocrinologist, Department of Pediatrics, Shands Hospital and Clinics, Gainesville, Florida.

Hyperlipoproteinemias.

David L. Rimoin, M.D., Ph.D.

Professor of Pediatrics and Medicine, University of California at Los Angeles School of Medicine; Chief, Division of Medical Genetics, Los Angeles County Harbor-UCLA Medical Center, Torrance, California.

Genetic Diseases.

A. Kim Ritchey, M.D.

Assistant Professor of Pediatrics, Yale University School of Medicine; Attending Pediatrician, Yale-New Haven Hospital, New Haven, Connecticut.

Leukopenia, Neutropenia, and Agranulocytosis. Disorders of the Spleen. The Postsplenectomy Syndrome.

Alan M. Robson, M.D.

Professor of Pediatrics, Washington University School of Medicine, St. Louis; Director, Division of Nephrology, St. Louis Children's Hospital, St. Louis, Missouri.

Systemic Hypertension.

Fred S. Rosen, M.D.

James L. Gamble Professor of Pediatrics, Harvard Medical School; Chief, Division of Immunology, Children's Hospital Medical Center, Boston, Massachusetts.

Angioneurotic Edema.

Arthur L. Rosenbaum, M.D.

Professor, Department of Ophthalmology, University of California at Los Angeles School of Medicine, Jules Stein Eye Institute, Los Angeles, California.

The Eye.

Philip Rosenthal, M.D.

Assistant Professor of Pediatrics, University of Southern California School of Medicine; Assistant Director, Division of Gastroenterology and Nutrition, Children's Hospital of Los Angeles, California.

Disorders of Porphyrin, Purine, and Pyrimidine Metabolism.

Thomas M. Rossi, M.D.

Assistant Professor of Pediatrics, State University of New York at Buffalo; Assistant Attending, Division of Gastroenterology and Nutrition, Children's Hospital, Buffalo, New York.

Intractable Diarrhea of Infancy.

Marc I. Rowe, M.D.

Professor of Pediatric Surgery, University of Pittsburgh; Chief of Surgery, Children's Hospital of Pittsburgh, Pennsylvania.

Hirschsprung's Disease. Disorders of the Anus and Rectum. Chest Wall Deformities.

Robert J. Ruben, M.D., F.A.C.S.

Professor and Chairman, Department of Otorhinolaryngology, Albert Einstein College of Medicine of Yeshiva University and Montefiore Hospital and Medical Center; Attending Otolaryngologist, Hospital of the Albert Einstein College of Medicine, Montefiore Hospital and Medical Center, Bronx Municipal Hospital Center, and North Central Bronx Hospital, New York, New York.

Labyrinthitis.

Barry H. Rumack, M.D.

Associate Professor of Pediatrics and Head, Section of Pediatric Clinical Pharmacology and Toxicology, University of Colorado Health Sciences Center; Director, Rocky Mountain Poison Center, Denver General Hospital, Denver, Colorado; President, American Association of Poison Control Centers.

Botulinal Food Poisoning. Acute Poisoning. Salicylate Poisoning. Acetaminophen Overdose.

Abdollah Sadeghi-Nejad, M.D.

Associate Professor of Pediatrics, Tufts University School of Medicine; Pediatric Endocrinologist, New England Medical Center, Boston Floating Hospital for Infants and Children, Boston, Massachusetts.

Undescended Testes.

Frederick J. Samaha, M.D.

Professor and Chairman, Neurology Depart-

ment, University of Cincinnati Medical Center, Cincinnati, Ohio.

Fibroplasia Ossificans Progressiva (Myositis Ossificans Progressiva). Myasthenia Gravis.

Julio V. Santiago, M.D.

Professor of Pediatrics, Washington University School of Medicine; Physician, St. Louis Children's Hospital, St. Louis, Missouri.

Systemic Hypertension.

Lawrence Schachner, M.D.

Associate Professor of Pediatrics, Associate Professor of Dermatology, Director of Division of Pediatric Dermatology, University of Miami School of Medicine, Miami, Florida.

Erythema Nodosum. Drug Reactions and the Skin.

Melvin D. Schloss, M.D., F.R.C.S. (Can)

Associate Professor, Department of Otolaryngology, McGill University; Director, Division of Otolaryngology, Montreal Children's Hospital, Montreal, Quebec, Canada.

Foreign Bodies in the Ear.

Edgar J. Schoen, M.D.

Assistant Clinical Professor, Department of Pediatrics, University of California at San Francisco; Chief, Department of Pediatrics, Kaiser-Permanente Medical Center, Oakland, California.

Tall Stature.

Martin L. Schulkind, M.D.

Associate Professor of Pediatrics and Community Health and Family Medicine, University of Florida College of Medicine; Attending Physician, Shands Teaching Hospital; Pediatric Consultant, Alachua General Hospital, Gainesville, Florida.

Cat-Scratch Disease.

Arthur D. Schwabe, M.D.

Professor of Medicine, Chief, Division of Gastroenterology, University of California at Los Angeles School of Medicine, Los Angeles, California.

Familial Mediterranean Fever.

Richard H. Schwartz, M.D.

Clinical Associate Professor, Child Health and Development, George Washington University; Clinical Associate Professor of Pediatrics; Georgetown University, Washington, D.C.; Attending Pediatrician, Fairfax Hospital, Falls Church, Virginia.

Otologic Infections.

R. Michael Scott, M.D.

Professor, Department of Neurosurgery, Tufts University School of Medicine; Neurosurgeon, New England Medical Center, Boston, Massachusetts.

Brain Abscess. Hydrocephalus. Spinal Epidural Abscess. Brain Tumor.

Roland B. Scott, M.D.

Distinguished Professor of Pediatrics and Child Health, Howard University College of Medicine; Attending Pediatrician, Howard University Hospital; Director, the Howard University Center for Sickle Cell Disease, Washington, D.C.

Sickle Cell Disease.

John H. Seashore, M.D.

Professor of Surgery and Pediatrics, Yale University School of Medicine; Attending Physician, Yale-New Haven Hospital, New Haven, Connecticut.

Total Parenteral Nutrition.

Boris Senior, M.D.

Professor of Pediatrics, Tufts University School of Medicine; Chief, Pediatric Endocrinology and Metabolism, New England Medical Center, Inc., Boston, Massachusetts.

Hypopituitarism.

Daniel C. Shannon, M.D.

Associate Professor of Pediatrics, Harvard-MIT School of Health Science and Technology; Pediatrician, Massachusetts General Hospital, Boston, Massachusetts.

Sudden Infant Death Syndrome. Childhood Sleep Disorders.

Bruce K. Shapiro, M.D.

Assistant Professor of Pediatrics, Johns Hopkins University School of Medicine; Developmental Pediatrician, John F. Kennedy Institute, Baltimore, Maryland.

Mental Retardation.

Harvey L. Sharp, M.D.

Professor of Pediatrics, University of Minnesota School of Medicine, Minneapolis, Minnesota.

Gastroesophageal Reflux and Hiatal Hernia.

Philip Shaul, M.D.

Pediatric Resident, Children's Hospital of Cincinnati, Ohio.

Magnesium Deficiency.

Bennett A. Shaywitz, M.D.

Associate Professor of Pediatrics and Neurology, and Director, Child Neurology Section, Yale University School of Medicine; Attending Physician, Yale-New Haven Hospital, New Haven, Connecticut.

Hypoxic Encephalopathy.

Sally E. Shaywitz, M.D.

Associate Professor of Pediatrics, Director, Learning Disorders Unit, Yale University School of Medicine; Attending Physician, Yale-New Haven Hospital, New Haven, Connecticut.

Attention Deficit Disorder.

I. Ronald Shenker, M.D.

Associate Professor of Pediatrics, Health Sciences Center, State University of New York at Stony Brook; Chief, Adolescent Medicine, Department of Pediatrics, Long Island Jewish-Hillside Medical Center, New Hyde Park, New York.

Obesity.

Sheila Sherlock, D.B.E., M.D.

Professor of Medicine, Royal Free Hospital School of Medicine (University of London); Consultant Physician, Royal Free Hospital, London, England.

Portal Hypertension. Chronic Active Hepatitis.

Henry H. Shinefield, M.D.

Clinical Professor of Pediatrics, University of California at San Francisco School of Medicine; Chief of Pediatrics, Kaiser-Permanente Medical Center, San Francisco, California.

Staphylococcal Infections.

Stanford T. Shulman, M.D.

Professor of Pediatrics, Chief of Pediatric Infectious Diseases, Northwestern University Medical School; Chief, Division of Infectious Diseases, Children's Memorial Hospital, Chicago, Illinois.

Streptococcal Infections.

Irwin M. Siegel, M.D.

Associate Professor, Departments of Orthopaedic Surgery and Neurological Sciences, Rush-Presbyterian-St. Luke's Medical Center; Attending, Orthopaedic Surgery, Louis A. Weiss Memorial Hospital, Assistant Attending, Orthopaedics and Department of Neurological Sciences, Presbyterian-St. Luke's Hospital, Chicago, Illinois.

Muscular Dystrophy and Related Myopathies.

Myron Siegel, M.D.

Assistant Professor of Pediatrics, State University of New York at Buffalo School of Medicine; Attending, Division of Pediatric Gastroenterology and Nutrition, Children's Hospital of Buffalo, New York.

Malabsorption Syndromes and Diarrhea.

Frank R. Sinatra, M.D.

Associate Professor of Pediatrics, University of Southern California School of Medicine; Director, Division of Gastroenterology and Nutrition, Children's Hospital of Los Angeles, California.
Necrotizing Enterocolitis.

William D. Singer, M.D.

Associate Professor of Pediatrics (Neurology), Tufts University School of Medicine; Pediatric Neurologist, New England Medical Center; Director, Boston Muscular Dystrophy Association Clinic, Lakeville Hospital, Lakeville, Massachusetts.
Spasmus Nutans. Infantile Spasms.

Sharanjeet Singh, M.D.

Associate Professor of Pediatrics (Cardiology) and Pharmacology, Department of Pediatrics, University of Miami School of Medicine; Attending Pediatric Cardiologist, University of Miami/Jackson Memorial Medical Center, Miami, Florida.
Cardiac Arrhythmias.

Lucius F. Sinks, M.D.

Professor of Pediatrics, Tufts University School of Medicine; Pediatrician, New England Medical Center, Boston, Massachusetts.
Acute Leukemia.

Arthur J. Sober, M.D.

Associate Professor of Dermatology, Harvard Medical School; Associate Dermatologist, Massachusetts General Hospital, Boston, Massachusetts.
Nevi and Nevoid Tumors.

Robert T. Soper, M.D.

Professor of Surgery, University of Iowa College of Medicine; Attending Staff, University of Iowa Hospitals and Clinics, Iowa City, Iowa.
Pyloric Stenosis. Disorders of the Esophagus.

Mark A. Sperling, M.D.

Professor of Pediatrics, Associate Professor of Medicine, University of Cincinnati College of Medicine; Director, Division of Endocrinology, Children's Hospital Medical Center, Cincinnati, Ohio.
Diabetes Mellitus.

Gopal Srinivasan, M.D.

Associate Professor of Pediatrics, Ohio Medical School; Attending Neonatologist, Cook County Hospital, Chicago, Illinois.
Infants of Drug Dependent Mothers.

Lynn T. Staheli, M.D.

Professor, Department of Orthopedics, University of Washington School of Medicine; Director, Department of Orthopedics, Children's Hospital and Medical Center, Seattle, Washington.
The Hip.

Joseph J. Stetz, M.D.

Associate Professor of Surgery, Tufts University School of Medicine; Assistant Surgeon, New England Medical Center, Inc., Boston, Massachusetts.
Pediatric Cardiac Tumors.

Joseph W. St. Geme, Jr., M.D.

Professor and Executive Chairman, Department of Pediatrics, University of California at Los Angeles School of Medicine; Attending Staff, Los Angeles County Harbor-UCLA Medical Center, Los Angeles, California.
Mumps. Herpes Simplex Virus Infections.

James A. Stockman III, M.D.

Professor of Pediatrics, State University of New York at Syracuse College of Medicine; Attending Physician, University Hospital and Crouse Irving Memorial Hospital, Syracuse, New York.
Hemolytic Anemia.

Robert C. Strunk, M.D.

Associate Professor of Pediatrics, University of Colorado School of Medicine; Director, Clinical Services, Department of Pediatrics, National Jewish Hospital/National Asthma Center, Denver, Colorado.
Serum Sickness.

Lawrence T. Taft, M.D.

Professor and Chairman, Department of Pediatrics, University of Medicine and Dentistry of New Jersey, Rutgers Medical School, Academic Health Science Center; Attending Staff, Middlesex General University Hospital, New Brunswick, New Jersey.
Cerebral Palsy.

Angelo Taranta, M.D.

Professor of Medicine, New York Medical College; Director of Medicine and Chief of Rheumatology, Cabrini Medical Center; Chief of Rheumatology/Immunology Section, New York Medical College, New York, New York.
Acute Rheumatic Fever.

Jean W. Temeck, M.D.

Fellow in Pediatric Endocrinology, Cornell Uni-

versity Medical College; Clinical Fellow, The New York Hospital, New York, New York.
Disorders of the Adrenal Gland.

M. Michael Thaler, M.D.
Professor of Pediatrics and Director, Pediatric Gastroenterology and Nutrition, University of California at San Francisco School of Medicine; Attending Physician, University of California, Medical Center, San Francisco, California.
Disorders of Porphyrin, Purine, and Pyrimidine Metabolism.

Reginald C. Tsang, M.B.B.S.
Professor of Pediatrics, Obstetrics, and Gynecology, University of Cincinnati College of Medicine; Director of Division of Neonatology, Attending Neonatologist, Children's Hospital of Cincinnati and University Hospital, Cincinnati, Ohio.
Magnesium Deficiency.

Charles S. Turner, M.D.
Assistant Professor of Surgery, Wake Forest University Bowman Gray School of Medicine, Winston-Salem, North Carolina.
Lymphedema.

J. A. Peter Turner, M.D.
Professor of Pediatrics, Faculty of Medicine, University of Toronto; Head, Division of Chest Diseases, The Hospital for Sick Children, Toronto, Ontario, Canada.
Aspiration Pneumonia. Atelectasis. Bronchiectasis. Emphysema.

John T. Twiggs, M.D.
Associate Staff Member, Subsection Allergy, Department of Medicine, Marshfield Clinic, Marshfield, Wisconsin.
Recurrent Acute Parotitis.

Russell Van Dyke, M.D.
Fellow, University of California at San Diego School of Medicine; Assistant Professor, Department of Pediatrics, Tulane University; Attending in Pediatric Infectious Diseases, Children's Hospital, New Orleans, Louisiana.
Plague.

W. Allan Walker, M.D.
Professor of Pediatrics, Harvard Medical School; Chief, Combined Division of Pediatric GI/Nutrition, Massachusetts General Hospital and Children's Hospital Medical Center, Boston, Massachusetts.
Ulcerative Colitis and Crohn's Disease.

David A. Waller, M.D.
Associate Professor of Psychiatry and Pediatrics and Director of Child and Adolescent Psychiatry, University of Texas Southwestern Medical School; Director, Pediatric-Psychiatry Liaison Service, Children's Medical Center of Dallas, Parkland Memorial Hospital, Dallas, Texas.
Psychosomatic Illness.

Diane W. Wara, M.D.
Associate Professor of Pediatrics, University of California, San Francisco School of Medicine, San Francisco, California.
Primary Immunodeficiency Disease.

H. James Wedner, M.D.
Associate Professor of Medicine, Washington University School of Medicine: Attending Physician, Barnes Hospital, St. Louis, Missouri.
Adverse Reactions to Drugs.

Paul F. Wehrle, M.D.
Hastings Professor of Pediatrics, University of Southern California School of Medicine; Director of Pediatrics, Los Angeles County-USC Medical Center, Los Angeles, California.
Influenza.

Allan J. Weinstein, M.D.
Lilly Research Laboratories, Indianapolis, Indiana.
Urinary Tract Infections.

Morris A. Wessel, M.D.
Clinical Professor of Pediatrics, Yale University School of Medicine; Attending Pediatrician, Yale-New Haven Hospital and St. Raphael Hospital, New Haven, Connecticut.
The Child and Death of a Loved One.

Milton Westphal, M.D.
Professor of Pediatrics, Medical University of South Carolina; Active Staff, Medical University Hospital, Charleston, South Carolina.
Alcohol and Drug Abuse.

Christopher B. Wilson, M.D.
Assistant Professor of Pediatrics, University of Washington School of Medicine; Associate, Division of Infectious Diseases, Children's Orthopedic Hospital and Medical Center, Seattle, Washington.
Toxoplasmosis.

Willis A. Wingert, M.D.
Professor of Pediatrics, Community Medicine, Public Health and Emergency Medicine, Univer-

sity of Southern California School of Medicine; Director, Pediatric Ambulatory Service, Los Angeles County – University of Southern California Medical Center, Los Angeles, California.
Animal and Human Bites and Bite-Related Infections.

Myron Winick, M.D.
R.R. Williams Professor of Nutrition, Professor of Pediatrics, Director, Institute of Human Nutrition, and Director, Center for Nutrition, Genetics and Human Development, College of Physicians and Surgeons, Columbia University, New York.
Treatment of Childhood Obesity.

Harland S. Winter, M.D.
Assistant Professor of Pediatrics, Harvard Medical School; Assistant in Medicine (Gastroenterology), Children's Hospital Medical Center, Boston, Massachusetts.
Nausea and Vomiting.

Joseph I. Wolfsdorf, M.D.
Instructor in Pediatrics, Harvard Medical School, Assistant in Medicine (Endocrinology), The Chil-

dren's Hospital Medical Center, Boston, Massachusetts.
Parathyroid Disease.

Calvin W. Woodruff, M.D.
Professor of Child Health, University of Missouri at Columbia School of Medicine; Attending Pediatrician, Health Sciences Center, Columbia, Missouri.
Pica.

Ram Yogev, M.D.
Associate Professor of Pediatrics, Northwestern University Medical School; Attending Physician, Division of Infectious Diseases, The Children's Memorial Hospital, Chicago, Illinois.
Streptococcal Infections.

John A. Zaia, M.D.
Associate Clinical Professor of Pediatrics, University of Southern California School of Medicine, Los Angeles; Director of Infectious Diseases, City of Hope Medical Center, Duarte, California.
Varicella and Herpes Zoster.

Preface

The regular biennial publication of *Current Pediatric Therapy* has over the course of time been greeted by a number of published reviews and commentaries, which have appeared in medical journals throughout the world. These, as well as letters from readers, testify to the wide awareness of the book and to its general usefulness. They also offer considerable help in our planning for new editions.

In the last few years, the observation has been made in published reviews that *Current Pediatric Therapy* has no references. We hope it is appropriate to use this opportunity to develop in some detail the essential purpose of this book.

As in so many spheres of human endeavor, it is in the nature of medicine that the gradual accumulation of experience and seasoning of clinical judgment over time provides a measure of knowledge and ability that is beyond the reach of someone equally skilled but having fewer chances to deal with a particular problem. The continuing specialization of pediatric practice only amplifies the difference.

Current Pediatric Therapy is a synthesis of advice developed from long experience with the continued studied application of informed evaluations of therapeutic advances. In their presentations, the authors have made use of many sources of information. The references themselves are easily found in the various cumulative indices.

We have consistently endeavored to make available to all who treat children the specific details of therapy that have been found effective by specialists who have extensive experience. We have consistently asked them to share not only those therapeutic approaches they have heard or read about but also, and more importantly, those that they themselves have used repeatedly. The authorities whose words fill these pages have devoted substantial effort to keeping abreast of the most current and complete information about treatment of sick children. Our task as editors is to identify them and to help direct their contributions toward specific therapeutic advice, so that readers can be confident that each volume measures up to the highest standard of completeness, currency and practicality.

Still, therapy is seldom final. Change may come gradually or suddenly. Consulting more than one edition of *Current Pediatric Therapy* is not only possible but may be desirable in order to make rational decisions. No edition will ever have the last word on any disease until, like smallpox, the disease is eradicated and the need for treatment disappears. In the meantime, our hope is that any physician will be able to depend on this book to be a quickly accessible compendium of currently acceptable therapeutic approaches.

It is obvious that editors and readers alike are deeply indebted to the experts who have taken the time to describe their methods. If readers find help in making decisions, the book will have accomplished its purpose.

SYDNEY S. GELLIS, M.D.
BENJAMIN M. KAGAN, M.D.

Contents

4 RESPIRATORY TRACT

1

Nutrition

General Malnutrition

RICHARD B. GOLDBLOOM, M.D.

The treatment of general malnutrition in infants and children requires scrupulous monitoring on a daily basis. An appreciation of three fundamental principles is essential to effective management:

1. In the short term, adequate total energy intake is a more critical determinant of rapid recovery than the balance of major nutrients.

2. The calorie intake required for rapid nutritional repair ("catch-up growth") markedly exceeds that required by children of the same age or height for normal rates of growth.

3. Few malnourished children will be capable of achieving the energy intake required for catch-up growth simply by being offered a "normal" diet and encouraged to consume as much as they wish. Therapeutic realimentation calls for an aggressive approach.

Although the caloric requirement for catch-up growth averages about 50 per cent above normal daily intake, there is considerable individual variation. Occasionally, as much as twice the normal requirement may be needed. In practice, the individual patient requirement will be determined simply by "how much it takes" to produce a satisfactory rate of recovery.

Caloric deficiency is the final common pathway in the pathogenesis of most instances of general malnutrition in pediatric patients, whether the malnutrition is associated with organic disease, dietary inadequacy, or psychosocial deprivation.

The ensuing comments emphasize the hospital treatment of children with malnutrition, since in North America it is frequently difficult to manage infants and children with significant degrees of malnutrition effectively on an outpatient basis. However, the basic principles are the same in either case.

The first step in managing the malnourished child is to determine the ideal weight for height. This is done by measuring the child's height and plotting the measurement on a standard growth chart. Extrapolation horizontally to the 50th percentile line will give the height age. The ideal weight is the 50th percentile weight for the child's height-age. The ideal weight for height is then used to calculate the total daily caloric requirement.

On the average, the diet should contain 2 to 3 grams of protein/kg/24 hr. The child should be weighed without clothing each morning before the first meal.

Working with a therapeutic nutritionist from the outset can be of inestimable value in determining how best to achieve the desired intake and in working out its composition.

In deciding the best feeding method for achieving the desired objective, a good rule is to begin with the simplest and least invasive route of administration. The choices, in increasing order of complexity, are

1. Supplementation of a normal diet in ways that will produce minimal increase in the volume of food to be consumed.

2. Nasogastric feeding, intermittent (e.g., nocturnal) or continuous.

3. Nasogastric feeding plus peripheral intravenous hyperalimentation.

4. Central intravenous hyperalimentation.

Normal diets may be supplemented with additional fat, carbohydrate, or both. For infants, medium-chain triglyceride (MCT) oil (8.3 kcal/gm) may be added in increasing quantities to the feeding in order to raise the fat content gradually to approximately 50 per cent of the total calorie intake.

In older children, the amount to be added, for

example, to a nasogastric feeding, must be determined by the amount required to achieve the desired caloric intake and by the child's tolerance.

Glucose polymer preparations (Polycose or Caloreen) are also useful as supplements to increase the caloric density of oral or nasogastric feedings without substantially increasing the volume fed. Again, the amount of supplementation should be calculated on the basis of the desired daily calorie intake, but attention should be paid to the contribution of the added glucose polymer preparation to the osmolality of the feeding. For undernourished infants and children with congenital heart disease or renal disease in whom sodium intake may need to be restricted, a low-sodium form of Caloreen is available.

Nasogastric feeding given as a continuous drip has the advantage of permitting feeding around the clock, thus eliminating the intermittent delivery of a large bolus of food to an enteric mucosa, the digestive and absorptive capacity of which may be reduced by the effects of malnutrition.

Recently available soft Silastic feeding tubes have greatly reduced the discomfort of continuous nasogastric feeding. Such tubes can be tolerated for long periods without being changed and with little interference with the child's activity. The child can also continue to eat comfortably despite the presence of the tube, if this is considered desirable.

Individuals inserting nasogastric tubes should always be cautioned not to advance the tube beyond the measured distance required to get the tip in the gastric lumen. One must resist the temptation to advance the tube "just an inch or two more to be sure it is in the stomach," since this maneuver may permit the tip of the tube to migrate through the pylorus. Introduction of a significant osmolar load then may cause diarrhea, which may be misinterpreted as intolerance of the feeding regimen, leading to unnecessary delays in recovery.

The composition of the food intake should be decided on an individual basis, taking into account the severity of the malnutrition and the observed tolerance of the infant or child. In more severe cases, both digestion and absorption may be impaired, and the use of elemental or lactose-free diet preparations, at least in the early days of treatment, may speed recovery. The major nutrient components of such preparations are protein hydrolysate, monosaccharide, and lipid in the form of corn oil, safflower oil, soy oil, or medium-chain triglyceride.

If the child is being fed nasogastrically, the physician should pay attention to the osmolality of the feeding mixture, and, if possible, should use a preparation the osmolality of which is not excessively high. This will reduce the risk of hyperosmolar diarrhea and permit a more rapid achievement of the desired daily energy intake.

The treatment program should be carefully reassessed every 24 hours, since it often takes several days to achieve the estimated requirement, and daily adjustments in feeding volume, caloric density, and rate of administration may be required.

If prolonged nasogastric feeding is contemplated, the physician should check the feeding composition carefully to ensure an adequate intake of vitamins and trace elements and add appropriate supplements where necessary. Total parenteral nutrition is discussed in the last article of this section.

Treatment of Childhood Obesity

MYRON WINICK, M.D.

Childhood obesity if not treated early is very likely to result in a form of adult obesity that is particularly refractory to treatment. Since the total number of fat cells are laid down during childhood and adolescence as the result of the multiplication of preadipocytes, obesity during the growing years is usually hyperplastic. The treatment goal is to have the child reach near desirable weight without compromising growth and development. The method of achieving this is calorie control and exercise.

In controlling calories it is important 1) to try to keep weight from increasing while allowing height to increase at its normal rate, and 2) to offer enough variety in food choices to ensure an adequate supply of vitamins and minerals.

To achieve the first objective, reduce the number of calories consumed *gradually* until you reach the point where the child's weight has stabilized. Keep the intake at that point and monitor the triceps and/or subscapular skinfold and the child's linear growth. The latter should continue normally, the former should remain unchanged. By using this approach you are allowing the child to gradually "grow out" of his or her obesity. While this approach may be slower in achieving results, it is safer than trying to induce actual weight reduction because it is much less likely to compromise growth, much easier for the child to comply with, and much more likely to avoid nutrient deficiencies.

Achieving the second goal may require the help of a trained dietitian. In principle, a diet should be offered that contains the daily requirement of all of the vitamins and minerals and is acceptable to the child. In practice, this may be very difficult. The major nutrients that are likely to be in short supply are iron, zinc, calcium, folate, and vitamin B_6. For this reason it is often wise to supplement a dieting child with a multivitamin combination and iron. This should be used as insurance and not in place of a varied diet.

Increasing the child's level of exercise is an excellent adjunct to controlling calories in a regimen to achieve weight reduction. Remember, however, that exercise, particularly strenuous exercise, may increase appetite. You may have to increase the caloric content of the diet somewhat as activity increases. However, it is possible to do this without inducing any weight gain by carefully monitoring the child's weight and skinfold thickness.

Although the overall results in the treatment of childhood obesity are far from satisfactory, the above approach offers the best possibility for long-term control and has the least risk for compromising the child's linear growth.

Vitamin Deficiencies and Excesses

RICHARD B. GOLDBLOOM, M.D.

FAT-SOLUBLE VITAMINS

Vitamin A. For children with chronic steatorrheic states, a daily supplement of 2000 IU of a water-miscible preparation of vitamin A is usually sufficient to maintain normal serum levels and to prevent clinical deficiency.

Night-blindness, conjunctival lesions, and Bitot spots may be treated by oral administration of vitamin A, 5000 to 10,000 IU daily for 10 days, or by a single massive intramuscular dose of 200,000 IU. If corneal xerosis is present, immediate intramuscular administration of 100,000 IU of a water-miscible vitamin A preparation is recommended, followed by oral administration of 200,000 IU one week later. Simultaneous use of an antibiotic ophthalmic ointment may be required, and associated protein-calorie malnutrition should be treated energetically, as outlined elsewhere.

When severe protein-calorie malnutrition is present, the clinical response of corneal xerophthalmia may be either delayed or (more dangerous) may be transient. It has been shown that the initial rise of holo-retinal-binding protein in response to vitamin A therapy is directly related to the adequacy of the antecedent serum albumin status. Relapses of corneal lesions usually respond to further treatment. Thus, in the presence of protein-calorie malnutrition, the dose of vitamin A should be repeated every one or two weeks until serum protein levels are normal.

Hypervitaminosis A may occur when doses of 20,000 IU or more are taken daily for protracted periods. The risk of intoxication has increased as a result of food faddism and of megavitamin therapy. Toxicity of vitamin A is heightened by marginal protein-calorie intake, parenchymal liver disease, or excessive alcohol intake. Acute vitamin A poisoning can occasionally lead to persistent deformities of the long bones as a result of premature closure of epiphyseal plates. Treatment consists of immediate discontinuance of vitamin A, after which signs and symptoms tend to disappear over days or

weeks. The time required for recovery is directly related to the duration of overdosage. For the unusual circumstance of the presence of hypercalcemia, treatment is described under hypervitaminosis D.

Vitamin D (Calciferol). Since the universal fortification of commercial cow's milk and infant formulas with vitamin D in North America, nutritional deficiency has been encountered only in special situations.

Vitamin D for therapeutic administration is currently available in three forms: 1) vitamin D_2 (ergocalciferol), the form included in commercial vitamin preparations and infant feeding products; 2) vitamin D_3 (calcitriol = 1,25-dihydroxycholecalciferol = 1,25$(OH)_2$-D_3) (Rocaltrol), the ultimate functional metabolite of vitamin D; 3) one alpha hydroxy vitamin D_3 (alphacalcidol = 1 α [OH]D_3) (One-Alpha).

PREVENTION. Ten μg (400 IU) of ergocalciferol daily is sufficient to prevent biochemical or clinical evidence of vitamin D deficiency in full-term, preterm, and low birth weight infants and in most children with steatorrheic disease.

The extent to which full-term, healthy, breast-fed infants require vitamin D supplementation is still unsettled. It seems clear that the concentration of vitamin D activity in human milk is low, about 40–50 IU/liter. However, detectable vitamin D deficiency in such children is rare unless unsupplemented breast-feeding is unusually prolonged and/or sun exposure is restricted. Human milk appears to supply calcium and phosphorus to young infants in a form utilizable for mineralization without the presence of a large amount of vitamin D. Until this paradox is elucidated further, vitamin D supplementation (as outlined above) is tentatively recommended for breast-fed infants. However, in view of the apparently very low risk to unsupplemented healthy full-term infants, it may be necessary to revise this recommendation in future.

TREATMENT. Most infants with vitamin D-deficient rickets can be treated safely and effectively with a vitamin D_2 (ergocalciferol) preparation in a dose of 5000 to 10,000 IU (125 to 250 μg) given once a day. Once biochemical and roentgenographic healing is complete, the dosage can usually be reduced to prophylactic levels.

Because commercially available 1,25$(OH)_2$-D_3 is expensive and requires close monitoring of dosage and of toxicity (hypercalcemia), its use is not recommended at present for the treatment of simple nutritional vitamin D deficiency.

Nutritional vitamin D deficiency has also been treated successfully and rapidly with a massive single dose (e.g., 600,000 IU, or 15,000 μg) of vitamin D_2*, but this approach is not required in most in-

---

*This massive dosage is not mentioned in manufacturer's official directive.

stances and may carry a potential risk of hypercalcemia due to vitamin D toxicity.

Different forms of vitamin D deficiency occur in association with chronic renal insufficiency and in the condition known as vitamin D dependency. Diffuse parenchymal renal disease, when sufficiently severe, is associated with low blood levels of $1,25(OH)_2$-D_3, and this deficiency is a major contributor to the development of renal osteodystrophy. Synthetic $1,25(OH)_2$-D_3 (Rocaltrol) has shown great promise in the treatment of renal osteodystrophy, but several cautions are required regarding its use in our current state of knowledge.

Before considering treatment with vitamin D metabolites, every effort should be made to normalize hyperphosphatemia, if present, through dietary restriction and the use of phosphate-binding agents. Correction of hyperphosphatemia in itself induces a rise in endogenous levels of $1,25(OH)_2$-D_3, a fall in elevated concentrations of parathyroid hormone, and an improvement in the response of serum calcium levels to parathyroid hormone.

Patients with moderate degrees of renal failure do not ordinarily require treatment with vitamin D metabolites, since serum levels of $1,25(OH)_2$-D_3 are usually normal if the glomerular filtration rate is in excess of 35 ml/min.

In severe renal failure with osteodystrophy, therapy with $1,25(OH)_2$-D_3 may be initiated with an oral dose of 0.25 to 0.5 μg/24 hr. Serum calcium levels must be followed closely throughout treatment, and the Ca X P product (mg/dl) should not be allowed to exceed 55.

If the serum calcium fails to increase by 0.5 mg/dl in 4 to 6 weeks, then the dose may be increased by 0.25 to 0.5 μg/24 hr. Dosage tolerance may decrease as treatment progresses, and the dose should be reduced somewhat as the serum calcium and alkaline phosphatase levels approach normal. Despite precautions, hypercalcemia may occur in a significant proportion of patients, and there is a possibility that hypercalcemia may induce a reversible or permanent further reduction in glomerular filtration rate. Dosages of the order of 0.5 μg/24 hr are generally regarded as safe if the patient is normophosphatemic.

An alternative to the use of $1,25(OH)_2$-D_3 is the use of the synthetic compound, alphacalcidol 1 $\alpha(OH)D_3$(One-Alpha).This compound is converted in the liver to $1,25(OH)_2$-D_3, thus bypassing the need for renal hydroxylation. Like $1,25(OH)_2$-D_3, it has a short half-life and may have a wider margin of safety as regards the risk of acute hypercalcemia.

In each patient the optimum dosage must be determined individually by "titration." The usual initial dose is 1 μg daily, with maintenance usually achieved with doses ranging between 0.25 and 1.0 μg daily or on alternate days.

If hypercalcemia should occur, treatment with vitamin D should be stopped and resumed at a lower dose when the serum calcium returns to normal. Some failures of treatment have been observed, but, in many children, healing of the bone lesions, disappearance of symptoms, and improvement in growth velocity and muscle strength have been the rewards of treatment.

Some patients with the nephrotic syndrome may develop vitamin D deficiency if they have prolonged proteinuria, which is associated with continuing loss of vitamin D_3 metabolites in the urine, leading to decreased intestinal absorption of calcium, secondary hyperparathyroidism, and skeletal resistance to parathyroid hormone. In such patients, administration of $1,25(OH)_2$-D_3 or 1 α OHD_3 can restore serum levels of the vitamin metabolite to normal.

Vitamin D-dependent rickets is due to a recessively inherited deficiency of the l-hydroxylase enzyme in the renal parenchyma required to convert hepatic 25-$(OH)D_3$ to the most active metabolite, $1,25(OH)_2$-D_3. Thus the resulting rickets can be completely cured by administration of the metabolite in physiologic amounts, that is, 1 to 2 μg daily, or by giving 1 α $(OH)D_3$ as described above. Prior to the availability of synthetic $1,25(OH)_2$-D_3, these children were treated successfully with vitamin D_2 (ergocalciferol) in doses on the order of 100 times the normal requirement, 40,000 to 50,000 IU daily. Because synthetic $1,25(OH)_2$-D_3 and $1\alpha(OH)D_3$ are expensive, vitamin D_2 may be the preferential treatment for many children. For all such children, vitamin D therapy must be maintained permanently.

HYPERVITAMINOSIS D. The first step in management is to stop administration of all forms of vitamin D immediately and to restrict dietary calcium intake. If the patient is being treated with $1,25$-$(OH)_2$-D_3, the serum calcium level will usually return to normal very rapidly when treatment is discontinued—within 2 or 3 days. In intoxication caused by vitamin D_2, correction of hypercalcemia may be much slower and may require more energetic intervention. The intensity of treatment and the number of agents used will have to be judged individually, depending on the severity of the hypercalcemia and the degree of resistance to initial treatment. The following additional modes of treatment of hypercalcemia can be used alone or in various combinations:

1. Maintain good hydration and urine output and correct any deficiency in serium sodium or potassium. Urinary sodium excretion enhances calcium excretion. Thus intravenous infusion of half strength saline is valuable.

2. Furosemide, 0.5 to 1.0 mg/kg initially, orally or parenterally, repeated at 6 to 12 hour intervals as required, depending on the response of the serum calcium level.

3. Prednisone, 2 mg/kg/24 hr.

In all but the most severe instances of hypercalcemia, these measures will usually suffice. However, other modes of lowering dangerously high serum calcium levels have been used successfully and may occasionally be required, such as 1) synthetic salmon calcitonin (Calcimar)*, 50 to 100 IU/24 hr, subcutaneously or intramuscularly (or 4 MRC units/kg every 12 hours, which may be increased to a maximum of 8 MRC units/kg every 6 hours, subcutaneously or intramuscularly); 2) sodium versenate (edetate disodium, USP) 15 to 50 mg/kg in half-isotonic saline or 5 per cent dextrose and water, given over a period of 4 hours. This treatment is contraindicated in children with renal disease.

Vitamin E (Tocopherol). The Recommended Dietary Allowance for tocopherol ranges from 3 mg of α-tocopherol equivalent (α-TE) per 24 hr in young infants to 10 mg of α-TE in adults. One International Unit (IU) is equivalent to the activity of 1 mg of dl-alpha tocopheryl acetate.

For most children with cystic fibrosis or other steatorrheic states, a daily oral dose of 1 mg/kg of a water-miscible preparation of alpha tocopheryl acetate will correct and maintain normal serum levels within a short period of time.

In children with cholestasis and diffuse liver disease (e.g., biliary atresia) much larger doses and intramuscular administration may be required to achieve normal serum tocopherol levels. In such patients the dose required should be determined by monitoring the serum level. This individualized approach to dosage and route of administration is especially important if neuromuscular disturbances are associated with very low serum tocopherol levels, as has now been described in some patients with cystic fibrosis and with biliary obstruction.

In very low birth weight infants, it now appears that the hemolytic anemia previously ascribed to tocopherol deficiency may be multifactorial in etiology. However, it has been suggested that administration of tocopheryl acetate in a dose of 16.5 mg daily to low birth weight infants (under 2000 gm) would result in significantly higher hemoglobin levels and lower reticulocyte counts than in infants receiving smaller amounts of tocopherol. The last word on tocopherol deficiency in very low birth weight infants has not yet been written. Thus, it is difficult to make dogmatic recommendations for or against routine supplementation of such infants' diets until further evidence becomes available.

Despite earlier claims, it now appears that tocopherol treatment has no significant protective value against the development of bronchopulmonary dysplasia in premature infants. Its efficacy for prophylaxis of retrolental fibroplasia is a matter of continuing debate and conflicting opinions.

---

*Manufacturer's precaution: There are no adequate data to support the use of Calcimar in children.

Vitamin K. The exact daily human requirement of vitamin K is unknown, since some of the vitamin is derived from synthesis in the intestinal lumen, though minimum dietary requirements have been estimated to be 1 to 5 μg/kg/24 hr for infants, and 0.03 μg/kg/24 hr for adults.

Prevention of vitamin K deficiency in the neonate is achieved by parenteral administration of 1 mg of water-soluble vitamin K_1 oxide (the natural form of vitamin K) at birth. Mild to moderate vitamin K deficiency, evidenced by prolonged prothrombin time without hemorrhagic manifestations, can usually be corrected by oral administration of 1 to 2 mg of vitamin K_1 per 24 hr. If signs of bleeding are present, parenteral administration of up to 5 mg of vitamin K_1 daily may be required. If the prothrombin deficiency is due to irreversible diffuse parenchymatous liver disease, then the prothrombin deficiency may fail to respond to vitamin K. In such cases, correction of the bleeding tendency may require transfusion of fresh frozen plasma.

Synthetic analogs of vitamin K may induce hemolysis in infants with glucose-6-phosphate dehydrogenase (G-6-PD) deficiency. Since such hemolysis does not occur with administration of vitamin K_1, the latter should be used preferentially.

In children with salicylate intoxication of any severity, parenteral vitamin K_1 oxide in a dose of 1 to 2 mg may be given as prophylaxis against prothrombin deficiency. Patients receiving total parenteral nutrition should be given vitamin K_1 oxide parenterally, 0.5 to 1 mg once weekly.

WATER-SOLUBLE VITAMINS

Thiamine (B_1). Thiamine combines with adenosine triphosphate (ATP) to form thiamine pyrophosphate (cocarboxylase). This compound is involved as a coenzyme in a number of intermediary metabolic reactions. The recommended daily dietary allowance for thiamine is 0.5 mg/1000 kcal. This is easily exceeded by most North American diets, and thus clinical thiamine deficiency in infancy and childhood is a rarity in North America.

Treatment consists of immediate parenteral (intravenous or intramuscular) administration of thiamine hydrochloride. Recommendations for initial dosage vary from 5 to 25 mg, depending on age and on the severity of the deficiency state. Treatment can be continued with oral thiamine, 5 to 10 mg daily, for 1 month.

In all forms of thiamine deficiency, the treatment regimen should include a diet that contains at least 1.5 gm protein/kg/day.

Riboflavin (B_2). Because riboflavin is widely distributed in the North American diet, clinical deficiency in children is rarely encountered. However, in less privileged parts of the world, clinical deficiency is seen, usually in association with protein-calorie malnutrition and deficiencies of other specific nutrients. The Recommended Dietary Allowance ranges from 0.4 mg/24 hr in young infants to 1.8 mg daily in young adults (based on an average allowance of 0.6 mg/1000 kcal/24 hr).

Treatment of clinical deficiency is oral administration of riboflavin in a dose of 6 to 20 mg/24 hr. In severe cases, an initial intramuscular dose of 25 mg may be given. At the same time, a diet containing adequate amounts of riboflavin should be prescribed. Principal dietary sources include milk, eggs, cereals, enriched bread, leafy green vegetables, and dried yeast. Recovery should be rapid, without sequelae, provided associated nutritional deficiencies are also treated vigorously.

Nicotinic Acid (Niacin). Treatment of clinical deficiency should begin with administration of nicotinamide (niacinamide) 50 mg subcutaneously three times daily until considerable clinical improvement has occurred. Thereafter supplementation with 10 to 20 mg per 24 hr by mouth will suffice. The diet should contain an adequate amount of tryptophan, which is metabolized to nicotinic acid. High concentrations of tryptophan are present in eggs, lean meat, and milk.

Pyridoxine (B_6). The generic term vitamin B_6 includes pyridoxine and its two derivatives, pyridoxal and pyridoxamine. The Recommended Dietary Allowance ranges from 0.3 mg/24 hr for infants under 6 months to 2.0 mg/24 hr for adults.

Satisfactory treatment of pyridoxine deficiency can usually be achieved with a dose of 10 to 20 mg daily for 3 weeks, following which the dose can be reduced to 2 to 5 mg daily for several weeks. In older children receiving antituberculous therapy with isoniazid, a dose of pyridoxine, 10 mg/100 mg INH per 24 hours is recommended.

Folic Acid (Folate, Folacin, Pteroylglutamic Acid). Recommended Dietary Allowances range from 50 μg daily in infants and 100 to 300 μg in children 1 to 10 years of age to 400 μg in older children and adults.

Megaloblastic anemia due to folic acid deficiency may be treated by giving 5 mg of folic acid orally per 24 hr for 2 to 3 weeks. Folic acid also can be given parenterally (IM, IV, or SC), as required. If there is any possibility of concomitant ascorbic acid deficiency, then ascorbic acid should be given concurrently in a dose of 200 mg daily.

Cyanocobalamin (B_{12}). The Recommended Dietary Allowances of vitamin B_{12} vary from 0.3 μg/24 hr for infants to 3.0 μg/24 hr for adults. The chief dietary source is animal protein. Primary dietary deficiency of vitamin B_{12} occurs in North America only when the diet structure has been very unusual.

The dose of vitamin B_{12} required to correct deficiency states must be determined on an individual basis. Congenital and juvenile pernicious anemias —both rare entities—require treatment for life. Treatment of these conditions may be initiated with intramuscular B_{12} in a dose of 15 to 50 μg every 1 to 2 days for 2 to 4 weeks. Thereafter, a single monthly intramuscular injection of 30 to 100 μg will usually provide satisfactory maintenance therapy.

Oral treatment with vitamin B_{12} should probably be used only for prophylaxis of deficiency in individuals on strict vegetarian diets. In such circumstances, a dose of 5 μg daily is adequate.

In uncomplicated B_{12} deficiency (without neurologic manifestations), a parenteral dose of 1 μg per 24 hr for 10 days is usually sufficient to induce clinical and hematologic remission, to be followed by 1 to 2 μg at monthly intervals, if required. If a Schilling test has been done, the loading dose of vitamin B_{12} will usually serve as adequate therapy for the first month.

Ascorbic Acid (Vitamin C). The Recommended Dietary Allowance is 35 mg/24 hr for infants, 40 mg/24 hr for young children, and 45 mg/24 hr for older children and adults. Breast milk normally contains adequate amounts (40 to 55 mg/liter), as do commercially prepared fruit juices and all commercial infant formulas.

In the newborn premature infant, a relative deficiency of ascorbic acid has been described in association with transient tyrosinemia. Although this phenomenon appears to lack serious ill effects or sequelae, the tyrosinemia will usually be corrected rapidly by administration of ascorbic acid, 50 to 100 mg daily, and by reducing the protein intake to 2 to 3 mg/kg/24 hr.

Scurvy is treated by oral administration of ascorbic acid, 100 to 200 mg daily for 1 to 2 weeks. At the same time, steps should be taken to insure that the subsequent diet meets the Recommended Dietary Allowance for ascorbic acid.

Total Parenteral Nutrition

JOHN H. SEASHORE, M.D.

Nutritional support is an essential part of management for 5–10% of hospitalized children. Inappropriate use, wasted resources, and complications can be minimized by careful patient selection and strict adherence to a protocol. A nutrition team (physician, nurse, pharmacist, and dietitian) should be responsible for establishing policies and guidelines, educating colleagues, and monitoring therapy.

Total parenteral nutrition (TPN) is an established technique that should be an integral part of good pediatric care. However, the potential complications and expense of TPN mandate careful patient selection. Many children who need nutritional support can be fed enterally, which is safer, less expensive, and more effective than TPN. The standard practice of including 5% dextrose in all intravenous solutions significantly decreases the rate of protein catabolism and is adequate for short periods of starvation. The addition of protein to the 5% dextrose further reduces nitrogen loss, but the patient is still in negative nitrogen balance and there is no evidence that this type of "protein-sparing" therapy has any significant clinical advantage over dextrose alone except in small premature infants. *Total* parenteral nutrition provides both protein and energy requirements and, in general, is indicated if a child will be fasting for more than 5–7 days. There is no evidence that TPN provides benefit for shorter time periods. However, it is much easier to *maintain* lean body mass than to replenish it. Therefore, we try to identify children who are likely to be fasting for more than 5 to 7 days and to start TPN before they become depleted.

CHOICE OF ROUTE

TPN can be given by central vein using protein and hypertonic dextrose (20–25%) or by peripheral vein with protein, 5–12.5% dextrose, and fat. Peripheral vein administration of protein and glucose alone does not meet the nutritional needs of children and is not indicated except in small, premature infants as noted above. The addition of appropriate quantities of an intravenous fat emulsion will provide *maintenance* energy requirements for most children and a modest increment for growth in some (Table 1). Since peripheral TPN is technically easier and somewhat safer than central TPN, it is usually preferred. However, there are some caveats to its use. The major risk of peripheral TPN is inadequate nutrition. A relatively high fluid volume (1.5 times maintenance) is necessary to give sufficient calories. The fat emulsion also must be infused at or near maximal allowable amounts to

ensure adequate calories (4 gm/kg/day in infants; 3 gm/kg/day in children). Interruptions of the flow of nutrients because of infiltration or the need to administer intravenous medications may make it impossible to administer the total amount of nutrients ordered for the day. Despite efforts to "catch up," actual caloric intake is often less than ideal. Other problems with peripheral TPN are limited venous access, skin sloughs from infiltrated solutions, and thrombophlebitis, which may cause sepsis. Peripheral intravenous sites *must be changed every 48 hours* to minimize the risk of phlebitis.

Central venous TPN obviates many of the problems of peripheral TPN but introduces mechanical, catheter-related complications and entails a higher risk of sepsis. Hypertonic glucose solutions provide about 1 kcal/ml (Table 1); therefore, maintenance caloric requirements can be provided in maintenance fluid volumes and the extra calories required by depleted or hypermetabolic patients can be given in acceptable volume.

In our experience, peripheral TPN is the appropriate choice for about 75% of children. Central TPN is indicated in patients who 1) require more than maintenance calories because they are wasted and/or hypermetabolic; 2) are fluid-restricted because of renal, cardiac, or pulmonary disease; 3) have no peripheral venous access; or 4) require long-term TPN (more than two weeks), particularly if growth is an important goal.

NUTRIENT SOLUTIONS

Our pharmacy provides three standard solutions, for infants, children, and adolescents (Table 2), which have proven to be suitable for about 75% of pediatric patients. At recommended rates of infusion (1–1.5 X maintenance) infants receive 2.5–3.0 gm/kg/day of protein and older children receive 1.5–2.0 gm/kg/day. Central TPN is initiated with a solution containing 10% glucose, increased to 20 or 25% dextrose over 48–72 hours in the absence of glycosuria. For peripheral TPN, glucose concentration is limited to 10–12.5%. The electrolyte content, including phosphate, is appropriate to the different age groups. Vitamins are supplied in a commercial mixture that is not ideal for children and must be supplemented with folate and vitamin K. However, clinical evidence of vitamin excess or deficiency has been rare, even during long-term TPN. There are at least 13 trace minerals known to be essential for humans. The requirements for 5 of these (zinc, copper, manganese, chromium and iodine) are reasonably well established for children, and these are routinely added to the solutions. As more data and clinical reports of deficiency states accumulate, selenium, molybdenum, and others may also be incorporated into standard TPN solutions.

Table 1. SAMPLE TPN REGIMENS

	ml/kg/day	Infants kcal/ml*	kcal/kg/day
D 12.5 P2	110	0.5	55
10% fat	40	1.1	44
Total	150		99
D 20 P2	150	0.75	114

	ml/day	30-Kg Child kcal/ml*	kcal/day
D 10 P3	1600	0.45	736
10% fat	900	1.1	990
Total	2500		1726
D 25 P3	2500	0.95	2375

*Hydrous glucose provides 3.4 kcal/gm.

Table 2. TPN SOLUTIONS

| | Contents per 1000 ml | | |
	Infants	*Children*	*Adolescents*
Dextrose	200 gm	250 gm	250 gm
Protein equivalent	20 gm	30 gm	40 gm
Kilocalories*	760	970	1110
Sodium	25 mEq	35 mEq	40 mEq
Potassium	24 mEq	36 mEq	36 mEq
Chloride	35 mEq	62 mEq	77 mEq
Calcium	11.3 mEq	8 mEq	4.8 mEq
Magnesium	4.8 mEq	4 mEq	8 mEq
Phosphate	7.8 mMol	7.8 mMol	21 mEq
Lactate	10 mEq	10 mEq	—
Acetate	12 mEq	18.7 mEq	26 mEq
Zinc	2.2 mg	3 mg	4.5 mg**
Copper	150 µg	200 µg	300 µg
Manganese	110 µg	150 µg	225 µg
Chromium	1.5 µg	2 µg	3 µg
Iodine	37 µg	50 µg	75 µg
Vitamins			
A	5000 units	3000 units	5000 units**
D	500 units	300 units	500 units
E	2.5 units	1.5 units	2.5 units
K	0.2 mg	0.2 mg	5 mg
Folate	0.25 mg	0.25 mg	1 mg

*Hydrous dextrose provides 3.4 kcal/gm.
**In adolescents, these amounts of trace minerals and vitamins are added to *1 liter* each day.

About 25% of pediatric TPN solutions must be modified to meet individual requirements. Alteration of electrolyte composition is common. Protein and/or glucose content may need to be decreased in children who do not tolerate the usual amount. Glucose content may be increased to provide adequate calories to children who require severe fluid restriction.

The solutions are prepared in the pharmacy under laminar flow hoods, using meticulous sterile technique. They are prepared and dispensed in appropriate-sized containers to minimize waste and to avoid the temptation to allow a bottle of solution to hang at room temperature for more than 24 hours.

TECHNIQUES OF ADMINISTRATION

Steel butterfly needles are preferred for peripheral TPN. Plastic cannulas are more thrombogenic and, because they are less likely to infiltrate, the temptation to leave them in place for more than 24 hours is too great. Venous cutdowns are also avoided, since it is prohibitive to change cutdown sites every 48 hours. Furthermore, the tip of the cutdown catheter may be in a deep and inaccessible vein where phlebitis is not recognized until sepsis supervenes. If a patient has no venous access except by cutdown, central TPN should be instituted.

The intravenous fat emulsion is administered by "piggyback" into the intravenous tubing near the point of entrance into the vein. Both solutions are delivered by pumps to ensure constant rates and prevent back-up of one solution into the other. Because venous access may be limited, it is often necessary to administer medications and other fluids through the same line. This is acceptable if the line is flushed with normal saline before and after medications are given, to prevent incompatibility reactions. Because frequent interruption of the TPN solutions to give medications may compound the problem of achieving adequate caloric intake, the importance of frequent checking that the child is receiving the amount of nutrient ordered cannot be overemphasized.

The preferred route for central TPN in older children is percutaneous catheterization of the subclavian vein. Although this technique can be used even in very small infants, it should be attempted only by experienced individuals. In most cases we catheterize the external jugular, common facial, or internal jugular vein by cutdown in small infants. The free end of the catheter is tunneled subcutaneously to exit the skin of the scalp or anterior chest wall, to protect against sepsis and provide a flat surface for the dressing. We use silicone rubber catheters, since they are soft, flexible, and less thrombogenic than others. The catheter is fixed in place by applying several short strips of tape directly to the skin with the aid of benzoin, and then taped securely to this patch of tape. This tape-to-tape method is more effective than sutures. Povidone-iodine ointment and a sterile occlusive dressing are applied. The dressing is changed by meticulous sterile technique 3 times a week.

The Broviac-type catheter, which is used routinely for home TPN, is worth considering even for short-term TPN. Although these catheters usually must be implanted under general anesthesia in children, the risk of sepsis is much lower. Evidence is accumulating that they are also safer for short-term use, probably because fibrous ingrowth into the Dacron cuff in the long subcutaneous tunnel provides excellent fixation of the catheter and minimizes to and fro motion of the catheter, which may cause local cellulitis and sepsis.

In general, central venous catheters are used only for the TPN solution, to decrease the risk of contamination. The Broviac-type catheter may be an exception to this rule because of its apparent safety and the accumulating experience with these catheters for TPN, fat emulsion, chemotherapy, and blood sampling. Our current policy is to allow multiple use of Broviac-type catheters in selected patients but to use conventional catheters only for TPN.

If fat is not given daily as a course of nonprotein calories, it is administered twice a week (2–3 gm/kg) to prevent essential fatty acid deficiency.

ESTIMATING ENERGY REQUIREMENTS

Numerous formulas have been proposed to estimate caloric needs. We prefer the simple formula:

Table 3. ESTIMATION OF ENERGY REQUIREMENTS

Basal = (55 – 2 × age) × kg	=	_____
Maintenance 20% × basal	=	_____
Activity 0–25% × basal	=	_____
Sepsis 13%/1°C × basal	=	_____
Simple trauma 20% × basal	=	_____
Multiple injuries 40% × basal	=	_____
Burns 50–100% × basal	=	_____
Growth/Anabolism 50% × basal	=	_____
Total	=	_____

estimated basal metabolic rate = 55–2 × (age in years) × wt in kg. The value obtained closely approximates measured BMR in children who are between the 10th and 90th percentile for age. Twenty per cent is added to the BMR to approximate resting metabolic expenditure, and additional increments are added for activity and various types of stress, as shown in Table 3. Another 50% of BMR is added to allow for growth, or for anabolism in the depleted patient. It should be emphasized that the resulting figure for caloric requirement is only an initial estimate. It is adjusted as indicated by the patient's clinical status, weight gain, serum albumin, and nitrogen balance.

COMPLICATIONS AND MONITORING

A complete discussion of the many potential complications of TPN is beyond the scope of this review but a few points should be mentioned. *Mechanical complications* related to the central catheter (pneumothorax, hydrothorax, venous thrombosis, cardiac arrhythmias, and perforation) can be eliminated or minimized by care in catheter placement and by radiographic confirmation of proper position before TPN solutions are infused.

Catheter-related *sepsis* is rightly the most feared complication of TPN, and occurs in 5–10% of pediatric patients. Sepsis is most frequently caused by *Staphylococcus aureus* or *S. epidermidis,* as a result of breaks in technique or local skin infection at the catheter insertion site. Gram-negative sepsis usually arises from a remote focus in the patient and the catheter serves to perpetuate bacteremia. Fungal sepsis is no longer common in TPN patients. The only way to know whether sepsis is related to the catheter is to remove and culture the catheter.

It is also nearly impossible to eradicate sepsis if an infected foreign body remains in the bloodstream. Therefore, the catheter is removed if the patient develops septic shock, a positive blood culture, or persistent, unexplained fever for more than 24 hours. Sepsis usually resolves promptly once the infected catheter is removed, and further treatment may not be necessary. However, if blood cultures are positive, we treat the patient with an appropriate course of antibiotics. Fatal sepsis is extremely rare if these guidelines are followed.

Potential *metabolic* complications are legion but most (glucose and electrolyte derangement, acidosis, fluid imbalance, vitamin and mineral deficiencies) can be prevented by appropriate formulation of solutions, or anticipated and corrected early by careful monitoring. Our protocol for clinical and laboratory monitoring is shown in Table 4. Hyperammonemia and cholestasis are common problems in pediatric TPN, particularly in premature infants. The etiology is unknown. The only effective treatment is to discontinue TPN and resume oral feedings. If that is not possible, a modest reduction of protein intake and substitution of fat for some of the glucose calories is beneficial in some children.

Fat emulsions are generally very safe in recommended doses but may not be effectively cleared from the serum or metabolized in sick patients, especially premature infants or older children who are stressed or septic. Determination of serum fat concentration by nephelometry is simple and more accurate than visual inspection and should be performed frequently. Even if the fat emulsion is cleared, fat may not be metabolized, so serum triglyceride concentration should be measured periodically.

Table 4. TPN MONITORING

Clinical	
Vital signs	q 4H
Intake and output	q 8H
Urine sp. gr. and glucose	q 8H
Weight	q d
Length and head circumference (infants)	1 ×/week
Laboratory	
Hematocrit, BUN, glucose, electrolytes	Daily × 4 then 2 ×/week
Bilirubin, SGOT, NH_3, alkaline phosphatase	1 ×/week
Ca, Mg, P, Protein, albumin	1 ×/week (optional in infants)
Patients receiving fat emulsion	
Serum fat emulsion level	Daily × 4 then 1 ×/week
Cholesterol, triglycerides	1 ×/week

2

Mental and Emotional Disturbances

Mental Retardation

MARK L. BATSHAW, M.D.,
and BRUCE K. SHAPIRO, M.D.

Mental retardation is defined as significant subaverage general intellectual functioning associated with impairment of adaptive behavior and manifested during the developmental period (AAMD, 1973). Treatment is palliative, as the underlying defect cannot be corrected. However, there are many ways pediatricians can help the mentally retarded child reach his potential, aid the family in coping and, in some cases, prevent the occurrence of mental retardation in future children. The first step is correct and early diagnosis to provide genetic counseling. Next, the pediatrician needs to advise the parents about appropriate expectations. Then, therapy must be directed at the child's educational needs, behavioral problems, and other associated deficits. Finally, there needs to be a periodic review of progress.

Early Diagnosis. Early diagnosis allows for the easing of parental anxiety, realistic goal setting, and greater acceptance of the child. Severely retarded children demonstrate major developmental delays at an early age, making the diagnosis straightforward. However, many mildly retarded children will not have significant developmental delays during the first year of life. Certain groups of children are at increased risk: premature infants, children who are small for gestational age, and infants who have suffered perinatal insults. However, most retarded children do not fall into an identifiable "at risk" group. Thus taking a complete developmental history is important for all children with developmental delays.

The parents will usually bring the retarded child to a pediatrician because the child is failing to fulfill developmental expectations. In early infancy, these include questions about hearing or vision and problems in feeding or swallowing. After six months of age, motor delay is the most common complaint. Language and behavior problems become prominent between two and four years, and school failure becomes evident in nursery school or in the early primary grades. Once identified, the child should be referred to an interdisciplinary evaluation center —e.g., school, university affiliated facility (UAF), or state diagnostic and evaluation center. Evaluation should include an examination by a developmental pediatrician and formal psychological testing. In addition to medical consultations, evaluations may be required from experts in behavioral psychology, special education, social work, speech, language and audiology, nursing, and physical and occupational therapies.

Etiology. Most cases of mental retardation remain idiopathic, especially in the mildly retarded group, which composes over 85% of the total mental retardation population. However, among retarded individuals with IQ < 50, determination of etiology is often possible. A diagnosis allows the parents to know why their child is retarded. It helps to reduce the guilt of "what could I have done differently to prevent this child's handicap" and allows association with other parents who have children with a similar diagnosis. It also permits prediction of future outcome based on reported experience with other children having similar diagnoses. Finally, it is important for genetic counseling. Among idiopathic cases of severe-profound mental retardation, the empiric recurrence risk is 3–5%. However in chromosomal or single gene defects, recurrence risks can be as high as 25–50%. Because of the diversity of conditions leading to mental retardation, there is no screening evaluation possible. A complete history and physical may give leads which should then be fully investigated, but fishing expeditions should be avoided. For example, skull x-rays, metabolic screens, and CT scans have not proven useful as diagnostic screening techniques in children with mental retardation. Various techniques of prenatal diagnosis are available for families with children having mental retardation of genetic origin.

Genetic Counseling. There are even a few examples of fetal therapy that may prevent mental retardation. For prenatal diagnosis to be successful, three conditions must be met. First, a correct diagnosis must be established. Second, the mother must be known to be at an increased risk for having a handicapped child; e.g., the increased risk of Down syndrome in a mother over 35 years old, the recurrence risk in a mother who has borne a Down child or a child with fragile-X syndrome, or a mother who is a translocation carrier. Third, the disorder must be identifiable by amniocentesis or other prenatal diagnostic techniques. For example, classic phenylketonuria cannot be diagnosed prenatally because phenylalanine hydroxylase, the deficient enzyme, is not expressed in amniocytes.

The most common form of prenatal diagnosis involves amniocentesis. The amniotic fluid can be used for alpha-fetoprotein determination of neural tube defects. The amniocytes are cultured for karyotyping, to determine the sex of the fetus or to detect chromosomal anomalies. Enzyme assays for inborn errors of metabolism can also be performed on the amniocytes. A second technique of prenatal diagnosis involves fetoscopy, which allows direct visualization of body parts so that syndromes associated with absent or deformed limbs can be identified. Fetal skin and liver biopsy have also been performed during fetoscopy. Fetal ultrasound, a method of indirect visualization, is now being used for definition of neural tube defects, microcephaly, and congenital heart defects.

The primary purpose of prenatal diagnosis has been to identify an affected fetus and offer therapeutic abortion. However, it may also influence the timing and mode of delivery or the perinatal care of the infant. For instance, a child with a complete urea cycle enzyme deficiency, organic acidemia, or maple syrup urine disease will become comatose during the first week of life. If diagnosed prenatally or at birth, the child can be started on appropriate therapy, and coma can be avoided. We are even approaching a time when fetal therapy may be possible. The classic example is the use of intrauterine transfusion for erythroblastosis fetalis. However, recently ventricular shunts have been placed in hydrocephalic fetuses, thyroxine has been injected into a hypothyroid fetus, and vitamin B_{12} has been given to a fetus with methylmalonic acidemia.

Associated Dysfunctions. Mental retardation is often accompanied by associated deficits that further limit the child's adaptive abilities. In their most obvious forms, associated dysfunctions can be considered additional diagnoses—cerebral palsy, visual deficits, seizure disorders, speech disorders, autism, and other disorders of language, behavior, and perception. *Formes frustes* of these disorders have also been recognized—clumsiness, attentional peculiarities, articulation disorders, hyperactivity, and school underachievement. The severity and frequency of the associated dysfunctions tend to be proportional to the degree of mental retardation but may be more incapacitating than the mental retardation itself. Failure to appreciate the effects of associated deficits usually results in unsuccessful habilitation and may heighten behavioral problems.

Educational Placement. If a mentally retarded child is placed in an inappropriate educational setting, his progress will be slowed, and behavioral problems are likely to increase. In 1975, Public Law 94–142, the Education for all Handicapped Childrens Act, came into force to ensure education for the retarded. The provisions of this law include identification, location, and evaluation of all handicapped children; provision of a full, appropriate public education for all handicapped children; and preparation and implementation of an individualized educational plan (IEP).

The goals for education should be based on the child's developmental level and the future goals for independence. If the child is mildly retarded (IQ 55–69), his prognosis for independence is good. Most of these individuals marry and hold jobs, although they are generally the last hired and first fired. Social-adaptive skills are also impaired, and this results in greater risks of deviant behavior and the need for assistance from social agencies. In school, these children need to gain basic academic and vocational skills and training in social interactions. Some may attain functional literacy (defined as a fourth grade education). The moderately retarded child (IQ 40–54) can look toward independence in self-care skills and partial social independence in a sheltered environment. Education needs to stress "survival" vocabulary and arithmetic and self-care skills. These children will not read for information. The severely–profoundly retarded child (I.Q. less than 40) may develop some language and self-help skills; however, he will remain basically dependent throughout life. If the child has associated deficits such as cerebral palsy or seizures, his function will be further impaired.

The appropriate placement for each of these groups of children should primarily be guided by their developmental level rather than by their chronological age. Although mainstreaming into homeroom, art, music, and physical education may be appropriate for the mildly retarded child, it has little benefit for children with more severe handicaps. The pediatrician should examine the individual educational program (IEP) to see if it appears appropriate in relation to the child's developmental level, especially if behavioral problems or poor school performance become evident.

Recreation is important to the mentally retarded child. Athletics should be encouraged. In general, retarded children do better in individual or small group activities than in the more complicated team sports. Activities requiring gross motor skills rather than fine motor coordination are most appropriate. Examples include track and field, swimming, and hiking. Although some physical limitations may be medically necessary, they should be as few as possible.

Behavior Management. Behavioral problems occur with greater frequency in retarded children than in normal children. The causes are complex and may result from the interaction of a variety of factors, including 1) inappropriate expectations of the child's developmental level; 2) organic behaviors: hyperactivity, short attention span, perseverance, self-injurious or self-directed behaviors; and 3) family problems.

These factors are not mutually exclusive and multiple causes are the rule. The majority of behavioral problems can be ameliorated by altering the child's environment, e.g., changing him to a more appropriate classroom setting and helping the parents understand that although he is 15 years old, he may not have the judgment to cross the street unsupervised. However, behaviors arising from organic deficits are less amenable to treatment by simple means. Two additional methodologies are employed to treat behavior problems: behavior modification and/or psychotropic drugs.

Behavior modification has proven effective in the control of various behavioral problems: hyperactivity, self-stimulatory, self-injurious, aggressive, and noncompliant behaviors. The basic premise in behavior modification is that behavior is controlled by its consequences. Thus, if a behavior is reinforced, it will occur with greater frequency in the future. If it is not reinforced, it will be less likely to recur. This theory leads to three basic methods of controlling behavior: reinforcement, punishment, and extinction.

Reinforcement leads to an increase in the frequency of a desired behavior. In positive reinforcement, food or social reinforcers, such as hugs, food or money, are given contingent on compliant behavior. Punishment differs from reinforcement in that it reduces the frequency of a behavior by use of aversive consequences or by the withdrawal of positive reinforcement. Aversive approaches, ranging from shouting "No" to electric shock, are used to control noncompliant or self-injurious behaviors. The other form of punishment, "timing out," involves placing the child in a situation or room that lacks anything of interest to him. This isolates him for 5–10 minutes from any social activity that would provide positive reinforcement.

Extinction involves the removal of positive reinforcement from a situation that was previously rewarding. In effect, the prior relationship between the behavior and the consequence is disconnected. An example is ignoring self-stimulatory behavior while providing positive reinforcement as soon as the child stops. Usually, the targeted behavior will increase initially and then gradually diminish. Often extinction is paired with a procedure called differential reinforcement of other behaviors (DRO). While the self-stimulatory behavior is being extinguished, an incompatible behavior such as stringing beads, is being reinforced. As a group, these behavioral approaches appear to be as effective as psychotropic drugs, although they obviously take more time and effort and long term outcome studies have not been performed.

Mental retardation does not necessarily mandate the use of *psychotropic agents.* Drugs should not be used as a substitute for programming but rather to facilitate learning and social interactions or to suppress behaviors that are harmful to the patient or others. The drugs most commonly used to control behavior fall into the groups of phenothiazines, butyrophenones, and amphetamines. Phenothiazines include chlorpromazine (Thorazine), thioridazine (Mellaril), and trifluoperazine (Stelazine). These drugs act as dopamine antagonists. They result in sedation and decreased levels of motor activity, anxiety, combativeness, and hyperactivity. They also impair attention span. The usual dose in childhood for chlorpromazine or thioridazine is 25–200 mg/day but this dosage needs to be individually titrated. The peak drug levels following oral intake occur in 2–3 hours. The half-life varies from 2–5 days. Common side effects include hyperphagia and lethargy. Uncommon toxic effects include blood dyscrasias, cholestatic jaundice, dermatitis, and increased seizure frequency. After long term therapy, tardive dyskinesia and akathesia may occur. These symptoms do not always disappear following termination of drug therapy. Haloperidol (Haldol), a butyrophenone, has similar therapeutic effects. However, it produces more frequent extrapyramidal side effects. The usual dosage range is 1–5 mg/day.

Stimulants such as methylphenidate (Ritalin) or dextroamphetamine (Dexedrine) have been shown to be effective in the short term control of hyperactivity and attentional problems in children with normal intellectual functioning. However, they are much less effective in controlling hyperactivity in mentally retarded children. Because they have fewer or less severe side effects than phenylthiazines, stimulants are still worth trying in the mentally retarded child. Dosage ranges from 0.5–2.0 mg/kg/day for methylphenidate and 0.25–1.0 mg/kg/day for dextroamphetamine. Peak levels occur in 2 hours, and the half life is 2–4 hours.

A 1–2 week trial should be sufficient to evaluate the effectiveness of a medication in controlling behavior. Preferably, the study should be done with the teacher remaining unaware of the drug condition and keeping records of attention, behavior, and hyperactivity. Drug holidays should be attempted at least yearly to evaluate the need for continued medication. Psychotropic approaches using antihistamines, megavitamin therapy, and caffeine have been found to be ineffective.

Thus, the benefits of psychotropic drugs in mentally retarded children are modest and the risks, especially of phenothiazines and butyrophenones, are not inconsiderable. The risk-benefit ratio is not clearly positive in many children. Psychotropic drugs should then be used as a last resort, on a short term basis, and only in combination with an appropriate behavior modification and educational program.

Family Counseling. The emotional impact of having a mentally retarded child is enormous. The stages of grief the family passes through are similar to those of parents who have lost a child. The initial response is one of disbelief. The parents will rarely hear what you say after the words mental retardation are mentioned. Thus, the parents may find it difficult to absorb medical information about their child at this time.

After the initial shock and denial, the parents start to feel guilty. The mother especially may feel that she could have done something during her pregnancy to prevent the handicap or could have given better care to the child or sought medical attention sooner. Accompanying these are feelings of anger, "Why us?" The parents may direct their anger at each other, at God, at the pediatrician, or even at their child. The risk of child abuse is increased. The parents also feel isolated. They may feel they are the only ones with this problem. They need reassurance from the pediatrician and may also benefit from a parents' support group.*

The next step in coping involves bargaining: "If only we try harder, perhaps he will be normal." The pediatrician needs to help the parents maintain realistic expectations during this time. Some parents may intellectualize, accumulating a great deal of medical information about the child instead of confronting their own feelings. Some parents remain in this stage forever. Others move on eventually to a stage of acceptance.

Having a mentally retarded child also affects the

*Batshaw M, Perret Y: *Children with Handicaps,* Brookes Publishing Co., 1981.

stability of a marriage and the emotional health of the siblings. It is not uncommon for parents to be at different stages of coping. Further, one parent may want to talk about his or her feelings while the other does not; this leads to feelings of frustration and isolation. The siblings may share this anxiety. They are stigmatized as being the brother or sister of the "mental kid" and they may worry that they can "catch" the mental retardation. While feeling relieved that they are not retarded themselves the siblings may also feel guilty about being normal. They may also feel resentful that the parents spend more time with the mentally retarded child than with them. They may even be worried that they will have to care for their handicapped sibling when they grow up. The grandparents need also to be considered as they may assume some of the care of the child and will certainly influence the attitudes of the parents. Thus, counseling of the entire family is needed.

Re-evaluations. Although mental retardation is considered a static encephalopathy, there is a need for periodic review. As the child and family grow, new information must be imparted, goals readjusted, and habilitation programming altered. A review requires information about health status, family functioning, child functioning at home and at school, and the nature of the school programs. Other information, such as formal psychological or educational testing, may be needed. Annual reviews are generally necessary until school age. These reviews should also be undertaken any time the child is not meeting previous expectations.

As the child grows, he moves from one service provision system to another. This also marks the time for a review. Re-evaluation is necessary with the move from preschool to primary grades, from primary to intermediate grades, from intermediate to senior programming, and at the conclusion of school. By this time, the child has been abandoned by other adolescents. The disparity between cognitive abilities and chronologic age prevents the retarded adolescent from fitting in. This isolation promotes social awkwardness and diminishes the adolescent's self-esteem. Many parents feel incompetent to deal with issues of emerging sexuality in their retarded children.

The teaching of sexuality, dealing with menses, masturbation, and inappropriate closeness are some of the more common issues brought up by parents of retarded adolescents. In the severely retarded patients, sexual drive is limited, and few problems other than masturbation develop. These youngsters should be taught that masturbation is acceptable behavior in the privacy of their room but not in public. In the moderately retarded patient, sexual drive may be normal, although late in developing. As judgment is limited, close parental supervision is essential. Contraception should be afforded to all retarded individuals who are sexually active. Although controversy regarding reversible versus irreversible methods of contraception continues to exist, the present legal climate precludes irreversible contraception in most cases.

Late adolescence coincides with the transition from intermediate to senior programs. School will be ending, and long term planning concerning vocation, living situation, and independence should be in progress. Such planning needs to be based more on achievement than on potential. It is not uncommon to see a leveling off of academic abilities, and this should not be confused with a progressive neurologic disorder. Heterosexual activities, marriage, contraception, and social intergration are all common concerns at this age. With the completion of school, there is no clearly identified service system for the retarded person. Plans for living arrangements and vocational pursuits should be in place and able to be activated when school is completed.

In the past, the answer to placement for the retarded patient was institutionalization. Many of those individuals are now being de-institutionalized and placed into group homes or smaller institutions or returned to their families. In general, the only patient who will be institutionalized in the foreseeable future is the multiply handicapped child whose parents cannot cope with the combined medical, behavioral and intellectual problems. Most moderately–severely retarded individuals will remain at home and attend activity centers or sheltered workshops. Alternate living situations, such as group homes, are gaining acceptance but are still few in number.

General Pediatric Care. Besides these special services, the mentally retarded child requires the same basic pediatric supervision as the child with normal intelligence. This includes following immunization schedules, growth parameters, and treating intercurrent infections. However, there may be additional concerns under certain circumstances. Mentally retarded children in classes or institutions where hepatitis B antigen has been identified may require the hepatitis B vaccine. Multiply handicapped children with recurrent respiratory infections may benefit from influenza vaccine. Weight gain may be deficient or excessive and requires nutritional intervention. Also counseling of parents concerning reduced growth potential is necessary. Dental hygiene needs to be addressed, especially for children receiving phenytoin or who are incapable of self-brushing. Preventive dental measures include decreasing the intake of sucrose-containing sweets by substituting noncariogenic snacks such as fruits and potato chips for candy and sugar-laden cereals. Toothbrushing and the use of fluoride should also be emphasized.

Psychiatric Disorders

DENNIS P. CANTWELL, M.D.

Treatment planning in child psychiatry depends partly on the nature of the psychiatric syndrome of the child. Treatment of various clinical psychiatric syndromes that *regularly begin* and *first manifest* themselves in infancy and childhood, such as schizophrenia, will be reviewed, but those that generally are seen in adult life will not be discussed or will be mentioned only briefly. Developmental disorders are covered later.

The various types of therapy available in child psychiatry may be broadly classified into the following categories: psychodynamic psychotherapies, which include individual psychotherapy with the child and play therapy, and marital and family therapies (most of which have a psychodynamic orientation); various forms of behavior therapy; and biologic therapies (primarily psychopharmacologic agents).

OVERT BEHAVIORAL DISORDERS

Attention Deficit Disorder (ADD)

This disorder is discussed separately in this chapter.

Conduct Disorders

Although this group of disorders has the strongest correlation with disturbed behavior in later life, treatment of conduct disorders has proved to be notoriously difficult. There is no solid evidence that psychotropic medication of any kind has any positive benefit in conduct disorder. Some children with conduct symptoms have an underlying attention deficit disorder with hyperactivity and may benefit from stimulant medication. Likewise, some children with conduct symptoms may have an associated affective disorder, and some children with affective disorder may develop conduct symptomatology after they become depressed. In both cases, the use of antidepressant medication may be beneficial. For the general run of children with conduct disorders, psychotropic medication will play little or no role.

Evidence for successful treatment of conduct-disordered children with individual dynamic psychotherapy is lacking. Many reports stress anxiety-reducing therapeutic techniques and imposed restraints and controls within a therapeutic setting for conduct-disordered children. This does not mean that individual psychotherapy may not be indicated and successful for certain cases. But outpatient treatment of conduct-disordered children using individual dynamic psychotherapy alone is not likely to produce major changes in behavior for the majority. Family therapists have described certain family dynamics that lead to conduct disorder behavior in children. These include such things as the "super ego lacunae," in which the child is conceptualized as acting out the wishes of the parent. In such cases family therapy may be effective in reducing the acting-out behavior of the conduct-disordered child.

Much of the literature on dynamic psychotherapy with conduct-disordered children has come from institutional settings that impose strong limits and controls on the children while providing individual and possibly family dynamically oriented psychotherapy. It is quite common for children to stay for several years in such institutions, especially during early adolescence.

The greatest advances in the treatment of conduct disorders have come in the area of various behavioral programs at home, school, and inpatient settings. Successful modification of such antisocial behaviors as destructiveness, aggression toward peers, stealing, fire setting, and running away by the use of behavior modification programs has been carried out in the home by parents and in classrooms by teachers and peers.

As with other psychiatric disorders of childhood, many conduct-disordered children suffer from a variety of academic deficits as well. Remediation of these deficits can in fact lead to improved self-esteem, and the provision of other "success experiences" is likewise likely to lead to increased self-esteem. Nevertheless, the treatment of conduct-disordered children remains a very difficult and perplexing problem with no easy solution.

EMOTIONAL DISORDERS

Separation Anxiety Disorder

This disorder is characterized by predominant, excessive anxiety occurring on separation from major attachment figures or from home or other familiar surroundings. When such separation occurs, the child experiences anxiety to the point of panic. This reaction is beyond what would be expected considering the child's developmental level.

School refusal is one of the most predominant manifestations of separation anxiety disorder in younger children, and the disorder has often been erroneously called "school phobia." Not all cases of school refusal are due to separation anxiety, but when separation is at the root of school refusal it is not a true phobia. In true school phobia, children fear the school situation whether or not they are accompanied by a parent. Many mild cases of separation anxiety with school refusal are handled by school personnel. School staff, including teachers, nurses, principals, and others, by blending a combination of emotional support for the child and emotional support for the parent (usually the mother) with coercion of the child to return to school may

be successful in mild cases. Psychotherapists in general also use a combination of coercion and emotional support.

The most successful management of school refusal with separation anxiety seems to employ a combination of dynamically oriented therapy for the child and/or family (especially when parents encourage dependent behavior) and behavior therapy techniques. Both implosion and systematic desensitization have brought a successful return of children to the school and decreased separation anxiety. Rapid return to school with a program involving lack of emphasis on somatic complaints, rewards for school attendance, and support for both parent and child has been described. A physician, parent, older sibling, teacher, or other individual may be a therapeutic ally. Imipramine in combination with a behavioral program was successful in abating the panic attack of children with separation anxiety disorder and leading them to return to school.

While there may be periods of exacerbation over a period of several years, separation anxiety disorder generally disappears with age. Only in rare cases, anxiety caused by a possible separation, and the avoidance of situations involving separations (such as going away to college), may persist into adult life.

Avoidant Disorder

Avoidant disorder is characterized by a predominant, persistent, and excessive shrinking from contact with strangers of sufficient severity that it interferes with social functioning and peer relationships. However, this is coupled with a clear desire for affection and acceptance, and relationships with family members and other familiar figures are warm and satisfying. This disorder has a variable course, with some children improving spontaneously. What percentage improve spontaneously and what percentage continue into adult life as avoidant personality disorder is unknown, but the latter generally is felt to be a rare occurrence.

Nondirective play therapy techniques have been used to overcome social inhibition in children with this type of problem. In general, these techniques have been shown to work best in younger children whose home environment is fairly restrictive. By developing a relationship with the therapist and growing in self-confidence, the child begins to do things independently.

Likewise, a variety of behavioral programs have been successful in modifying the social isolation of avoidant-disordered children. Modeling with guided participation, in which a therapist leads a child through tasks the child had been unable to do previously because of fear, has been used. The tasks are arranged in a hierarchy of difficulty, and the therapist first demonstrates, then practices with, then participates with the child in performing the task. Eventually the child is able to perform the feared response alone. Social reinforcement by teachers to modify isolated behavior and training in the use of social skills by videotape demonstration have also been found effective with this type of problem.

When parents and other family members consciously or unconsciously reinforce the child's dependency and isolated behavior, concurrent family work or a more dynamic family therapy approach will be necessary. In some cases this reinforcement of the child's socially isolated behavior by the parents may indicate an underlying parental depression or other disorder, which may have to be treated in addition to the work done with the child.

Overanxious Disorder

Treatment of anxiety must take into account a variety of factors. "Slow to warm up children" who take a long time to adapt to new situations and do so with excess anxiety should be allowed to move at their own pace into new settings and to make adaptations to environmental change. In these children treatment will be directed toward support and reassurance to overcome feelings of insecurity or failure. Parents will have to be helped to understand the nature of their child's temperamental style and to try to minimize or remove relevant stresses in the child's environment. When an acute anxiety state is precipitated by an actual or frightening experience, treatment may take the form of behavioral methods such as teaching the child to relax, or by desensitization to overcome the situation-specific anxiety.

When chronically anxious parents induce stress in the parent-child interaction and prolong their child's anxiety by their own insecurity and anxiety, treatment may require a more family-oriented approach.

In some children the treatment of choice will be individual, dynamically oriented psychotherapy, which aims at delineating the actual origins of the anxiety. Time-limited, focused therapy is particularly useful in these situations. In contrast to their use with anxiety disorders in adult life, the antianxiety drugs play little role in the treatment of generalized anxiety in childhood.

Phobic Disorders

Although there is a very large body of research comparing different methods of treatment for phobic disorders in adults, there are fewer systematic studies of treatment of phobic disorders using different therapeutic methods in children. As with generalized anxiety disorders, psychotropic drugs play little or no role in treatment. Generally, treatment involves a combination of dynamically oriented psychotherapy and various forms of behavior therapy. In simple, circumscribed phobias, behav-

ior therapy seems to be the first choice. The four basic essentials involved in any type of treatment of phobia are (1) establishing a therapeutic relationship with the child and the family; (2) clarifying the phobic stimulus; (3) desensitization to the phobic stimulus by a variety of mechanisms, including modeling, interpretation in psychotherapy, reciprocal inhibition, graded change, or implosion; and finally (4) confrontation with the feared object, which seems to be an essential part of the treatment. Families must also be helped to develop better mechanisms in dealing with the situation they fear and to refrain from allowing the child to manipulate them with avoidance behaviors to the phobic stimulus. These behaviors then become rewarding to the child in themselves.

Obsessive-Compulsive Disorder

This disorder usually begins in adolescence or early adulthood, but may begin in childhood. Individual psychotherapy of the child coupled with parental counseling has been the main technique used with obsessional children for the longest period of time. More recently, behavioral approaches have been used with this disorder in childhood and seem to be the most promising method of treatment. These include modeling of appropriate behavior, response prevention (to prevent the child from carrying out the compulsive act), and real life exposure to feared stimuli. With both adults and children, psychotropic drugs have been found to play little or no role in treatment. Recently, chlorimipramine, developed as a treatment for depressive disorders in adults, has been found to be effective in obsessive-compulsive disorder in adults. To date no such studies have been carried out with children.

In all the disorders described above, anxiety either is the predominant symptom or occurs if the child attempts to master the symptoms. Thus in phobic disorder anxiety occurs if the child confronts the feared object or attempts to resist the obsessions and compulsions in obsessive-compulsive disorder. These disorders are described as classic "neurotic disorders" in psychodynamic terminology. The term "emotional disorders" is used here as a purely descriptive term to denote the entire set of disorders, with no implication that etiologically they are all due to unconscious psychodynamic conflict, which the term "neurosis" or "neurotic disorder" often implies.

Affective Disorders

Affective disorders are characterized by disturbance of mood accompanied by a complete or partial manic or depressive syndrome. Manic episodes, that is, episodes with a predominantly elevated, expansive, or irritable mood accompanied by other characteristic symptoms, do occur in children but only rarely. A depressive syndrome is characterized by dysphoric mood and a pervasive loss of interest or pleasure in almost all or usual activities, accompanied by other characteristic symptoms; this occurs more commonly in children than do manic episodes.

The availability of lithium carbonate has changed the treatment of manic syndromes in adults drastically over the last 10 years. Lithium is thought to be not only effective for ameliorating the active phase of the manic syndrome but also prophylactic for both future manic and depressive episodes in susceptible individuals. There are very few studies of children with manic syndromes, but lithium seems to be an effective mode of treatment for them as well. It should be coupled with individual psychotherapy for the child, with a clear explanation so that the child can understand the nature of the disorder, what factors may precipitate a manic episode, and better ways of coping with those factors. Work with the parents should focus on similar aspects.

The treatment of depressive *syndromes* in children should be distinguished from the treatment of depressive *symptoms,* particularly the symptom of demoralization. Depressive symptoms are very common in a wide variety of psychiatric disorders in children. Demoralization as a syndrome is very similar to the depressive syndrome, and it is also quite common in children with a variety of different psychiatric disorders. However, these depressive symptoms and the demoralization syndrome are not accompanied by the *pervasive anhedonia* that characterizes the depressive syndrome. It is important to make this distinction because tricyclic antidepressant medication has been shown to be as effective in the treatment of the depressive syndrome in childhood as it is in the treatment of the depressive syndrome in adults. The demoralization syndrome does not respond to tricyclic medication.

Both individual and family psychotherapy should be utilized with children who have a significant depressive syndrome. Psychotherapy should aim at helping the child recognize the nature of the condition and find more appropriate and more successful ways of coping with everyday stress. Promoting self-esteem and alleviating excessive guilt are also goals of individual therapy. Work with the parents should focus on more appropriate ways of dealing with certain environmental stresses that may provoke the depressive syndrome in the child.

A significant number of parents may be depressed themselves, suggesting both environmental and possible genetic predisposing factors to the depression in the child. Intense family conflicts also may lead to depressed feelings in the child. Helping the parents toward open communication in the family and helping them to promote sources of self-esteem in the child are goals of family work with parents of depressed children.

Pervasive Developmental Disorders (Childhood Psychoses)

More is known about the treatment of infantile autism than that of other types of pervasive developmental disorders. Conceptualization of the nature of infantile autism has changed radically over the last few years, and the treatment has changed accordingly. Probably the single, most important aspect of the treatment is skilled special educational techniques. Those techniques involving specific teaching of specific skills in a very structured and organized program are more effective than those that are permissive or regressive. Techniques designed to overcome the children's handicaps should be stressed. Since a cognitive deficit in receptive language is one of the key, if not the cardinal, symptoms of infantile autism, skilled speech and language therapy is an important part of any treatment program. However, simple parroting of language is not the desired goal. It is important that the child's understanding of language be increased, and, in this context, increasing imitative behavior and increasing the range of play may be very useful. Developing gestural techniques may be appropriate in children who cannot develop useful degrees of spoken language after extensive speech therapy. Nevertheless, even with the best of special education and language techniques, the ultimate prognosis depends on the level of IQ. Those children below the IQ level of 50 make considerably less progress than those with IQs of 50 and above.

Most modern therapeutic programs also emphasize working directly with the parents of autistic children. Several factors are important here. Stresses caused by having an autistic child in the family can be very great. Helping parents cope with these stresses as well as giving them skills to modify the child's behavior and involving them directly in language programs and other therapeutic programs has been found to be effective. A structured environment and using short sentences which are more appropriate to the child's level of verbal comprehension are useful techniques.

Most studies of behavioral programs have shown that a variety of behavior modification techniques may be useful in reducing various types of deviant and destructive behavior, including aggressive behavior, self-injury, and stereotypes. However, it is important to recognize that any improvement in behavior will tend to be very specific to the situation in which the children have been treated. Behavior change successfully induced in a hospital setting will not generalize to the home or school setting unless parents and teachers are involved to insure it.

Because in the past infantile autism was thought to be the earliest manifestation of adult-onset schizophrenia, it was felt that the major antipsychotic drugs so useful in the treatment of adult schizophrenia would be useful in a similar fashion with autistic children. Most studies of psychotropic drug management have failed to separate autism from other pervasive developmental disorders and from schizophrenia that may occur in childhood. However, it is generally recognized that major tranquilizers such as the phenothiazines do not have an antipsychotic effect in the true sense of the word as they do with adults with schizophrenia. They may play a contributory role in lessening certain aspects of deviant behavior. Because of possible side effects their use should be judicious and only for the enhancement of the child's response to other aspects of the therapeutic program. No drug has been found to be specific for the cardinal symptoms of autism itself.

While less is known about treatment of other types of pervasive developmental disorders, the same principles probably can be enunciated for them. The treatment of schizophrenia that begins only rarely in childhood is basically no different from its treatment in adult life except that it has to be geared to the developmental context of the child.

PSYCHIATRIC DISORDERS WITH PRIMARILY PHYSICAL MANIFESTATIONS

Eating Disorders

Anorexia Nervosa and Bulimia. The management of anorexia nervosa involves a combination of treatment modalities. Individual psychotherapy for the patient is necessary to explore underlying factors relating to the disturbed body image and eating behavior. Family therapy, generally coupled with direct intervention using behavior modification procedures, is also generally used in conjunction with individual psychotherapy for the patient. The eating behavior of the patient no longer should be the concern of the whole family, but rather a problem between the patient and the treating physician. Behavior modification procedures aimed at obtaining greater rewards for maintenance of body weight and normal eating behavior are most effective in reaching and maintaining a normal body weight. Severe cases generally have to be hospitalized because of the risk of death by starvation, infection, or metabolic disturbances such as hypokalemia.

Active drug treatment with phenothiazines has been advocated, and antidepressants have recently become popular because of the relationship between anorexia and affective disorder. There is some question whether the addition of drug treatment adds anything to these regimens. Cyproheptadine and insulin treatment to produce an artificial hypoglycemia and create appetite have also been advocated, but the data to support such treatment are lacking. Studies of the outcome of anorexia nervosa indicate a significant mortality rate, especially in the older reports. Psychopathology, particularly of the affective type, may still be present in recovered anorexics. Thus treatment should be vigorous and consist of a multimodal approach.

Pica. This is discussed later in this section.

Stereotyped Movement Disorders

Stereotyped movement disorders involve abnormalities of gross motor movement and all involve tics. Three stereotyped movement disorders may be distinguished: transient tic disorder, chronic motor tic disorder, and Tourette disorder. These may represent three distinct conditions or they may be considered to be a continuum of severity. Treatment of motor tics, both transient and chronic, has generally emphasized psychotherapy for the child coupled with behavioral approaches such as massed practice, operant techniques, negative practice, and aversive techniques.

A wide variety of approaches to the treatment of Tourette disorder have been used, including psychotherapy, behavior therapy, hypnosis, shock, isolation, and other approaches. However, in the past few years haloperidol has become the mainstay of treatment. This may be used in conjunction with other forms of therapeutic intervention. Because of lack of comparative studies, it is unclear whether combinations of psychotherapy or behavior modification or other treatments with haloperidol would produce more lasting results than haloperidol alone. Clonidine recently has been found to be an effective therapeutic agent for Tourette disorder in those patients who have had a poor response to haloperidol.

Enuresis

Enuresis is *primary* if it has not been preceded by a period of urinary continence for at least a year and *secondary* if there has been a period of urinary continence for at least 1 year. The onset of primary enuresis is generally before the age of 5 years; most cases of secondary enuresis begin between ages 5 and 8 years. Psychotherapy has not been shown to be effective in controlled studies in the treatment of enuresis. Generally, treatment entails the use of simple measures such as restricting fluid intake before the child goes to bed and night lifting, which has had variable success; teaching children to defer micturition during the day—a procedure called daytime training, which has been shown to be effective; conditioning treatment such as the buzzer and pad; and the use of tricyclic antidepressants like imipramine. The buzzer and pad are most likely to be the most effective treatment. Use of this reduces the enuretic rate in a greater number of children than does drug treatment, and also there are fewer relapses when the conditioning treatment is removed. No drugs other than tricyclic antidepressants have been shown to be consistently effective in the treatment of enuresis.

The treatment of daytime wetting usually involves giving the child an increased fluid load and forcing the appropriate use of the toilet when the child recognizes the urge to pass urine. Habit training has also been used. In this approach the child is taught to go to the toilet regularly at predetermined intervals during the day even though he or she does not feel the urge to void.

Systematic epidemiologic studies show that most enuretics do *not* have other psychiatric disturbances and that most bedwetters never receive treatment.

Encopresis

Treatment of encopresis depends on understanding the physiologic mechanisms involved. Hersov distinguished three types of enopresis. (1) The child has demonstrated control of the physiologic process of defecation but deposits his or her normal feces in inappropriate places. (2) There is true failure to gain bowel control. The child is unaware of soiling or is unable to control the bowels. (3) Soiling is due to feces that are excessively fluid. This type may result from diarrhea or may arise from constipation leading to retention with overflow.

In the third type of encopresis, treatment involves clearing any blockage of feces in the bowel, which serves the dual purpose of preventing a large impaction and also removes anxiety and fear in the young child, and putting the child on a regular bowel training program, using stool softeners and laxatives. Special care must be given to insure that the bowel training program does not perpetuate any battle between the parent and child over toilet training.

In the second type, the proper approach is a consistent bowel training program. This may involve simple behavioral rewards for using the toilet successfully and regularly or more complex schemes of reinforcement that involve not only material rewards but also social reinforcement from the parents. These families may exhibit a disturbed parent-child interaction that must receive attention.

In the first type, there is more likely to be a more generalized psychiatric disorder, of which the encopresis is part. Families of these children may also have a more deviant parent-child interaction. This type of encopresis is more difficult to treat and requires a multimodal approach involving treatment of the child's general psychiatric disorder, restoration of a more normal parent-child interaction, as well as the more pragmatic aspects of simple rewards in a behavioral sense for nonsoiling and relief of constipation.

Sleep Terrors (Pavor Nocturnus) and Sleep Walking (Somnambulism)

Treatment of sleep walking can generally be carried out by the parents. A child who is found sleep walking should be led back to bed. A system can be set up to confine sleep walking to the bedroom by securely fastening bedroom doors or gates. In some cases, giving a child direct suggestion that he or she will awaken fully as soon as his foot touches the floor is helpful. Imipramine has also been used for treatment.

Both imipramine and diazepam have been used successfully to treat sleep terrors. Psychotherapy to allay the child's anxiety and fears, which may underlie some of the night terrors, has been found to be effective. The parents should be instructed to provide a warm, quiet atmosphere prior to bedtime to help prevent occurrences; during an episode they should be comforting, help orient the child to reality, and stay until the episode is over.

OTHER PSYCHIATRIC DISORDERS OF CHILDHOOD

Elective Mutism

Elective mutism is characterized by a continuous refusal to speak in almost all social situations by children who have the ability to comprehend spoken language and to speak normally. A wide variety of therapeutic modalities have been tried, with mixed results. These include inpatient treatment, long-term psychotherapy (both verbal and nonverbal), behavior modification procedures such as desensitization, social relearning, reciprocal inhibition, and systematic reinforcement of speaking in social situations.

Schizoid Disorder

Schizoid disorder is characterized by a defect in the capacity to form social relationships. Depending on the etiologic factors, treatment involves a combination of individual and family therapy and teaching of specific social skills to the child by the parent. Behavioral programs in which the parents actively encourage and promote group participation and social interaction with the appropriate awards are also effective.

Autism

ALAN N. MARKS, M.D.

Primary symptoms of autism are a lack of social interest, delayed or deviant development of speech and language, and resistance to changing a repeated simple pattern of behavior. About half of autistic children do not have meaningful speech by the age of 5 years, and the proportion is roughly the same among autistic adolescents. Recent work suggests that some of these children may be taught to communicate by sign language, but it is too early to judge how effective this approach will be. Among autistic children who do talk, speech and language tend to be impoverished and odd. The speech is like that of a robot, lacking the usual inflections and changes in tone.

Resistance to change, odd preoccupations or attachments, and repeated simple patterns of behavior together make up one of the defining characteristics of the syndrome. These characteristics could be loosely described as compulsive or ritualistic behavior. Any one of these items may be seen in only about one third of autistic children, but a characteristic seen in nearly all such children is a resistance to learning or practicing a new activity. They need direction and external reinforcement or even to be postured through an activity before they will reluctantly go down a slide, put on their socks, or name an object in a picture for the first time. A common observation is that autistic children are capable of such behavior as talking or communicating by gesture, but they simply do not exercise these skills.

The specific problems of autistic children can be grouped into the categories of self-help, speech and language development, social skills, and formal education. Painstaking behavioral treatments do seem to improve self-help and social skills in almost all children and to accelerate development in the other two areas for brighter autistic children, but the effectiveness of behavioral methods has not yet been established experimentally. Many reports have illustrated ways of reducing self-abuse or self-stimulation and of building language, attention, and responsiveness, but, for all the apparent rigor of behavior therapy, large scale control studies are remarkably absent.

From the practical point of view, it is most efficient to train parents and local teachers to carry out whatever behavioral approaches are found effective by the professionals who evaluate an autistic child. Apart from this efficiency, this plan ensures that children spend as much time as possible in normal settings building their own self-reliance, and understanding and realistic optimism among parents, siblings, and teachers. Whether autistic children are first studied in treatment plans worked out during a brief hospital stay or in a local special school will depend on geography and local services, but there is a definite drawback to long-term residential treatment. Autistic children are handicapped in generalizing from one situation to another, so that skills that they have learned in a hospital or school tend not to transfer to home.

Virtually all psychotropic drugs have been tried in order to sedate or energize autistic children. Again, there is a remarkable lack of research involving large groups of autistic children, proper controls, and adequate experimental design. Most studies seem tentative, possibly because the results are disappointing.

Pica

CALVIN W. WOODRUFF, M.D.

Pica is defined as the eating of inedible substances such as newspaper, toilet paper, cleansing tissue, dirt, plaster, wood, cigarettes, matches, starch, paint, powder, crayons, grass, leaves, soap, clay, hair, ice, and bugs. Infants begin to have hand to mouth behavior as early as five months of age and it tends to disappear by 18 to 36 months. During this time a certain amount of ingesting of foreign substances is considered to be normal in most cultures. Persistence of pica beyond the age of 18 months has been attributed to inadequate patterns of parental control of mouthing behavior. Psychiatric teaching suggests that unavailability of the mother, excessive oral gratification because of maternal overstimulation, and aggression toward the mother at the time of introduction of solid foods may be factors in the development of abnormal cravings. Pica is apt to be more severe in brain damaged children. In one study, 63% of the mothers also had pica and often introduced their children to this behavioral variant.

In the past, lead poisoning was the pediatric focus on pica because at least half of children having pica had elevated blood lead levels and many were symptomatic from eating plaster and paint with a high lead content. More recently, it has been observed that half of the children having accidental ingestion of poisons also had pica, suggesting that the serious consequences of this behavior vary in time and place, depending upon the toxic substances present in the environment.

The association of pica with iron deficiency has a long and confusing history. There are no well designed studies to answer the question as to whether iron deficiency is the result of pica or whether pica is a response to the deficient state. *Pagophagia* (ice eating) in women is the clearest example, since it disappears when treatment with iron is instituted.

With clay and starch eating, the role of the abnormal substance in the absorption of iron and trace elements such as zinc has been postulated, since intakes may be in the normal range. The recent literature has an increasing number of papers on biochemical evidence of iron and zinc deficiency in children and adults having pica. Of 23 references to pica in the Index Medicus for 1981 and 1982, 12 were on altered mineral metabolism while only 3 were on lead poisoning. This trend suggests that newer diagnostic techniques for trace element status are showing that they may play a significant role in this type of behavior and may also influence the persistence or aggravation of a normally transient phase of development.

Treatment of pica must consist of both physiologic and psychologic components. A family history of similar practices is important. Such factors as the quality of parenting and adequacy of the environment should be evaluated. Brain damage and retardation should be suspected. Hematologic and biochemical assessment for iron and zinc deficiency (see appropriate sections) should be carried out. Lead poisoning (see that section) should be suspected and treated when found. Since the best tool for the diagnosis of iron deficiency is treatment with 4.5 mg/kg/day of elemental iron in divided doses, this regimen plus 5 to 10 mg of elemental zinc daily as zinc acetate solution may be given for one month as a diagnostic test. Whatever the presumed etiology, the immediate environment of the child should be kept free of poisons such as lead and the common agents found in accidental poisoning. The child's behavior should be modified by reorientation of caretakers concerning the development of more appropriate uses for his or her mouth. This may be accomplished by a preschool program, nursing, or social work intervention in the home, or, in more advanced cases, by psychiatric care.

Psychosomatic Illness

DAVID A. WALLER, M.D.

The concept of psychosomatic illness has been broadened in the new psychiatric classification system to include any situation in which a physical condition appears to be affected by psychological factors. Examples in pediatrics might include a child with nonspecific physical symptoms that appear to be related to a recent environmental stress, or a child with asthma whose attacks appear related in terms of timing and severity to emotional factors, or an adolescent with diabetes whose recent illness is related to inappropriate behavior (i.e. noncompliance).

The author of this section, who is board certified in both pediatrics and child psychiatry, is still waiting for the first child or parent to come to him wondering whether psychological factors are playing an important role in some physical problem and wanting help from him in sorting this out. To be sure, as pediatricians we frequently think along these lines, and all of us have seen instances where good psychiatric intervention seemed to have helped certain children with physical symptoms and disorders. But the children and families in question almost never share these concerns, at least not initially. They may even actively resist the idea, creating a situation very different from the usual instant partnership that exists between family and pediatrician when the problem is strictly medical. It is essential to understand these family concerns and to address them, if treatment is to proceed.

One concern is that once attention is directed toward psychological factors there will be less interest in the medical or physical side of the problem. This is a legitimate concern, especially when there is diagnostic uncertainty. Most families have heard of cases where doctors said the problem was psychological, only to find out later that an important and perhaps obscure or difficult medical diagnosis had been missed. As pediatricians we share this concern, and would probably sooner make any error than that one.

For this reason, the author favors exhaustive diagnostic work-ups in such cases, and even when nothing is found, a continuing open-minded approach based on the idea that perhaps something is being missed or has yet to reveal itself. This does not mean that, because there is some uncertainty, the child should function as an invalid. It is usually possible at least to reassure parents that the child does *not* have certain serious or dire diseases they may have been concerned about. Periodic outpatient medical re-evaluations can and should be scheduled with the pediatrician. Attention can then be directed at having the child function in a manner appropriate to his or her current situation. This generally includes going to school and participating in extracurricular activities as the pediatrician sees fit. Psychiatric evaluation and intervention may be helpful in achieving this goal.

Sometimes it turns out that a problem is psychosomatic in the sense that there is symptom exaggeration. The child may have a very real medical problem that is being experienced in an exaggerated form because of various psychosocial factors. It is especially important in such cases that both the biologic and psychosocial aspects of the case be approached in a sophisticated manner. A pediatric-psychiatric team is ideal.

A second reason that a psychosomatic approach is problematic for children and their families has to do with the implications that such an approach has for the child's and/or family's self-esteem. It may appear to the child that he or she is being accused of being "crazy," "weak," or of "faking," or to a parent that he or she is being held responsible in some way for the child's illness (or the severity of it). This is particularly a problem when we suspect this is the case! The question is how to help our patients and their families to feel comfortable in receiving the help they need.

Most of us know a psychiatrist or two that we feel confident will help the child or family feel *better* about themselves, not worse. We can refer a child or family to such an individual in a way that lessens their anxieties. Children and families can be reassured that we know the problem is "real," but that various stresses can play a part in producing very real symptoms, as in individuals who develop headaches as a response to tension (or diarrhea or constipation). Psychological help is thus presented as an attempt to "round out" treatment, so as not to neglect any aspect of the child's problem. Moreover, medical problems of any type are generally stressful. It is reasonable for this aspect of a medical problem to receive careful attention.

Even when it is made clear that medical factors will continue to be attended to, and even when psychiatric help is proposed in a nonthreatening manner, as part of a comprehensive approach, it is still not unusual for children and families to have difficulty cooperating with treatment plans. There is often a kind of entrenched quality to the problem, the best explanation for which may be in one instance biological, in another, behavioral or psychodynamic. For example, a biologic mood disorder (depression, or affective illness) may be responsible for the difficulty certain children and/or their parents are having in coping with what would otherwise be a manageable physical problem. From a learning theory perspective, physical symptoms or illness in the child may have become associated with specific kinds of secondary gain, which reinforce the child in the sick role. In psychodynamic terms, exaggerated or unduly perpetuated physical illness in a child may serve the role of paradoxically stabilizing a family with other, psychological problems. Minuchin has demonstrated that physical illness in a child can detour other, more threatening family problems, such as marital conflict.

The net result is that when there appears to be a psychosomatic dimension to a child's medical problem, we need to first try to make sense out of it, *then* fashion an intervention based on our hypothesized explanation. For example, a bright adolescent female patient with diabetes who is admitted nearly dead after three weeks of ketoacidosis may turn out (as happened in our recent experience) to have a specific problem in calling the clinic for help because of what it means to her in terms of who is controlling her. Her apparently irrational behavior may serve a useful purpose, given certain of her psychological concerns. When treatment is set up in a way that is more colleagual, one friend to another, the patient's problem with authority figures (which may be primarily a problem between her and her parents) is circumvented.

All too often, interventions are designed for such patients on a basis of blind assumptions rather than careful assessment. For example it might be inferred that the patient referred to above must not be aware of how serious her diabetes is, and that the solution is to parade her through wards of patients with diabetic complications. In fact, however, our preliminary work in this area suggests, as did the careful evaluation of this patient, that the adolescent's perception of the severity of his or her illness is not nearly so important to successful adherence to the medical regimen as are family relationships.

In summary, medical problems in pediatrics that are complicated by psychological factors can be frustrating to deal with but are also challenging, like a detective story, and rewarding in those instances when we hit upon the key that seems to unlock the problem. Too often these children and adolescents fail to receive the help they need, either because resources are inadequate or too costly, or, more commonly, because the internal barriers to accepting help have not been successfully hurdled.

Childhood Sleep Disorders

DANIEL C. SHANNON, M.D.

Sleep-related symptoms that are brought by parents to pediatricians generally represent behaviors or physiologic alterations not visible by day. Perhaps this explains why evaluation tends to be delayed; not seeing the physical basis for symptoms in the awake child, the pediatrician may not take them seriously. Indeed, most such symptoms appear to represent self-limiting behavioral changes for which only reassurance is necessary. Thus, in most cases, a delay becomes therapeutic.

Behavioral symptoms such as fears, bad dreams, enuresis, or rocking need little more than reassurance of parents by the physician and of children by their parents. With this approach, they will generally be replaced by restful sleep. When these symptoms persist, the physician should consider that the child is mirroring family instability.

Table 1 lists symptoms that warrant special attention. Enuresis that persists beyond toilet training or is accompanied by other symptoms should prompt consideration of obstructive uropathy or obligate diuresis seen in diabetes mellitus or insipidus. Choking or gagging that occurs repeatedly may indicate repeated aspiration or excessive tracheobronchial secretions—the former from gastroesophageal reflux or an abnormal communication from the gastrointestinal to the respiratory tract, the latter from cystic fibrosis or asthma.

Insomnia and hypersomnia are unusual complaints for a child and generally reflect abnormal

Table 1. SLEEP DISORDER SYMPTOMS

Neurologic	insomnia hypersomnia narcolepsy
Pulmonary/Airway	color of skin pattern of breathing snoring or stridor sweats
Gastrointestinal	gagging, choking
Genitourinary	enuresis

physiology. Sleep is particularly disturbed in children with severe respiratory tract disease so that they are excessively tired and sleep during the day. Recognition and adequate treatment of the underlying conditions will quickly relieve these symptoms. Hypoglycemia should be considered in the child who awakens repeatedly in the early morning hours. While drug or alcohol abuse is the most likely cause of hypersomnia in the adolescent, narcolepsy usually should be considered.

The symptoms that are potentially serious and are most frequently overlooked by practitioners are snoring, apnea, and color change. In each instance, the infant or child is usually normal when seen by the physician even an hour following such observations by the parents. Snoring represents apposition of tongue, palate, and posterior pharynx. The noise is generally louder on inspiration when a transmural collapsing pressure develops in the trachea. In order to generate airflow, there must be a more negative pressure in the airway than in the surrounding air. At points of turbulent flow, a choke point develops and if the tissues are very compliant, they will collapse, obstruct breathing, and occasion noise when airflow reaches sonic frequencies. If the diaphragm responds appropriately, it will contract more forcibly; with obstruction in the hypopharynx, the membranous portion of the trachea will now collapse and contribute to the obstruction. This is important to recognize for several reasons. First, because of the sleep-related changes in skeletal muscle tone, obstruction of oral airflow when the tongue abuts the palate, or of nasal airflow when the soft palate meets the posterior pharynx, obstruction may be present in active but not in quiet sleep. Second, once seen, it is tempting to make a diagnosis of tracheomalacia. It must be appreciated that any lesion obstructing the airway above the larynx will be associated with inspiratory narrowing of the normal tracheal air column to the point of airlessness.

When tonsillar, adenoid, or adipose tissue is added to this functional change in airway anatomy, a spectrum of symptoms will be seen. Many infants and children will have no apparent obstructed breathing, some will snore without physiologic consequence, and a few will become hypoxemic and hypercapnic. Although excessive sweating during sleep, probably from cholinergic stimulation due to altered gas exchange, should indicate cause for concern, its absence should not prompt complacency. On occasion, parents will volunteer that the child develops an "odd," "pale," "funny," or "bluish" color when asleep. All such infants and children should be evaluated for the cause of obstruction. Even 3-month-old infants are not immune to obstructive apnea from enlarged adenoids. If evaluation is delayed, the medical literature attests to psychomotor retardation, obesity, and cardiac failure as late complications.

The most subtle symptoms are sleep-related apnea and color change. As noted, parents will observe that color is abnormal but may not see the child as "blue." Apnea associated with such color change should always prompt immediate investigation. Apnea alone, when greater than 15 seconds in duration, is abnormal at any time during the first year of life. When parents complain of these signs, the physician will occasionally see an obvious cause, such as unsuspected cardiac or pulmonary disease. Most often, a thorough evaluation is required to look for subtle neurologic, cardiac, or pulmonary causes. These include a seizure disorder, brain stem encephalitis, absent corpus callosum, congenital central hypoventilation, idiopathic sleep apnea, and cardiac arrhythmia. Diagnostic evaluation should include a lumbar puncture, polygraph examination during sleep to include electroencephalogram, electrocardiogram, respiratory movements of chest and abdomen, and preferably exhaled P_{CO_2} and transcutaneous P_{O_2} or oxygen saturation. A computed tomographic scan may be needed to identify an absent corpus callosum.

Because of their potential to affect respiratory control adversely, anticonvulsants should be used more cautiously than usual in patients with apnea or hypoventilation syndromes. Infants with idiopathic sleep apnea respond well to theophylline given to achieve a serum trough level of 10 to 15 μg/ml. Those with congenital sleep hypoventilation will need mechanical support of breathing for an indefinite duration during sleep with either a volume-cycled ventilator or electrophrenic stimulators. For all infants and children to whom curative therapy cannot be given, electronic monitoring of respirations and heart rate should be considered. When used, this should not be attempted without a medical, technical, and psychosocial support program.

Voice, Speech, and Language Disorders

SYLVIA ONESTI RICHARDSON, M.D.

Therapy for voice, speech, and language disorders should be administered by qualified speech clinicians (also called speech-language pathologists). The physician's primary responsibilities are in the prevention and early diagnosis of speech, language, and voice problems; in parent counseling; and in the appropriate, timely referral of patients to qualified speech therapists and clinics.

VOICE DYSFUNCTIONS

Hypernasality of voice quality usually is associated with the velopharyngeal incompetence of a child with a cleft palate, even a submucous cleft. Such a child should be followed by a speech therapist who can supervise the home program from the age of 3 months to 2 years, regardless of the type of operative or nonoperative treatment. The parents must be taught how to help the child develop non-nasal speech.

If the hypernasality is not due to anatomic defect (functional) and is serious enough to create a problem for the child, a speech clinician can teach the patient to use the soft palate by doing blowing exercises. Parents also can help at home. To learn to direct the breath stream through the mouth and to help strengthen the palatal muscles, the child should spend several periods a day in blowing activities such as blowing soap bubbles, keeping a feather aloft, blowing boats in the bath-tube, and blowing a Ping-Pong ball across a table.

Hyponasality, or "adenoidal speech," in which "n" sounds like "d," "m" sounds like "b," and "ng" sounds like "g," can be caused by excessively enlarged adenoids or any nasal or nasopharyngeal obstruction. This usually disappears if the adenoidal mass becomes smaller or if adenoidectomy is performed. If excessive nasality occurs post-adenoidectomy and persists for more than 8 weeks, speech therapy should be considered to help the child relearn to use the soft palate correctly.

Hoarseness may appear in children 8 to 10 years of age, especially boys, because of development of tiny nodules between the anterior and middle thirds of the vocal cords. These may be due to prepubescent endocrine changes, allergy, or too much yelling in the Little League outfield. Treating any allergy or requiring the child to stop yelling or singing loudly is usually successful, though difficult to enforce in the latter case. If such hoarseness persists and the nodule shows a slow reduction in size, a speech clinician can teach the child to alter vocal pitch until healing is effected. This disturbance usually disappears spontaneously when change of voice occurs around the age of 12 and 13 years.

DISORDERS OF ARTICULATION

Dysarthria is due to neuromotor involvement of the muscles used for articulation, phonation, or respiration. The child with *articulatory dyspraxia* is able to carry out the movements necessary for articulation spontaneously but has difficulty in directing them for voluntary imitation of movements (motor planning) or for reproduction of the correct articulatory sounds when hearing is normal. *Dyslalia* includes those defects of articulation which appear to be functional in origin rather than attributable to damage to the brain or failure of neurologic maturation for speech. In this article we are concerned with the latter.

Indications for the physician's referral to a speech and hearing clinic for further evaluation and possible therapy are as follows: 1) Articulation is mostly unintelligible after age 3 years. If the causes appear to be chiefly environmental or functional, a good nursery school can be therapeutic if recommended by a speech clinician. 2) There are many substitutions of easy sounds for difficult ones after age 5 years. In such cases, psychologic evaluation may be sought to determine mental age or reasons for retention of infantile speech patterns. Speech therapy is influenced by the cause of the disorder, as is parent counseling. 3) The child is omitting, distorting, or substituting any sound past age 7 years. Speech therapy consists largely of ear training and teaching the child to produce the sounds correctly in isolation and then in combination with other sounds.

Audiologic evaluation is important in *every* case and is particularly indicated when the speech is characterized by omission of sounds or word endings or if there has been a history of chronic otitis media. Assuming that hearing is normal and the problem is one of dyslalia, the majority of articulatory defects in children under 7 years of age can be handled at home by the mother, in nursery school, or in the classroom. However, such management should be recommended and supervised by a qualified speech clinician.

Home management must be handled skillfully without pressure, or not at all. All members of the family are instructed to use clear, precise speech to provide suitable models. At first, two or three 15-minute periods can be set aside daily when one member of the family reads aloud, leafs through picture books naming the pictures, plays games involving imitation of different animal sounds, and engages in similar activities. As the child begins to identify pictures correctly, these may be cut out and placed in a scrapbook for review. As stated above, the parents should confer with a speech therapist for guidance.

Most children show marked improvement in articulation between the first and second grades and some between the second and third grades. Thus the child's maturation within a good speech environment is often the best course of therapy for simple articulatory defects.

A note on "tonguetie": Parents and others still seem to think a child is "tonguetied" if there is any kind of speech problem. If a child can articulate t, d, n, or l; can say "no," "ta-ta," and "da-da"; or can lick a lollipop, the speech problem is not due to tonguetie alone, if at all. If there is a true tonguetie and the lingual frenulum is bound down to the lower central incisors, the treatment is surgical—not a scar tissue-producing snip with a pair of scissors.

STUTTERING

The physician's ability to determine the child's position in the continuum from developmental nonfluency to established stuttering is important in planning treatment.

Effective parent counseling by the physician is the first step in treatment of the problem of nonfluency. He can explain to the parents the developmental nature of early nonfluency and provide instructive reading for them.

Treatment of nonfluency in pre-school children is indirect, aimed at the child's environment rather than the child. The parents must help to change the conditions that precipitate or perseverate stuttering episodes, including problems in the home that tend to produce anxiety in the child. The parents are advised to encourage the child to speak during fluent periods, to allow ample time for him or her to speak, to maintain eye contact when the child speaks, and to be responsive listeners. Comments like "Slow down, Johnny," or "For heaven's sake, stop and think before you try to talk" are to be discouraged—as is any suggestion that the child modify his speaking.

The effectiveness of the treatment is directly proportionate to the consistency the parents are able to maintain. For this reason, counseling with a speech therapist must be regular and must continue until the problem is resolved.

When nonfluency has progressed to the point at which children think of themselves as stutterers and develop struggle reactions to speech, such as circumlocutions to avoid a sound on which they usually block, facial tics, and grimaces or other evidence of avoidance or anxiety reactions, the treatment is direct and may involve combined speech therapy and psychotherapy.

SPEECH AND LANGUAGE DELAY

Treatment of speech and language delay depends upon definitive dignosis, and this may be considered one of the most difficult diagnostic problems in pediatrics.

Treatment for delayed speech development may vary from counseling parents to sending the child to a good preschool, or to play therapy in a speech clinic. Psychiatric treatment may be indicated before speech therapy is attempted. Direct speech therapy is usually not recommended before a child has reached a general developmental level of about 4 years.

Deafness and mental retardation must be ruled out. Mentally retarded children usually present a picture of retardation in all areas of development, especially when the IQ level is below 70. Improvement in speech and language may occur with development and maturation, but training in prelinguistic sensory-motor skills is most helpful. The parents of these children often need to understand that speech therapy per se is of no value to the child until he or she has had adequate prelinguistic experience and has developed the necessary motor coordination of the articulatory muscles to produce speech.

The term language disorder is used to include dysphasia, dyslexia, and dysgraphia. Dysphasia is the inability or limited ability of a child to use spoken symbols for communication. To plan treatment for the young dysphasic child, one must determine whether the primary problem is receptive (understanding speech), expressive (self-expression with speech), some combination of these two, or global (lacking "inner language"). The last condition represents a severe disorder in which the child cannot use symbols internally for thinking, and prognosis is poor regardless of therapy.

The dyslexic child has a problem in the reception of written symbols, and the dysgraphic child has a problem with expression of written symbols. Developmental dysphasia, dyslexia, and dysgraphia are closely related conditions and may be found together in the same patient or in members of the same family. Some children learn to speak adequately and are not recognized to be dyslexic until they fail to learn to read in school.

Therapy for any language disorder requires a total program in which the environment can be suitably structured and the therapy can be tailored to suite the child's individual needs. Speech therapy alone, or any other single kind of therapy, is inadequate and unsuitable for such a child. An experienced team of specialists is usually required for reaching a diagnosis and for recommending appropriate language therapy.

Treatment plans for very young children with language disorders usually include sensory-motor activities: training in the motor bases of behavior, such as posture, the development of laterality and directionality, and the development of body image; training in perceptual skills, such as form perception, space discrimination, stereognosis, and recognition of texture, size, and structure; and training in auditory perception (listening), visual perception (looking), and kinesthetic perception (muscular memory of movements, positions, and posture). The child with a language disorder usually requires assistance in learning these skills, which are developmentally antecedent to language production per se.

Speech and hearing clinicians are now involved in the development and application of new assessment and intervention techniques for high risk and developmentally delayed infants. They are valuable members of the interdisciplinary teams involved with parent-infant programming.

For those with severe communicative disorders, a number of augmentative systems are available. Manual communication using signs has been employed with mentally retarded, cerebral palsied, and autistic children. Communication boards may be used to facilitate communication for those with extensive motor problems. When such systems are used, the speech and language clinician's task is essentially the same as when oral language is taught —to train comprehension and production of language using the augmentative system.

The American Speech-Language-Hearing Association (ASHA) can provide information concerning speech correction facilities throughout the United States. Speech, language, and hearing specialists who are certified by ASHA are listed in its annual directory, which is available at The American Speech-Language-Hearing Association, 10801 Rockville Pike, Rockville, Maryland 20852.

Disorders of Learning and Attention

MELVIN D. LEVINE, M.D.

In recent years there has been growing recognition of a series of central nervous system disabilities affecting children and known to constrain academic performance and, in some cases, behavioral adjustment. These so-called "low severity-high prevalence" disorders consist of a varied group of handicaps that can be described and classified according to different conceptual models. Table 1 shows one such model to delineate the most frequently encountered clinical disorders of learning, including those handicapping conditions that limit the concentration or selective attention of school children. The therapeutics of these disorders necessarily depends upon the antecedent description of individual children. The treatment of a particular deficit depends, at least in part, upon the availability and mobilization of compensatory strengths in other aspects of a child's development. By compiling a broad "functional profile," one can design and implement services that include appropriate counseling, educational intervention, and other forms of treatment.

The management of children with learning and attention disorders is intrinsically multifaceted and almost always multidisciplinary. It is becoming increasingly common for general pediatricians or specialists in developmental pediatrics to serve as coordinators of intervention. In doing so, the clinician endeavors to integrate eight areas of service, including 1) counseling and "demystification"; 2) educational intervention; 3) home management; 4) medical treatments; 5) special services; 6) advocacy; 7) follow-up (i.e., assessments of progress and the effectiveness of service).

COUNSELING AND DEMYSTIFICATION

It is common for children who are failing in school to harbor fantasies about why they are doing poorly. Most often they overestimate their degree of handicap, frequently believing they are retarded

or "dumb." An even broader array of misconceptions is found in parents who may attribute their child's difficulties to laziness, generalized "slowness," or indifference. Even teachers may misunderstand the plight of a child with a learning disorder. They may construe the phenomenon as poor motivation, primary emotional disturbance, or an aberration of attitude. Therefore, a critical initial therapeutic step is the process of education or demystification.

First, the child's handicaps must be carefully delineated and demarcated. Simple explanations, using nontechnical language as well as helpful analogies, should be employed. For example, in describing a child with difficulty in processing language, one might explain: "Although you really don't have any trouble thinking about things or remembering, it is very hard for you to figure things out when people explain them to you in long sentences with a lot of words. This is because you have trouble learning well through your ears. You do much better at understanding what you see. It is as if you were a television set whose picture was very clear but whose sound has too much static." In providing such explanations, the clinician should highlight the youngster's strengths while instilling optimism with respect to the managability of problems. It should be made clear to the child and parents that the deficit is not primarily one of motivation, that the child is not "dumb," and that there *are* ways to help. A nonaccusatory approach that is supportive and sufficiently optimistic is likely to be most effective.

Either by letter, through a conference, or by telephone, the clinician needs also to present his view of the child's disabilities and strengths to school personnel. This too can dispel misunderstandings and establish a good alliance between the health care provider, the school, the parents, and the child.

EDUCATIONAL INTERVENTION

It is obvious that much of the rehabilitation of a child with a learning disorder must take place in an educational setting. Schools have a major role to play, although their effort should not be viewed as the exclusive modality of intervention. Within the school, three delivery systems can be identified: *special education, regular education,* and *special services.*

Special Education. Special education input for children with learning problems includes interventions that generally take place outside of a regular classroom and are aimed at remedying or overcoming the deficits impairing progress. The initial step in such intervention is the selection of a service prototype. Five common prototypes are summarized below in order of their magnitude:

A. SPECIAL ASSISTANCE WITHIN THE REGULAR CLASSROOM. In this model a teacher's aide or some

Table 1. COMMON DEVELOPMENTAL DYSFUNCTIONS (LOW
SEVERITY DISABILITIES) IN SCHOOL CHILDREN

Dysfunction	Common Cognitive Impacts	Common Academic Impacts	Circumvention	Intervention
Selective attention	Weak reflection, poor planning Poor monitoring Inattention to detail Inconsistency Easy cognitive fatigue Erratic memory	Carelessness Impersistence Poor classroom adjustment Trouble following instructions Inconsistency	Demystification Accommodation Small "chunks" Preferential seating Feedback	Stimulant medication Remedial help—small group or 1:1 Behavioral modification
Visual-spatial	Confusion over: figure-ground, size, shape, relative position Poor appreciation of detail	Poor letter, word recognition Possible math problems Phonetic spelling	Auditory inputs Multisensory linguistic approach to reading, spelling	Proofreading for detail Visual-spatial activities Auditory-visual integration
Temporal-sequential	Poor sequential memory Trouble with multistep processes Secondary inattention	Trouble following instructions Trouble with multisyllable words Poor multiplication, spelling Disorganization	One or two step inputs, repetition Teach to strong channel Note-taking	Diaries, calendars, clocks Mastery over larger chunks Practice recall with feedback
Receptive language	Poor or slow language interpretation Secondary inattention Impaired verbal reasoning	Trouble following instructions Reading, writing weaknesses—math word problem problems	Visual inputs Repetition, short sentences Visual approaches to skills	Language therapy: Use of tapes, other language enhancers
Expressive language	Possible "dysphasia" Diminished vocabulary Articulation problems Poor sentence formulation	Trouble participating in class discussions Delayed reading Poor written expression	Verbal volunteering Strong visual inputs Less stress on oral expression	Speech therapy Dictionary work Expressive exercises
Memory	Difficulty registering, storing, or retrieving specific types of data	Variable, depending on impairment Spelling, math problems Trouble retaining new skills	Subvocalization, mnemonics, rules/generalizations Underlining Note-taking	Specific gradual exercises to enhance weak modality using strong area
Gross motor	None	Social withdrawal Fearfulness Low self-esteem	Avoidance of certain sports Privacy	Adaptive physical education
Fine motor	None	Nonspecific	Reduced output demand More time Prioritization Typing	Overlearning motor patterns, pencil control Extensive writing exercises Work on grasp
Social	Poor feedback from and "titration" of relationships	Indirect	Fostering individuality	Social "tutoring" Parent support Small group work
Higher order cognition	Poor comprehension of new concepts Impaired inference, generalization Concreteness	Delayed acquisition of skill and knowledge, generalized	Use of concrete manipulative materials Use of strengths	"Cognitive Therapy" Work with rules, logic, abstract reasoning

other individual observes and periodically offers assistance to the child with a learning problem. The youngster is not removed from the regular classroom, but is helped during the school day at times when difficulty is noted or anticipated.

B. RESOURCE ROOM OR LEARNING CENTER HELP. In this model, the child receives assistance usually in a small group setting (ranging from 1–7 other students in most cases). A specially trained educator works with the students to remedy specific deficits. Often the effort is aimed at helping a child catch up in areas of delayed skill acquisition. Alternatively, the special educator may wish to work specifically to strengthen a child's developmental weaknesses rather than skill delays. For example, there may be an effort to provide the youngster with exercises aimed at enhancing visual-perception, language, attention, or memory. In such cases, the goal is to work on functions thought to be prerequisites of skill acquisition rather than on the skills themselves. It is not uncommon for both strategies to be employed, namely a combined program of skill-building with intervention to strengthen areas of developmental weakness.

C. TUTORING. Tutorial services often are provided on a one-to-one basis. For economic reasons, schools may find this impractical to implement. When feasible, parents may seek tutoring outside of school. Most often such intervention is aimed at the enhancement of academic skills. Specific drill in spelling, mathematics, reading, or writing may be offered. Some tutors may wish to work specifically to help a youngster with organization or study skills.

D. FULL-TIME CLASS FOR LEARNING DISORDERS. Some school systems offer special classes for children with learning problems. Often these contain less students or at least a more favorable teacher: student ratio than do regular classrooms. Special curriculum materials may be employed. Work may be presented at a slower rate, with reduced volume expectations (for homework and tests), and with more repetition. While such classrooms usually offer a considerable degree of expertise geared to the needs of the student, recently there has been some concern about their possible stigmatizing impact. It is not unusual for children in such programs to refer to the special class as "the mental room."

E. PRIVATE SCHOOLS FOR LEARNING DISABILITIES. In North America there has been a proliferation of private schools that specialize in the management of children with learning disorders. Such schools are staffed by people who have the training, experience, and sensitivity to deal with children afflicted with learning disorders. Specialized curriculum materials often are employed. Classes tend to be small. Because of this, tuition fees are beyond the reach of many families. In some instances, however, school systems will pay the tuition for youngsters whom they feel they cannot teach adequately within the community. Special schools for learning disabilities have the advantage of allowing children to associate with other youngsters who have the same problems, thereby feeling less different. On the other hand, attendance at such an institution could make a child feel that he is not a part of the community or neighborhood, he is in educational "exile." Special schools for learning disabilities may be either residential or day programs.

Many factors enter into the choice of a special educational prototype. Among these are the child's own strengths and weaknesses, the extent of academic delay, the availability and quality of the various prototypes within a community, and the desires and values of the parents and child.

In the United States, Public Law 94–142 has mandated that communities must provide adequate education for children with handicapping conditions, including those with learning disorders. An individualized educational plan is developed, and this specifies the prototype along with specific educational goals and the quantity of service to be offered (e.g., the amount of time per week in a resource room). As part of this law, there has been a growing emphasis on what is called the "least restrictive alternative": while it is deemed important for children to have an appropriate education, serious consideration is given to "mainstreaming" or allowing the youngster to be part of a program that is as close as possible to that of normal children in the community. In this context, sending a child off to a special school for learning disabilities might be considered "restrictive," the least desirable alternative, or "a last resort."

Regular Education. Unless a child is in a full-time learning disability program his or her regular educational program (i.e., the school day minus the special educational component) is just as important, and in some cases more, than the special intervention. Daily management in a regular classroom is critical to ongoing skill development as well as self-esteem and motivation.

It is essential that the regular classroom teacher have a good understanding of the child's problems. Insensitivity of the teacher to the child's plight can result in a counterproductive experience marked by diminishing incentive, effort, and self-esteem.

Within the regular classroom, the emphasis is on compensation or "bypass strategies." While the special educational program is geared to help youngsters *overcome deficits,* the regular classroom should be a place where children are encouraged to *circumvent their weaknesses.* For example, a teacher may need to accommodate to the fact that a youngster cannot process a long series of verbal instructions. Succinct directions, visual reinforcement of instructions, and some repetition may be needed. A child who has attention deficits and is highly distractible may need to sit close to the teacher. A youngster who has fine motor problems impairing writing may need to be allowed to type, to write less, to be spared excessive criticism of his poor handwriting, and to not have to recopy papers. A child with memory weaknesses may need help in taking notes, using mnemonics, and developing flashcards to help bypass retention weaknesses. Many other examples of such strategies could be cited. Their selection depends largely upon the child's strengths and weaknesses. Wherever possible, a student's assets should be used in trying to work around handicaps.

The choice of curriculum is another important aspect of regular education for a child with learning difficulties. This is exemplified in reading. A child with language processing problems may need a strong visual approach (a so-called "sight word" method) to reading. Many of these youngsters require a multisensory reading curriculum that uses several modalities simultaneously to reinforce word recognition and analysis. An example is the Orton Gillingham Method, which is widely applied. Some approaches to reading stress language. A child who has difficulty with visual perception or visual memory may benefit from a reading curriculum that emphasizes the *phonetic analysis* of words rather than their *visual configuration.*

Many children with learning disorders require more time than other children to finish tests, to complete assignments, and to assimilate and integrate new skills or knowledge. The classroom teacher must recognize this. In order to accommodate to such time-related constraints, some assignments may need to be shorter. It now is possible for youngsters with learning disorders to take college entrance examinations or secondary school admission tests on an untimed basis. Such allowances can make an enormous difference for an affected student.

Many children with learning problems are dreadfully ashamed of their lack of academic success. In particular, they fear exposure in front of their peers. They are obsessed with maintaining a good reputation, with looking good. It is important that adults not humiliate disabled students in front of their peers. A certain amount of privacy is critical. For example, if a youngster has a writing problem such that his papers are chronically messy and disorganized, it is cruel to allow other students to correct his work. If a child has expressive language problems, one should be careful and sensitive about calling upon him in a classroom. If a child has difficulty with reading, one may wish to minimize the requirement for oral reading.

As children progress through school, course selection becomes important. Here it is helpful to anticipate the natural history of a child's disability. Many youngsters with language disorders tend to do quite poorly when they are expected to learn a foreign language. One might wish to postpone or even obtain an exemption from such courses. In selecting subjects, however, it is important not to create self-fulfilling prophecies. Many children with learning disorders are extraordinarily resilient and seem to "come to life" academically late in junior high or high school. One should avoid therefore selection of a curriculum that will constrain future opportunities.

SPECIAL SERVICES

In addition to special educational input and modifications in regular education, some youngsters with learning disorders require more specialized services. A wide range of options is available, although there is considerable variation from school system to school system, and even between schools in the same community. A practicing physician needs to develop a good understanding of available resources. Among the special services are the following: speech and language therapy for children with either receptive or expressive disorders; guidance or school adjustment counseling for children with social, motivational, or behavioral concomitants of their learning problems; occupational therapy for those with significant motor handicaps; adaptive physical education to enhance motor skills; and social service, particularly useful when family problems complicate the clinical picture.

HOME MANAGEMENT

Frequently parents want to know what *they* can do to help. It is a mistake to minimize their role. Parents can be a reliable "labor force" to help a failing youngster. If they sense their role is minimal, feelings of hopelessness or futility may supervene. Parents can be of direct assistance with homework and with the establishment of study skills. While they should not actually perform the child's assignments, they can be invaluable with regard to organizational skills. Many youngsters with learning problems are disorganized. Parents can help a child "get started" with homework; they can find and prepare the appropriate place to study and set up a work schedule; they can coordinate assignments with teachers; they can help the youngster allocate time effectively; and they can be helpful in pursuing certain games and activities that can enhance a child's learning. For example, reading to a child at bedtime and then asking questions about the story might enhance receptive language abilities. Listening to the child read can be helpful for a youngster with delays in reading skills.

Home management is a major issue for parents of children who have behavioral difficulties along with their learning problems. This is seen most commonly in those with attention deficits. In addition to their poor concentration in school, such youngsters may be overactive, provocative in their behaviors, difficult to satisfy, impulsive, and irresponsible with regard to chores at home. Parents may need help in establishing a system of accountability for such a youngster. Distinct priorities need to be established and short-range incremental goals set. Parents need to be helped to be consistent with such children, to avoid unattainable goals, and to try not to be too moralistic about the youngster's difficulties.

A critical component of home management is the planning and organization of a child's recreational and social life. It is not uncommon to encounter children with learning problems who are seriously "success-deprived." Their parents cannot recall any recent incident in which the child was able to display mastery in any area. This may be the closest thing to a developmental emergency, and there is a serious need for "success induction." Utilizing a child's natural strengths and inclinations, parents should be encouraged to program experiences in which the youngster can feel successful. A child who is failing in school but who likes to draw cartoons might benefit from art lessons and having his works displayed prominently both at home and in school. A youngster whose mechanical skills are excellent but who, because of language difficulties, is having inordinate problems in school, might thrive on computers, on fixing engines, or building model airplanes. Chronic success deprivation is one of the major complications of learning disorders. A critical part of intervention rests in its reversal.

A number of children with learning problems also have difficulties with socialization. They may experience undue rejection by peers. In other instances, they seem to isolate themselves. Parents can help by encouraging social experiences at home, by coaching in the formation and maintenance of relationships with peers.

MEDICAL TREATMENTS

The standard medical treatment for a learning problem generally entails two modalities: the correction of any complicating, underlying, or secondary medical problems and pharmacotherapy.

It is important for the physician to recognize and treat any medical disorders or symptoms complicating a child's learning problems. In this group one frequently encounters chronic somatic symptoms, such as enuresis, encopresis, recurrent abdominal pain, tics, or sleep difficulties. These require medical attention, treatment, and follow-up. In some instances, reassurance can be helpful in alleviating the anxiety these symptoms promote. In some cases direct therapy is necessary.

A number of chronic conditions can complicate learning problems. Most common are seizures, allergies, recurrent ear infections, and sinusitis. Any or all of these can compromise a child's ability to concentrate and acquire skills. Further problems ensue from extended periods of school absence and side effects of medication. The latter is particularly common with the use of antihistamines, theophylline-containing compounds, and some seizure medications (such as barbiturates and primidone).

Various pharmacologic agents are used to help children with learning disorders. Most commonly prescribed are the stimulants. These are summarized in Table 2. Their appropriate use is in children with attention deficits. Stimulant medication appears to strengthen selective attention, diminish impulsivity, curb restlessness and overactivity, and result in some improved learning. Enhanced socialization also can be observed. Stimulants are not beneficial in correcting specific learning disabilities, nor are they appropriately thought of as "tranquilizers." Instead, they appear to affect arousal and alertness probably through regulation of neurotransmission in the reticular activating system of the brain stem. In prescribing stimulant drugs, the clinician should use as small a dose as possible. In most cases, it is best to administer the drug only on school days (the exception being the youngster who is so frenetic that serious behavioral problems occur on weekends and vacations). Periodic "drug

Table 2. STIMULANT MEDICATIONS FOR USE IN CHILDREN WITH ATTENTION DEFICITS

Generic Name	Brand Name	Preparations	Range of Daily Dose (average)	Onset of Action	Duration of Action	Comments
Methylphenidate	Ritalin	Tablets: 5, 10, 20 mg*	5–60 mg (10–30) (0.3–1.0 mg/kg)	30 min	3–5 hr	Not recommended below 6 years
Dextroamphetamine	Dexedrine	Tablets: 5 mg; sustained release capsules: 5, 10, 15 mg	5–40 mg (5–20)	30 min	3–5 hr (longer in sustained release form)	Not recommended below 3 years
Pemoline	Cylert	Tablets: 18.75, 37.5, 75 mg	18.75–112.5 mg (56.25–75)	2–4 hr (may not see clinical results until 3–4 weeks of therapy)	"Long-acting"	Not recommended below 6 years

*Methylphendiate also is available in a sustained release tablet (Ritalin SR 20 mg), which is the equivalent of 10 mg b.i.d. of the regular form.

holidays" should be attempted. These are days or weeks off medication, designed ultimately to wean the youngster from the drug. It is important that the child, the parents, and the teachers all understand the justifications, therapeutic effects, and possible side effects of the medication.

In recent years many forms of poorly evaluated medical therapy and medically related interventions have been advanced and supported (generally by the providers). These include physical exercise programs, optometric training, special diets, allergic hyposensitization programs, and drugs to correct vestibular dysfunction. Varying degrees of research have been directed toward proving the efficacy of such interventions. Although further investigation is warranted, at the time of this writing none of the above has been shown in scientifically replicable and rigorous research to be effective.

OUTSIDE REFERRALS

A child with learning disorders may need services within the community but outside of the school. Selection obviously depends upon what is available in a given area. In addition, the quality and accessibility of interventions *in school* will influence the choice of outside services. Although numerous programs exist, the more common ones include psychotherapy (from a child psychiatrist or psychologist), speech and language therapy, private tutoring, specialized medical help (e.g., neurology, otolaryngology, ophthalmology), and recreational programs.

ADVOCACY

The clinician has a crucial role to play in advocating for the rights and needs of children with learning disorders. Helping parents obtain appropriate services, informing them of their legal entitlements (such as those guaranteed under Public Law 94–142), and helping to insure that interventions of high quality actually occur are all components of the advocacy role of the clinician. In addition, physicians can be critical in helping parents and schools determine the scientific efficacy (or lack thereof) of various attractive interventions that may tempt them. Scientific consumer advocacy can prevent parents and schools from going to great expense to pursue unsound treatments that replace or delay appropriate intervention.

FOLLOW-UP AND MONITORING

A learning disorder must be perceived by the clinician as a chronic disease. Long term follow-up and the monitoring of progress is essential. The physician constitutes an objective professional who has continuity with the child and family and who possesses no conflicts of interest or strong disciplinary biases.

In treating a child with a learning disorder, it is important to agree upon a mechanism for periodic review of progress. If possible, educational testing of skills should be done regularly by an objective specialist *outside* of the school. Based on the results of such periodic re-evaluations, the physician can determine the need for alterations in the amount or type of service, and at the same time be constantly fortifying an alliance with the child and family, which can help to minimize the secondary effects of failure on affect, socialization, self-image, and aspiration.

Attention Deficit Disorder

SALLY E. SHAYWITZ, M.D.,
BENNETT A. SHAYWITZ, M.D.,
and DONALD J. COHEN, M.D.

The term attention deficit disorder (ADD) represents a diagnostic term designed to encompass and replace minimal brain dysfunction (MBD), minimal cerebral dysfunction, clumsy child syndrome, and hyperactive child syndrome. Two subtypes of the disorder are recognized: ADD with hyperactivity, by far the more common, and ADD without hyperactivity. Cardinal features of ADD with hyperactivity are inattention, hyperactive motor behavior, and impulsivity; ADD without hyperactivity describes children with inattention and impulsivity.

Most of these children exhibit a variety of associated features that may, in fact, be the primary reason for referral. These include school learning difficulties and conduct disorders. Many evidence neurological dysfunction, as demonstrated by abnormalities on special neurological examination ("soft signs"). Laboratory studies are generally not helpful, though nonspecific EEG abnormalities are evident in perhaps half of affected children. They may also demonstrate abnormalities on tests of cognition, arousal, habituation, reaction time, vigilance, distractibility, and motor speed, though none is diagnostic of the disorder. Some also have abnormal concentrations of monoamines or their metabolites in urine or cerebrospinal fluid, though again, none of these biochemical studies alone is sufficient for a diagnosis of ADD.

ADD is a common disorder, perhaps the most frequently observed neurobehavioral problem in the pediatric age group. Prevalence rates have been estimated to range between 5–10%, and boys are affected much more often than girls, in ratios of 3–4 : 1.

While this review will focus on the pharmacotherapy of ADD, we emphasize that drugs are only one component of a management plan that always incorporates educational therapy, and frequently employs behavioral therapy and psychotherapy as well. We believe that educational therapy is the cornerstone of management, whether used alone or with medications, behavior therapy, or psychotherapy. The pediatrician should become familiar with such general principles as providing a structured classroom environment, removing the child from distracting stimuli, and making curriculum modifications when appropriate.

Behavior therapy is an alternative to stimulant medication, and several investigations suggest that the combination of behavior therapy and stimulants is more effective than either alone. Although such treatment avoids the potential side effects of medication, it is often difficult and expensive to implement. Individual psychotherapy may be an important component of therapy in some children, providing support for the emotional lability, immaturity, and disturbed interpersonal relationships that characterize many children with ADD.

Any discussion of the pharmacotherapy of ADD must focus primarily on the effects of the stimulants amphetamine and methylphenidate, which are the most effective medications for the treatment of ADD, with drug response rates averaging between 70 and 80%. Stimulants help improve attention regulation and modulate hyperactive motor activity, and, on rare occasions, may also help to improve fine motor activity, such as handwriting. Stimulants will not improve academic skills but, by increasing attention span, should help create the atmosphere that will make the child more receptive to learning. Stimulants affect the child and his immediate environment, his community, and society in general.

To a great extent, the pediatrician's clinical judgment, understanding of the child, family, and school environment, and knowledge of educational practices within the community are the most important elements in deciding whether stimulant medication should begin immediately or be deferred until nonpharmacologic approaches have been tried. The pediatrician may be particularly influential in making certain that the school system has evaluated the child, and insuring that the most appropriate school placement has been effected. Stimulant therapy will almost certainly be ineffective unless the child's educational placement is satisfactory.

Before beginning medication the pediatrician must determine which symptoms are the targets of treatment, and decide at which times these symptoms are most troublesome. In general, stimulant therapy will be more effective in ameliorating attentional difficulties in school than in improving the child's behavior at home. In part, this reflects the biological availability of the stimulant, but it also reflects the fact that school is the best environment to assess those attentional processes that respond best to stimulants.

In most cases medication should not be initiated simultaneously with the child's beginning a new school year or with his entrance into a classroom setting that has just been changed. Such a practice not only allows the physician to determine the child's baseline functioning without medication, but more importantly, gives the child an opportunity to adjust to the new environment prior to beginning stimulant therapy.

A positive pharmacologic response depends upon the physician's skill in deciding upon the appropriate dose and whether the drug needs to be administered more than once each day. The recent development of a gas chromatographic assay for methylphenidate (MPH) has facilitated the determination of blood levels and permitted an examination of the pharmacokinetics of MPH and the relationship between MPH concentrations and behavioral response. After a lag phase of 0.5–1 hour, MPH reaches a peak plasma concentration 2.5 hours after administration, with maximal concentrations averaging 11.2 ng/ml at a dose of 0.34 mg/kg and 20.2 ng/ml at a dose of 0.65 mg/kg; terminal half life averages 2.5 hours. Comparable doses of amphetamine demonstrate a higher peak concentration (65.9 ng/ml) and a longer half-life (about 7 hours). However, blood levels of MPH are not yet generally available and the pediatrician must decide empirically upon dosage and modify the initial dosage on the basis of the clinical situation.

Although both d-amphetamine and MPH have comparable effects, many investigators believe that MPH produces fewer side effects and is the drug of choice. We begin with an initial dose of 0.3 mg/kg 30 minutes before breakfast because absorption of the drug is more complete on an empty stomach. By the time the child reaches school, MPH should be absorbed and peak levels attained within 2–3 hours. We encourage the school to place the child in academic subjects during these morning hours so that the effects of the drug on attentional processes will be maximal when the child needs the most help. Thus, by lunchtime, and in afternoon classes, which we hope will be nonacademic subjects (physical education, music, etc.), the medication's effect will be waning but the need for the drug will not be as great. We follow the clinical response by obtaining weekly feedback from the parents and, most importantly, from the school system. We obtain weekly ratings from the child's primary academic teachers using standardized assessment instruments (Conner's Abbreviated Parent-Teacher Rating Scale and the Yale Behavior Rating Scale).

If the child is not responding satisfactorily after

2 weeks of treatment we raise the dose by 0.1 mg/kg, and continue this procedure until 0.6 mg/kg is reached. If the child fails to respond satisfactorily to the 0.6 mg/kg dose, we obtain 2 and 3 hour plasma MPH levels, and if they are in the 15–20 ng/ml range at the 0.6 mg/kg dose, will consider switching to another medication. If the levels are low we will continue increasing dosage in 0.1 mg/kg increments every 2 weeks. On many occasions the child will do well in the morning at the 0.3 mg/kg dose but the effects wear off by early afternoon. In this situation we add another 0.3 mg/kg dose at lunchtime.

Another important issue that must be considered is whether medication should be administered daily, or just on school days, with drug holidays when the child is away from school. Administration only during school offers the advantage of limiting potential toxicity while maximizing the effect of MPH when it is most needed, i.e., during the school day. We give MPH each school day but not on weekends or school holidays, and not during the summer months. However, on rare occasions when the child's impulsivity and activity prevent optimum peer and family interaction, we continue MPH on weekends.

The decision to stop medication is easier if the drug is discontinued during the summer. We stop the drug not only during the summer months but also during the first 4–6 weeks of school. Thus, we are able to evaluate how the child will do off medications once school has begun. If he is doing well without medication during the first 4–6 weeks of school, we do not resume pharmacotherapy. However, the child still needs to have careful follow-up, since as the school year continues and academic pressures increase, initial sanguine assumptions about the lack of a need for medication may not be valid. Clearly such a procedure may need to be modified in specific situations. For example, if the physician believes that the child's response to medication has been so dramatic and that starting a new school year without medication would be detrimental to the child, he or she may initiate medication as soon as school begins.

Insomnia or sleep disturbances and decreased appetite are the most frequently observed side effects of stimulants, with weight loss, irritability, and abdominal pains almost as common. These and a host of other, less frequent side effects (e.g., headaches, nausea, dizziness, dry mouth, constipation) usually disappear as the child becomes tolerant to the medication, or resolve if the dosage is reduced. However, two other potential side effects are of much more concern: growth retardation and precipitation of Gilles de la Tourette's syndrome (TS).

Recent evidence indicates that chronic administration of stimulant drugs will produce a moderate reduction of weight, with perhaps a minor suppres-

sion of growth in stature. The effects appear to be dose related, with higher doses administered for prolonged duration producing the greatest effects. This problem may be minimized if the drug is discontinued over the summer, allowing some catch-up growth to occur.

In contrast to the other side effects, which are either transient or reversed by a reduction in drug dosage, the precipitation of TS poses serious consequences. We have observed several children with TS whose symptoms appeared in association with the administration of MPH. Since MPH acts via central catecholaminergic mechanisms, and TS may result from stimulation of supersensitive DA or NE neurons, it is reasonable to believe that the onset of the tics after MPH was more than coincidental. Good evidence suggests that TS occurs more frequently in the offspring of parents with TS and in the siblings of affected individuals. Thus we do not administer stimulants to children with ADD whose parents or siblings have a history of tics.

Various other pharmacological agents have been employed in the therapy of ADD. Pemoline* is a CNS stimulant that differs in structure from either amphetamines or MPH. It is believed to act via central DA mechanisms, but the exact mechanism is unknown. It appears to be as effective as amphetamine and MPH when administered at a dose of 2.25 mg/kg and the effects may be observed for several weeks after discontinuation of the drug. The principal advantage of pemoline is its relatively prolonged duration of action, allowing the administration of a single dose in the morning. However, hypersensitivity reactions, usually involving the liver and occurring after several months of therapy, present a major obstacle to its use. This possibility necessitates checking liver function tests periodically in children taking pemoline, adding to the cost and complexity of monitoring children.

Tricyclic antidepressants have been successful in the treatment of enuresis, and some studies have shown them to be effective in ADD as well, though not to the same degree as stimulants. Like the stimulants, they exert their actions via central catecholaminergic systems. Unfortunately, death from cardiac arrhythmia has been reported in rare instances at relatively low dosages, making their use risky. The usual effective dosage is 5–14 mg/kg given in divided dosages.

Our experience with clonidine in the treatment of TS prompted us to examine the effects of this agent in ADD. Clonidine is begun at low dosages (1 μg/kg or 0.05 mg/day) and slowly titrated over several weeks to 3 μg/kg (0.15–0.3 mg/day). Dosages above 0.5 mg/day are more likely to lead to

---

*Manufacturer's warning: Safety and efficacy of Pemoline in children under 6 years of age have not been established.

side effects. Though our experience is still limited, we have been impressed that both behavior and attentional difficulties improve significantly and that side effects are minimal (rare hypotension, nausea). Clonidine may eventually prove particularly useful in children with ADD who have a family history of tics, or who have developed abnormal movements while taking stimulants.

A wide variety of pharmacologic agents have been employed in the treatment of ADD, including antipsychotic agents such as haloperidol, phenothiazines, lithium, deanol, and levodopa. To date, none has proven superior to stimulants and all have significant side effects that limit their use.

3

Nervous System

Head Injury

RAYMOND W. M. CHUN, M.D.

Thousands of Americans each year suffer injuries of the scalp, cranium, and intracranial contents. According to the National Safety Council, in 1979 130,000 head injuries occurred in the workplace alone. Add to this the number of head injuries sustained in automobile and motorcycle accidents, in sports, during birth, and in other situations and it becomes obvious that head injury is a major public health problem. In children, head injury is one of the most frequent causes of death.

The basic physical forces producing head injury —sudden acceleration, deceleration, or deformation of the cranium and its contents—may shear, tear, rotate, or compress the intracranial contents. Because of the serious sequelae of these injuries, prompt and correct diagnosis and treatment are essential.

INJURIES INVOLVING THE SCALP

The scalp is extremely vascular and bleeds profusely when cut; nevertheless, minor lacerations of the scalp should be thoroughly cleansed. Foreign debris should be removed and the skull inspected for fractures or the presence of cerebrospinal fluid (CSF). Prior to suturing, the hair around the laceration should be shaved. With contaminated wounds, tetanus toxoid booster should be administered if previous immunization was more than 5 years ago. With cleaner wounds, immunization every 10 years should suffice.

The scalp of the newborn infant may undergo bruising in the process of labor and delivery, causing several kinds of head injury. Caput succedaneum is a collection of fluid in the loose areolar tissue of the scalp. This soft, fluctuant mass may extend over a wide area, but is frequently located over the biparietal area. It is usually self-limiting and will be reabsorbed in several days. Cephalohematoma, on the other hand, is a subperiosteal collection of blood. It is limited by the suture lines and is frequently unilateral. The site most often involved is the parietal bone. Linear skull fractures are frequently present under the hematomas. The hematoma should not be routinely aspirated, but only when an infection is suspected. Cephalohematoma will generally resolve over several months.

SKULL FRACTURES

Skull fractures are classified as linear, comminuted, or depressed. Depending on the nature of the wound, the fracture may be open or closed. Open or compound fractures require operative management and are not discussed further in these sections.

The child with a head injury that has a potential of skull fracture should be carefully evaluated. If there is a history of unconsciousness or signs of basilar or depressed skull fracture, focal neurologic deficit, or other suspicious signs, radiologic examination of the skull should be done. If signs of spinal cord compression are evident, spinal films, especially of the cervical region, should be obtained.

Linear Fractures

Most skull fractures are linear and occur over the vertex of the skull. The simple closed fracture per se requires no treatment. When fracture lines cross the middle meningeal groove or the major venous sinuses, the patient should be hospitalized and observed for early signs of neurologic impairment due to a possible intracranial bleed. Fractures involving the basilar portion of the skull are sometimes associated with ecchymosis over the mastoid area (Battle sign), or around the eyes (raccoon sign). Basilar skull fractures may be complicated by CSF otorrhea or rhinorrhea, which provide a potential source of CSF infection. If otorrhea or rhinorrhea persists beyond several days, radionucleotide or tomographic studies should be done to identify the site of CSF leakage so that the dural rent can be repaired. A young child or infant with a linear skull fracture in association with a dural tear should undergo a followup radiographic evaluation of the skull 3 or 4 months later to look for a "growing fracture." If a leptomeningeal or cerebromeningeal cicatrix is demonstrated, surgical repair is indicated at the time of diagnosis.

Depressed Fractures

Blows to the head with a blunt instrument are particularly likely to cause depressed fractures. Focal neurologic signs accompanied by a palpable skull defect are symptomatic. Simple depressed skull fractures may readily be diagnosed by skull x-ray films, especially on tangential views.

Depressed skull fractures should be surgically elevated if the depression is more than 5 to 10 mm deep or if signs of dural involvement or focal neurologic deficits are present. The rationale for the elevation of the depressed fracture is to prevent further damage to the underlying brain and leptomeningeal tissue, and early repair of the depressed skull fracture may decrease the incidence of post-traumatic epilepsy.

MINOR CLOSED HEAD INJURY

Cerebral concussion is characterized by a brief loss of consciousness and usually is the result of a nonpenetrating closed head injury. The associated amnesia may be retrograde or anterograde. Vomiting, paleness, irritability, or other autonomic manifestations may be present. At times, cerebral concussion is associated with linear skull fractures.

The child with a concussion or mild closed head injury usually has a short, uneventful course. Most such children can be observed at home after the parents have been instructed to note and to report the presence of pernicious vomiting, increasing lethargy, or changes in pupils, pulse, or respirations.

However, if mild head injury is associated with focal neurologic deficits or with a skull fracture crossing the middle meningeal groove or large dural vessels, the child should be hospitalized for observation. Disorientation or persistent changes in levels of consciousness warrant serial neurologic evaluations stressing mental status and motor and pupillary signs. If an intracranial bleed cannot be ruled out, computed tomography (CT) scanning should be done. Otherwise, general supportive therapy is indicated. The restless or combative child should be calmed to prevent any further personal injury. Paraldehyde or small dosages of antihistamines or chlorpromazine may be helpful, but should be used sparingly so as not to confuse the neurologic assessment.

SEVERE CLOSED HEAD INJURY

The management of a child with severe closed head injury begins with a careful but rapid neurologic examination assessing levels of consciousness, and cranial nerve and motor functions. The physician should determine whether there is primarily cerebral injury, or whether brain stem deficits are also present. Tonically deviated eyes indicate the presence of focal cerebral cortical deficits. Pupillary size and reaction may indicate the presence of brain stem deficits. A unilaterally fixed pupil that does not react either directly or consensually to light usually denotes a third nerve compression due to uncal herniation. Other brain stem lesions tend to cause either bilaterally small or fixed dilated pupils. Abnormal reflex movements of the eyes (oculocephalic or oculovestibular reflexes) are also indices of brain stem lesions. Unilateral motor deficits are more likely to be related to cortical lesions, while bilateral motor deficits, such as decerebrate posturing, are suggestive of brain stem involvement. The more caudal the involvement, the worse the long-term prognosis.

Various scales quantify the level of consciousness, and are also useful for following the course of the patient. The Glasgow Coma Scale assesses the major areas of eye opening and verbal and motor responses. Each of these areas is subdivided into four or five stages ranging from alert to no responses. Serial determinations of changes of level of consciousness are helpful to evaluate progression of the CNS deficit.

The CT scan—now routine with severe closed head injury—has largely replaced arteriography or ventriculography as the initial neurodiagnostic procedure. It should be done in head-injured patients with unconsciousness or unexplained focal neurologic deficits. Diffuse swelling, hemorrhagic parenchymal lesions, or the presence of subdural or epidural hematomas is detectable by this noninvasive procedure. If symptoms progress, serial CT scans may be done.

An important step in the management of the child with severe head injury is to maintain factors necessary for cerebral metabolic activity. An adequate airway should be established early and the airway maintained by suctioning to remove secretions. Mechanical respiration following intubation may be necessary for patients with respiratory embarrassment or no spontaneous respiration, or those requiring hyperventilation to control increased intracranial pressure.

Deeply comatose children or those having a rapidly progressive course should have continuous monitoring of their intracranial pressure. While lumbar puncture may measure the ICP, the performance of a lumbar puncture is usually not warranted in a child with severe head injury. Continuous monitoring of intracranial pressure is best done with the sensors placed in the lateral ventricle or implanted in the subarachnoid, subdural, or epidural space. These monitors coupled to transducers will alert the physician instantaneously to intracranial pressure fluctuations.

Most of the patients with severe head injuries are comatose due to a combination of direct injury, cerebral edema, and increased intracranial pressure. In these cases, the edema is treated with hypertonic solutions. Mannitol (1.0 gm/kg) or urea (0.25 gm/kg) may be given every 4 to 6 hours as necessary. Large doses of these agents (1.0 to 2.0 gm/kg of urea) have sometimes been recommended, but the small doses seem to be as effective. Some investigators also have recommended diuretics such as furosemide (1 mg/kg) to help reduce cerebral edema. Intravenous fluid therapy should be guided by the monitoring of intake and output volumes and electrolyte concentrations. Fluids should be administered at about two thirds the volume required for normal maintenance. Serum osmolality should be measured when hypertonic agents are given.

The value of steroids in the treatment of increased intracranial pressure from severe head injuries has not been confirmed in controlled studies. Both low doses (15 mg per 24 hr) and high doses (96 mg per 24 hr) of dexamethasone have been variously advocated by different investigators. The effect of steroids upon brain edema due to tumors is rarely noted until 10 to 12 hours after it is given, and its use in severe head injuries remains controversial. Hypothermia as an adjunctive therapy to reduce the metabolic rate of the brain is rarely employed because of the exceptional efforts required to reduce core temperature.

Barbiturate treatment of increased intracranial pressure in head injury is currently being studied. It has been shown that barbiturate therapy [pentobarbital (3 to 5 mg/kg), thiopental (3 to 5 mg/kg), or phenobarbital (5 to 10 mg/kg)] will reduce persistent intracranial pressure in some cases of severe head injury, but adverse side effects, such as decreased cardiac output and impairment of immunologic defense systems, require constant vigilance. Serum barbiturate levels should be determined.

The management of increased intracranial pressure in a child with severe head injury is very complex. Cerebral perfusion should be maintained at 40 to 50 mm Hg pressure to assure adequate cerebral blood flow. Serial neurologic evaluations may be needed to assess the condition of the child. However, if barbiturate therapy or curarization has been initiated, clinical neurodiagnostic signs are lost. Serial CT scans, continuous monitoring of the intracranial pressure, blood gases, and cardiovascular and respiratory changes are the data which must be relied on to make further changes in patient care. It is essential, therefore, that such patients be managed in intensive care units.

When seizures are present, slow intravenous phenytoin is administered in loading doses of 18 mg/kg and then subsequently in maintenance doses of 7 mg/kg. Anticonvulsant therapy should be continued for several years after the head injury.

Cerebral Edema

JEROME S. HALLER, M.D.

There is little doubt that the edema surrounding a brain tumor or abscess will recede with steroid therapy, with remarkable clinical improvement. What other causes of edema need to be treated and how to treat are questions that are not easily resolved. For example, there is evidence in pediatric closed head injury that, initially, the swollen brain is produced by an increased blood volume that will respond to controlled ventilation/hyperventilation with $Paco_2$ at 20 to 25 torr. If edema develops, it seems to appear 3 or more days following the injury and then patchily beneath contused cortex. If we are to be guided by experimental data, mannitol is inappropriate during the first phase of this condition. Steroids might be used during the second phase, but the clinical literature is divided on the results of steroid therapy.

Treatment must be based on the clinical state of the patient. If the child is unconscious, or if there is neurologic deterioration and the CT scan does not reveal an operative lesion, then intracranial pressure monitoring should be instituted and the patient managed much the same as is outlined in the section on Reye syndrome. If the child is rapidly deteriorating, a bolus of mannitol should be given at a dose of 1.5 gm/kg over a 20-minute period. Rapid deterioration suggests the presence of a hematoma and the need for surgical intervention.

These same issues must be addressed when the disease process is an infection of the central nervous system, bacterial or viral meningoencephalitis. Might the neurologic status be related solely to the infection or in association with edema, or is increased intracranial pressure a contributory factor? There is no indication for steroid therapy in bacterial meningitis; indeed, it may be contraindicated except in meningococcal meningitis. A trial dose of mannitol might be given, but, without ICP monitoring, dosage and response will be difficult to ascertain.

Supportive management of children with viral meningoencephalitis who are comatose, that is, demonstrating nondirected motor activity in response to painful stimulation or decorticate or decerebrate posturing, should be in the manner described in the section on Reye syndrome. They require intubation, controlled respiration, and ICP monitoring. Steroid therapy is warranted, using dexamethasone, 0.2 mg/kg/24 hr. Half of the calculated dose should be given intravenously initially and then four divided doses every six hours thereafter. Mannitol should be administered as noted in the Reye syndrome section. Along with institution of steroid therapy, antacids have been recommended.

If cerebral edema is primarily a disturbance of vascular permeability, there can be little rationale in restricting fluids to two thirds of maintenance. More important is avoiding fluid overload. It is my contention that maintenance fluid amounts are appropriate, whether calculated by body surface or insensible loss plus urinary output. Practically, the use of humidified air when a patient is on a respirator makes either method only a guideline. Weight, electrolytes, and urinary output must be carefully observed.

Treatment of cerebral edema cannot be discussed in a recipe format to cover all contingencies. The presence of edema does not necessarily correlate directly with increased intracranial pressure. Intervention should be determined not only by the presumed disease but also by the patient's clinical condition.

Epidural Hematoma and Subdural Hematoma

PAUL R. DYKEN, M.D.

EPIDURAL HEMATOMA

In the treatment of epidural hematoma, it is extremely important to be able to make a quick and accurate diagnosis of the location, type, and extent of the hematoma while at the same time initiating treatment. It is of utmost importance to take care of the vital body functions while arranging as rapidly as possible ultimate specific surgery. Support treatment includes maintenance of an open airway, sedation, support of vital signs, and initial attempts to control increased intracranial pressure. Control of epileptic seizures is also important, even though seizures are relatively uncommon in acute epidural hematoma contrasted to other forms of head trauma. One must always be aware that a patient who is reasonably stable might rapidly deteriorate within minutes. In some instances with careful monitoring, however, one can obtain skull x-rays and computer-assisted tomography while the operating room is being prepared. Seldom is it necessary to go further than this in diagnostic work-up,

and the patient should never be left without skilled intensive observation. Certain procedures, such as lumbar puncture, are contraindicated in the presurgical period.

Some controversy exists concerning the use of antiedema agents in the presurgical treatment of epidural hematoma. Some have used intravenous mannitol (0.25–1.5 mg/kg) in an effort to retard the cerebral pathophysiology until surgery can be accomplished. However, mannitol and other agents such as glycerol and urea act by creating an osmotic gradient causing water to be drawn from the brain through the capillary wall into blood, thereby reducing intracranial pressure. This effect may be immediate and great but produces disturbances that tend to potentiate intracranial bleeding. In the period immediately prior to surgery such agents are appropriate but, unless surgery is imminent, they should not be used. Steroids, on the other hand, which do not potentiate intracranial bleeding, have not been demonstrated to be effective in the acute treatment of the increased intracranial pressure associated with epidural hematoma because they are slower in action. Steroids may be useful in the follow-up period, however. Passive hyperventilation is prompt and does not potentiate intracranial bleeding. This is accomplished by reducing $Paco_2$ from 40 torr to 25–28 torr (using either face mask or endotracheal tube). Passive hyperventilation lowers intracranial pressure by inducing vasoconstriction and is, therefore, a useful adjunctive therapy for the immediate control of increased intracranial pressure. Barbiturate coma may be another way to decrease intracranial pressure by producing vasoconstriction and restricted cerebral blood flow in a fashion similar to passive hyperventilation. One gives an initial dose of 3–5 mg/kg of pentobarbital intravenously over 10–20 minutes, followed by 1–3 mg/kg every 1–2 hours. Barbiturates, in general, also reduce cerebral metabolism by as much as 50%. They do not potentiate intracranial bleeding. Hypothermia (27–31°C) may be an additional form of treatment of the increased intracranial pressure associated with epidural hematoma but has a disadvantage compared to both barbiturate coma and passive hyperventilation in that its peak effectiveness may be several hours. Barbiturate coma and hypothermia are not commonly used prior to surgery in epidural hematoma but they have a greater utility in the postoperative care of such patients.

Regardless of the form of supportive treatment for epidrual hematoma, the ultimate and most important definitive therapy is evacuation. An epidural hematoma of significant size should be treated as an acute surgical emergency with the most rapid surgical intervention possible. Although the residual effects of an acute epidural hematoma are relatively infrequent, they do occasionally occur in the form of lingering motor and sensory abnormalities, mental dysfunctions, and seizures. These must be considered in the long term treatment of this condition.

SUBDURAL HEMATOMA

Subdural hematoma is due to the collection of free blood or serosanguinous fluid and membranes beneath the dura mater. The original blood collection is produced by the tearing of a bridging cortical vein(s), which drains into the large dural sinuses. Usually the bleeding is caused by head trauma. In infants especially, it is probable that nutritional and fluid disturbances contribute to the mechanical factors that result in bleeding. Although free blood initiates the process, the blood accumulation is later enclosed by membranes and altered by the body's attempt at resolution. The two basic types of subdural hematomas encountered are distinguished by clinical as well as pathophysiologic mechanisms. Acute subdural hematoma reflects the period when there is a mass of free blood within the subdural space and is a greater threat to life and morbidity, owing to other neurological dysfunctions resulting from associated brain concussion, contusion, hematoma, and laceration. Chronic subdural hematoma occurs after the free blood has been altered and compartmentalized by neovascularized membrane formation, a process that usually takes weeks. Certainly, both conditions may be medical and surgical emergencies but since different therapies exist, they will be discussed separately.

Acute Subdural Hematoma. This condition is usually associated with severe head injury and considerable coexisting parenchymal disturbance and a wide range of neurological dysfunctions. Occasionally, a single bridging vein is torn and no or minimal coexisting neurological symptoms are encountered. These later presentations are associated with small subdural blood collections. In this instance, the hematoma may resolve totally or develop later into chronic subdural hematoma.

In the therapy of acute subdural hematoma, it is important to emphasize that it is not the blood in the subdural space that produces the major neurologic symptoms. Symptoms are produced by the effect of the blood accumulation on the surrounding brain and by direct brain injury. As with all acute neurological emergencies, it is important to take special care of the vital body functions. Maintenance of an open airway, adequate respiratory exchange and oxygenation, blood pressure and other vital sign regulation, careful fluid and electrolyte therapy using restricted water load, protection against infection, replacement of blood loss, bladder and bowel care, sedation, control of epileptic seizures, which are more frequent than in epidural

hematoma, and therapy to combat increased intracranial pressure are indicated.

Treatment for increased intracranial pressure deserves special consideration. Probably the most effective methods of combating increased intracranial pressure in acute subdural hematoma is passive hyperventilation (reducing Pa_{CO_2} to 25–28 torr). Pentobarbital anesthesia (initial dosage of 3–5 mg/kg intravenously over 10–20 minutes followed by 1–3 mg/kg every 1–2 hours) and hypothermia (27–31°C) are also potentially useful means of treatment. The osmotic gradient agents such as mannitol and glycerol are probably contraindicated in acute subdural hematoma management because of their tendency to promote intracranial bleeding and rebound increased pressure unless they are used in the immediate period before surgical intervention. Steroids may have a more appropriate use in the treatment of acute subdural hematoma than in epidural hematoma. Dexamethasone given intravenously in a 0.1 to 0.2 mg/kg dose acts by stabilizing the blood-brain barrier and promoting renal excretion of sodium. Steroids do not produce rebound and do not promote intracranial bleeding, although complicating gastrointestinal bleeding may occur. Steroids, however, act slowly and this could explain why their use in acute subdural hematoma is still controversial. There has been no confirmation that they are totally effective in the treatment of any form of acute head trauma. If used, one should carefully monitor for gastrointestinal bleeding and use antacid therapy.

Seizures occur acutely in from 50–70% of those with acute subdural hematomas. Thus, anticonvulsant therapy is an important adjunct to the management of those patients who have seizures. Choice of an anticonvulsant depends upon the type of seizure and the condition of the patient. If the patient is in major status epilepticus, which, however, is rare, phenobarbital given by slow intravenous infusion at a dosage ranging from 15–20 mg/kg is indicated. Patients must be carefully monitored and careful seizure frequency documentation is required. Other forms of treatment of status epilepticus may be used also, such as slowly administered intravenous diazepam (0.1–0.3 mg/kg) and phenytoin (15–20 mg/kg). Usually in acute subdural hematoma, seizures are not continuous. When frequent convulsions occur, a loading dose of 10 mg/kg phenobarbital can be given intravenously. This is best followed by a daily maintenance dosage of 3–4 mg/kg/day titrated so as to reach blood levels of around 40 μg/ml. Barbiturates are preferred in the management of seizures in acute subdural hematoma because they are known to decrease brain metabolism. Other anticonvulsants can also be used, such as phenytoin at 5 mg/kg/day maintenance dosage both with and without loading dosages initially.

Acute subdural hematomas sufficiently large enough to produce a mass effect should be evacuated by way of craniotomy. Since subdurals may be bilateral, either a bilateral or unilateral craniotomy with multiple burr holes on the other side are often performed. Occasionally, shunting procedures may be necessary before definitive surgery. Subdural taps for therapy are probably not indicated even in infants with open fontanels unless the infant is only mildly symptomatic with relatively small collections of subdural fluid.

Neurological residuals from acute subdural hematoma may be extensive. Treatment includes prevention of recurrence (especially important in child abuse cases), the long term management of seizures, psychoeducational planning and therapy, and rehabilitation in the form of speech and physical and occupational therapy.

Chronic Subdural Hematoma. Chronic subdural hematoma represents, in most instances, a late effect from acute subdural bleeding and thus usually is a reflection of head trauma as well. In this instance, however, the body's defense mechanisms have come into play and the fresh blood has been replaced by serosanguinous fluid and membrane formation that usually has a fairly well developed inner and outer portion, both of which show considerable neovascularization. The subdural fluid has a high osmotic density, which allows an internal gradient system, important in the production of many of the symptoms associated with this entity. Although nutritional and fluid factors may also play a role in the development of subdural hematoma in infants, trauma is usually believed to be the initiator of the process. Yet, a history of significant head trauma may not be elicited because the hematoma may be caused by relatively minor forms of trauma, such as shaking, or be denied, as in child abuse. Characteristic symptoms are pallor, irritability, seizures, failure to thrive, anemia, fever, macrocrania, "box-shaped" crania, bulging anterior fontanel, other signs of increased intracranial pressure, and a variety of other neurologic and systemic disabilities. In the process of diagnostic work-up, symptomatic treatment should be initiated, to combat infection, control seizures, alleviate headache and pain, produce sedation, correct anemia and nutritional state, and overcome increased intracranial pressure.

In some mildly symptomatic infantile cases with small fluid collection, subdural taps not only may confirm the diagnosis but also may be of therapeutic benefit. It must be emphasized that subdural taps are fraught with problems and complications and should be reserved for special situations and then only with careful precautions. Since the procedure is still used in therapy of subdural hematoma, a recommended procedure will be listed here. The subdural puncture is performed through the coronal suture immediately lateral to the most lateral aspect of the anterior fontanel. Subdural taps are always performed with assistance and by using strict asepsis after shaving the head. While an assistant stabilizes the head in a supine position at the edge of the table, the skin of the scalp is pulled taut to form a "Z" tract. A number 20 subdural needle with a guard is inserted perpendicularly to the scalp and is then directed toward the inner canthus of the ipsilateral eye. If subdural needles are not available, a 20 gauge lumbar puncture needle with a short bevel may be used, clamping a sterile forceps about 5–8 mm from the tip. When the needle penetrates the dura mater, a "pop" is felt. This occurs usually when the needle tip is several millimeters beneath the inner table of the skull. A few drops of clear fluid will normally be present. If no fluid is evident, the tap is repeated 1.5 to 2.0 cm immediately lateral to the fontanel through the coronal suture. Once abnormal fluid is encountered, fluid should be allowed to flow out spontaneously. No more than 15 ml should be removed at one time to help prevent hypovolemic shock. Aspiration should never be performed, owing to the risk of rebleeding and injuring the underlying brain. After the tap is completed, firm pressure should be applied to the puncture site with sterile gauze for a minimum of two minutes, after which sterile collodion is applied. Subdural taps are hazardous unless done properly and may be complicated by infection, rebleeding, subgaleal hemorrhage, and trauma to the underlying cerebral cortex.

Some patients become asymptomatic after one subdural puncture or burr hole and there is no reaccumulation of fluid. More often, however, repeated subdural tapping or repeated tapping of the burr hole is necessary. If the child continues to have symptoms, and in particular continues to manifest signs of increased intracranial pressure, surgical intervention is usually necessary. In such cases, shunting procedures drawing the subdural space may be performed as a means of correcting for the reaccumulation of fluid and chronic protein loss.

The treatment of chronic subdural hematoma continues well into convalescence and even later. In child abuse particularly, measures must be taken to prevent recurrent traumatic episodes. Those with chronic subdural hematoma may also have residual brain damage. Not only must we be concerned with the social aspects of the various causes of subdural hematoma but also we must have facilities available for long-term follow-up to include expert modern seizure management, speech, physical and occupational therapy, and psychoeducational management if these residuals are present.

Intracranial Hemorrhage

PAUL G. MOE, M.D.

Intracranial hemorrhage, or bleeding into the head, includes subarachnoid, subdural, and epidural bleeding, in addition to intraparenchymal bleeding into the cerebrum or cerebellum. Bleeding at any of these sites can be due to trauma, vascular malformation, congenital berry or mycotic aneurysm, or hemorrhagic stroke, or it can be associated with clotting disorders (leukemia, thrombocytopenic purpura, hemophilia).

Newborns

In the newborn, birth trauma/hypoxia, especially in the premature infant, is the most common cause of intracranial hemorrhage. The diagnosis is suggested by the history, e.g., deteriorating fetal heart rate during labor, poor Apgar scores, or necessity for resuscitation at birth. Signs of fetal distress include hypotonia, poor suck, seizures, lethargy, and tremulousness. Increased intracranial pressure with bulging fontanel and/or rapidly enlarging head often reflects, in varying combinations, hypoxic cerebral edema, intracranial hemorrhage, and hydrocephalus. Any distressed infant deserves study to rule out intracerebral hemorrhage. Immediate B-mode ultrasound is the most available safe test and is usually diagnostic with subependymal and intraventricular hemorrhages, and often can diagnose the more rare intracerebellar and subdural bleeds. Small amounts of subarachnoid blood may be missed but are of little importance. Computed tomography (CT) scans should be done if ultrasound is inconclusive and there remains high clinical suspicion of hemorrhage. Spinal fluid examination is less helpful. Many newborns will have xanthochromic or even bloody spinal fluid from unimportant subarachnoid bleeding secondary to the "normal" trauma of birth. Spinal fluid must, however, be examined if there is any suspicion of infection; thus a lumbar puncture is often done in a distressed newborn, even when hemorrhage is strongly suspected or proved. Unless the baby is acutely deteriorating, treatment is supportive. Thus, if brainstem herniation is suggested by bulging fontanel or worsening vital signs or level of consciousness, accessible (subdural) or strategically located (posterior fossa) hematomas may need surgical drainage. Bloody subdural hematoma can be tapped with a short-bevel, 18 or 20 gauge needle through the corner of the fontanel. In an emergency this can be done as a diagnostic/therapeutic procedure prior to CT or ultrasound. If subdural taps are "dry" or negative, a single needle pass can be continued on either side to try to release intraventricular fluid under pressure.

Intracerebellar and epidural hematomas (both rare) often require craniotomy for removal.

The usual, less heroic supportive treatment may include controlled respiration to ensure oxygenation and low P_{CO_2} (22–25 mm Hg) for its vasoconstrictive/anticerebral edema effect. Blood pressure maintenance is vital to prevent hypertensive surges and hypotension, either of which may cause rebleeds, or infarction. Vitamin K prophylaxis (for clotting) decreased handling, anticonvulsant prophylaxis (phenobarbital 10–20 μg/kg load, 5 μg/kg/day daily maintenance monitored by everyday blood phenobarbital levels), transfusions, and careful fluid balance are prosaic but important therapies. Nonstandard therapies include low dose phenobarbital (5 μg/kg/day) to prevent blood pressure fluctuations, and high dose barbiturate (pentobarbital, phenobarbital) to reduce cerebral edema. Serial lumbar punctures are used to remove spinal fluid, or acetazolamide* (100 mg/kg/day), furosemide (1 mg/kg/dose) or oral glycerol (1–2 gm/kg/day) to reduce spinal fluid production. Serial head measurements and ultrasound (or CT) scans should be done to diagnose progressive hydrocephalus. Treatment for rapidly progressive ventriculomegaly may include external ventriculostomy if fluid is very bloody, or if the infant is critically ill or too tiny to tolerate an internal shunt. The more usual standard treatment is ventriculoperitoneal shunt with a valve that will tolerate high protein ventricular fluid (e.g., Denver shunt).

Infants, Toddlers, and Older Children

In infants and toddlers intracranial bleeding is most often due to trauma. If after history and physical, the etiology is still obscure, nonaccidental trauma ("NAT") should be considered. The history will often not explain the findings; for example, subdural hematomas and intraocular hemorrhages seen in the context of "rolling off the bed." Examination must include inspection of the skin for cigarette burns or bruises. Radiologic survey for overt fractures or subtle periosteal or epiphyseal changes should be done. The infant/toddler must be hospitalized both for medical reasons and for searching social investigation. After informing the parents or caretaker of the necessity, social service or "nonaccidental trauma team" consultation should be sought. CT scan should be obtained for any child who has sustained enough trauma to cause more than brief unconsciousness. Spinal tap is inadvisable in clear-cut trauma, but if done, should be deferred until the CT scan has ruled out a mass lesion (e.g., hematoma or swelled hemisphere). A

---

*This use is not listed by the manufacturer

spinal tap should be done only if meningitis is suspected. Patients with traumatic intracerebral hemorrhage may have normal or bloody spinal fluid; the results seldom influence therapy.

Most trauma-associated intracerebral hemorrhages can be managed conservatively with mild (30°) head-up position and rest, and charting of neurologic and vital signs in an intensive care unit. Serial CT scans are often necessary to follow the course. More vigorous management of intracranial pressure may be necessary with intracranial monitoring devices, controlled ventilation, blood gas monitoring, blood pressure control, fluid restriction, even iatrogenic barbiturate coma. Occasionally, mannitol (1–2 gm/kg of 20% solution over 20 to 30 minutes intravenously), and furosemide (1–2 mg/kg intravenously) may be necessary for associated cerebral edema. (The latter agents perhaps should not be used with an enclosed hematoma—unless in conjunction with surgical evacuation of the hematoma. Some believe the resultant shrinking of the brain may remove the tamponade effect on the hematoma and cause rebleeding.)

In the deteriorating patient, epidural, and posterior fossa hematomas, and sometimes subdural hematomas, may need surgical removal.

Other causes of intracerebral bleeding in children of all ages include arteriovenous malformations (AVM), congenital berry aneurysms (very rare prior to adolescence), or mycotic aneurysms (e.g., in immunocompromised patients with bacterial or fungal meningitis). Bleeding can be a result of hemorrhagic strokes, for example in cyanotic congenital heart disease or in severely dehydrated infants with venous thrombosis. Blood dyscrasias are a final possible cause of hemorrhage.

Rarely is there a historical clue to the AVM's: seizures may be present, but usually the bleed is the initial event. Acute or subacute cause of severe headache, stiff neck, clouding of consciousness, and fundal hemorrhages are seen in severe bleeds. CT scan with contrast is almost always positive; rapid infusion (venous) subtraction angiography, or aortic arch arterial angiography is often necessary to delineate the site and fine anatomy. Conservative treatment (as above) is usual. Accessible (surface), and small malformations should be surgically removed; the timing depends on the patient's condition. Usually the operation is done after the acute event has stabilized. In a deteriorating patient, removal of clot, and embolization or ligation of feeding vessels may "buy time" for a second-stage definitive operation.

Congenital berry aneurysms are similar treated. Mycotic aneurysms (usually small, distally located) often heal with diagnosis and treatment of the underlying infection or other cause. Examples include subacute bacterial endocarditis and heroin or phencyclidine injection. In teenagers, intravenous drug abuse can lead to intracranial hemorrhage, more often without visible aneurysm. The therapeutic implications are obvious.

In children with cyanotic congenital heart disease, hemorrhagic strokes may reflect hyper- or hypocoagulability or high viscosity (high hematocrit/dehydration). Drugs to affect coagulation (e.g. platelet-inhibitory agents) or phlebotomy occasionally have a therapeutic role.

In blood dyscrasias (e.g., leukemia, thrombocytopenic purpura), there will "always" be bleeding elsewhere, such as in the skin, to herald an intracranial bleed. Platelet transfusions are a therapeutic mainstay; the other treatment is beyond the scope of this article. Hemophiliacs may present with "headache"; this is "intracranial bleed" until proven otherwise, and should be treated as an emergency with antihemophilic globulin, and hematologic consultation.

Rarely, brain tumors in children present as an intracranial bleed: choroid plexus papillomas and ependymomas are two examples. The CT scan will usually be diagnostic. Treatment is surgical and/or radiation therapy.

Hydrocephalus

J. T. JABBOUR, M.D.

The treatment of hydrocephalus usually requires a surgical procedure and on occasion medical treatments, which are currently available. Management and treatment are often an emergency because of the intracranial hypertension, which produces vomiting, dehydration, alteration of consciousness, and rarely, cerebral and/or brain stem dysfunction, which leads to death.

The medical treatment of hydrocephalus should alter the rate of production of cerebrospinal fluid and can be achieved with acetazolamide (Diamox) or other osmotic agents for short periods of time.

There are few surgically correctable brain lesions. On occasion, one will find a tumor obstructing the foramen magnum or the third ventricle. An arachnoid cyst or a Dandy-Walker cyst can be drained and thus provide relief from ventricular enlargement. Choroid plexus papillomas within the ventricular spaces are occasionally found, and their removal may result in normalization of cerebrospinal fluid production.

The most important approach to the treatment of hydrocephalus is the ventricular shunt, which diverts the cerebrospinal fluid to the peritoneal cavity or to the auricle of the heart. Various shunts have greatly improved the lives of children with hydrocephalus, and the prognosis has improved in spite of recurrent infections and shunt obstructions, which infrequently occur.

Extracranial ventricular shunts are extremely valuable in patients with communicating hydrocephalus or obstructive lesions such as aqueductal stenosis, arachnoid cyst, or tumors.

The shunts that have been developed consist of 1) a ventricular catheter, 2) a connecting cylindrical pump or valve, and 3) a distal catheter. The devices most often are placed in the lateral region of the head, usually behind the ear, and the tubing is directed posterior along the lateral aspect of the neck and under the skin across the lateral chest into the peritoneal cavity. The device for pumping is usually located behind the ear, most often on the right side, and provides easy access for the physician to evaluate the patency of the proximal or distal catheter.

The pressure valves on the connecting shunt portions vary in pressure from 40 to 110 mm of water and can be utilized under various conditions of increased intracranial pressure. The shunts can be gauged according to the subjective and/or objective pressure measurements suspected in each child who will be shunted.

Shunt selection is usually dictated by the patient's need for a first shunt or replacement of an obstructed and/or infected shunt.

Placement of a peritoneal shunt is the best procedure, and is utilized in most patients initially. The procedure is less likely to be associated with the complications of bacteremia and is not as difficult as placement in the auricle of the heart. Such complications include bacterial infection (usually *Staphylococcus epidermidis*), shunt tube obstruction by debris, a peritoneal cyst about the distal end of the catheter, or a hydrocele or hernia. A ventriculoatrial shunt is used as an alternate shunt because of abdominal infection, perforation, or thrombotic disease.

DIAGNOSIS OF SHUNT OBSTRUCTION

In order to determine the location and obstruction of a shunt, a radiopaque material is injected into both the proximal and the distal ends, and a radiograph of the area is obtained. By pumping the valve, the obstruction can often be determined when the pump does not refill. When a shunt is obstructed, immediate removal and replacement is mandatory in order to prevent intracranial hypertension. When the shuntogram is performed, a sample of ventricular fluid should be obtained for analysis of white blood cells, protein, glucose, and culture of the more common bacteria that may cause the obstruction. If there is evidence of an infection, a continuous ventricular drainage is placed when intracranial pressure is excessive, while the patient receives systemic and/or ventricular antibiotics until placement of a new shunt is undertaken.

Shunt infections may be associated with ventriculitis, meningitis, wound infection, or evidence of endocarditis or a shunt nephritis. Antibiotics are usually administered intravenously as well as into the ventricular cavity. Culture of these fluids should dictate the antibiotic to be used, and the dosage and length of treatment by such antibiotics is dictated by serial analyses of ventricular and/or cerebrospinal fluid.

On occasion, the child may require serial CT scans in order to determine if there is a nidus of infection (cerebritis, subdural effusion) contributing to the shunt infection. In addition, in patients who have intraventricular hemorrhage or hematomas, there will be a need to define the extent of such hemorrhage and to determine if there is a secondary focus of infection.

Effective treatment of *S. epidermidis* and *S. aureus,* as well as other organisms, is dependent on cerebrospinal or ventricular fluid cultures. The antibiotics of choice are gentamicin, vancomycin, cephalosporins, and nafcillin, and are dictated by culture and sensitivities.

The rare complication of subdural hematoma, although serious, is carefully monitored by CT scans. The selection of the appropriate pressure valve is most important in order to prevent this complication. On occasion, a subdural hematoma may occur after trauma to the head; fortunately this is very rare, but one must be ready to evacuate such hematomas.

The need for elective revision is dictated by suspected obstruction of the shunt and observation of a patient who has early signs of intracranial hypertension. Shunt revision may be necessary when the catheter length is too short for the patient.

PROGNOSIS AND FOLLOW-UP

While the prognosis in patients prior to the era of the more functional ventricular shunts and the newer antibiotics was much poorer, there is now evidence that patients can achieve greater control of their motor, mental, and academic abilities than in the past. If the shunt functions properly, the child can be normal, with no cerebral dysfunction. On occasion, with obstructions which go unrecognized, cerebral injury may result from infections and intracranial hypertension, and thus result in neurological dysfunction and impairment. All patients should be followed carefully by the pediatrician, neurologist, and neurosurgeon in an effort to prevent any compromise of cerebral function.

Myelodysplasia

DAVID W. BAILEY, M.D.

The major structural birth defects which fall under the classification of myelodysplasia (MDP) include spina bifida cystica, myelomeningocele, lipomeningocele, and caudal regression syndromes. Because the term implies the clinical variability seen among these infants, MDP will be defined as any congenital spinal neurectodermal malformation with associated immediate and/or remote neurological deficit(s). Anencephaly, a neural tube defect often included in studies and biostatistics with MDP, will not be discussed here.

Recent experience suggests a decline in the incidence of MDP, at least in some areas of the country. Currently, it occurs in approximately 1 per 1000 live births in the general population. Recurrence in siblings and incidence in offspring of a parent with MDP is sharply increased to the range of 20 to 40 per 1000 live births. The incidence in offspring of aunts and uncles of an affected child is only slightly increased (2 to 3 per 1000 live births), and approaches that seen in the offspring of mothers over 35 years of age.

Preliminary evidence suggests that the risk of recurrence of MDP in siblings, and perhaps the basic incidence, can be reduced sharply by administering certain vitamins (especially folic acid) to the mother for a month before and after conception. Amniocentesis can be performed early in pregnancy to measure the alpha-fetoprotein level in the amniotic fluid; this will be elevated if the fetus has a defect leaking cerebrospinal fluid. After confirmatory ultrasound studies, voluntary interruption of pregnancy can be performed. Currently, most informed high-risk mothers are following these procedures.

The implications of the previous two paragraphs in regard to causation are clear. The polygenic factors that influence the development of MDP occur with varying prevalence throughout the world, and are most common among Celtic peoples. Operating in conjunction with these genetic predilections are environmental factors, some of which appear to be related to folic acid metabolism (alcoholism, malnutrition, certain drugs).

INITIAL ASSESSMENT AND MANAGEMENT

The diagnosis of MDP is usually made post partum because most afflicted infants are born at community hospitals lacking the specialized personnel and facilities these infants usually require. It is the responsibility of the pediatrician or generalist called to see the baby to complete an assessment that will allow him/her to inform and counsel the family, guide them in their initial referral decisions, and properly prepare the receiving facility's personnel.

Detailed prenatal and perinatal histories are essential to the recognition of other associated acquired problems (sepsis, anoxia, hemorrhage), which have a major bearing on prognosis. The details of family history and possible teratogenic factors should not be dwelt upon at this stage in order to avoid exacerbation of the parents' guilt feelings.

The initial examination of the infant focuses on four main areas. First, the spinal lesion itself is carefully inspected. If there appears to have been membrane rupture with exposure of the neural plaque, cultures of the surface are taken, using care not to further damage the plaque, which is then covered with a generous layer of silver sulfadiazine (Silvadene) cream followed by a moist saline dressing. If the sac is intact and bulging, a needle aspirate (approaching from the edge through normal skin) is obtained for Gram stain and culture. The size and shape (sessile, pedunculated, cystic) of the lesion and any associated bony anomalies (kyphosis, diastematomyelia, protuberant alae) are noted.

Secondly, the examiner's attention is directed to the infant's head, looking particularly for signs of hydrocephalus. The occipitofrontal circumference is recorded, and transillumination may be carried out. Skull x-rays that reveal lükenschädel (lacunar skull deformity) are diagnostic of hydrocephalus even if the baby is normocephalic. Notation of cranial nerve and/or brain stem deficits (oculomotor palsies, stridor, dysphagia, apneic spells) will alert the receiving facility as to the likelihood of problems related to a severe associated Arnold-Chiari malformation.

The third area of emphasis is the level and symmetry of paresis in the lower extremities, which may not correlate well with either the level of bony defects on the spine x-rays or the sensory level. Also, it can be difficult to distinguish voluntary movements from those arising on a reflex basis via an isolated lower cord segment, especially in infants with higher thoracolumbar lesions. Suspension by a hand under the mid-trunk in the prone position, or attempts to elicit other postural reflexes (Moro, asymmetric tonic neck) may facilitate this important distinction.

Lastly, a careful look at the whole infant is very important. Infants with MDP who also have severe inoperable cardiac malformations, anencephaly, or trisomy 13 may be better served by avoiding the stress to them and their families of transfer to a strange, distant medical center. Conspicuous commonly associated malformations such as polydactyly, radial ray hypoplasia, arthrogryposis, and/or cloacal exstrophy should be discussed with the family prior to transfer. Both parents need the opportunity to ask questions while seeing and holding their baby.

SUBSEQUENT ASSESSMENT AND MANAGEMENT

The receiving group at the referral center includes the pediatrician, social worker or nurse, and neurosurgeon from the myelodysplasia center team plus the NICU nurse and resident. Each member of the team must review the data from the referring facility and accomplish his/her own comprehensive evaluation. Additional immediate studies include cranial ultrasound to assess hydrocephalus and to look for intracranial hemorrhage. Urgent consultations, e.g. cardiology or urology, may be suggested by initial clinical findings such as a cardiac murmur or abnormal kidneys on palpation. Orders must be written for scrupulous topical care and protection of the spinal lesion, with Silvadene cream and systemic antibiotics if the sac is leaking or the neural plaque exposed.

When these preliminary steps are completed, as many of the team as possible must sit down and fully discuss their findings with responsible family members (usually father and one or more grandparents). Efforts to convey information to the mother, directly by phone and indirectly via the father or referring physician, are essential. Written materials, both general pamphlets and lists of items dealing with the particular infant, should be provided to supplement the verbal discussions.

After fully informing the family of the nature and severity of their baby's problems, the team must provide unified and consistent recommendations regarding management, based on the interests of the child. Parents appreciate being fully informed and will only rarely fail to accept the team's recommendations. When that failure appears to stem from family dynamics not based on the baby's own interests, it may be necessary to adopt an official advocacy role with involvement of the courts. Fortunately, this is rarely necessary, provided that the other steps outlined above have been taken.

When confronted by a newborn infant with a large thoracolumbar myelomeningocele, severe hydrocephalus, and other major anomalies, the team and family may concur that aggressive intervention is inappropriate. With time, some of these infants stabilize and a shift in management to definitive surgical intervention becomes appropriate. Daily reassessment of the baby and ongoing counseling of the family are essential.

The vast majority of MDP babies undergo closure in layers of the spinal defect as soon as possible after birth. The closure may require removal of bony spurs, but correction of an associated kyphosis at the initial surgery is not indicated. Every effort is made to return the neural plaque contents to the spinal canal without further injury. The family must understand that the degree of paraplegia may appear to have increased or decreased postoperatively, but that it usually persists unchanged. The closure must not allow CSF leak. Systemic antibiotics pre-, intra-, and post-operatively are indicated.

The timing of the CSF shunting procedure, usually ventriculoperitoneal, is determined by a number of factors. A trial period without shunting after back closure is justifiable if there is reasonable hope that the baby will be among the minority who do not develop progressive hydrocephalus. Those with lower spinal lesions and little or no hydroceph-

alus on ultrasound are most likely to escape shunt procedures. Serial ultrasound exams are easily obtained and help allay concern when a baby with a full fontanel and increasing head circumference is being followed post-closure. Of course, intracranial hypertension which is causing pain or threatening the integrity of the back closure demands immediate surgical intervention.

In the minority of cases where the baby's interests are best served by nonintervention, it becomes the task of the family and care team to consider timely, pain-free death as the desired outcome. Care should be limited to humane measures intended to keep the baby warm, dry, clean, fed, and free of pain. Changing circumstances may dictate a change in treatment plan. Those individuals with the greatest experience in caring for infants with MDP are convinced that there are no criteria which can reliably predict the quality in any meaningful sense of the infant's future life. A flexible, cautiously optimistic approach to the early management of these children is therefore appropriate.

LONG-TERM MANAGEMENT

An interdisciplinary team is essential to the ongoing care of these children. The MDP team members from the urology and orthopaedic services should accomplish their baseline evaluations, perform any urgent studies or treatment, and contribute to the management planning and family counseling prior to the baby's discharge from the newborn unit. Occupational and physical therapists will have instructed the parents in stimulation and range of motion interactions. A clinical nurse specialist may have assessed, and augmented as necessary, their parenting and health promotion/maintenance capabilities. Detailed, up-to-date briefing of the baby's primary care physician is a prerequisite to discharge.

In each of the discussions that follow in this section, a basic principle or goal is to maximize the child's potential for learning self-care at the various stages of his/her development. Adherence to this principle stems from the conviction that the MDP child's eventual social adjustment and level of achievement depend on his/her intellect, attitudes, personal hygiene, and mobility.

Stool Toilet Training. Early measures must be undertaken to assist children with MDP in establishing social continence so that they can join in the group setting of school and other peer gatherings. The pathophysiology of colonic and of anorectal sphincter dysfunction is complex, and the degree of dysfunction correlates only to a limited extent with the level of the spinal lesion. A dietary program designed to avoid severe constipation, together with a compulsive bowel regimen that takes advantage of the gastrocolic reflex and includes the use of bisacodyl suppositories if necessary to ensure daily rectal emptying, can with early implementation and meticulous attention to detail be successful in nearly all cases.

Urinary Toilet Training. The pathophysiology of urinary incontinence in MDP children is far more complex than its colonic counterpart. Added to this greater complexity are the life-threatening implications of urinary tract mismanagement. A successful genitourinary program must include measures which will 1) maintain drainage and preserve renal structure and function; 2) minimize the risk of pyelonephritis; 3) provide hygienic care of the skin in the diaper area; 4) teach self-care, which will avoid the malodorous "outhouse syndrome"; 5) assure continence with or without chemical (drugs), mechanical (clean intermittent catheterization), and/or surgical (artificial sphincter, diversion) adjuncts; and 6) counsel and treat to maximize sexual potential.

These objectives can be reached only with the assistance of an experienced pediatric urologist who functions as a regular member of the myelodysplasia center team. With such skillful care and with the cooperation of the patient, parents, and school, a basic program of clean intermittent catheterization with or without pharmacotherapy to enhance bladder storage and continence will be successful in most children. For the others, modifications of the program such as timed voiding, panty inserts, penile collectors, or even surgical procedures may be needed. With good compliance, the appropriate program should consistently result in social continence and renal preservation.

The parents' and/or patient's concerns about sexuality issues are rarely brought up without timely, direct encouragement. The potential for normal sexual activity and reproduction in people with myelodysplasia is better than most expect. Males may encounter problems with dysfunctional erections or retrograde ejaculations, both of which can be dealt with urologically. Females should be raised with the expectation of being fully capable sexual partners. Complications can be anticipated during pregnancy, particularly involving the spine and the urinary tract. Genetic counseling prior to conception is essential when either prospective parent has myelodysplasia.

Mobility. The timing and amount of orthopedic intervention in patients with MDP are determined by the level, symmetry, and type of paraplegia. Many children with thoracic or high lumbar lesions who "walk" in therapy or special school settings with various supportive devices will voluntarily choose a wheelchair as a less conspicuous and more practical alternative when they reach adolescence. They and their care providers must realize that such an outcome does not represent failure on anyone's part.

Supportive devices and/or surgery as necessary to allow sitting with both hands free by 4 to 6 months of age and standing by 12 to 18 months of age are appropriate goals for all MDP children. Those with thoracic or high lumbar levels may ambulate around the house in long braces with or without crutches, but generally prefer a wheelchair for community ambulation. Most children with lower lumbar paraplegia (functional quadriceps) are ambulatory in the community with short braces, and a sacral level lesion is usually compatible with full ambulation. A pragmatic approach aimed at efficient, functional, independent mobility yields the best results.

Skilled orthopedic care is required for the commonly associated spinal curvatures (kyphosis, scoliosis). The lower extremity fractures to which these patients are prone require prompt recognition and treatment.

MISCELLANEOUS

Obesity. Children with limited mobility have sharply reduced caloric needs, yet often look upon eating as one of the few enjoyable pastimes available. To be successful, weight control measures must begin in infancy and involve the full cooperation of the entire family. The primary physician has a key supportive role. The height and weight of the child must be recorded at each office visit, and the caloric intake adjusted as required to keep the weight within one standard deviation of the height (length).

Decubiti. The only successful management of this problem is prevention. The key measures are scrupulous hygiene, avoidance of obesity, and assurance of mobility. Patients in wheelchairs must use special cushions and learn to shift their weight to their arms at regular intervals through training or the use of a signaling device. Pressure decubiti over the sacrum or ischial tuberosities are major multispecialty surgical problems and even after healing or grafting will always be susceptible to recurrence.

Progressive Neuromuscular Loss. This can result from such complications as tethering of the spinal cord, pressure on the cord from a lipoma or teratoma, pressure on the nerve roots from a herniated disc, and hydromyelia related to shunt dysfunction. The progressive functional loss in each case may be insidious but must be promptly recognized, since surgical intervention only prevents further regression and usually does not restore lost function.

Epilepsy. The incidence of recurrent seizures in children with MDP may be as high as 15%, probably due to the commonly associated brain malformations, CNS infections, and/or neurosurgical procedures. Recognition and pharmacologic control of the seizures follows established principles covered elsewhere in this text.

School Problems. Although the majority of children with MDP are not mentally retarded, they often manifest specific learning disabilities, particularly of the visuomotor perceptual variety. Early recognition and treatment of these disabilities will go a long way toward improving overall prognosis and outcome. The services of a psychologist skilled in the objective evaluation of developmentally disabled, physically handicapped children can be invaluable.

Brain Tumor

R. MICHAEL SCOTT, M.D.

HYDROCEPHALUS ASSOCIATED WITH BRAIN TUMORS

Most pediatric brain tumors are located in the posterior fossa, and their primary presenting symptoms are often related to hydrocephalus caused by obstruction of cerebrospinal fluid flow at the fourth ventricle or aqueduct. The surgeon must decide initially whether to treat the hydrocephalus prior to attacking the tumor by either ventriculoperitoneal shunting or external ventricular drainage, or to proceed directly to removing the tumor, hoping that the hydrocephalus will resolve following surgery.

A ventriculoperitoneal shunt will often relieve the child's symptoms immediately, lowering intracranial pressure, relieving headache, and improving neurologic function. Postoperative care of the child may be simplified because the craniectomy incision heals under no tension; in general, postoperative morbidity seems lessened. The disadvantages of preoperative shunting include all the complications seen with shunting of non-neoplastic-induced hydrocephalus, including infection, shunt malfunction, subdural hematoma, and, particularly important in this group of patients, shunt dependency even when the CSF pathways are effectively unblocked by subsequent tumor removal. Certain tumors that can metastasize via the CSF, including cerebellar medulloblastomas and pineal germinomas, may seed the peritoneum by way of the shunt, although this is a relatively infrequent occurrence. Rarely, a very large posterior fossa tumor may herniate upward through the tentorium or hemorrhage following shunting, presumably due to shifts in pressure differential between the supra- and infratentorial compartments, necessitating emergency surgery in a gravely ill patient.

An alternate plan is the placement of an external ventricular drain through a burr or twist drill hole to permit temporary decompression of the ventricles to a closed drainage system. Intracranial pressure can be measured through the catheter during this time, and the eventual need for a shunt assessed by following the pressure measurements postoperatively. The major problem with this technique is infection, and ventriculitis with hospital-acquired organisms in a postoperative patient may be extremely difficult to treat. In general, we try to avoid both shunting and ventricular drainage if at all possible in these patients, treating them with high-dose steroids (dexamethasone, 0.2 mg/kg every 4 hours) as soon as the diagnosis of posterior fossa tumor is made. Often the steroids alone will dramatically improve the patient's symptoms, rendering the posterior fossa surgery less emergent. Following surgery, the need for shunting is assessed on the basis of clinical course, bulging of the incision, and CT scan evidence of progressive or continuing symptomatic hydrocephalus.

SURGERY AND ADJUVANT THERAPY

Certain posterior fossa tumors can be completely excised at surgery; these include cerebellar astrocytomas, particularly the cystic variety, and some ependymomas. I believe that medulloblastomas should be grossly totally removed as well, since evidence is accumulating that total excision, if possible, leads to a more favorable long-term prognosis. Postoperative CT scanning has been a great help in evaluating completeness of removal of all tumor types, and surgical statistics based on this information are now being accumulated.

Although radiation therapy should not be given to the patient with the totally excised cystic cerebellar astrocytoma, there is no question that it improves survival in the medulloblastoma patient. Because the medulloblastoma can seed the subarachnoid spaces, and because a certain percentage of these patients at the time of surgery will already have demonstrable but asymptomatic spinal metastases, craniospinal axis irradiation is routinely administered. The physician must be aware of the potential side effects of this treatment, which include growth retardation, endocrinopathies, and, in younger children, possible long-term mentation disturbances. The role of chemotherapy at present as an adjuvant to radiation therapy following diagnosis is uncertain; numerous trial protocols are in progress. Late central nervous system or systemic metastases may respond spectacularly to chemotherapy, but are never cured. Radiation therapy is often recommended for ependymomas, particularly if total excision has not been achieved. If postoperative CSF cytology is positive, spinal axis irradiation is also administered, since the ependymoma and the more rapidly growing ependymoblastoma can seed throughout the CSF spaces.

Brain stem tumors remain particularly difficult to treat. They are frequently low-grade gliomas, but occasionally are rapidly growing glioblastomas. With the aid of improved CT scanning for localization purposes, these neoplasms are being biopsied more and more frequently, especially if they are partially cystic or growing exophytically out of the brain stem. Survival data remain bleak. We will usually employ radiation and steroid therapy for these tumors, expecting a brief remission and survival in terms of months after surgery or diagnosis.

Debate continues regarding the appropriate treatment of craniopharyngiomas. These tumors, often heavily calcified and partially cystic, may be tightly adherent to optic nerves, pituitary stalk, vessels in the circle of Willis, and the hypothalamus; their total removal represents a surgical tour de force, a feat greatly aided by recent refinements in microneurosurgical techniques. Nevertheless, pursuing total removal of this tumor in the face of adherence to vital structures may lead to severe postoperative endocrinologic or neurologic deficits. Our policy has been total removal when possible, using radiation therapy when this cannot be done, since the results in some series with radiotherapy alone are quite good. When recurrent, these lesions are difficult to deal with surgically because of distortion of tissue planes and scarring induced by the initial surgery. Recurrent cyst aspirations may need to be carried out, and, occasionally, trans-sphenoidal removal or drainage can be performed if the bulk of the lesion is intrasellar. Careful postoperative endocrinologic management is essential for these children, who may have long-term hormone deficiencies.

Hypothalamic gliomas are not curable by surgery, and often only a biopsy can be carried out. Again, postoperative radiation is employed. The pure optic gliomas, involving the optic nerve, chiasm, or tract, however, should be dealt with surgically if the lesion can be demonstrated to be confined to a single optic nerve. Excision of the nerve lesion just proximal to the normal chiasm is curative. Any lesion involving tract or chiasm is irradiated. Controversy regarding this group of tumors continues, with some physicians maintaining that radiation alone is sufficient to deal with gliomas of the optic system even if confined to the nerve alone and others believing that some tumors' growth will be self-limited and not extend to the chiasm regardless of therapy.

Pineal region tumors have been the center of renewed interest over the past decade. Most of these patients will have signs and symptoms of hydrocephalus at diagnosis, since the location of these lesions in the posterior third ventricle and above the aqueduct may lead to early obstruction of CSF pathways as the tumor grows. Although the germinomas (previously called atypical teratomas) and other primitive types of pineal tumors have the potential to seed the subarachnoid spaces and ventricular system, the primary treatment of these patients usually is a ventriculoperitoneal shunt to control hydrocephalus. The next decision involves whether to proceed empirically with radiation therapy to the neoplasm, since the germinoma group is quite sensitive to radiation therapy, or to perform surgery for biopsy and perhaps total removal of the mass. Our practice has been to obtain CSF from the shunt and lumbar puncture (if the ventricles are decompressed by CT scan) for cytology and hormone tumor markers, including alpha-fetoprotein and human chorionic gonadotropin. These substances may be elevated in certain subtypes of pineal region neoplasms; the measurements can be repeated postoperatively and following treatment, when their levels help ascertain the effect of the treatment on the neoplasm. If cytology is positive or if there is evidence of other CNS metastasis upon CT scan or myelography, radiation therapy alone will be administered to the craniospinal axis. Otherwise, we carry out a direct approach to the pineal region, since a certain number of these lesions are benign, removable, and not affected by radiation therapy.

Numerous other tumors may occur in both supratentorial and infratentorial compartments in children. The goal of treatment remains surgical excision, if possible; radiation therapy is often administered for palliative purposes in the nonremovable lesions. In certain slow-growing lesions, which may represent hamartomas (e.g., gangliogliomas and certain low grade astrocytomas), a case can be made for withholding radiation therapy in the nonresectable lesion, using progress of the tumor on CT scanning as a guide to whether or not radiation therapy should be administered subsequently.

GENERAL POSTOPERATIVE PRINCIPLES

Intraoperative and postoperative antibiotics have greatly reduced the incidence of surgical infection on many neurosurgical services, and we routinely administer oxacillin, 50 mg/kg IV prior to surgery, and 25 mg/kg every 4 hours for 24 hours postoperatively. The antibiotic regimen in a given institution may vary and should be based on past experience with surgical infection in the particular surgical unit.

Steroids have become a routine medication in the postoperative care of all brain tumor patients because of their demonstrated ability to reduce cerebral edema. We use 0.1 to 0.2 mg per kg of dexamethasone every 4 hours for 3 to 5 days postoperatively, reducing the dose gradually thereafter depending on the patient's course. Following posterior fossa surgery, children frequently develop high fevers and complain of headache and stiff neck, and their craniectomy incision may bulge; the CSF may contain inflammatory cells but repeated cultures are sterile. These children have the syndrome of "aseptic meningitis," which is often exquisitely steroid-sensitive, promptly resolving when steroids are initiated or the dosage increased. Dilantin (5 to 8 mg/kg/24 hr) or phenobarbital (3 to 5 mg/kg/24 hr) is given for seizure prophylaxis following supratentorial surgery; the medication may be rapidly tapered postoperatively if no cortical damage was felt to occur intraoperatively, for example, following subfrontal surgery for optic glioma. We continue anticonvulsants in most patients for 6 months to a year postoperatively; an electroencephalogram often may help assess whether the medication needs to be continued thereafter.

The physicians caring for these patients postoperatively must pay close attention to all principles of management of increased intracranial pressure, including airway protection, maintenance of the head elevated position to avoid jugular venous distension, avoidance of overhydration of the patient, and so on. CT scanning as needed in the postoperative period and in long-term followup has been a major advance in the postoperative care and assessment of these children.

Brain Abscess

R. MICHAEL SCOTT, M.D.

The primary treatment of brain abscess is surgical, although there are certain exceptions to this rule. The appearance of the abscess on CT scanning and the general condition of the patient have been the primary determinants of the order and type of treatment used.

We usually operate directly on a large abscess having a well-defined capsule associated with significant mass effect, attempting to excise the lesion completely if it is located in a relatively silent area of the brain. The abscess cavity is tapped at surgery to provide material for immediate Gram stain and culture; since many brain abscesses occur in children with complicating medical illness or who are already on antibiotics or immunosuppressive agents, anaerobic, fungal, and acid-fast cultures are obtained when appropriate. If there is considerable cerebral edema associated with the abscess, steroids (dexamethasone, 0.1 mg/kg) should be given without hesitation; the reduction in brain swelling and associated morbidity following their administration more than outweighs the very small risk of reduced resistance to infection often mentioned as a reason for not administering them. Cerebral edema may in fact be the primary cause of neurologic morbidity and mortality in acute abscess and may require vigorous measures, including intermittent intravenous mannitol in doses of 0.25 to 2 gm/kg/dose as needed, intubation and hyperventilation, and, finally, the induction of barbiturate coma. Barbiturate coma may be life-saving in certain patients and is discussed elsewhere in this text.

If the patient requires mannitol to control edema, we implant an intracranial pressure monitoring device to observe the patient's response to therapy. Certain abscesses should not be excised, either because they are associated with a great deal of encephalitis and are poorly defined, or because of their location deep in the cerebrum or brain stem or in eloquent areas of the cortex. These lesions can be dealt with by periodic tapping through a twist drill or standard burr hole. Again, the CT scan will be useful in providing the coordinates for the aspirating needle as well as for following the size of the abscess with therapy. We usually irrigate the interior of the abscess with antibiotic solution whenever tapping is carried out, but occasionally leave irrigating catheters in the abscess cavity for periodic irrigation and instillation of antibiotics at the bedside in particularly refractory cases.

Multiple brain abscesses, often associated with subacute bacterial endocarditis, require medical management, using massive doses of appropriate antibiotics as directed by the results of blood and other cultures. Occasional large abscesses may have to be tapped. There have been several recent reports of complete resolution of what appeared to be both multiple and isolated brain abscesses during antibiotic therapy, and certainly such treatment should be continued until complete resolution of the lesions by CT scanning.

Anticonvulsants should be administered routinely since associated cortical scarring, meningoencephalitis, and cortical vein phlebitis may cause seizures in the acute and chronic phase of illness. Finally, lumbar punctures should not be employed in the management of these children unless absolutely necessary; the cerebrospinal fluid is often sterile in brain abscess and the lumbar puncture may be dangerous, precipitating uncal or tonsillar herniation if brain edema is significant.

Spinal Epidural Abscess

R. MICHAEL SCOTT, M.D.

Spinal epidural abscess is treated by prompt surgical drainage via laminectomy. The surgeon obtains a Gram stain of the material in the epidural space, so that the appropriate antibiotic therapy can be begun immediately, and requests routine, anaerobic, and fungal cultures so that the organisms can be correctly identified. If the initial Gram stain is negative, antibiotic therapy is directed against staphylococcus, the most frequent cause of spinal epidural abscess. At surgery, I place irrigation and drainage catheters in the epidural space, close the wound, and irrigate the epidural space with either antibiotic or povidone-iodine solution for up to a week postoperatively. If the infection has been extensive and involves the paravertebral or dorsal soft tissues, I leave the wound open, performing daily irrigations and closing the wound secondarily at a later date. The laminectomy may be extensive if there has been considerable rostral and caudal extension of the abscess, and postoperatively spinal instability may be a problem if there has been considerable involvement of the vertebral bodies by osteomyelitis. Orthopedic consultation and regular radiographic followup of the involved area of the spine should be obtained to detect evidence of progressive scoliosis, kyphosis, or instability. Deteriorating neurologic status following laminectomy suggests inadequate decompression, inappropriate antibiotic regimen with extension of the abscess, or spinal instability, and immediate spine x-ray films and repeat myelography or spinal CT scanning must be obtained. For this reason, we use Pantopaque—a nonabsorbable contrast material—for the initial myelogram, rather than the rapidly absorbed water-soluble agent metrizamide; the contrast medium can be left in place following the first study so that the patient need only be refluoroscoped if the postoperative neurologic course is not satisfactory. Pantopaque should not be used, however, if spinal CT scanning is to be employed, since this radio-dense contrast agent interferes with the resolution of the CT image.

Recovery of the preoperative neurologic deficit, as in most conditions in which spinal cord compression occurs, is directly related to the degree of preoperative neurologic deficit. Young children with virtually any evidence of neurologic function below the level of compression may have a relatively good prognosis for return of strength and sensation. With total loss of all neurologic function below the level of compression, prognosis for recovery is poor; however, because of the difficulty in ascertaining degree of neurologic deficit in young children, firm statements to the parents regarding prognosis should not be made. If bladder dysfunction occurs secondary to the cord compression, intermittent catheterization should be utilized postoperatively until recovery occurs; these and other routine measures in the care of a patient with a spinal cord deficit are discussed in the section on spinal cord injury. The length of postoperative antibiotic treatment is best determined by considering the organism involved, its antibiotic sensitivity, and the recommendations of an infectious disease consultant; most infections require a minimum of 3 weeks of parenteral antibiotic administration.

Cerebrovascular Disease in Infancy and Childhood

EDWARD F. RABE, M.D.

Strokes are spontaneous cerebrovascular events due to thrombosis or embolization of vessels, or to intracranial bleeding in the subarachnoid or intracerebral compartments. Management of these ictal events is dependent upon the diagnosis of what has occurred, and of where and how the events are moving in time. The spectrum of signs and symptoms is wide, ranging from recurrent headaches with or without stiff neck and mild focal neurological deficits to sudden ictus with hemiconvulsions, hemiplegia, and coma. These occur if the pathology is in the anterior or middle cranial fossa. If the pathology is in the posterior fossa, then vertebrobasilar symptoms appear, with headache, dizziness, ataxia, diplopia, dysarthria, and unilateral or bilateral motor and/or sensory symptoms.

The major pathology is cerebrovascular occlusion, spontaneous intracranial bleeding, or vascular spasm. *Arterial occlusions* in children occur most often in the carotid vessels as well as the anterior cerebral and middle cerebral arteries. Less frequently they occur in the vertebrobasilar system. They are often idiopathic and occur on the background of a mild antecedent illness. Occasionally, internal carotid occlusions are secondary to trauma of the pharynx or pharyngomaxillary space infections. Vertebrobasilar occlusions can occur after chiropractic or athletic-induced traction and turning of the neck leading to vertebral artery intimal tears with thrombosis and embolism. The treatment and prognosis of supratentorial arterial occlusions are influenced by the presence or absence of multiple telangiectasias in the region of the basal ganglia. If these are present, the term "moya-moya" disease is affixed, implying that the syndrome is progressive and may be immunologically based. Without telangiectasias, with an onset after 2 years, and without seizures as a presenting complaint, the patient is unlikely to develop epilepsy, intellectual deficit, or a restricting motor deficit.

Cortical vein thromboses may occur secondary to congenital heart disease, and *venous sinus thrombosis,* secondary to dehydration or local infections of the scalp, mastoid, or middle ear in older children (sagittal or transverse sinus disease, respectively). Small vessel occlusions occur in sickle cell disease and homocystinuria, while intracranial arterial occlusions are seen in fibromuscular dysplasia in children. Necrotizing arteritis causing beading of small arteries can occur after ingestion of street drugs, such as the amphetamines and pseudoephedrine.

Spontaneous intracerebral hematomas occur secondary to ruptures of arteriovenous malformations (AVM's), intracranial aneurysms (uncommon in children), as late sequelae of cranial trauma, in association with bleeding diathesis in leukemia, thrombotic thrombocytopenic purpura, or hemophilia, and very uncommonly as the presenting symptom of intracerebral tumor. Multiple small intracerebral perivascular hemorrhages occur with hyperosmolar states, and this may also produce venous sinus thromboses.

Diffuse vasoconstriction, which may be reversible, occurs as the result of ingestion of phencyclidine (angel dust), LSD, or mescaline. This may be reversed or prevented by a nonapproved drug, a Ca antagonist, verapamil.

The holistic approach to infants and children with strokes is important so as to alert the physician to the cause of the stroke. For example coarctation of the aorta or polycystic kidneys suggests intracranial aneurysm, inflammation of the ears, mastoiditis, and/or lateral sinus thrombosis. A careful neurologic examination will suggest the vascular area involved, and repeated observations will determine the pace of the evolving pathology.

The major ancillary tests, besides the routine tests of blood count, urine, blood electrolytes, and appropriate blood chemistries, are the CT scan, with and without contrast, followed when indicated by an arch arteriogram to demonstrate all four major cerebral vessels.

The child with a stroke should be closely monitored in an ICU until the cause of symptoms is known and the direction and pace of the physiologic changes are understood. Cardiopulmonary and renal status must be known and supported. If Hgb S disease is present, the patient should be transfused to reduce the percent of Hgb S to less than 20 before arteriography is performed. Hydration at a rate not to exceed 1200 ml/M^2/24 hours, with 0.2 to 0.4% saline and 10% glucose and, when renal function is adequate, 20 mEq per liter of potassium should be started. If febrile, appropriate wide spectrum antibiotics should be used until a definite etiologic diagnosis is reached. Cardiac arrhythmias should be appropriately managed.

Seizures should be stopped as quickly as possible. If status epilepticus occurs, sodium phenobarbital in a dose of 12 mg/kg (300 mg/M^2 in children larger than 25 kg) should be given slowly intravenously over 5 minutes. If the seizures continue longer than 15 minutes, a repeat dose of 6 mg/kg (in children larger than 25 kg, 150 mg/M^2/dose) should be given slowly. If the seizure is not controlled within 15 to 20 minutes phenytoin in a dose of 14 mg/kg at a rate not to exceed 50 mg/min in a concentration of 10 to 15 mg/ml should be given. Subsequent doses of phenobarbital should be given at 6 to 8 hour intervals to maintain a level between 30 and 55 μg/ml, and if phenytoin is also used, IV doses should be given every 12 hours to maintain a level between 15 and 20 μg/ml.

Diazepam (Valium) may be used intravenously to treat the seizures initially, in place of phenobarbital, in a dose of 0.2 mg/kg, not to exceed 10 mg/dose in patients 50 kg or more. The dose should be given slowly IV, never diluted. The dose may be repeated if seizures are not stopped in 15 to 20 minutes. If by then the seizures are not stopped, intravenous phenytoin or phenobarbital as described above may be given. The combination of diazepam and phenobarbital is alleged to produce respiratory depression, although if each is injected slowly, we have not observed this. If diazepam is used initially and controls the seizures, it will still have to be followed by either long-acting anticonvulsant (phenytoin or phenobarbital as described above), since the t$_{1/2}$ of IV diazepam is only 15 to 24 minutes.

Some children with strokes will have signs of increased ICP due to the mass effect of the blood and/or the brain swelling, which occurs secondary to free blood in the brain. Immediate reduction of pressure can be obtained with IV mannitol, 20%, in a dose of 0.5 to 1.5 gm/kg, given over 20 to 30 minutes. The dose may be repeated in 4 to 6 hours, and the smaller dose is recommended if repeated administration appears necessary. An effect upon the blood-brain barrier (BBB), which helps to minimize brain edema, occurs with steroid administration. This effect takes up to 12 hours to develop. IV dexamethasone (Decadron) in doses of 0.25 mg/kg q 8 h following a loading dose of 0.5 mg/kg may be used concomitantly with mannitol. Decadron may be used for 7 to 10 days without apparent serious side effects, but the dose should be gradually decreased as soon as increased ICP is no longer a clinical problem.

Further management of strokes in children is handled in conjunction with a neurosurgeon, who may work with the neuroradiologist. Large subdural hemorrhages, ruptured intracranial aneurysms, and accessible AVM's with significant symptoms are best handled surgically. Some large AVM's or AVM's in surgically inaccessible areas are now managed by controlled embolization through the internal carotid artery with plastic spherules, reducing the size of the AVM and then reassessing the value and safety of surgical removal. Some cases of thrombosis of the extracranial common, or internal carotid, artery are surgically amenable to treatment.

Children with strokes have recognized sequelae that must be dealt with as soon as the acute event subsides. Motor deficits with developing spasticity must be treated with PT and OT. In infants with onset under 2 years of age, seizure disorders are often chronic and are sometimes difficult to control medically. Behavior problems, especially the hyperactivity syndrome, may be treated successfully with CNS stimulants. Intellectual assessment, as well as achievement test results, should be used to monitor the progress of these children in school, for it is often irregular occasionally, and appropriate intervention can be guided by such repeated testing.

Benign Intracranial Hypertension

(Pseudotumor Cerebri)

ABE M. CHUTORIAN, M.D.

This essentially benign disorder requires treatment to prevent permanent loss of vision resulting from optic nerve compression secondary to prolonged, unrelieved, raised intracranial pressure. Blindness has been documented to occur in an occasional affected child even with continued alertness, and even in the absence of headache, vomiting, or sixth cranial nerve palsy.

Treatment should begin with the most conservative measures and should proceed to modalities that carry more serious risk only when the conservative measures fail to provide relief from raised intracranial pressure, as determined chiefly by the appearance of the fundi and by the determination of manometric cerebrospinal fluid pressure on lumbar puncture. It is emphasized that visual loss or optic atrophy may denote permanent optic nerve damage and cannot therefore be used as a guide to the implementation of more vigorous therapeutic modalities. Since duration and degree of intracranial hypertension do not, singly or in combination, constitute reliable prognostic criteria in regard to anticipated visual integrity, the proposals offered below concerning progression through the various therapeutic regimens are of necessity somewhat arbitrary.

Since the majority of children with benign intracranial hypertension do not have an associated disorder that, however obscurely, underlies the development of raised intracranial pressure, treatment is symptomatic rather than specific for most. All children, however, require diagnostic appraisal in regard to the possibility of the known underlying disorders so that specific, rather than purely symptomatic, treatment can be offered when appropriate. Examples abound, and include the treatment of lateral venous sinus occlusion, hypoparathyroidism, hypervitaminosis A, chronic anemia, polycythemia, and so on. Obesity-related pseudotumor is common in children and requires a strict and rapidly implemented diet in addition to the symptomatic treatment outlined below. Intracranial hypertension occurring during corticosteroid withdrawal, following treatment for a variety of unrelated disorders such as chronic asthma or collagen-vascular disorders, requires elevation of corticosteroid dosage and more gradual withdrawal, as in corticosteroid therapy for idiopathic benign intracranial hypertension.

When there is no indication for specific treatment, the following therapeutic measures are indicated, in order of optimal safety and efficacy.

Sequential Lumbar Puncture. The majority of affected children respond to one or several lumbar punctures, probably reflecting early spontaneous resolution in most, rather than the therapeutic benefit of lumbar puncture. In those who ultimately respond to sequential lumbar puncture, the presumed therapeutic mechanism is prolonged effusion of cerebrospinal fluid into the subdural or epidural space through the apertures created by puncture of the arachnoid and dural membranes (this mechanism is responsible for the occasionally protracted "drainage headache" following lumbar puncture in any individual).

Following the first lumbar puncture, a combined diagnostic and therapeutic procedure, a significant minority of children have lasting remission. A second lumbar puncture should be done 48 hours after the first. If CSF pressure is over 200 mm of water and/or vascular pulsations overlying the optic disc on fundoscopic inspection are not re-established, a third lumbar puncture should be done 48 hours after the second. If there has not been a progressive decline in cerebrospinal fluid pressure, lumbar punctures at 24-hour intervals are warranted. Progressive decline in cerebrospinal fluid pressure is sought by sequential lumbar punctures until the CSF pressure is below 200 mm of water, at which time additional 24-hour intervals may be added to the time intervening between lumbar punctures. No further immediate lumbar punctures are indicated when either three successive procedures are each rewarded by normal cerebrospinal fluid pressure or there is progressive resolution of papilledema. Daily examinations of the fundi and visual acuity determinations are warranted during this time and may be conducted at weekly intervals after successful response to sequential lumbar punctures, until resolution of papilledema is documented.

Sequential lumbar punctures may be abandoned as a therapeutic failure if raised intracranial pressure persists after 12 punctures have been performed. Occasionally, persistence beyond this level is rewarded by remission in some patients, and occasionally cessation of this treatment modality is required because of mechanical failure of puncture due to persistent subdural or epidural cerebrospinal fluid effusion without remission, or because of poor tolerance for the procedure.

If strict aseptic technique is employed, the risk of introducing infection by repeated lumbar puncture is extremely remote.

Pharmacotherapy. ACETAZOLAMIDE. Acute lowering of cerebrospinal fluid pressure following administration of acetazolamide has been documented, presumably as a result of decreased cerebrospinal fluid secretion following carbonic anhydrase inhibition. However, a systematic or controlled study of its chronic use in intracranial hypertension has not been carried out, and experience suggests that compensatory mechanisms come into play with re-elevation of cerebrospinal fluid pressure, which limits the usefulness of the drug.

Dosage of 10 to 30 mg/kg of body weight per 24 hr may be tried, up to 1 gram per day, given in 3 divided doses. Dose-related side effects include drowsiness and tingling of the extremities. Potentially more serious toxicity includes allergic manifestations and bone marrow depression.

CORTICOSTEROIDS. Dexamethasone (Decadron) has a rapid effect in lowering intracranial pressure, by mechanisms that are still obscure and under dispute. Clinical and quantitative manometric effects can be demonstrated within 12 hours of administration, and progressive dose-related lowering of intracranial pressure can be documented. The oft-related precaution concerning the use of corticosteroid therapy, namely, that use of the drug will create steroid dependency and thus result in protracted use of the drug with attendant increase in risk, does not occur with proper administration. Indeed, the duration of the disorder in children with benign intracranial hypertension can be reduced by employing Decadron at the outset, but this does not constitute an indication for routine or indiscriminate use of corticosteroid therapy in this disorder, owing to its brief duration in most children and because of the potential hazards associated with the use of corticosteroids. Eight mg of Decadron, given in 2 divided doses, may be administered to children refractory to sequential lumbar puncture. Occasionally, a dose of 12 mg per 24 hr is required in children who continue to have elevated cerebrospinal fluid pressure, which is measured by lumbar puncture 72 hours after treatment has been initiated. The dose is maintained for 5 to 7 days after normal cerebrospinal fluid pressure is documented. Thereafter, it is gradually tapered by 1 mg per day at intervals of 72 hours; lumbar puncture is performed 72 hours after each drop in dosage and withdrawal is continued if cerebrospinal fluid pressure is normal. However, if cerebrospinal fluid pressure rises above 200 mm of water, the previous dose is restored and maintained for 1 week before lumbar puncture is renewed. Thereafter, withdrawal of 1.0 mg increments is effected at weekly intervals as long as remission persists. In this manner the lowest effective dose and duration of therapy are sought in each patient.

Unusually refractory patients will be encountered whose disorder persists for 6 months or longer. Alternate-day corticosteroid therapy may be effective in such patients, justifying a trial of such management before surgical therapy is warranted. In these instances, dexamethasone is inappropriate becuase of its prolonged half-life and attendant continued adrenal suppression through the treatment cycle.

Prednisone should be used, in a dose of 80 to 120 mg, given as a single early morning dose on alternate days, permitting recovery from adrenal suppression prior to each successive dose, thus reducing related side effects and complications of therapy. Most children treated in this manner will demonstrate significant transient escape from therapeutic effect on the morning of the day of treatment, and remission on the treatment-free day. However, in my experience, continued management on an alternate-day regimen has been rewarded by ultimate remission if papilledema improves progressively and cerebrospinal fluid pressure becomes normal on the morning following administration of prednisone. Attempted withdrawal of prednisone should be more gradual in these cases, beginning with a 5 mg drop in alternate-day dosage at weekly intervals when normal cerebrospinal fluid pressure has been achieved.

Surgical Treatment. Ventricular shunts are to be avoided because the small ventricular volume in this disorder not only creates difficulties for shunt installation but is often associated with early shunt failure.

Although similar mechanisms conspire against effective lumboperitoneal shunting, the demonstrated efficacy of this type of shunt in benign intracranial hypertension and the lack of need for cerebral penetration make lumboperitoneal shunting a viable option in the rare child who does not respond to more conservative management.

Lumboperitoneal shunting seems preferable to subtemporal or suboccipital decompression by craniectomy—in the former instance because of the risk of temporal lobe damage by impaction against the craniectomy site, and in the latter case because experience has been too limited to permit reliable appraisal of therapeutic results. On the other hand, cranial decompression requires consideration in the rare child with pseudotumor cerebri who requires surgical therapy, and in whom early shunt failure occurs following lumboperitoneal shunting.

It is emphasized that surgical treatment is required exceedingly rarely and should be employed as the treatment of last resort.

Neurocutaneous Syndromes

BRUCE O. BERG, M.D.

The principal members of this disease category are inherently dysplastic in nature and tend to form tumors of the peripheral and central nervous systems, skin, and viscera. Bielschowsky believed tuberous sclerosis and neurofibromatosis to be similar in this regard, and van der Hoeve introduced the term "phacomatoses" (Gr—*phakos*, "round, mother-spot, freckle") for the commonly occurring retinal tumors. Von Hippel-Lindau disease and Sturge-Weber syndrome were later included in this group of disorders, and more recently ataxia-telangiectasia was added.

These are the five most commonly encountered neurocutaneous syndromes in clinical practice and, except for Sturge-Weber syndrome, all have a genetic basis. Many other syndromes have been added to this group, and the reader is referred to standard neurology texts for identification of lesser known entities. There are reports describing the coexistence of two separate neurocutaneous syndromes, but this can be explained on a chance basis rather than "overlap" of disease processes.

Tuberous Sclerosis

Tuberous sclerosis, an inherited autosomal dominant trait, commonly affects multiple organ systems; the clinical presentation depends upon the age of the patient and the organs involved. The mutation rate is about 80%. Early studies suggested that the triad of mental retardation, adenoma sebaceum, and fits were diagnostic of the disease, but it has become apparent that there is a wide spectrum of clinical findings.

Characteristic skin lesions are adenoma sebaceum, hypopigmented "ash-leaf" spots, fibromas, and the leathery "shagreen" patch usually found in the lumbosacral region. Subungual and periungual fibromas often appear late in the first decade and may be single or multiple, affecting toes more often than fingers. Oral fibromas or papillomas have been found in about 10% of patients, usually in the anterior aspect of the gingiva. Pitting or "indentation craters" are found on the dental enamel.

The cerebral lesions for which the disease is named—the tubera—are found within the cortical gyri, more commonly near the sulcus terminalis or embedded within the basal ganglia or thalamus, projecting into the ventricle. These subependymal hamartomas are usually indolent tumors but may undergo neoplastic changes.

Retinal lesions are common and are either a flat, yellow-gray glial patch located centrally or peripherally or a nodular mass that may be cystic, often seen in the optic disc area. The lesions do not impair vision and require no treatment. Renal tumors, usually angioleiomyomas, are reported in 80% of patients, and cardiac rhabdomyomas are found in one third to one half of patients. Cystic lesions of the digital bones and the lung also occur, and hamartomas have been occasionally found in the pancreas, thyroid, and adrenal glands.

Adenomata sebacea are usually found on or about the nose, nasolabial folds, and chin. These angiofibromatous lesions appear during the first few years of life as a faint erythematous, papular rash, but in time the lesions become larger and involve greater facial area. Some result in significant deformity and should be surgically removed. There is no effective treatment for removal of the skin lesions, however. Periungual fibromas are surgically removed only if they are a source of discomfort to the patient.

Neuroradiologic studies confirm the clinical diagnosis, and intracranial calcifications have been found in about 60% of skull radiographs. Computed tomographic (CT) brain scans are most valuable in demonstrating intracranial pathology, including hamartomas, ventriculomegaly, and subependymal tumors. Mineralization of the hamartomas may develop as early as 5 months of age and become more prominent with time. Areas of diffuse demyelination have also been described, but the mineralized subependymal nodules are the most reliable of all CT brain scan findings.

Removal of cerebral tubers is inappropriate unless they significantly enlarge to cause obstructive hydrocephalus with increased intracranial pressure. Any neurosurgical procedure depends upon the state of the patient and the extent and location of the tumor mass. Occasionally, a shunting procedure may suffice.

Convulsions may be present from birth or any time thereafter and occurred in 88% of one large series of patients. Infantile spasms are very common in the young patient and later become generalized or partial seizures. Usually, patients who are mentally deficient have fits, but there is no clear relationship between the severity of the convulsive disorder and the degree of mental subnormality. Adrenocorticotropic hormone (ACTH) or prednisone is recommended as the initial treatment of spasms. ACTH is given daily at a dosage of 40–80 units IM for about 4 weeks, then gradually tapered over several more weeks for a total treatment period of 6 to 8 weeks. If prednisone is selected rather than ACTH, the oral dosage is 2 mg/kg/day for the same period of time, gradually tapering the dosage during the last several weeks. Other anticonvulsants used include valproic acid, clonazepam, or nitrazepam, when available.

The renal tumors are usually indolent, and biopsy should be avoided. Since the tumors are so frequently bilateral, nephrectomy is not performed unless absolutely necessary. Cardiac rhabdomyomas are also common and are best demonstrated by echocardiography. These may cause heart failure and at times sudden death, but there is no universally accepted treatment at this time.

Pulmonary cysts are usually found in adult female patients but may occur in children, declaring their presence by hemoptysis or spontaneous pneumothorax. Similarly, the cyst changes found in roentgenograms of digital bones are usually present in adult patients but may occur in children also.

Moderate to severe mental retardation is found in about two thirds of patients. Some, particularly those with convulsive disorders recalcitrant to treatment, have significant behavioral abnormalities and, regardless of the amount of parental care and love, and careful follow-up by physicians and education specialists, are most difficult to manage. Attention deficit disorders are often present and may not respond to medications such as methylphenidate and thioridazine. One cannot predict the patient's response to these medications, however. Special class placement is recommended, particularly where the staff is expert in behavioral modification techniques.

The overall management of children with tuberous sclerosis is difficult, and all available medical, educational, and social services should be mobilized to help support the child and family.

Neurofibromatosis (von Recklinghausen's Disease)

Neurofibromatosis, transmitted as an autosomal dominant trait, is characterized by tumors of the peripheral and/or central nervous system, skin lesions, and musculoskeletal, vascular, and endocrine abnormalities. Clinical findings vary greatly. Patients generally have either a peripheral type with skin lesions and/or tumors of the peripheral nerves or a central type with tumors involving the central nervous system. Both sexes are affected but there is a reported male preponderance.

The café au lait spot ranges in size from millimeters to several centimeters and appears more frequently on the trunk than the limbs. It is generally believed that persons with six or more spots greater than 1.5 cm in the largest diameter have a presumptive diagnosis of neurofibromatosis. Axillary freckling is commonly found; other lesions include fibroma molluscum, diffuse areas of hyperpigmentation, and hypopigmented spots.

Neurofibromatosis may affect any peripheral nerve, with tumor size ranging from millimeters to centimeters. They are usually subcutaneous and are more commonly found on the trunk than the limbs. Plexiform neuromas usually involve the limbs and are often associated with hypertrophy of the soft tissues and bone. The autonomic nervous system may be affected, and in about 10% of patients the gastrointestinal tract is involved. Other sites affected are the tongue, mediastinum, and adrenal medulla; ganglioneuromas sometimes originate in the sympathetic ganglia in the posterior mediastinum. Approximately 3 to 5% of patients with neurofibromatosis have lesions that undergo sarcomatous change.

Evidence of the disease may be apparent in the neonate. The diversity of lesions may affect different organ systems, and one must anticipate a variety of potential problems. This makes the initial and later evaluations more difficult, for the clinician must conscientiously care for the patient while, at the same time, avoiding unnecessary anxiety in parents and child. Most patients with this disorder lead relatively normal lives and the risk of severe complications is less than earlier believed.

Initial evaluation should be complete and well documented. Blood pressures should be determined because of the increased incidence of pheochromocytomas in this disease (5–23%) and/or dysplastic changes of the renal arterial walls, both of which may result in hypertension. Particular attention should be directed to the visual system because of the increased incidence of optic gliomas, and visual fields, acuity, and evaluation of the optic disc must be well described. The optic glioma of childhood is relatively slow-growing and may be unrecognized unless carefully pursued. An increased incidence of acoustic neuroma is also found in this disease, and a complete hearing assessment is mandatory. A CT brain scan should be performed to assess intracranial structures, particularly the optic and acoustic nerves, as well as to identify the presence of other possible intracranial tumors.

Patients with skeletal abnormalities require a radiographic bone survey, particularly of the skull and vertebral column. Dysplastic bone changes are common, including "punched-out" lesions of the skull, scoliosis, and/or kyphosis, anterior meningoceles, and enlargement of the intervertebral foramina. Macrocrania is sometimes present.

Scoliosis or kyphosis may be secondary to neurofibromas of spinal nerves, spinal cord or spinal meningeal tumors, syringomyelia, or vertebral bone anomalies. One should consult with a child neurologist and a neurosurgeon, and myelography and CT of the spine may be required to rule out tumor. Occasionally there is a bowing of the tibia and fibula, and spontaneous fractures occur in the region of the mid to lower third of bony shafts. Pseudarthroses often develop; orthopedic consultation is required.

Mental retardation is present in about 10% of patients, and at least 10% have specific learning disabilities. Cortical heterotopias and cytoarchitectonic abnormalities have been demonstrated, the more severe abnormalities being found in mentally subnormal patients. Convulsive disorders also occur (8–13%), and about half are associated with intracranial tumors.

One should be cautious when evaluating the patient with learning problems and/or behavioral abnormalities, for the problems may be secondary to increased intracranial pressure as a result of optic nerve/chiasmal gliomas or other intracranial tumors. Impaired vision associated with optic gliomas may be unrecognized for a long time, resulting in abnormal behavior and poor school performance.

These tumors sometimes involve the floor of the third ventricle, resulting in precocious puberty or the diencephalic syndrome of infancy. Endocrine consultation should be obtained in these cases.

Management of childhood optic gliomas is as yet unsettled. There has been a conservative approach, carefully evaluating the child at periodic intervals, and shunting in case of secondary hydrocephalus. The commonly recommended treatment is radiation to the tumor site. One should consult with a child neurologist, neuro-ophthalmologist, neurosurgeon, and radiation therapist. Acoustic neuromas should be surgically removed by persons who are expert in this neuroanatomical area.

The less frequent patient with plexiform neuroma or localized hypertrophy of digits or limb may greatly benefit from reconstructive surgery. Some peripheral neurofibromas, particularly those that are disfiguring or subjected to repeated abrasion, should be removed. Cautious judgment is required.

von Hippel-Lindau Disease

von Hippel-Lindau disease, inherited as an autosomal dominant trait with variable penetrance, is characterized by the presence of retinal and/or cerebellar hemangioblastomas. Patients may also have cystic tumors of the pancreas, kidney, or epididymis, and there is an increased incidence of pheochromocytoma. Spinal cord angiomas may be present, sometimes associated with a syrinx. Skin lesions are uncommon.

Retinal hemangioblastomas, found most often in the periphery, occur at any age but are usually first recognized in adults. Patients may have no visual symptoms unless the macula is affected; retinal detachment may occur, however. Cerebellar hemangioblastomas, which can be found in any part of the cerebellum but most often in the paramedial region near the cortical surface, have also been rarely found in the cerebral hemisphere, medulla oblongata, and pituitary gland. Signs of cerebellar dysfunction are apparent, and occasionally there is evidence of increased intracranial pressure. Polycythemia is found in 10 to 20% of patients, and the cerebrospinal fluid protein is commonly elevated.

Patients with retinal hemangioblastomas require ophthalmologic consultation. Treatment methods vary but include photocoagulation techniques and cryotherapy. A CT brain scan should be obtained and consultation with a child neurologist and a neurosurgeon is mandatory. Vertebral angiography may be required to clearly demonstrate the cerebellar lesion. Those tumors are surgically removed. Patients must be examined periodically. The blood pressure must be documented and complete general, neurologic, and ophthalmologic examinations performed.

Sturge-Weber Syndrome

This sporadic syndrome is characterized by a facial nevus, contralateral partial or generalized convulsions, contralateral hemiparesis, intracranial calcification, and mental retardation. The facial nevus is congenital and is most commonly unilateral, involving at least the supraorbital region. The eye is sometimes involved with choroidal angioma, glaucoma, or buphthalmos. Cavernous angiomas may also occur in the nasopharyngeal mucosa. The essential components of the syndrome are facial nevus and leptomeningeal angioma.

Most patients have seizure onset before the end of the first year. Motor development is generally satisfactory until that time, but with the onset of seizures development becomes delayed and some children may actually regress. Seizures are usually simple partial (focal) but may become generalized with tonic/clonic activity. Computed brain tomography has improved our ability to demonstrate intracranial lesions, and brain mineralization may occur as early as the neonatal period.

Phenobarbital, phenytoin, and/or carbamazepine is usually given for convulsive control. Management of patients may be difficult for all because the convulsive activity may be intractable despite varying anticonvulsant regimens. Recently interest has increased in surgically removing the affected hemisphere early in the course of the convulsive disorder. It would seem that such a major procedure would be considered only after thoughtful consideration.

Orthopedic evaluation may be required to assess and treat hemiparesis with concomitant hemiatrophy. Ophthalmologic consultation is also required, particularly in children with glaucoma or buphthalmos.

Ataxia-Telangiectasia

Ataxia-telangiectasia, an inherited autosomal recessive trait, affects multiple organ systems. It is characterized by ataxia, oculocutaneous telangiectasiae, recurrent sinopulmonary infections, immunoincompetency associated with underdeveloped or absent thymus gland, and lymphoreticular neoplasia.

Ataxia presents during the first few years of life, usually before the appearance of telangiectasias, and progresses insidiously. Patients are hypotonic and weak, with decreased to absent stretch reflexes. Choreoathetotic movements are common, as is oculomotor apraxia. Telangiectasiae appear from 2 to 6 years of age, usually with the bulbar conjunctivae affected first, and eyelids, nasal bridge, and cheeks later. Other skin changes include café au lait spots, vitiligo, and sclerodermoid and progeric changes of the skin and hair. Hypogonadism is common in both sexes, and growth retardation is seen in most patients. There are abnormalities of both humoral and cell mediated immunity systems, and immunodeficiency states vary among affected patients. In most patients IgA and IgE concentrations are decreased or absent as a result of their reduced synthesis, with normal to increased levels of IgM and normal to low IgG content. One striking feature is an abnormally developed or absent thymus gland. There is increased incidence of lymphoreticular neoplasia, particularly malignant lymphomas, reticulum cell sarcomas, and Hodgkin's disease. Alpha-fetoprotein is abnormally elevated in most cases.

Patients should receive vigorous supportive therapy, with particular attention to recurrent infection and pulmonary function. Despite vigorous attempts to improve the immunologic status of patients, including plasma transfusions, administration of IgA, thymosin, and/or fetal thymic transplants, there has been no substantive improvement in the immunologic neurologic status.

Patients are unusually hypersensitive to immunosuppressive agents and radiation therapy, which may result in ulcerative dermatitis, severe esophagitis, dysphagia, and deep tissue necrosis. Thus, one must use caution in approaching treatment methods for the lymphoreticular malignancies so commonly found. Most patients do not survive beyond the third decade.

Acute Ataxia

BRUCE O. BERG, M.D.

Ataxia generally refers to incoordination secondary to abnormal cerebellar modulation of movement and posture. Incoordination may also be caused by impairment of sensory input (proprioception) and muscle weakness. It is useful to consider cerebellar function within a developmental frame of reference: the flocculonodular lobe, uvula, and nodulus concerned with maintenance of equilibrium (archicerebellum); the midline anterior and posterior lobes regulating input and output from the spinal cord and vestibular nuclei (paleocerebellum); and the cerebellar hemispheres (neocerebellum) reciprocally connected with cerebral cortex and ultimately the final motor pathway. Each component has its own neural circuitry but all are elegantly integrated with one another.

Careful assessment of the quality of incoordination and time course of symptom onset will usually enable one to place the site of the lesion and categorize its nature. Onset may be acute, subacute, or chronic; processes with acute or subacute onset are more likely to be remediable. Causes of acute or subacute ataxia include infection, intoxication, metabolic (endocrine), trauma, tumor, or vascular. Chronic ataxia may be secondary to anomalous development, degenerative diseases, or metabolic disorders.

Infection

Viral agents associated with acute ataxia include Coxsackie type B, echo type B, influenza types A and B, mumps, polio, rubeola, and varicella. Of these, varicella is probably most often identified, and ataxia has been reported in the pre-eruptive phase of the disease. An acute ataxic syndrome may be apparent at any time during infancy and childhood, but one syndrome, *acute cerebellar ataxia,* is thought to primarily affect children 1 to 2 years of age. About half of these children experience nonspecific illness several weeks before the onset of marked truncal ataxia and severe gait disturbance. Tremors may accompany the ataxia, involving the head, trunk, and limbs. Approximately 50% of children with acute cerebellar ataxia have nystagmus, and some demonstrate a transient dysarthria. Headaches and nuchal rigidity are seldom apparent.

Some patients improve within several weeks and about two thirds have good recovery within several months. About one third of patients have chronic neurologic sequelae, including ataxia, dysarthria, and mental subnormality with associated behavioral abnormalities. Symptoms may be exacerbated during the ensuing several years as a result of febrile illness, but recovery is usually realized. The relationship of acute cerebellar ataxia to other acute ataxic syndromes, idiopathic or associated with an identified viral infection, is unclear and any difference may be more apparent than real. There is no specific therapy for these ataxic syndromes aside from general supportive measures; however, the clinician should be generally optimistic regarding recovery.

One syndrome of acute ataxia is additionally characterized by myoclonus and opsoclonus. Myoclonus is present at rest with gross tremors of trunk and limb, and volitional movements are severely disorganized. Marked truncal instability is apparent, and opsoclonus (recurring intermittent gross conjugate eye movements) occurs in agitated bursts during sleep as well as alert wakefulness. Many of these children have occult neuroblastomas, and a careful diagnostic search for the tumor should be made with roentgenograms of the chest and abdomen, computed tomography (CT), and intravenous pyelography. Assay for urinary vanillylmandelic acid should also be performed. Because the tumor may not be apparent at onset of symptoms, periodic evaluations at 4- to 6-month intervals should be performed for 18 to 24 months after onset of symptoms.

Surgical removal of the tumor and/or administration of chemotherapy may result in significant lessening of abnormal neurological signs and symptoms, but improvement is measured in terms of months to years. In some cases, the administration of adrenocorticotropic hormone (ACTH) or prednisone has been useful in lessening opsoclonus. For reasons unclear, ACTH is preferred by most clinicians and is given at a dosage of 40 units IM daily for a period of 2 to 4 weeks, then slowly tapering the dosage over another several weeks. If prednisone is preferred, it is administered orally at a daily dosage of 2 mg/kg/body weight. After 2 to 4 weeks of treatment the drug is similarly tapered. Despite an improvement of neurological status, a number of patients are left with neurological, intellectual, and/or behavioral sequelae.

Intoxication

One of the common causes of acute ataxia is intoxication by a number of chemical agents including heavy metals and thallium, anticonvulsant drugs, sedatives, psychotropic drugs, alcohol, and combinations thereof. Heavy metals, most notably lead and thallium, are potential causes of ataxia and one must carefully screen for these substances. Children with lead poisoning commonly have an ataxic gait and tremors of the limbs, but it is not established that the ataxia is specifically related to cerebellar lesions. Young children usually have signs of increased intracranial pressure, with a bulging fontanelle in infants, papilledema, and possible suture separation. The skull is abnormally tympanitic to percussion. Important clues suggesting thallium intoxication are alopecia, headache, and painful, symmetrical distal neuropathy.

Ataxia is a particularly prominent adverse effect of most anticonvulsant medications commonly administered, including barbiturates, benzodiazepines, carbamazepine, hydantoins, succinimides, and valproic acid. Patients known to regularly take anticonvulsants should have periodic determinations of serum levels of the drug(s) ingested to avoid this circumstance. Clinicians must be aware of potential drug interactions that may effect ataxia, even though drugs are administered in the usually recommended doses.

Alcohol ingestion, both acute and chronic, affects the paleocerebellum (anterior-midline syndrome), resulting in a broadbased, reeling gait and incoordination, particularly of the lower limbs. In acute alcoholic intoxication, dysarthria and ataxia are both lessened with decreasing serum alcohol levels. This occurs over a period of hours, usually without specific therapeutic manipulation. Whenever intoxication is considered a possible cause of acute ataxia, the clinician must pay particular attention to the history of drugs ingested and drugs that are potentially available to the patient. Drugs may be prescribed and taken appropriately as well as inappropriately; one should not overlook the possibility of attempted suicide. As part of that careful history, the clinician may be required to visit the home to see what drugs and other chemical agents are available to the patient. Urine and blood specimens should be obtained as quickly as possible, and, whether or not assays are performed at that time for heavy metals, thallium, anticonvulsants, and psychotropic drugs, those specimens or adequate portions thereof should be carefully stored so that an assay may be obtained later if needed.

Patients must be carefully monitored with particular regard to respiration, blood pressure, and level of consciousness. Every effort should be made to remove the noxious agent from the patient. This may require gavage, administration of specific antidotes, use of cathartics and other techniques to enhance elimination of the material.

Metabolic Disorders

Several forms of intermittent acute ataxia are known, including Leigh disease, Hartnup disease, an intermittent form of maple syrup urine disease, and abnormalities of the urea cycle. Patients are relatively well between attacks, which may persist for weeks to months. Some attacks may be provoked by concomitant infectious processes. An ataxic syndrome has been seen in hypothyroidism, the symptoms of which are generally reversed with treatment.

Tumors

Brain tumors in the cerebral posterior fossa are more common in children than in adults. Signs and symptoms though usually subacute or chronic in onset, may be acute, particularly in cases of midline tumors such as medulloblastoma affecting the flocculonodular lobe and resulting in acute gait ataxia, vertigo, and nystagmus. Brain stem tumors and hemangioblastomas as well as cerebellar hemispheric tumors usually have a subacute onset but these, too, may abruptly declare their presence. The quality of the history suggests increased intracranial pressure and the neurologic examination will clarify the site of the lesion. Neurodiagnostic studies include CT, cerebral angiography and radionuclide scans. Treatment is generally nuerosurgical and/or radiation therapy directed to the tumor site.

Trauma/Vascular

Trauma to the cerebellum and vascular lesions (congenital vascular malformations, hemorrhage, or infarction) may also be the basis for an acute ataxic syndrome. Cerebellar ischemic attacks and/or hemorrhage are uncommon in childhood, but occur in some systemic disorders such as subacute bacterial endocarditis and homocystinuria. Rarely, occlusive disease of the vertebrobasilar system has been reported in children, presenting with acute ataxia, dysarthria, vertigo, and occasionally alterations of consciousness. Aside from the circumstances of trauma, which may require debridement and control of bleeding, therapeutic measures are generally supportive.

Impairment of Proprioception

Abnormalities of peripheral nerve, dorsal root ganglion, and/or the dorsal columns of the spinal cord result in ataxia. Without normal sensory input, one has difficulty in perceiving where body members are in space, resulting in a steppage or high, slapping gait. Most pathophysiological processes affecting these neural components have a subacute or chronic onset. Acute trauma to the spinal cord may affect proprioception but this is uncommon.

Guillain-Barré syndrome, idiopathic polyneuritis, is one of the most frequent forms of acute polyneuropathy, and though weakness may sometimes be confused with ataxia, decreased muscle power is generally the overriding symptom. Fisher syndrome, thought to be a variant of Guillain-Barré syndrome, is characterized by ataxia, areflexia and external ophthalmoplegia. These conditions are treated by general supportive measures with particular attention to monitoring pulse, blood pressure, and respiration. The value of steroid administration is yet not clear.

Degenerative Diseases of the Nervous System

GERALD S. GOLDEN, M.D.

Degenerative diseases of the central nervous system form a heterogeneous group of conditions characterized by progressive loss of one or more of the functional abilities mediated by the brain and spinal cord. These include all higher cerebral functions (language, cognition, emotion, etc), motor abilities, special sensory function, and somatic sensation. Common usage excludes from this classification those conditions caused by an exogenous agent such as a toxin or slow virus infection. By definition, the impairment becomes progressively severe, although the rate varies with the specific disorder and between families with the same condition. Within families the course shows less variability.

Most degenerative disorders are hereditary, implying the presence of specific biochemical deficits. Unfortunately, however, these defects have been determined in only a limited number of conditions. In the absence of consistent biochemical markers for the majority of the degenerative disorders, a useful classification is based on clinicopathologic correlations.

1. *Gray matter diseases.* These present clinically with the onset of dementia, behavioral abnormalities, and seizures, often myoclonic. There may be an associated movement disorder or ataxia. Pigmentary degeneration of the retina, macular degeneration, or a macular "cherry red" spot are often present. Pathologically, there is either neuronal storage of ceroid-lipofuscin, or diffuse loss of neurons without evidence of inflammation or acute necrosis.
2. *White matter diseases.* The initial clinical presentation is usually the development of spasticity, although cortical blindness, ataxia, and behavioral changes can be seen. The most typical ocular finding is optic atrophy. Pathologically, there is demyelination with or without sparing of axons.
3. *System degenerations.* There is progressive degeneration of specific neuronal systems and tracts. Classification and symptoms depend entirely on the systems involved.
4. *Metabolic diseases.* Some generalized metabolic diseases present with progressive degeneration of the central nervous system.

PRIMARY PREVENTION

No specific treatment exists for the majority of the degenerative diseases. If a firm diagnosis can be made, the mode of inheritance will usually be known and genetic counseling is mandatory. Carrier detection is possible in many of the conditions with defined metabolic defects. In these disorders amniocentesis can be used to document fetal involvement, giving the parents the option of termination of pregnancy.

If a specific diagnosis is not available, genetic counseling should involve a worst-case assumption of autosomal recessive inheritance with a 25% risk for each subsequent pregnancy. Before this assumption is made, however, it is mandatory that a complete three-generation pedigree be constructed and parents and siblings carefully examined. This is the only way to rule out autosomal dominant inheritance with a recurrence risk of 50%.

SPECIFIC THERAPY

Specific therapy depends on detailed definition of the underlying metabolic defect. When such knowledge is available, various strategies can be used. Enzyme replacement is the most straightforward, but the problems are many. If the enzyme is not of human origin, hypersensitivity would be expected to develop. The enzyme must enter the proper cells and become active within the appropriate subcellular compartment, or therapeutic efficacy would not be expected. Finally, significant damage may have been done prenatally (e.g., Tay-

Sachs disease), and even if the condition is arrested, the functional outcome would be limited.

Genetic engineering, introducing the gene for production of the missing enzyme into the patient's genome, would seem to be an ideal solution but is not yet practical. This would have to be done in the early prenatal period in order to minimize central nervous system damage.

In some cases enzyme function can be improved by the use of pharmacologic doses of a vitamin or other cofactor. In these disorders the enzyme is present but has limited activity, possibly due to structural abnormalities. Reducing the intake of a substrate not metabolized because of a metabolic block can prevent damage due to the accumulation of this substance or its alternate metabolites. This approach also may require provision of additional quantities of one or more substances beyond the block. Abnormal accumulation of naturally occurring substances can be partially prevented by dietary reduction or changing the offending substance so that it is not absorbed from the gastrointestinal tract.

Various strategies have been attempted to replace a substance, such as a neurotransmitter, which is reduced as a result of failure of production or loss of specific neuronal systems. As many of these neurotransmitters are amines which do not cross the blood-brain barrier, precursors are used, which upon entering the nervous system are converted into the desired compound. Drugs that prevent the degradation of a neurotransmitter or prevent its reuptake at the presynaptic membrane can enhance activity. Agonists can mimic its action at the receptor site. Activity can be decreased by preventing storage in presynaptic vesicles or by blocking receptors. These manipulations allow the balance between transmitters to be changed, which is often more important than the absolute level of either.

A somewhat more radical approach, limited to only a few specific conditions, is neurosurgical ablation of certain brain nuclei or pathways.

Gray Matter Diseases. Systemic and intrathecal administration of purified enzyme has been used in gray matter diseases with defined metabolic defects. Although circulating levels of the storage product are reduced, no clinical improvement has been reported. Treatment of ceroid-lipofuscinosis with large doses of antioxidants such as vitamin E is of unproven benefit.

White Matter Diseases. Attempts to treat adrenoleukodystrophy by dietary restriction of long-chain fatty acids have been instituted. It is too early to evaluate the results. Metachromatic leukodystrophy has not improved clinically with restriction of vitamin A or infusion of purified arysulfatase A.

Administration of aspirin increases the serum level of the enzyme, but not into an effective range. Refsum disease responds favorably to dietary elimination of all dairy products and meat and fats from ruminants. These foods contain high levels of phytanic acid.

System Degeneration. Juvenile parkinsonism responds to levodopa* or carbidopa-levodopa (Sinemet)** therapy, titrated slowly against the patient's symptoms. Stereotactic cryothalamotomy improves symptoms of dystonia musculorum deformans in some patients. Complications include hemiparesis or, following bilateral procedures, pseudobulbar speech.

Metabolic Diseases. Leigh disease (subacute necrotizing encephalomyelopathy) may respond transiently to administration of large doses of thiamine or thiamine derivatives, but sustained improvement has not been observed.

GENERAL MANAGEMENT

The absence of effective treatment for the majority of degenerative diseases of the central nervous system does not mean that a nihilistic view need be taken. Three general principles can be applied to all cases:

1. *Maintain function to the greatest extent possible.* Despite the progressive nature of the disorder, loss of motor function can be delayed by physical and occupational therapy, and loss of language function by speech therapy. Intellectual and social skills will deteriorate much more rapidly if the patient is allowed to become withdrawn and isolated. A supportive, helpful approach should be taken, and as dementia progresses, the patient needs to be constantly reoriented and reassured.

2. *Use compensatory techniques and adaptive equipment.* This approach, used routinely for people with static handicaps, is often neglected if the disorder is progressive. As an example, the time between independent ambulation and the patient being bedridden can be prolonged by use of an electric wheelchair.

3. *Provide attention to the family's needs.* The growing child normally becomes increasingly self-sufficient. In the face of a degenerative disease this does not occur or, in most cases, regression occurs so that the individual becomes increasingly dependent. All families need counseling and support, and will eventually require increasing contact with social and government agencies. The social worker can provide these services. Many children will, at some time, require institu-

---

*The safety of levodopa in children under 12 years of age has not been established.

**The safety of Sinemet in patients under 18 years of age has not been established.

tional or chronic nursing facility placement. The family's needs and desires should be carefully assessed, and they should then be given support in carrying out the appropriate plan.

Medical aspects of management are complex and involve every organ system. In each case the general principles of maintaining function and then using compensatory techniques and adaptive devices a useful framework.

Motor Function

Motor function becomes limited because of weakness, spasticity, progressive contractures, ataxia, adventitious movements, or loss of sensory function. Ambulation can be maintained by the addition, as needed, of one or two canes and then a tripod cane or four-legged walker. Traditional braces provide little benefit, although lightweight plastic orthotic devices to correct foot drop are useful. Physical therapy is used to maintain motor strength and normal motor patterns and to slow down the progression of joint contractures. It is most important to establish a home program, as the benefit of a brief therapy session several days each week is limited. Passive range of motion, and active resistive exercises for older children, need to be carried out several times each day. As the ability to walk is lost, the physical therapist can be of assistance in ordering an appropriate wheelchair. The parents will need instruction in helping the child to transfer from chair to bed, tub, and toilet. With larger children, mechanical devices such as lifts may be required.

Occupational therapy concentrates on maintaining fine motor function, adaptive skills, and activities of daily living. A large number of simple adaptive devices will allow the patient to continue independent feeding, dressing, grooming, and toileting activities despite major motor disability.

Speech therapy has a traditional role in correcting abnormal speech patterns and articulation disorders. More important is the maintenance of communication by any means available. Standard sign language, idiosyncratic gestures, and communication boards of varying complexity are all acceptable if some level of communication can be maintained. This gives the patient essential social contact and eases the task of the caretakers.

Visual loss due to retinal degeneration or optic atrophy cannot be corrected by refractive lenses. Large print, magnifying glasses, and strong illumination will help maintain some functioning vision. Night blindness is frequently the first sign of retinal degeneration, and it is important to maintain enough light for the patient to be able to move about. If visual loss significantly precedes intellectual deterioration, recorded books and magazines are useful. Some older children can learn braille.

Hearing loss also can occur before there is signifi-

cant cognitive disability. Amplification may allow maintenance of auditory communication. If deafness is profound, alternate communication systems should be developed.

Orthopedic surgery, used with discretion, has a limited role. Muscle transplantation and surgical release of contractures should be considered if there is good assurance of an increase in functional ability for a reasonable period of time. Scoliosis is common, either as a primary part of the degenerative disease or due to muscle weakness. Progression of the scoliosis can limit pulmonary reserve, already compromised by the neuromuscular problems, cause pain and, rarely, produce spinal cord compression. If conservative treatment with a brace or lightweight jacket does not slow progression, surgical correction should be considered. Newer procedures using flexible rods wired to the spinal column at each level allow ambulation within days following surgery. This procedure has been effective even when used in the face of degenerative disease.

Skin care becomes a problem when the patient is confined to a wheelchair or bed, or if sensation is lost. Skin breakdown can be minimized by padding over pressure points on bony prominences, by frequent changes in position, and by use of air or water mattresses. Skin must be kept dry and clean. The treatment of decubitus ulcers in general is unsatisfactory. Prevention is crucial.

Feeding becomes a problem at some point for almost all patients because of neuromuscular dysfunction or loss of cognitive function and alertness. If the patient can swallow, a blenderized diet, fed from a spoon or syringe, is the best way to ensure a balanced diet. Strict attention should be paid to adequate fluid intake. If swallowing is poor or aspiration a problem, a nasogastric tube can be used. This may be a problem if the patient is at home, as frequent reintubation is required and the parents may find placement of the tube difficult. A tube left in place for long periods of time increases the likelihood of gastroesophageal incompetence and aspiration. Management of a feeding gastrostomy is often easier and preferable. Many patients do not require fundal plication if care is taken to not overfill and distend the stomach.

Constipation, a major problem in all non-ambulatory patients, can be partially ameliorated by ensuring adequate fluid intake and including high fiber foods in the feedings. A stool softener such as docusate sodium (Colace) 10–40 mg/day for children under 3 years of age and 50–200 mg/day for older children is useful. Mineral oil should be avoided because of the danger of aspiration. Occasional use of enemas and bisacodyl (Dulcolax) or other contact laxative suppositories will be required. Seriously debilitated patients still can be expected to develop fecal impactions and require repeated enemas or manual disimpaction to clear them. Fecal soiling requires prompt attention to prevent skin breakdown.

Behavior disorders frequently accompany all of the degenerative diseases, probably because of organic and psychological factors. Behavior management techniques can be quite useful, although specific applications will change as the condition progresses. The parents need to be instructed in the principles of developing a behavior management plan, which can be applied to novel situations as they arise. Psychotic or aggressive behavior presents major problems with some patients. Although many psychotropic drugs have been used, the largest experience is with thioridazine (Mellaril). Initial doses of 10 mg twice a day can be gradually increased, as necessary, to levels of 30–120 mg per day, or as limited by sedation. Addition of an antiparkinsonian drug is required only if an extrapyramidal reaction or parkinsonian symptoms occur. An acute dystonic reaction is treated with intravenous diphenhydramine (Benadryl) 25 to 50 mg Benztropine mesylate (Cogentin)* can then be started and maintained at a dose of 1 to 2 mg per day. Tardive dyskinesia is not a major concern unless the disorder is expected to have a prolonged course. In such a case, the dose of the psychotropic drug should be kept at the minimum needed for a therapeutic effect and drug holidays attempted periodically. An uncommon side effect of tranquilizers is a decrease in the seizure threshold with recurrence of previously controlled seizures.

Cardiorespiratory problems including pulmonary infections and atelectasis are important and often fatal complications. These result from the interaction of a large number of factors including repeated aspiration, limited respiratory excursions due to muscle weakness, decreased cough reflex, and reduced pulmonary reserve due to scoliosis. Prevention of aspiration requires frequent suctioning of the oropharynx, attention to the volume of feedings, and proper positioning of the patient. Postural drainage, in combination with suctioning, is an important part of daily therapy. If atelectasis does not respond to conservative treatment, bronchosocopy is required. Cardiomyopathy is a primary part of some of the degenerative diseases. Heart failure is treated in standard fashion.

Urinary incontinence helps to cause skin breakdown and is a major social handicap. A condom catheter and bag can be used with males, but there are not adequate external urinary appliances for females. If there is incomplete bladder emptying, intermittent catheterization is preferable to the use of an in-

dwelling catheter. Although parents may initially find this a disturbing technique, it is much less likely to produce a urinary tract infection.

Renal calculi are a problem in some nonambulatory patients. Adequate fluid intake is important and foods containing high levels of calcium should be limited.

Hypothermia or episodic *hyperthermia* occurs in some patients who are severely involved. Abnormalities of body temperature should always trigger a search for sepsis, which is common. Potential foci of the infection are decubitus ulcers, lungs, and urinary tract. Some patients respond to variations in environmental temperature and act as if they were poikilothermic. Use of thermostatically controlled heating or cooling blankets may be required.

Drug Treatment

Seizures are frequently associated with the degenerative diseases and should be treated as outlined in the article on seizure disorders.

Pharmacologic treatment of spasticity is not fully satisfactory. Diazepam (Valium) in doses as high as 2.5 to 5 mg two to three times a day can be used.* Lower doses are initially begun, and the drug is increased as tolerated. The only serious side effect is sedation. Dantrolene sodium (Dantrium) has an initial dosage of 1.0 mg/kg/day in divided doses, and then can be increased weekly to a maximum level of 3 mg/kg/day or 400 mg/day.** Side effects include drowsiness, bowel disturbances, and serious hepatotoxicity. Baclofen (Lioresal) is not recommended for use in children under 12 years of age.

Adventitious movements are also difficult to treat, and unpredictable in their response to any drug. Diazepam, in doses as outlined above, and haloperidol have been the most useful. This is begun at a 0.5 mg daily and increased by 0.5 mg every 4–5 days to a maximum dose of 5–10 mg/day. Important side effects are lethargy, depression, and irritability. An anticholinergic agent is not used concomitantly unless an acute dystonic reaction or parkinsonian symptoms appear. Amantadine (Symmetrel†) is occasionally helpful. A maximum dose of 1–2 mg/kg/day or 150 mg/day is given in divided doses. Severe side effects include an increase in seizures, depression, and congestive heart failure.

---

*The manufacturer states that Valium is contraindicated in children under 6 months of age because of lack of clinical experience.

**The long-term safety of Dantrium in children under the age of 5 years has not been established.

†The safety and efficacy of Symmetrel in newborn infants and infants below 1 year of age have not been established.

---

*Cogentin is contraindicated in children under 3 years of age.

Cerebral Palsy

LAWRENCE T. TAFT, M.D.

Although cerebral palsy per se is a motor disorder, associated nonmotor handicaps, such as mental retardation, often prove more disabling. The specific strategies necessary for the child to develop to his full potential are but partly determined by the type and extent of the cerebral dysfunction. At least as important in the selection of optimal strategies are the child's family and social milieu.

The first goal in pediatric management should be to maximize the coping abilities of the child and family. Several general principles are particularly important in achieving this goal: 1) Past success is a powerful motivator for future effort. Thus, whenever possible the child should be placed in situations that optimize his chances for success. Failure depresses and tends to lessen motivation; failure must be avoided. 2) The importance of achieving functional motor improvements, such as independent ambulation, should not be unduly stressed. 3) Coordination of the diagnostic and treatment modalities involved is essential. 4) Achievement of the rights of the child and his family vis-à-vis governmental and other institutional support may require active advocacy on the part of the health care provider.

INITIAL DIAGNOSIS

The parents must be told of the problem in a compassionate and empathetic manner as soon as the diagnosis is suspected or confirmed. They should be given as much information about the cause, treatment, and prognosis as is available. When, as frequently occurs, the prognosis for independent ambulation and/or functioning cannot be accurately stated, the parents should be told of the limitations of early prognosis. Upon hearing the words "Your child has cerebral palsy," the initial reaction of the parents is commonly extreme grief. Listening may continue but comprehension often suffers. Thus it is often necessary to repeat the explanations and to answer the same questions over several subsequent sessions to ensure that the parents understand the situation and have no misconceptions.

At the time of the informing interview, let the parents know that you will be referring the child to a nearby "early intervention center." Many of these programs are home-based. If center-based, they require the parent to bring the child to only one session per week. Explain that the center will educate the parents further about cerebral palsy, will explore the problems the infant and the family usually have in coping, and will offer intervention strategies that will optimize the child's intellectual and motor functioning. The parents will act as therapists, under the tutelage of the intervention center staff. The advantage of immediate referral is that it does not leave the parents with a sense of complete hopelessness after they are informed of the diagnosis. It offers immediate, essential family support.

The Committee on Children with Handicaps of the American Academy of Pediatrics has concluded that early intervention programs mitigate the denial that families experience after learning of the diagnosis and, consequently, allow for an earlier adaptation.

SPECIFIC INTERVENTION STRATEGIES

Motor Performances. Many techniques are used to improve motor function or prevent complications. The purpose may be to modify the dyskinetic movements, to decrease the hypertonus, or to develop specific skills. Treatment includes physical therapy, adaptive devices such as braces, medications, chemical neurolysis to decrease tone, and orthopedic intervention to correct the musculoskeletal abnormalities that develop in the growing child with cerebral palsy.

Physical Therapy. Physical therapy for cerebral palsy can be broadly categorized into two major types: the first is to maintain the range of motion of the joints and to increase muscle strength; the second is to favorably modify the abnormal tone and movements.

The first, most traditional, type includes passive and active stretching of joints to maintain a full range of motion and prevent musculoskeletal deformities; strengthening exercises by active movements against increasingly greater resistance to counteract the weakness of specific muscle groups; and the teaching and encouragement of the voluntarily performance of specific tasks, especially those related to daily living. Parents can be taught to be "therapists." As the child gets older he himself can assume responsibility for many of these therapies.

Techniques that attempt to favorably influence tone and posture are more controversial. They are best known by the name of the individuals who have described them, e.g., Bobath, Rood, Kabat, Bronstrum, Fay. The Bobath neuromuscular facilitative technique appears to be the most commonly used by physiatrists and physical therapists. It attempts to inhibit persistent primitive reflexes and to modify tone by the use of applied sensory stimuli, tactile, vestibular, and proprioceptive. An example of the inhibition of a primitive reflex would be modification of the dysfunctional posture caused by a persistent obligatory symmetric tonic neck reflex. When this reflex is present, the trunk extension that often occurs in these children activates extension of the upper extremities. This latter posture does not allow the child to engage in hand-to-mouth activities or to learn eye-hand coordination. With the Bobath technique, the child is placed in a position that encourages trunk flexion. This activates the symmetric tonic neck reflex in a manner to cause flexion of the upper extremities, thereby facilitating the child's use of his hands and, hopefully, making him more functional. With active use of his hands, he can improve eye-hand coordination and also increase his sensory experiences.

Drug Modification of Tone. Successful use of medication to decrease tone (to improve voluntary control of movement) has been limited by drug side effects. Diazepam (Valium) will usually have a marked sedative effect before it favorably ameliorates hypertonus. However, when anxiety increases involuntary movements, especially athetoid, Valium may be beneficial. Dantrolene, which acts directly on the muscle to limit its contractility, also may cause sedation. However, the major concern with dantrolene is that the desired decrease in muscle tone is often associated with marked muscle weakness. In addition, dantrolene is hepatotoxic, and liver function must be carefully monitored while the child is on this drug. Baclofen, a gamma-aminobutyric acid derivative, is believed to inhibit neurotransmitter impulses. It has mild sedative effects with no significant toxic effects. Studies in children are limited and have not proved its effectiveness. A trial of therapy may be indicated, especially in children with severe hypertonus. Use of a muscle relaxant may also benefit the caretaker of the cerebral palsied child. For instance, a child with severe adductor spasticity will be difficult to diaper. The spasticity may be minimized with the use of the appropriate drug.

Local therapy to improve tone has included the use of phenol. Because of phenol's neurolytic properties, injection of the drug around the motor nerve will result in partial denervation. This effect may last from a few weeks to a few months. It may especially help to alleviate a spastic equinus foot or severe hip adductor spasm. However, repeated injection of the solution is contraindicated, and surgical correction may then be considered. Use of the phenol solution may allow a more accurate prediction of the functional result achievable through surgery.

Orthotic and Adaptive Equipment. Bracing is used for two purposes: to prevent contractures and to maintain joint stability as an aid in achieving an erect posture. Although lightweight braces are now available, bracing is becoming a less popular mode of therapy.

There are numerous adaptive devices to aid in independent functioning. Occupational and physical therapists can evaluate the patient to determine the need for these devices, and the type that would provide more independent self-care abilities.

Wheelchairs may be self-driven or propelled by caretakers. The latter are called travel-chairs, and usually are most appropriate for the severely handicapped child. The chair can be aligned to permit maximal stability of the trunk and to minimize reflexive spastic responses such as hyperextension. The traditional, independently propelled wheelchair has independent segments to support the leg, seat, and back. These can be adjusted to minimize abnormal postures. The specific type of wheelchair and adaptive equipment should be prescribed by an experienced professional.

Biofeedback. Biofeedback involves the patient's active participation in an attempt to control motor activity through sensory feedback mechanisms. There are very few controlled or long-term studies of the duration of the effects achieved. However, there have been some suggestions that biofeedback has helped hemiplegic cerebral palsied children of normal intelligence to attain a more symmetrical, more cosmetic gait.

Inhibitory Casting. Attempts have been made to realign partially deformed ankles by use of a walking cast, applied for a period of 4 to 6 weeks. The foot is maintained in a more normal anatomical position which, in spastic cerebral palsy, necessitates sustained stretching. It is hoped that short-term casting will prevent spastic deformities and avoid surgery. Its value remains questionable.

Surgery. Orthopedic surgery is often recommended to correct deformities due to the neuromuscular imbalance of cerebral palsy. Heel-cord lengthening, adductor tenotomies, and hip flexor and hamstring releases are done to improve posture and function. Unfortunately, there is still controversy regarding the optimal timing of these procedures, as well as which procedures are most effective.

Neurosurgery. Chronic cerebellar stimulation to modify hypertonus has been attempted. Not enough is known about its short- and long-term effects to justify its use except in special cases, such as in spastic children with normal intelligence who are so severely involved that they have virtually no voluntary motor control.

HEALTH MAINTENANCE

Cerebral palsied children should benefit from the health maintenance routines offered to children without handicaps. For example, they should be immunized according to the standard recommended schedule. However, there are a number of screening tests and areas of anticipatory guidance that are particularly relevant to the care of disabled children.

Routine screening for auditory abilities is essential. Over 70% of athetoid cerebral palsied youngsters, secondary to bilirubin encephalopathy, have high-frequency hearing loss. Thirty per cent of all other cerebral palsied children have sensorineural hearing impairment. Early recognition of and appropriate intervention for these problems are important for the prevention of additional difficulties.

Vision screening should be stressed during routine exams. Strabismus is present in over 75% of cerebral palsied individuals. Early recognition and referral to an ophthalmologist will help prevent amblyopia exanopsia. Ophthalmoscopic examination should be done to evaluate for cataracts and to judge whether a refractive error exists. Nearsightedness is commonly found. When the child is cognitively ready, visual acuity should be tested with the use of "E" or Snellen charts.

There should be routine assessments of the range of motion of spastic joints. Tightness or limitation in the full range of joint motion indicates referral to a physical therapist. The parents can be taught to passively stretch the child's joints to prevent irreversible contractures.

The presence of scoliosis must be monitored. A high prevalence is noted, especially in quadriplegic patients.

Leg-length discrepancies should be assessed in hemiplegic infants and children. Over 50% of patients with hemiparesis due to congenital insult will have a leg-length discrepancy. In an ambulatory child, early recognition and correction of an inequality of leg length by the use of a sole lift will help prevent the development of scoliosis.

Advice must be given to parents regarding the importance of preventing obesity in the child. The limitation of physical activity that results from a neuromotor handicap often results in excessive weight gain.

During each health maintenance visit, the parents should be asked if there are any recurrent episodes in which the child appears to be unaware of his surroundings. These may be seizure manifestations. Over one half of children with cerebral palsy develop epilepsy. Some types of psychomotor seizures may not be recognized as such, being attributed to aberrant behavior.

Assisting Psychosocial Adjustment. Anticipatory guidance of the parents might help minimize adverse psychosocial adjustment of the child and family members. Parents should be advised not to act solicitously toward the child. Doing so can cause the child to develop a self-concept of dependency and helplessness. Parents should be encouraged to discipline the child as they would a healthy youngster.

Preschool children frequently believe their handicap is punishment for some wrongdoing. The pediatrician should explore this issue with the child and, if there is evidence that this is the case, the youngster should be informed that his problem is not related to a punishment or previous bad behavior. As the child grows older, his inability to compete motorically and socially may lead to isolation from his peers. Attempts should be made to find recreational or social activities in which the youngster might successfully interact with peers and, it is hoped, develop more positive social relationships.

Education. Early intervention centers for infants are quite abundant. In almost all states mandatory education for handicapped youngsters must be offered from 3 years of age. Parents of young cerebral palsied children should be encouraged to have their child enrolled in these preschool programs. However, if the disability is minimal, as is often found in hemiplegic patients, and if the youngster does not have a significant cognitive deficit, a normal nursery school placement is preferable.

Mainstreaming children who are capable of competing with their normal peers is preferable to special class placement. However, if there is any suggestion that the child is finding it difficult to maintain his self-esteem because of an inability to compete academically with his peers, he should be placed where he can experience success and better maintain his self-esteem. Children in wheelchairs can be successfully mainstreamed if they have the necessary cognitive abilities.

Nonverbal Communication. Many children with cerebral palsy have difficulties with expressive language, owing to severe dysarthria, verbal dyspraxia, or expressive aphasia. The inability to control one's environment through the use of language can be very depressing. With the use of communication devices as substitutes for spoken or written language, significantly language-impaired children can make themselves understood. There are many devices that resemble calculators, which the child can use to make selected inquiries or responses. The use of nonverbal communication has had amazing success. Many children who are thought to be retarded or withdrawn have demonstrated unexpectedly high cognitive abilities. Successful nonverbal communication has also resulted in positive personality changes. The children become more interested in relating to their peers and caretakers. An infant who has evidence of a severe motor dysfunction of the oropharyngeal muscles should be offered non-verbal communication aids. This will not inhibit later development of the ability to communicate verbally.

Recreation. Recreational and social programs geared to the handicapped are necessary so that the child does not become homebound. Parents should be referred to the regional voluntary health agency, such as the United Cerebral Palsy Association or the state Developmental Disability Council, to learn where and what programs exist.

Day-care and sleep-away camps are also available and should be utilized.

Vocational Training. Adolescents should receive vocational training. Parents should be advised to urge their child's educators to find a suitable vocational training program. This should not be delayed until graduation. If the handicap is so great as to preclude functioning in competitive employment, sheltered workshops should be considered.

Spinal Diseases

DAVID W. BAILEY, M.D.

When considered collectively, the disorders associated with spinal cord dysfunction are quite common. However, except for myelodysplasia, the individual entities within the group are uncommon or rare. They also tend to be insidious in their onset and atypical in their clinical presentation, which accounts for the frequently seen delays and/or errors in diagnosis and management of spinal diseases in children.

Treatment of spinal diseases can often only prevent further progression, not restore lost function. Primary care providers must therefore have a high index of suspicion when confronted with an infant or child whose symptoms include back pain, disturbance of gait, refusal to walk, or bowel/bladder dysfunction.

HEREDITARY DISORDERS

Spinal muscular atrophy is an autosomal recessive disease associated with absent or reduced anterior horn cells and progressive weakness. Whereas the infantile form is usually fatal by a year of age, the juvenile variety more closely mimics muscular dystrophy and therefore calls for a multidisciplinary supportive treatment program.

Most *spinocerebellar degenerative disorders* do not become clinically evident until well into childhood or even adolescence. Recognizable entities within this group include Friedreich's ataxia, peroneal muscular atrophy, spastic paraplegia/ataxia, and juvenile-onset metachromatic leukodystrophy. The mode of inheritance is variable among, and sometimes within, the various so-called entities. Treatment is limited to counseling and symptomatic measures. Surgery for associated deformities is generally contraindicated because of the likelihood of functional regression during postoperative immobilization.

Neurofibromatosis is the most common phakomatosis, and also the one most likely to be associated with spinal disorders. Neurofibromas of the spinal nerve roots can induce scoliosis, and an intraspinal tumor may lead to signs of cord compression.

CONGENITAL MALFORMATIONS

Spina bifida occulta is a common finding on x-ray and by itself is of little or no significance. However, when it occurs in conjunction with an overlying cutaneous abnormality (port wine stain, dimple, tuft of hair, lipoma), it must be taken more seriously. A midline dimple above the gluteal crease may portend a dermal sinus that communicates with the meninges or an intraspinal dermoid. Neurosurgical exploration on an urgent basis is indicated, in order to prevent bacterial (usually gram-negative) meningitis. Other conditions associated with occult dysraphism that require neurosurgical intervention include diastematomyelia and tethered cord with or without a lipoma. When delays in the diagnosis and treatment of these conditions occur, they can usually be attributed to failure to include careful inspection of the spine in the general examination.

An *arteriovenous malformation* of the spinal vasculature can be associated with any form of spinal cord dysfunction depending on its level and extent. Diagnosis and surgical treatment are challenging and only feasible at major referral centers.

Children with Down or Morquio syndromes have an increased incidence of recurrent *atlantoaxial dislocation,* with compression of the cord by the odontoid process. Immobilization in extension is followed by surgical stabilization.

TRAUMA

Babies delivered by breech extraction may suffer *traction injury* to the cervical cord. If the level is sufficiently low, the characteristic upper extremity postures, together with flaccid paraplegia, make diagnosis relatively simple. If the level is high enough to cause flaccid quadriplegia and respiratory distress, the clinical picture can resemble cerebral hypotonia or transient myasthenia gravis. Myelography is usually not required, and treatment is supportive and expectant.

Later on in childhood, cord trauma is a common component of deceleration injuries. *Cord contusion* usually causes a transient paraparesis, and may be associated with a simple spinal fracture. *Fracture dislocations* are always associated with cord dysfunction and require immediate immobilization, traction as soon as possible, and in some cases respiratory support and surgical intervention.

Intervertebral disc herniations are unusual in children and nearly always complicate an acute injury. Because of their rarity, and since the link between trauma and symptoms may be more apparent than real, myelography to confirm the diagnosis and rule out tumor is indicated in most cases. Conservative treatment, with analgesics and bed rest, is usually effective.

INFECTIONS

Osteomyelitis of the spine, and particularly tuberculous spondylitis, may present obscurely in early childhood with vague symptoms including fussiness and inactivity. Careful examination may reveal kyphosis and/or focal spinal tenderness to percussion. With radiologic confirmation and the results of skin tests and cultures in hand, treatment is straightforward.

Epidural abscess, because it causes rapidly progressive cord dysfunction, is a medical and surgical emergency. It occurs most commonly as a complication of a dermal sinus. Immediate drainage and concomitant and aggressive antibiotic treatment are mandatory.

Intervertebral disc space infection ("discitis") is a difficult to diagnose and poorly understood disorder of young children. Once suspected, the diagnosis can be confirmed radiologically, with narrowing of the affected intervertebral space on plain films and a positive bone scan. The need for confirmatory needle aspiration is debatable, but a positive culture of the aspirate (usually *Staphyloccus aureus*) may help guide antibiotic treatment. Most orthopedists do not advocate open biopsy or myelography. Treatment includes bed rest, analgesics, and a 10- to 14-day course of antibiotics. The erythrocyte sedimentation rate, which is consistently elevated in these patients, can be used along with clinical course as a guide to the efficacy and continued need for therapy. Long-term outcome is generally good, and recurrence extremely uncommon.

Transverse myelitis is usually an idiopathic, post-, or parainfectious phenomenon. It quite often results in permanent cord dysfunction.

TUMORS

Most *spinal tumors* in children are slow-growing and insidious in nature. Clinical findings are confusing but include some degree of weakness in all cases with sensory changes in at least half. A high index of suspicion will reduce the delays and errors in diagnosis in these children.

Intraspinal tumors are generally benign and include gliomas and ependymomas. Extradural tumors are more malignant and include medulloblastoma, lymphoma, and sacrococcygeal teratoma.

Plain x-rays of the spine usually reveal interpedicular widening at the level of the tumor. Computed tomography together with intrathecal metrizimide is replacing traditional myelography as the confirmatory study of choice. Treatment includes surgical removal followed by irradiation and/or chemotherapy as appropriate.

Seizure Disorders

JOHN H. MENKES, M.D.

The objective in the treatment of the epileptic patient is complete control of seizures, or at least reduction in their frequency to the point at which they no longer interfere with physical and social well-being. At the same time, therapy or its side effects should not disrupt the child's life.

The first question to be considered is whether the patient requires treatment. Although agreement is unanimous that all patients with recurrent seizures should be treated as soon as the diagnosis is established, considerable controversy exists regarding the optimum method of dealing with certain groups of patients.

1. An isolated major motor seizure. In the absence of structural brain abnormalities, we believe treatment of this type is optional and largely dependent on social factors. In view of a recurrence risk of some 20% for idiopathic grand mal convulsions, I am reluctant to treat the youngster with his first seizure whose EEG is normal and who has a negative family history of epilepsy.

2. Breath-holding spells. We have found antiepileptic drugs to be of no value in preventing recurrences of these attacks. Reassuring the parents that these attacks are benign and presage neither epilepsy nor major behavior disturbances is usually sufficient.

3. Syncopal attacks. Anticonvulsant therapy is of little use in prevention of either the attack or the brief clonic seizure that sometimes terminates it.

4. One or more episodes of which the epileptic nature cannot be established with certainty. One should either defer therapy until the clinical picture has become clear or use an anticonvulsant as a therapeutic trial if it is more likely than not that the child has experienced a seizure. Repeated electroencephalographic tracings or ambulatory cassette recordings may assist in the diagnosis.

5. Febrile convulsions. This is discussed in a subsequent article.

Once treatment has been decided upon, several therapeutic principles should be kept in mind:

1. The selection of the drug of first choice is based on the type of seizure and on the drug's potential side effects.

2. Treatment should begin with one drug. Dosage is increased until seizures are controlled or the child develops toxicity. If the drug does not control seizures, it is discontinued gradually while a second drug is started and its dosage slowly increased.

This preferential use of a single anticonvulsant in the treatment of seizures has gained considerable support from a number of clinical studies. These have documented the following disadvantages of polytherapy:

A. Chronic toxicity is directly related to the number of drugs consumed. Even though none may be present in toxic level, their effect, particularly on sensorium and intellectual performance, is cumulative.

B. Drug interactions may not only enhance toxicity but may also lead to loss of seizure control.

C. Polytherapy may aggravate seizures in some patients.

3. Alterations in drug dosage should be made gradually, usually not more frequently than once every 5 to 7 days.

4. The number of truly effective anticonvulsants is small, and there is little likelihood of controlling a patient with a lesser-known drug when the usual medications have failed. Conversely, the chances of inducing toxic side reactions when trying out a new or rarely used drug are great.

5. Once seizures are controlled, the medication should be continued for a prolonged period without altering its dosage unless this is dictated by changes in the child's body weight.

6. Frequent determinations of anticonvulsant blood levels are necessary in all patients. This becomes particularly important when the child is not responding to therapy, or when there is question about the presence of drug toxicity. Therapeutic and toxic blood levels for the more commonly employed anticonvulsants are listed in Table 1.

7. Anticonvulsants should be withdrawn gradu-

Table 1. THERAPEUTIC AND TOXIC BLOOD LEVELS FOR MAJOR ANTICONVULSANTS

Drug	Days to Achieve Steady State Blood Level	Serum Half-Life (hours)	Therapeutic Blood Levels (μg/ml)	Toxic Blood Levels (μg/ml)
Phenobarbital	14–21	96 ± 12	10–30	>40
Phenytoin (Dilantin)	7–21	13–46	10–20	>20
Primidone* (Mysoline)	4–7	12 ± 6	>5	>12
Ethosuximide (Zarontin)	5–8	30 ± 6	>40	>100
Carbamazepine (Tegretol)	5–10	8–20	4–12	>8 §
Clonazepam† (Clonopin)	up to 14	22–33	>0.013	>0.013
Valproic acid‡ (Depakene)	4	6–15	—	—

*Primidone is converted to phenobarbital and phenylethylmalonamide. Ratio of phenobarbital to primidone blood levels ranges from 2–4 to 1.

†Relationship of blood levels to therapeutic and toxic effects has been questioned.

‡Correlation between blood levels and therapeutic effects or adverse reactions cannot be demonstrated.

§The relationship of toxic effects of blood levels is not clear-cut, inasmuch as carbamazepine is converted to a pharmacologically active epoxide.

(From Menkes, J. H.: Textbook of Child Neurology, Philadelphia, Lea and Febiger, 1985, 3rd ed.)

Table 2. PREFERRED TREATMENT OF THE VARIOUS CONVULSIVE DISORDERS*

Grand Mal	Petit Mal	Psychomotor	Minor Motor	Focal Seizures	Infantile Spasms
Phenobarbital	Ethosuximide (Zarontin)	Carbamazepine (Tegretol)	Valproic acid (Depakene)	Carbamazepine (Tegretol)	ACTH or corticosteroids
Carbamazepine (Tegretol)	Valproic acid (Depakene)	Valproic acid (Depakene)	Clonazepam (Clonopin)	Phenobarbital	Nitrazepam (Mogadon)
Phenytoin (Dilantin)	Clonazepam (Clonopin)	Phenytoin (Dilantin)	Ethosuximide (Zarontin)	Phenytoin (Dilantin)	Valproate (Depakene)
Valproic acid (Depakene)	Trimethadione (Tridione)	Primidone (Mysoline)	Primidone (Mysoline)	Primidone (Mysoline)	
Primidone (Mysoline)	Paramethadione (Paradione)	Phenobarbital	ACTH	Valproic acid (Depakene)	
Mephenytoin (Mesantoin)	Methsuximide (Celontin)	Mephobarbital (Mebaral)	Diazepam† (Valium)		
Mephobarbital (Mebaral)			Ketogenic diet		

*In this table drugs are arranged in order of personal preference. A number of other anticonvulsants that we have usually found less effective have not been listed.

†Preferred drug for minor motor (petit mal) status.

(From Menkes, J. H.: Textbook of Child Neurology, Philadelphia, Lea and Febiger, 1985, 3rd ed.)

ally. Sudden withdrawal of medication, particularly of barbiturates, is the most common cause of status epilepticus.

The drugs of choice for the various types of paroxysmal disorders are presented in Table 2.

ANTICONVULSANT THERAPY

Phenobarbital. This is an effective anticonvulsant in the treatment of grand mal epilepsy and partial seizures of elementary symptomatology (focal seizures). The therapeutic dosage varies among patients; the starting dose should be about 5 mg/kg/24 hr. Since the drug equilibrates slowly, 2 to 3 weeks are required to achieve 95 per cent of the maximum serum levels. In most patients with grand mal seizures controllable with phenobarbital, the drug is effective at serum levels of 10 to 15 μg/ml, and a level of 15 μg/ml or higher is generally considered to be therapeutic. The maximum variation in serum concentration with one daily dose of the drug is between 7 and 14 per cent. Therefore, even in small children, two daily doses suffice for maintenance of therapeutic blood levels.

Toxic levels of phenobarbital vary from one individual to another, but as a rule no permanent sedation is seen with levels below 35 μg/ml. The principal toxic sign is sedation. Hyperkinetic behavior is encountered in about a third of patients. Most of these have some pre-existing evidence of a behavior disorder or known structural abnormalities of the brain.

The long-term effect of phenobarbital as well as of the other anticonvulsants on intellectual performance is a matter of much debate. Some authors have found that the drug induces disturbances in sleep, fussiness, and impaired concentration, whereas others, confirming an initial impairment in cognitive functions, show that these side effects disappear after the first year of therapy.

Mephobarbital (Mebaral). This drug is commonly used in place of phenobarbital, as it is believed to have fewer side effects. However, its gastrointestinal absorption appears less reliable than that of phenobarbital, and frequent determinations of anticonvulsant blood levels are therefore imperative.

Primidone (Mysoline). This drug is an effective anticonvulsant for major motor and focal seizures caused by organic disease of the brain. It is less effective against partial seizures of complex symptomatology (temporal lobe or psychomotor seizures).

In children, primidone is started at low levels, generally 50 mg/24 hr, given in two divided doses. The daily dosage is gradually increased until the average effective dose (150 to 500 mg/24 hr) is reached. This procedure is intended to circumvent marked sedation, which often occurs when the drug is started at higher levels. As a rule, prior exposure to phenobarbital makes the subject less likely to develop primidone toxicity. The drug is converted into two active metabolites whose potencies relative to primidone are unknown. Thus monitoring of blood levels can be used only to determine compliance.

Phenytoin (Dilantin). Phenytoin is as effective as phenobarbital and carbamazepine in the control of tonic-clonic (grand mal) seizures, but because of the wide variability in its absorption and the effect of other anticonvulsants and even mild intercurrent illnesses on its rate of metabolism, and because of the relatively high incidence of side reactions, it has lost much favor as a long-term anticonvulsant for use in children.

The average therapeutic dose in children ranges between 5 and 10 mg/kg/24 hr. The drug is only slowly absorbed from the gastrointestinal tract, and, at the above dosages, blood levels do not equilibrate until 7 to 10 days after the initiation of therapy. The drug is given twice daily to older children; in those under 30 kg, administration at approximately 8-hour intervals is generally necessary.

Clinically effective phenytoin levels usually range from 10 to 20 μg/ml. At these concentrations, relatively small dose increments will induce large increments in blood anticonvulsant levels, so these must be monitored frequently, particularly in smaller children, in order not to overdose the patient.

Phenytoin produces a number of untoward reactions; in most instances these are related to overdosage and are relieved by reducing drug intake. Nystagmus at lateral gaze appears at blood levels of 15 to 30 μg/ml, frank ataxia above 30 μg/ml, and lethargy or aggravation of seizures at levels above 40 μg/ml. Irreversible degeneration of the cerebellar Purkinje cells may occur after chronic or severe acute intoxication. In these instances, a CT scan may demonstrate cerebellar atrophy. The rate of phenytoin metabolism is greatly variable and appears to be under polygenetic control. A few patients have a defect in the para-hydroxylation of phenytoin and readily develop toxic symptoms. Small infants, likewise, only eliminate 1 to 20 per cent of the drug in a 24-hour period and frequently develop toxicity.

About 2 to 5 per cent of patients receiving phenytoin develop fever, a morbilliform rash, and lymphadenopathy within 2 weeks of the start of therapy. Blood levels at the time of the reaction are in the therapeutic range. Symptoms clear after discontinuation of the drug. Phenytoin is also known to induce antinuclear antibodies (ANA) and a lupus-like disease. ANA have also been detected in those receiving phenobarbital or ethosuximide exclusively. Although the presence of ANA in asymptomatic children has aroused considerable concern, it is not an indication for discontinuation of anticonvulsants. However, the incidence of malignant lymphomas and Hodgkin disease in patients who had received long-term hydantoin therapy is four to ten times greater than in the general population.

In a significant proportion of patients, phenytoin causes gum hyperplasia, and 75 per cent of patients develop hirsutism. The former complication usually appears 2 to 3 months after initiation of the drug and is seen at therapeutic blood levels in as many as 93 per cent of patients. Gum changes can be reduced by strict oral hygiene, daily massage of the gums, and repeated excision of hyperplastic tissue. Another consequence of long-term phenytoin therapy is coarsening of facial features, also a result of the drug's action on connective tissue.

Patients on prolonged phenytoin therapy may develop megaloblastic anemia and lowered serum folate concentrations, which respond to folic acid therapy. The mechanism by which the drug alters folate metabolism is still uncertain, and this complication may, in part at least, reflect inadequate food composition or intake. Although prolonged folate deficiency may induce an organic brain syndrome, folate therapy has had no effect on the behavior or mental deterioration of some chronic seizure patients.

A disturbed vitamin D metabolism, resulting in hypocalcemic rickets, decreased serum calcium and phosphorus, and increased alkaline phosphatases, is seen in some ambulatory, noninstitutionalized patients after long-term therapy with phenytoin, primidone, or phenobarbital. This observation suggests that children who are on long-term anticonvulsant therapy should receive vitamin D supplementation and be encouraged in outdoor activities to ensure adequate exposure to sunlight.

A phenytoin encephalopathy is encountered at toxic blood levels, but has rarely been seen at therapeutic levels as an idiosyncratic reaction. Mentally retarded subjects are particularly vulnerable to this syndrome. Like phenobarbital, phenytoin may aggravate any underlying behavior disorder or hyperkinesis.

A significant incidence of major congenital malformations in children of women who received anticonvulsants occurs. In particular, phenytoin may induce a syndrome characterized by a short, broad nose, hypertelorism, and phalangeal hypoplasia.

Carbamazepine (Tegretol). Carbamazepine is an iminostilbene, chemically unrelated to any of the other major anticonvulsants. Children with psychomotor and grand mal seizures are most likely to benefit from the drug. The starting dosage in children aged 6 to 12 years is 200 mg/24 hr, and the maximum dosage for effective seizure control is in the neighborhood of 800 mg/24 hr. The suggested starting dose for children under age 6 years is 100 mg/24 hr. Although optimal therapeutic levels generally lie between 4 and 12 μg/ml, carbamazepine-plasma protein binding and the conversion of carbamazepine to a pharmacologically active 10,11-epoxide, which cannot readily be assayed, complicates the interpretation of serum concentrations. Ratios of carbamazepine to its epoxide range from 5:1 in subjects receiving only carbamazepine to 2:1 for those receiving other anticonvulsants as well.

The most common untoward reaction encountered is diplopia, which is usually a toxic effect. It may disappear with reduction of the total daily dosage, or upon giving the drug oftener and in smaller amounts. Other side reactions, in order of frequency, include rashes, chemical evidence of hepatic dysfunction, leukopenia, and hyponatremia.

As with phenytoin, carbamazepine may induce an increase in the levels of liver enzymes. Generally, this reflects enzyme induction rather than an incipient hepatotoxic reaction, as supported by the microscopic finding of proliferation of the smooth endoplasmic reticulum within the liver.

Leukopenia consequent to carbamazepine administration is exceedingly rare, although a significant number of individuals experience a depression in red and white cell series which improves spontaneously even when the drug is continued. In some, a minor viral illness may induce the fall of white cells.

Because of these potential side reactions, routine hematologic and hepatic evaluations are necessary. We conduct these every 2 weeks during the period of increasing carbamazepine dosage, and then at intervals of 1 to 3 months depending on social and geographic circumstances. Generally, GGT (gamma-glutamyl transferase) and, to a lesser degree, the serum transaminases become elevated most readily. Their elevation is not necessarily an indication for cessation or reduction of drug therapy since transaminase levels have been shown to return to normal within 8 to 14 months on the same drug dosage.

Despite these inconveniences, most neurologists now consider carbamazepine superior to phenytoin because of a lower incidence of side effects and the fact that carbamazepine does not produce behavioral disorders; in fact, in some instances it may even improve cognitive function.

Ethosuximide (Zarontin). The most effective drug in the treatment of primary generalized epilepsy (petit mal absence seizures) is ethosuximide. Starting doses for children are 250 mg two times a day, or approximately 20 mg/kg/24 hr. The drug is given two to four times daily. Optimal therapeutic plasma levels range between 40 and 100 μg/ml. We use ethosuximide alone in the treatment of petit mal attacks, unless the patient has a history of other seizure types or has an electroencephalogram with abnormalities other than the 3 per second spike and wave discharges. Then, combined phenobarbital and ethosuximide therapy is used, with the phenobarbital being started first, and ethosuximide added to the regimen about 1 week later. Occasionally, phenobarbital controls petit mal attacks and under these circumstances the drug should be continued as the sole anticonvulsant.

Side effects of ethosuximide include gastrointestinal upsets, usually during the first few days of drug therapy, rashes, headaches, and rarely hematologic abnormalities, principally a reversible leukopenia. An increase in the levels of hepatic enzymes is also encountered.

Valproic Acid. The treatment of minor motor seizures (Lennox-Gastaut syndrome, myoclonic epilepsies, atonic-akinetic attacks) is truly perplexing.

Valproic acid (VPA), either as its sodium or magnesium salt, or as the free acid, is a highly effective drug, not only for minor motor seizures but also for tonic-clonic (grand mal), absence (petit mal), and simple partial seizures.

The drug inhibits GABA-transferase and succinic semialdehyde activities, and in this manner elevates GABA concentrations within the brain. Whether this is the actual mechanism of its anticonvulsant action is the subject of considerable investigation.

Starting dosages for children are 15 to 20 mg/kg/day given once or twice daily, with the dose increased at weekly intervals to a level that provides seizure control, usually around 20 to 70 mg/kg/day.

The dose-serum concentration relationship is complex, in part because of the short half-life of VPA and in part because of the high degree of plasma protein binding. At low plasma VPA levels, protein binding is 90 to 95%, but with increasing dosages, the proportion of protein binding falls progressively, and as a consequence the total serum concentration of VPA does not rise proportionately to the dose.

Although plasma half-life is short, 6 to 15 hours when VPA is administered alone, and even less when given in combination with other anticonvulsants, the practice of administering the drugs in two to four daily doses may not be required, and once-daily administration of enteric-coated drug appears to provide equally good seizure control.

As a consequence of the widespread use of VPA, numerous side reactions have been encountered. The most common of these are gastrointestinal upsets. These may be reduced by taking the medication with food, or by the use of an enteric-coated preparation. Increased appetite is also common. It has been our experience that significant weight gain is encountered in patients who respond best to the drug. Less often, one encounters thinning of hair.

The effects of VPA on liver function have been of serious concern. Raised serum transaminase concentrations are seen in some 3% of patients receiving VPA as the sole anticonvulsant. Generally, these abnormalities are transient. Far more serious is a Reye syndrome-like hepatic failure occurring during the first 6 months of therapy. This complication is unrelated to VPA dosage, and nearly 90% of patients had been on polytherapy. The cause for VPA induced acute hepatic failure is unknown, but it is clear that there is not a continuum between patients who show an elevation in serum liver enzymes and those who develop hepatic failure. Thus, routine monitoring of liver function will probably not prevent the latter complication.

Sedation due to VPA is rare and, when it occurs, is usually attributable to other, concurrently administered anticonvulsants. Episodes of stupor have also been encountered, almost invariably in children being treated for complex partial (psychomotor) seizures, either VPA exclusively or in combination with other anticonvulsants. Whether hyperammonemia has a role in the development of stupor is unclear. What has been amply demonstrated is that VPA elevates serum levels of some anticonvulsants, notably phenobarbital, ethosuximide, primidone, and carbamazepine. VPA lowers total phenytoin concentrations, but by displacing it from its plasma binding sites increases the proportion of free phenytoin; thus toxicity will be encountered at lower phenytoin levels. The combination of VPA and clonazepam results in strong hypnotic effects, and in some instances, induces absence states. These complex anticonvulsant drug interactions underline the advisability of monotherapy.

Tremor and, less commonly, asterixis have been encountered. It has been our experience and that of others that in most instances it is only seen at doses greater than 40 to 50 mg/kg/day, and is reduced if not cleared by dosage reduction. Asterixis is quite rare and is associated with polytherapy. A fall in platelet count, often transient, is dose related. It appears to be on an autoimmune basis, and generally is not sufficiently severe to require reduction or withdrawal of VPA. The thrombocytopenia may become aggravated with infections, and at such times may result in bruising or minor bleeding. Pancreatitis and hyperglycinemia are much rarer side reactions to VPA therapy.

Recent reports implicate VPA in the development of neural tube defects. Although these observations have yet to be confirmed, determinations of alpha-fetoprotein levels on pregnant women receiving VPA appear indicated.

Despite the variety of side reactions, VPA is an excellent anticonvulsant, not only because it provides better seizure control but also because it does so without sedating the child. Nevertheless, patients on this drug should be followed at 2 to 3 month intervals, and routine blood studies, liver function tests, and platelet counts should be obtained at every visit.

Clonazepam (Clonopin). Clonazepam, a benzodiazepine, is an effective anticonvulsant for most types of minor motor seizures. It is instituted in gradually increasing dosages, beginning at 0.05 mg/kg/24 hr in three or four divided doses, and increased by 0.05 mg/kg every fifth to seventh day until seizures are controlled or until a dose of 0.25 mg/kg/24 hr is reached. Thereafter, the dose is raised more slowly to 0.5 mg/kg/24 hr* if needed, or until side effects are encountered. These include ataxia, drowsiness, dysarthria, and excessive weight gain. The side effect we have found to be the most limiting is an alteration in the behavior of children receiving the drug. Hyperactivity, irritability, and belligerence are encountered in at least one third of children, and pre-existing emotional disturbances are often aggravated, particularly when clonazepam is administered in conjunction with barbiturates or other benzodiazepines.

Although seizure control is exceedingly good when clonazepam is first initiated, drug effectiveness is lost within a few weeks or months in about one third to one half of subjects.

Blood clonazepam levels are not readily available.

Clonazepam is most effective in akinetic seizures and in atypical petit mal. It is ineffective in infantile spasms.

Nitrazepam (Mogadon). Nitrazepam is a fairly useful drug for the treatment of all varieties of minor motor seizures. It is also the most effective drug

---

*This dose may exceed the manufacturer's recommended dosage.

in the treatment of infantile spasms. Since laboratory evidence of hepatotoxicity has been encountered in about half of subjects receiving the anticonvulsant, it has been kept off the U.S. market by the FDA. Currently, nitrazepam is readily available in Europe and Latin America.

Clorazepate (Tranxene) appears to be another potentially useful drug for the treatment of seizure disorders. At present, it appears to be most effective when given in conjunction with phenobarbital or other anticonvulsants. Strict advocates of monotherapy will therefore be reluctant to use the drug.

Other Anticonvulsants. Other anticonvulsants, notably mephenytoin (Mesantoin), phenacemide (Phenurone), acetazolamide (Diamox), paramethadione (Paradione), methsuximide (Celontin), and clorazepate (Tranxene), are less commonly used in the treatment of seizures. Blood level determinations are not readily available for any of these; therefore, starting and maximum dosages are presented in Table 3.

Ketogenic Diet. This diet involves restricting protein and carbohydrate intake and supplying 88 per cent of total caloric requirements in the form of fats. The mechanism by which this regimen controls convulsions is still unknown.

The diet is most effective in children between 2 and 5 years of age. Older children do not respond as well, in part because they fail to maintain an

Table 3. DOSAGES OF SOME LESS COMMONLY USED ANTIEPILEPTIC DRUGS

		Starting Dosage		Maximum Dosage	
	Age in Years	mg	Times/day	mg	Times/day
Bromides	Under 6	320	2	640	3
	Over 6	320	3	1000	3
Metharbital (Gemonil)	Under 6	50	3	100	3
	Over 6	100	3	200	3
Ethotoin (Peganone)	Under 6	250	3	750	4
	Over 6	500	3	1000	4
Dextroamphetamine (Dexedrine)	Under 6	2.5	1	2.5	3
	Over 6	2.5	2	7.5	3
Paramethadione (Paradione)	Under 6	150	2	300	3
	Over 6	300	2	600	3
Phensuximide (Milontin)	Under 6	250	2	500	3
	Over 6	500	2	1000	4
Methsuximide (Celontin)	Under 6	150	3	300	4
	Over 6	300	2	600	4
Acetazolamide (Diamox)	Under 6	125	3	250	3
	Over 6	250	2	250	4
Phenacemide (Phenurone)	Under 6	250	3	1000	3
	Over 6	500	3	2000	3
Clorazepate (Tranxene)*		7.5	3	—	—

*A specific anticonvulsant action of clorazepate has been questioned. This specific use is not listed by the manufacturer of Tranxene.

(From Menkes, J. H.: Textbook of Child Neurology, Philadelphia, Lea and Febiger, 1985, 3rd ed.)

adequate degree of ketosis. The best therapeutic results are seen in minor motor seizures, particularly in those unassociated with obvious organic pathology. Grand mal seizures and psychomotor attacks may also respond. Petit mal attacks are usually not influenced.

It is now our practice to reserve the ketogenic diet for children who have been unable to tolerate anticonvulsant drugs because of multiple allergies. A diet not as restricted in carbohydrate and protein and supplemented by the addition of medium-chain triglycerides is sometimes found more palatable.

In summarizing medical therapy for seizure disorders, we believe that the following are the most common mistakes incurred:

1. The physician fails to diagnose correctly the type of seizure experienced by the child, almost always because of an inadequate history.

2. Anticonvulsants are not given in sufficiently high dosage. No drug should be abandoned unless the physician is certain that it has no beneficial effect and toxic symptoms (verified, if possible, by blood level determinations) are encountered.

3. Too much reliance is placed on uncommonly used drugs in the hope that one of them will "turn off" the seizures.

4. Medications are altered too frequently, and the dosage of more than one drug is changed at the same time.

5. Blood anticonvulsant levels are not monitored.

6. The tendency for polytherapy to increase seizure frequency has been insufficiently appreciated. We have found that complete discontinuation of anticonvulsant medication may produce significant improvement in about a third of patients with intractable minor motor seizures, and we therefore advocate periodic withdrawal or reduction of anticonvulsants in patients whose seizures are poorly controlled.

Considerable controversy exists as to when, if ever, anticonvulsant therapy should be terminated. Because of their potentially serious long-term effects, we believe that anticonvulsants should be terminated as soon as feasible, and consider gradual reduction of medication after about 2 years of seizure control.

When anticonvulsants are discontinued after 4 years of seizure control, a relapse rate of approximately 30% is encountered. More than half of recurrences are seen during the first year following anticonvulsant withdrawal, and 85% by 5 years. Other studies have come up with a similar recurrence risk. As a rule, the earlier the onset of seizures, the more likely is relapse. Neither the sex of the patient nor the age when drugs are withdrawn affects the relapse rate. Children with neurologic dysfunction have a higher incidence of recurrence. The relapse rate is highest in children with simple partial (jacksonian) seizures (58%) and lowest in grand mal (14%) and absence (petit mal) seizures (12%). Whether the EEG is predictive of a relapse is still unresolved.

SURGICAL THERAPY

When drug therapy has been unsuccessful, and there is evidence for a single, distinct epileptic focus in a surgically removable area of the brain, excision of the involved tissue may be considered as a therapeutic approach.

The effectiveness of surgery is in direct proportion to the care in patient selection. The following steps should be followed prior to surgery:

1. Establish a diagnosis. As indicated, this requires a careful history and physical examination. Patients with subnormal intelligence usually are unsuitable for surgical ablations.

2. Rule out a structural lesion. A CT scan is the most suitable radiologic procedure. Preliminary studies to seek evidence of a focal lesion include standard ictal and interictal EEG's.

3. Trial of anticonvulsant therapy over the course of at least 2 years. This implies the use of the proper drug, and documenting patient compliance and adequacy of anticonvulsant blood levels.

4. If drug therapy is unsuccessful, the patient is hospitalized, serial EEG's are performed, as is telemetry monitoring and, if available, a PET scan.

5. If these studies do not reveal a focus, or if multiple foci are uncovered, chronic recordings from stereotactically implanted depth electrodes may be desired. These can localize the site of the earliest ictal discharge with far greater accuracy than is possible with scalp recordings, and complement the localization derived from the PET scan.

6. If a single focus is established, lateralization of cerebral dominance may be established by intracarotid injection of sodium amytal (Wada test).

In patients with intractable complex partial seizures, surgery consists of removal of the anterior portion of the temporal lobe, usually 4 to 5 cm of the dominant lobe, or 6 to 7 cm when the epileptic focus is on the nondominant side. Anticonvulsants are continued for at least 2 years.

TREATMENT OF SPECIAL SEIZURE CONDITIONS

Mixed Seizure Forms. As a rule, children presenting a mixed seizure disorder are difficult to handle. With a combination of grand mal and minor motor seizures, the most commonly encountered mixed seizure disorder, valproic acid is the best starting drug. Often a combination of two anticonvulsants will be necessary. Under no circumstances, however, should both be started concurrently. In our experience, the combination of carbamazepine and valproic acid is exceptionally good, as is phenobarbital and ethosuximide.

Infantile Spasms. This topic is discussed in a separate article in this section.

Status Epilepticus. There are four sequential aspects to the management of this patient: maintenance of vital functions, drug therapy to control convulsions, assigning a cause for the condition, and, lastly, prevention of further convulsions.

The physician treating a child in status epilepticus should act promptly to maintain an adequate airway, prevent aspiration of mucus, and secure the child from injury induced by the violence of the convulsive movements. Hyperthermia, hypoxia, and hypotension must also be corrected.

The most favored current mode of therapy is diazepam (Valium). The drug is best administered intravenously at a dosage of 0.3 mg/kg to 1 mg/kg, at a rate of 1 mg/minute. Rectal diazepam, by means of a rubber tube inserted 4 to 5 cm beyond the anus, is a simple and safe means of controlling prolonged grand-mal seizures. Considerable individual variability in the amount of the drug required for seizure control is apparent. The principal advantages of diazepam are rapid effectiveness, margin of safety, and its ability to control seizures of cortical as well as centrencephalic origin. The principal side effects is respiratory depression, most likely to occur in patients receiving a combination of drugs, particularly diazepam and phenobarbital. Hypotension is also encountered with this combination. Another drawback is that redistribution of diazepam within the body terminates the anticonvulsant effects within 30 to 60 minutes.

The escape from diazepam may require a repeat dosage, or can be prevented by the concurrent administration of intravenous phenytoin (20 to 30 mg/kg). Phenytoin enters the brain more rapidly than phenobarbital but not as rapidly as diazepam. Once phenytoin has controlled seizures, the likelihood of immediate recurrence is small. The drug is generally preferred for patients with status epilepticus following a head injury, in whom preservation of consciousness is desirable. Phenytoin should not be administered intramuscularly, since it is absorbed too slowly to result in effective anticonvulsant serum and tissue levels.

Another means of controlling status epilepticus is with sodium phenobarbital. The initial dose of 10 mg/kg is administered intravenously, intramuscularly, or even subcutaneously. Since the drug requires 15 minutes to penetrate the blood-brain barrier, regardless of its mode of administration, the rate at which seizures are controlled by this means is slower than with diazepam. If seizures continue for 20 or 30 more minutes, a second dose of phenobarbital (10 mg/kg) is given.

Intravenous phenobarbital can also be used as an adjunct to diazepam, if the latter has failed to control seizures within 15 to 40 minutes following its administration. If phenobarbital is to be used as a backup to diazepam, the child will first need to be intubated. Paraldehyde can be used as an adjunct to the treatment of status epilepticus when phenobarbital has been the drug of choice. It is given by muscular injection within 15 to 30 minutes of the administration of phenobarbital, in a dosage of 1 ml per year of age, not exceeding a total dosage of 0.35 ml/kg or 5 ml for a single injection site.

Lorazepam (4 mg IV in large children) has recently proven extremely useful in the control of status epilepticus. There has not been much experience with the drug. It is, however, becoming clear that it has advantages over both diazepam and phenobarbital. The anticonvulsant effect becomes apparent within 5 minutes or less after injection, but because of a half-life that is significantly longer than diazepam, repeated injections are generally unnecessary. Lorazepam could become the drug of choice for the treatment of status epilepticus.

In some instances convulsions remain refractory to the above drugs. This is of grave import and requires extreme measures. When brain edema is suspected, as when status epilepticus follows a head injury, steroids or antiedematous agents should be given. In other instances, one may have to resort to generalized anesthesia, curarizing the patient to reduce hyperthermia and hypoxia. Although it is always advantageous to monitor the electrical activity of the brain whenever a patient is in status epilepticus, this measure becomes mandatory in the child with refractory status.

Whatever the means of treatment, the physician must keep several principles in mind:

1. The intravenous route is the preferred way to administer anticonvulsants.

2. The most common mistake is to give repeated yet insufficient doses of anticonvulsants.

3. With the exception of the combination of phenobarbital and paraldehyde, the physician should avoid using more than one anticonvulsant drug.

Following termination of status epilepticus, the patient is continued on intramuscular anticonvulsant therapy, usually sodium phenobarbital (4 to 6 mg/kg/24 hr), until consciousness returns. Oral medication is then resumed. Plasma levels should be assessed at least daily for the first 5 to 10 days, the time required to reach a steady-state equilibrium. Diazepam should not be used for seizure control after the first 24 to 48 hours.

FEBRILE CONVULSIONS

The treatment of the febrile convulsion consists of controlling the convulsion itself by sodium phenobarbital or diazepam in dosages analogous to those recommended for the treatment of status epilepticus, reducing body temperature by conductive or evaporative cooling of the child, and treating the acute infection responsible for the fever.

Whether the infant who has just suffered his first febrile convulsion should undergo lumbar puncture has been a matter of debate. We believe that it is best to err on the side of safety and to perform the procedure.

There also is considerable controversy as to whether a child who has experienced his or her first febrile convulsion should receive continuous prophylactic anticonvulsant therapy. Controlled prospective studies suggest that the incidence of recurrent febrile convulsions is not significantly less in patients who have been placed on phenobarbital to be given at the onset of fever than in those who receive no medication. Although a number of anticonvulsants, notably valproate, have been used overseas for this purpose, phenobarbital given daily in dosages adequate to yield blood levels of 15 μg/ml or above is effective in preventing recurrences of febrile convulsions. However, behavior disorders are common in children who receive long-term phenobarbital, particularly when there has been an antecedent history for these. Hyperkinesis and distractibility are often sufficiently severe to require discontinuation of the prophylactic medication.

In reconciling the various viewpoints with respect to prophylactic therapy of a child following the first febrile convulsion, we suggest that patients be treated who have one or more of the following risk factors:

1. Antecedent neurologic or developmental abnormality.
2. Severe febrile seizures (generalized or focal convulsions of longer than 15 minutes' duration or more than one seizure per 24 hours).
3. Onset of febrile convulsions prior to 1 year of age.
4. Multiple recurrences of febrile convulsions.
5. A positive family history of epilepsy.

Children who have none of these risk factors need not be treated with continuous prophylactic anticonvulsants until a second or third seizure has occurred. If treatment is decided upon, in all instances blood barbiturate levels must be monitored.

NEONATAL CONVULSIONS

Phenobarbital is the best anticonvulsant for use during the neonatal period. The drug is administered in an intramuscular loading dose of 15 to 20 mg/kg. Peak concentrations are reached within 1.5 to 6 hours, and maintenance doses of 3–4 mg/kg/day, generally given orally, are deferred until the blood barbiturate level falls below 15 to 20 μg/ml. Because of the very long half-life of the drug in the neonate, this usually does not occur until 5 to 7 days following the loading dose.

These drug schedules are irrespective of gestational age. Nevertheless, it is imperative that for optimal seizure control, daily or twice daily barbiturate levels be secured.

We have not had much success in the control of neonatal convulsions using oral or parenteral phenytoin. As a rule, the relation between drug dosage and serum levels is unpredictable, and there is a high incidence of toxic reactions, probably because of the immaturity of the hepatic hydroxylating system responsible for phenytoin detoxication. The drug is administered orally or parenterally in doses of 5 to 15 mg/kg/day.

Diazepam has also been suggested as an anticonvulsant in the newborn infant. This drug, in our experience and that of others, is no better than phenobarbital for the treatment of neonatal seizures. On the other hand, its short duration of action makes it a poor drug for maintenance. Furthermore, we have found that whenever seizures are not controlled by phenobarbital, they are usually poorly controlled by other drugs.

THE EPILEPTIC CHILD AND HIS WORLD

The physician who treats the child with epilepsy is dealing with a chronic, often life-long condition, which profoundly affects the way the child is viewed by the family, peers, the school, and, most importantly, the self.

The best antidote to the feelings of anger and depression evoked by the diagnosis of epilepsy is a frank, unhurried discussion by doctor, parents, and child of the various problems likely to be encountered. The epileptic child will feel different from peers regardless of what is being said and done. However, the feeling of having been singled out can be minimized by insisting that the child participate in all normal activities, including sports. The hyperventilation incurred in the more strenuous athletics is not of the degree to induce seizures. However, the more hazardous contact sports, such as high school football, are best avoided as they should be for nonepileptic youngsters, and swimming should be done under competent adult supervision.

There is no reason why the youngster with epilepsy should not obtain a driver's license. However, the ingestion of alcoholic beverages is contraindicated.

Febrile Convulsions

EDWARD F. RABE, M.D.

Febrile convulsions occur in infants or children with fever due to an infection in any organ or tissue except the brain or meninges. They occur commonly between the ages of 6 months and 5 years, with a peak incidence at 23 months. It is estimated that between 3 and 4% of children 5 years of age and under have had febrile seizures. Twenty per cent of the siblings or parents have also had febrile seizures.

One third of patients who have had febrile convulsions will have at least one recurrence. The recurrence rate is mainly affected by the age at onset; thus, if the first febrile seizure occurs before 13 months of age, there is a 2.3:1 chance of recurrence; if between 14 and 32 months, a 1:2 chance of recurrence; and if after 32 months, a 1:5 chance of recurrence. It is equally important to know that one third of recurrences appear within 6 months of the first seizure, one half within 13 months, and 88% within 30 months.

The complications most commonly noted are epilepsy, mental retardation, and permanent motor and coordination defects. Death from febrile convulsions occurs only when status epilepticus (seizures lasting more than one hour, or repeated seizures without regaining consciousness between them for more than one hour) complicates the convulsions. Incidence of most of these complications is not definitely known, but they occur more frequently in children with a complicated perinatal course, onset of febrile convulsions before 13 months of age, or in those with an abnormal neurological or developmental status before the first febrile convulsion.

Epilepsy occurs in 2 to 3% of children with febrile convulsions. This is four times the incidence in other children but epilepsy does not occur equally in all children who have had febrile convulsions. Rather, it occurs more frequently in those with certain "high risk factors." These are a family history of afebrile seizures, occurrence of more than one febrile convulsion in the first 24 hours of the febrile illness, or the febrile convulsion being complex, i.e., it was focal, it lasted more than 15 minutes, or the patient had abnormal neurologic or developmental status before the seizure. If two of these factors occur there is a 13% incidence of epilepsy in such children before 7 years of age. Other factors that are reported to cause an increased likelihood of significant sequelae are severe febrile convulsion (more than 30 minutes in length) and multiple febrile convulsions.

Infants and children with febrile convulsions of any duration need systematic medical evaluation. This includes a history and a physical and neurological examination. Infants less than 2 years of age, or any child in whom the cause of fever is not apparent, should have a lumbar puncture. There are rare clinical exceptions. Other laboratory tests may be obtained if deemed appropriate, but none of the "routine tests" in these children have provided evidence not suspected clinically.

The usefulness of the EEG in these children is moot. In a single, widely accepted study on this subject, children with febrile convulsions who developed recurrent afebrile seizures (epilepsy) developed epileptiform EEG tracings *after* the clinical epilepsy. More information is needed.

Children who have had febrile convulsions are treated to prevent recurrence, and by so doing prevent prolonged seizures, recurrent multiple seizures, development of mental retardation or learning disorders, epilepsy, and other chronic debilitating neurological sequelae. In truth, the only proved value of appropriate chronic medication is that it prevents the occurrence of febrile convulsions. The previously cited data imply that more is accomplished by preventing these convulsions and their concurrent sequelae, but this is not proved.

Who should receive chronic anticonvulsant medication to prevent recurrence? Simple, brief febrile convulsions in infants and children over 18 months of age seem to be benign. Since febrile convulsions may appear with the onset of a febrile illness, only chronic ongoing medication would be effective. Based upon the foregoing information, infants and children who have had one febrile convulsion, and any of the following, appear to deserve chronic anticonvulsant medication: infants under 15 to 18 months of age; patients who have had a complex seizure; patients who are neurologically or developmentally abnormal; patients who are neurologically normal but have a family history of afebrile seizures; and patients who are normal but have had two febrile convulsions.

Management is concerned with treatment of the acute convulsion followed by treatment of the potential chronic state, i.e., prevention of recurrent febrile seizures in those who are at high risk for complications. Simple febrile convulsions are usually terminated spontaneously within a few to 15 minutes. Although convulsions longer than 15 minutes have been shown in one study to be almost devoid of serious sequelae, many other reports state that prolonged febrile convulsions are the ones most frequently followed by serious sequelae. It is prudent, then, to treat patients whose seizures have lasted more than 15 minutes, both to stop the seizure and then to prevent recurrent convulsions. A patient with a febrile convulsion lasting more than 15 minutes should receive an anticonvulsant to stop the seizure. Several options exist. They are as follows:

1. *Sodium phenobarbital,* 10 mg/kg IV or IM (250 mg/m^2 in patients weighing more than 25 kg). An IV dose will produce a rapidly attained level, while an IM dose will take from 30 to 90 minutes to reach a therapeutic plateau. The latter route will prevent a recurrent convulsion, but will not quickly terminate an ongoing status epilepticus. The IV dose may be repeated at 15 to 20 minute intervals up to three doses, if needed to stop the convulsions.

2. *Diazepam,* 0.2 mg/kg IV (never IM), not to exceed 5 mg in a patient weighing 25 kg or 10 mg in a patient weighing 50 kg or more. The dose should be given slowly, never diluted. The dose may be repeated every 15 minutes, if needed, up to two or as many as four times.

3. *Phenytoin,* intravenously, 14 mg/kg, at a rate

not to exceed 50 mg/min. Blood pressure and cardiac rhythm should be monitored during administration. Rarely, IV phenytoin produces hypotension, which is the result of a high level secondary to too rapid administration. Phenytoin should never be given IM, since it is painful and the absorption from this site is inconstant. If the seizure is not stopped by the IV dose within 20 minutes, another anticonvulsant may have to be used.

4. *Lorazepam,** a recently issued anticonvulsant, is not available for general use. In doses of 0.05 mg/kg, given IV slowly, it promises to be less toxic and have a much longer t½ than its benzodiazepine predecessor, diazepam.

The need to treat a prolonged seizure in a patient with febrile convulsions indicates that this is a complex seizure and the patient requires chronic medication. Whatever drug is thereafter used, the necessity to reach a therapeutic plateau level quickly must be recognized and an appropriate dose and route should be used to prevent rapid recurrence of febrile seizures.

Chronic anticonvulsant medication, such as phenobarbital, valproic acid, or rectal diazepam, is given to prevent recurrent febrile convulsions. Rectal suppositories of diazepam are not available in the United States, and since one report of its use abroad noted poor compliance by parents, this is a poor option for treatment. Valproic acid in a minimum of two divided doses daily and in amounts from 30 to 60 mg/kg/day, aiming at a serum level between 50 and 100 μg/ml, has been comparable in effectiveness to phenobarbital. However, with its tendency to produce as many early side effects as phenobarbital, and its proclivity to produce hepatic toxicity, with death, and with no satisfactory indicators to predict these serious side effects, advocacy for this therapy has not grown rapidly. Phenobarbital is the most commonly used anticonvulsant to prevent recurrent febrile seizures. It is given in two or rarely three divided doses and in amounts to produce a serum level between 15 and 21 μg/ml (4 to 6 mg/kg/day). Chronic treatment has produced hyperactivity and poor sleeping in from 10 to 20% of children, with a tendency to note these effects as an exaggeration of pretreatment personality. There is no convincing evidence that phenobarbital produces adverse effects on intellectual development or school performance in children. Studies of adverse effects of phenobarbital upon the behavior and development of experimental animals are not directly applicable to children.

Whatever anticonvulsant is used to prevent recurrent febrile convulsions, it should be given for at least 2½ asymptomatic years. At the end of this interval, medication, especially phenobarbital,

*Lorazepan (Ativan is available in the U.S. but use as an anticonvulsant is not listed by the manufacturer.

should be gradually discontinued over a period of 4–6 weeks.

If, during the period of chronic treatment, the patient does not tolerate phenobarbital, and valproic acid is either not tolerated or deemed unacceptable, are there other drugs to use? Dilantin may be considered. It has been shown to decrease the severity of febrile convulsions in young children and possibly prevent them in children over 3 years of age. Its use needs further evaluation. Primidone may be considered, since it is metabolized to phenobarbital and one other effective anticonvulsant metabolite. One should measure and obtain appropriate phenobarbital serum levels when using primidone. A better tolerance to primidone than to phenobarbital alone has been suggested by some, but this has not been proven.

Infantile Spasms

WILLIAM SINGER, M.D.

Infantile spasms usually begin within the first year of life (peak incidence between 4 and 8 months) with occasional cases reported to begin as late as 2 years. The seizures consist of brief spasms of the neck, trunk, or extremities, in flexion or extension, or, most commonly, as a combination of the two. Spasms are usually bilaterally symmetrical, but some children may have asymmetrical movements. They may occur as single spasms or as a series of rapidly recurring spasms lasting up to several minutes. Preceding or following the spasms, the child may cry out as if in pain, leading to a misdiagnosis of colic attacks. Accompanying the spasms is a characteristic electroencephalographic pattern of hypsarrhythmia. EEG's should be performed in awake, drowsy, and sleep states, as the features of hypsarrhythmia may only be seen in the latter two states.

Up to 80% of these children exhibit signs of mental retardation and/or motor abnormalities resulting from intrauterine or perinatal insults, CNS infections, or have inherited disorders affecting the brain (e.g., tuberous sclerosis, Down syndrome). Up to 50% of the children who have normal clinical examinations and normal development until spasms begin will on CT scan of the head have structural abnormalities consistent with a preceding neurologic insult (e.g., atrophy, porencephaly) or malformations (e.g., agenesis of the corpus callosum). Therefore, only 10% will be free of preexisting neurologic abnormalities associated with infantile spasms. Thus, infantile spasms can be thought of as the response of an immature brain to a variety of insults.

Only ACTH and corticosteroids have been

shown to have a significant effect on these seziures. Comparisons of these two agents suggest that ACTH may be more effective. Treatment with benzodiazepines (clonazepam and nitrazepam), valproic acid, and the ketogenic diet has produced variable, but generally poor, seizure control. Conventional anticonvulsants such as phenobarbital and phenytoin have been ineffective.

Various regimens using ACTH have been advocated. Using the following treatment plan, up to 87% of children will be brought under complete control. Initial treatment consists of intramuscular aqueous ACTH, 40 units once daily. During this time, the parents are taught to administer intramuscular medication. Upon discharge from the hospital, longer acting ACTH gel is given in a dose of 80 units every other day. This dose is maintained for a minimum of 3 months or for 1 month after complete spasm control is achieved. Since 60% of patients will show complete spasm control by the end of 1 month of treatment, 71% after 3 months, and 87% after 6 months, short treatment courses of ACTH may fail to control a significant percentage of children whose spasms will be responsive if treatment is carried out for a longer period. Therefore, treatment at initial dosages should be carried out for 3 months, and preferably 6 months, before it is deemed unsuccessful. The ACTH dosage is then gradually taped by 20 units at monthly intervals. The change at 20 units q.o.d. is to 10 units q.o.d. for 1 month, then 5 units q.o.d. for 1 month, then the ACTH is discontinued. If spasms recur, the ACTH dose should be raised to 80 units q.o.d. until spasms are controlled for 1 month before restarting the tapering. Since transient hypocortisolism has been reported, those children who become ill during the first month after ACTH is discontinued should receive supplementary corticosteroids.

If no response to this regimen occurs, treatment with clonazepam, nitrazepam, valproic acid, or the ketogenic diet should be considered, but such treatment is unlikely to alter the natural history of the spasms.

Early diagnosis and treatment are significant determinants of outcome, as up to 85% of patients treated within 1 month of spasm onset will be free of spasms, compared to less than 60% of patients treated after 1 month of spasm onset. The recurrence rates are 3% and 21% for the respective treatment groups.

Thirty per cent of patients will have seizures predating the onset of infantile spasms. These seizures will not be affected by ACTH; therefore, previously prescribed anticonvulsants should be continued. Twenty-five to 30% of patients will develop additional types of seizures after spasms begin. These should be treated with anticonvulsants. (See section on seizures/epilepsy).

The developmental outcome for children with infantile spasms is not affected by treatment with ACTH. In our experience, no child who was even mildly retarded at the time treatment was begun improved to the point to be considered normal at long-term follow-up. Even among children whose development was normal at the time of diagnosis, only 50% will have normal intellectual levels after followup of 5 years or more. In this group, abnormalities on CT scan (e.g., atrophy, porencephaly, congenital malformation) generally indicated a poor developmental prognosis, in spite of rapid and complete spasm control.

In our experience, clinical signs of hypercortisolism, (cushingoid facies, acneiform eruptions, etc) were the most frequent side effects of ACTH therapy, occurring in over 50% of patients. Although hypertension occurred in one half of cases, none became symptomatic. In all instances, these manifestations of hypercortisolism, including hypertension, resolved as ACTH was tapered. Long-term follow-up of patients revealed none to be hypertensive.

Electrolyte imbalance, congestive heart and impaired immunologic responses are reportedly rare.

Spasmus Nutans

WILLIAM D. SINGER, M.D.

This unusual benign condition begins between 3 and 12 months of age and is characterized by head nodding, nystagmus, and head tilt. Unexplainedly, it begins most frequently during winter months. It is a self-limited disorder with spontaneous remission occurring 4 to 36 months after onset. There is no sex preference. The reported incidence is declining, making this a rare disorder.

Head nodding, often the first symptom noted, may be intermittent or constant and may be either from side to side or forward to back. The nodding is not compensatory for nystagmus. It is accentuated when the child is upright and during ocular fixation, decreasing when supine, and disappearing during sleep. Nystagmus, when present, may be unilateral or bilateral but is more marked in one eye. The movements are rapid and of small amplitude, horizontal, vertical, rotatory or pendular in character. Combinations of these movements may be seen. The abnormal eye movements disappear when the eyes are covered and during sleep. Head tilt is the least constant finding, occurring in approximately one third of cases.

The diagnosis of spasmus nutans should be reserved for children who are neurologically normal and have no structural or functional abnormality of the eyes. It may be differentiated from the bilateral searching nystagmus associated with marked visual impairment and congenital nystagmus. The latter two are bilateral and do not disappear with advancing age. Congenital nystagmus may be accompanied by head nodding compensating for the abnormal eye movements. The head tilt must be distinguished from that associated with structural abnormalities of the neck, cerebellar hemisphere tumors, and abnormalities of extraocular muscles with malalignment of the eyes.

Computed tomography of the head should be performed because of the occurrence of symptoms resembling spasmus nutans associated with optic gliomas and frontal lobe tumors.

No treatment is necessary for this self-limited disorder.

Headache

PETER R. HUTTENLOCHER, M.D.

Headache is a common symptom in a large variety of illnesses, especially when there is increase in intracranial pressure, hypertension, fever, or nasal sinus involvement. This discussion is limited to the management of chronic, recurrent headache in the child who is free of such underlying medical illnesses. Often, recurrent headache in the otherwise well child can be classified in one of the following categories: 1) migraine; 2) tension (muscle contraction) headache; 3) headache as a manifestation of psychiatric illness. However, there is a group of residual cases which cannot be easily assigned to any one group. Exact diagnostic criteria are lacking.

Migraine. This is a common cause of vascular (throbbing or pounding) headache in childhood. Attacks may recur several times weekly or they may be rare with many symptom-free months. The head pain typically is unilateral, associated with nausea and often with vomiting. There may be a prodrome or aura consisting of visual phenomena (scintillating lights or scotomata, hemianopsia, or total obscuration of vision), vertigo, and rarely other transient neurologic manifestations such as oculomotor palsy ("ophthalmoplegic migraine"), hemiparesis, numbness, or aphasia.

The management of migraine should include a detailed discussion of the problem with the parents and child. This should include mention of the benign nature of the condition and of its tendency to improve with age. It also must be emphasized that there is no evidence of a causal relationship between psychiatric disorders and migraine. It may be helpful to point out that migraine tends to occur on a familial basis, suggesting a genetically determined susceptibility. Reassurance that there is no serious, life-threatening illness may be of greater benefit than medications. Follow-up studies indicate that childhood migraine often improves after initial medical consultation, no matter what medication is prescribed.

Drug Therapy. A simple analgesic such as acetylsalicylic acid should be tried first (60 mg per year of age up to 900 mg at the onset of an attack and repeated in 6 hours if needed). The following agents may also be useful when administered at the first sign of an attack:

Cafergot (1 mg ergotamine tartrate plus 100 mg caffeine). One tablet is given at the onset, followed by a second tablet 1 hour later if needed. This drug should be used only in children over age 12 years.

Fiorinal (50 mg butalbital, 200 mg acetylsalicylic acid, 130 mg phenacetin, 40 mg caffeine) is given as a single tablet at the onset of an attack. Fiorinal has been established to be safe only in children age 12 years or above.

Continuous (prophylactic) therapy with phenobarbital may be indicated in the young child, especially when attacks are frequent and incapacitating, as in migraine complicated by transient neurologic impairment. Up to 3 mg/kg/day are given in a single daily dosage or in two divided doses. Treatment is continued until the patient has been free of severe attacks for 3 to 6 months, and the medication is then tapered over a period of 2 to 4 weeks. Phenobarbital administered at this dosage is well tolerated by children, except for rare allergic reactions and occasional subtle effects on attention span and on school learning.

Prophylactic therapy with propranolol, a beta-adrenergic blocking agent, has also been reported to be effective in childhood migraine. The usual starting dosage in a child over 10 years of age is 10 mg t i d; this may be increased up to 20 mg q i d if the lower dosage fails to provide relief. The drug is contraindicated if there is a history of bronchial asthma. It should not be used in conjunction with psychotropic drugs. The occurrence of postural hypotension is indication for reduction in dosage.

Cyproheptadine hydrochloride (Periactin) has been reported to be an effective agent in adults with migraine. Its effectiveness in childhood migraine is not yet established.

Drugs to be avoided include narcotics, phenothiazine antiemetics, and the serotonin antagonist methysergide. The risks of these medications outweigh any benefit that might be derived from the control of migraine symptoms. Desensitization injections are of no proven value. Both migraine and allergies are common conditions and therefore may occur simultaneously in the same patient, but there is no proof of a cause-effect relationship. Special diets are of no proven value. However, the child should be encouraged to eat regular meals. Prolonged fasting may trigger an attack in some patients.

Tension Headache. Tension headache or muscle contraction headache may occur in the school-age child or adolescent. The headache has a gradual onset during the day, usually reaching its peak by afternoon or evening. It is rarely severe and is described as a steady, dull ache over the occiput, neck, or temples. The aura and nausea characteristic of migraine are absent. Treatment is directed toward identification of factors in the environment that may be stressful to the child. School failure, peer pressures, and family discord are common factors underlying this symptom in the pediatric age group. Drug therapy should be limited to the use of simple analgesic agents such as acetylsalicylic acid, 60 mg per year of age up to 900 mg, repeated in 6 hours if needed. Drugs with muscle-relaxing and tranquillizing actions such as diazepam are often effective, but their chronic use should be avoided.

Headache as a Manifestation of Psychiatric Illness. Headache may be the major manifestation in hysteria or conversion reaction. It may also be a prominent symptom in the child or adolescent with depressive illness. The head pain in hysteria is often bizarre and it is always described as being extremely severe and incapacitating. For example, the patient may describe a sensation that the head is exploding. In the depressed child, the headache tends to be continuous; associated symptoms include withdrawal from peers, school, and other activities. Marked incapacitation in the absence of any objective findings is characteristic of both syndromes. These children often have histories of prolonged absences from school. Major recent family discord such as impending divorce or separation is a frequent factor, especially in the child with hysteria. Early recognition is important, since it may prevent extensive and unnecessary medical and neurologic studies. Proper management usually involves psychiatric referral and family therapy. Drugs other than simple analgesics such as acetylsalicylic acid should be avoided. In particular, the use of narcotics is strictly contraindicated. Antidepressant agents such as amitriptylene, up to 50 mg daily, may be useful in the adolescent with headache due to depressive illness when used in conjunction with psychotherapy.

Guillain-Barré Syndrome

JOHN W. BENTON, M.D.

Guillain-Barré syndrome (GBS) is progressive weakness that usually appears a few days after a mild nonspecific infection. The weakness progresses symmetrically from distal to central muscle groups. Sensory abnormalities are frequent and variable in clinical severity.

Epstein-Barr, influenzae A and B, and cytomegalovirus infections are common antecedents. Although the diagnosis is usually obvious, other possible causes of acute progressive neuropathy must be excluded by appropriate testing.

Treatment. Therapy is symptomatic and rehabilitative. Potential paralysis of respiratory muscles must be considered in each patient. The onset of dyspnea or weakness in muscles of the shoulder requires immediate preparation for respirator support. Serial vital capacity measurements are of value in following progress of muscles affecting respiration. A nasotracheal tube or tracheostomy should be placed under controlled conditions in patients who will require ventilator support.

The role of corticosteroids in therapy is still unclear. At present, steroids should be reserved for the rare patient with recurrent GBS. Inconsistent responses have been reported following plasmapheresis, and its role in therapy requires further investigation.

Involvement of the autonomic nervous system may lead to unstable blood pressure and heart rates. Antihypertensive or vasopressor drugs may be required to maintain normal blood pressure. If so, the response to medication must be closely monitored because of unpredictable and exaggerated reactions to small doses of vasoactive drugs.

Attention must be given to the nutritional requirements of each patient. Bladder and bowel functions are usually spared, but should be closely monitored in the acute phase.

Recovery progresses at variable rates and is not related to disease severity. Physical therapy including active and passive exercises are important until recovery is ensured. In all phases of the illness, attention to psychological factors should be monitored. The prognosis for recovery is excellent in the pediatric patient with GBS who receives good supportive care.

Chronic Relapsing Polyneuropathy

GUY M. McKHANN, M.D.

Chronic relapsing polyneuropathy may present much in the same way as Guillain-Barré syndrome but it usually is more insidious in onset. Patients are similar to patients with acute Guillain-Barré disease in that sensory findings are minimal and motor weakness is marked. The disease is usually quite symmetrical, beginning in the lower extremities and then moving upward. There are often spontaneous relapses and remissions, the relapses lasting many weeks.

Unlike patients with acute Guillain-Barré syndrome, patients with chronic relapsing polyneuropathy often will respond to steroid administration. The problem, however, is in finding a way to wean them from the steroids. In young children, the rate of complications related to steroids has led to the utilization of other therapeutic approaches.

We have had some success with plasmapheresis in therapy of chronic relapsing polyneuropathy patients, but the number of these patients is not large and it is still too soon to tell whether this willl be effective treatment. In other instances we have used more potent forms of immunosuppression such as cyclophosphamide* (Cytoxan) or azathioprine* (Imuran). The doses we use are similar to those used for other forms of immunosuppression, that is, doses required to keep the white blood cell count down around 1000 to 1500. Obviously, one uses these forms of therapy only as a last resort in these cases. The cases of chronic relapsing polyneuropathy are relatively rare and it is not clear whether they are a variant of acute Guillain-Barré syndrome or actually represent a more distinct entity.

Familial Dysautonomia

FELICIA B. AXELROD, M.D.

Many of the clinical manifestations of familial dysautonomia are caused by a deficit in autonomic homeostatic function and sensory appreciation of peripheral pain and temperature. Both deficiencies can be accounted for by the decreased number of unmyelinated neurons noted in sural nerve biopsies and autopsies. Prominent early manifestations include feeding difficulties, hypotonia, delayed developmental milestones, labile body temperature and blood pressure, absence of overflowing tears and corneal anesthesia, marked diaphoresis with excitement, recurrent aspiration pneumonia, breath-holding episodes, ataxia, spinal curvature, and intractable vomiting.

Treatment is directed to specific symptoms and complications.

FEEDING

Breastfeeding is usually impossible owing to the infant's poor suck, uncoordinated swallow, and misdirection of liquids. Experimentation with different nipples and thickening feedings should be tried before deciding to eliminate oral liquids completely from the infant's diet. For infants completely unable to suck and thus unable to maintain hydration, gavage feedings are used as a temporary measure. If the infant accepts spoon feedings well, the gavage feedings can be discontinued. However, if the problem persists, a gastrostomy is indicated to maintain nutrition and avoid dehydration and prevent aspiration.

FEVERS

Labile body temperatures result in brief episodic fevers in response to dehydration, mucus plugs in the bronchi, excessive external temperature, and even stress. Fever often is accompanied by shaking chills, cold extremities, and lack of sweating. Antipyretics may not suffice. Cool extremities should be massaged while cooling the trunk by sponging or even with a hypothermic mattress.

A muscle relaxant often is helpful in reducing anxiety and muscular spasms during hyperpyrexia. Diazepam** (0.1 mg/kg/dose) or chlorpromazine (0.5 mg/kg/dose) has been found effective.

A persistent fever lasting more than 24 hours requires a search for a source of infection.

VOMITING

Dysautonomic patients have abnormal gastrointestinal motility patterns, making them prone to vomiting. Vomiting occurs intermittently in some patients as part of a systemic reaction to infection or stress. In another group of patients (40 per cent), vomiting assumes a cyclical pattern. These vomiting crises often are associated with hypertension, tachycardia, diffuse sweating, personality changes, and, occasionally, hyperpyrexia. The cyclical pattern can be quite marked and is usually characteristic for that patient. The vomiting may occur once a month or even once a week. The crises can last from 3 to 72 hours and can lead to severe dehydration. Aspiration is an ever-present risk.

Management has five goals: (1) maintenance of adequate hydration; (2) relief of gastric distention to prevent gastroesophageal reflux and aspiration; (3) cessation of clinical vomiting with antiemetics; (4) relief of hypertension; and (5) induction of sleep, which seem to be necessary for resolution of the crisis. Despite the loss of copious amounts of gastric fluid, the dehydration is characteristically isotonic. A volume expander, such as Ringer lactate, should be given rapidly upon hospital admission at 10 ml/kg for mild dehydration and 20 ml/kg for severe dehydration. Maintenance and calculated rehydration are given with a solution of one-third normal saline in 5 per cent glucose. Dehydration is best estimated on the basis of weight change. A nasogastric tube should be placed and set on low intermittent suction and continued until the vital signs are stable and nausea has abated.

---

*This use of cyclophosphamide and azathioprine is not listed by the manufacturer.

**Manufacturer's Precaution: Oral diazepam is not for use in infants under 6 months of age. IV diazepam is not for use in the neonate.

Diazepam is now considered to be an effective antiemetic for the dysautonomic vomiting crisis. The initial dose is 0.1 to 0.2 mg/kg/dose IV. The dose should be effective in normalizing the blood pressure and producing sleep. *If hypertension is still present 15 minutes after the diazepam,* then chlorpromazine, 0.5 to 1 mg/kg, IM or by rectal suppository should be given. If hypertension is not present but the patient is not sleeping, then chloral hydrate, 30 mg/kg, can be given as a rectal suppository. Subsequent doses of diazepam are repeated at 3-hour intervals until the crisis resolves. Chlorpromazine and chloral hydrate can be repeated at 6-hour intervals. Frequent monitoring of blood pressure is indicated, because the choice of subsequent antiemetics will be influenced by the absence or presence of hypertension. Cimetidine (20 mg/kg/24 hr) IV is a useful adjunct in reducing emesis volume. The crisis usually resolves abruptly and is marked by normalization of personality and return of appetite. At this point the patient may be allowed to resume a normal diet.

PNEUMONIA

Recurrent pneumonias are frequent. Repeated aspiration is probably the major factor in causing pulmonary disease, with most of the damage to the lung occurring during infancy and early childhood. Gastroesophageal reflux also may be a contributing factor. The signs of pneumonia may be subtle. Cough is not consistently present and is rarely productive. The child is more likely to vomit increased pulmonary secretions. Tachypnea is generally not evident and auscultation may be unrevealing because of decreased chest excursion. Radiographic examination is often necessary for diagnosis. Pathogens cultured from tracheal aspirations are often uncommon agents, such as *Escherichia coli, S. proteus,* or *Serratia.* Broad-spectrum antibiotics should be used until bacteriologic study permits more specific therapy. In the seriously ill child, blood gases must be monitored to detect CO_2 accumulation, which may be severe enough to cause coma and require assisted ventilation.

Bronchiectasis is a common sequela of repeated pneumonias. Pulmonary hygiene, consisting of postural drainage and intermittent positive pressure breathing, is helpful not only in the acute situation but also as a daily routine for children with chronic lung disease. Suctioning is often required because of ineffective cough. Chest therapy should be administered at home by the parents on a regular basis. Chest surgery is rarely indicated, as the disease usually is diffuse. In patients with gastroesophageal reflux, fundoplications have been performed if medical management has been unsuccessful.

SPINAL CURVATURE

Spinal curvature (kyphosis or scoliosis or both) will develop in 95 per cent of dysautonomic patients by adolescence. Spinal curvature may start as early as 3.5 years or as late as 14 years. There may be rapid progression at any time. The completion of puberty generally halts the progression of scoliosis as it does in the idiopathic adolescent form, but puberty is commonly delayed in dysautonomia. Spinal curvature further compromises respiratory function, adding the component of restrictive lung disease to bronchiectatic disease.

Annual radiographic examination of the spine is recommended after the child starts to walk. Splinting with a brace is the only effective conservative treatment. The brace must be carefully fitted and the skin inspected daily at pressure points because of the risk of ulceration as a result of decreased sensitivity to pain. The brace may also impair pulmonary ventilation. Most patients rely primarily on the use of their abdominal muscles for adequate pulmonary excursion. A high anterior projection on a brace, compressing the epigastric area, may restrict breathing and even contribute to esophageal reflux. The orthopedist should be alerted to the possibility of these problems. If the brace is not successful in halting progression, or if the patient has a severe curve, spinal fusion is recommended.

CORNEAL ABRASIONS

Corneal complications have been decreasing with the regular use of artificial tear solutions containing methylcellulose. Artificial tears are instilled three to six times daily, depending on the child's own baseline eye moisture, environmental conditions, and whether or not the child is febrile or dehydrated. Moisture chamber spectacle attachments help to maintain eye moisture and protect the eye from wind and foreign bodies. If an ulcer occurs, the eye should be patched. Tarsorrhaphy of the medial or lateral part of the palpebral fissure has been reserved for unresponsive and chronic situations. Soft contact lenses have been found recently to be very effective in promoting corneal healing.

BREATH-HOLDING (SEIZURES)

The phenomenon of prolonged breath-holding with crying in the early years can result in actual cyanosis, syncope, and seizure activity. This is due to lack of awareness that it is necessary for the next inspiration to be initiated, i.e., the patients are manifesting insensitivity to hypoxia and hypercapnea. This may become a manipulative maneuver with some children. Such an episode is frightening but self-limited and, in our experience, has never been fatal. The cyanosis of breath-holding must be differentiated from that which occurs with mucus plugs. Both types of cyanotic spells can produce seizure-like movements and decerebrate posturing. Electroencephalograms usually are normal or nonspecific, and the frequency of either type of spell is unaffected by anticonvulsant therapy.

Owing to the lack of appropriate response to hypoxia and hypercapnea. diving, underwater swimming, and air travel at high altitudes are potential hazards. If the plane's altitude exceeds 39,-000 feet, the cabin pressure will be equivalent to >6000 feet, and supplemental oxygen probably will be necessary.

AZOTEMIA

A large proportion of patients have a moderate degree of azotemia (20 to 30 mg/dl) and variable values for creatinine clearance. Although these patients do not exhibit clinical signs of dehydration, the urea nitrogen often may be reduced by simple hydration. In four patients whose urea nitrogen was consistently greater than 40 mg/dl and unalterable by IV hydration, renal biopsies were performed. These showed significant ischemic-type glomerulosclerosis. The high prevalence of this renal lesion has been confirmed by retrospective analysis of autopsy material. It has been suggested that these slowly progressive lesions are associated with labile blood pressure. Patients are being encouraged to maintain adequate hydration, especially during warm weather. Treatment of postural hypotension is becoming more aggressive (see below).

POSTURAL HYPOTENSION

Episodes of postural hypotension may be associated with actual syncope, complaints of "dizziness," brief loss of vision, or leg cramps. These episodes may also occur with micturition or with sudden change in position, such as after sitting for extended periods in a car or theater.

In addition to increasing dietary salt and fluids, the addition of caffeinated beverages has been very helpful. Elasticized waist-high stockings also are beneficial.

ANESTHESIA

Anesthesia for surgical procedures is associated with an increased risk because of extreme lability of blood pressure and diminished responsiveness to variations in blood gases. Local anesthesia with diazepam as preoperative sedation is preferred whenever possible. Large amounts of epinephrine should not be infiltrated because of the exaggerated response to sympathomimetic drugs. If general anesthesia is indicated, the gas anesthetics are preferred because of the rapid reversibility of their effects. An intravenous drip is maintained to assure adequate hydration and to permit the rapid administration of volume expanders and/or norepinephrine to combat profound hypotension. The amount and duration of norepinephrine administration is determined by the blood pressure response. In lengthy surgical procedures, an arterial line should be inserted for frequent monitoring of blood gases and blood pressure. If the patient is going to have

a prolonged postoperative course, as in spinal fusions, elective tracheostomy may be performed 1 week before the major surgery, as it is during this period of inactivity that the patient is most likely to aspirate and develop mucus plugs and pneumonia.

Because dysautonomia is a multisystem disorder, the physician can render the family a great deal of support and comfort by becoming thoroughly familiar with its varied manifestations. Living with the dysautonomic child imposes a great burden upon the parents, who are aware of the serious prognosis and are faced with the care of a chronically handicapped child with repeated life-threatening crises. A sympathetic, artful physician can provide needed reassurance.

Injuries to the Brachial Plexus, Facial Nerve, and Sciatic Nerve

JEROME S. HALLER, M.D.

FACIAL NERVE PALSY IN THE NEWBORN

Peripheral facial nerve palsy, partial or complete, in the newborn results from compression of the nerve in utero by dint of facial position against pelvic prominences or from misapplied forceps during the delivery process. Facial nerve electrodiagnostic tests are usually normal during the first 3 days even with complete paralysis. There is no therapy for this form of facial palsy. Spontaneous recovery is the usual course beginning within 3 to 6 weeks of delivery. Rarely will there be a permanent paresis.

Neonatal peripheral facial palsy should not be confused with the asymmetric crying-face syndrome or hypoplasia of the trangularis muscle. In this situation, there is no inferolateral movement of the corner of the mouth with crying, but there is normal deepening of the nasolabial fold. This anomaly is important because of its association with cardiac and renal anomalies.

Bell's palsy, or idiopathic facial paralysis, is an inflammatory neuropathy believed by some to be a component of a cranial nerve polyneuropathy most frequently caused by a viral infection. In adults, the most likely agent is herpes zoster. This may well account for the complaints of facial and retroauricular pain reported commonly in adults but infrequently in children. As with the newborn facial palsy, electrodiagnostic testing will initially be normal and of little value in predicting the degree of recovery. Children tend to recover more completely than adults.

Before considering treatment, it is necessary to have established that the paralysis is not associated with an active otitis media and mastoiditis or one manifestation of a postinfectious polyradiculoneuropathy or brain stem tumor.

Although touted for use in adults, there is no

clear indication for steroid therapy in the pediatric-age patient with Bell's palsy.

A very small percentage of patients have a recurrent facial palsy. Repeated bouts may result in permanent residua. It is conceivable that such a patient might be beneficially treated with prednisone, 2 mg/kg/day, for 10 days, beginning as soon as possible following the appearance of palsy.

BRACHIAL PLEXUS PALSY OF THE NEWBORN

Obstetric injury of the newborn infant's brachial plexus by excessive traction on the shoulder or neck may take one of three patterns, an upper plexus paralysis (C5, C6 and to a lesser degree C7, Erb-Duchenne), a lower plexus palsy (C8, T1 with or without Horner's syndrome, Klumpke), or total plexus palsy. If respiratory distress is present, C3 and C4 spinal nerves may also be involved, with a resultant hemidiaphragmatic paralysis.

The posture of the involved arm indicates the initial acute injury, but not necessarily the eventual recovered state. A flaccid limb without response to pin prick or to Moro reflex corresponds to a total paralysis. An arm inwardly rotated, elbow extended, and with fingers flexed and in the pronated position represents an upper plexus palsy. Abduction of the shoulder and flexion of the elbow are lost; therefore, the Moro response will be asymmetric or even absent. The lower plexus of Klumpke's palsy results in loss of function of the triceps, wrist extensors, and some of the finger flexors. Since the proximal musculature is unaffected, shoulder abduction is possible with a Moro response. X-rays of the involved extremity and the clavicle should be done to exclude fracture of the involved bony structures.

Therapy is directed toward preserving joint function and preventing contractures. Range of motion activity can begin 2–3 days after delivery. Splinting is used only to maintain functional hand position.

Recovery can begin within 2–3 weeks of birth. Limited return can be anticipated with a complete paralysis. Useful functional recovery of an upper or lower plexus palsy depends on intact sensation of the involved hand. Recovery may continue for as much as the first 3 years of life. The upper plexus palsy has the greatest likelihood of recovery, with almost full function, the residua being mild weakness of the most proximal musculature of the shoulder.

A brachial plexus palsy in the older child or adolescent resulting from penetrating injuries of the plexus is best managed by neurosurgical and orthopedic specialists.

Brachial plexopathy is an acute onset paralysis and atrophy of several muscles enervated by trunks, divisions, and nerves of the brachial plexus. Immediately preceding paralysis, there is rather significant, but transient shoulder and arm pain, leaving behind an area of hypesthesia or anesthesia over the deltoid, C5 root. The disorder may be unilateral, bilateral, or present sequentially on one side and then the other. Antecedents to this disorder have been viral infections, immunizations (not necessarily in the afflicted extremity) and surgery. Although steroid therapy has been recommended, it may not be effective and prognosis for a complete recovery is uncertain.

INJURY TO THE SCIATIC NERVE

This injury is most commonly iatrogenic, from a misplaced injection into the gluteal muscles. Irreversible injury to the sciatic nerve may be caused by direct injection of material, usually an antibiotic, into the nerve sheath or into the immediately surrounding tissue.

The sciatic nerve has three major branches: the lateralmost, making up the perineal nerve; the middle branch the tibial nerve; and the most medial branch, which innervates the hamstring muscles. The least injury to a child may be a foot drop and sensory impairment over the dorsum of the foot and lateral aspect of the leg. Dorsiflexion weakness, sensory loss of the sole of the foot, and hamstring weakness indicate deeper penetration of the neurotoxic substance.

The only treatment of such an injury is to prevent its occurrence. If necessary, injections into the gluteal muscle might be directed into an area bounded by the anterior superior iliac spine, the iliac crest, and the greater trochanter, using the palm of one's hand to locate the latter, and placing the widespread second and third fingertips on the other two points. This area is free of major nerves and vasculature, providing a relatively safe segment of musculature for injections.

Hypoxic Encephalopathy

BENNETT A. SHAYWITZ, M.D.

In pediatric practice hypoxic-ischemic encephalopathy is seen at all ages. In the newborn period its pathogenesis is usually intrauterine asphyxia, though this may be complicated by postnatal difficulties including recurrent apnea, congenital heart disease, sepsis, and, in premature infants, hyaline membrane disease. Intrauterine asphyxia is typically diagnosed by low Apgar scores at birth, depressed level of consciousness, seizures beginning 6-12 hours after birth, and often, frequent apneic spells, Other clinical features are weakness in the hip-shoulder distribution in full-term newborns and lower limb weakness in premature newborns, and disturbances in feeding and persistent hypotonia. Neuronal necrosis is evident in the cerebral and cerebellar cortices, thalamus, brainstem, basal ganglia, and, perhaps, in the parasagittal and periventricular areas.

While postnatal events may exacerbate pre-existing problems, in most cases, hypoxic-ischemic encepalopathy is a consequence of intrauterine factors. Thus, effective treatment depends upon the identification of the woman who is at high risk for the development of hypoxic-ischemic encephalopathy and the subsequent careful intrauterine monitoring of the fetus. If signs of intrauterine asphyxia become evident, measures must be taken to deliver the infant by cesarean section as quickly as possible. After birth, the primary focus is prevention of an exacerbation of the hypoxic-ischemic events. Good supportive care must include maintenance of adequate ventilation; this may necessitate intubation and controlled positive pressure ventilatory support. Measures must be taken to treat such common sequelae of hypoxia-ischemia as seizures, myocardial failure, and acute tubular necrosis. Seizures should be treated with phenobarbital given as an intravenous loading dose (10-20 mg/kg) and then at 5 mg/kg/day to maintain phenobarbital blood levels at 20–30 $\mu g/dl$. If seizures continue, phenytoin should be added at an intravenous loading dose of 15 mg/kg and a daily maintenance dose of 5–7 mg/kg, designed to maintain blood levels between 10–20 $\mu g/dl$. Myocardial failure is treated with agents to improve cardiac contractility and prevent arrhythmias. Acute tubular necrosis is managed by appropriate fluid therapy, and, at times, dialysis. Sepsis, too, may complicate the immediate postnatal course, and appropriate antibiotics are frequently employed. More specific measures in the treatment of the hypoxic-ischemic insult itself, such as the prevention and treatment of associated brain edema, the use of barbiturates, and the role of glucose therapy, remain controversial in the newborn period. Their role in hypoxic-ischemic encephalopathy in older individuals is discussed below. A significant and often the most difficult part of the management of hypoxic-ischemic encephalopathy in the newborn period is determination of severity of the insult. Such an estimate is critical in providing the physician with a rationale for counseling the parents of the affected infant about the prognosis and potential complications. Thus, the mortality rate ranges between 10 and 20% and the incidence of neurological sequelae in survivors is estimated at 25-45%. These include a variety of spastic motor deficits (cerebral palsy), psychomotor retardation, bulbar difficulties, and seizure disorders. The treatment of each of these complications is formidable and includes, in addition to anticonvulsant agents to treat seizures, physical and occupational therapy, speech therapy, and supportive counseling to the parents. Details of each of these are discussed elsewhere in this volume.

In contrast to hypoxic-ischemic encephalopathy in the newborn period, which nearly always results from intrauterine asphyxia, the disorder in older children may occur after a variety of insults. Thus hypoxic-ischemic encepalopathy is seen in disorders resulting in airway obstruction, such as suffocation and drowning; as a consequence of obstruction of blood flow in the cerebral vessels in strangulation, severe brain edema from a closed head injury, or disseminated intravascular coagulation from sepsis or leukemia; and in sudden decreases in cardiac output, as in myocarditis or hemorrhagic shock. Such an insult immediately deprives the brain of substrate and oxygen for the formation of high energy phosphate, which is necessary for maintenance of the integrity of the brain. The clinical consequences are immediate and are characterized by sudden loss of consciousness, pupillary dilatation, and, often, generalized convulsions. Although survival with good neurologic functioning has been reported in rare instances (associated with drowning in ice cold water) of prolonged asphyxia (10–20 minutes), several minutes (2–4) of anoxia will usually result in significant neurologic sequelae, with damage first to mitochondria and neuronal cell body. The neuronal injury is compounded by the development of brain edema and local circulatory disturbances, which further exacerbate the hypoxic-ischemic insult.

As was the case in the infant with a hypoxic-ischemic insult, prevention of further hypoxia by attention to ventilatory support and maintenance of circulatory parameters is critical in these older children. Management of brain edema often plays a critical role in reducing mortality and minimizing neurologic sequelae. Cerebral edema is often difficult to recognize. Papilledema may be observed, but it is far more common after an hypoxic-ischemic insult for brain edema to be suspected and then confirmed after intracranial pressure monitoring. We accomplish this by insertion of a ventricular catheter led to a transducer. Intracranial pressures are maintained below 20 mm/Hg, a pressure chosen to maintain cerebral perfusion pressure (calculated as the difference between mean arterial blood pressure usually approximately 100 mm Hg, and intracranial pressure) above 60-70 mm Hg. Measures taken to reduce intracranial pressure include careful monitoring of fluid intake; administration of decadron at a loading dose of 1 mg/kg and then a daily maintenance dose of 0.25-0.5 mg/kg; and periodic intravenous infusion of mannitol at doses ranging between 0.25-1 gm/kg. Mannitol infusion usually results in reductions in intracranial pressure within 5-10 minutes and a duration of effect between 30 minutes and 4 hours.

In addition to the treatment of the complications of hypoxic-ischemic encephalopathy described, investigators have attempted to mitigate the effects of the insult by measures designed to increase the tolerance of the brain to hypoxia. The first such attempt was the use of hypothermia to reduce the energy requirements of the brain. For example, with body temperatures as low as 16 degrees C, cardiac arrest can be tolerated for as long as 30 minutes; this technique has been employed for many years in patients undergoing open heart surgery. However, such extreme hypothermia is accompanied by major systemic complications, and thus is not practical, even in intensive care situations. A less severe degree of hypothermia, though effective in experimental paradigms of hypoxia, has proven to be disappointing in the usual clinical situation.

More recent studies have focused on the observation that administration of barbiturates either before or shortly after an insult may offer some degree of protection against the hypoxic-ischemic episode. Their mechanism of action is not altogether clear. Barbiturates may act to reduce cerebral metabolism and reduce elevated intracranial pressure by reducing cerebral blood flow. Recent evidence suggests that a significant portion of the residua of a hypoxic-ischemia may be related to the action of free radicals released during the insult which damage the lipids of cell membranes. Barbiturates are believed to inactivate these free radicals and thus limit the extent of the brain injury. More recent studies, using animal models, suggest that barbiturates have little effect on cerebral metabolism or inactivation of free radicals, but rather help by ameliorating the seizures that often complicate the hypoxic-ischemic episode. Until the issue is resolved in well-controlled clinical studies, we advocate the use of barbiturates in cases of hypoxic-ischemic encephalopathy complicated by increased intracranial pressure. We use phenobarbital in doses calculated to achieve blood levels of 20-30 μg/dl. Other investigators employ pentobarbital in doses of 5 mg/kg/24 hrs.

Prognosticating the effects of hypoxic-ischemic encephalopathy remains a difficult problem and, to date, such laboratory procedures as computed tomography, EEG, and brain stem evoked responses have provided little help. In general, rapid initial improvement remains the most reasonable gauge of further recovery; children who remain unresponsive to painful stimuli for 2 weeks after the insult have a bleak outcome.

Reye Syndrome

JEROME S. HALLER, M.D.

The diagnosis of Reye syndrome should be based on the medical history of a viral syndrome followed by vomiting, altered consciousness, and biochemical hallmarks of elevated blood (arterial, if possible) ammonia, SGOT, SGPT, and prolonged prothrombin time. In infants under 1 year of age, tachypnea and seizures are prominent features and hypoglycemia a frequent finding. Liver biopsy is not essential for diagnostic purposes. Patient care consists of maintenance of fluid and electrolyte balance and treatment of increased intracranial pressure by monitoring pressure, controlling respiration, and infusing mannitol and, if necessary, barbiturates.

FLUID AND ELECTROLYTES

At the time of admission, serum electrolytes, glucose, BUN, and serum osmolality should be determined. An intravenous solution of 10 per cent dextrose and one-half normal saline solution should be given at a rate of 1200 to 1500 ml/m²/24 hr. Fluid deficits of more than 10 per cent dehydration should be corrected. Potassium chloride can be added in the usual manner once urination has commenced. Urinary output must be monitored. If the patient is unable to void spontaneously, either condom drainage or catheterization is necessary. Although there continues to be controversy about fluid restriction versus normal maintenance, fluid overload should be absolutely avoided. An alternative method of fluid management is to use the same intravenous solution at a rate that produces a urinary output of 1.5 to 2 ml/kg/hr. Hypoglycemia must be corrected with a 50 per cent glucose solution, making certain that the intravenous needle is well placed in a large peripheral vein. Though there is no proof of cellular depletion of glucose, recognized biochemical disturbances of gluconeogenesis and other enzymes related to glucose metabolism support the recommendation of maintaining high serum glucose levels. I have found that the 10 per cent dextrose solution has been generally effective, obtaining levels of 150 to 200 mg per cent.

INTRACRANIAL PRESSURE MANAGEMENT

Rather than use the stages of coma, I prefer to discuss intervention in terms of neurologic status at the time of admission or neurologic deterioration afterwards. Vague terms such as stupor or semicoma are of little help in the sequential evaluation of children with this syndrome. If the child can respond to his or her name, can carry out a simple command although sleepy, or is agitated and disoriented though still able to push away painful stimuli, watchful waiting is recommended. Should the child fail to respond to verbal commands, become quiet, react to painful stimuli with nondirected motor activity, or show decorticate or decerebrate posturing, the patient is obviously deteriorating and intervention is necessary. Papilledema need not be present. If it is, or if the patient is deteriorating rapidly, an infusion of 20 per cent mannitol at 1 gm/kg should be given over a 10- to 15-minute time span. The child should be prepared for intracranial pressure monitoring. Because of the clotting defects associated with Reye syndrome, 10 ml/kg of fresh frozen plasma must be administered. A CVP line, an arterial line for blood pressure monitoring as well as for arterial blood gases, and an intravenous line are required.

The patient should be intubated and respirations controlled to maintain $PaCO_2$ at 20 to 25 torr and PaO_2 at 90 to 100 torr. Muscle relaxation is maintained with pancuronium bromide (Pavulon), given at a dosage that will cause diaphragmatic paralysis, 0.05 to 0.1 mg/kg every 2 hours. To prevent additional intracranial pressure from venous stasis, the patient's head should be elevated to 30 degrees.

The method by which intracranial pressure monitoring is carried out is not important. We have been using a subarachnoid bolt, adapted for pediatric patients by the Department of Neurosurgery at The University of Pennsylvania, since it is shorter than the Richmond bolt and has a metal collar and Silastic gasket that forms a tight seal with the skull and prevents leaking of CSF. The transducer should be placed at the level of the patient's ear. The intent of intracranial pressure monitoring and treatment is to maintain pressure below 15 torr concomitant with a cerebral perfusion pressure (CPP) of greater than 45 torr.

CPP = mean systemic arterial pressure (MSAP)- ICP

MSAP = diastolic pressure
$$+ \frac{(systolic-diastolic\ pressure)}{3}$$

The implications of these formulae are that severely increased intracranial pressure can reduce cerebral blood flow and secondarily produce ischemic damage, or, alternatively, systemic hypotension should be prevented because it may have the same effect. Pressure waves of over 15 to 20 torr, which rise and fall rapidly, probably have little effect on cerebral circulation. For pressure waves that fall slowly over a period of longer than 2 minutes, or for pressure plateaus over 15 but less than 20 torr, hyperventilation for 2 minutes may be satisfactory treatment. With plateaus of 20 torr or greater, 20 per cent mannitol is recommended, starting with a dose of 250 mg/kg infused over a 10- to 20-minute period.

The advantage of monitoring is that the effectiveness of the mannitol dosage can be seen. Thus, one can use the smallest dose possible and at 30- to 60-minute intervals, if necessary. If the lowest dose fails, the amount can be increased to 500 mg/kg or to as much as 1.5 gm/kg. If there is a recurrence of a pressure rise, the lowest effective dosage should be repeated. Serum osmolality should be monitored 2 hours after the last dose of mannitol or before the administration of the next. An osmolality of 320 milliosmoles or more precludes the use of this agent temporarily. Renal failure, either as a component of Reye syndrome or as a complication of mannitol therapy, must be watched for.

Suctioning or frequent position changes can easily provoke pressure spikes during the first 24 to 48 hours and should be carried out as infrequently as possible. Should ICP be unresponsive to mannitol or if serum osmolality exceeds 320 milliosmoles, barbiturate infusions using phenobarbital or pentobarbital to maintain a level of 25 to 35 μg/ml have been recommended. We have had only one occasion to use pentobarbital. The recommended loading dose is 20 mg/kg infused at a rate of 10 mg/kg/hr over a 2-hour period. The recommended maintenance dose is 2 mg/kg/hr. A level should be obtained at the end of the loading infusion, and periodically thereafter every 8 to 12 hours. An additional loading dose of 10 mg/kg can be given over a second 2-hour period if maintenance level has not been achieved.

When the ICP has been stable at less than 15 torr for 24 hours, the patient may be weaned from the support system. The pentobarbital infusion can be stopped without tapering dosages. The respirator is next adjusted to permit pCO_2 to return to normal. If there is no change in ICP, Pavulon can be discontinued.

If, over the next 24 hours, the pressure remains normal, the monitoring system can be removed and the patient extubated.

Steroids are not felt to be of any use in this disorder, nor has any attempt to reduce intestinal flora —i.e., reduction of NH_3—been undertaken.

This regimen has significantly reduced mortality and morbidity during the past 3 years. Any pediatric unit unprepared to manage a child with this or a similar protocol would be advised to transfer the patient.

4

Respiratory Tract

Malformations of the Nose

COLLIN S. KARMODY, M.D.

Malformations of the nose are uncommon except when they are associated with clefting of the lip and palate.

Midline nasal dermoids, a small pit in the midline of the dorsum of the nose, require excision, particularly if there is secondary infection. Approach can be made via a midline incision or an incision along the lateral border of the nose. The surgeon must be prepared for the possibility of intracranial extension, which will require excision via craniotomy.

Bifidity of the nose usually requires no treatment. Severe deformity, however, is managed surgically and much improvement can be obtained by rhinoplastic procedures.

Atresia of both posterior choanae of the nasal passages results in a severe respiratory obstruction because the neonate is an obligatory nasal breather. This presents a dire emergency for the neonate. Immediate treatment is with an oral airway, a McGovern nipple, or a large gavage tube. If this is satisfactory for breathing and feeding and if efficient nursing care is available, the child is allowed to grow for a few weeks or months. Mouth breathing is usually mastered in 3 to 4 weeks. The choanae are then opened by a transnasal approach, using microsurgical techniques. Obstructing tissue is removed with instruments or with a laser beam. The openings are splinted with silicone tubes, which are left in place for a minimum of 6 weeks. Periodic dilatation might be necessary afterward. Alternatively, a transpalatal approach might be necessary, but this is more applicable in the older child. In an emergency the atresia can be opened by a sharp instrument passed through the nose and guided by a finger in the nasopharynx. The opening is then dilated with graduated bougies and finally splinted with silicone tubes.

Nasal meningoencephaloceles require excision by combined nasal and transcranial approaches for excision of the intranasal sac and sealing of the dural defect.

Spontaneous leakage of cerebrospinal fluid can occur through a congenital defect in the cribriform plate. This, however, is a very rare problem. Surgical repair is necessary and the defect in the cribriform plate can be sealed via an inferior approach using a flap of septal mucoperichondrium. Alternatively, a craniotomy and repair with fascia might be necessary.

Congenital nasal hemangiomas might be internal or external. Congenital hemangiomas may regress spontaneously and should be allowed to do so. If they do not regress or if they expand rapidly, a course of corticosteroids should be given in a weight-related dosage. Radiation therapy is used only if absolutely necessary. Surgical excision of these lesions is hazardous and is a last resort used only if there is substantial cosmetic deformity.

Congenital cystic hygromas are rare and usually affect the neck. They tend to increase in size and should be excised with great care.

Congenital anosmia is caused by aplasia of the olfactory bulb and tracts, and treatment is not effective.

Tumors and Polyps of the Nose

COLLIN S. KARMODY, M.D.

BENIGN TUMORS

Polypoid degeneration of the nasal mucosa might be secondary to allergy or infection, and the underlying allergy or infection must be treated. Large obstructing polyps require removal, which is probably best done under general anesthesia in children.

Antrochoanal polyps are single, large, usually unilateral, smooth masses that originate in the maxillary sinus and eventually extend into the posterior nasal passage and through the posterior choana into the nasopharynx. They are removed by simultaneous transnasal and transantral approaches. If the intrasinus part of the polyp is not removed, it will regrow into the nose.

Simple squamous papillomas occur on the skin of the nasal vestibule and are best treated by application of podophyllin or a silver nitrate stick. Excision is possible, but recurrence and seeding of the incision might occur.

Inverting papillomas are locally invasive, and a few will become malignant. They are treated by wide surgical excision, which usually requires exenteration of the ethmoid labyrinth and excision of the middle turbinate via a lateral rhinotomy. Radiation therapy should not be used because of the tendency to malignant degeneration.

Osteomas are more common in the frontal and ethmoid sinuses and are removed only if they cause symptoms. They are rare in children.

Juvenile angiofibroma is a vascular tumor of the nasopharynx that is confined to pubescent boys. The patients complain of nasal obstruction or may present massive epistaxis. These tumors tend to spread in all directions into the adjacent areas and might even extend intracranially. Investigation must include tomography and angiography. Juvenile angiofibromas are treated surgically. There is evidence, however, that some can be controlled by radiation therapy.

MALIGNANT TUMORS

The commonest malignant tumor of the nose in children is a rhabdomyosarcoma. At present, rhabdomyosarcomas are treated with a combination of chemotherapy—doxorubicin hydrochloride (Adriamycin), vincristine—and radiation therapy. If possible, the tumors should be excised prior to initiation of treatment, but wide mutilating surgery generally has not controlled these lesions and is not recommended.

An esthesioneuroblastoma is rare in children and is treated by excision and radiation therapy. Similarly, malignant melanomas of the nose are exceedingly rare in children; however, when they do occur they should be treated with wide surgical excision followed by chemotherapy.

Squamous cell carcinoma and adenocarcinoma are very rare in children, but sporadic cases have been reported in teenagers. Treatment is by wide surgical resection followed by radiation therapy. The surgical defect is closed with a removable prosthesis.

Nasal Injuries
COLLIN S. KARMODY, M.D.

FRACTURES OF THE NASAL BONES AND NASAL SEPTUM

The nasal skeleton is vulnerable to injury, usually by blunt trauma. Fractures of the nasal bones in children should be manipulated into normal alignment under general anesthesia as soon as possible, because children's bones heal very rapidly. The usual practice in adults of waiting 6 to 7 days for subsidence of swelling is not advisable. Very mobile fragments might require splinting.

Fractures of the facial bones occur rarely in children. LeForte Types II and III fractures are uncommon but require manipulation and interosseous wiring. Injuries are usually secondary to massive trauma, and facial fractures should take second place to head injuries and other life-threatening problems. Fractures can be treated a few days later. Interdental wiring in children should be avoided because of the softness and vulnerability of the deciduous teeth.

Hematomas of the nasal septum may occur in children, frequently secondary to trauma but occasionally spontaneously. The nasal passage is obstructed by a smooth septal swelling that is easily seen by elevation of the tip of the nose. A uni- or bilateral subperichondrial collection of blood and serous fluid jeopardizes the vitality of the septal cartilage. The hematoma must be evacuated as soon as possible by making a vertical incision into the septal mucosa. After evacuation, both sides of the nose are firmly packed with iodoform-impregnated gauze, which is left in place for at least 5 days. Occasionally, a septal hematoma becomes infected. The same incisions are used for evacuation but, in addition, all dead cartilage should be removed. The pus is sampled for culture and sensitivity studies and the appropriate antibiotic given systemically.

Open soft tissue injuries of the nose should be repaired immediately. The wound must be scrubbed clean to remove foreign material and to prevent tattooing, and nonviable soft tissue and skin are excised. Absorbable sutures are used to approximate deeper tissues. If good subdermal approximation is achieved, the skin can be closed with 6-0 catgut, which does not require removal. If the wound breaches the nasal mucosa, the nasal cavity must be packed with iodoform-impregnated gauze for about 6 days to minimize stenosis of the lumen.

FOREIGN BODIES

Nasal foreign bodies may be recent or longstanding. Longstanding foreign bodies cause suppuration and irritation of the mucosa and usually require general anesthesia for removal. Most recent foreign bodies can be removed after topical applications of drops of 2 per cent cocaine. The child is wrapped in a sheet and is held in a sitting position by an experienced nurse, with the head firmly anchored. The foreign body is removed under direct vision, using an instrument that can be passed behind the object, which is then drawn forward. An old-fashioned hernia director or eustachian tube catheter or even a bent hairpin is useful. If general anesthesia is required, the child should be intubated and the pharynx packed to prevent aspiration of the foreign body.

Epistaxis

DANIEL D. BROUGHTON, M.D.

Nosebleeds are among the most common complaints encountered in childhood. Fortunately, serious bleeding is rare. Generally, the bleeding resolves spontaneously or by the application of pressure and does not come to the attention of a physician. Parents may be instructed by telephone to apply firm pressure to both sides of the nose with the thumb and forefinger for 5 to 10 minutes. The child usually will be more comfortable if sitting upright with the head slightly forward in order to prevent blood from dripping down the throat.

When bleeding cannot be quickly controlled, the patient and family often become anxious. Reassurance that the problem can be easily handled is important. Often just calming the patient down results in resolution of the bleeding without the need for further intervention.

Most of the bleeding sites will be anterior, with 90 per cent being limited to the nasal septum. Generally, a single bleeding site is responsible; bilateral bleeding is uncommon. Initial efforts should be made with this in mind. Because pressure usually has been tried unsuccessfully before the patient is seen by the physician, a topical vasoconstrictor, such as phenylephrine (0.25 to 0.5%), is helpful, either by direct spray or by inserting a soaked cotton swab or pledget into the nostril and leaving it in place. Pressure is then applied for 5 to 10 minutes.

If the bleeding persists, an attempt to visualize the bleeding site should be made. The child should be adequately restrained, and unnecessary movement must be prevented. The nose should not be traumatized further by attempts at treatment. Restraint may be accomplished by having the child sit on a parent's lap. If possible, the child should be seated with the head slightly forward during this procedure. Frequently, more vigorous restraint such as the use of a "papoose" board will be necessary. General anesthesia is needed rarely.

For adequate visualization, a good light source is needed. A head lamp or a mirror provides good light and allows the physician the use of both hands for any necessary manipulation; an otoscope is not adequate. The nose should be cleared by suction or, if the child can cooperate, by blowing the nose.

If a single bleeding site is identified, direct cautery should be tried. Before this procedure is attempted, the nose should be anesthetized by applying lidocaine (2%). The bleeding site is then cauterized by applying a silver nitrate stick held in place for 15 to 30 seconds. Electrocautery is more difficult and should be used only by those with considerable experience.

Occasionally, packing will be necessary. If the bleeding is anterior, the procedure is relatively straightforward but will cause considerable discomfort. Individual strips of petrolatum or iodoform gauze impregnated with antibiotic ointment can be layered; the first strip should be advanced with bayonet forceps until it reaches the posterior pharyngeal wall, with subsequent layers added until an adequate pack is formed. The pack should cover the bleeding site and may need to fill the entire nasal fossa. It should be left in place for 48 hours.

Oxidized cellulose also can be used as packing, and such packs will increase in size as blood is absorbed, thus applying more pressure to the site. The cellulose pack does not need to be removed. Analgesia usually will be necessary when packing is used, and antibiotics, either penicillin or erythromycin, should be considered.

If bleeding persists despite anterior packing or if posterior bleeding is apparent, a posterior nasal pack may be necessary. These packs are much more difficult to insert and are associated with a significant risk of morbidity. Therefore, consultation with someone who has considerable experience with this technique should be sought at this time. If bleeding is heavy and intervention is necessary before such consultation can be obtained, an initial pack can be constructed out of a finger cot or the finger of a rubber glove filled with gauze impregnated with petrolatum. The size of this pack can be varied as needed, and it should conform to the shape of the cavity. Various balloons, such as the Stevens, Brighton, or Nasostat, have been designed to provide easy tamponade, and these may be helpful in an emergency. All of these devices should be lubricated before insertion.

Once the bleeding has been controlled, the cause of the bleeding should be sought and preventive measures initiated. Most nosebleeds in children are caused by trauma, such as nosepicking or noserubbing. Nosebleeds are more common in cold, dry weather and frequently are seen in children with rhinitis.

Obviously, the child should be counseled to

avoid picking or rubbing the nose as much as possible, but often the trauma occurs while the child is sleeping or unaware. The nose should be lubricated with petrolatum, and adequate humidity should be provided by using a vaporizer or humidifier in the patient's room. Any accompanying nasal condition, such as allergic or vasomotor rhinitis or upper respiratory infection, should be treated. Also, parents should be trained in the use of cotton or gauze plugs soaked with phenylephrine for the treatment of future episodes.

Bleeding rarely is due to a specific entity, such as a bleeding dyscrasia, neoplasm in the nose, or hypertension; if this is found, the underlying disorder must be treated.

Foreign Bodies in the Nose and Pharynx

DANIEL D. BROUGHTON, M.D.

A large variety of foreign objects have been found in the noses of children. These objects can be hard or soft, organic or inorganic, small or large. The nose generally reacts to a foreign body by developing edema, congestion, and hyperemia. A unilateral nasal discharge, often with a foul odor, is common, although a bilateral discharge can be seen if the object is far enough posterior.

Although the diagnosis can be difficult, once it is made the treatment can seem deceptively easy. Rarely does a foreign body in the nose represent a true emergency. However, aggressive attempts at removal can cause serious injury to the nasal tissue. Sudden dislodging of the object posteriorly can result in aspiration and in a much more serious problem.

To avoid unnecessary apprehension, the patient and the parents must be carefully prepared for the procedure. The child must be immobilized to prevent any unnecesssary movement. A "papoose" board is often needed, or the child may be wrapped tightly in a sheet to prevent thrashing about. Sedation may be advisable with chloral hydrate, 25 to 50 mg/kg, which may be repeated once if necessary, or a combination of meperidine (2 mg/kg), promethazine (1 mg/kg), and chlorpromazine (1 mg/kg), with a maximum dose of meperidine 50 mg, promethazine 25 mg, and chlorpromazine 25 mg. Occasionally general anesthesia is needed.

An adequate light source is critical and is best supplied by a head lamp or mirror that will leave both hands of the physician available for maneuvering the foreign body. Spraying the nares with a topical vasoconstrictor such as phenylephrine (0.25 to 0.50 per cent) or epinephrine (1 per cent) and an anesthetic such as lidocaine (2 per cent) helps in visualization while providing local anesthesia.

Once the patient is prepared, many different techniques are available. The method chosen should depend on the location, size, and consistency of the object.

If the object is small or can be easily grasped, bayonet forceps and alligator forceps are often useful. If a soft object is wedged anteriorly and superiorly, a hemostat can be inserted into the nasal cavity, gently following the anterior surface until the foreign body is encountered. Care must be taken to grasp only the foreign body, not the nasal mucosa.

Larger foreign bodies often can be removed by inserting a blunt hook or wire loop around the object and carefully pulling it out. An ear curette also can be used. A similar method involves passing a small Fogarty catheter past the object, filling the bulb with fluid, and gently pulling the catheter back to remove the object. The size of the bulb can be varied as needed. The catheter can be cleaned and used for this procedure on subsequent patients.

If the foreign body is round, a suction catheter may be constructed by flanging one end of intravenous tubing and connecting the other end to a suction device. The flanged end is inserted and placed against the object. Suction is applied, and the tubing is withdrawn from the nose, pulling the object with it. If the foreign body cannot be removed quickly and easily, consultation should be obtained and referral may be necessary.

A foreign body in the nasopharynx is a much more serious problem. The oropharynx should be inspected with a laryngoscope. Indirect laryngoscopy also may be helpful in locating the object. Palpation should be avoided because of the risk of advancing the foreign body. Although the foreign object frequently may be easily visualized and removed, there is always the risk of airway obstruction. In order to successfully remove nasopharyngeal foreign bodies, precaution must be exercised. General anesthesia is often necessary. Before doing this procedure, the physician should be prepared to provide an emergency airway, if necessary, by tracheotomy. The inexperienced physician should not attempt to do this procedure, and consultation should be promptly sought.

Nasopharyngitis

(The Common Cold)

RICHARD B. GOLDBLOOM, M.D.

The symptom complex of the common cold may be produced by infection with rhinoviruses, respiratory syncytial virus, adenovirus, influenza virus, or parainfluenza virus. The lack of any specific or particularly effective treatment for these infections or their symptoms is emphasized by the variety of remedies promoted for the purpose.

Very preliminary studies have suggested that rhinovirus colds may be preventable by use of nasal spraying of human interferon alpha-2 from *Escherichia coli,* and that antiviral agents effective against rhinovirus may reduce cold symptoms in infected individuals. At present these are no more than attractive experimental possibilities.

Irrespective of its cause, the common cold is normally self-limited. Younger children in large groups, as in day-care centers, are especially susceptible. Prevalence increases with the opening of school and remains high through winter and spring.

These infections may cause fever, especially in younger patients. Other signs and symptoms are sneezing, sore throat, mucoid or mucopurulent nasal discharge with nasal obstruction, cough, conjunctivitis, headache, chills, and malaise. The acute symptoms usually last 3 or 4 days, often followed by several days of nasal catarrh and cough. Secondary complications, which may be bacterial, can include otitis media, cervical adenitis, sinusitis, and pneumonia.

The course of the viral illness is completely unaltered by antibiotics, and these should be reserved for infants and children with strong evidence of bacterial infection, such as otitis or pneumonia. Fever alone does not constitute such evidence. Antibiotics are of no value as prophylaxis against the bacterial complications of viral respiratory illness, and the practice of prescribing antibiotics over the telephone for infants and children with nonspecific respiratory illness when the child has not been examined must be condemned.

Treatment is directed at the relief of symptoms, of which nasal obstruction is one of the most bothersome, often interfering with an infant's ability to feed or sleep. Some relief can often be provided by using an inexpensive rubber bulb type of infant nasal aspirator. Parents should be instructed in the correct use of the aspirator, which can be effective in clearing the nasal airway. The procedure is best performed 15 minutes or so before feedings.

If nasal obstruction is severe, the nose can be irrigated with 2 or 3 drops of lukewarm normal saline before using the aspirator. Alternatively or additionally, decongestant nose drops may improve patency of the nasal airway temporarily and facilitate feeding. Phenylephrine (Neo-Synephrine), 0.25%, or xylometazoline (Otrivin Pediatric Nasal Solution), 0.05%, 2 drops in each nostril every 4 hours, may be used in infants over 3 or 4 months of age. In younger infants, it is best to avoid these sympathomimetic decongestants, since they may cause irritability and tachycardia, and to use only

saline irrigation and the aspirator. For children over 2 years of age, 0.25% phenylephrine drops may be used, and 1% xylometazoline drops or spray may be used for children over the age of 12 years. Decongestant nose drops should never be used for more than 4 or 5 days, because progressively increasing rebound swelling of the nasal mucosa develops with continuing use.

Because otitis media is a complication of viral upper respiratory infection, one should remember that in infants the supine position during feedings (and possibly at other times, such as during sleep) allows fluid direct access via the eustachian tube to the middle ear during the act of swallowing. It follows that infants should never be fed in the supine position, and that moderate elevation of the head may be helpful during respiratory infections in preventing or relieving earache, which occurs most commonly at night.

When the onset of infection is associated with fever and anorexia, mild degrees of ketoacidosis are common, especially in young children and when fever is present. This phenomenon is often evidenced by irritability and acetone breath. The association of ketosis with minor infections is often overlooked, which is a pity, because the symptoms often can be prevented or treated by the temporary administration of any form of concentrated carbohydrate (clear candy, honey, lollipops, soft drinks) and by encouraging a good fluid intake. In this situation the same soft drinks and candy that are looked upon with horror by our dental colleagues may constitute simple but valuable therapeutic adjuncts, which can effectively lessen the crankiness that so often accompanies minor infections in young children.

A cool, humidified atmosphere, best achieved with a cold water home nebulizer may give some relief, especially if the house is abnormally dry.

Bed rest is advisable only if significant fever is present. Concern has been expressed recently over the use of acetylsalicylic acid in the treatment of influenza virus infections and varicella in children, because of an epidemiologic association that has suggested that salicylates may enhance the susceptibility of young children to the developemnt of Reye's syndrome. The validity and causal significance of such an association is still unsettled. Until the matter is clarified, a conservative approach to antipyretic medication seems prudent, especially if the illness has features suggestive of influenza.

Minor temperature elevations do not require medication, and may be treated if necessary with tepid water sponging and encouragement of a good fluid intake. Pending settlement of the salicylate–Reye's syndrome controversy, acetaminophen may be given orally in the following dosage: under 1 year, 60 mg four times daily; 1–3 years, 60–120 mg four times daily; 3–6 years, 120 mg four times daily;

6–12 years, 150–300 mg four times daily. Or dosage may be calculated on the basis of surface area, giving 700 mg/M²/24 hours, divided into 4–6 doses.

Alternatively, and in the absence of influenza-like features (and of chickenpox), acetylsalicylic acid may be given in a dose of 65 mg/kg/24 hours, divided in 4–6 doses. Antipyretics are rarely required for more than one or two days.

Innumerable cold remedies are available over the counter and are prescribed widely by physicians. These include assorted combinations of vitamin C, sympathomimetics ("oral decongestants"), antihistamines, antitussives, analgesics and/or belladonna alkaloids.

Vitamin C has not been shown to have significant therapeutic or prophylactic value. Orally administered sympathomimetics are of questionable or limited value in diminishing nasal congestion. The dose sufficient to do so may also cause some degree of general vasoconstriction and a rise in blood pressure.

As for antihistamines, the few studies that have been well designed and controlled show no benefit attributable to antihistamine administration for prevention or relief of the common cold. These compounds may have some drying and inspissating effect on secretions; they also commonly have a pronounced sedative effect—a consideration that may have special importance for adolescents of driving age in whom drowsiness may render driving dangerous. Antihistamines may be expected to provide some relief to nasal congestion only if allergic rhinitis is present.

Oral decongestant mixtures, with or without antihistamines do not reduce the frequency of otitis as a complication of colds, nor do they improve the course or outcome of otitis itself.

Sympathomimetic-antihistamine mixtures are even available in oral drop dosage form. These may carry particular risks for young infants, in whom we have observed hypercapnia attributable to respiratory depression following their use, especially if the infant happened to be mildly dehydrated. Too often these mixtures are prescribed principally as a result of advertising pressure or as the easiest way to deal with parental pressure to "do something." This sort of parental anxiety is normal and should be dealt with more directly through reassurance and explanation of what can be expected in the normal course of the illness. The emotional tolerance of different families for the normal frequency of respiratory illness in their children is variable. Many parents are unaware of the fact that the average North American preschooler or young school-age child has 5 or 6 minor respiratory infections per year.

Removal of the tonsils and adenoids is without effect on the frequency of viral upper respiratory infections, and the empirical administration of gamma globulin under such circumstances is completely without logical foundation or demonstrated value. Kleenex and "tincture of time" remain the bulwarks of treatment of the common cold.

Rhinitis and Sinusitis

BESS G. GOLD, M.D.

RHINITIS

Rhinitis is one of the most common childhood illnesses. Although often considered trivial, rhinitis is associated with significant discomfort and morbidity.

Before initiating treatment, it is important that the clinician review the multiple causes of rhinorrhea. Obviously, some modalities of therapy may not be appropriate in all situations. There are three major causes of severe rhinitis; infections, allergies, and vasomotor instability.

Infections. Viruses cause most upper respiratory tract infections (URIs). No specific antiviral agents have been shown to be effective in treating the common cold. Furthermore, there is no evidence to support the use of antibiotics to reduce the frequency of bacterial complications such as pneumonia and otitis media. Data suggest, however, that a single daily dose of antibiotic (usually a sulfonamide) decreases subsequent episodes of acute otitis media in the otitis prone child. In this specific group of children, antibiotic prophylaxis during the winter and spring months (the peak period for incidence of otitis media) may be warranted. Nevertheless, data on chronic antibiotic prophylaxis for the child with recurrent otitis media is not directly applicable to the normal child with a viral URI. Future vaccines, and such new drugs as interferon, may modulate the severity of many viral respiratory illnesses, but at present, these possibilities seem remote. The development of effective vaccines will be hindered by the fact that immunity to most respiratory viruses is of limited duration and that there are a multitude of viral agents that can produce a URI symptom complex. Additionally, vaccine production is tedious and costly, thus the management of the viral URI should remain largely symptomatic in the near future.

Purulent rhinitis is poorly differentiated and inadequately studied. Although bacterial infections can cause rhinorrhea, it may actually be an early phase of acute sinusitis. Pathogens include *Streptococcus pneumoniae*, *S. pyogenes*, *Hemophilus influenzae*, and *Staphylococcus aureus*. The physician should perform careful pneumatic otoscopy to assess whether there is an associated acute otitis media. It is also essential to rule out other, more serious associated illness. High fever and URI may be the sole symptoms of walk-in bacteremia in young children. A CBC and erythrocyte sedimentation rate are useful in determining which of those patients are at risk of bacteremia.

After more serious illness is excluded, a trial of oral antibiotics may be warranted if fever is present or purulent rhinorrhea has persisted for longer than 2 weeks, even in the absence of fever. Amoxicillin (40 mg/kg daily in 3 divided doses) is effective against the probable bacterial pathogens. Atlhough *Mycoplasma pneumoniae* can be cultured from young children with isolated rhinitis, no evidence exists to suggest that the illness responds to or requires antimicrobial treatment. To answer these questions, a rapid method to establish this diagnosis will be needed.

Decongestants may make the patient more comfortable and may promote sinus drainage. In general, because of problems of dosage in the small infant and paradoxical CNS stimulation, they should be used sparingly in infants less than one year of age. Symptomatic relief is often provided by humidifying the environment of the child with rhinitis, regardless of etiology.

Allergies. These are four major steps in treating the child with allergic rhinitis: 1) identification; 2) symptomatic treatment of the allergic response itself, including efforts to block the response; 3) elimination or reduction of exposure to the allergen; and 4) reduction of the patient's hypersensitivity. Successful management and sustained results require a comprehensive approach and careful, and consistent follow-up.

Often, in children, allergic rhinitis is misidentified as recurrent URI. A family history of allergic disease and physical stigmata such as "allergic shiners" and the transverse nasal crease should always suggest an allergic etiology. The allergic response cannot be modified if it goes undetected.

Five major types of drugs have proved useful in the symptomatic management of allergic rhinitis: 1) antihistamines, 2) alpha-adrenergics, 3) anticholinergics, 4) corticosteroids, and 5) cromolyn sodium. Symptomatic treatment with antihistamines often relieves sneezing, nasal itching, nasal discharge, and the cough frequently associated with postnasal drip. Because antihistamines are competitive inhibitors of histamine, maximum benefit is achieved when the drug is administered before histamine is released. Thus, antihistamines are ideally suited to long-term use during pollen seasons for patients with pollinosis and to continuous use for patients with perennial rhinitis. Chronic usage of a single drug may cause tachyphylaxis, which may require

changing to another type of antihistamine. Although children do tolerate antihistamines better than adults, untoward side effects of drowsiness (and, occasionally paradoxical central nervous system stimulation) precludes prolonged antihistamine therapy in many patients. Generally, sedation is more frequent in patients who are taking antihistamines from the ethanolamine or phenothiazine series. Clinicians should familiarize themselves with a few drugs from each major class of antihistamines so that they can maintain a therapeutic effect by switching to a different class when tachyphylaxis or unacceptable side effects develop (Table 1).

Table 1. ORAL ANTIHISTAMINES

Drug Group	Trade Name	Usual Daily Dose (in mg/kg)
(1) Ethylenediamines	Histadyl,	5
	Neo-Antergin,	5
	Pyribenzamine	5
(2) Ethanolamines	Benadryl,	5
	Clistin,	0.4
	Decapryn	2
(3) Alkylamines	Actidil,	0.2
	Chlor-Trimeton,	0.35
	Dimetane,	0.5
	Teldrin	0.35
(4) Piperazines	Bonine,	1.5
	Marezine	3
(5) Piperidines	Optimine,	0.1
	Periactin	0.25
(6) Phenothiazines	Phenergan,	0.5
	Tacaryl	0.3

Alpha-adrenergic drugs (decongestants) are useful because they constrict the vessels of the nasal mucosa. They are most effective when used in the form of nose drops or sprays. Topical application should be limited to 3–5 days, since prolonged use can damage the mucosa and lead to rebound congestion (rhinitis medicamentosa). Several different alpha-adrenergic agents, such as phenylephrine, ephedrine, isoephedrine, phenylpropanolamine, and cyclopentamine, are available for oral administration. Although not as effective as topical agents, they may be used for prolonged periods with fewer side effects.

Additionally, several preformulated combinations of antihistamine and sympathomimetic drugs are available (Table 2).

Anticholinergics such as atropine are not generally useful in managing rhinitis in children. Although these drugs can relieve rhinitis, the doses required are too frequently associated with unac-

Table 2. ANTIHISTAMINE/SYMPATHOMIMETIC COMBINATIONS

Trade Name	Ingredients	Directions Provided for Use in Children			
		<1 Year	1–6 Years	>6 Years	>12 Years
Actifed	Triprolidine, pseudoephedrine		X	X	X
Co-Pyronil	Pyrrobutamine, methapyrilene, cyclopentamine			X	X
Demazin	Chlorpheniramine, phenylephrine			X	X
Dimetapp Extentabs	Brompheniramine, phenylephrine				X
Dimetapp Elixir	Phenylpropanolamine, phenylephrine		X	X	X
Novahistine	Chlorpheniramine, phenylephrine			X	X
Novafed A	Chlorpheniramine, pseudoephedrine				X
Pyribenzamine	Tripelennamine, ephedrine				X
Rondec	Carbinoxamine, pseudoephedrine	X	X	X	X
Triaminic	Phenylpropanolamine, pheniramine maleate, pyrilamine maleate	X	X	X	X

ceptable side effects such as drying of secretions, drying of the mouth, blurred vision, and tachycardia.

Because of their potential for serious side effects and toxicity, systemic corticosteroids are not generally recommended. There are, however, occasional situations in which a short course of steroids may be indicated. If a patient who has used topical sympathomimetic agents excessively develops rebound nasal congestion, a brief (1–2 week) course of steroids combined with oral decongestants may be required to alleviate severe nasal obstruction until the effects of the topical vasoconstrictors are eliminated. When steroids are needed, beclomethasone dipropionate* nasal aerosol or flunisolide** may be used topically. Dexamethasone phosphate should not be used, because these new agents are safer. The clinician must remember, however, that some degree of systemic absorption does occur even with this route of administration. However, short term use in recommended doses of flunisolide or beclomethasone nasal spray has not been reported to cause adrenal suppression. There are rare reports of superinfections following the use of

topical steroids. Nasal corticosteroids should not be used in patients with untreated infections of the respiratory tract, nor should they be used immediately after surgery or significant trauma involving the nasal mucosa.

Cromolyn sodium, applied topically, also relieves the symptoms of allergic rhinitis. Because it must be applied to the nasal mucosa before the onset of symptoms, it is most beneficial when allergens have already been identified and the allergic stimulus can be anticipated. Cromolyn sodium can be used for prolonged periods of time and has not been associated with significant adverse effects. Its use is more limited in younger children because of difficulties with administration.

Efforts to reduce the patient's exposure to the allergens that precipitate symptoms are equally if not more important in the management of the child with allergic rhinitis. Patients with seasonal allergic rhinitis can be taught to avoid the out-of-doors during periods when pollen counts are highest. Use of air conditioners and humidifiers to maintain internal humidity at 30–40%, and frequent changing of furnace and air conditioner filters often provide symptomatic improvement. The most important area is the child's bedroom. Furnishing should be simple, with bare floors that can be easily kept dust free and window coverings that do not trap dust. Shelving should be enclosed in glass, and stuffed

*Manufacturer's precaution: Not recommended for children under 12 years of age.
**Manufacturer's precaution: Not recommended for children under 6 years of age.

toys and animals should not be kept in the bedroom.

The allergens that provoke perennial rhinitis are frequently multiple and more difficult to avoid. Although respiratory allergens such as dust and mites are frequently at fault, dietary allergens also play a prominent role. Trials of dietary elimination and subsequent challenge feedings can be used to identify dietary causes. Such trials involve caution in implementation and interpretation, and a child's diet should never be restricted for prolonged periods without convincing evidence of significant clinical improvement. If dietary restrictions are introduced, the physician must make sure that the diet is nutritionally sound.

Hyposensitivity is the third mainstay in the management of the child with allergic rhinitis. A full discussion of extract preparation and immunization schedules is beyond the scope of this chapter and should be undertaken only by someone with specific training and experience in these areas. The pediatrician should remember that patients should be retested periodically during desensitization to discover any shifts in antigen pattern.

Vasomotor Instability. Vasomotor rhinitis is caused by an overactivity of the parasympathetic system. These patients must be taught to avoid changes in temperature, exposure to spicy foods, and other stimuli that trigger rhinorrhea. Pseudoephedrine (anticholine) or propantheline bromide (antivagal) are generally useful. In general, antihistamines and cromolyn sodium are not effective; however, a subgroup of patients who have no other evidence of allergic disease but who have significant numbers (greater than 25%) of eosinophils on smears of nasal secretions often do respond well to antihistamines.

Other Causes. Remember, poor nasal and sinus airflow secondary to any kind of obstruction can cause rhinorrhea. Adenoidal hyperplasia is one of the most frequent causes of chronic rhinitis in patients referred to otolaryngologists. It is most often seen in the child between 2 and 7 years of age. Other anatomic causes of chronic rhinitis are less common but should be considered. Trauma can cause deviation of the nasal septum and will require surgical correction to alleviate symptoms. Blood-stained nasal discharge suggests a possibile neoplasm. Persistent unilateral nasal discharge, even without a supportive clinical history, suggests a foreign body. Evaluation under anesthesia may be required to rule this out because hypertrophic changes in the nasal mucosa may obscure visualization. Nasal polyps should always suggest possible cystic fibrosis.

All rhinorrhea patients can benefit from learning that nasal symptoms are worse on lying down, because of increased venous congestion of nasal tissues. Even a small infant with nasal obstruction will be more comfortable if his head is elevated. The older child can be taught that deep diaphragmatic breathing, causing reflex dilatation of the nasal passages, can help overcome transient nasal obstruction.

SINUSITIS

It is often impossible for the clinician to differentiate between purulent rhinitis and early sinusitis and perhaps there is really no difference. Certainly, sinusitis should be considered in any child in whom rhinorrhea or unexplained coughing has continued for longer than 2 weeks.

Unless complications are present, the treatment of acute sinusitis is primarily medical. The patient should be advised to avoid forceful blowing of the nose, flying, and swimming. Specific therapy is aimed at promoting sinus drainage, eradicating infection, and alleviating discomfort. Topical nasal decongestants such as oxymetazoline HCl (0.05% for children > 6 years and 0.025% for children 2–5 years, 2–3 drops) are useful at first; however they should not be continued for longer than 5 to 7 days because of the danger of rebound nasal congestion. Systemic decongestants are generally used. Many preparations are combined with an antihistamine, although no clinical trials have shown better results when a combination drug is used. Some specialists believe that antihistamine-decongestant combinations are too drying and that they make sinus secretions more tenacious and, therefore, more difficult to drain. To promote drainage, the environment should be kept warm and well humidified.

Antibiotics of choice are those that are active against the major pathogens implicated in acute sinusitis in childhood. These include *S. pneumoniae, H. influenzae* (predominantly nontypable isolates), and *S. pyogenes.* Ampicillin (75–100 mg/kg/day) or amoxicillin (in equivalent doses) are usually the drugs of choice. Alternatives are trimethoprim/sulfamethoxazole (12 mg TMP/60 mg SMX/kg/day in 2 divided doses), a combination of erythromycin (50 mg/kg/day) and sulfisoxazole (150 mg/kg/day) both in 4 divided doses, or cefaclor (40 mg/kg/day in 3 divided doses). The alternative regimens are effective against ampicillin-resistant hemophilus. As many as 15% of nontypable strains of *H. influenzae* produce beta-lactamase and will be resistant to ampicillin and amoxicillin. However, no clinical studies have shown superiority of these drugs over ampicillin. Cost considerations therefore preclude a change in the recommendation for initial antimicrobial therapy at this time.

Preliminary reports from ongoing clinical studies suggest that *Branhamella catarrhalis* may be a more prominent pathogen than previously suspected. Because these organisms are frequently resistant to ampicillin and cephalosporins, results of clinical trials may ultimately prove the superiority of antimicrobial regimens that combine a penicillin with a beta-lactamase inhibitor. Examples of such new drug combinations are Augmentin and Sulbactam. Antibiotics should be administered for 10–14 days for acute, uncomplicated sinusitis.

Analgesics should be given to alleviate discomfort. In most cases, acetaminophen is sufficient. Local heat should be applied to the involved sinus.

The pediatric patient with acute sinusitis should be followed carefully to assess whether clinical response is satisfactory. Any patient with sinusitis involving the frontal sinus should be seen *daily* until significant clinical improvement is noted. Repeat sinus radiographs are usually indicated in the child who does not respond well to therapy. Despite traditional teaching, recent studies and personal experience confirm the usefullness of sinus radiographs in children older than 1 year of age.

Patients with acute sinusitis must occasionally be hospitalized for initial management. Any child presenting with a complication of sinusitis, ranging from periorbital or orbital cellulitis to a soft tissue swelling overlying the frontal sinus suggestive of a Pott's puffy tumor, should be hospitalized for thorough evaluation and management, as should patients who appear extremely toxic. The frontal sinusitis patient who does not respond in 48 hours to outpatient management should also be hospitalized. A more aggressive approach is justified in these patients, since frontal sinusitis is more frequently associated with life-threatening complications than is disease limited to the ethmoid or maxillary sinuses. This propensity may be partially due to the tortuous course of the nasofrontal duct and the fact that the posterior wall of the frontal sinus is a common wall to the anterior cranial fossa.

The possibility of a central nervous system (CNS) complication should be excluded in any child hospitalized with sinusitis. The young child with ethmoid sinusitis and periorbital cellulitis often has bacteremia, and coexistent meningitis is not uncommon. A lumbar puncture should be performed in such children who are less than 2 years of age to exclude this possibility. Although meningitis is an infrequent complication in the older child, localized CNS complications must be excluded in those who require hospitalization. The risk of such complications is greatest in the child with frontal sinusitis, and, therefore, they are seen primarily in the adolescent patient. Localized CNS complications include epidural and subdural empyema, cerebritis, brain abscess, and cavernous sinus thrombosis. The computerized tomogram (CT) often provides useful information about the extent of sinus disease and also may identify such CNS complications. A lumbar puncture should not be performed if a localized CNS complication is demonstrated on the CT scan. When the CT scan fails to reveal a CNS complication, a lumbar puncture is usually indicated. An increased opening pressure and pleocytosis of the spinal fluid may be the only findings in the patient with early CNS complications.

Bacterial cultures play no role in the management of the usual outpatient with sinusitis. Several studies have shown that the only reliable cultures to determine the etiologic agents are those obtained by direct aspiration from the sinus. It is appropriate, however, to obtain cultures from any patient requiring hospitalization. Cultures should also be obtained when sinusitis develops in a debilitated or immunodeficient patient. Samples should be submitted for aerobic, anaerobic, and, if quantity permits, fungal cultures. The importance of obtaining suitable stains (such as the Gram stain) cannot be overemphasized, since they may provide immediate diagnostic data; provide information on the relative importance of various organisms subsequently identified in culture; and implicate organisms that are never recovered from the cultures. Since sinusitis is frequently a polymicrobial infection and different pathogens may be isolated from different sinuses in a single patient, culture results are more often useful in indicating the need of expanding rather than narrowing antimicrobial coverage.

Antimicrobial therapy of the sinusitis patient who requires hospitalization should be broad in its coverage. Because of the risk of associated bacteremia in the young child with ethmoiditis and periorbital cellulitis, and potential intracranial complications in the older patient (especially in those with frontal sinusitis), antibiotics that diffuse well into the cerebrospinal fluid should be used. A semisynthetic penicillin and chloramphenicol combination is frequently a good choice. Duration of parenteral therapy will depend on the nature and extent of disease. Parenteral therapy for the patient without complications should be continued until the patient is improved and has been afebrile a minimum of 72 hours. Such children should complete therapy with oral antibiotics. In general, a total of 2 weeks is sufficient for treatment of acute uncomplicated sinusitis. The child with associated bacteremia and/or meningitis will require at least 10 to 14 days of parenteral therapy. The child with osteomyelitis or central nervous system complications other than meningitis will require a minimum of 4–6 weeks of parenteral therapy.

The patient with complicated sinusitis almost invariably requires aggressive surgical drainage of the involved sinuses. One exception is in young children with preseptal cellulitis complicating ethmoiditis. Surgical approach will depend on the sinuses involved. An experienced otolaryngologist will aid in the selection of appropriate techniques.

The team approach is essential in the management of the patient with complicated sinusitis. Ophthalmologic examinations should be obtained early in treatment to establish a baseline of visual function, even in children without obvious involvement of the periorbital space. The otolaryngologist must follow each patient closely to ascertain that sinus drainage is prompt and complete. The pediatrician, sometimes with the help of an infectious disease specialist, should monitor antimicrobial therapy. Since antimicrobial therapy is often prolonged, the pediatrician should ensure that the patient is monitored for possible side effects. Perhaps the most important functions of the pediatrician are to provide counseling for the patient and family and to coordinate the efforts of the specialists involved in the patient's care.

Retropharyngeal and Lateral Pharyngeal Abscesses

ELLEN MAE FRIEDMAN, M.D.

Retropharyngeal cellulitis may respond to vigorous parenteral antibiotic therapy. Most otolaryngologists concur, however, that abscesses require incision and drainage. Controversy exists as to whether an intraoral or an external approach is more useful. This decision is usually dictated by the size, location, and extent of the abscess cavity. The computed tomography scan plays an important role in the decision-making process.

Small retropharyngeal abscesses may be drained intraorally. The patient should be gently intubated to avoid iatrogenic rupture of the abscess. The patient should be placed in the Trendelenburg position. With a headlight for illumination, a midline incision should be made, with suction in hand. Aerobic and anaerobic specimens should be sent for culture and sensitivity and a swab sent for acid-fast bacilli. A blunt curved clamp is used to break septate pockets within the cavity and promote prolonged drainage. Naturally, one must bear in mind the position of the carotid arteries at all times.

Larger abscesses require an external approach for drainage. Similar care with intubation is exercised. A transverse incision is made at the level of the anterior border of the sternocleidomastoid muscle. The muscle and the carotid sheath are retracted laterally, and the abscess cavity is usually identified at the level of the hypopharynx. Again, culture and sensitivity specimens are crucial in determining appropriate antimicrobial management. The full extent of the abscess cavity must be appreciated and opened by evaluating the entire length of the carotid sheath. External drains should be inserted and kept in place for several postoperative days.

Postoperative care includes vigorous parenteral antibiotic therapy. Ampicillin, 100 mg/kg/24 hr in four divided doses, and oxacillin, 200 mg/kg/24 hours in four divided doses, given initially. The predominant organism is a beta-hemolytic streptococcus, although staphylococcus and anaerobic organisms have been isolated. It is wise to employ broad-spectrum antibiotic coverage pending the results of the intraoperative cultures and sensitivities, following which the choice of antibiotic coverage can most accurately be determined. Warm saline irrigations as well as local heat can add to the patient's comfort.

The Tonsil and Adenoid Problem

TREVOR J. I. McGILL, M.D.

Controversy still surrounds the indications for tonsillectomy and adenoidectomy. This is due to the striking paucity of well-controlled clinical trials in this area. Surgical attitudes have changed considerably during the past 10 years; surgical intervention is advocated in very specific clinical situations. Definite indications include 1) corpulmonale secondary to chronic upper airway obstruction. Lymphoid hyperplasia resulting in hypoventilation and pulmonary hypertension may require either tonsillectomy or adenoidectomy or both, depending on the relative size of the adenoids and nasopharynx and the tonsils and oropharynx; or 2) the peripheral sleep apnea syndrome, secondary to severe adenotonsillar hyperplasia. Patients with this syndrome do not display hypercarbia while awake but have profound apneic episodes with oxygen desaturation during sleep. The oxygen desaturation observed in these patients during sleep may be associated with cardiac irregularities. The hypothesis that sudden death may occur in patients with severe tonsillar and adenoid enlargement and associated apneic episodes has evolved from this observation.

Tonsillectomy is also indicated under the following circumstances: 1) seven episodes of recurrent streptococcal tonsillitis occurring during the previous 12 months or ten episodes of recurrent streptococcal tonsillitis occurring during the previous 24 months. Each episode should be confirmed by a positive culture for group A beta-hemolytic streptococci or it should be a clearly defined bacterial illness with temperature over 38.3° C (101° F), exudative tonsillitis, cervical adenopathy, and a positive response to antimicrobial therapy; or 2) peritonsillar abscess occurring in adolescents. Under certain circumstances the operation of drainage of the abscess and removal of the tonsils can be combined.

Adenoidectomy alone should be considered when significant obstruction of the posterior choana by adenoid hypertrophy exists. The situation can be confirmed by a lateral radiograph of the neck in which complete obstruction of the nasal airflow is seen to result in stagnation of secretions and persistent rhinorrhea. Patients with recurrent bacterial rhinitis and sinusitis commonly benefit from an adenoidectomy.

Disorders of the Larynx

VICTOR E. CALCATERRA, M.D.

The three major roles of the larynx are airway control, sphincteric closure, and phonation. In disease, dysfunction of these roles results in the symptoms of stridor, aspiration, and hoarseness, respectively. Each laryngeal disorder affects function in a unique and predictable way. Careful attention to the subtle variability of symptoms, such as the acoustic character of stridor and hoarseness in different laryngeal diseases, can provide the clinician with valuable information in making a diagnosis.

CONGENITAL

Laryngomalacia is the most common cause of stridor in the neonate and infant. The diagnosis is confirmed by the observation of collapse of the supraglottic structures during inspiration, for which the flexible fiberoptic laryngoscope is ideally suited. Treatment consists of assuring the parents that their child will outgrow the stridor in anywhere from a few months to a few years. Occasionally placement of the patient in the prone position is helpful. A tracheostomy is rarely required.

Congenital neurologic impairments of laryngeal function usually occur as part of a larger neurologic disorder. If the vocal cords are paralyzed in a paramedian position, airway obstruction with stridor will be present, and a tracheostomy is needed. If there is inadequate laryngeal closure or pharyngeal dysfunction, aspiration occurs, necessitating a gastrostomy and possibly a tracheostomy. Isolated vocal cord paralysis and congenital subglottic stenosis will be discussed later.

Congenital webs and cysts are best treated endoscopically by surgical excision. If the web is thin, midline division is usually adequate, but subsequent dilatations may be necessary. In thicker webs, excision of tissue becomes necessary, followed by soft intraluminal stenting for 6 weeks.

In the last few years, the carbon dioxide laser has proved effective in the treatment of *subglottic hemangioma*. The lesion can be totally removed endoscopically at the time of diagnosis without performing a tracheostomy. The success of this method has greatly reduced the need for long-term steroid therapy. Radiotherapy should be avoided.

TRAUMATIC

Laryngeal fractures, although uncommon in children, represent life-threatening emergencies. Because edema and hemorrhage will almost certainly reduce the laryngeal airway, a tracheostomy is mandatory once the condition is recognized. Subsequent repair will not be discussed except to say that it usually involves open reduction.

Vocal cord nodules are the result of vocal abuse. These cases should be referred to a speech pathologist for evaluation and possible treatment. One should keep in mind that vocal cord nodules tend to disappear at puberty, possibly due to improved vocal habits. Surgical removal is rarely required.

IATROGENIC

The first stage of *acquired subglottic stenosis* is acute mucosal injury, usually from prolonged or poorly managed endotracheal intubation resulting in mucosal denudation, edema, granulation tissue, and sometimes chondritis. Airway obstruction following extubation usually alerts the clinician to the existence of the stenosis. If the airway is reasonably safe, direct laryngoscopy may be performed to assess the injury and to determine whether a tracheostomy is needed. At the same time, exuberant granulation tissue and necrotic debris can be removed, improving the airway and possibly avoiding a tracheostomy. In such cases the child should be closely monitored and treated with steroids, antibiotics, and a mist tent. Except for airway control prior to a tracheostomy, tracheal reintubation for an additional length of time is to be avoided because it will only worsen the subglottic injury.

In patients requiring a tracheostomy, subsequent treatment should include systemic antibiotics and steroids to reduce granulation tissue and prevent scarring. Topical antibiotic ointment should be applied to the tracheostomy site to control stomal bacteria and lessen tracheobronchial contamination. In a few weeks, the subglottic inflammation will subside, leaving behind either a normal subglottic lumen or a cicatricial, stenotic subglottic space. During this period of healing, direct laryngoscopy with dilatation and intralesional steroid injection should be performed. If a partial stenosis finally results but the airway is adequate, allowing decannulation, nothing further should be done as the subglottic lumen will increase in size as the child becomes older.

If cicatricial subglottic stenosis results and decannulation cannot be achieved, scar tissue excision should be performed. This is best accomplished endoscopically, using the carbon dioxide laser. Following excision, a soft intraluminal stent is left in place for approximately 6 weeks. If an adequate subglottic airway is not obtained after this procedure, an external laryngeal approach is necessary. Various techniques have been devised to deal with this surgical challenge. Most of the procedures include dividing the cricoid either anteriorly or posteriorly, depending on the position of the stenosis, and, if necessary, the upper tracheal rings. A free graft of bone or cartilage is then interposed to maintain the surgically enlarged subglottic space.

Congenital subglottic stenosis results in varying degrees of airway obstruction, and approximately 50 per cent of patients will require a tracheostomy. Treatment is based on the fact that the obstruction typically decreases with age because of subglottic growth. Direct laryngoscopy and dilatation are performed every 4 months until an adequate airway is attained. In children with tracheostomies, the smallest possible tube is used, to encourage function of the larynx and permit speech development. Most children can be decannulated by 2 years of age.

In a *unilateral vocal cord paralysis* secondary to recurrent laryngeal nerve injury, the paralyzed vocal cord assumes a paramedian position. The nonparalyzed vocal cord is capable of approximating the paralyzed cord during phonation, resulting in a near-normal voice. Dysphagia or aspiration or both are unlikely, and usually the airway is adequate. As a result, unilateral vocal cord paralysis will probably not require treatment; however, occasionally in neonates the narrowed glottic airway is inadequate, and a tracheostomy is necessary. When a unilateral vocal cord paralysis is secondary to a lesion in the proximal portion of the vagus nerve near its exit from the base of the skull, pharyngeal dysfunction occurs with dysphagia and aspiration, requiring a gastrostomy and possibly a tracheostomy.

In *bilateral vocal cord paralysis,* both vocal cords assume a paramedian position, resulting in airway obstruction necessitating a tracheostomy. Swallowing is usually unaffected.

INFECTION

The medical treatment of *epiglottitis* and *laryngotracheobronchitis with subglottic edema* (croup) is discussed in the following section. The method used for airway intervention in severe epiglottitis and croup has been controversial and is worthy of comment. For many years tracheostomy was the only procedure used, but recently endotracheal intubation has been shown to be a safe and effective method and is now the procedure of choice. Minimal laryngeal or tracheal damage occurs if the endotracheal tube is sufficiently small and properly managed. However, a staff experienced in pediatric intubation and an intensive care unit familiar with proper management of indwelling endotracheal tubes are needed. In their absence, the time-honored tracheostomy is preferred.

NEOPLASIA

Juvenile laryngeal papilloma (also known as recurrent respiratory papilloma) is the most common laryngeal neoplasm in children, and evidence so far suggests a viral etiology. Although immunotherapy, chemotherapy, and radiotherapy have been used, meticulous endoscopic excision is the mainstay of treatment. The goal is thorough removal of the lesions to maintain phonatory and airway function of the larynx while avoiding damage to normal laryngeal tissues. Treatment results should be viewed in terms of remissions and not cures since recurrences may develop after a disease-free interval of 10 years. A tracheostomy should be avoided as it appears to promote the spread of the papillomas into the tracheobronchial tree.

The Croup Syndrome: Laryngotracheobronchitis and Epiglottitis

RICHARD B. GOLDBLOOM, M.D.

The term croup denotes a symptom complex characterized by a barking cough and varying degrees of inspiratory stridor. The symptoms can result from any condition that irritates the supraglottis, glottis, or subglottic trachea or from any disorder that compromises the lumen of the upper airway.

The commonest and most benign variety of croup syndrome is so-called spasmodic croup. Typically, the child goes to bed apparently well and awakens suddenly a few hours later with a characteristic cough, reminiscent of a seal's bark. This may be accompanied by varying degrees of stridor. Symptomatic relief is often obtained by exposure to cold air and high levels of humidity. The latter is best achieved by the use of a cold-water home nebulizer. If not available, a humidifier may be used or the child may be taken into a bathroom humidified by letting the hot shower run. In most children with spasmodic croup, symptoms will disappear or be markedly improved within a few hours but may recure intermittently thereafter, especially at night. Often there is no obvious antecedent respiratory infection. Provided stridor is not severe, these children can usually be managed successfully at home without medication.

Several types of infection can produce combinations of supraglottic, glottic, and/or subglottic swelling with the potential for acute upper respiratory obstruction. Management plans for this group of conditions should be well worked out in advance, by both individual physicians and emergency room teams.

Until recently, the chief representatives of the infective croup syndromes were felt to be epiglottitis due to *Hemophilus influenzae* and subglottic croup of viral origin, of which parainfluenza Type I and respiratory syncytial virus are the commonest agents. A less common but important condition, membranous laryngotracheobronchitis, usually caused by *Staphylococcus aureus* must now be added to the list. This infection involves chiefly the larynx and subglottic area, producing a membrane of inflammatory debris on the tracheal wall.

The therapeutic priorities in all these conditions are 1) the assurance and maintenance of a secure and adequate airway, and 2) specific treatment of the infecting organism, when possible. Treatment should be modified in accordance with the skill and experience of the caretakers and the nature of available facilities.

Upper respiratory obstruction induces acute anxiety in both the child and family, thus it is important that the anxiety not be compounded by frantic behavior on the part of emergency room staff. All concerned should be soft-spoken, outwardly calm, and reassuring. All painful procedures such as fingerpricks for blood counts or venipuncture for blood cultures should be postponed until a satisfactory airway is assured.

VIRAL LARYNGOTRACHEOBRONCHITIS (SUBGLOTTIC CROUP)

In treating any child with acute infectious croup, the physician must first determine whether the obstructive swelling is supraglottic or subglottic. The risk of sudden, life-threatening obstruction is chiefly associated with supraglottic obstruction, especially epiglottitis; in viral laryngotracheobronchitis, obstruction sufficient to require an artificial airway is uncommon.

Many children with viral croup obtain significant relief from exposure to cool water vapor. At home a cold-water nebulizer may be used, or in hospital a mist tent, with or without oxygen, as required.

Children with upper respiratory obstruction should not be sedated unless it has been clearly established that restlessness, if present, is *not* due to cerebral hypoxia. The administration of sedation to a child who is anxious and restless as a result of cerebral hypoxia can worsen the hypoxic state.

Nebulized racemic epinephrine and/or corticosteroids may offer transient benefit in reducing edema and mucosal swelling in the upper respiratory tract.

Nebulized racemic epinephrine 2.25% in a dose of 0.2 to 0.4 ml added to 3 ml of water or normal saline may be administered by mask inhalation with oxygen prior to endotracheal intubation. There appears to be no particular advantage to administering racemic epinephrine with intermittent positive pressure breathing (IPPB), as opposed to simple nebulization alone. Nebulization without IPPB may be better tolerated by younger patients. The beneficial effects of racemic epinephrine are transient (generally less than two hours). Also, some degree of rebound phenomenon is possible. Thus, it should be given only to children who are under close observation in hospital, and not as a means of alleviating croup in emergency rooms.

The evidence of benefit from corticosteroid administration in the croup syndrome is still equivocal. Short-term usage (1 or 2 days at most) does not appear to carry significant adverse side effects, but should be regarded as no more than adjunctive therapy. Steroids should probably be used only in children who are sufficiently ill to require hospitalization. Dexamethasone may be given intramuscularly in a dose of 0.5–1.5 mg/kg, or methylprednisolone 4–6 mg/kg. There is evidence to suggest that suppression of the inflammatory response is directly proportional to the dose of steroid given.

ACUTE EPIGLOTTITIS

Among the croup syndromes, epiglottitis carries the highest risk of sudden, life-threatening respiratory obstruction. Sometimes the diagnosis can be strongly suspected from information provided by the parents or referring physician over the telephone. Sudden onset of illness with high fever, dysphagia, sore throat, the child wishing to sit up with the chin pushed forward, and drooling are the hallmarks of epiglottitis. If transport to an emergency room is required, careful instructions for management during transport should be given. If possible, the child should be accompanied by a physician who is capable of orotracheal intubation. The youngster should be transported in the sitting position. Oxygen and a bag and mask should be available. The child may get some transient relief from exposure to cold air, e.g., keeping the car window open.

On arrival at hospital, if there is doubt about the diagnosis, lateral soft tissue radiographs of the neck may be desired. No attempt should be made to insert a tongue depressor in the mouth. Prior to establishment of a secure airway, the child should be constantly accompanied by an individual capable and equipped to deal with sudden airway obstruction. Radiographs, if required, should be taken on a portable machine in an intensive care area, always with the child in a sitting position, never recumbent. If there is little doubt about the diagnosis and endotracheal intubation is already considered essential, then there is little to be gained by performing radiographs, and valuable time may be lost in the process.

The crux of management in epiglottitis is early establishment of an adequate, secure airway until the worst of the inflammation has subsided. The preferred management is orotracheal intubation by a competent physician, followed by substitution of a nasotracheal tube. Nasotracheal intubation carries much less risk of spontaneous extubation than does orotracheal intubation.

Induction of inhalation anesthesia should be carried out with the child in the sitting position, under ECG monitoring, using halothane and 100% oxygen. When consciousness is lost, the child is placed in the "sniffing" position, using several folded towels under the neck.

Premature attempts at intubation are dangerous —thus anesthesia is deepened for at least 10 minutes. Laryngospasm and airway obstruction are managed with good bag and mask technique, using continuous positive airway pressure (CPAP) ± assistance.

When full anesthesia is reached, the laryngeal opening is identified and an endotracheal tube inserted. The epiglottis is often unrecognizable and the vocal cords not seen due to marked swelling of the false cords. Following orotracheal intubation, the airway is cleared of secretions and the patient is given several minutes of good spontaneous or assisted ventilation prior to insertion of a nasotracheal tube.

Cultures taken from the throat or epiglottis are of little value, since they are frequently negative despite the presence of *H. influenzae* infection. The organism is much more likely to be isolated from blood cultures, which are best taken while the child is under anesthesia.

Following intubation, a high level of humidification and adequate oxygenation of the inspired air should be maintained. Humidified 30% O_2 will suffice in most cases. In most cases, extubation can be safely carried out within 24–48 hours. Demonstration of air leakage around the nasotracheal tube, lack of fever, and the presence of clear secretions are good indicators that the tube can be safely removed.

Tracheostomy is very rarely necessary. It should never be attempted as an heroic "kitchen table" emergency procedure unless there is failure of intubation, but should only be carried out following orotracheal intubation and complete stabilization of the child's condition.

It is possible that a few cases of epiglottitis can be managed successfully without establishing an artificial airway. However, one should be acutely aware of the risk of sudden, acute obstruction in any child with epiglottitis. Management without inserting an endotracheal airway should be considered only in a well-equipped tertiary care center when a physician skilled in intubation will remain close to the child's bedside around the clock until all danger of obstruction is past.

Most instances of epiglottitis are due to *H. influenzae* infection. Since as many as 10–15% of *H. influenzae* isolates may be ampicillin-resistant, treatment should be initiated with intravenous ampicillin, 200 mg/kg/24 hours, and IV chloramphenicol, 100 mg/kg/24 hours. If the organism is isolated from the blood culture and proves sensitive to ampicillin in vitro, then chloramphenicol should be discontinued. Antibiotic therapy should be maintained orally as soon as feasible for 7–10 days.

If *H. influenzae* is isolated from the patient, any siblings under the age of 4 years should be given prophylaxis with rifampin, 20 mg/kg, given once daily for 4 days (maximum dose 600 mg daily).*

MEMBRANOUS LARYNGOTRACHEOBRONCHITIS

At its onset membranous laryngotracheobronchitis or membranous tracheitis, usually due to infection with *S. aureus,* may be difficult to distinguish clinically from epiglottitis or viral laryngotracheobronchitis. The degree of stridor in membranous tracheitis is variable, and hoarseness may be prominent. Lateral soft-tissue radiographs of the neck, taken in inspiration, may help to make the distinction, in that the involvement is chiefly subglottic in membranous tracheitis and the epiglottis and aryepiglottic folds appear normal radiographically and by endoscopy. In this condition, endoscopy may be necessary to establish the diagnosis and to remove the inspissated secretions and debris that form the so-called membrane. Based on the degree of obstruction, a judgment will have to be made whether short-term intubation is required or whether maintenance of good hydration with intravenous fluids, humidified oxygen or air, and nebulized racemic epinephrine are required. The other important therapeutic reason for distinguishing this form of laryngotracheobronchitis is the need to select an antibiotic effective against *S. aureus.* Treatment may be initiated with cloxacillin, 150 mg/kg/24 hours intravenously in 4 doses.

Pneumothorax and Pneumomediastinum

KEITH W. ASHCRAFT, M.D.

Air in the pleural space compromises the expansion of the lung. A disruption of the integrity of a bronchiole or of integrity in the visceral pleura is the usual cause of pneumothorax, although a penetrating chest wall injury may allow air in without

---

*This use of rifampin is not listed by the manufacturer.

damage to the lung itself. A small, transient air leak need not be treated, because the air will resorb if the leak is stopped. A large pneumothorax or a continuous leak that compromises re-expansion of the lung will need to be treated by placement of a pleural drainage tube to underwater seal. Underwater seal or negative pressure (suction) applied to the tube will expand the lung approximating visceral and parietal pleura, which will usually allow the leak to seal within a short time.

In patients with chronic lung disease such as cystic fibrosis a small pneumothorax may be exceedingly serious and require chest tube drainage. A massive air leak may shift the mediastinum toward the undamaged lung, compromising its ability to expand. A tension pneumothorax is thus a life-threatening lesion and must be treated as an emergency. Placement of a trocar or a large bore needle into the pleural space may be life-saving until satisfactory chest tube drainage can be established.

Treatment of the pneumothorax should fit the severity of the lesion. Judgment must be made as to the etiology of the pneumothorax and its potential for producing serious trouble. It is best to err on the side of safety by placing a chest tube unnecessarily than to assume the pneumothorax will be of little consequence until dire circumstances develop.

Placement of a chest tube for simple pneumothorax is probably best done in the anterior, superior portion of the chest wall. The tube for treatment of traumatic pneumothorax is probably best placed through the seventh or eighth intercostal space in the midaxillary line, directed posteriorly because it will then be capable of draining associated blood or fluid, which may be accumulating in the pleural space. Local anesthesia consisting of 1% lidocaine infiltrated into the area of skin incision and along the proposed subcutaneous tunnel into the intercostal space, where the tube will penetrate the pleura is sufficient. In the newborn infant, lidocaine may be toxic, even in small doses, and local anesthesia, if any, should consist of 0.5% procaine (Novocaine) in very small amounts. It is important, particularly in the small infant with very little subcutaneous fat, that the skin entry site be two interspaces below the intercostal space used for insertion of the tube into the pleura so that upon withdrawal of the tube the tract may easily be compressed from outside without the use of a purse-string skin suture or further surgical manipulation. After the skin incision has been made to the anesthetized area, a curved hemostat is inserted under the skin up to the interspace selected, punched through the pleural space, and spread slightly. By grasping the tube between the jaws of the same hemostat, repetition of this maneuver will allow delivery of the chest tube into the pleural space with

little problem. Sterile technique is indicated, both on insertion and removal of this chest tube. It is important that the tube not be pushed too far into the pleural space in order to prevent bending and kinking of the tube, which tend to reduce its effectiveness. Some estimate of length should be made prior to the insertion of the tube so that the most proximal hole in the chest tube will be just barely inside the pleural space. A silk ligature tied around the tube as an indicator will help identify the depth to which the tube should be placed. The chest tube, varying from 12 to 24 F, can be used in children, depending upon the size of the patient and the amount of air leak anticipated. An occlusive dressing of petrolatum gauze ought to be placed at the skin entry site because at times a leak into the pleural space from the penetrating wound will produce a continued pneumothorax.

Placement of a chest tube may be complicated by injury to an intercostal artery. The bleeding that results can be massive. This complication must always be kept in mind and some facility for surgical treatment should be available.

The chest tube is connected to a waterseal with or without the use of suction device to help the lung expand. Chronic pneumothorax in an older patient may resolve slowly while an acute pneumothorax in almost any patient will resolve very quickly most times. If the waterseal is maintained and the air leak is not massive, negative pressure is often not necessary and frequently not is desirable in treatment of the pneumothorax.

When the chest tube has ceased bubbling and the radiograph indicates that the lung is fully expanded, the chest tube is probably ready for removal. As a test prior to removal of the chest tube, the tube should be clamped for 4 to 24 hours. A chest radiograph is taken just prior to anticipated removal. If a pneumothorax reaccumulates while the tube is clamped, the tube is certainly not ready to be removed. The tube should then be reopened to waterseal drainage and/or suction.

Recurrent Pneumothorax

Some patients with chronic respiratory problems such as cystic fibrosis or pulmonary blebs may have recurrent pneumothorax on one or both sides. A relatively minor pneumothorax in a patient with chronic pulmonary disease may well be life-threatening, and therefore tube thoracostomy is indicated prior to establishment of some form of pleurodesis. Pleural fusion to prevent further collapse may be produced by instillation of intrapleural tetracycline. Two or three instillations may be necessary. Open thoracotomy with abrasive handling of the lung surface and parietal pleura often produces enough postoperative adhesions to keep the lung attached to the parietal pleura from that point onward and prevent life-threatening recurrent pneumothorax. Pleural stripping or instillation of talc are additional methods of producing adhesions between the pleural surfaces.

Pneumomediastinum

Pneumomediastinum almost always occurs as a ventilatory complication when small pulmonary parenchymal leaks dissect back along the bronchus to the mediastinum and produce dissection of air. Air may dissect into the pericardium or down along tissue planes to the abdominal cavity and produce pneumoperitoneum from this same lesion. In the very ill, ventilator-dependent patient, it is often difficult to determine whether a perforation of the intestinal tract has occurred. Contrast study of the upper gastrointestinal tract may well be indicated. Demonstration of an intact gastrointestinal tract will avoid an unnecessary operation in a critically ill infant, while intraperitoneal spill of contrast will lead to prompt laparotomy. Most often pneumomediastinum is not associated with excessive pressure and is a self-limiting disorder. At times it may require needle aspiration, either by the subxiphoid route or through the sternal notch. Occasionally, insertion of a chest tube by either of these routes will be needed to relieve tension.

Complete resolution of the pneumomediastinum will not occur immediately because air may have dissected into many small tissue planes, not all of which readily communicate with the inserted mediastinal tube. As long as the tension is relieved, however, the patient should be improved. Once the need for high ventilatory pressures is over, the mediastinal tube can be removed. It is not necessary to go through a period of clamping of the tube prior to its removal.

Pneumomediastinum that occurs as the result of an acute perforation of the esophagus by a foreign body usually requires surgical drainage and the administration of antibiotics. It may even be best to consider open surgical closure of the esophageal laceration once the etiology has been established.

and, as with pneumothorax, expansion of the lung is the physiologic parameter that is compromised.

In the early postoperative patient who has straw-colored fluid draining from his chest tube, chylothorax may be difficult if not impossible to diagnose. Only with the resumption of oral fat intake does the chyle take on its characteristic creamy nature. Most often by this time the postoperative chest drainage tube has been removed. Intrapleural accumulation of fluid signals that all is not well. Thoracentesis may be the first step in diagnosis and treatment of chylothorax but it is very unlikely that this alone will suffice as definitive treatment. Even repeated thoracentesis over a period of days, unless the amount of fluid accumulating is markedly diminished each day, is likely to be unsuccessful. Most chylothoraces require placement of a chest tube and continuous drainage.

The amount of chyle produced is related somewhat to the intake of fat, and therefore the more elemental the diet the less chyle will be produced. Elemental diets often must be fed by nasogastric tube. Even under these circumstances, the production of chyle may not be diminished, in which case total parenteral nutrition will be required.

Dietary restriction and tube drainage treatment of chylothorax may require from 7 to 21 days. If there seems to be little or no resolution in the chyle leak by the beginning of the fourth week re-exploration of the chest is probably warranted. At operation the identification of the chyle leak may be facilitated by the administration of cream by nasogastric tube after the patient has been anesthetized and intubated. The chyle leak can be oversewn or ligated. We have seen one patient whose tension chylothorax was resistant even to two attempts at suture ligation and responded only to a modified thoracoplasty wherein the lateral chest wall pleura was taken down from the top four ribs and used to oversew the mediastinum superiorly. This child had had a pneumonectomy because of a congenital malformation of his lung and pulmonary vessels.

Chylothorax

KEITH W. ASHCRAFT, M.D.

Chylothorax is usually a complication of thoracic surgery but it sometimes occurs spontaneously in the presence of lymphangioma of the mediastinum. It most often follows operations in the lower posterior mediastinum on the right side or the upper posterior mediastinum on the left side of the chest. At either point, major thoracic lymphatic channels can be interrupted, producing leak of intestinal chyle into the pleural space. The negative intrapleural pressure allows for accumulation of chyle

Intrathoracic Cysts

KEITH W. ASHCRAFT, M.D.

A variety of cysts can occur within the chest cavity. The congenital lesions that occur most commonly in the mediastinum are duplication cysts of the esophagus, bronchogenic cysts, cystic teratomas or dermoids, thymic cysts, pericardial cysts, and cystic hygromas. Simple lung cysts are probably congenital in origin, as are cystic adenomatoid malformations. Lung parenchymal cysts, which result from infection such as pneumatocele or lung abscess must also be considered.

All congenital cysts that occur within the thoracic cavity are surgical lesions and should be removed. Even though the lesion may be asymptomatic at the time of discovery, the natural history of all of these lesions is to produce symptoms at some time. Thoracotomy with removal of the cyst is usually a very benign procedure in the proper hands.

Esophageal *duplication cysts* are usually but not always located in continuity with the esophagus. They are often located in the lower portion of the mediastinum, sharing a common muscular wall with the esophagus. Symptoms usually arise as a result of pressure upon the lumen of the esophagus producing dysphagia. Ulceration of the esophageal mucosa adjacent to the cyst may produce gastrointestinal bleeding. Surgical extirpation of the cyst lining may be accomplished by opening the muscle coat and dissecting out the cyst mucosa. Often this is a very simple procedure.

Some mediastinal cysts are extensions from below the diaphragm of foregut duplications. These may be gastric, duodenal, or upper jejunal duplications. Removal of these lesions requires both laparotomy and thoracotomy and may be difficult because of their posterior location in the upper abdomen.

Bronchogenic cysts are mediastinal cysts filled with mucus but with respiratory epithelium and sometimes small bits of cartilage. They may be located in the lower mediastinum, as are many of the esophageal duplication cysts, or they may be located up in the upper mediastinum adjacent to the trachea or either of the major bronchi. Removal of these cysts is usually a simple procedure.

Cystic teratomas or dermoids are located in the upper, anterior mediastinum, producing symptoms by compression of the airway. Calcification may be seen in a mediastinal teratoma, but it is not seen in those cysts that have only two germ-cell layers represented (dermoids). Mediastinal teratomas may be benign or malignant. Most teratomas that are mainly cystic lesions are found to be benign, but this is not an invariable rule. Whether the best approach is right thoracotomy, left thoracotomy, or median sternotomy depends upon the size of the tumor and other investigations that may indicate its extent.

Thymic cysts are unusual lesions that are also located in and about the thymus. They are usually easily removed from a lateral thoracotomy and tend not to recur.

Pericardial cysts are located on the pericardium and are often diagnosed by echocardiography and elimination of other possibilities by barium study. Whether they all need to be removed is somewhat questionable but excision is so simple that probably it is best to treat them surgically.

Cystic hygromas are among the most difficult childhood tumors to remove, for even though completely benign they may produce compromise of major mediastinal structures by infiltration and even produce death. The dissection is tedious, often bloody, frequently unsuccessful the first time or two, and probably best left to the expert. Enlargement at time of regional infection can produce acute stress and even abscess formation.

Simple lung cysts are usually rounded, are often located in the upper lobes of either the right or left lung, and are often discovered in the child who has a chest x-ray done for chronic wheezing. They are probably best treated by segmental resection of the lung or by lobectomy, depending upon the size and location. The most likely major complication of an untreated simple lung cyst is a pneumothorax.

Cystic adenomatoid malformation of the lung usually involves an entire lobe. Satisfactory treatment requires resection of the entire lobe or whatever tissue is involved. There is little or no functioning lung tissue involved, so that removal does not compromise ventilatory ability but, indeed, improves it.

Pneumatocele occurs most commonly in conjunction with staphylococcal pneumonitis. Fortunately pneumatoceles seem to be associated with enough pleural reaction that, even though they may rupture into the pleural space, acute pneumothorax does not often occur. The possibility of a pneumothorax must be kept in mind should acute respiratory distress develop in a person who has had a parenchymal infection with pneumatocele. The facility for insertion of a chest tube as an urgent procedure should be readily available. Surgical treatment other than tube thoracotomy is rarely required.

Lung abscess can occur with pneumonitis of bacterial etiology. The abscess is often large, occupying 20 to 25% of the lung volume. An air-fluid level indicates that there is bronchial communication. Once this communication becomes free enough to allow the liquid content to be coughed out or to be induced by transbronchial catheter drainage using a stiff catheter placed endoscopically or fluoroscopically, the lung abscess will resolve. It can, however, rupture into the pleural space, producing an acute empyema that may require insertion of a chest tube as an urgent procedure. Careful observation to determine the size and progression of the lesion is required.

Tumors of the Chest

KEITH W. ASHCRAFT, M.D.

A presumptive diagnosis of a chest tumor in childhood can often be made by the region in which the tumor is located. Tumors of the upper anterior mediastinum are thymic or teratomas. *Thymomas* are usually benign tumors. They produce symptoms by means of their bulk, usually compressing the airway. They are usually associated with a benign course and should be removed. There is little or no involvement of other structures. The tumor can be removed by thoracotomy on the side of its predominant location.

Both Hodgkin's and non-Hodgkin's *lymphomas* occur in the chest. Hodgkin's disease often is an extension of disease in the cervical lymph nodes and is identified by biopsy of the nodes in the neck. Non-Hodgkin's lymphoma usually occurs in the upper mediastinum, producing symptoms by pressure upon the trachea. The onset of symptoms is often insidious and the tumor may have reached an alarming size by the time a chest radiograph is obtained. Although the need for tissue diagnosis is acute, the anesthetic complications of a large mediastinal tumor may be fatal. Several days of prednisone in a dose of 2 mg/kg/day will often result in impressive shrinkage of the tumor, allowing for a much safer thoracotomy for biopsy. Multidrug chemotherapy is the mainstay of definitive therapy, and cure may be anticipated in a large percentage of patients.

Mediastinal teratomas are unusual lesions that also produce symptoms by means of airway compression. The diagnosis is difficult to establish with certainty, except when calcification is seen in the lesion. Teratomas sometimes involve the pericardium or are pedunculated on the surface of the heart. A solid tumor in this location should be considered to be a teratoma until proven otherwise. Obviously surgical removal of these lesions is indicated. The incidence of malignancy in mediastinal teratomas is about 20 to 25%.

Neural crest tumors are solid lesions that may be located anywhere from the apex of the chest to the diaphragm on either side. They may be benign, malignant, or mixed. There is evidence to suggest that malignant neuroblastomas spontaneously undergo maturation to benign paraganglioneuromas. Surgical removal is indicated, but often incomplete resection is the only thing possible, regardless of whether the lesion is benign or malignant.

Bronchial adenomas produce symptoms by causing hemoptysis or distal airway obstruction. Rarely, *sarcoma* or *carcinoma* of the lung may produce much the same picture in the child. Any obstructive lesion should be endoscopically evaluated, biopsied, and removed as if it were malignant. Parenchymal pulmonary lesions in children are often *metastatic* osteogenic sarcoma, Wilm's tumor, or rhabdomyosarcoma. Osteogenic sarcoma metastases should be surgically removed by wedge resection. Metastatic Wilm's tumors or rhabdomyosarcomas are usually multiple and are best treated by chemotherapy.

Chest wall tumors include hemangiomas, lymphangiomas, and desmoid tumors. Hemangiomas and lymphangiomas are often extensive but superficial and can be removed surgically when they are small in order to reduce the need for skin grafting. Capillary hemangiomas of the skin may resolve spontaneously. This process may be enhanced by the administration of systemic steroids. Cavernous hemangiomas, however, do not resolve, may be platelet trapping, and may bleed from repeated trauma. Most of the time these can be surgically removed without much difficulty or blood loss.

Desmoid tumors of the chest wall are much more difficult to manage and often require extensive resection of intercostal muscle and ribs. Extensive chest wall reconstruction may be necessary.

Pulmonary Sequestration

KEITH W. ASHCRAFT, M.D.

Pulmonary sequestration is a developmental anomaly in which a portion of pulmonary tissue is isolated from the tracheobronchial tree and the normal pulmonary circulation. Occasionally, the sequestration will communicate with the esophagus via a primitive bronchus. The involved pulmonary parenchyma is often cystic and degenerative, serving no useful purpose. The mechanism by which bacteria gain access to such an area is usually unknown, but occasionally infection may be a presenting symptom.

The lesion most often occurs in the lower lobes and is sometimes associated with Bochdalek's hernia of the diaphragm, although we have never seen the two lesions simultaneously. The sequestered segment of lung may be located within the pleura that invests a particular lobe, in which case it is referred to as an intralobar sequestration, or it may be completely enclosed in its own pleura, in which case it is known as an extralobar sequestration.

Surgical removal is indicated. The blood supply to the sequestered segment of lung usually comes directly off of the aorta, and on occasion will come from below the diaphragm through the inferior pulmonary ligament to supply the sequestration. Division of this ligament could cause much bleeding if the surgeon is not familiar with the lesion and its blood supply. The bronchial communication with the foregut, if present, is divided and oversewn close to the esophagus.

Only the sequestered segment of the lung should be removed. The remaining portions of the involved lobe are normal and should be carefully preserved. It is probably not necessary to do preoperative arteriography on these lesions if the surgeon is aware that the blood supply is systemic and approaches the lesion from that point of view. The most likely postoperative complication will be persistent air leak, which would be treated by leaving the chest drainage catheter in place until the leak stops.

Middle Lobe Syndrome

KEITH W. ASHCRAFT, M.D.

The natural relationship of hilar lymph nodes to the right middle lobe bronchus may cause a condition known as the middle lobe syndrome. An inflammatory process in the middle lobe of the right lung will produce a reaction in the lymph nodes and lymphatics that drain the middle lobe and surround the bronchus to the middle lobe. Enlargement of these nodes and organizing lymphangitis compresses the bronchus, which produces atelectasis and interferes with the process of clearing pneumonitis involving the middle lobe. Persistence of this pneumonitis enhances the lymphadenopathy, lymphangitis, and perilymphatic fibrosis and further prevents clearing of the middle lobe parenchyma. Even though the inflammatory process may have been resolved, the mechanical obstruction of the middle lobe bronchus by these enlarged lymph nodes may persist for months. Determination as to whether there is an active inflammatory process or whether it is simple mechanical obstruction will in large measure be decided by the patient's clinical course. Fever, productive cough, and chest pain may indicate an active pneumonitis but the absence of these with only radiographic findings of middle lobe atelectasis suggest that the inflammatory process has resolved and only the mechanical process remains. It is often difficult to convince the medical colleague caring for the patient with middle lobe atelectasis that bronchoscopy and bronchograms are very unlikely to be of benefit. The asymptomatic patient should be observed for months. We have never seen a patient who required resection of the middle lobe for persistent atelectasis due to adenopathy, nor have we seen one who was benefited by bronchoscopy or bronchography. Perhaps only after the process is continued unchanged for a period of 9 to 12 months should endoscopy be seriously considered.

Bronchitis and Bronchiolitis

FRED W. HENDERSON, M.D.

Bronchitis, or preferably *tracheobronchitis*, refers to inflammation of the trachea and larger central intrapulmonary airways; illness is characterized by an increased volume of lower respiratory tract secretions. *Bronchiolitis* refers to inflammation of smaller peripheral pulmonary airways; wheezing is the cardinal clinical sign of this syndrome. Acute respiratory tract infection is the major cause of these illnesses in childhood; this discussion will focus on the management of illness due to infection.

The majority of cases of bronchitis and bronchiolitis occur in otherwise healthy children. These illnesses are usually uncomplicated, and hospitalization is required relatively infrequently. Occasionally, normal children less than 1 year of age will require hospitalization for bronchiolitis; life-threatening illness is most often observed in children with associated abnormalities, usually of the cardiac or respiratory systems.

In formulating a therapeutic plan for children with bronchitis or bronchiolitis, a decision must be made regarding the probable cause of infection. Respiratory viral infection is responsible for most episodes of bronchitis and bronchiolitis throughout childhood; in school-age children, *Mycoplasma pneumoniae* infection becomes an important cause of these illnesses, in addition to its role as a cause of pneumonia. Viral and mycoplasmal infections are the most common causes of exacerbations of asthma requiring physician visits. Antibiotic therapy for *Streptococcus pneumoniae* and *Hemophilus influenzae* should not be used routinely for the treatment of bronchitis, bronchiolitis, or exacerbations of asthma.

Clinically useful antiviral chemotherapy is currently restricted to amantadine for influenza A infections. Pre-exposure prophylactic use of amantadine is approximately 70 per cent effective in preventing influenza A infection. There is some evidence that administration of amantadine early in the course of influenza A infection will reduce illness severity; however, it is not recommended for this purpose clinically.

Likewise, prevention of respiratory viral infection by immunization is only available for influenza A and B viruses; annual immunization with killed-virus vaccine (split product) is recommended for children with established chronic cardiorespiratory disease.

Antibiotic therapy is effective in shortening the course of clinical symptoms in patients with *Mycoplasma pneumoniae* and *Chlamydia trachomatis* infections. Erythromycin (35 to 50 mg/kg/24 hr for 2 weeks) is effective for either infection. Tetracycline (25 to 50 mg/kg/24 hr) may be used for mycoplasmal infections in children over 8 years of age; sulfisoxazole* (150 mg/kg/24 hr) may be substituted for erythromycin for treatment of chlamydial infection in infants. Antibacterial therapy does not alter symptoms in *Bordetella pertussis* infections although

---

*Not recommended for children less than 2 months of age.

colonization is terminated with erythromycin therapy, and the risk of transmission of infection to susceptible persons is reduced.

Children with single episodes of uncomplicated viral bronchitis or bronchiolitis who will be managed as outpatients require no therapy. Antihistamines, decongestants, and expectorants are of no value in ameliorating respiratory symptoms due to viral infection.

Children who require hospitalization for bronchiolitis are at risk of respiratory failure because of severe peripheral airway obstruction in the presence of an adequate ventilatory effort, or caused by hypoventilation, periodic breathing, and apnea. Mechanical ventilatory support must be available to manage respiratory insufficiency of either cause. Arterial hypoxemia is present in all children with bronchiolitis ill enough to be hospitalized; an arterial pO_2 of 50 to 60 mm Hg in room air would be typical. Supplemental inspired oxygen should be provided to maintain the arterial pO_2 between 80 and 100 mg Hg. Controlled studies of steroid therapy in bronchiolitis have been performed; no benefit related to steroid therapy was observed. These agents should not be employed in the management of bronchiolitis.

Occlusion or partial occlusion of small airways by secretions, sloughed epithelial cell debris, and airway wall edema accounts for most of the airflow obstruction observed in bronchiolitis of infants. Generally, bronchodilator therapy is thought to be ineffective in this clinical setting. However, bronchodilator therapy has not been systematically studied in bronchiolitis of infants. In children with good ventilatory effort and severe airway obstruction (particularly when respiratory failure appears imminent), a trial of bronchodilator therapy should be given. Aminophylline (2 to 3 mg/kg IV over 20 minutes) followed by an aerosolized beta 2 agonist (isoetharine hydrochloride 1 per cent, 0.25 ml in 0.75 ml saline administered through a loosely applied face mask over 10 minutes) is an appropriate therapeutic trial. If convincing physiologic benefit is achieved, continued bronchodilator therapy is reasonable. The aminophylline dose varies during the first year of life, ranging from 5 to 8 mg/kg/24 hr in 3- to 4-month-old children to 10 to 12 mg/kg/24 hr in 6- to 9-month-olds to 15 to 20 mg/kg/24 hr in 12- to 15-month-old children. Theophylline levels should be monitored to avoid toxicity, especially in children less than 9 months old. The therapeutic range of serum theophylline levels is 10 to 20 μg/ml.

The most common decision to be made by those managing children with recurrent symptomatic lower respiratory infections is whether illness is likely to represent a manifestation of the asthma syndrome. Our data show that the occurrence of three separate wheezing illnesses suggests strongly that reversible bronchoconstriction is contributing to the clinical illness. Oral theophylline therapy should be considered beginning with the third wheezing illness. I would not recommend bronchodilators in the outpatient management of children with first or second episodes of wheezing with respiratory infection.

Since there is a strong association between asthma and allergy in childhood, environmental control measures to minimize aeroallergen exposure should be instituted in an attempt at preventive intervention in children with recurrent wheezing illness. Recurrent nonwheezing lower respiratory infections are not as closely linked to asthma and allergy as recurrent wheezing illnesses. Occasionally children with bronchial hyperreactivity will have chronic cough without wheezing. A history of exercise limitation or exercise-induced shortness of breath, not necessarily with wheezing, may suggest the diagnosis of reversible bronchoconstriction in these individuals. The management of asthma is discussed more completely in a separate chapter.

Aspiration Pneumonia

J. A. PETER TURNER, M.D.

This is defined as inflammatory reaction in the lung due to the entrance of foreign matter into the respiratory passages.

Hydrocarbon aspiration, a common cause of chemical pneumonia in childhood, is related to accidental ingestion/aspiration of petroleum distillates such as gasoline, kerosene, turpentine, or furniture polish. The usual episode consists of fluid intake into the mouth, followed by gagging and primary aspiration of the hydrocarbon with simultaneous ingestion of the substance. If the child has had a significant choking and coughing episode at the time of ingestion or if he has signs of tachypnea, dyspnea, and/or cough when seen, the likelihood of aspiration pneumonia is strong. Initial chest radiographs may be deceptively clear, only to show progressive changes usually in the lung bases over 48 to 96 hours. If significant amounts are aspirated initially, the patient may be profoundly affected, with signs of ventilatory insufficiency.

In mild cases observation over several days will suffice. If there are pneumonic signs, bronchodilation with intravenous theophylline 20 mg/kg/24 hours and the inhalation of beta 2 agonists are helpful. The role of steroids is not well established and routine antibiotic therapy on a prophylactic basis is not indicated. If there are signs of respiratory insufficiency, supplemental oxygen and ventilatory support are necessary. When chemical pneumonitis is severe and protracted in time, secondary bacterial infection may become a problem, at which point appropriate antibiotic therapy may be specifically indicated.

Initial routine gastric lavage is no longer utilized. Indeed, even ipecac-induced vomiting has been recently questioned, since evidence is accumulating that absorption of hydrocarbon from the GI tract is not as great a potential as once believed.

Aspiration of stomach contents may occur in the unconscious patient or in alcoholic or drug induced states. Establishment of an airway by means of bronchoscopy or endotracheal intubation is essential as an initial procedure. Where the resulting pneumonitis is extensive, supplemental oxygen and assisted ventilation may be required. Bronchodilator therapy with theophylline and beta agonists is useful in improving airway patency. Steroid therapy is of questionable benefit in reducing the immediate inflammatory response occasioned by aspirated gastric contents. Broad spectrum antibiotic therapy is indicated if the clinical course is protracted or if pneumonic changes are progressive. Organisms commonly associated with secondary infection are anaerobic and gram-negative bacteria and *Staphylococcus aureus.*

Milk aspiration in infancy is a common aspiration phenomenon. If the amount aspirated is large, the application of continuous positive airway pressure (CPAP) by face mask or head box may be utilized. If the patient is unconscious and requires mechanical ventilation, positive end-expiratory pressure (PEEP) is helpful in maintaining patency of the airways. Close attention to arterial blood gases is important. Bronchodilator therapy using theophylline and beta agonists is helpful. Steroids and prophylactic antibiotics are not indicated.

If episodes of milk aspiration are recurrent, underlying functional or anatomic abnormalities must be considered. Subjects with neurologic impairment may exhibit primary pharyngoesophageal dyskinesia, which is responsible for incoordinate swallowing and recurrent aspiration episodes. Gastroesophageal reflux because of incomplete cardiac sphincter function may allow for recurrent aspiration related to regurgitation from the stomach. Anatomic malformations such as H-type tracheoesophageal fistula, and vascular ring anomalies such as double aortic arch should be considered. Detection of these anatomic malformations depends upon cineradiographic studies and requires surgical intervention. When anatomic malformations do not exist and recurrent aspiration is related to either pharyngoesophageal incoordination or gastroesophageal reflux, simple thickening of the milk feedings using cereal in the proportion of 4 tablespoons to each 8 oz of milk may result in more efficient swallowing function and hence a reduction in the aspiration potential. Propping the infant after feeding is helpful. In more severely compromised patients, gastrostomy tube feeding or fundal plication surgery may be necessary. Although recurrent feeding by nasogastric tube is sometimes advocated, this is not an easy procedure for many parents of affected infants.

Bronchiectasis

J. A. PETER TURNER, M.D.

Bronchiectasis occurs when bronchial obstruction persists to the point that distal airways become dilated, secretions are static, and infection supervenes, setting the stage for bronchial wall destruction and a series of events progressing from cylindrical or reversible bronchiectasis to saccular or irreversible bronchiectasis.

Unresolved pneumonia involving one segment of lung is probably the commonest event leading to bronchiectasis. More widespread involvement occurs after infection with pathogenic adenovirus infections. Tuberculous hilar lymphadenopathy with extrusion of caseous material into a contiguous bronchus may eventually produce bronchiectatic change, frequently involving the right middle lobe or either of the upper lobes. Unrecognized foreign body aspiration invariably leads to bronchiectatic change.

Underlying problems commonly associated with bronchiectasis are cystic fibrosis, immune deficiency states, and immotile cilia syndrome. The last category includes cases formerly diagnosed as Kartagener's syndrome.

Although bronchiectasis may be strongly suggested in plain chest radiographs, confirmation depends upon the bronchogram. The extent of involvement determined by this examination is particularly important when surgery is contemplated.

Medical management is indicated for cylindrical bronchiectasis. Chest physiotherapy with the addition of bronchodilator agents such as beta agonists or theophylline is directed against the obstructive component of the condition, so that ectatic change may be reversed. Surgical resection is indicated for segmental saccular bronchiectasis, provided that the remainder of lung is not extensively involved from underlying problems as noted above.

Atelectasis

J. A. PETER TURNER, M.D.

Atelectasis may be defined as reduction in alveolar aeration due to collapse of previously expanded alveoli. This occurs as a result of obstruction of the airway by intraluminal or extraluminal factors. The area involved may be subsegmental, lobar, or multilobar in distribution. Intraluminal obstruction causes are mucus, granulation tissue, or foreign body. Extraluminal compression results from hilar lymph node enlargement, cystic malformation, or tumor masses.

Mucus in the airway is the usual cause of obstruction and occurs in inflammatory conditions such as pneumonia. In asthma, atelectasis is a common problem, again related to mucus secretions. The lobe most frequently involved in asthma is the right middle lobe because of the anatomic nature of the middle lobe bronchus and because of the relative paucity of collateral ventilating channels in that lobe. For most endobronchial obstructions due to mucus, a combination of bronchodilator therapy using inhaled beta agonists and theophylline plus physiotherapy to the affected segment of lung is sufficient to improve aeration. If endobronchial foreign body is suspected as a cause, bronchoscopic aspiration is necessary using a rigid bronchoscope.

In rare instances in which atelectasis is related to compression due to fluid accumulation in the pleural space, removal of fluid is the obvious method of management. Where extrabronchial compression is due to hilar nodes, tumor masses, or cystic malformations, therapy is directed toward the underlying cause.

Atelectasis may persist for extended periods of time before irreversible bronchiectasis ensues. Therefore, observation of an affected lung over a period of one year may be appropriate before surgical management is considered.

Emphysema

J. A. PETER TURNER, M.D.

The term emphysema has been applied to a number of pulmonary conditions in the pediatric patient. For the sake of simplicity, it may be categorized as intra-alveolar emphysema and extra-alveolar emphysema.

INTRA-ALVEOLAR EMPHYSEMA

Panacinar emphysema, more commonly recognized in the adult, occurs rarely in childhood as a result of alpha-1 antitrypsin deficiency. Lack of this specific serum protein usually produces progressive liver disease in the pediatric age group but it may occasionally cause progressive dyspnea related to destruction of elastin in the alveolar septa. This in turn will produce the characteristic changes of panacinar emphysema. No specific therapy is available. However, it is well recognized that the emphysema associated with alpha-1 antitrypsin deficiency may progress more rapidly with cigarette smoking. The patient therefore should be urged to avoid any contact with tobacco smoke. The prompt treatment of pulmonary infections with broad spectrum antibiotics is also important, since it is speculated that an increase in inflammatory cells in the lung may enhance progression of the disorder.

Congenital lobar emphysema implies overdistention of one lobe of lung resulting in compromise of adjacent ipsilateral lung lobes. The affected lobe may herniate through the mediastinum to cause disruption of function in contralateral pulmonary structures. The nature of this disorder is not well recognized. Occasionally incomplete obstructive phenomena have been described in the bronchus to the affected lobe, such as deficiency of cartilaginous rings. However, in most instances no such pathology is apparent. Management usually involves surgical resection of the affected lobe. This is an emergency procedure in the neonatal period where the affected infant may develop significant respiratory embarrassment. Removal also should be considered where involvement of surrounding normal lung threatens function and development of normal tissues. Under no circumstances should needle aspiration of lobar emphysema be considered.

Compensatory emphysema is a phrase used to describe enlargement of normal lung to compensate for such loss of adjacent lung tissue as hypoplasia, atelectasis, or surgical removal of lung substance. There is rarely any indication for specific therapy except for management of atelectasis, which is a remedial primary problem.

Emphysema due to air trapping exists because of a check-valve obstruction in the air passage leading to the affected portion of lung. The commonly associated mechanisms are a mucus-plug phenomenon in asthma or an aspirated foreign body. For the former, treatment is by bronchodilator agents. For the latter, rigid bronchoscopy and removal of the foreign body are mandatory.

Extra-alveolar emphysema implies the presence of air in tissues such as the interstitium of lung or in subcutaneous spaces. This can occur by trauma to the lung or such air-containing structures as the esophagus or bronchus. The usual sequence of events is overdistention and rupture of a marginal alveolus because of incomplete mucus-plug obstruction in the airways. As a result, air escapes into the adjacent interstitium and tracks upward, giving rise to interstitial pulmonary emphysema, mediastinal emphysema, and finally subcutaneous emphysema in the neck. The pattern is not infrequently seen as a complication of asthma.

Management of these conditions relates to cause. If there is a history of trauma, then investigation for bronchial or esophageal air leak should be carried out by bronchoscopy, esophagoscopy, and barium swallow radiography.

If asthma is the underlying problem, conservative management using bronchodilator therapy with theophylline and inhaled beta agonists is indicated. In severely compromised asthmatics, intravenous isoproterenol or albuterol is necessary. High concentrations of oxygen by mask will aid in resolution of extra-alveolar air. Where ventilatory support is necessary, positive pressure ventilation may aggravate the original air leak. If high ventilatory pressures are required to adequately ventilate the patient, the potential for pneumothorax is considerable. If such pressures are contemplated, the placement of bilateral intercostal chest tubes will minimize the effects of that complication should it occur.

Pulmonary Edema

RICHARD D. BLAND, M.D.

Effective treatment of pulmonary edema includes measures designed to reduce hydraulic pressure in the pulmonary microcirculation and increase intravascular protein osmotic pressure. When edema results from increased microvascular permeability to protein, supportive therapy should be provided, thereby allowing time for the pulmonary endothelium to heal, with resolution of edema.

Whatever the cause of the edema, fluid and salt intake should not exceed insensible losses. In cases of cardiogenic edema, treatment with digitalis is often useful. The total digitalizing dose, given IM, is 30 μg/kg of body weight in premature infants, 60 μg/kg in full-term infants up to about 6 months of age, 40 μg/kg for infants from 6 months of age to about 2 years, and 30 μg/kg for children beyond 2 years of age. Usually one half of the digitalizing dose is given initially, followed by one quarter at two 8-hour intervals thereafter. Daily maintenance therapy should provide approximately one quarter of the digitalizing dose. Morphine sulfate, given IM in a dose of 0.1 to 0.2 mg/kg of body weight, may be useful for treating acute pulmonary edema, but it must be administered cautiously because of its potential depressant effect on ventilation.

Diuretics are the mainstay of therapy for pulmonary edema. In cases of severe edema, furosemide may be injected IV in a dose of 1 to 2 mg/kg of body weight. This usually produces an abrupt diuresis, which decreases pulmonary microvascular pressure and increases the concentration of protein in plasma. These two changes inhibit fluid filtration into the lungs and hasten the entry of water into the pulmonary microcirculation from the interstitium.

Patients who require prolonged diuretic therapy often lose a considerable amount of potassium chloride in their urine. Depletion of these electrolytes usually can be prevented by treatment with supplemental potassium chloride, 3 to 5 meq/kg of body weight daily. Spironolactone, 1 to 2 mg/kg daily, is sometimes useful in conjunction with furosemide to reduce potassium losses. In the presence of anuria or oliguria from kidney failure, pulmonary edema must be treated with peritoneal dialysis, in which the dialysis fluid should be hypertonic or protein-rich to facilitate extraction of water.

Although hypoproteinemia may predispose patients to pulmonary edema, infusions of salt-poor albumin (0.25 gm/ml) or plasma usually do not benefit infants and children with severe pulmonary edema. Such infusions tend to increase pulmonary microvascular pressure, and this offsets the effect of increased intravascular protein osmotic pressure. Furthermore, the infused protein leaks into the interstitium of the lungs within a short period of time, and this frequently aggravates the edema.

If there is cyanosis or arterial oxygen desaturation, supplemental oxygen should be provided to maintain a normal partial pressure of oxygen in arterial blood. If anemia and severe pulmonary edema coexist, a partial exchange transfusion with packed red blood cells may be safer and offer more benefit than a simple transfusion. Conditions that may impair myocardial performance, such as hypoglycemia, hypocalcemia, or infection, require specific therapy, which usually restores normal myocardial contractility. Conditions that increase pulmonary blood flow, such as hypoxia, pain, and fever, should be avoided or treated promptly. Environmental conditions should remain comfortable to minimize oxygen consumption. A semi-upright position sometimes lessens respiratory distress in infants with pulmonary edema.

If these measures are not successful in substantially reducing edema, ventilatory support with positive end-expiratory pressure is often beneficial. Positive end-expiratory pressure does not reduce lung water content, but it does redistribute fluid in the air spaces and improve respiratory gas exchange. Ventilation also spares energy reserves by reducing the work of breathing. If ventilatory assistance becomes necessary, sedation may further decrease oxygen consumption and thereby facilitate recovery. When intractable pulmonary edema complicates the course of infants and children with congenital abnormalities of the heart, surgical correction or palliation at one of several regional cardiovascular centers should be considered.

Pulmonary Embolism

BURTON H. HARRIS, M.D.

Pulmonary embolism, while rare in children, remains a life-threatening disease requiring aggressive treatment with potent drugs. There is so little recorded experience with these drugs in children that dosages, side effects, safety, and efficacy are not certain, and many of them have not earned specific regulatory approval for pediatric use.

Pulmonary embolism is a complication of venous thrombosis. The primary thrombus may be in any venous bed, but the usual site is the deep veins of the lower extremity. Deep venous thrombosis (DVT) is associated with trauma, immobilization, invasive devices, wasting diseases, and hypercoagulable states. Therapy must be started in three simultaneous directions—control of the basic disease, prevention of further clot at the site of origin, and treatment of acute cardiopulmonary insufficiency due to emboli in the pulmonary artery.

Pulmonary Artery Occlusion. Treatment begins with supportive emergency measures common to critical care situations. Airway control, assisted ventilation, supplemental oxygen, vascular access, and volume augmentation are used as indicated. Emergency pulmonary embolectomy (Trendelenburg procedure) has been abandoned because of an unacceptable mortality, and replaced with attempts at pharmacologic dissolution of the embolus with parenteral streptokinase.

The dangers of streptokinase are allergic reactions and induction of a serious bleeding diathesis. Prior to using the drug, a control prothrombin time (PT), partial thromboplastin time (PTT), and thrombin time or euglobulin lysis is performed. Next, a single intravenous dose of hydrocortisone, 1.5 mg/kg, is given as prophylaxis against hypersensitivity reactions. Streptokinase* is then given in peripheral intravenous infusion for 30 minutes of each hour. The initial dose is 3000 units/kg, then 1500 units/kg/hr for the first 12 hours of treatment, followed by 1000 units/kg/hr. Treatment is limited to 36–48 hours. Doses can be adjusted to keep the thrombin time between two and four times the control value, but empiric doses with a single check of accelerated euglobulin lysis during the first 12 hours are more appropriate for pediatric patients. Streptokinase dissolves clots by enhancing thrombolysis, so no anticoagulant can be used with it and venipuncture and invasive procedures must be minimized. New techniques to reduce the systemic effects by delivering the drug near or in the clot through an intravascular catheter are being developed.

Venous Thrombosis. Six hours after the last dose of streptokinase, direct anticoagulation with heparin should begin. Continuous intravenous infusion is the preferred method. After an initial dose of 25 units/kg/hr, a PTT is done every 4 hours and the dose adjusted to keep the PTT two to three times the control value. A steady state is usually reached in the first 24–36 hours of treatment, and then the PTT can be checked once every 24 hours. Heparin remains effective for 10–14 days, and should be continued for at least two weeks.

Surgical interruption of the inferior vena cava sometimes becomes necessary despite adequate drug therapy. The indications for surgery are continuing embolism or extending or recurrent thrombophlebitis in the face of complete anticoagulation. The normal reticence to commit such critically ill patients to operation must be overcome. Percutaneous intravascular partial occlusion devices cannot be used because the vessel of entry, the internal jugular vein, is too small to accommodate them. The inferior cava must be ligated or partitioned with a fenestrated clip just below the renal veins through a trans- or retroperitoneal approach. The effects of heparin are reversed with protamine during the procedure, and heparin is started again after operation.

Prophylaxis. The incidence of recurrent DVT is lessened by the use of warfarin (Coumadin) for 3–6 months. Warfarin interferes with the production of clotting factors in the liver, so its full effect is seen 4–5 days after the first dose. It should be started 5–6 days before cessation of heparin is contemplated. Treatment is begun with a once-daily oral dose of 1–2 mg/kg for 2 days, followed by a daily maintenance dose of 2.5–10 mg (total, *not* per kilogram) controlled by daily prothrombin time (PT) determinations. The therapeutic range for the PT is 1.5–2.5 times the control value. Once reproducible results are obtained, the PT can be repeated 2–3 times each week, then weekly, then biweekly. The antidote for acute prothrombinemia is vitamin K.

The wisdom of prophylactic anticoagulation requires a delicate judgment based on promptness of recovery, physical activity, age, return to school, and control of the underlying disease. If true anticoagulation is considered too risky for an active child, daily aspirin use to reduce platelet adhesiveness may be a reasonable compromise.

Primary Pulmonary Hemosiderosis

DOUGLAS C. HEINER, M.D.

Primary pulmonary hemosiderosis is a severe form of pulmonary disease in which there is diffuse bleeding into the alveoli but no known underlying disease such as heart failure, collagen vascular disease (e.g., pulmonary polyarteritis or disseminated lupus), anomaly of the pulmonary vascular system, elevated pulmonary venous pressure, or a primary bleeding disorder. The diagnosis must be confirmed by the demonstration of iron-laden macro-

---

*Manufacturer's precaution: Safety and effectiveness of streptokinase in children have not been established.

phages in gastric or bronchial washes or in the alveoli at pulmonary biopsy. Unexplained pulmonary hemosiderosis probably has diverse etiologies. In a significant proportion of infants with this diagnosis, there appears to be an abnormal immunologic and clinical response to dietary constituents —most commonly cow's milk proteins. Rational treatment requires a careful search for etiologic agents which can be eliminated from the diet or from the environment. Contributing factors include: 1) upper or lower esophageal dysfunction with aspiration of food or gastric contents; 2) immunologic disturbances including both selective IgA deficiency and high levels of precipitating antibodies to cow's milk proteins which may predispose to the deposition of immune complexes in the lungs.

Once the diagnosis is established, I recommend a trial on a milk-free diet, since the likelihood of benefit far outweighs the risks of psychologic or nutritional deprivation, problems which can be avoided by skilled physicians. About two thirds of infants with primary pulmonary hemosiderosis respond favorably to the elimination of cow's milk and milk products from the diet. Perhaps one third of patients 4 to 10 years of age also respond to this measure, as do about one tenth of those in later childhood and adolescence. A trial milk-free diet must be maintained for a minimum of 1 month in subjects who are experiencing continuous symptoms, since a favorable response may not be apparent until that time. In addition, strict milk elimination must be continued for a period exceeding the length of any spontaneous remission that has occurred prior to the time of beginning the milk-free diet. Thus, if a patient has had persistent symptoms for many months and there is no response following 1 month of a milk-free diet, it is unlikely that a response will occur, and other measures should be taken. However, if there have been intermittent pulmonary symptoms with remissions, for example, of up to 6 months' duration, the milk-free diet must be contineud for at least 7 months in order to provide some assurance that any remission observed is not a spontaneous one, unrelated to the diet. I have seen a number of children who provided no evidence by history or laboratory studies of an etiologic role for milk, yet in 3 of them remissions of greater than 2 years followed the institution of a milk-free diet. On the other hand, I am aware of a greater number of subjects without clues that milk played a contributory role who continued to have persistent or recurrent pulmonary disease in spite of a milk-free diet. Some subjects seem to improve not at all or incompletely on a milk-free diet, yet when milk is reintroduced into the diet it induces an exacerbation. Only by dietary challenge following a period of milk elimination does it become apparent that milk intake should be prohibited.

The initial period of milk elimination should include all milk-containing products. Beef and gelatin share bovine serum proteins with cow's milk and are to be avoided, as are goat's milk, cheeses of all kinds, chocolate and all products containing milk or whey solids. After prolonged remission has been established, a trial of well-cooked beef and foods containing boiled or canned milk can be made. A food known to aggravate the disease may cause no trouble if eaten in small quantities on infrequent occasions. However, caution must be exercised in ever allowing unrestricted use of a food once shown to cause clinical exacerbations. One must be quite certain that he is not contributing to the insidious development of chronic lung disease. Hence, at least yearly evaluation of pulmonary function by a competent specialist is necessary if milk or another incriminated food is again permitted. Similar comprehensive pulmonary follow-up studies are required in subjects who have had a progression of pulmonary symptoms or infiltrates in the previous year. If there is an unavoidable exposure to milk or another offending food, symptoms can sometimes be minimized or averted by the administration of antihistaminics or corticosteroids or both for a period of 48 hours.

When a patient is critically ill with respiratory distress or massive bleeding, I recommend treatment with generous doses of corticosteroids. I prefer IV methylprednisolone (Medrol) 0.5 mg/kg every 6 hours, continued until active bleeding has ceased and the patient's condition has stabilized for 48 hours. I follow this by daily, then alternate-day, steroids in the amounts needed to minimize or abolish ongoing symptoms. If fresh bleeding continues after 3 days of adequate corticosteroid therapy, or if the patient's status deteriorates in spite of therapy, either azathioprine,* 3 mg/kg/day po, or cyclophosphomide (Cytoxan),* 2 mg/kg/day IV for 1 week, may be given in addition to continuing the corticosteroids. If either of these drugs is used, WBC and platelet counts should be determined once or twice weekly and the physician must be familiar with the use of the drug, including side effects which might mitigate against its continued use.

Oxygen is administered when there is hypoxemia. Positive pressure respiration may be helpful during severe exacerbations since it may diminish active bleeding. Whole blood transfusions should be given to replace blood loss and to correct anemia. On two separate occasions following whole blood transfusions, one patient with primary pulmonary hemosiderosis and marked IgA deficiency in both plasma and secretions had dramatic reversal of severe pulmonary bleeding and near fatal respir-

---

*This use is not listed in the manufacturer's official directive.

atory distress. It was tempting to speculate that a deficiency was repaired or a more normal immunologic balance attained following transfusion in this child, yet extensive investigations revealed no deficiency other than a lack of serum and secretory IgA. Plasma or whole blood infusions of 10 ml/kg IV may have particular value in patients with a deficiency of serum IgA (10 per cent of children with primary pulmonary hemosiderosis are IgA deficient). A word of caution should be given against overloading the circulation with large amounts of fluid, particularly saline, since this may aggravate pulmonary congestion. Usually no greater than one quarter normal saline (in 5 per cent dextrose) is used for patients with active pulmonary disease who require IV fluid therapy.

It is always essential that a patent airway be ensured, especially if there is evident airway obstruction due to tracheal blood, secretions or tonsillar or adenoidal hypertrophy, or if cardiomegaly, pulmonary hypertension or ECG evidence of right ventricular strain is found. An endotracheal tube or a tracheostomy occasionally may be needed.

In patients in whom there is a history of swallowing difficulty or tracheal aspiration in early childhood or in whom there is current clinical evidence of esophageal dysfunction, appropriate studies of lower esophageal sphincter competence and of swallowing function should be made. In infants with postprandial regurgitation or demonstrable esophageal dysfunction, continuous propping in a semi-upright position may help. If simple measures such as propping and frequent small feedings spaced throughout the day are of insufficient value, surgical measures should be considered. Even if the history is negative for esophageal symptoms, it is wise to evaluate esophageal function carefully and institute appropriate treatment in children with primary pulmonary hemosiderosis who fail to respond to a milk-free diet.

Congenital Diaphragmatic Hernia

MAX L. RAMENOFSKY, M.D.

There are two commonly recognized types of congenital diaphragmatic hernia, the most serious being the hernia through the foramen of Bochdalek, the second being of the foramen of Morgagni.

BOCHDALEK HERNIA

Congenital diaphragmatic hernia through the foramen of Bochdalek continues to be a defect of major importance because of the exceptionally high mortality rate associated with its presence. The foramen of Bochdalek, although a misnomer for the site of the hernia, is taken in context to mean the pleuroperitoneal canal, located anatomically at the posterolateral aspect of the developing diaphragm, and is the last portion of the diaphragm to close, thus separating the pleural from the peritoneal cavity.

Neonates with congenital diaphragmatic hernia are usually full term with anomalies associated only with the hernia. Occasionally an intracardiac defect is present. Anomalies related to the congenital diaphragmatic hernia include bilateral pulmonary hypoplasia (both endodermal and mesenchymal derivates), malrotation of the intestine, and a small peritoneal cavity. Also encountered are pathophysiologic abnormalities such as patent ductus arteriosus and patent foramen ovale. The hernia is located on the left side in 80%, is on the right side in 10–15%, and is bilateral in 5% of cases.

The time at which the hernia causes symptoms is of greatest prognostic value for ultimate outcome. Most patients present at delivery, as soon as the umbilical cord is clamped. Mortality in this group varies from 50–70%. Patients whose symptoms occur after leaving the delivery room but before 24 hours of age have a 40% mortality, and infants presenting after 24 hours of age approach 0% mortality. The mortality appears to be most closely related to the degree of pulmonary hypoplasia. The most severe degrees are manifested by very early presentation and result from inability of the hypoplastic lungs to sustain adequate ventilation.

From the outset, diagnosis and treatment are inseparable. This congenital disease represents the ultimate pediatric surgical emergency! The time from the onset of symptoms to treatment must be minimized to maximize the chances of survival.

Treatment of patients with congenital diaphragmatic hernia can be separated into three phases: preoperative, operative, and postoperative.

Preoperative Treatment. The full-term newborn with respiratory distress in the delivery room when the cord is clamped requires prompt diagnosis and treatment. Once respiratory distress has been noted, oxygen must be started and an orogastric tube (12 F) inserted into the stomach. An immediate upright and lateral chest/abdominal x-ray is obtained. This diagnostic/therapeutic maneuver will show the hernia, frequently with the orogastric tube coursing into the hernia in the chest. The tube will allow evacuation of swallowed air, allowing the intrinsically compromised pulmonary parenchyma more room for expansion and ventilation.

Most of these infants are not born in hospitals where there are pediatric surgical expertise and a neonatal ICU. Consequently, transfer is necessary. Time should not be wasted attempting to resuscitate these infants, as the ultimate resuscitation must occur in the operating room.

Ventilation is difficult. If the infant is able to self-ventilate, oxygen should be continued. However, if the infant remains tachypneic and cyanotic, an endotracheal tube (3.5) should be inserted and assisted ventilation started. Maximal ventilatory pressure should not exceed 25 cm H_2O. It is often necessary to use positive end-expiratory pressure (PEEP) of 4–6 cm H_2O to overcome the high intrapleural and consequently transpulmonary pressures generated by the herniated viscera. All further resuscitative efforts should be performed in the operating room, where conditions can be more rigidly controlled.

An umbilical arterial line is inserted and arterial blood gases obtained. Respiratory acidosis is managed by correcting the ventilatory defect. Metabolic acidosis is often present as well and should be corrected by the use of a buffer, usually sodium bicarbonate. The following formula has proven useful: meq $NaHCO_3$ = BE X weight (kg) X 0.3 BE = a negative base excess. The bicarbonate is diluted and given over a 3–5 minute period. If the P_{CO_2} is greater than 55 torr, bicarbonate should not be given; rather the ventilatory rate should be increased.

The period of resuscitation should last only as long as the patient shows improvement but not longer than one hour. Should no improvement occur or should the patient start to deteriorate, the operation should be started immediately.

Operative Treatment. Most pediatric surgeons prefer a transverse left upper quadrant abdominal incision for left-sided defects. However, the incision must be made rapidly. If the hernia is on the right side, most prefer a right posterolateral thoracotomy. However, if intestine, in addition to liver, is in the defect on the right side, an abdominal incision is often favored. The herniated viscera are reduced, and a sac, if present, is excised. The lung, as visualized through the hernial defect, appears to be very small and hypoplastic. The anesthesiologist should *not* try to inflate this lung. A thoracostomy tube is placed into the chest on the side of the defect but *not* attached to waterseal drainage. A second prophylactic chest tube is placed into the opposite pleural cavity at the end of the operation and is attached to waterseal. The hernia defect is closed. The hernia defect itself may be closed primarily, as there is usually a posterior rim of muscle which can be used for closure, but on occasion a silicone coated nylon patch is required.

At the end of the operative procedure, a right radial or right temporal arterial line should be inserted. If an umbilical arterial line was not inserted prior to the start of the procedure, one should be inserted at this point. If technically feasible, a pulmonary arterial catheter should be inserted postoperatively, as this is very helpful in the management of the rapid changes in these patients' pulmonary arterial pressures.

Postoperative Treatment. The postoperative care of the neonate with congenital diaphragmatic hernia requires constant attention to the details of ventilatory therapy, acid-base balance–pulmonary arterial pressure, and mediastinal positioning. In essence, the management involves treatment of a persistent or recurring fetal circulation. Although the details of management will be discussed under the separate topics of ventilatory management, acid-base balance–pulmonary arterial pressure, and mediastinal stabilization, in practice simultaneous evaluation and treatment is necessary.

Ventilatory Management. Most neonates will require ventilatory assistance. The most common mistake is the use of an inspiratory pressure that is too high. Because the hemithorax on the side of the hernia is empty because of the hypoplastic lung, the use of a high inspiratory pressure causes the contralateral lung to overexpand into the empty hemithorax. The use of a low ventilatory pressure with a rapid ventilatory rate is preferred. Positive end-expiratory pressure is contraindicated.

The initial FiO_2 should be 100%. When the arterial blood gases, both pre- and postductal, are normal, the FiO_2 should be decreased but not at increments greater than 5% per setting change. Too great or too rapid change results in rebound pulmonary hypertension and progressive return of the fetal circulation.

Acid-Base Management–Pulmonary Arterial Pressure. Right-to-left shunting occurs in these patients. Three loci of shunting have been identified, all associated with the development of pulmonary hypertension: the foramen ovale, the ductus arteriosus, and within the lung. Monitoring pulmonary arterial pressure is the ideal way to identify pulmonary hypertension. However, simultaneous pre- and postductal arterial blood gas determinations via the right radial and umbilical arterial catheters can be used to estimate the degree of right-to-left shunting through the ductus arteriosus, which indicates pulmonary hypertension. For example, if a right-to-left shunt through the ductus arteriosus is present, the preductal pH and Pa_{O_2} will be higher than the postductal pH and Pa_{O_2}, indicating that the preductal blood has traversed ventilated lung whereas the postductal blood had not. Additionally, a preductal arterial blood gas gives important information regarding the oxygen tension of the blood perfusing the brain.

Simultaneous pre- and postductal blood gases do not give information about shunts through the foramen ovale. A preductal arterial blood gas and the use of a shunt equation or a shunt nomogram provides useful information about the degree of right to left shunting through the foramen ovale. There is normally an 18–20% physiologic right-to-left shunt in the neonate. When a 25% shunt is present, the pulmonary arterial hypertension causing the increased shunt should be treated.

Pulmonary hypertension is treated with dopamine (10 μg/kg/min) and chlorpromazine* (1 mg/kg/8 hours). It is important that the neonate's intravascular volume be in the normal range before starting these drugs, as severe systemic hypotension may result if the patient is hypovolemic. Normovolemia can best be estimated by a normal urine output and a normal pulse and blood pressure. Once these drugs have been started they should *not* be stopped abruptly but should be tapered over a period of several days.

Acidosis is one cause of pulmonary hypertension. Thus, if the patient becomes acidotic, it is vitally important to bring the pH back into the appropriate range. If the $Paco_2$ is less than 55 torr, sodium bicarbonate can be given by the formula noted previously. However, if the $Paco_2$ is greater than 55 torr, another buffer such as THAM or TRIS should be given. The use of sodium bicarbonate when the $Paco_2$ is elevated results in a further increase of the $Paco_2$. The ideal arterial pH in such a patient is 7.46–7.50. At this pH range the ductus is neither solidly closed or widely patent, owing to the degree of oxygen saturation. This is the ideal situation, since any pulmonary overload can be shunted through the ductus, as the ductus will serve as a "pop-off" valve. For this reason, ligation of the patent ductus in these patients is contraindicated.

Mediastinal Stabilization. After repair of the hernia there is a period of relative pulmonary ventilatory stability. This may last up to 18 hours postoperatively. After that, progressive pulmonary insufficiency may occur. One cause of this deterioration is overexpansion of the contralateral lung. The lung expands because of the void on the side of the repaired hernia resulting from the long-delayed expansion of the lung on that side. Stated another way, the ventilatory pressure needed to expand one lung normally is counterbalanced by the expanding lung on the opposite side. If the opposite side is empty, the lung will overexpand into the empty side, particularly if the mediastinum is mobile, as it is in the neonate. The inspiratory pressure will serve only to overinflate the good lung into the empty space. Attaching the thoracostomy tube on the side of the hernia to waterseal serves only to keep the intrapleural pressure on that side negative, thus allowing overexpansion of the opposite lung. Rather, air should be injected into the empty hemithorax to stabilize the infant's mobile mediastinum in the midline radiographically. Occasionally the mediastinum may appear to be pushed or fixed in the chest opposite to the side of the hernia. In this situation the thoracostomy tube on the side of the hernia should be used to evacuate air from the side of the hernia and to pull the mediastinum toward the midline. This will allow the inspiratory pressure to effectively ventilate the lung instead of causing it to underexpand.

The length of time required for the patient's condition to stabilize and improve is 4–7 days. The end point should be spontaneous ventilation on room air, permanent resolution of the pulmonary hypertension, and stabilization of the mediastinum in the midline, which will occur when the lung on the opposite side of the hernia grows and expands.

MORGAGNI HERNIA

A hernia through the foramen of Morgagni is usually asymptomatic. However, symptoms may result should incarceration of the herniated viscera occur. Operative repair should be carried out when the diagnosis is made.

---

*Safety and effectiveness of chlorpromazine in children have not been established.

5

Cardiovascular System

Congestive Heart Failure

MARY ALLEN ENGLE, M.D.

When cardiac output is inadequate for bodily needs, the heart has failed. The heart, blood vessels, endocrine organs, kidneys, and sympathetic-parasympathetic nervous system are affected and are interrelated in ways that are increasingly coming to be understood and used in treatment to the patient's advantage. The physician's responsibilities are to recognize the condition; to tend to the acute needs of the infant or child to relieve the symptoms and reverse the signs; and to identify the underlying cause of the failure so that he or she may treat that, if possible, and if not, prepare for chronic, long-term therapy for congestive heart failure.

The cardinal signs of cardiac failure are dyspnea (from elevated pulmonary venous pressure) and fatigue (from inability to raise the low cardiac output and elevate the depressed maximum oxygen uptake). Since 90% of the instances of cardiac failure in pediatric subjects are in infants, feeding problems and failure to gain weight are the usual symptoms. Other signs we recognize are increased heart rate and size with pulmonary venous congestion (tachypnea, dyspnea, sometimes rales) and with systemic venous congestion (hepatomegaly and peripheral edema). A vicious cycle ensues: When blood flow to the kidneys is impaired, the renin-aldosterone-angiotensin system is activated, releasing angiotensin II and leading through vasoconstriction to an inappropriate increase in peripheral vascular resistance, and to sodium and fluid retention with volume overloading. The patient not only suffers from depressed myocardial contractility in the failing heart but has secondary problems of preload (fluid retention) and afterload

(increased systemic vascular resistance). In infants and children, primary problems of contractility, preload, and/or afterload may have caused the heart to fail in the first place. Treatment is directed at relief of the secondary and primary abnormalities. The immediate goal is to decrease the rapid heart rate and improve the contractile state. Unless there is strong contraindication, treatment is best carried out in the hospital.

ATTENTION TO ACUTE NEEDS

The physician should undertake some immediate specific pharmacologic interventions while ensuring that the patient is as comfortable as possible and that his general needs are met. Treatment begins promptly after the history, physical examination, and preliminary laboratory studies have been done: electrocardiogram, roentgenogram, electrolytes, blood count, cultures if there is evidence of infection, and sometimes an echocardiogram.

Diuretics. To reduce preload of elevated blood volume, diuretics are given. Furosemide (Lasix) is administered slowly intravenously, if needed as emergency treatment or if an intravenous line is in place for other aspects of the early treatment. The intravenous dose is 1 to 2 mg/kg (Table 1). If the patient is able to take oral medications and there is little chance of vomiting, *furosemide* may be given orally in a dose of 2 to 4 mg/kg daily. This agent should be given at outset of treatment and again

Table 1.

Route	Diuretic: Furosemide Acute	Chronic
IV	1–2 mg/kg	—
PO	2–4 mg/kg	2–4 mg/kg qd, qod, biweekly

each morning until edema has cleared. It is not necessary to divide the dose into two smaller doses each day. For the older child, it is especially inconvenient for diuresis to occur each night during sleep when a dose is given at night. Acute diuresis is already underway promptly while *digitalis,* the second agent of treatment, is administered. At the outset, when serum potassium is normal, it is not necessary to supplement with potassium chloride, but in chronic therapy potassium chloride should be given if furosemide is needed daily but not if it can be given as infrequently as every other day or less (twice weekly, e.g.). *Spironolactone* (Aldactone) 25 mg tid or qid can be added for chronic, long-term diuretic usage in order to spare potassium in children.

Digitalization. (Table 2). To improve contractility, digitalis has for nearly 200 years been the inotropic agent of choice. Digitoxin is not available in small dosage size for infants. Digoxin is readily and almost universally available in liquid form suitable for babies, and it is available in various sizes of tablets for children and adults. Digitalization can be either fast or slow. Then maintenance therapy follows.

Since most infants and young children with heart failure are acutely and sometimes desperately ill, traditionally pediatric cardiologists prefer loading in divided doses to achieve a therapeutic level quickly, followed by maintenance therapy. The digitalizing dose is based on age and dry body weight. If the child is markedly edematous, estimate the dry weight as 20–25% less than the measured weight on admission in failure, or use the last weight before onset of failure.

In the previously undigitalized patient, one can give half or two thirds of the calculated dose at once without fear of toxicity. In an emergency, the full dose can be given, but rarely is this necessary.

An early effect is experienced in half to one hour and the full effect of that dose in 4 to 6 hours. After observing the patient for relief of any signs or symptoms of failure, obtain a full electrocardio-gram (not just lead II "rhythm strip," for one could miss changes in ST-T waves that are apt to occur in chest leads). One completes the rapid digitalization.

Slow digitalization can be accomplished, usually in an ambulatory older child with mild congestive failure, by calculating the maintenance (chronic) dose and administering that twice daily by mouth. Take advantage of the pharmacokinetics of digoxin, which is eliminated by the kidney and has a relatively short half-life when compared with digitoxin.

Chronic therapy with digoxin is needed to keep the restored, or at least the less depressed, myocardial contractility functioning as effectively as possible. This is done by maintenance with one fourth of the dose each day that was required for full therapeutic effect with initial digitalization. In infants and young children and in most children who need this drug, maintenance therapy seems best carried out by dividing the daily dose in half and giving it twice daily.

Therapeutic effect in the patient is the goal for the drug. There is no advantage to using a higher dose than necessary to accomplish that effect. Indeed, there is a disadvantage. It is important to avoid digitalis toxicity and to recognize that in any digitalis preparation the range between efficacy and toxicity is narrow. The package insert for digoxin (Lanoxin) gives helpful information on the use of this drug.

Salt and Water Restriction. Until the renin-aldosterone-angiotensin system is restored to balance, one should restrict sodium and fluid intake. Babies who are nursing when they go into failure may continue to do so if hospital logistics permit. Usually they do not; so one chooses a formula similar to breast milk in its low-sodium content. For children, modest limitation comes from no added salt and use of fresh rather than canned fruits and vegetables. If stricter restriction is needed, the dietitian can help. Restriction of sodium intake helps in early treatment and may be needed in long-term care.

In acute treatment, fluids can be restricted to about 75% of maintenance, and for chronic, long-term care, some limitation is still desirable.

Attention to General Condition. To make the patient comfortable and to provide as much rest as possible are important. A parent's presence can provide a great deal of comfort, support, and help for the young child as well as for the medical and nursing staffs.

The dyspneic, orthopneic baby is made comfortable in an upright position in a reclinable baby seat, while the child is placed with the head of the bed elevated. Since hypoxia can depress already compromised myocardial contractility, humidified oxygen is helpful until diuretics and digitalis have had time to exert their beneficial effects.

Table 2.

Age	Oral Digoxin Acute (mg/kg)	Chronic
Newborn	0.03 –0.04	1/8 acute dose bid
Infant	0.035–0.06	1/8 acute dose bid
Toddler	0.025–0.035	1/8 acute dose bid
Child	0.02 –0.025	1/8 acute dose bid

Intravenous Digoxin

Since oral absorption is incomplete, the intravenous dose should be reduced to 2/3–4/5 of the oral dose.

If other conditions, such as anemia or infection coexist, they are treated appropriately.

TREATMENT OF UNDERLYING CAUSE

To identify the cause of the cardiac failure and to take care of the underlying condition are crucial steps to be undertaken as soon as the patient has improved, or if there is little relief of failure, to be undertaken without delay. Pediatricians are far more fortunate than those who care for adults during this phase of management. The treatable causes of cardiac failure occur with far greater frequency, and myocardial contractility is impaired for a shorter time than in adults.

Quite the opposite of adults, for whom Dr. Jay Cohn observed that 90% would be dead within a few years after onset of their cardiac failure, 90% of our infants and children can be salvaged, as a result of medical management supplemented in some instances by surgery. Long-term management of the patient, after attention to acute needs, depends on an accurate diagnosis of the underlying condition and the type of burden this has placed on the circulation from the standpoint of afterload, preload, and contractility. Precise diagnosis often requires cardiac catheterization, angiocardiography, and echocardiography.

Most of these cardiac failures occur during the first three or four months of life and most are due to severe congenital heart disease, a few to arrhythmia, and even fewer to myocardial abnormalities. We shall now consider common causes and management.

Afterload. Problems in this category relate chiefly to obstruction to ventricular outflow in the form of severe *coarctation of the aorta, aortic stenosis,* or *pulmonic stenosis.* A ventricle responds to a pressure load by hypertrophy. If the hypertophied ventricle in the last two conditions dilates, and fails, it is because the stenosis is severe and needs immediate surgical relief. However, if the infant with coarctation improves promptly on medical management and is not hypertensive, surgery may be postponed a few months or years to permit growth of the aorta and development of collateral circulation. Acute *hypertension* or chronic, longstanding hypertension can also cause the heart to fail and pulmonary edema to be manifest. Pharmacologic measures to lower the blood pressure acutely, such as intravenous *diazoxide* or *nitroprusside*, help in the emergency situation, while the patient with chronic hypertension needs long-term pharmacologic therapy, singly or in combination. Included in the armamentarium are *hydrochlorothiazide, diuretics, vasodilators* (Table 3), beta blockers (*propranolol*, 1–4 mg/kg/day), angiotensin-converting enzyme inhibitor (*captopril*), and a number of preparations recently approved by the FDA for use in adults.

Table 3. VASODILATOR THERAPY FOR HYPERTENSION

Agent	Dose	
	Acute	*Chronic, Daily*
Captopril	0.5 mg/kg PO	5–10 mg/kg ÷ 4
Diazoxide	5 mg/kg IV	
Hydralazine	0.25 mg/kg IV	1 mg/kg q 4–6 h
Nitroprusside	0.1–8 μg/kg/min IV	

Preload. A large volume load on one or both ventricles exerts a preloading effect that in the neonatal myocardium can cause failure, as can a smaller volume load over a long period of time. Congenital cardiac lesions in this category include conditions that cause a large left-to-right shunt after birth and opening up of the pulmonary arterial bed, such as *ventricular septal defect, patent ductus arteriosus,* and *atrioventricular canal*. Left-to-right shunt through an atrial septal defect takes a couple of decades before cardiac enlargement leads to cardiac failure. Valvular regurgitant lesions (*severe aortic insufficiency, mitral insufficiency*) similarly produce a volume overload on the left ventricle that can cause it to fail.

Early cardiac surgery is indicated for the premature or term infant with a large ductus and cardiac failure, although in the immature premature, one or two courses of *indomethacin* may be tried first if the infant is in the first week or so of life. The most recent recommendation from a cooperative study yet to be published calls for intravenous administration in three doses: 1) 0.2 mg/kg, 2) 0.1 mg/kg after 12 hours, and 3) 0.1 mg/kg 24 hours after the second dose. Oral administration of freshly prepared indomethacin has also been effective in a dose of 0.2 mg/kg, followed 12–24 hours later by a repeat dose.

Early surgery is called for if the baby with a large ventricular septal defect (VSD) does not improve on intensive medical management. If he does improve, he has a good chance for the VSD spontaneously to decrease in size or even to close altogether so that surgery might never be needed.

Children with severe valvular regurgitant lesions, congenital or acquired, may improve on the conventional treatment with digitalis and diuretics or may respond to use of vasodilators to improve forward flow into the systemic bed (see below and Table 4). Surgery to replace a regurgitant valve with a tissue valve or synthetic valve is not undertaken without strong indication, after failure to improve medically, for there are serious problems imposed in the growing child by inability of the artificial valve to increase in size, by deterioration of the valve, by thromboembolic risk and problems of anticoagulants as well as chance of infection of the valve. Nonetheless, when really needed, valve replacement can be life-saving and can cause considerable relief of signs and symptoms of cardiac failure.

When the child with cyanotic congenital heart disease and a volume-loaded heart goes into cardiac failure, his heart suffers not only from the problem of preload but also from problems of contractility that hypoxemia causes. *Total anomalous pulmonary venous return, transposition of the great arteries with large ventricular septal defect,* and *truncus arteriosus* are in this category. Treatment is surgical following initial medical management and diagnostic studies.

An uncommon condition associated with cardiac failure in some newborns is *congenital complete heart block* with a slow ventricular rate, usually below 40–45/minute. Greatest risk of heart failure is in the first few days of life. The problem of the ventricles falls in the category of preload, for the atria empty at a much more rapid rate into the ventricles, which become volume-loaded and which do not have the benefit of the atrial kick to promote emptying that normal sinus rhythm provides. Here medical management is in conjunction with use of a temporary or permanent cardiac pacemaker.

Contractility. In this third category are the problems of primary myocardial disorders such as *myocarditis, congestive cardiomyopathy,* and *endocardial fibroelastosis.*

Tachyrhythmias, such as paroxysmal supraventricular tachycardia and atrial flutter, probably belong in this category too. They cause the heart to fail because the rapid rate limits the period of ventricular diastole, when the ventricles fill and normally are nourished by coronary arterial flow. Contractility is impaired when the rate is sustained around 200/minute or higher. Such tachyrhythmias are most often encountered in the first weeks of life and sometimes even in fetal life. Obstetrical monitoring of fetal heart rate is identifying more such prenatal arrhythmias. Fortunately, most babies with supraventricular tachyrhythmias respond to *digitalization,* even transplacentally, from the digitalized mother to the fetus. Use of *verapamil* (a calcium or slow-channel blocker) may also be considered for acute conversion pharmacologically of the arrhythmia. Verapamil is given intravenously over two minutes in a dose of 0.1 mg/kg while monitoring the blood pressure. If tachycardia persists, the dose can be increased cautiously up to 0.4 mg/kg if necessary.

In the acutely distressed patient, electrical *cardioversion* is carried out. The shock delivered increases according to weight: 10 watt seconds for a weight of 5 kg, 20 up to 10 kg, 30 up to 20 kg, and 50 for a weight up to 50 kg.

If the tachycardia has caused cardiac failure, maintenance digitalis should be continued for the next 6 to 12 months (and sometimes longer) to prevent recurrences.

Table 4. VASODILATOR THERAPY FOR REFRACTORY CARDIAC FAILURE

Agent	Daily Dose
Captopril	5–10 mg/kg ÷ 4
Hydralazine	1 mg/kg q 4–6 h
Isosorbide dinitrate	20–40 mg
Nitroglycerin paste	1–2 inches on chest wall
Prazosin	1 mg tid and increase daily to effect up to 8 mg tid

Primary myocardial impairment is often more difficult to manage satisfactorily or successfully than any of the aforementioned conditions. Here the chronicity of the problem and the inability to achieve or maintain improvement make the situation more nearly comparable to adult cardiac failure in outlook and outcome. Additional measures and prolonged bed rest or marked limitation of activity, in addition to the traditional therapy already mentioned, may be needed.

PLANS FOR CHRONIC THERAPY

If the patient's cardiac failure is refractory to conventional therapy, then one can call on one or more of the additional modes of therapy that have recently come into use in adults in that same situation (Table 4). Some of these agents act as vasodilators to reduce afterload or preload, or both. They include oral agents such as *hydralazine* as a direct arterial vasodilator for afterload reduction, *nitrates* for venodilation and preload reduction, and *captopril* as an angiotensin-converting enzyme inhibitor for afterload reduction by relief of vasoconstriction. *Prazosin,* an arterial and venodilator, may call for increasing doses because of tachyphylaxis. In addition, a new category of drugs, the slow-channel (calcium-channel) blockers have just this past year been approved by the FDA for use in adults. Experience in children is quite limited. *Verapamil, nifedipine,* and *diltiazem* are in this category. They produce vascular dilatation. Side effects are noted on the package inserts. With growing experience in adults on chronic vasodilator therapy and with rapid pharmacologic developments in the field, it is likely that these and other agents yet to come will help those infants and children whose cardiac failure does not respond to traditional therapy.

Congenital Heart Disease

WILLIAM F. FRIEDMAN, M.D.,
and BARBARA L. GEORGE, M.D.

Congenital cardiovascular disease, an abnormality in cardiocirculatory structure or function present at birth, results from altered or arrested development of a normal structure in utero.

Approximately one third of all infants with congenital heart disease will die in the first months of life unless there is prompt recognition, accurate diagnosis, and treatment of their life-threatening anomaly. Heart failure and cyanosis are the two cardinal signs of heart disease in the infant or child. Other serious problems related to congenital heart disease are infective endocarditis and complications following cardiothoracic surgical procedures.

ACUTE CYANOSIS

Newborn. Cyanosis in the newborn often presents as an emergency and requires prompt diagnosis of the cause. Cyanosis is produced by reduced hemoglobin in cutaneous vessels in excess of 3 gm/dl. Hence, an infant with cyanotic heart disease who has significant anemia may not appear "blue," whereas an infant without heart disease but with polycythemia may. It is important to distinguish between three types of cyanosis—peripheral, differential, and central—and to recognize that cyanosis may accompany diseases of the central nervous, hematologic, respiratory, and cardiac systems. Figure 1 outlines a general approach to diagnosis.

Peripheral cyanosis is distinguished by normal arterial oxygen saturation and may be the result of altered capillary blood flow (acrocyanosis), septicemia associated with low cardiac output, exposure to cold, or polycythemia.

Differential cyanosis virtually always indicates congenital heart disease, often with patent ductus arteriosus and coarctation of the aorta; the upper part of the body will be pink and the lower part blue. In contrast, the patient with transposition of the great vessels and coarctation of the aorta will demonstrate the reverse, i.e., the lower part of the body will be pink and the upper part blue. Simultaneous determinations of oxygen saturation in the temporal or right brachial artery and the femoral artery will help to confirm the presence of differential cyanosis.

Central cyanosis results from arterial blood oxygen desaturation. Although noncardiopulmonary processes may produce cyanosis (e.g., central nervous system depression and methemoglobinemia), the physician's greatest challenge is to distinguish between cyanosis due to a primary pulmonary disorder and that due to cyanotic heart disease. Central cyanosis in a full term infant with minimal respiratory distress other than mild tachypnea, a chest radiograph showing no primary pulmonary disease, and an arterial pO_2 that does not rise significantly with the administration of 100% oxygen should be

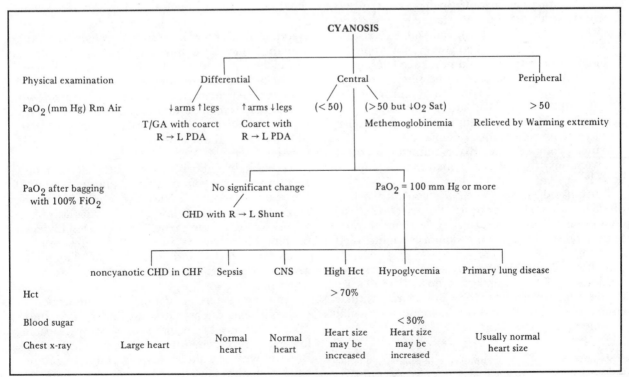

Figure 1.

considered to be cardiac cyanosis until proven otherwise. Generally, newborns with presumptive cyanotic heart disease require emergency cardiology consultation. This, in turn, frequently results in immediate cardiac catheterization, as there is considerable risk of rapid deterioration. In preparing such an infant for transport to a cardiac center or while awaiting cardiology consultation, the primary physician should consider infusing prostaglandin E_1 (0.1 μg/kg/min) to maintain patency of the ductus arteriosus. Prostaglandin E_1 infusion has been an effective short-term measure to correct hypoxemia and acidemia in many newborns with cyanotic heart disease.

Infant/Child. Hypercyanotic or hypoxemic spells commonly complicate the clinical course in older infants and children with certain types of cyanotic heart disease, especially tetralogy of Fallot. Spells are characterized by anxiety, hyperpnea, a sudden and marked increase in cyanosis, and a sudden decrease or disappearance of the previously loud systolic ejection murmur, and are often followed by irritability, lethargy, or frank syncope. These "blue spells" result from an abrupt reduction in pulmonary blood flow. Unless terminated, the hypercyanotic episodes may lead to convulsions and death. The sudden reduction in pulmonary blood flow may be precipitated by fluctuations in arterial P_{CO_2} and pH, a sudden fall in systemic or increase in pulmonary vascular resistance, or both, or an acute increase in the severity of right ventricular outflow tract obstruction. Spells occur typically upon arising in the morning, immediately after a meal (particularly breakfast), and with exercise.

Medical treatment of the hypercyanotic episode includes 1) placing the child in a knee-chest position with the head turned to one side; 2) oxygen administration; 3) administration of morphine sulfate (0.1–0.2 mg/kg/IM); and 4) intravenous administration of sodium bicarbonate (1–2 meq/kg) to correct any significant acidemia.

With a prolonged spell that is refractory to these interventions, the following medications may be useful:

1. Alpha-adrenergic receptor stimulants such as phenylephrine (1–5 μg/kg IV bolus followed by continuous IV infusion of 0.1 μg/kg/min) to raise peripheral resistance and diminish right-to-left shunting.

2. Beta-adrenergic blocking agents such as propranolol (0.15–0.25 mg/kg per dose, IV)* that reduce cardiac sympathetic tone and depress cardiac contractility directly, and that increase ventricular volume by reducing heart rate.

*Manufacturer's note: Data on the use of propranolol in the pediatrics age group are too limited to permit adequate directions for use.

Additional measures should be considered:

1. Transfusion of packed red blood cells if anemia is present.

2. Intravenous volume expanders (colloid or crystalloid) if there is evidence of decreased circulating blood volume.

3. Intravenous glucose because increased metabolic demands during profound hypoxemia may result in significant hypoglycemia.

4. Referral to a cardiac center for definitive therapy; which, in most instances, will involve surgical intervention. When immediate surgical intervention is not possible, oral propranolol (1–2 mg/kg per dose given q 6 h)* may decrease the number and severity of the hypercyanotic episodes.

CHRONIC CYANOSIS

Other therapeutic measures are necessary in chronically hypoxemic patients. Administration of iron may be necessary if a "relative" iron deficiency anemia is present. Chronic hypoxemia stimulates erythrocytosis and results in polycythemia. The increased red cell volume provides an increased oxygen-carrying capacity and enhanced oxygen supply to the tissues. However, the compensatory polycythemia may be so severe that it produces adverse physiologic effects, including thrombotic and hemorrhagic episodes. Oral steroid contraceptives are contraindicated in the adolescent cyanotic female because of the enhanced risk of cerebral thrombosis. Erythrophoresis (red cell volume reduction and replacement with fresh frozen plasma or 5% albumin) lowers blood viscosity, increases systemic blood flow and systemic oxygen transport, and thus may be helpful in patients with severe polycythemia (hematocrit $\geq$ 65%). A final hematocrit of 55 to 63% should be the goal; the higher than normal hematocrit is necessary in patients with low initial oxygen saturation in order to avoid a severe reduction in arterial oxygen. Acute phlebotomy without fluid replacement is contraindicated.

Cerebral thrombosis is a complication commonly seen in severely cyanotic children under 2 years of age. Such thromboses may occur even when the hematocrit is relatively low, and is particularly likely when oxygen requirements are increased by fever, or blood viscosity is increased by dehydration. Therefore, fever and dehydration should be avoided whenever possible, and treated promptly, when present.

Brain abscess is an important complication of cyanotic heart disease. It is rare under 18 months of age; and onset is insidious marked by headache, low-grade fever, vomiting, and personality change. Brain abscess should be suspected in any cyanotic child who develops focal neurological signs. Abscesses are thought to occur in approximately 2%

of those with cyanotic heart disease. Prompt recognition and treatment are mandatory because the 30 to 40% mortality rate is often related to delay in diagnosis and treatment.

INFECTIVE ENDOCARDITIS

Infective endocarditis is uncommon before age 2 years, and most often occurs in children with tetralogy of Fallot (especially if there has been a prior systemic-pulmonary anastomosis), aortic stenosis, and patent ductus arteriosus. The presence of intracardiac or intravascular foreign material (prosthetic heterograft or homograft valves, or conduits) is a significant risk factor for infective endocarditis. Other factors predisposing to endocarditis are cardiovascular surgery with infection during the perioperative period; respiratory tract infections; and ear, nose, throat, and dental procedures. Less frequently implicated are transient bacteremia as a consequence of contamination during a surgical procedure or cardiac catheterization, and infection involving the skin, genitourinary tract, or other organ system. Prompt treatment is necessary. Routine antimicrobial prophylaxis is recommended for all children with congenital heart disease. Antibiotic prophylaxis is recommended for all dental procedures (except minor readjustments of braces), trauma, tonsillectomy, gastrointestinal surgery, genitourinary surgery, and diagnostic procedures such as proctosigmoidoscopy and cystoscopy. The risk of endocarditis is undoubtedly related to the magnitude of bacteremia, type of organism, and the type of underlying heart disease. Because infection of a prosthetic heart valve or conduit may be devastating, parenteral administration of a combination of antibiotics is advisable. The American Heart Association publishes a wallet-sized card with specific recommendations. These cards are usually available from the local Heart Association. The specific recommendations are as follows.

For dental procedures, tonsillectomy, adenoidectomy, and bronchoscopy:

I. For most patients: *Penicillin.*
   a. *Intramuscular (IM) plus oral:*
      30,000 U aqueous penicillin G/kg (not to exceed 1,000,000 U) mixed with 600,000 U of procaine penicillin IM, followed by 250 mg penicillin V every 6 hours for 8 doses (children under 60 lb). Children over 60 lb, the dose of penicillin V is 500 mg every 6 hours for 8 doses.
   b. *Oral only:*
      Children under 60 lb: 1.0 gm of penicillin V orally 30 minutes to 1 hour prior to procedure and then 250 mg orally every 6 hours for 8 doses. For children over 60 lb, the doses are 2.0 gm initially followed by 500 mg every 6 hours.

II. For those allergic to penicillin: *erythromcin* 20 mg/kg (not to exceed 1.0 gm) orally 1 1/2 to 2 hours prior to procedure and then 10 mg/kg (not to exceed 500 mg) every 6 hours for 8 doses.

III. For patients at higher risk: *penicillin plus streptomycin* IM penicillin is outlined in I.a. Streptomycin dose is 20 mg/kg (not to exceed 1.0 gm) IM. This is followed by the oral penicillin doses outlined in I.a.

IV. High-risk patients allergic to penicillin: *vancomycin* intravenously (IV) and *erythromycin* orally. Vancomycin dose is 20 mg/kg (not to exceed 1.0 gm) IV over 30–60 minutes, begun 30–60 minutes before procedure; then erythromycin, 10 mg/kg (not to exceed 500 mg) every 6 hours for 8 doses, orally.

For GI, GU surgery and instrumentation, and for surgery of infected tissues:

I. For most patients: *penicillin* or *ampicillin* plus *streptomycin* or *gentamicin.* Aqueous penicillin G dose is 30,000 U/kg IM or IV (not to exceed 2 million units) *or* ampicillin 50 mg/kg IM or IV (not to exceed 1.0 gm); gentamicin 2.0 mg/kg (not to exceed 80 mg) IM or IV. This should be given 30–60 minutes before procedure. Repeat every 8 hours for 2 additional doses if gentamicin is used, or every 12 hours for 2 additional doses if streptomycin is used.

II. Patients allergic to penicillin: *vancomycin* plus *streptomycin.* Vancomycin dose is 20 mg/kg (not to exceed 1.0 gm) IV given over 30–60 minutes plus streptomycin 20 mg/kg (not to exceed 1.0 gm) IM given 30–60 minutes before procedure. Doses may be repeated in 12 hours.

POSTOPERATIVE COMPLICATIONS

Three postoperative complications that may occur after the patient has been discharged from the hospital are of particular importance to the primary physician.

Postpericardiotomy Syndrome. This most frequently occurs within a few days to a few weeks after cardiac surgery in which the pericardium has been opened. It is uncommon in children under 2 years of age. The syndrome is characterized by fever, chest pain, pericardial and/or pleural effusions, occasionally a friction rub, leukocytosis with polymorphonuclear predominance, and an elevated erythrocyte sedimentation rate. Although usually a mild self-limited illness, it can be so severe as to produce cardiac tamponade. Once the diagnosis is considered, cardiology consultation should be obtained. Effective treatment usually consists of bed rest and aspirin, but corticosteroid administration and even emergency pericardiocentesis may be required. Relapse can occur months after the first episode.

Postperfusion Syndrome. This usually occurs later (2 to 7 weeks postoperatively) than the post-pericardiotomy syndrome, but there is significant overlap. The etiology is believed to be a cyto-megalovirus infection. It occurs almost exclusively in patients who have had cardiopulmonary bypass, and is characterized by fever, anorexia, hepatos-plenomegaly, pleural effusion, and atypical lym-phocytosis. Like the postpericardiotomy syndrome, this is usually self-limited and mild. If symptoms are significant, treatment is the same as outlined for the postpericardiotomy syndome.

Infective Endocarditis. Infective endocarditis in the late postoperative period is less frequent than the postpericardiotomy or postperfusion syn-drome, but is always life-threatening. Therefore, blood cultures and other appropriate diagnostic tests must be done whenever there is unexplained, persistent fever, new constitutional symptoms, evi-dence of embolization, brain abscess, or sudden cardiac decompensation.

GENETIC COUNSELING

Malformations appear to result from an interac-tion between multiple genetic and environmental factors that are too complex to allow a single speci-fication of etiology. Less than 5–10% of all cardiac malformations can be attributed to recognized chromosomal aberrations or transmission of a ge-netic mutation.

Family studies indicate a two- to five-fold in-crease in incidence of congenital heart disease in siblings of affected patients or offspring of an affected parent. Table 1 provides the recurrence risks observed in 3400 siblings of probands with various congenital heart lesions. The incidence of congenital heart disease in the offspring or siblings of an index patient is only 2 to 5%; hence, it is rarely wise to discourage the parents of an affected child from having additional children (unless both parents are known to have a cardiovascular abnor-

mality). Moreover, the low recurrence rate and in-creasing possibilities for effective treatment or cor-rection of nearly all cardiac lesions usually justify a positive approach to family counseling. However, when two or more members of the family are affected, the recurrence risk may be high, and a pedigree should be obtained before further coun-seling. If a dominant or recessive mendelian pat-tern is established, the mendelian laws apply, and the risk of recurrence in each pregnancy is equal.

The Child at Risk of Coronary Disease as an Adult

JAMES J. NORA, M.D.

Because of lively debate on the issue of pediatric preventive programs for coronary disease, it must be stated that the following recommendations may be opposed by some. In the absence of 70-year longitudinal studies, one can always assert that the evidence for the efficacy of a specific or even a gen-eral preventive program is not available. With this disclaimer, I present the approach we follow on our service.

1. For the majority of children and families, specific preventive programs are not required beyond a general commitment to a life-style that embraces exercise, ideal weight, stress control, a reason-ably prudent diet (but not necessarily adhering consistently to the prudent diet shown in Table 1), and abrogation of smoking. However, it

Table 1. RECURRENCE RISK IN SIBLINGS OF PROBANDS WITH CONGENITAL HEART LESIONS

Defect	Affected Siblings (%)
Ventricular septal defect	4.4
Patent ductus arteriosus	3.4
Tetralogy of Fallot	2.7
Atrial septal defect	3.2
Pulmonic stenosis	2.9
Atrioventricular canal	2.6
Transposition of great arteries	1.9
Coarctation of aorta	1.8

Modified from Nora, J. J., et al.: Etiologic aspects of cardio-vascular disease and pre-disposition detectable in the infant and child. *In* Friedman, W. F., et al. (eds.): Neonatal Heart Disease. New York, Grune and Stratton, 1973, p. 279.

Table 1. A PRUDENT DIET

1. Avoid overweight, consume only as many calories as you ex-pend: if overweight, decrease calories and increase expendi-ture.
2. Increase consumption of fruits, vegetables, and whole grains (complex carbohydrates and "naturally occurring" sugars) from the present 28 per cent of calories in the average diet to about half (48 per cent) of your caloric intake.
3. Decrease consumption of refined and other processed sugars and foods high in such sugar by almost half (about 45 per cent) to account for only about 10 per cent of total calories.
4. Decrease consumption of foods high in total fat from 42 per cent of calories to 30 per cent.
5. Specifically reduce saturated fat in the diet (from the present 16 per cent to 10 per cent) and partially replace this with polyunsaturated and monounsaturated fat to account for the remaining 20 per cent of fat intake, by reducing intake of animal fat from meats and high fat dairy products. Eat more fish and poultry, and select lean means low in fat (e.g., trimmed ground round in place of hamburger). Low fat and non-fat milk may be substituted for whole milk except in those in-fants whose diet is almost entirely milk.
6. Reduce cholesterol to about 300 milligrams per day. (The major dietary sources of cholesterol are egg yolks, meats, whole milk, and high fat dairy products.) For children, the major dietary source of cholesterol is whole milk.
7. Decrease your consumption of salt and foods high in salt content.

Table 2. High-Risk Diet for Those with High Cholesterol Levels That Do Not Respond Adequately to the Prudent Diet

1. Avoid overweight, as in the prudent diet.
2. Increase consumption of complex carbohydrates (fruits, vegetables, grains) to about half (48 per cent) of total caloric intake, as in the prudent diet.
3. Decrease refined sugar and other processed sugar to about 10 per cent of total calories, as in the prudent diet.
4. Decrease total fat intake to 30 per cent of calories, as in the prudent diet.
5. Reduce saturated fat and take twice as much polyunsaturated fat (P/S = 2/1), as in the prudent diet.
6. Reduce cholesterol to 100 mg; this is lower than in the prudent diet.
7. Reduce salt consumption, as in the prudent diet.

should be noted that this prudent diet is the diet recommended by the U.S. Senate committee on nutrition for *all* Americans.

2. For high-risk children from high-risk families, the commitment to prevention cannot be casual. Those at high risk should be deliberately sought out at an early age and should have a preventive program designed to attack the specific risk factors. We recommend that at between 1 and 2 years of age (or at later pediatric ages if necessary) the following be done.

   a. Obtain a family history of onset of coronary disease or stroke in first- and second-degree relatives before age 65.
   b. Obtain family history of hypertension in first- and second-degree relatives and begin annual "tracking" of patient's blood pressure.
   c. Obtain serum cholesterol level.
   d. For those with a family history of early-onset coronary heart disease or stroke and a cholesterol level above 190 mg/dl, the cholesterol study should be repeated and the prudent diet initiated if the cholesterol level is found to be above 190 mg/dl on the second determination.

Table 3. High-Risk Diet for Those Who Have Both High Cholesterol and High Triglycerides That Do Not Respond Adequately to the Prudent Diet

1. Reduce weight to the lower limits of the desirable weight range.
2. Maintain complex carbohydrate consumption (fruits, vegetables, grains) at about half (48 per cent) of total calories, as in the prudent diet.
3. Eliminate as much as possible refined sugars and processed foods high in sugar—certainly hold this to less than 5 per cent of calories. This is lower than in the prudent diet.
4. Decrease total fat intake to 30 per cent of calories, as in the prudent diet.
5. Reduce saturated fat, as done in the other diets, to the point that twice as much polyunsaturated fat is consumed as saturated (P/S = 2/1).
6. Reduce cholesterol to 100 milligrams per day, much lower than in the prudent diet.
7. Reduce salt intake, as in the prudent diet.

e. For those without a family history, the cholesterol level may be "tracked" at annual visits for 2 years. If the elevated level persists over 190 mg/dl, the prudent diet should be instituted and consistently adhered to.

f. Young children *with a positive (or unknown) family history* who do not respond to a prudent diet by lowering cholesterol (being sure that the prudent diet is truly being followed) should receive the following additional evaluation and therapeutic approach.

   (1) A study of total cholesterol, high-density lipoprotein (HDL) cholesterol, triglycerides, and lipoprotein fractions in the child for phenotyping.
   (2) An initial study of cholesterol levels in first-degree family members (parents, siblings) to help distinguish between the dietary-resistant monogenic and the dietary-responsive polygenic forms. This differential diagnosis will be discussed in the next section.
   (3) If the family pattern is compatible with the polygenic forms, diet alone (with the healthful life-style indicated in Item 1) is all that is necessary. However, a diet stricter than the prudent diet may be required for some families. These diets are provided in Tables 2 and 3. Diets for elevated triglycerides alone are rarely needed for polygenic forms, and the contribution of high triglycerides to coronary disease is small compared with cholesterol. If a child has elevated triglycerides in spite of being ideal weight, but does not simultaneously have high cholesterol, we do not usually suggest a special diet beyond the prudent diet.

3. Distinguishing monogenic from polygenic forms of hyperlipoproteinemia.

   a. Monogenic forms in heterozygotes generally have the following features.
      (1) Higher levels (e.g., cholesterol in childhood of 260 mg/dl rather than 200 mg/dl).
      (2) Do not respond well to diet alone.
      (3) Show bimodality in cholesterol values in family studies. A "classic" monogenic family of six first-degree relatives (adults and children) would have the following cholesterol values: 300, 290, 310, 180, 195, 175—as though the cholesterol levels were coming from two different populations or families.
   b. A "classic" polygenic family of six first-degree relatives (adults and children) would have the following cholesterol levels: 220, 240, 255, 215, 260, 205—as though the cholesterol levels were all from the same bell-shaped distribution curve.

Table 4. Phenotyping Hyperlipoproteinemias

Phenotype	Cholesterol	Triglycerides	Serum	Electrophoresis	Ultracentrifugation
I	↑	↑	creamy	Chylomicrons	Chylomicrons
II (IIa)	↑		clear	Beta ↑	LDL ↑
III	↑	↑	± cloudy	Broad beta	Intermediates
IV		↑	± cloudy	Pre-beta ↑	VLDL ↑
V	↑	↑	creamy	Chylo, pre-beta ↑	Chylo, VLDL ↑
VI (IIb)	↑	↑	± cloudy	Beta ↑, pre-beta ↑	LDL ↑, VLDL ↑

c. The monogenic forms should fit comfortably into the lipoprotein phenotype classification of Fredrickson and the W.H.O., with the caution that possible underlying diseases such as hypothyroidism and lupus must be eliminated before concluding that the lipoproteinemia is a primary rather than a secondary disorder. See Table 4 for a classification of phenotypes.

4. Treating monogenic hyperlipoproteinemias in heterozygotes.
   a. This is the most difficult and controversial area.
   b. Even strict dietary measures are usually insufficient.
   c. We do not usually consider medication except for patients with cholesterol levels above 240 in children and 270 in young adults on a 100-mg cholesterol diet.
   d. If medications are then used, we first consider what medications are showing successful results in the parents and older siblings, because there is doubtless considerable heterogeneity among the monogenic disorders. If a regimen works well for one family member, it is more likely to work in first-degree relatives.
   e. A resin (such as cholestyramine or colestipol) in combination with nicotinic acid, or either agent alone are regimens we use in children (with considerable caution, starting with very low doses, looking for adverse reactions, and being prepared to discontinue if results are unsatisfactory). A dosage schedule will not be offered for these drugs because one has not been established for children. If management with drugs is undertaken as the lesser of two unfavorable alternatives, it may be wise for the primary physician to work with a consultant experienced in this area.
5. Treating monogenic hyperlipoproteinemia IIa in homozygotes. These rare conditions require intensive diagnostic evaluation at the hands of experienced consultants. Portacaval shunt has been the most efficacious approach in our experience.

Cardiac Arrhythmias

HENRY GELBAND, M.D.,
SHARANJEET SINGH, M.D.,
and ARTHUR S. PICKOFF, M.D.

Over the past 10 years significant advances in the diagnosis and therapeutic management of cardiac rhythm disturbances in the pediatric patient have been made. Prior to this time, the therapy of cardiac arrhythmias in infants and children was largely empiric and anecdotal and, for the most part, utilized antiarrhythmic drug regimens based entirely on experience in adults. Two major advances are primarily responsible for the rational approach to proper therapy for cardiac arrhythmias: 1) technologic advances, including intracardiac electrophysiologic studies that have resulted in an accurate delineation of the mechanisms of cardiac arrhythmias, and 2) utilization of the principles of pharmacokinetics and electropharmacology of the antiarrhythmic agents as a guide to effective drug therapy.

The realization that the basic clinical pharmacology and pharmacokinetics of the antiarrhythmic drugs in pediatric patients differ significantly from those in adults has significantly affected therapy. Thus, pharmacologic information derived from adults may be inappropriate when applied to the pediatric patient. For example, it has been shown that when using propranolol or quinidine, much higher doses (on a mg/kg basis) are occasionally necessary to achieve the desired therapeutic blood level to suppress a given cardiac arrhythmia. These observations raise many unanswered questions about the basic underlying differences in the pharmacokinetics of pediatric and adult patients. The measurement of blood levels of the common antiarrhythmic agents is now available in many hospital laboratories on a routine basis. The availability of such information affords the physician an excellent guideline upon which to base adjustments in dosage schedules.

GENERAL PRINCIPLES OF THERAPY

Cardiac rhythm disturbances have to be approached and considered in the framework of the clinical setting in which they appear and the natural history of the abnormal rhythm in order to assure proper management. The child with congenital complete heart block has a different anatomic lesion, prognosis, and approach to therapy than the child with surgically induced complete heart block. In the former, as long as the patient is hemodynamically stable and asymptomatic, there is a relatively good prognosis and the use of pacemaker therapy can generally be put off for a number of years. In comparison, the child with surgically induced complete heart block frequently has some residual intracardiac hemodynamic abnormality, and pacemaker therapy is indicated before significant symptomatology occurs.

While the failure to recognize and treat lifethreatening dysrhythmias and conduction disturbances in patients can result in a tragedy, inappropriate aggressiveness with pacemaker therapy and potential toxic antiarrhythmic agents can be equally disastrous.

The choice of the proper modality in the treatment of a cardiac rhythm disturbance is based on the nature of the disturbance as well as the physician's personal experience and expertise (Table 1). The physician must make a choice as to drug therapy, electrical therapy, or surgery. Occasionally the physician will have to utilize two modes of therapy for the same patient: cardioversion or electrical pacing to interrupt a life-threatening cardiac arrhythmia (e.g., supraventricular tachycardia) as an acute mode of therapy, followed by the oral antiarrhythmic agents for chronic suppressive therapy.

Table 1. MODALITIES OF CARDIAC ARRHYTHMIA THERAPY

Pharmacologic Agents
  Available
    Digitalis
    Quinidine
    Procainamide
    Propranolol (Inderal)
    Phenytoin (Dilantin)
    Lidocaine
    Atropine
    Disopyramide (Norpace)
    Bretylium
  Investigational
    Verapamil
    Ajmaline
    Aprindine
    Amiodarone
    Mexiletine
    Tocainide
Electrical
    Cardioversion
    Pacing, overdrive suppression
    Pacemaker
Surgery
Combinations

Managing antiarrhythmic drug therapy (see Table 2) in the pediatric patient can often be a frustrating therapeutic undertaking unless some knowledge of the mechanism responsible for the arrhythmia and a judgment of the relative risk of the arrhythmia versus the risk of drug therapy are known. This includes consideration of the pharmacologic agent's electrophysiologic effects, cardiovascular effects, and actions on organ systems other than the cardiovascular system.

If an abnormality of cardiac rhythm is secondary to an etiology extrinsic to the heart, treatment should be directed toward correcting that etiology primarily. For example, ventricular extrasystoles resulting from congestive heart failure often can be eliminated by improving cardiac compensation, while those resulting from abnormalities of electrolyte or acid-base imbalances are best treated by appropriate control of these metabolic factors.

In general, it is best to initiate drug therapy with one agent instead of the simultaneous use of more than one agent. When initiating combinations of drugs, it is often impossible to determine which drug is responsible for the achieved therapeutic effect and, more importantly, which drug may be responsible for any undesirable side effect that may occur. The selected antiarrhythmic agent should be administered until either there is termination of the arrhythmia or toxic manifestations occur. Maximal single drug therapy should be monitored with frequent electrocardiographic and clinical evaluations, as well as blood concentration determinations of the drug whenever possible, as a guide to the management. When one specific single drug fails to control the arrhythmia, only then should combined pharmacologic therapy be employed.

Sinus Tachycardia and Sinus Bradycardia. Both sinus tachycardia and sinus bradycardia are generally well tolerated in the pediatric patient and usually do not require therapy since hemodynamic compromise from impairment of diastolic filling time, in the case of sinus tachycardia, or low cardiac output secondary to severe bradycardia, is distinctly uncommon.

Sinus bradycardia may require treatment if cardiac output and perfusion are compromised by the rhythm. This requires clinical judgment and should not be based solely upon the degree of sinus bradycardia. In the preterm infant, clearing the pharynx of secretions or simple tactile stimulation may result in termination of a period of sinus bradycardia. In the presence of acute severe sinus bradycardia with circulatory compromise, atropine, 0.01 mg/kg IV, or an isoproterenol infusion, 0.05 to 0.2 μg/kg/min, may be used to restore the heart rate to normal. In all cases of severe sinus bradycardia, a search for a correctable underlying cause, including metabolic abnormalities, should be instituted.

Sinus Arrhythmia. Sinus arrhythmia is mentioned here because it is the most common cause, in the pediatric patient, of an irregular heart rate. This rhythm results from autonomic reflexes consequent upon respiration. The rhythm may be suspected clinically by auscultation. With inspiration, the heart rate will be appreciated to gradually increase and with expiration, decrease. This arrhythmia is benign and no further evaluation of the patient is necessary. If doubt exists, an electrocardiogram can be obtained to exclude extrasystoles and conduction disorders as a cause of the irregular rhythm.

Sinus Node Dysfunction. The syndrome of sinus node dysfunction or sick sinus syndrome has been increasingly recognized in the pediatric patient. In the symptomatic child with significant bradyarrhythmias associated with sinus node dysfunction or in the postoperative patient with evidence of significant sinus node depression, insertion of an artificial pacemaker is the treatment of choice. When tachycardias complicate the clinical picture, specific antiarrhythmic therapy is initiated, depending on the associated arrhythmia. Since many of the antiarrhythmic drugs (i.e., propranolol, quinidine) can adversely affect sinus node function, concomitant insertion of a prophylactic artificial pacemaker in these patients is often indicated.

Premature Supraventricular Extrasystoles. In the vast majority of pediatric patients with premature supraventricular extrasystoles, no underlying etiology for the arrhythmia can be detected and no specific therapy is indicated since the arrhythmia is considered benign. As noted, specific antiarrhythmic therapy for premature supraventricular extrasystoles is, in the overwhelming majority of

Table 2. DRUG THERAPY IN CARDIAC ARRHYTHMIAS

Drug	Indications	Half-life (hr)	Protein-binding (%)	Blood Levels Effective	Toxic
Digoxin	Supraventricular tachycardia; atrial flutter-fibrillation (without WPW)	24–48†	25	0.8–3.5 ng/ml‡	>2.5 ng/ml
Quinidine	Ventricular arrhythmias; supraventricular tachycardia and atrial flutter-fibrillation, especially in presence of WPW	6–72	80–90 (adult) 60–70 (neonate)	2–7 µg/ml‡	>9 µg/ml
Procainamide	Ventricular arrhythmias; supraventricular tachycardia	2.5–5.0†	15–20	3–10 µg/ml‡	>10 µg/ml
Lidocaine	Ventricular arrhythmias (acute)	1.5	20–60	2–6 µg/ml	>10 µg/ml
Propranolol	Ventricular arrhythmias; supraventricular tachycardias (especially A-V nodal re-entry)	2–4.5	95	20–150 ng/ml‡	—
Phenytoin	Ventricular arrhythmias; supraventricular arrhythmias when digoxin-induced	8–60 (dose-dependent)	80–95	10–20 µg/ml	>20 µg/ml
Verapamil*	Supraventricular tachycardia; atrial flutter-fibrillation (to slow ventricular rate)	3–7	90	—	—
Disopyramide*	Drug-resistant ventricular arrhythmias	6–8	30–65	2.5–7.5 µg/ml	—
Bretylium*	Ventricular fibrillation	6–10	—	0.5–1.5 µg/ml	—

* Not approved for use in children.
† Evidence to suggest shorter half-life in children (except in neonate).
‡ Some patients may require and tolerate higher levels for control of arrhythmias.
§ Depends on age and weight of child.
‖ Pediatric dose not established by manufacturer.

pediatric patients, not indicated. A possible exception to this is the patient with dilated atria secondary to acquired or congenital heart disease. In this select group, the onset of frequent supraventricular extrasystoles may herald the onset of atrial flutter-fibrillation. Reduction in the excitability of the ectopic agrial focus with agents such as procainamide or quinidine, which decrease automaticity of the ectopic site, is indicated.

Supraventricular Tachycardia. The acute treatment of the critically ill infant or child presenting with a supraventricular tachycardia can be approached in the following manner. If there is severe hemodynamic compromise (congestive heart failure, shock), DC countershock (1 to 2 watt-sec/kg) can be employed to terminate the arrhythmia. If the patient is clinically stable at the time of presentation, rapid digitalization or the use of intravenous

verapamil (0.15mg/kg up to 5 mg) is recommended. The classic vagal maneuvers such as unilateral carotid massage and the gag reflex can also be employed to acutely slow conduction within the AV node and terminate the arrhythmia. Recently, it has been reported that immersion of the face in ice water, making use of the "diving seal" reflex, is often successful in provoking an effective vagal discharge within the AV node.

Enhanced vagal tone can also be established by pharmacologic means. Edrophonium hydrochloride (Tensilon), an anticholinesterase inhibitor, in a dose of 0.2 mg/kg IV, or phenylephrine (Neo-Synephrine) (0.1 mg/kg/dose IV) can interrupt the tachycardia by slowing conduction through the AV node, either by directly increasing the concentration of acetylcholine (edrophonium) or by inducing a reflex vagal response to a controlled elevation in

Table 2. DRUG THERAPY IN CARDIAC ARRHYTHMIAS *(Continued)*

Dosage				
		IV		
Oral/24 hr	Dosing Interval	Initial	Maintenance	Major Side Effects
10–25 μg/kg (following digitalization)	once or twice daily	§	1/3–1/4 total digitalization dose	Vomiting, premature atrial and ventricular contractions, A-V block, atrial tachycardia (with block)
15–60 mg/kg	q 6–8 hr	contraindicated	contraindicated	GI disturbances, QRS interval prolongation, premature ventricular contractions, syncope, thrombocytopenia, hypotension
15–50 mg/kg	q 4–6 hr	3–6 mg/kg (over 5 min)	20–50 μg/kg/min	Hypotension, lupus-like syndrome
—	—	1 mg/kg (may be repeated in 10 min)	10–50 μg/kg/min	Drowsiness, muscle twitching, convulsions
0.5–14 mg/kg‖	q 6 hr	0.05–0.2 mg/kg (over 10 min)	—	Bradycardia, hypotension, hypoglycemia, bronchospasm
3–8 mg/kg	q 12 hr	5 mg/kg (over 5 min)	—	Ataxia, nystagmus, tremor, confusion
80–120 mg (adult) 10–20 mg/kg (child) (180 mg/24 hr max)	q 6–8 hr	0.15 mg/kg (may be repeated) (5 mg max)	—	Bradycardia, hypotension, worsening heart failure
9–12 mg/kg	q 6 hr	—	—	Dry mouth, constipation, urinary retention, decreased cardiac output
—	—	5–10 mg/kg (over 10 min)	5 mg/kg q 6–8 hr	Hypotension

systemic blood pressure. These vagal maneuvers are often more effective when partial digitalization has occurred.

Finally, a most effective method of terminating the tachycardia acutely is by pacing techniques. If one has expertise with introducing a pacing catheter into the right atrium, the delivery of random extrastimuli or rapid bursts can almost always disrupt the arrhythmia.

Electrocardiographically, a broad definition of supraventricular tachycardia consists of any regular tachyarrhythmia with (usually) narrow QRS complexes where P waves are either not visible or occur, with retrograde activation, following each QRS complex. Close scrutiny of the relationship of the P wave to the QRS complex can suggest an underlying mechanism. When P waves are not visible or occur almost immediately following the QRS complex on the ECG, the underlying mechanism is most likely to be AV nodal re-entry with almost simultaneous activation of the ventricle and atria. In such patients, drugs that suppress conduction within the AV node (digoxin) are most likely to be successful in the chronic treatment of this arrhythmia. In patients failing to respond to an adequate trial of digoxin therapy, either substitution or addition of propranolol* or verapamil, which also results in slow conduction within the AV node, may be required for chronic suppression. Patients with supraventricular tachycardia who are not controlled with a combination of digoxin and propranolol should undergo intracardiac electrophysiologic study to definitely delineate the mechanism of the arrhythmia.

Recently, a second variety of AV nodal reentry in the pediatric patient has been described. This form occurs much less frequently, but is important because it is recognizable by the surface ECG and often requires more aggressive doses of digoxin and propranolol for control. In this form of supraventricular tachycardia, a very slow conducting AV nodal pathway is utilized to carry the impulse back to the atria and, thus, retrograde P waves are recorded on the ECG and tend to occur at long intervals after the QRS complex.

In infants and children utilizing accessory Kent connections to complete a tachycardia circuit (atria → AV node → ventricles → Kent connection → atria) retrograde P waves are often recorded a short but clear interval following the QRS complex. If the patient is known to have a Wolff-Parkinson-White pattern on the electrocardiogram during regular sinus rhythm, this too would alert one to the possibility that the patient is utilizing the Kent connection during tachycardia. The chronic pharma-

cologic management of these patients can be directed to blocking the tachycardia circuit, either with drugs that preferentially slow conduction within the AV node (digoxin, propranolol) or, if this fails, by employing agents that depress conduction within the Kent connection (procainamide or quinidine). Rarely, re-entry can occur within the sinus node itself. Quinidine may have a role in the management of this arrhythmia. Hence, the chronic pharmacologic management of children with supraventricular tachycardia is best undertaken after an attempt is made to understand the mechanism, then selecting antiarrhythmic agents that are most appropriate for that mechanism.

Several antiarrhythmic agents may eventually assume an important role in the management of supraventricular tachycardia in children. Verapamil, a calcium antagonist that results in delay of AV node conduction and has been extensively used in Europe in the acute and chronic management of supraventricular tachycardia with considerable success, is now an approved drug. Amiodarone (investigational) is an agent that appears to be extremely useful in children with supraventricular tachycardia associated with Kent connections.

While re-entry is the most important mechanism for childhood supraventricular tachycardia, an occasional patient will have supraventricular tachycardia due to an enhanced ectopic atrial or junctional pacemaker. This is most often encountered in the postoperative cardiac patient. The arrhythmia is characterized by a narrow QRS tachycardia and dissociation of P waves and QRS complexes. The rhythm is frequently resistant to chronic suppression. Pharmacologic agents that have been proposed as useful in treating this arrhythmia in children include digoxin alone or in combination with propranolol, phenytoin, reserpine (0.07 mg/kg q 12 hr IM) or chlorpromazine (0.5 to 1 mg/kg IM).

Atrial Flutter-Fibrillation. Electrophysiologic investigations suggest that re-entry within the atrium is responsible for the genesis of atrial flutter and probably fibrillation. In some patients with very rapid conduction, atrial flutter may not be discernible on the electrocardiogram and the possibility of a re-entrant supraventricular tachycardia may be entertained. In such instances, the performance of vagal maneuvers often can slow the ventricular rate enough to uncover the underlying atrial rhythm, and thus disclose the correct diagnosis.

Digoxin is considered the first drug of choice in treating atrial flutter and fibrillation. Should digoxin alone fail to control the arrhythmia, verapamil may be substituted or quinidine may be added. In the acute situation, countershock or intracardiac pacing techniques are particularly effective in the case of atrial flutter.

Special consideration needs to be directed to the

---

*The manufacturer of brands of this product comments that data on the use of propranolol in children are too limited to permit adequate directions for use.

treatment of pediatric patients with atrial flutter or fibrillation associated with an accessory Kent connection. If critically ill upon presentation, or if unsure as to the correct diagnosis, DC countershock (1 to 2 watt-sec/kg) should be used to terminate the arrhythmia. For chronic pharmacologic suppression of this arrhythmia, it has been recommended that digoxin be avoided. It has been shown in children that digoxin can result in electrophysiologic improvement of the conduction properties in the Kent connection and worsen the arrhythmia. In such an instance, a combination of propranolol or verapamil (to block the arrhythmia from conducting over the AV node) and quinidine (to block conduction over the Kent connection) is effective in treating children with this arrhythmia.

Premature Ventricular Contractions. Premature ventricular contractions are a frequent occurrence in otherwise healthy children. When the ventricular extrasystoles are unifocal and disappear with exercise, no treatment is recommended. However, multifocal extrasystoles, or extrasystoles induced by exercise, particularly in the postoperative patient, require therapy. Correction of an underlying hemodynamic or metabolic derangement if present is mandatory, and antiarrhythmic drug therapy is then indicated if an underlying cause cannot be identified or satisfactorily corrected. Phenytoin, propranolol, quinidine, procainamide, and disopyramide have all been effective in the suppression of ventricular extrasystoles with varying degrees of success. Propranolol should not be used when the myocardium is depressed as in cases of myocarditis, postoperative patients with significant residual lesions, or patients with sinus node depression. Phenytoin is perhaps the most benign oral agent and is recommended for use in those patients with ventricular extrasystoles following cardiac surgery or digitalis intoxication. Quinidine and procainamide are also quite effective orally for chronic suppression of ventricular extrasystoles. These drugs should be used cautiously in patients with poor myocardial contractility or conduction disease. Disopyramide, though similar electrophysiologically to quinidine and procainamide, is at times useful when other conventional drug therapy fails.

Ventricular Tachycardia. Ventricular tachycardia, an uncommon arrhythmia during childhood, is life-threatening and requires prompt treatment since hypotension and degeneration to ventricular fibrillation are common. Synchronized DC electrical cardioversion using 1 to 2 watt-sec/kg is the treatment of choice if significant hypotension is present. Suppression of ventricular tachycardia can then be maintained by IV lidocaine infusion (1 to 2 mg/kg bolus followed by 20 to 50 μg/kg/min). Prophylaxis against recurrent attacks of ventricular tachycardia is mandatory in virtually every case.

Digitalis is relatively contraindicated in ventricular tachycardia but may be used along with other agents if congestive heart failure is present. It is recommended that procainamide or quinidine be initially utilized unless ventricular tachycardia occurs in the postoperative child, when phenytoin is the drug of choice. Ventricular tachycardia associated with increased catecholamine stimulation (exercise-induced) is best treated with propranolol. Electrical pacing of the atrium or ventricle may prevent recurrence in rare cases of ventricular tachycardia that do not respond to drug treatment.

In those few patients who persist with ventricular tachycardia, in spite of attempts at adequate control of their arrhythmia with the usual pharmacologic measures, there is evidence to suggest that a combined invasive electrophysiologic-pharmacologic study may be of considerable benefit. Experience in children suggests that electrophysiologic studies can localize the region of ventricular myocardium generating the arrhythmia by reproducing the arrhythmia in the laboratory, using stimulation and recording techniques. Once this has been accomplished, a pharmacologic agent can be administered (procainamide, propranolol), in gradually increasing doses, until the arrhythmia can no longer be reproduced. The drug levels measured during these studies may serve as a guideline to the levels necessary to be achieved with chronic oral dosing to effectively control the rhythm disturbance.

Rarely, the pediatrician will see a child who is asymptomatic, with no underlying heart disease, but with ventricular tachycardia documented electrocardiographically. The etiology of the arrhythmia is often occult, and the long-term prognosis of this small group of children is not well defined. At this time, most centers would agree that such children do merit clinical and invasive electrophysiologic investigation as well as an attempt to suppress the arrhythmia pharmacologically.

Ventricular Fibrillation. Ventricular fibrillation is uniformly fatal if left untreated. Cardiopulmonary resuscitation should be immediately instituted. DC countershock (1 to 2 watt-sec/kg) is the treatment of choice. Bretylium (5–10 mg/kg over 10 minutes) is an antiarrhythmic drug, not as yet approved for use in children, that can acutely convert ventricular fibrillation to sinus rhythm. Recurrences of ventricular fibrillation need to be prevented by intravenous infusion of lidocaine in the immediate cardioversion period. Chronic prophylaxis against recurrence of ventricular fibrillation can be achieved by the orally administered antiarrhythmic agents—procainamide, quinidine, or disopyramide.

Arrhythmias in Patients with Mitral Valve Prolapse. Atrial and ventricular arrhythmias are frequent in patients with mitral valve prolapse.

Frequent PVCs, APCs, supraventricular tachycardia, ventricular tachycardia, or rarely fibrillation may occur. Syncope, palpitations, and the occurrence of exercise-induced arrhythmias are useful in deciding upon the need for antiarrhythmic therapy. Propranolol is the most frequent antiarrhythmic agent employed.

Arrhythmias in Patients with Long Q-T Syndrome. Prolonged Q-T interval with (Jervell and Lange-Nielsen syndrome) or without (Romano-Ward syndrome) congenital deafness is associated with syncopal episodes due to ventricular arrhythmias, including fibrillation. In selected patients, left stellate ganglion blockade has been effective in reducing the Q-T interval and eliminating symptoms, lending support to the hypothesis that the pathogenesis is related to abnormalities in ventricular refractoriness secondary to an imbalance of cardiac sympathetic innervation. It also has been suggested that β-blockade with propranolol is effective in reducing the risk of sudden death.

Atrioventricular (A-V) Block. First-degree A-V block is a benign conduction abnormality and usually requires no therapy. Cautious medical observation is indicated if this conduction abnormality occurs following cardiac surgery, to determine whether higher degrees of A-V block will ensue.

Second-degree A-V block is characterized by intermittent failure of A-V conduction. Mobitz type I (Wenckebach) A-V block has been described in otherwise normal pediatric patients and, in this setting, is usually of little significance. However, it can be seen in any condition resulting in anatomic or functional impairment of the A-V node. When Wenckebach periodicity occurs secondary to digitalis toxicity, phenytoin can be used to accelerate A-V conduction if patients are symptomatic. Alternatively, beta agonists (isoproterenol) can be utilized to enhance A-V conduction and increase the cardiac rate.

Mobitz type II second-degree A-V block consists of intermittent cessation of A-V conduction, usually due to a block in the distal A-V conduction system. This form of A-V block is more serious and can progress to complete heart block. Sympathomimetic drugs and temporary pacing are indicated for acute emergencies, followed by chronic pacemaker therapy.

Congenital third-degree A-V block usually results from block within the A-V node. When this conduction disturbance is associated with a structural cardiac defect, it is frequently poorly tolerated. Permanent pacemaker therapy is indicated as soon as symptomatology (syncope, dizziness), cardiomegaly or early signs of congestive heart failure are present, to increase the heart rate and improve cardiac output.

Surgically acquired third-degree heart block requires a permanent pacemaker. The site of block in these cases is usually below the A-V node, and the risk of sudden death is significant unless prophylactic pacemaker therapy is instituted. It has been reported that patients with intact A-V conduction but who develop right bundle branch block with left anterior block postoperatively are at a greater risk for sudden death. At the present time, only close medical observation is indicated in this group of patients for progression of their conduction abnormality or symptomatology before pacemaker insertion is recommended.

Electrical Management of Cardiac Arrhythmias

Electrical therapy for the treatment of cardiac rhythm disturbances includes 1) cardioversion, 2) overdrive electrical stimulation of the atrium or ventricle, and 3) pacemakers. Cardioversion is a safe, rapid method and is most frequently utilized in patients with ventricular fibrillation, chronic atrial fibrillation, and supraventricular or ventricular tachycardia in which the rate is very rapid and the patient's clinical condition is deteriorating. Dosage guidelines should be adhered to in order to deliver effective energy to the heart as well as to prevent possible myocardial injury. One word of caution: all patients on prior digitalis therapy may have postcardioversion arrhythmias that may be more difficult to control than the primary arrhythmia for which the cardioversion was utilized.

Direct programmed electrical stimulation of the heart with random or burst pacing (overdrive suppression) delivered to the atria or ventricle is an excellent means for acute control of supraventricular and ventricular arrhythmias. The same catheter utilized for endocardial conversion of the arrhythmia also can be utilized for intracardiac recording to document the mechanism or origin of an arrhythmia, if necessary. When utilizing overdrive suppression, one generally has to pace the atrium or ventricle at a rate fast enough to capture the atrium or ventricle for at least 30 seconds. Discontinuation of pacing usually results in termination of the arrhythmia. This principle has resulted in the development of new permanent implantable pacemakers to provide electrical conversion of tachyarrhythmias on a chronic basis in patients who do not respond to conventional medical treatment. There is early successful experience in the pediatric patient with such devices.

Epicardial and endocardial pacemakers are utilized in the permanent treatment of conduction disorders (complete heart block, sick sinus syndrome). The type of pacemaker to be utilized must be decided upon after careful consideration of the patient's age, general condition, disease, and availability of cardiologic and surgical expertise. One has to weigh the risks of an epicardial pacemaker, which requires a thoracotomy, against a permanent transvenous pacemaker, which carries the risk of ventricular perforation or catheter and electrode displacement.

Surgical Management of Cardiac Arrhythmias

This represents a rather new approach to the treatment of cardiac arrhythmias in the pediatric patient. The specific applications and methodology are still being developed. Surgical treatment of cardiac arrhythmias is currently limited to three areas: 1) resection of a cardiac aneurysm or tumors when associated with cardiac arrhythmias, which will frequently alleviate the cardiac rhythm disturbance, 2) ventricular arrhythmias associated with chronic scarring secondary to prior cardiac surgery, and 3) those incessant supraventricular arrhythmias associated with accessory bypass tracts, which are resistant to all conventional means of medical therapy. In such cases, a surgical cure can be obtained either by interruption of the accessory pathway that is part of the re-entrant circuit, or by inducing complete heart block (interrupt the His bundle) with the placement of a permanent pacemaker.

Cardiomyopathies and Pericardial Diseases

IAIN F. S. BLACK, M.D.

THE CARDIOMYOPATHIES

Cardiomyopathy is a general term describing diseases of the muscle of the heart, which can be conveniently divided into primary and secondary groups, recognizing that some cases of secondary cardiomyopathy will be mislabeled as primary because the cause was not apparent at the time of diagnosis. Since the purpose of this review is to emphasize treatment, the primary group is subdivided according to clinical presentation, with the appropriate management of each category being discussed in detail.

Primary

Hypertrophic Cardiomyopathy. In this disease there is either concentric or asymmetric diffuse hypertrophy of the muscle fibers. The asymmetric form is characterized by disproportionate septal hypertrophy with or without left ventricular outflow tract obstruction. This is considered a familial inherited disorder, although documentation may be difficult if the number of family members affected is small.

In the early stages of the *nonobstructed form* there is no dilatation of the cavities, and muscle function is adequate. Early fatigue and dyspnea are rare but may occur with exercise because of an impairment of cardiac reserve. There is no specific treatment.

Progression of the disease may result in the development of asymmetric septal hypertrophy with left ventricular outflow tract obstruction or ventricular dilatation with congestive heart failure. Treatment is the same as for patients in those groups.

The severity of the outflow tract obstruction in the *obstructed form* is determined by the size of the left ventricular cavity during systole, and any reduction in its size intensifies the gradient. For this reason positive inotropic agents such as isoproterenol (Isuprel) or digoxin are contraindicated. In contrast, an expansion of blood volume or the use of a peripheral vasoconstrictor such as phenylephrine hydrochloride (Neo-Synephrine) (0.1 mg/kg SC or IV) or methoxamine hydrochloride (Vasoxyl) (0.5 mg/kg IM or 0.15 mg/kg IV) increases left ventricular size and reduces the severity of the obstruction.

The beta-adrenergic receptor blocking drugs are still the drugs of choice for obstructive hypertrophic cardiomyopathy. Not only do they cause slowing of the heart rate, which increases diastolic filling of the left ventricle, but they also suppress sympathetic activity, which intensifies the degree of obstruction, particularly during exercise. The drug of choice is propranolol hydrochloride (Inderal), the starting dose being 1 mg/kg/day divided into four doses. This may not always be practical for the adolescent, in whom an eight hourly schedule may be tried. A maximum dosage has not been established for children. It is recommended that the dosage be gradually increased until there is a satisfactory clinical response or the side effects of hypotension or marked bradycardia occur. The therapeutic blood level range is 100–200 ng/dl, although higher levels can be tolerated without the appearance of toxic side effects. Therapy must be continued indefinitely. Propranolol hydrochloride is contraindicated in bronchial asthma, hypoglycemia-prone patients, first and second degree A-V block and in congestive heart failure except as outlined in this chapter.

Research work with calcium blockers such as verapamil hydrochloride and nifedipine indicates that they may be useful for the treatment of this condition. Both are now approved for use in the U.S.A.; however, pediatric dosages are not listed for nifedipine in the Physicians' Drug Reference. Both have reduced symptoms and improved exercise capacity in patients with obstructive hypertrophic cardiomyopathy. The mechanism of their effect is not clear; although there is inhibition of slow-channel ion flux and improved diastolic function, the end result is a reduction in the severity of the gradient allowing the ventricle to empty more efficiently.

If the obstruction is severe or symptoms are un-relieved by medical management, surgery may have to be considered. Relief, significant at times, has been obtained by making a longitudinal incision through the septal hypertrophy with or without removal of a part of the ventricular septum. However, although this may reduce or abolish the gradient, the primary muscular hypertrophy is unchanged. Surgery of this type is associated with significant mortality and should be reserved for the most serious cases.

Patients with hypertrophic cardiomyopathy have an increased incidence of Wolff-Parkinson-White syndrome as well as supraventricular and ventricular arrhythmias and are at risk for sudden death. Twenty-four hour ambulatory electrocardiographic monitoring is advisable for all children with obstructive or nonobstructive hypertrophic cardiomyopathy. The occurrence of premature ventricular contractions or ventricular tachycardia justifies treatment with an antiarrhythmic agent to minimize the risk of sudden death. The recommended drug is propranolol hydrochloride* starting at 1.0 mg/kg/day divided into four doses. Should atrial flutter or atrial fibrillation be present, then quinidine gluconate should be added, starting at 10 mg/kg/day, divided into three doses, to a maximum of 40 mg/kg/day. The ideal serum level is 2–5 μg/dl. Signs of toxicity are tinnitus, blurred vision, nausea, vomiting, and widening of the QRS interval of the electrocardiogram by more than 25%.

A transient form of hypertrophic cardiomyopathy occurs in infants of diabetic mothers. In some there is septal hypertrophy with or without left ventricular outflow tract obstruction but others have large hearts and develop congestive heart failure. The severity of the failure is aggravated by a low blood sugar which may justify the use of corticosteroids. Rarely surgery may be necessary to remove part of the pancreas. For children who survive, the disease is self-limiting with gradual improvement over the first 2 years of life. Propranolol hydrochloride has been used for the left ventricular outflow tract obstruction but only in infants with a normal blood sugar, since it can increase the severity of the hypoglycemia. Digoxin is contraindicated because of its inotropic effect.

Congestive Cardiomyopathy. The patient presents with an enlarged heart due to dilatation of the ventricular cavities. There is nonspecific myocardial degeneration, with intercellular edema and hypertrophy of the muscle fibers being a frequent finding. As a result of impaired ventricular compliance there is systolic dysfunction, with the development of congestive heart failure. The etiology of the myocardial degeneration is not known and may be due to a number of different factors. It is reasonable to assume that some of these patients may in fact have a secondary form of cardiomyopathy that was unrecognized or subclinical at the time of its occurrence.

Endocardial fibroelastosis is considered to be a primary cardiomyopathy and belongs in this group because the deterioration of myocardial function leads to left ventricular dilatation and cardiac failure. This occurs despite the proliferation of fibroelastotic tissue in an attempt to strengthen and protect ventricular function.

Management is as for congestive heart failure, with digoxin being the most effective drug. The doses for children are listed in Table 1. The total digitalization dose is given as three doses over 16 to 24 hours. Half initially then one quarter twice at intervals of 8 to 12 hours. The maximum oral digitalizing dose is 1.5 mg, and the maximum daily maintenance dose is 0.25 mg. The intramuscular route is not recommended because of slow and uneven absorption. If digoxin is to be given intravenously each dose is reduced by one third. The therapeutic serum level is 0.7–2.0 ng/dl, with levels of 2.5 ng/dl or higher considered to be in the toxic range. In infants, the therapeutic range is wider, with toxicity rarely being seen under 4.0 ng/dl. Arrhythmias due to digoxin toxicity are treated by giving phenytoin intravenously in a bolus of 1–2 mg/kg over 2 to 3 minutes. Diuretics such as chlorothiazide (Diuril), 20–40 mg/kg/day divided into two doses, and furosemide (Lasix), 1–2 mg/kg/dose, are useful if the cardiac failure is severe. Both drugs can cause electrolyte depletion with the development of hypokalemia, which in turn may precipitate digitalis toxicity. Furosemide potentiates the hypotensive effect of antihypotensive medications and increases the risk of salicylate toxicity in patients requiring high doses of salicylates. Spironolactone (Aldactone) is an aldosterone antagonist that is helpful in counteracting the increase in potassium excretion due to the prolonged use of diuretics. The dose is 1 mg/kg 3 times a day.

Despite the presence of congestive heart failure, beta-receptor blocking agents have been shown to noticeably improve systolic and diastolic myocardial function. The beneficial effect is believed to be due to the neutralizing effect the beta-blocker has

---

*Manufacturer's note: Data on the use of propranolol in the pediatric age group are too limited to permit adequate directions for use.

Table 1.   DIGOXIN DOSAGES—ORAL ROUTE

	Digitalization	Maintenance
Birth to 2 months of age	0.04 mg/kg	0.01 mg/kg
2 months to 2 years of age	0.06 mg/kg	0.01–0.015 mg/kg
2 years to 6 years of age	0.04 mg/kg	0.01 mg/kg
Over 6 years of age	0.02 mg/kg	0.01 mg/kg

on either a hypersensitivity to sympathetic stimulation or on an inappropriate sympathetic response to cardiac stimulation. It is recommended that a beta-blocking agent such as propranolol be added to the conventional treatment with digitalis and diuretics if there is persistence of severe congestive heart failure.

Vasodilators have a role in the management of severe congestive heart failure. Sodium nitroprusside (Nipride), which decreases both preload and afterload, is most helpful in the acute management of severe heart failure. The intravenous dose range is from 0.5–8 μg/kg/min. A suitable starting dose is 3 μg/kg/min, adjusting the dose up or down according to blood pressure response. Since exposure to light causes degradation of the sodium nitroprusside, a prepared solution must not be kept for longer than 4 hours. To minimize deterioration, the infusion solution and all tubing should be wrapped in aluminum foil. A complication of using sodium nitroprusside is retention of thiocyanate in the body. The blood level of thiocyanate should be checked daily, with the infusion being reduced or stopped if the value approaches the toxic level as determined by your own laboratory. No specific figure is recommended, since what is considered to be the toxic level varies from one laboratory to another according to the method of analysis. Adverse reactions to the drug are caused by too rapid a drop in blood pressure.

Our experience with oral vasodilator drugs is with hydralazine hydrochloride (Apresoline), an afterload reducing agent, 1 mg/kg/day in four divided doses up to a maximum of 7 mg/kg/day, and prazosin hydrochloride (Minipress),* a preload and afterload reducing agent, 0.03 to 0.04 mg/kg/day in three divided doses to a maximum of 0.4 mg/kg/day. If prazosin hydrochloride is used, it is necessary to monitor the first dose closely, since a marked hypotensive response is not uncommon. The effects of the drug are potentiated if it is used simultaneously with diuretics or with propranolol hydrochloride. A further disadvantage of the drug is that in time tolerance develops. A complication of hydralazine hydrochloride therapy is the risk of developing systemic lupus erythematosus. Terbutaline (Brethine), which has been used in adults, is a oral beta-agonist with both vasodilatory and inotropic properties. It has yet to be established if this drug is beneficial in the treatment of children with this lesion.

Marked dilatation of the left ventricular cavity associated with poor contraction predisposes to the development of thrombosis and the risk of embolism. Anticoagulants such as intravenous heparin or oral coumadin should be prescribed for these patients. Despite aggressive medical management the prognosis is poor for children with congestive cardiomyopathy. The ultimate hope for these children is cardiac transplantation, which is currently being undertaken at several centers in the United States.

Restrictive Cardiomyopathy. The restrictive cardiomyopathies are probably the least well understood and the least common in children. There are three groups, Löffler's endocarditis, primary restrictive cardiomyopathy, and tropical and nontropical endomyocardial fibrosis, all of which have a guarded prognosis. There is usually extensive fibrosis scattered throughout the deep layers of the myocardium, especially in the subendocardium, and endocardial fibrosis is prominent but variable. The result is impaired diastolic function preventing adequate filling of the ventricle. Typically the patient has mild or moderate cardiac enlargement with variable right-sided failure.

Medical management with digitalis and a diuretic is usually unsuccessful. Surgical removal of the thickened and fibrotic ventricular endocardium is known to be helpful in tropical endomyocardial fibrosis but the tricuspid and mitral valves may also need to be replaced. Current research suggests that the calcium blockers may be helpful because of their ability to improve diastolic dysfunction, but further study is needed to determine if these drugs will be beneficial for clinical use in this condition.

Secondary

Infectious. Myocarditis is the most common of all the heart muscle diseases and is associated with almost every known virus, bacterium, rickettsia, spirochete, and parasite.

The more common of the identified viruses are the coxsackie B group. Less common are the cytomegaloviruses, herpes viruses, other enteroviruses, and certain of the adenoviruses. Myocarditis may also occur as a complication of mumps, measles, varicella, and variola. Rheumatic fever and diphtheria are the best known bacterial causes, but abscess formation in the myocardium as a complication of septicemia should not be overlooked. The rickettsial diseases include typhus, Rocky Mountain spotted fever, and Q fever. Rare parasitic and protozoal infections include toxoplasmosis, Chagas disease, amebiasis, trichinosis, and visceral larva migrans. Other rare causes are tuberculosis, leptospirosis and fungal diseases such as histoplasmosis and actinomycosis.

The first priority of management is identification and treatment of the causal infection. In many cases the specific treatment of the primary disease is also the treatment of choice for the cardiac findings. Discussion of the treatment of these primary diseases is beyond the scope of this text.

If there is significant myocardial involvement,

---

*Manufacturer's note: No clinical experience is available with the use of prazosin hydrochloride in children.

dilatation of the heart occurs with the development of congestive heart failure. With some modifications, treatment is as for congestive cardiomyopathy. There is still controversy as to the optimal dose of digoxin to be given to a patient with acute infective myocarditis. Some believe the myocardium to be more sensitive to digoxin during the acute phase and that the dose should be reduced accordingly. I recommend that two thirds of the digitalizing dose be given only if digitalization must be completed within 24 hours. If the plan is to digitalize for a longer period, the total digitalizing dose should be given. In either case, the electrocardiogram (ECG) must be watched closely for signs of toxicity. There should be no reduction in the maintenance dose if digitalization is well tolerated and there are no irregularities of rhythm. Diuretics (Diuril or Lasix) are indicated if there is retention of fluid. Anticoagulants are necessary if there is a risk of clots developing in the dilated ventricular cavity.

Dysrhythmias are a complication of myocarditis. The incidence is highest in diphtheria, where complete heart block may also occur. It is important that the ECG be monitored continuously in any patient with myocarditis and that antiarrhythmic therapy be started if premature ventricular contractions occur. Phenytoin (Dilantin) 3–8 mg/kg/day is preferred to propranolol hydrochloride, which may precipitate congestive heart failure. Optimal therapy is at the dosage required to maintain a blood level of 10–20 μg/ml. A side effect is the early development of fever with either a scarlatiniform or morbilliform rash, requiring the drug to be stopped. Gingival hypertrophy is a complication of continued therapy that can be minimized, but not prevented, by good dental care with regular brushing. If complete heart block occurs, a temporary transvenous pacemaker should be inserted.

In the majority of centers all patients with severe rheumatic carditis are treated with corticosteroids, but in mild cases of carditis some authorities consider acetylsalicylic acid to be a suitable alternative. My own decision has been to use corticosteroids for all cases of rheumatic carditis, but this is a personal preference and should not be interpreted as a criticism of the role of salicylates in this disease.

There is even more controversy as to the dose and the duration of treatment. Some centers give corticosteroids in large doses for only a few days while others select more moderate doses to be given for a number of weeks. I give 60 mg of prednisone a day in four divided doses for 2 weeks. During the third week the dose is rapidly reduced and therapy is stopped on the twenty-first day. If the disease is still active at that time, the corticosteroids are restarted for a further 2 weeks. The dosage is a repeat of the second and third week of the initial course.

An appropriate dosage schedule for acetylsalicylic acid (aspirin) is 120 mg/kg/day, in 4–6 doses, for 48 hours then 60 mg/kg/day for 3–5 weeks. If the clinical response is poor, the dose may be increased, provided the serum salicylate level is kept below 20 mg/dl. Some centers continue therapy for longer than 6 weeks. I do not think this is justified, since the active phase is usually of short duration. However, if the disease is still active, I restart the aspirin at 60 mg/kg/day for a further 3 weeks. The symptoms and signs of toxicity are tinnitus, nausea, vomiting, headache, and hyperpnea. Bed rest is necessary during the initial febrile stage and early ambulation is encouraged except during a second attack of carditis or if there is a slow response to therapy.

Although the use of steroids for rheumatic carditis is accepted, there is disagreement as to their role in viral infections. There is concern, supported by clinical studies, that corticosteroids increase susceptibility to, as well as the severity of, acute viral infections. On the other hand, there are reports of patients with coxsackie B myocarditis who appear to have been helped by corticosteroid therapy. The consensus of opinion is that corticosteroid therapy is justified only in life-threatening situations such as shock due to poor cardiac output or complete heart block with syncope.

Ischemic. Anomalous origin of the left coronary artery from the pulmonary trunk is the most common congenital cause of myocardial ischemia. Symptoms most frequently occur in the young infant. As the pulmonary artery pressure falls after birth, flow from the aorta to the pulmonary artery is encouraged through the connecting system. If the intercoronary anastomoses are well developed, the left coronary artery is likely to be well perfused. More commonly, the communications are limited, perfusion of the left ventricular myocardium is inadequate, and dilatation with cardiac failure develops. The impaired perfusion leads to ischemic episodes resembling anginal attacks. Although the use of digitalis and diuretics help in the management of the congestive heart failure, significant improvement can be brought about only by surgery. If good collaterals are present between the coronary arteries, ligation of the left coronary artery at its entrance into the pulmonary artery should improve myocardial perfusion. If the anastomoses are not adequate, ligation of the left coronary artery can cause sudden myocardial infarction; for these children, the operation of choice is transplantation of the left coronary artery to the ascending aorta. Although successful, this surgery is associated with a high mortality.

Metabolic and Endocrine. This group is characterized by cardiac dilatation with congestive heart failure. Only the more common lesions will be discussed.

Glycogen storage disease (Pompe's disease) of the heart occurs in the young infant, and survival beyond a year is rare. Infiltration of the myocardium with glycogen results in hypertrophy, impaired function, dilatation, and failure. Medical or surgical treatment is of no real help. Caution should be used in prescribing digitalis, since the myocardium is sensitive to the drug and arrhythmias may result.

Although thyrotoxicosis in adults is associated with significant cardiac findings these are rare in children. The exception is the neonate in whom hyperthyroidism can cause marked cardiac enlargement with severe congestive heart failure. Most patients respond well to antithyroid medication. Propranolol hydrochloride,* 1 mg/kg/day, has been used to control the increased blood pressure and heart rate. Hypothyroidism causes cardiac enlargement, poor myocardial contractility, and a decreased cardiac output; however, failure is rare. The condition improves with thyroid medication.

Acromegaly is associated with pronounced cardiac hypertrophy, especially of the left ventricle. This in turn leads to chronic congestive heart failure. The only treatment is directed to the control of the excessive secretion of growth hormone. Equally of concern is the mucopolysaccharide invasion of the myocardial muscle fibers in children with the Hunter-Hurler syndrome. Deterioration of myocardial function leads to dilatation of the heart and the development of congestive heart failure. There is no specific treatment available.

Infantile beriberi, in contrast to the juvenile or adult forms, is associated with cardiac dilatation and congestive heart failure. There is usually an excellent response to thiamine (vitamin B$_1$) therapy. Digoxin is not contraindicated but appears to have little benefit.

Persistent marked hypocalcemia, such as is seen with hypoparathyroidism, can result in cardiac decompensation. Myocardial function returns to normal with the restoration of a normal serum calcium.

Neoplastic and Infiltrative. Malignant tumors of the heart are rare in children. Sarcomas are the usual primary form, having been reported in children as young as three days. The clinical findings depend on the nature of the involvement and the location of the tumor. If it is diffuse, a restrictive cardiomyopathy will result. If localized, it may extend into a cavity and cause valvular or outflow tract obstruction. Treatment is of the tumor itself.

Infiltrative diseases such as amyloidosis and sarcoidosis are the most common causes of restrictive cardiomyopathy in adults but are rare in children.

Neuromuscular and Muscular. This group is characterized by cardiac dilatation with the late development of congestive heart failure.

In Friedreich's ataxia there is a diffuse concentric hypertrophy of both ventricles with degeneration of individual fibers and diffuse fibrosis throughout the myocardium. Dilatation of the heart is common but failure is rare. Dysrhythmias are not uncommon and when present require the usual therapeutic measures. Progressive muscular dystrophy is associated with atrophy of the myocardial fibers and the development of fibrosis. Mild cardiac enlargement may occur but failure rarely occurs in childhood. There is no specific treatment for either condition.

Miscellaneous. In systemic lupus erythematosus, fibrinoid degeneration of the myocardium with atrophy can occur. Rarely does this lead to congestive heart failure. In such cases, corticosteroids can be added to the usual anticongestive regimen of digoxin and diuretics. Occasionally a supraventricular arrhythmia or complete heart block is the presenting feature of an underlying myocarditis. The treatment is described above.

In children with mucocutaneous lymph node syndrome (Kawasaki's disease), congestive myocarditis may complicate the acute stage. There is no specific therapy but anti-inflammatory agents are used because of the accompanying vasculitis. Acetylsalicylic acid is the drug of choice and has the advantage of also inhibiting platelet aggregation. It is recommended to start with 80–100 mg/kg/day, dropping this to 10 mg/kg/day when the fever is under control. The treatment should be continued until the platelet count and sedimentation rate have returned to normal (6 to 10 weeks). There is no decision as to how long the acetylsalicylic acid therapy should be continued if aneurysms are found on the coronary arteries. Some authors believe this justifies continuing the drug for 1 year after the acute illness, others believe it can be stopped after 4 to 6 months. Corticosteroids are contraindicated, since they are thought to increase the incidence of aneurysm formation and may increase the platelet count without decreasing the platelet adhesiveness.

Congestive cardiac failure has been reported in children under 2 years of age who have cystic fibrosis. The deterioration of left ventricular function is due to the development of multifocal fibrosis in the myocardium.

Mention should be made of the cardiomyopathy associated with sickle cell anemia, in which the persistent chronic anemia leads to cardiac dilatation and congestive heart failure. Although digitalis and diuretics are helpful in treating the congestive heart failure, clinical improvement is best achieved by a blood transfusion. Congestive heart failure may also occur in thalassemia. It is not clear if this is secondary to myocardial damage from transfusion

---

*Manufacturer's note: Data on the use of propranolol in the pediatric age group are too limited to permit adequate directions for use.

hemosiderosis or due to another cause. Attempts to eliminate the excessive stores of iron by chelation have not been successful. Other metals such as cobalt and copper may also cause cardiomyopathy.

Daunorubicin (Cerubidine) and doxorubicin (Adriamycin), drugs used to treat leukemia and lymphoma, have a cumulative toxic effect on the myocardium, depressing ventricular function. This is considered to be at a toxic level if an echocardiographic evaluation shows that the shortening fraction of the left ventricular myocardium has fallen to 20%. If it is essential to continue the medication, it is recommended that digitalis be given for support. Cyclophosphamide, which is used in preparation for bone marrow transplantation, also has a toxic effect on the myocardium.

Cardiomyopathy with asymmetric septal hypertrophy and obstruction has been reported in children with end stage renal disease and hypertension. In our experience working with a busy nephrology service, the cardiomyopathy is easily explained on the basis of chronic hypertension, and we have not seen any patients with this form of asymmetric septal hypertrophy.

PERICARDIAL DISEASES

Congenital

Congenital absence of the pericardium is a rare finding and is seldom diagnosed clinically. Left-sided absence constitutes the majority of cases, while right-sided and complete absence are extremely rare. It is usually a benign lesion with symptoms occurring only if the heart herniates through a partial defect. The only treatment for this is surgical.

Tumors

Pericardial tumors are extremely rare in children, and when present are cause for concern, since over 50% are malignant.

The benign tumors include simple cysts, angiomas, fibromas, lipomas, leiomyomas, and teratomas. These rarely interfere with cardiac function and are usually discovered during routine chest x-ray. Malignant tumors are either primary, such as sarcomas and mesotheliomas, or, more commonly, metastatic and due to leukemia or lymphosarcoma.

Because tumors are so rare, there is no specific plan of treatment. In theory, many of the benign tumors may not need to be removed, but often the diagnosis is not made until there is pathologic examination after surgery to identify the cause of an unidentified mediastinal shadow or mass. Metastatic tumors are treated as part of the therapy for the primary source, although there may be a pericardial effusion which requires drainage.

Pericarditis

Two important clinical features of pericarditis are chest pain and pericardial effusion. The pain, sharp in character, is usually present over the precordium, and patients may find some relief by sitting upright and leaning forward. Occasionally pain is referred to the abdomen, with the patient having tenderness and guarding. In infants, unusual restlessness or orthopnea may be the only manifestation of the pain. Treatment is symptomatic with acetylsalicylic acid; if the pain is very severe, morphine sulfate may be required. Many pericardial effusions are small and if left alone resolve spontaneously. However, if a bacterial infection is suspected a drain should be inserted by surgery rather than attempting pericardiocentesis. The drain should be left in place until all drainage has stopped, to minimize the risk of adhesions and the late complication of constrictive pericarditis. Pericardiocentesis is justified only in an emergency for immediate relief of an acute tamponade. It is the policy in our institution to insert a surgical drain for patients with recurrent effusions rather than to consider repeated needle aspirations. The choice of antibiotics and the decision to use corticosteroids is dealt with in more detail under the specific lesions.

Rheumatic fever, bacterial infections, rheumatoid arthritis and the viral/idiopathic group account for approximately 70% of the cases seen in children. It is convenient to divide the cases up into groups: 1) rheumatic fever; 2) purulent; 3) rheumatoid; 4) viral/idiopathic; 5) miscellaneous; 6) chronic effusive; and 7) traumatic.

Rheumatic fever. Pericarditis is not seen until after 2 years of age and then it is almost always associated with acute carditis. Pericardial effusion and subsequent tamponade rarely occur. Treatment is with acetylsalicylic acid unless there are cardiac findings that justify the use of corticosteroids. The dosage recommendations are the same as listed for rheumatic carditis.

Purulent. This is the most serious group in childhood and is responsible for most of the cases of pericarditis under 2 years of age. Pericardial involvement is usually secondary to a primary source such as pneumonia, empyema, osteomyelitis, or pyelonephritis but may occur in a primary form as a complication of a bacteremia. In the older child the causal organism is most commonly the *Staphylococcus aureus,* with pneumococcus, streptococcus and meningococcus following in that order. In the 1 month to 6 year age group, *Hemophilus influenzae* type b is the most common cause. Gram-negative organisms such as *Escherichia coli, Klebsiella, Proteus,* and *Bacteroides* are all rare causes but have to be considered in infections under 1 month of age. Since successful treatment depends on early diagnosis, it is important to remember that half the cases of pyogenic pericarditis in childhood occur under 2 years of age and can be seen in the first few weeks of life.

The selection of an antibiotic is important (Table 2). If the organism and its sensitivity are known, the appropriate antibiotic is easily selected. However, in most cases, this information is not immediately available, and a combination of two antibiotics is selected to give the broadest possible coverage in the initial stages of the illness. In infants under 1 month of age an appropriate combination is nafcillin (100 mg/kg/day) combined with gentamicin (7.5 mg/kg/day) or kanamycin (20 mg/kg/day). Between 1 month and 6 years of age there must be adequate coverage for *H. influenzae* type b. If the child is not critically ill a combination of nafcillin and ampicillin (200 mg/kg/day) is started. Because of the fact that 10 to 30% of *H. influenzae* type b are resistant to ampicillin if the child is critically ill then the nafcillin is combined with chloramphenicol (75 mg/kg/day). Since chloramphenicol is a toxic drug known to cause aplastic anemia, thrombocytopenia, and granulocytopenia, it should be discontinued as soon as the organism is found to be sensitive to ampicillin. For children over 6 years of age the combination of nafcillin and ampicillin is preferred. The duration of parental treatment depends on the response in the individual case but rarely should be less than 3 weeks.

In purulent pericarditis a varying degree of effusion occurs, with the risk of developing adhesions and loculation of pus. The recommendation for prompt insertion of a drain to prevent this has already been stressed. Until that is done the patient should be watched closely for the development of cardiac tamponade, which can occur acutely with sudden deterioration in the clinical picture over a couple of hours.

Rheumatoid. Pericarditis occurs in approximately 10% of patients with rheumatoid arthritis. The inflammation is serofibrinous and can form dense, fibrous adhesions similar to those in rheumatic fever. Occasionally an effusion is present, but it is usually not large enough to cause tamponade. Treatment is symptomatic, and acetylsalicylic acid is the drug of choice. Although corticosteroids have been used, most physicians believe that they have no role in this lesion and recommend that they not be used except in life-threatening situations, and then only for a short period of time.

Viral/Idiopathic. Only in recent years has viral pericarditis been accepted as a separate entity. The most important viruses are those of the coxsackie group B, with cases due to influenza, mumps, herpes zoster, varicella and other viruses having been reported. Also, there is indirect evidence of an etiologic relationship between pericarditis and other viruses, such as the adenoviruses and the echo viruses. The number of cases grouped under the classification of idiopathic pericarditis is diminishing as virology techniques improve. However, it would be a mistake to assume that all cases of idiopathic pericarditis must have a viral etiology. The diagnosis of idiopathic pericarditis is one of exclusion, and it is important to remember that pericardial involvement with effusion can occur in the absence of a specific infection, such as in uremia and blood dyscrasias. The term viral pericarditis should be reserved for cases of proven viral origin.

Although viral and idiopathic pericarditis are etiologically different they are discussed together, since their management is the same. No specific therapy is available. Treatment is symptomatic, with acetylsalicylic acid (60–80 mg/kg/day) usually being sufficient for the relief of any fever or pain. Therapy rarely needs to be continued longer than four weeks. Corticosteroids are rarely if ever indicated for treatment in the pediatric age group. There is no documentation that they are of help and they appear to be contraindicated because they might increase the severity of a viral infection if that is the cause. Some centers use corticosteroids to help in the management of the acutely ill child or the patient who is having recurrent attacks of pericarditis. There is no evidence that the drug is beneficial in either of these situations.

Less than 5% of children have effusions large enough to cause tamponade. Nevertheless, this should be kept in mind as a life-threatening complication for the acutely sick infant or newborn. Treatment is by insertion of a surgical drain if it is a rapidly accumulating effusion, although pericardiocentesis may be necessary for emergency care of acute tamponade. The aspirated fluid shows a lymphocytic picture.

Miscellaneous. Pericarditis occurs as a secondary complication in a number of other infections. Tuberculous pericarditis is uncommon in children and is a result of either spread of the infection from the tracheobronchial lymph nodes or direct extension from a pulmonary lesion. Effusions occur and occasionally may result in cardiac tamponade. In most cases there is a rapid response to antituberculous medication but if the effusion persists, and particularly if signs of chronic tamponade develop, partial pericardiectomy should be performed.

Table 2. **ANTIBIOTIC DOSAGES—PARENTAL ROUTE**

Nafcillin	100 mg/kg/day	Q4–6H
Gentamicin	7.5 mg/kg/day	Q6–8H
Kanamycin	20 mg/kg/day*	Q 8 H
Ampicillin	200 mg/kg/day	Q 6 H
Chloramphenicol	75 mg/kg/day	Q 6 H

*Exceeds the dose recommended by the manufacturer.

Other causes of granulomatous pericarditis are rare and include toxoplasma infection, coccidioidomycosis, histoplasmosis, candida infection, aspergillosis, and amebic infection.

Pericarditis occurs in lupus erythematosus, and in fact may present as the first manifestation of the disease. It also occurs in scleroderma, periarteritis nodosa, and mucocutaneous lymph node syndrome. Pericarditis is a rare finding in brucellosis, tularemia and glycogen storage disease.

Chronic Effusive. The major characteristic of this group is the tendency to develop large persistent effusions in the absence of acute pericarditis. In many cases the cause of the effusion cannot be identified. Rarely is the patient symptomatic, but tamponade and failure may occur. In such cases, pericardiectomy is indicated for relief.

Chronic effusions occur in some metabolic disorders. In myxedema the effusion disappears after thyroid therapy is started. In uremia the effusion occurs late in the disease and there is no specific therapy other than treatment of the lesion causing the uremia. Chronic effusions occasionally occur as a complication of other cardiomyopathies in children such as Friedreich's ataxia and endocardial fibroelastosis. They may also be present in thalassemia, sickle cell disease, and congenital hypoplastic anemia.

Traumatic. Penetration of the chest with a knife or similar sharp instrument requires that bleeding into the pericardium be considered, since cardiac tamponade of rapid onset is a serious complication. Less obvious is the bleeding into the pericardium that can occur after chest surgery or as a complication of a cardiac catheterization. During a catheterization, if the catheter perforates the ventricular wall, it can be withdrawn and any significant effusion aspirated with a needle. This is usually sufficient, since further bleeding rarely occurs. There is some controversy as to how to manage atrial perforation. Atrial perforation occurs occasionally with no complications developing after the catheter is withdrawn. Nevertheless, there is a high risk of bleeding, with the development of acute cardiac tamponade. If perforation is recognized to have occurred while the catheter tip is still through the atrial wall it is recommended that it be left in that position and used to aspirate blood until it is removed at surgery.

Children who have been involved in road traffic accidents in which there is likely to have been compression of the thorax can have major trauma to the heart with minimal external signs. Since the cause of a developing effusion is likely to be due to rupture of the heart or a major vessel, the need for emergency thoracotomy with direct inspection of the heart should be considered before attempting to drain any pericardial effusion.

Postpericardiotomy Syndrome

This form of pericarditis is seen in a small percentage of children who have had open heart surgery. The etiology is unknown but it is thought that it may be an immunologic response to damaged autologous tissue within the pericardium. Its onset may be as early as a week after surgery or delayed for a number of months. The presenting findings are chest pain, fever, and pericarditis with or without an effusion.

Early diagnosis is essential since it is believed that bed rest in the early stages of the disease can prevent the development of the full picture; this should be for 1 to 2 weeks followed by slow ambulation. In the more severe cases with chest pain or pericardial effusion, acetylsalicylic acid should be given. The starting dose is 80 mg/kg/day, continued for a week to 10 days and then tapered slowly over the next 6 to 8 weeks. Corticosteroids are indicated if the symptoms are severe and there is little or no response to acetylsalicylic acid. Signs of congestive heart failure, which are rare, justify the use of digoxin and diuretics; these are stopped as soon as the patient recovers.

The differential diagnosis includes pericarditis of the postperfusion syndrome, which is thought to be a separate syndrome characterized by fever, lymphocytosis, splenomegaly, and occasional hepatomegaly. The characteristic lymphocytosis with the tendency for seasonable outbreaks makes a strong case for a viral etiology, with the cytomegalovirus being implicated as the likely causal agent. Treatment is with acetylsalicylic acid, the dosage being the same as for the postpericardiotomy syndrome.

Constrictive Pericarditis

Constrictive pericarditis is rare in children. No cause can be found in 60% of the cases, which are called idiopathic. The most commonly identified cause is tuberculosis, which accounts for approximately 30% of cases. About 10% of cases have been identified as secondary complications of trauma, malignant tumor, and mycotic and parasitic infections. It is a very rare complication of bacterial or viral pericarditis.

In this condition the visceral and parietal layers of the pericardium become thickened and adhere to each other as well as to the underlying myocardium. As the pericardium becomes thickened, rigid restriction of diastolic ventricular filling occurs, leading to the development of right heart failure without dyspnea. Treatment is surgical and consists of stripping as much pericardium as possible off the heart, particularly from around both ventricles. If an active infection, such as tuberculosis, is present, then it should be treated medically.

Systemic Hypertension

DAVID GOLDRING, M.D.,
ALAN M. ROBSON, M.D.,
and JULIO V. SANTIAGO, M.D.

Hypertension is the major health problem in our country, because it has been estimated that approximately 20 to 25 million people have hypertension and that about 250,000 die each year from the complications of this disease. Traditionally, hypertension has been classified as either primary or essential when the cause is unknown and as secondary when it is associated with or a consequence of renal, endocrine, or congenital vascular disease. Even in secondary hypertension, the specific cause is incompletely understood. The above classification profoundly affects the decision and results of therapy. For example, treatment for primary hypertension is usually effective, but it must be emphasized that the therapy is symptomatic. By contrast, for some forms of secondary hypertension the treatment may be curative. One must also keep in mind that the decision to treat a hypertensive patient depends upon the level of blood pressure which justifies a diagnosis of hypertension. This level of blood pressure is arbitrary. For example the World Health Organization has recommended that 140/90 mm Hg be designated borderline hypertension and 160/95 mm Hg and higher as definite hypertension in adults. These values are inappropriate for infants and children, whose blood pressure is lower than that of the adult and increases progressively with growth. A reasonable working guideline might be as follows: The pediatric patients whose blood pressure is persistently between the 90th and 95th percentile for age and sex be considered as suspect and those individuals whose pressures are persistently above the 95th percentile for age and sex be classified as hypertensives. Suggested blood pressure levels which we have used to identify suspect hypertensives are shown in Table 1.

Table 1. APPROXIMATE GUIDELINES FOR SUSPECT BLOOD PRESSURE VALUES

Supine Position—Lowest of 3 Readings *Boys and Girls*		
Age in years	3–5	6–9	10–14
Blood pressure mm Hg	>110/70	>120/75	>130/80

Seated Position—Average of Second and Third Readings			
	Girls	*Boys*		
Age in years	14–18	14	15	16–18
Blood pressure mm Hg	>125/80	>130/75	>130/80	>135/85

PRIMARY HYPERTENSION

If the above arbitrary definitions of hypertension are used, the most common type in the pediatric population is primary hypertension. During a 5 year period, we measured the blood pressures in approximately 20,000 subjects, 14–18 years of age, in the St. Louis metropolitan area; one student was found with coarctation of the aorta, and one with hypertension due to hyperthyroidism, but approximately 1000 suspected primary hypertensives were found.

Although the cause is unknown, effective symptomatic therapy is available.

The decision to use pharmacologic therapy in asymptomatic primary hypertensive pediatric patients must be examined from a different perspective than that used for the adult. Therapy may be more effective in the young, early hypertensive, and it may be possible to arrest or even cure the disease in the pediatric patient; this has not been possible in the adult. On the negative side, the undesirable, sometimes serious side effects of all antihypertensive drugs are well known, so that the risk-benefit ratio must be very carefully considered. The drug therapy must be a lifetime commitment, and there is no information about what serious untoward effects these drugs may have upon a young, growing subject. Finally, in a 10-year follow-up of approximately 100 young primary hypertensives we found that in 30% the blood pressure spontaneously returned to normal levels. In the light of the above, we feel that the nonthreatening, safe, therapeutic regimen discussed below is the preferred course to follow in the young primary hypertensive.

Weight Reduction. It has been shown in studies that at least 50% of young primary hypertensives are obese. The pathogenesis of the hypertension with obesity in unknown. In recent studies of adult obese hypertensives, significant reduction in systolic and diastolic pressures was achieved. There are no reported similar studies in pediatric patients, but we would recommend this approach in view of the above experience with hypertensive adults. Patient compliance would be difficult. Expert guidance by the physician is important, and the effectiveness of a weight reduction program would be enhanced by consultation with a nutritionist, a social worker, and in some instances a psychiatrist.

Exercise. Regimens of dynamic exercise have been shown to normalize blood pressure in some adult primary hypertensives. We have just completed a study on a group of 30 adolescent primary hypertensives who all experienced a drop in systolic and diastolic pressures during and after an exercise regimen of 6–8 months. The mechanism for lowering blood pressure with dynamic exercise is incompletely understood. It has been suggested that several months of dynamic exercising produces a relatively hypokinetic circulatory state, which is probably due to the negative inotropic effect of reduction in heart rate and to adaptations in the neuroendocrine system, which results in increased vagal tone and decreased release of norepinephrine and epinephrine.

The regimen we suggest to our young patients is summarized in the following instruction sheet. Supervision and surveillance are provided by weekly visits to the physician. This helps with patient compliance in this dramatic change in their lifestyle.

ENDURANCE EXERCISE TRAINING

For endurance exercise training to be effective in helping to lower your blood pressure, a few simple guidelines must be followed:

1. The activity should exercise a large amount of your muscle mass. Exercises which meet this requirement are running, cycling, and swimming.
2. The activity must elevate your heart rate to at least approximately 160 beats per minute. This can be measured by taking your pulse for 6 seconds *immediately after exercise* and multiplying by 10. The pulse can be felt either at the wrist or in the neck below the angle of the jaw. Your doctor can help you locate the pulse if needed.
3. The activity must continue for 30–45 minutes at least every other day but preferably 5 times per week. If you select running, you should build up your endurance so that you run approximately 3 to 5 miles a day 5 times per week. If you select bicycling, you should build up your endurance so that you ride 10 to 15 miles a day 5 times a week. If you select swimming, you should build up your endurance so that you swim 1 to 2 miles a day 5 times per week.

The tendency is to start out much too quickly which will elevate your heart rate too much and not allow you to continue for 40 minutes. The idea is to start slowly. Find the running, swimming, or cycling pace which results in a heart rate of approximately 160 beats/minute.

Eventually you will have to increase your pace as your fitness level begins to increase. At this point, it is still essential that you attain a heart rate of approximately 160 beats/minute.

There are no shortcuts to physical fitness. It requires a sincere and serious promise to stick with the program, but it offers a way to lower your blood pressure without taking medicine.

Isometric exercise such as hand-grip and certain forms of weight lifting are not recommended for the adult primary hypertensive who may have in addition either known or silent coronary artery disease. In the young primary hypertensive the incidence of coronary artery disease is very low, therefore, isometric exercise does not pose a risk. However, more studies are needed before these exercises should be recommended for the young primary hypertensive.

Diet Modification (Blood Lipids). Some years ago a number of investigators proposed that elevated blood lipids predisposed an individual to the development of atheromatous coronary artery disease. Elevated blood lipids as well as hypertension were thus considered risk factors. Reducing the intake of foods with a high cholesterol content and drug therapy such as clofibrate, colestipol, and nicotinic acid to lower the blood cholesterol has been recommended for adults with hypertension to protect them against the development of atheromatous coronary artery disease. This subject is still controversial for the adult subjects. Therefore, advising radical changes in the diet for infants and children with primary hypertension to reduce the risk of developing coronary artery disease in adulthood is not justified, because we do not know what serious harm may come to the young individual from this drastic modification of the diet.

Dietary Salt Restriction. There is considerable circumstantial evidence suggesting a link between a high dietary salt intake and hypertension in genetically predisposed individuals. The degree of salt restriction required to produce a significant reduction in blood pressure is unknown. It is believed by some that a diet containing 50 mEq of salt per day may be effective in reducing blood pressure. The degree of salt restriction would be unpalatable and most children would not comply. We, therefore, suggest that mothers do not add salt to food in cooking and that they restrict food with high salt content.

Other Forms of Therapy. Smoking should be prohibited, and contraceptive drugs, steroids, amphetamines, and liberal use of nose drugs should be discontinued. Behavior modification methods such as biofeedback, relaxation techniques, and psychotherapy are of questionable benefit.

An occasional patient might be considered a candidate for drug therapy as described below under renal hypertension; e.g., a young primary hypertensive who is obese and has a strong family history of hypertension who has not responded to nonpharmacologic therapy and whose pressure is progressively rising.

Unfortunately, the treatment of hypertension in the young will continue to be symptomatic and weakly effective until the pathogenesis of primary hypertension is better understood.

SECONDARY HYPERTENSION

Renal Disorders

Secondary hypertension most often is the consequence of a renal lesion. It may present as an acute event, sometimes requiring treatment as a medical emergency. Alternatively, it may represent a problem of long-term management. Since the approaches to these two situations are different and the drugs used also differ, each will be discussed separately.

Management of Acute Hypertension and Hypertensive Crises. Patients who fit into these categories have no previous history of hypertension or have an acute increase in blood pressure above their previous stable values. Typically, blood pressure levels are elevated well above the 95th percentiles for age. When such an increase is associated with symptoms or signs of an encephalopathy or heart failure, it must be treated as a medical emergency. However, it is important to remember that children are more susceptible to the changes of malignant hypertension at lower blood pressure levels than are adults. Thus, we consider any child who presents with a systolic pressure of 170 mm Hg or greater or a diastolic pressure of 120 mm Hg or greater to be at risk of major complications and to require urgent treatment. Such urgent treatment may be indicated at even lower blood pressure values in the neonate or infant. The only exception to this general rule would be the patient with coarctation presenting in childhood, without heart failure.

Causes of such acute severe elevations in blood pressure include acute poststreptococcal and other acute glomerulonephritides, hemolytic uremic syndrome, collagen vascular diseases, especially when affecting the renal vasculature, chronic pyelonephritis, segmental renal hypoplasia, infantile polycystic kidneys, and renovascular diseases. The initial approach to treatment is the same, regardless of the underlying etiology.

Sodium retention plays an important role in the genesis of the hypertension in many of these patients. Thus, attempting to decrease body sodium content by limiting sodium intake and by increasing urinary sodium losses with diuretics often represents an important adjunct to therapy with antihypertensive drugs. However, it is inappropriate to rely upon this approach alone to treat severe acute hypertension. These measures take too long, frequently days, to become effective. Dietary sodium restriction alone can only prevent sodium retention from becoming worse, and the kidney typically responds poorly to diuretics in many of the renal diseases causing acute severe hypertension. The loop diuretics are the most potent. Our preference is to use furosemide 0.5 to 1.0 mg/kg given either orally or parenterally. On occasion we have used larger doses without problems. The thiazide diuretics are less effective.

The drug that we usually use first is hydralazine. It is a vasodilator which also increases cardiac output and has the advantage of not decreasing renal blood flow even when blood pressure is lowered. Side effects are those seen with vasodilators, namely flushing of the skin, headaches, tachycardia, and palpitations. They occur infrequently in children. The drug is well absorbed when given by mouth, and an effect typically is seen within 1 to 2 hours. The initial oral dose is 0.25 mg/kg and can be repeated every 4 to 6 hours. The total daily dose can be as high as 4.5 mg/kg. An effect from a dose of hydralazine of 0.15 mg/kg may be seen within a few minutes when given intravenously and within 15 to 30 minutes when given intramuscularly. Doses may be repeated within 30 to 90 minutes, but oral therapy should be implemented as soon as possible. The intravenous injection of hydralazine often is effective in reducing blood pressure in patients refractory to the drug given orally.

The combination of reserpine, 0.02 mg/kg per day to a maximum dose of 1 mg given intramuscularly every 12 hours, with hydralazine may be effective if hydralazine alone does not lower blood pressure satisfactorily. When reserpine is used, the dose of this drug is kept constant and the frequency of dosage of hydralazine is modified according to the patient's response. Some begin therapy with this combination of drugs. We avoid reserpine when possible because of its side effects, which include symptoms of depression in older children, drowsiness, nasal congestion, and stimulation of gastric secretion, which may result in peptic ulceration and bleeding from the gastrointestinal tract. It should not be used in patients in whom surgery is anticipated.

Patients who do not respond to the regimens outlined above should be treated next with diazoxide.*The initial dose is 5 to 10 given by rapid intravenous infusion over 1 to 2 minutes. A slower rate of administration usually is ineffective, because the drug is protein bound. The dose can be repeated 30 minutes later if there is no response. The length of action of the drug, typically, is from 4 to 24 hours, although an effect for 36 hours or longer may be seen. Side effects are rare, although nausea and hyperglycemia have been reported. Hypotension does not occur unless frequent repeated small doses of the drug are given, usually in combination with other antihypertensive drugs.

Sodium nitroprusside is an effective intravenous antihypertensive agent which we use in patients who do not respond to any of the above drugs. Its onset of effect is immediate, and the response lasts for as long as the drug is infused. To prepare it for use, 50 mg are diluted in 1 liter of 5% dextrose in water (50 μg/ml). The solution is infused at a rate of from 0.5 to 8.0 μg/kg/min. The rate of infusion is titrated according to the blood pressure response. The drug is not stable when exposed to sunlight so that the bottle and infusion lines should be wrapped with aluminum foil throughout the infusion. Blood pressure should be monitored constantly throughout the infusion. Whenever possible the drug should not be administered for longer than 48 hours, especially in patients with renal failure, since the drug is metabolized to cyanide, which

---

*Manufacturer's warning: The safety of diazoxide injection in children has not been established.

normally would be excreted by the kidney. If the drug has to be administered for 48 hours or longer, blood thiocyanate levels should be monitored after this period of time.

Very few patients do not respond to the preceding approach. Those who do not respond, typically have hypertension in association with markedly elevated levels of plasma renin activity (PRA) and do respond to the angiotensin-converting enzyme inhibitor, captopril. The recommended starting dose is approximately 0.33 mg/kg three times a day. The drug is not stable in solution and should be given in tablet, or crushed-tablet, form. If response is poor, the dose is increased in stepwise fashion, usually at 24 hour intervals, until a satisfactory response is obtained. The total daily dose should not exceed 6 mg/kg. The effectiveness of the drug often can be potentiated by the use of furosemide (1 mg/kg/day in 2 divided doses) and propranolol* (1 mg/kg/day in 4 divided doses, increasing to a maximum of 5 mg/kg/day). We prefer, however, to use a single drug, rather than a combination of drugs, when possible. Few acute side effects have been observed with captopril. Long term complications include proteinuria and a decrease in the white blood cell count. If either abnormality develops, the drug should be discontinued.

The preceding, sequential approach to therapy is designed to control acute hypertension and to reduce the risk of major complications developing from the elevated blood pressure. Once blood pressures have been reduced below the 95th percentile for age, the physician should consider whether there may be a surgically treatable cause for the hypertension and, in those patients in whom hypertension is likely to be chronic, begin to introduce the appropriate drugs for long term control of blood pressure.

Renovascular lesions are the most likely cause of secondary hypertension that can be controlled by surgery. They should be considered in any patient with very severe hypertension and in those with elevated PRA levels. Nowadays, such lesions can usually be demonstrated most satisfactorily after an intravenous injection of contrast agent and digital vascular imagining in centers where the appropriate equipment is available. This methodology avoids the much more invasive technique of renal arteriography. There has been considerable interest in the use of percutaneous transluminal angioplasty (PTLA) to treat patients with vascular stenoses, including those of the renal artery. This method appears to have limited value in children, since many of the renal artery lesions occur at the origin of the renal vessels and typically involve the

*Manufacturer's note: Data on the use of propranolol in the pediatric age group are too limited to permit adequate directions for use.

abdominal aorta. There have been reports of successful treatment of mid-artery lesions in children using PTLA. It is not clear, however, whether such stenoses will return with time. Treatment of segmental lesions within the renal parenchyma can be particularly difficult. Successful selective embolization of a stenotic intrarenal artery in a child has been reported and would appear preferable to nephrectomy. In all cases, the surgical success depends on the experience of the surgeon in this kind of work.

Management of Chronic Hypertension. The major difficulty in managing hypertension on a long term basis is patient compliance. It is self-evident that if a drug is to be effective it must be taken regularly. Compliance is less a problem in the younger child, since most mothers ensure that the physicians advice is followed closely. Most problems are experienced in teenage patients. Compliance can be improved if the drug regimen is simple, is free from side effects, and is relatively inexpensive. A suitable regimen must be supplemented by extensive education of the patient and the family about hypertension, about the prescribed drugs, and about the reasons for prescribing those drugs. It is sometimes very hard to convince asymptomatic patients that they need to take potent drugs, usually for the rest of their lives. Follow-up should be as convenient for the patient as possible.

Antihypertensive drugs can be considered in three basic groups: vasodilators, diuretics that reduce volume, and those that modify release, metabolism, or function of pressor systems such as the renin-angiotensin system. The same principles about determining whether hypertension is volume or pressor related and treating with a drug that has an appropriate action applies to children as well as to adults. Again, as in adults if a drug from one major group is ineffective and a second drug is to be added, it is better to use a drug from a different group than from the same group. Thus, if a patient has a less than satisfactory response to a vasodilator and has a component of volume expansion, it is usually better to add a diuretic to the therapeutic regimen than another vasodilator. If secondary hyperreninism develops, the addition of a drug such as propranolol would be appropriate. However, such an approach often results in a confusing or cumbersome regimen that contributes to poor patient compliance. Thus, we prefer, whenever possible, to use maximum doses of a single drug rather than to use multiple drugs.

It is difficult to recommend specific regimens to treat hypertension. Each patient must have an approach individualized to his or her needs. Below we consider the major groups of drugs and our experience with them.

Vasodilator Drugs. Hydralazine may be used on a chronic as well as on an acute basis. Its effectiveness, however, is limited in most patients with secondary hypertension. Its major value in our clinic is to treat night-time hypertension in patients treated primarily with guanethidine. Dosage and side effects have already been outlined. The protracted use of hydralazine in high doses may result in a syndrome resembling systemic lupus erythematosus (SLE). Typically, but not always, this reverses when hydralazine is discontinued. For this reason we do not like to use this drug in patients with SLE even though there is no evidence that hydralazine exacerbates SLE in patients on concomitant immunosuppressive therapy.

Minoxidil is a vasodilator that is a valuable addition to our armamentarium, since patients resistant to other drugs frequently respond to it. The recommended initial dose is 0.2 mg/kg as a single daily dose. This may be increased in increments of 50 to 100% every 2 or 3 days until blood pressure control is achieved. The effective dosage range usually is between 0.25 and 1.0 mg/kg/day with a recommended maximum daily dose of 50 mg. It is advised that a patient receive a beta-blocker such as propranolol before starting minoxidil. Since minoxidil induces fluid retention, which can be severe and result in pericardial effusions and tamponade, a diuretic such as furosemide should be used concurrently. The side effect that is most distressing to patients and their families is hypertrichosis. Many patients are unwilling to accept the severe overgrowth of hair over their face and forehead, and female patients dislike this growth on other parts of their bodies. Because of its side effects and the inability to use minoxidil as a single drug, we reserve this drug for patients who are resistant to other drugs.

Prazosin has a direct effect on vascular smooth muscle and also has features of an alpha-adrenergic blocking agent. Therefore, reflex tachycardia typically is not a major complication when prazosin is used to lower blood pressure. The initial dose in older children is 1 mg 2 or 3 times a day. This may be increased slowly until an adequate response is obtained. Daily doses above 20 mg rarely increase the efficacy of the drug, although some patients may benefit from doses as high as 40 mg/day. There has been relatively little experience with this drug in younger children, and the size of the smallest capsules (1 mg) makes it difficult to provide a suitable starting dose for very small children. The effects of the drug are enhanced by simultaneous use of diuretics and beta-adrenergic blocking agents. Postural hypotension has been the most important side effect. Blood pressure should be monitored with the patient in the supine and in the upright positions. The patient should be alerted to the possibility of postural symptoms, and if they do occur, the patient should be advised to assume the recumbent position. Such side effects should alert the physician to the need to modify drug dosage. The major advantages of prazosin are the few side effects experienced with its use and the need for only twice a day dosage. However, in our experience, it is not as potent as other drugs. When used in large dosage, tachycardia and fluid retention may occur.

Drugs Affecting Adrenergic Activity. Propranolol* has been found to be an effective antihypertensive agent in children. It is thought to act as a beta-adrenergic blocking agent. Since the renin-angiotensin system is regulated in part by beta-adrenergic activity, it was thought originally that propranolol worked through this mechanism. More recent studies have indicated that other modes of action must be involved too. The drug is readily absorbed from the gastrointestinal tract. The initial dose should be between 0.5 and 1.0 mg/kg/day. Originally it was advised that the total dose should be divided into 4 doses a day; more recently, twice-daily doses have been found to be effective. Doses can be increased on a daily or every-other-day basis until a suitable response occurs. Daily doses as high as 16 mg/kg/day have been used. The major complication has been the development of heart failure. The drug should not be used, therefore, in any patient with heart disease or pulmonary disease, especially if heart failure is present. We do not use propranolol as a drug of first choice when treating chronic hypertension, because we have been disappointed with it when used alone. However, it is a most useful and effective adjunct to other antihypertensive agents.

Several other beta-adrenergic blocking agents have been developed. The one that might offer definite advantages for children is nadolol,** since it is effective when taken once a day. We have, however, little personal experience with its use.

Guanethidine blocks sympathetic activity and has a prolonged serum half-life, which permits a single daily dose. This is a major advantage when treating hypertension in children. It works only when the patient assumes the upright position and therefore is of very limited value in neonates and infants. In children between the ages of 2 and 10 years we usually use a single daily dose of 5 mg to start. In older children this dose should be 10 mg/day. Effects are rarely seen for 3 or more days. Thereafter, the dose can be increased in increments of 5 or 10 mg/day at weekly intervals. Most patients respond to a dose of 25 mg/day or less, occasional patients require up to 50 mg/day. The major side effect is postural hypotension, typically when the

---

*Manufacturer's note: Data on the use of propranolol in the pediatric age group are too limited to permit adequate directions for use.

**Safety and effectiveness in children have not been established.

patient arises in the morning or stands up abruptly. Sitting with legs over the edge of the bed for a few seconds before standing up or standing up slowly usually eliminates this side effect. Diarrhea is a side effect in a small minority of children. Fluid retention has been reported with the drug but has not been a problem in our experience. The drug should not be used in any patient receiving an monoamine oxidase (MAO) inhibitor. When monitoring the effectiveness of guanethidine, blood pressure should be taken with the patient in the supine and the upright positions as well as after exercise to determine its postural effect. One major disadvantage of the drug is that it has little effect when the patient is asleep. This can be rectified by having the patient propped up on pillows when asleep. Alternatively, a small dose of hydralazine can be added to the regimen in the evening. Recently we have found that some teenage male patients in whom blood pressure is controlled by guanethidine have discontinued this drug when they became sexually active because of its side effect on inhibiting ejaculation. We now warn teenage males about this problem and convert their control, usually to prazosin, if it appears that this side effect may pose a problem. Extensive experience with guanethidine has convinced me that this drug often is a most effective agent which can be used alone and requires only a single morning dose, helping to ensure compliance.

Methyldopa is a moderately potent antihypertensive agent that probably works by interfering with the production of the neurotransmitter norepinephrine. Its absorption is very variable, and it results in a positive direct Coombs' test in 20% of patients. The first two patients we treated with this drug developed hemolytic anemia. Although this is a rare occurrence, it limited our enthusiasm for the drug. Other patients complain of a sedative effect when starting methyldopa, an effect that may or may not lessen with time. Methyldopa has been reported to be effective in controlling hypertension in children, especially when taken with a diuretic to limit sodium and water retention, which is sometimes seen when the drug is taken alone. The recommended starting dose is 10 mg/kg/day taken in 3 divided doses. The dose can be increased in stepwise fashion every 3 to 5 days up to 40 mg/kg/day. The maximum recommended daily dose in 2 gm.

Other drugs in this group include reserpine and clonidine. Used on a long term basis, reserpine produces drowsiness, symptoms of depression, and nasal stuffiness. It must be stopped several days in advance of any operation requiring a general anesthetic. Its routine use is not recommended, although it may have a role in some patients resistant to or unable to take other drugs. Clonidine is a much newer drug which acts on alpha-adrenergic receptors. It too may produce drowsiness. Other side effects include dryness of the mouth and rebound hypertension if the drug is stopped abruptly. We have had limited experience with the drug but have not found any advantage to recommend it in preference to guanethidine or prazosin.

Drugs Modifying Renin-Angiotensin System. Beta-adrenergic blocking agents such as propranolol interfere with renin release, and at least part of their action is through this mechanism. More recently, drugs have been developed that inhibit the enzyme responsible for the conversion of angiotensin I to angiotensin II, which is the pressor substance. The drug in this category which is absorbed when taken by mouth and which is now available by prescription is captopril. Recent observations suggest that it is effective by acting on both the renin-angiotensin and the kinin systems. Its use in acute hypertension has been detailed already. We have found it to be an extremely valuable agent in the management of chronic hypertension too, expecially that which is renin mediated. The initial dose is 1 mg/kg/day divided into three doses, and this is increased in stepwise manner, at 8 hour intervals if necessary, until effective blood pressure response is observed. The maximum dose should not exceed 6 mg/kg/day. The use of beta-adrenergic blocking agents and diuretics will often potentiate the effect of captopril, and all antihypertensive agents other than those in these two groups should be discontinued before captopril is used. We have been most pleased by the effectiveness of the drug and by patient acceptance. To date, we have not seen proteinuria nor decreased white blood cell count, the two complications that require that the drug's use be discontinued.

Drugs Acting on Volume. Hypervolemia may contribute to chronic hypertension in many patients, or fluid and sodium retention may occur secondary to the use of several of the vasodilator drugs. Thus, the use of diuretics has an important role in the management of hypertension.

The most frequently prescribed diuretics are the thiazides. Their effect in hypertension appears to be through their action to increase urinary losses of sodium and water. The drugs are well absorbed when taken by mouth and are relatively free of side effects. Potassium wasting with or without hypokalemia may occur with prolonged use. Hyperuricemia, a common complication of using thiazides in adults, is seen infrequently in children. Nor have hyperglycemia and hypercalcemia been reported as a complication of thiazide use in children. Hydrochlorothiazide will be used as an example of a typical thiazide. The starting dose is 2 mg/kg/day taken in two equally divided doses, the second one of which should be given no later than early afternoon to avoid nocturia. The dose may be doubled, but one should wait for at least 7 to 14 days before increasing the dose, since the maximum therapeutic response may take this long to develop. Unfortunately many children with secondary hypertension have a renal cause for their elevated blood pressure and therefore do not respond optimally to the thiazides.

Chlorthalidone is chemically unrelated to the thiazides but has very similar actions. Its major advantage is that it has a longer length of action and is effective when taken only once a day.

Furosemide acts on the ascending limb of the loop of Henle and thus is referred to as a loop diuretic. It and ethacrynic acid are the most potent diuretics known. Although furosemide has a short plasma half-life, it needs to be given only once a day, in the morning. The usual starting dose is 0.5 to 1 mg/kg/day. There has been little published experience to show that larger doses given for protracted periods of time in children are safe but to date we have not experienced any problems. The major complication is potassium wasting, necessitating oral potassium supplements. Most effective potassium preparations are extremely unpalatable. We have found that the use of a salt substitute on foods is best tolerated by our patients. Caution in administering any potassium supplement must be exercised in any patient with renal insufficiency in case hyperkalemia develops. Concern has been expressed that furosemide may be ototoxic, but there is little evidence to support this concern when the drug is used as outlined above.

Spironolactone is a competitive inhibitor of aldosterone. When used in conjunction with a thiazide diuretic or furosemide, it potentiates the diuresis and may have a slight potassium-sparing effect. We sometimes use it for this purpose, but do not believe that it is an effective antihypertensive agent when used alone. The starting dose may be up to 3.3 mg/kg/day in single or divided doses. Effects from the drug may not be seen for 3 or more days, and maximum effectiveness may take up to 14 days to develop.

Triamterene is a nonsteroidal potassium-sparing diuretic. We do not use it, since most of our hypertensive patients have renal disease, and we are concerned about the potential of this drug to induce significant hyperkalemia.

Any patient in whom a diuretic is indicated should also receive a salt-restricted diet. It is not practical to restrict sodium intake to levels as low as 0.5 gm (20 meq) per day in nonhospitalized patients. We have found that usually the best one can accomplish is to restrict intake to around 35 to 50 meq/day. It is important to emphasize to parents that the higher the sodium intake, the greater will be the dose of diuretics needed. We do not recommend attempting to control chronic severe or moderately severe hypertension with dietary sodium restriction alone. It rarely works; if a benefit is seen, this usually is short lived, since most patients find that adhering to a low salt diet is extremely arduous.

Summary. The therapeutic regimen that is developed should be as simple and as free from side effects as possible. Preferably, a single drug should be used. Those that we use most are guanethidine or prazosin. We are now using captopril more often, especially in patients with renin-mediated hypertension. Minoxidil may prove effective in patients resistant to other drugs. When a second drug is needed, we use a diuretic and dietary sodium restriction if volume expansion or sodium retention appears to be an etiologic factor in the hypertension. A thiazide diuretic or chlorthalidone is used if a moderate diuresis is required; furosemide for a more vigorous diuresis. If secondary hyperreninemia appears to be responsible for a reduced effect of the primary antihypertensive drug, we add propranolol to the regimen, but have begun to use naldolol, because it is effective when taken once a day.

Endocrine Disorders

Since some children with hypertension caused by endocrine disorders can be cured with appropriate surgical or medical therapy, consideration should be given early in the course of diagnosis or therapy to the possibility that hypertension may have an endocrine cause in all hypertensive children. Some of the more important causes of endocrine hypertension are briefly outlined in Table 2.

Pheochromocytoma usually presents as sustained rather than intermittent hypertension. Pheochromocytomas may present as isolated cases or in association with Sipple's syndrome (medullary carcinoma of the thyroid and bilateral pheochromocytomas). High perioperative morbidity requires expert use of alpha- and beta-adrenergic blocking agents as well as careful monitoring of the hydration status. Surgical removal is the treatment of choice.

Two syndromes associated with congenital adrenal hyperplasia can cause hypertension in young children. They are caused by the accumulation of desoxycorticosterone (11-B-OH deficiency) or mineralocorticoids (17 α-OH deficiency) due to an increased secretion of ACTH secondary to deficient cortisol production.

Approximately 80% of children with Cushing's syndrome due to bilateral adrenal stimulation by ACTH or to an isolated adrenal tumor will be hypertensive. Treatment consists of surgical removal of the tumor responsible for excess cortisol or ACTH production.

The presence of a low plasma renin in a salt-repleted patient with hypertension should lead to a suspicion that the patient has a form of congenital adrenal hyperplasia or hyperaldosteronism. These disorders are often responsive to appropriate glucocorticoid or spironolactone or to surgical removal of an aldosterone-producing tumor.

Systolic hypertension is sometimes a manifestation of hyperthyroidism, and treatment may either be surgical or medical, as noted in Table 2.

Congenital Vascular Disease

Coarctation of the Aorta. Coarctation of the aorta is a congenital malformation characterized by constriction of the aorta distal to the origin of the left subclavian artery. Characteristically, there is hypertension in the upper limbs and hypotension in the lower extremities. It is generally agreed that surgical correction be carried out in the infant who presents with congestive heart failure due to coarctation of the aorta, and a left-to-right shunt such as a patent ductus arteriosus or a ventricular or atrial septal defect. Thus, a volume overload is imposed upon a pressure overloaded left ventricle. The critically ill infant in congestive heart failure should be started upon treatment for the heart failure. The baby should then be evaluated by cardiac catheterization and angiocardiography. If the diagnosis of coarctation of the aorta is verified, the baby should be operated upon. The time elapsed from admittance to operation should be 24–48 hours.

There is also general agreement that surgical correction is imperative in patients with isolated coarctation in the age range of 5 to 8 when the aortic lumen has achieved approximately 50% of the cross-sectional area of the adult aorta. A second operation will therefore not be needed in adulthood, even if the anastomotic site does not grow with age. Most patients have generalized hypertension postoperatively, which spontaneously returns to normal values in 2 or 3 weeks in approximately 90% of patients. Although some authors have advocated antihypertensive therapy during this period, I have seen no evidence to support the reason for such treatment. Nor is there evidence to support the suggestion that antihypertensive drug treatment is of any value in the preoperative state. About 10% of patients have persistent generalized hypertension even if the aortic obstruction is completely relieved. The reason for this is unknown. It may be that these patients are destined to develop primary hypertension.

Hypotension

HERBERT S. HARNED, Jr., M.D.

The pediatric practitioner must be able to judge very rapidly the severity of hypotensive states. To recognize hypotension, he must be aware of the normal range of blood pressures in children of differing age groups and be knowledgeable about the proper cuff sizes, manometric techniques, and interpretations of Korotkoff and Doppler sounds and flush methods. Recognition of shock must be

Table 2.

Endocrine Disorder	Clinical Presentation	Therapy
1. Pheochromocytoma	90% sustained hypertension 80% headache, 65% sweating 35% intermittent abdominal pain	Alpha-adrenergic blockade (phenoxybenzamine, phentolamine) Beta-adrenergic blockade (propranolol) Careful monitoring of hydration status intraoperatively
2. Congenital adrenal hyperplasias (a) 11-B hydroxylase deficiency	Hypertension Rapid growth Virilization in females Elevated 11-desoxycortisol and DOC	Replacement glucocorticoids
(b) 17-α hydroxylase deficiency	Hypertension Hypokalemic alkalosis Ambiguous genitalia in males Delayed puberty in girls	Replacement glucocorticoids
3. Cushing's syndrome	Growth failure Signs of glucocorticoid excess	Surgical removal of adrenal or pituitary tumor
4. Hyperaldosteronism	Hypokalemia in sodium repleted state Low renin, high aldosterone	Surgery (for isolated tumor) or spironalactone
5. Hyperthyroidism	Systolic hypertension, emotional lability, increased sweating, increased height for age, weakness, tremor, tachycardia, elevated T_4, T_3, FT_4, and RT_3U	Surgical excision of thyroid gland or medical treatment with propranolol, propylthiouracil, or methimazole (Tapazole).

made from observing tachycardia, thready pulses, venous collapse, delayed capillary filling, pallor, coldness and moisture of the skin, obtunded consciousness, and oliguria. These findings indicate inadequate oxygenation and perfusion of vital organs and call for immediate action.

Although the various etiologies of severe hypotension with shock require certain specific therapies, especially with septic, anaphylactic, or neurogenic shock, certain general measures must be directed toward the rapid reversal of this life-threatening state. An understanding of recently developed knowledge of treatment of shock handled under ideal circumstances in an ICU setting will be presented. From this perspective, the practitioner can extrapolate appropriate therapeutic measures and monitoring techniques which might apply in his particular circumstances. An organized approach is needed, with one person as the leader. The more assistants one can mobilize, the better the chance of reversal of a case of severe hypotension. At least four active physicians or knowledgeable ancillary intensivists are desired to handle a severe hypotensive episode.

Shock often is the precursor of cardiopulmonary arrest, and similar therapeutic measures are initiated to those needed for the latter condition. An approach using the initials VIP for "ventilation-infusion-pump" has set proper priorities.

First, immediate attention to ventilation is vital, with realization that the Trendelenburg position (head down) is often detrimental. Improving the state of ventilation, by ensuring a proper airway, administration of oxygen, and hyperventilating to lower P_{CO_2} and combat detrimental acidosis, offers a direct treatment of the basic problem in shock, i.e., decreased cellular oxidation. In an ICU setting, the person most skilled in endotracheal intubation and ventilatory management should immediately be assigned to this task.

Suctioning, use of an oral airway, passage of a nasogastric tube for gastric decompression, mouth-to-mouth insufflation, use of self-inflating and reservoir-type resuscitation bags, use of face masks, and use of 100% oxygen need to be applied as necessary if ventilation is inadequate. The decision concerning endotracheal intubation may be difficult, but this must be done if the severely compromised patient is not improved within minutes.

If the heart rate falls below 40 and severe shock is apparent, external cardiac massage is indicated. Immediate ECG monitoring needs to be instituted and systematic blood pressure recordings taken. An arterial sample for P_{O_2}, P_{CO_2}, and pH determinations may be taken. Additional, more precise monitoring techniques are to be instituted and proper intravascular lines established for administering fluids and drugs. Lack of access for giving drugs limits immediate treatment to such nonsclerosing medications as epinephrine and atropine, which can be injected intramuscularly, lingually, or endotracheally as well as by stat IV injection. The stat doses of these medications are as follows: epinephrine (0.1 ml/kg/dose of a 1:10,000 solution or 10 μg/kg) and atropine sulfate (0.01–0.03 mg/kg/dose).

The first line to be placed is a venous line preferably, using the most propitious site. Soon after this is in place, a central venous pressure line must be established and, concurrently, an arterial catheter for manometric recording of intra-arterial pressures and periodic sampling for blood gases and electrolytes, especially valuable if the course is protracted. A 12 lead EKG and chest x-ray are done as soon as possible.

With the establishment of a venous line, the therapeutic options are greatly enhanced, for it is now possible to administer emergency medications optimally. Also, isotonic crystalloid solutions such as 0.9% NaCl solution or Ringer's lactate (20 ml/kg) or colloids such as 25% salt-poor albumin (1 gm/kg) diluted to 5% with isotonic saline preferably, plasma or whole blood (10 ml/kg) infused over 15 minutes can be administered as a CVP line is being placed. These infusions are given to combat the second major feature of shock, poor peripheral perfusion.

While fluids are being administered through the venous line, the CVP and arterial lines should become activated. With the CVP for guidance, one can ascertain rapidly whether there is a cardiogenic element in the shock state of the patient. The bolus of crystalloids or colloids, presumably already underway and to be repeated if necessary, can indicate the degree of myocardial failure while the CVP is raised to as high as 15 mm Hg. The bolus increases cardiac filling in all states where decreased circulating blood volume is the cause of decreased cardiac output. It may act as a pump-priming to invoke the Frank-Starling response to increased end-diastolic myocardial fiber length and may produce improved cardiac output in states where myocardial function is impaired to a degree. On the other hand, if the bolus does not result in any improvement in the hypotension and peripheral perfusion, one must be very concerned about the cardiogenic nature of the shock state. In addition, the CVP indicates right ventricular filling pressures that may differ widely from those on the left side, which may be estimated better by placement of a pulmonary wedge pressure line.

In many cases, poor cardiac function may be a temporary condition caused by metabolic acidosis, hypoglycemia, hypocalcemia, or hyperkalemia, and these possible factors should be considered and appropriately treated. If peripheral perfusion has been poor, one can assume the presence of lactic acidosis from anaerobic glycolysis and give NaHCO$_3$ solution (1–2 mEq/kg IV). This NaHCO$_3$ therapy has several immediate favorable effects, including 1) improvement of cardiac contractility, 2) potentiation of the sympathetic-adrenal responses to shock and of the actions of administered sympathomimetic drugs, 3) reversal of local acidosis with improved vasoconstriction of small arterioles, and 4) amelioration of the myocardial effects of potassium toxicity if this exists. Administration of NaHCO$_3$ may need to be repeated if the state of shock remains profound and if blood gas determinations continue to show severe acidosis. Adequate ventilation must be maintained to eliminate excessive CO$_2$ with this bicarbonate loading. Also, NaHCO$_3$ solutions chemically neutralize sympathomimetic drugs and must never be given in the same line without proper measures to avoid such a deleterious reaction. NaHCO$_3$ solutions are sclerosing and should only be given through adequate intravascular lines, as is the case with calcium and glucose solutions. Use of glucose to supply needed substrate for myocardial metabolism is an agent often forgotten in the melee of resuscitative efforts. If a blood Dextrostix determination shows less than 45 mg/dl, then 50% glucose (1–2 mg/kg IV) is given, followed by an infusion of 10% glucose.

All of the measures described above should have been completed within 20 minutes. In addition, after several bolus doses of epinephrine have been given at 5 minute intervals, selection of effective inotropic agents for use during the ensuing hours must be considered if a precarious state continues. Decisions as to the preferred agent can be complex and may require consultations with cardiologists and anesthesiologists.

As the most widely used treatment, a continuous epinephrine infusion, administered by an accurate infusion pump, has several advantages, including stimulation of cardiac rate and contractility and increase of peripheral vascular resistance with improved coronary flow. The infusion can be prepared rapidly by adding 5 ml of 1:1000 aqueous epinephrine to a 250 ml bottle of 5% dextrose to make up a solution of 20 μg/ml. The infusion is started at 0.1 μg/kg/min (or 6 μg/kg/hr) and increased to as much as 1.5 μg/kg/min. An infusion chart must be prepared and kept current by one member of the ICU team responsible for recording and calculating the drug dosages. Disadvantages of epinephrine include its tendency to cause tachycardia with increased myocardial O$_2$ consumption and its arrhythmogenic effects in severe hypoxic states.

Isoproterenol (Isuprel), a very strong positive inotropic agent, may be given in the same dosages as epinephrine, but should not be infused with epinephrine because of their potentiated tendency to produce arrhythmias. In contrast to epinephrine, isoproterenol decreases systemic and pulmonary resistance. Other, newer, positive inotropic agents are now being more widely used.

Dopamine (Inotropin),* in doses below 5 μg/kg/min, has the valuable property of redistributing blood flow to renal, mesenteric, coronary, and cerebral arteries. It has been especially useful in combating poor renal perfusion, but when doses are as high as 15 μg/kg/min, α-receptor activity predominates and this desirable effect is reversed.

Dobutamine (Dobutrex),* in doses below 7.5 μg/kg/min, has properties similar to dopamine and can increase cardiac stroke volume without significantly altering heart rate.

Digoxin is a slower-acting inotropic agent that is not as potent as the sympathomimetic drugs. It is also a dangerous drug in acute hypotensive states and has well-established toxic properties. Its primary effectiveness is in conditions where prolonged action is desired, as in low cardiac output states from cardiac failure.

When vasoconstrictor effects are desired primarily, norepinephrine (levarterenol, Levophed) infusions, starting at 0.1 μg/kg/min with stepwise increased doses, or phenylephrine (Neo-Synephrine) infusions in the same dosage may be used. These drugs constrict the renal and mesenteric vessels so that their prolonged use causes progressive impairment of perfusion of these regions.

When left ventricular pump failure is the major factor in hypotension, outflow resistance can be decreased effectively by primary vasodilator therapy. Special attention must be paid to the intra-arterial pressures, which must be monitored closely to maintain a pressure adequate for coronary perfusion. The systolic pressure should be maintained not lower than 3/4 that expected for the child's age as a guideline for dosage of these powerful agents. Sodium nitroprusside (Nipride) infusions, starting a 1 μg/kg/min and increasing to as high as 12 μg/kg/min are widely used, especially in adults with severe myocardial dysfunction. With high doses, one must be aware of inducing thiocyanate toxicity manifested by vomiting, sweating, and muscle twitching or of cyanide poisoning causing intractable acidosis. It is highly advisable to monitor the use of this agent by insertion of a Swan-Ganz catheter for continuous estimations of LV filling, as delineated by the pulmonary capillary wedge pressures. Passage of this flow-directed catheter is accomplished readily in the older child and adult but is often difficult to achieve in the young child without the assistance of a pediatric cardiologist or anesthesiologist. Fluoroscopic guidance may be

---

*Safety and effectiveness for use in children have not been established.

needed, but the catheter can be located in the RV outflow tract by echocardiography. Combined use of dopamine or dobutamine and sodium nitroprusside has been effective, especially in severe pump failure, but obviously needs particularly careful monitoring. Nitroglycerin solutions are under investigation as a safer substitute for nitroprusside infusions when preload reduction is desired.

If bradycardia develops in association with hypotension, a stat dosage of atropine (0.01–0.03 mg/kg/IV) may be useful, but emergency placement of a transvenous pacemaker by a cardiologist may be necessary. Calcium, most reliably given in the form of $CaCl_2$ (0.3 ml/kg of a 0.1 mg/ml 10% solution), must be administered IV with the aim of strengthening cardiac contraction through another mechanism than that of β-adrenergic stimulation. One must be aware that this agent should never be given in the same line as $NaHCO_3$ because calcium carbonate will be precipitated. Also, it should be given cautiously to digitalized patients, since these two drugs potentiate each other. It is also an extremely sclerosing material and should only be given through well-established intravenous lines.

Cardiac arrhythmias may cause pump failure and require specific diagnosis and treatment. A variety of causes for these disorders may be identified by using the procedures described. Electrolyte imbalance, especially potassium deficiency or excess, acidosis, alkalosis, digitalis toxicity, hypoxia, fever, hypovolemia, presence of pericardial fluid, and irritation from CVP or pulmonary wedge pressure catheters are treatable. Primary arrhythmias, such as paroxysmal tachyarrhythmias, may also require selective therapies, such as the drug regimens and external cardioversion and defibrillation discussed elsewhere. Not to be forgotten is the occasional effectiveness of sharp blows to the chest in reversing known ventricular tachyarrhythmias, and the vagal stimulating maneuvers (facial immersion, carotid massage, induced gagging, etc.) in reversing supraventricular tachyarrhythmias.

The effects of shock on various organ systems must be weighed in the therapeutic plan, especially if hypotension is persistent. Damage to endothelial cells and alveolar epithelial cells in the lung (shock lung) may result in permeability edema and decreased surfactant production (adult respiratory distress syndrome). Adequate ventilation by endotracheal intubation, use of pancuronium (Pavulon), 0.06–0.1 mg/kg/dose IV every 30–60 minutes and sedation (such as morphine 0.1–0.2 mg/kg/dose q 2–4 hours), appropriate supplemental O_2, proper airway pressure adjustments, and chest physiotherapy are often indicated. Furosemide (Lasix), 1 mg/kg, increasing to as high as 5 mg/kg/dose, and colloid therapy to raise oncotic pressure may be needed to handle this most difficult aspect of severe hypotension.

The renal blood flow and urinary output must be maintained if possible. Low dose dopamine*infusions, mannitol (0.5–1.0 gm/kg over 30 minutes every 4–6 hours), and furosemide are used to combat oliguric renal failure.

If paralytic ileus has occurred, the stomach contents need to be emptied by nasogastric tube. Stress ulcers and erosive gastritis may develop from mucosal ischemia. Antacids such as aluminum hydroxide (Maalox or Amphojel, 5–20 ml q 4 h po) are given to raise the pH to 4.0.

Adequate nutrition must be maintained to provide liver substrates, as well as nutrition, for host defenses against infection. The catabolic effects of shock need special attention if the patient has been nutritionally deficient before hypotension develops. Intravenous alimentation may be needed under these circumstances. Glucose therapy may result in increased glycogen synthesis with lipogenesis causing hepatomegaly and abnormal liver function. Infusions of glucose with insulin and potassium have favorably improved cell membrane function and can improve cardiac carbohydrate metabolism.

If treatment is prolonged, concerns will arise about infection from catheters which act as foreign bodies, and difficult decisions must be made concerning antibiotic therapy. Patients with severe hypotension have lowered resistance to infection from a variety of causes. At present, prevention or early treatment with antibiotics aimed at preventing bacteremia is the best therapeutic approach, but treatments to specifically stimulate host defense mechanisms and granulocyte transfusions may find wider use soon.

Special mention must be made of hypotension from sepsis, anaphylaxis, and neurogenic causes. Early in septic shock, increased vascular capacity with peripheral vasodilation produces a picture different from other forms of shock. The skin may be warm and flushed, blood pressure may be normal with wide pulse pressure, and the patient may be febrile, hyperventilating, and having chills. Alpha stimulators, such as epinephrine, norepinephrine, and Neo-Synephrine are usually ineffective. The preferred treatment as the condition progresses to systemic vasoconstriction appears to be vigorous volume expansion initially and then use of an agent such as isoproterenol or nitroprusside. Concurrent antibiotic therapy, platelet concentrates, fresh plasma or blood, exchange transfusions, and steroids (dexamethasone, 5 mg/kg, or methylprednisolone, 30 mg/kg IV in form of a bolus) must be considered in this shock state especially. This corticosteroid treatment may be re-

---

*Safety and effectiveness in children have not been established.

peated every 4–6 hours in the severely compromised patient but has not been shown to be effective after 3 days. Another controversial but promising agent is naloxone (Narcan), an endorphin blocker (given in repeated doses of 0.01 mg/kg IV), which may counteract the deleterious cellular effects of these intrinsic substances. Naloxone is also an effective stimulator of central respiratory drive.

Disseminated intravenous coagulation, present as a major complication of sepsis, may exist to a degree in most severe nonseptic shock states. Treatment is directed against the associated conditions (hypotension, anoxemia, acidosis, and infection), but platelet and fresh frozen plasma transfusions are also indicated. Vitamin K (1–5 mg IM or IV) should also be administered. Heparin (100 units/kg/dose q 4 h or 10–25 units/kg/hour as an IV infusion) is only advised where thromboses have been demonstrated.

Anaphylactic shock is to be expected in the office as well as hospital setting because of the variety of drugs now being administered and other allergens patients may contact. The practitioner must be aware of the variable nature and time of occurrence of this condition, the latter varying from minutes to hours after exposure. Usually, symptoms with parenteral drug administration will occur within 30 minutes, hopefully while the child is still under observation. The treatment is clear-cut—epinephrine should be given, 0.1 ml/kg IM or IV of a 1 : 10,000 dilution (or 10 μg/kg), as soon as the diagnosis has been made. Withdrawal of the offending antigen or isolation of its site of injection by a tourniquet should be accomplished. Prophylactic administration of diphenhydramine HCl (Benadryl), 0.5–1.5 mg/kg po or IV may be useful. Concern for maintaining an adequate airway, use of aminophylline for persistent bronchospasm, and general circulatory support with fluids and vasopressors have a role in severe cases of anaphylaxis, as they do in other forms of shock.

Many hypotensive episodes can be reversed readily. Gradual development of hypotension can often be reversed by crystalloid infusions, with the realization that these may leave the vascular compartments significantly within minutes or with plasma infusions. Attention to maintenance of the hematocrit at 35–40%, continuous monitoring of blood pressure, heart rate, ECG, urinary output (by indwelling catheter), and arterial blood gas determinations are needed. In refractory cases, withdrawal of inotropic agents and decisions as to when respiratory support and monitoring may be discontinued require artful judgments, often involving empirical trials. At least, these decisions can be made deliberately and after discussions with colleagues with special expertise.

Simple syncope can present major problems in differential diagnosis, but can usually be identified by its postural nature resulting in inadequate cerebral perfusion and by its rapid recovery when the patient's head is brought to or below heart level. Other neurogenic causes of hypotension, such as head injury and seizures, require special measures detailed elsewhere.

The practitioner must tailor the idealized treatments possible in an ICU setting to his own practice with the realization that patients with severe hypotensive epidoses will present under suboptimal conditions, often without warning. Since acute shock states require similar equipment and drugs to those needed for other forms of emergency such as primary respiratory arrest states, it would seem wise to establish a "crash cart" in the office with the drugs and equipment detailed in the early part of the above treatment plan for severe shock. The desired equipment, techniques for ventilation, placement of intravascular lines, and emergency drugs are detailed elegantly in the Textbook of Advanced Cardiac Life Support, available through the American and local Heart Associations. This should be required reading by the pediatrician and his support personnel. It would be most desirable for many pediatricians, especially those not familiar with intensive care as it is now practiced in most teaching centers, to participate in the Advanced Cardiac Life Support teaching programs and other similar programs at their hospitals. Organization of the office personnel so that each has a defined role in such emergencies is important, as is a thorough knowledge of the effectiveness of the local rescue squad and hospital emergency room. Decisions as to adequacy of equipment and drugs in the office can also be made by knowing the equipment on the hospital crash carts in locations away from the ER and ICU areas.

Peripheral Vascular Disease

BEVERLY C. MORGAN, M.D.

A rational approach to the therapy of peripheral vascular disease requires an understanding of the vessels involved and of the pathophysiology affecting them. This discussion will be limited to the diseases affecting the arteries, veins, and lymphatics of vessels distal to the major component trunks and will include the vasospastic disorders and frostbite.

PERIPHERAL ARTERIAL DISEASE

Occlusive disease of the lower extremities in adults is usually atherosclerotic in etiology, but the most common cause in pediatric patients is iatrogenic, because of placement of aortic catheters, primarily in sick neonates and in cardiac patients undergoing arterial catheterization. The major therapy is obvious: limit the use of indwelling arterial catheters to situations in which the information obtained from their use is essential to the management of the patient's course. Should any evidence of occlusion of an aortic branch (to internal organs or to the extremities) be noted, the catheter must immediately be withdrawn. Aneurysms or pseudoaneurysms may occur, and a number of cases of mycotic aneurysms following umbilical arterial catheterization have been reported.

Arterial trauma is not rare in children; therapy depends upon the location and nature of the injury. Acute arterial thrombosis in pediatric patients occurs most commonly as a complication of introduction of catheters for cardiac diagnostic procedures (catheterization or angiocardiography) or for placement of arterial catheter monitors, often in young patients following drowning, cardiac arrest, and so on. Surgical removal of an acute arterial thrombosis may be indicated, but operative intervention is not always indicated. Improvement of the circulatory status, together with thrombolytic agents (streptokinase, urokinase) or anticoagulants, may be sufficient therapy. Acute arterial thrombosis and embolus are emergencies, however, and treatment must be initiated as soon as the diagnosis is made. Delay may result in loss of an extremity.

Arterial embolization to peripheral vessels may occur. In the vast majority of cases the embolus originates in the heart, usually in patients with mitral stenosis, atrial fibrillation, or bacterial endocarditis affecting the left side of the heart. Treatment is of the underlying disease and the prevention of further embolization. Surgical removal of the emboli should be considered, if in an accessible area and causing impairment of function. Anticoagulation may be indicated as well.

Severe aortic coarctation, while representing a proximal abnormality in a major vessel, may present claudication of the lower extremities. Surgical repair of the coarctation is the obvious treatment for this condition.

ARTERIOVENOUS FISTULAS

Congenital arteriovenous fistulas are uncommon, but may result in severe local and even systemic abnormalities. Extremities are a common site for such fistulas. The keystone of therapy is conservatism. Surgical intervention should be undertaken only when the lesion is of sufficient size to threaten ulceration or bleeding or when a vital structure is involved. Rarely, cardiovascular complications necessitate operative intervention. Because surgical excision must be considered palliative in the majority of patients and the lesion usually recurs, conservative therapy is strongly recommended. Traumatic arteriovenous fistulas may result from penetrating or even blunt injuries and should be borne in mind when seeing children following trauma. Venipuncture in the femoral area may produce an A-V fistula.

PERIPHERAL VENOUS DISEASE

Venous thrombosis is uncommon in the very young, but may occur in older children. Embolization to the pulmonary arteries is the major hazard. Conditions associated with a high risk of venous thromboembolism in the adolescent female include pregnancy, the postpartum state, and the use of oral contraceptives; in younger patients fractures and other trauma to the lower extremity may lead to this complication. Anticoagulation with heparin should be considered in all major episodes of venous thrombosis and is definitely indicated if significant pulmonary embolism occurs.

Varicose veins are uncommon in the pediatric age group, but may occasionally present a major problem in adolescence. If the disease is extensive, surgical consultation should be obtained; otherwise, conservative management is indicated.

PERIPHERAL LYMPHATIC DISEASE

Congenital or acquired abnormalities of the lymphatics may present in infancy and childhood. Persistent edema of the extremities may represent congenital lymphedema (Milroy disease) or may be associated with Turner syndrome. No therapy is indicated for lymphedema associated with these syndromes. Lymphangitis may occur with cellulitis, and the treatment should be directed at the primary disease (antibiotic therapy for the underlying infection).

VASOSPASTIC DISORDERS

Raynaud Phenomenon. Raynaud phenomenon may exist as a primary disorder termed Raynaud disease or may be secondary to more serious disease. Raynaud disease occurs more commonly in females and often has its onset during the teen years. The major therapy is avoiding cold or other stimuli that precipitate vasoconstriction. Tobacco should be avoided. Vasodilator drugs have been tried, but none have been of consistent benefit. In extreme cases with ulceration of the fingers and severe pain, methyldopa has been used with variable results. If persistent ulceration occurs, surgical consultation is indicated since cervicodorsal sympathectomy is occasionally indicated. It is important to consider the fact that Raynaud disease may be a forerunner of subsequent inflammatory vascular diseases such as systemic lupus erythematosus, periarteritis nodosa, and so on.

Livedo reticularis is a persistent cyanotic mottling of the skin, which may involve all parts of the extremities and the trunk. Acrocyanosis presents a diffuse cyanosis of the fingers and hands and the toes and feet. These disorders result primarily from vasoconstriction. Erythromelalgia is apparently a result of vasodilatation. Patients have warm, bright red feet and lower legs, and burning, tingling, and itching may be associated.

Disability with these conditions is usually mild and the importance lies in differentiating them from more serious underlying disease. Usually reassurance is sufficient therapy. For persistent or severe episodes of erythromelalgia, which is related to temperature, wearing sandals and avoiding stockings and heavy bedding are helpful. Aspirin may provide relief to some patients.

Frostbite may be considered a peripheral vascular disease and in severe cases prompt therapy is indicated. Prevention is the best therapy. If tissue injury has occurred, rapid warming of the tissue is the most important aspect of treatment. Core temperature should be restored and the frozen tissue placed in warm water, beginning with a temperature range of 10 to 15°C and increasing 5 degrees every 5 minutes to a maximum of 40°C. Following rewarming, the extremities should be elevated and carefully protected in a sterile environment. Most cold injuries do not require rewarming. Conservative therapy consists of bed rest, and elevation of the injured part will suffice.

Disseminated Intravascular Coagulation and Purpura Fulminans

WILLIAM E. HATHAWAY, M.D.

Treatment considerations in disseminated intravascular coagulation (DIC) include three points: 1) alleviation of the precipitating or triggering event, 2) replacement of depleted hemostatic factors, and 3) interruption of the intravascular clotting process by anticoagulants.

1. Probably the most important aspect of therapy is the identification and removal of the triggering event. Clinical examples include antibiotic therapy, volume replacement, and circulatory support (dopamine) in bacterial sepsis; relief of hypoxia and correction of acidosis in neonatal asphyxia and respiratory distress syndromes; restoration of blood volume in hemorrhagic shock; and use of antiviral agents in severe viral infections. If the precipitating event can be quickly removed (i.e., relief of hypoxia or shock), often no other therapy is needed. Serial determination of coagulation tests will help in deciding whether further therapy is indicated.

2. Replacement of depleted coagulation factors and platelets is frequently necessary in severe DIC, especially with an associated bleeding diathesis or potential severe hemorrhage. Depending on the triggering event, it is often possible to anticipate the kind of replacement necessary. Hypoxia-acidosis is most apt to produce consumption of fibrinogen without significant platelet depletion; on the other hand, viral syndromes and sepsis are frequently associated with severe thrombocytopenia with only minor fibrinogen consumption. Fibrinogen and other clotting factors can be replaced by fresh frozen plasma (FFP); the dose of 10 to 15 ml/kg of FFP will raise the clotting factor level by about 20%. Fibrinogen (and factor VIII) can be given in cryoprecipitates also; one cryoprecipitate per 3 kg in infants or one cryoprecipitate per 5 kg in older children will raise the fibrinogen by about 75 to 100 mg/dl. Platelets are replaced by use of platelet concentrates; in the neonate, 10 ml/kg of platelet concentrate will raise the platelet count by about 75,000 to 100,000 per μl. In older children, one concentrate per 5 to 6 kg is the usual dose. The minimal hemostatic levels of procoagulants are estimated by a platelet count of 30,000 to 50,000 per μl, a prothrombin time of 18 seconds, and a fibrinogen level of 100 mg/dl.

It should be remembered that less than the optimal response to transfusions may be seen in patients with DIC since they often have ongoing consumption (until the trigger is relieved) as well as the presence of circulating fibrin-fibrinogen degradation products that may alter the function of transfused platelets and fibrinogen. For these reasons, the optimal replacement therapy for the severely affected neonate or infant may be an exchange transfusion with relatively fresh whole CPD blood. Experience has indicated that repeated replacement therapy does not significantly aggravate DIC and therefore should be used to halt or prevent bleeding.

3. In specific instances, interruption of the clotting process by heparin may be necessary when the triggering event cannot be quickly removed, and the consumption coagulopathy or tissue necrosis is ongoing. Examples of these clinical situations include acute promyelocytic or monocytic leukemia, giant hemangioma, associated large vessel thrombosis, early tissue ischemia or gangrene in septic shock, and purpura fulminans. In these instances, heparin will frequently halt the DIC or allow it to be more effectively treated by replacement therapy while the primary disease is being specifically treated. The most effective and safest method of giving heparin is by continuous intravenous administration. A loading dose of 50 units/kg is followed by 10 to 15 units/kg per hour by continuous IV infusion. Unless there is significant tissue necrosis present, this dose is usually effective, and improvement in the coagulation screening tests should occur in 12 to 24 hours or less.

In purpura fulminans, where heparin is absolutely indicated, a higher dose (20 to 25 units/kg per hour) may be indicated in order to halt the gangrenous process. Alternatively, heparin can be given intermittently (75 to 100 units/kg every 4 hours) by intravenous push. Intermittent therapy may be indicated if continuous therapy cannot be achieved owing to technical difficulties. Monitoring of heparin effect is usually not necessary in DIC if the desired result on the coagulation process is obtained, that is, stabilization and improvement in the prothrombin time, fibrinogen level, and platelet count. In purpura fulminans, heparin effect on the partial thromboplastin time and/or activated whole blood clotting time should be achieved (prolongation of these tests to 1.5–2 times normal).

In DIC, heparin remains the drug of choice for anticoagulant action. Other anticoagulants, such as the coumarin compounds, are too slow in their action to be of use in DIC. Platelet inhibitors (aspirin, dipyridamole, sulfinpyrazone) may have specific uses in chronic intravascular coagulation syndromes in the future. In purpura fulminans, 6 percent dextran has been used with reported clinical benefit. Antifibrinolytic agents, such as epsilon aminocaproic acid (Amicar), are contraindicated in DIC.

Complications. The major complication of the use of heparin in DIC is aggravation of the bleeding tendency. If minimal hemostatic levels (especially of platelets) are achieved by replacement therapy, the doses of heparin recommended are safe and usually effective. If reversal of the heparinization process is desired, protamine sulfate given in a dose equivalent to the estimated blood level of heparin is indicated, that is, 100 units of heparin equal 1 mg of protamine sulfate. In severe and persistent DIC, the level of antithrombin III–heparin cofactor may need to be increased by infusions of FFP (10 ml/kg) in order to achieve an adequate heparin effect. Since heparin may rarely cause thrombocytopenia (on prolonged usage), the platelet count should be monitored at least daily in patients with DIC undergoing heparinization.

Acute Rheumatic Fever

ANGELO TARANTA, M.D.

Therapy of acute rheumatic fever still revolves around aspirin, steroids, and bed rest. Only a few points in therapy are buttressed by controlled studies: this article therefore reflects our biases as much as our knowledge.

GENERAL MEASURES AND BED REST

All patients with acute rheumatic fever should be placed at bed rest. They should be examined daily to detect carditis for the purpose of starting treatment promptly should heart failure or cardiomeg-

Table 1. GUIDE FOR BED REST AND AMBULATION IN PATIENTS WITH ACUTE RHEUMATIC FEVER

Cardiac Status	Management
No carditis	Bed rest for 2 weeks and gradual ambulation for 2 weeks even if on salicylates
Carditis, no cardiomegaly	Bed rest for 4 weeks and gradual ambulation for 4 weeks
Carditis, with cardiomegaly	Bed rest for 6 weeks and gradual ambulation for 6 weeks
Carditis, with heart failure	Strict bed rest for as long as heart failure is present and gradual ambulation for 3 months

aly appear. If carditis is going to appear, it will do so within 2 to 3 weeks after onset; therefore, close observation is needed only during this initial period. Thereafter, the duration and degree of bed rest vary with the nature and severity of the attack. Table 1 is a general guide.

ANALGESIC AND ANTI-INFLAMMATORY TREATMENT

Anti-inflammatory treatment is very effective in suppressing the acute inflammatory manifestations of rheumatic fever, so much so that prompt response of the arthritis to aspirin is helpful in supporting the diagnosis. More vigorous anti-inflammatory treatment, such as steroids, is useful in controlling pericarditis and the congestive failure of acute carditis; unfortunately, it has no effect on the long-term sequelae of active rheumatic fever, i.e., on the incidence of residual rheumatic heart disease. Steroids cannot be used as a therapeutic trial to confirm the diagnosis of rheumatic fever because other kinds of arthritis, including septic arthritis and juvenile rheumatoid arthritis, also "respond," at least initially, to steroids (although they should not be treated with them).

In patients with arthralgia only or with mild arthritis and no carditis, anti-inflammatory drugs (steroids and salicylates), should be withheld and analgesics used if needed. This is particularly wise when the diagnosis is not definite, because analgesics will not interfere with the full development of migratory polyarthritis, which may clinch the diagnosis. Patients with moderate or severe arthritis but no carditis, or with carditis but no cardiomegaly, should be treated with aspirin: 100 mg/kg/24 hr in divided doses for the first 2 weeks, and 75 mg/kg/ 24 hr for the following 4 to 6 weeks. Sometimes slightly larger doses may be necessary to control arthritis. One should be alert to the possibility of salicylate intoxication, usually manifested by tinnitus (ringing in the ears) and hyperpnea.

In patients with carditis and cardiomegaly, aspirin is often insufficient to control fever, discomfort, and tachycardia, or does so only at toxic or near-toxic doses. These patients should be treated with steroids. Prednisone is the steroid of choice, starting with a dose of 2 mg/kg/24 hr in divided doses. In cases of extreme acuteness and severity, therapy should be started by intravenous administration of methylprednisolone (10 to 40 mg) followed by oral prednisone. After 2 or 3 weeks, prednisone may be slowly withdrawn, decreasing the daily dose at the rate of 5 mg every 2 to 3 days. When tapering is started, aspirin at 75 mg/kg/24 hr should be added and continued for 6 weeks. This "overlap" therapy reduces the incidence of post-therapeutic clinical "rebounds" (that is, reappearance of clinical manifestations shortly after treatment is stopped, or while it is being tapered, and without a new streptococcal infection). See Table 2.

Steroids are recommended for patients with severe carditis because of the clinical impression that such patients tolerate steroids better and respond more consistently and more rapidly than with salicylates. Most clinicians feel that death from uncontrollable congestive heart failure during the acute attack may be avoided by steroid administration, but for long-term outcome, most well-controlled studies have failed to prove that treatment with steroids decreases the incidence of residual rheumatic heart disease.

The termination of anti-inflammatory treatment may be followed in rheumatic fever patients by the reappearance within 2 to 3 weeks of laboratory abnormalities, or of clinical abnormalities as well. All the "laboratory rebounds" and most of the "clinical rebounds" are best left untreated or should be treated symptomatically with analgesics or small doses of aspirin, lest the full treatment be followed by another rebound and the duration of the attack lengthened. Only the most severe clinical rebounds necessitate reinstitution of the full original treatment.

DIURETICS AND CARDIOTONIC MEDICATION

The heart failure of rheumatic carditis is often controlled with bed rest and steroids only. If it is not, diuretics may be added first, followed by digitalis if needed. Digitalis should be used with caution because its therapeutic index may be decreased in rheumatic carditis. The need for digitalis should be re-evaluated at the end of the rheumatic attack, and periodically thereafter. In assessing the effect of digitalis, one should distinguish cardiac tachycardia, present during sleep, from emotional tachycardia which subsides during sleep.

TREATMENT OF CHOREA

Patients with chorea may benefit from administration of barbiturates or tranquilizers. Since chorea often occurs as an isolated manifestation or a few months after arthritis or carditis, anti-inflammatory medication is not usually needed. Although steroids in large doses have been reported to control choreic movements, the course of chorea is unpredictable, and well-controlled studies are lacking. Since steroids (especially large doses) are not harmless, it would be unwise to use them in any but the most severe cases of chorea.

Pediatric Cardiac Tumors

RICHARD J. CLEVELAND, M.D.,
and JOSEPH J. STETZ, M.D.

Hardly common at any age, cardiac tumors are strikingly infrequent in childhood. The vast majority of all cardiac tumors are matastatic in origin and occur in adults, while pediatric malignancies, with the exception of the leukemias, do not commonly involve the heart.

The easiest general classification of cardiac tumors is to divide them into benign and malignant, with malignant tumors being subdivided into primary and secondary. Primary cardiac tumors in the pediatric age group are overwhelmingly benign, with rhabdomyomas, myxomas, and fibromas being the most common. However, even the histologically benign tumors may cause death by interfering with normal cardiac function. They may also cause life-threatening arrhythmias and conduction disturbances, pericardial effusions leading to tamponade, acute valvular obstruction, peripheral embolization, and cavitary obliteration by the mass lesion.

BENIGN TUMORS

Rhabdomyoma. The therapy for a solitary rhabdomyoma is resection, if possible. It may not be feasible, however, to resect all the tumor mass since it frequently arises in the intraventricular septum. Complete resection may well interfere significantly with the conduction system. Approximately 30 per cent of rhabdomyomas involve the atrium as well as the ventricle and often total section is not technically possible because of the involvement of the valvular annulus. Under these circumstances, par-

Table 2.   RECOMMENDED ANTI-INFLAMMATORY AGENTS FOR ACUTE RHEUMATIC FEVER

Clinical Manifestation	Treatment
Arthralgia	Analgesics only
Arthritis only, and/or carditis without cardiomegaly	Salicylates, 100 mg/kg/24 hr for 2 weeks and 75 mg/kg/24 hr for 4 to 6 weeks
Carditis with cardiomegaly or failure	Prednisone, 2 mg/kg/24 hr for 2 weeks; taper over 2 weeks. Add salicylates, 75 mg/kg/24 hr at 2 weeks, and continue for 6 weeks

tial resection may be necessary to reduce the size of the mass and improve intracavitary blood flow. The decision to operate on patients with this tumor must be tempered with the knowledge of the mortality rate of tuberous sclerosis, if this condition is also present in any given patient. Radiotherapy and chemotherapy are of no value in the treatment of the tumor.

Intramural Fibroma. In the symptomatic patient, surgical excision is indicated since continued growth can interfere with myocarial contraction or intraventricular conduction.

Myxoma. Because these are completely curable in their most common locations by surgical excision, they should be kept in mind whenever a patient has evidence of intermittent valvular obstruction or develops a cardiac murmur that changes in its characteristics with changes in position of the patient. Long-term postoperative followup after excision of a myxoma is important and should include echocardiography to provide continued evaluation about potential recurrence of the tumor.

Miscellaneous. Various other relatively rare benign intracardiac primary neoplasms have been reported. These include lipomas, congenital cysts, angiomas (both hemangiomas and lymphangiomas), teratomas, hamartomas, and mesotheliomas. Several valvar tumors are generally only incidental findings at autopsy and are rarely a problem in life. These include congenital blood cysts of the mitral and tricuspid valves, focal myomas of any cardiac valve, and Lambl excrescences. These three valvar tumors do not require any form of therapy. The first-mentioned group produce symptoms not unlike the major categories of primary cardiac tumors and, therefore, may require resection because of their location and size.

MALIGNANT TUMORS

Fortunately, malignant cardiac tumors of childhood are rare. Of this group, sarcomas are the most common.

Sarcomas. Various forms of sarcomas involving the heart have been reported in the pediatric age group, with the most common being rhabdomyosarcoma and fibrosarcoma. The therapy for these is extremely difficult and disappointing. Surgical resection for cure is rarely possible though, on occasion, if the tumor arises in a critical area—for example, near a valve annulus—a partial resection may provide symptomatic relief for a period of time. Most often, there is widespread infiltration of the myocardium with spread to the mediastinum and lung by the time of diagnosis. This situation precludes effective surgical therapy. Other forms of therapy, including combined chemotherapy and radiation, may be relatively successful in relieving symptoms for a short period of time, but there is no effective long-term therapy currently known for primary malignant cardiac neoplasms.

Secondary Tumors (Metastatic). In the pediatric group, cardiac metastases from noncardiac primary tumors are much less common than they are in adults, in whom approximately 10 to 20% of the patients dying of neoplastic disease show some evidence of cardiac involvement. Acute leukemias do involve the heart in a majority of the patients, but this is generally not a matter of clinical importance. The cardiac involvement responds to the same therapy as does the leukemia itself. Most of the patients who die of leukemia and who are found to have cardiac involvement at autopsy generally did not demonstrate any significant cardiac abnormalities during life.

The only other pediatric tumors that show a significant metastatic involvement of the heart are those belonging to the sarcoma group. These should be treated with whatever form of therapy is found to be most useful for the control of the primary lesion.

6

Digestive Tract

Dental Caries

STEVEN D. BUDNICK, D.D.S.

Many microorganisms can produce acid from the fermentation of sugar. This acid may lead to demineralization of tooth substance and the development of dental caries. Prevention of dental caries includes making the teeth more impervious to this acid demineralization, removal of these microbiological plaques and sugars, and minimizing the intake of fermentable substrates.

The incorporation of fluoride into the enamel during tooth development forms fluorapatite crystals, which are more resistent to demineralization than the hydroxyapatite crystals normally present. The main source of systemic fluoride is community water fluoridation. Optimal fluoride concentration in the public water supply is one part per million, which reduces the incidence of dental caries by 50–60%. Higher levels of fluoride concentration (greater than 2 ppm) may lead to staining and pitting of the teeth. For those using sources other than public drinking water, the concentration of fluoride can be determined by most state departments of health.

Supplementation of fluoride is necessary under two different circumstances: 1) when the water supply contains little natural or added fluoride, 2) in breast-fed and formula-fed infants. Since breast milk and most commercially prepared formulas contain little fluoride, supplementation is necessary. Daily dosage recommendations are as follows: less than 2 years, 0.25 mg; 2-3 years, 0.50 mg; greater than 3 years, 1.00 mg. These levels can be achieved by the use of fluoride drops or tablets. When the water supply provides 70% of the daily fluoride need, no supplementation is necessary. In formula-fed infants, compliance may be improved by the use of formula concentrates that must be mixed with water, rather than ready-to-feed convenience formulas that contain little fluoride and require active supplementation.

The topical use of fluoride has its greatest benefits in suboptimally fluoridated areas and reduces caries incidence by approximately 30%. Concentrated topical fluorides may be applied in the dental office semiannually, and supplemented at home by the use of commercial preparations. The use of fluoride-containing toothpaste also has an additive effect.

Nutritional and home care information to parents and children is essential in reducing the incidence of dental caries. The diet should be modified to minimize the intake of fermentable sugars (a full-time job for most parents). Information on proper home care should be given to both the child and the parent, and reinforced at regularly scheduled dental visits. The parents of young children should actively participate in home care, and the care of older children should be monitored closely. A special precaution should be given to parents about putting the child to sleep with a bottle. This is the most prevalent cause of caries in infants and toddlers. If a bottle is to be used at these times it should contain only water, and should be removed when the child falls asleep.

When dental caries develops, the caries must be removed and the teeth restored with appropriate materials. If the caries extends to the pulp of the tooth, periapical infection may ensue, with swelling, pain, and fistulous tract formation. Frequently, this infection is present with no discomfort to the child. Pulp treatment, root canal therapy, and the judicious use of antibiotics are necessary to remove the source of infection. Restoration with full coverage crowns is usually necessary after resolution of the infection. Prevention of dental caries and elimination of existing carious lesions can only be achieved via an ongoing interaction of parent, child, and dental practitioner.

Congenital Epulis of the Neonate

STEVEN D. BUDNICK, D.D.S.

Congenital epulis of the neonate presents as a pedunculated firm mass on the anterior alveolar ridge, the maxilla being more commonly involved than the mandible. This benign tumor, which is present at birth, has a normal mucosal surface. The lesion ranges in size from a few millimeters to several centimeters in diameter. Females are affected eight times more commonly than males. Differential diagnosis includes the neuroectodermal tumor of infancy, vascular lesions, and eruption cysts involving neonatal teeth.

Appropriate treatment of the lesion is simple surgical excision, as the lesion may lead to feeding and respiratory problems. Although incomplete excision does not appear to lead to recurrence, the base of the lesion should be included in the removal.

Diseases and Injuries of the Oral Region

HERMINE M. PASHAYAN, M.D., *and* MICHAEL B. LEWIS, M.D.

CLEFT OF THE LIP AND/OR PALATE

Cleft Lip. Cleft lip may be present alone but more frequently is associated with a cleft of the palate. It may also be uni- or bilateral, incomplete or complete, and extend into the nostril. When present alone, a cleft of the lip should not cause associated medical problems, such as feeding difficulty or serous otitis media and conductive hearing loss. Controversy about the ideal time to repair a cleft lip exists. Some plastic surgeons repair the cleft lip in the newborn period, but the majority prefer to close the defect some time between 3 and 5 months of age, when a child tolerates general anesthesia with less risk. In complete unilateral or bilateral cleft lip, secondary procedures such as scar and nasal revision may be necessary later.

Cleft Palate. The presence of a cleft of the palate causes specific problems in different age groups. In the newborn period, the infant with a cleft palate is unable to produce adequate intraoral pressure and is, therefore, unable to have an effective suck. The universal presence of middle ear fluid in these patients causes a mild to moderate conductive hearing loss and the superimposed middle ear infection, if it occurs, requires aggressive systemic antibiotic treatment. In certain patients, insertion of ventilation tubes is recommended to allow for drainage and aeration of the middle ear.

The management of the infant born with a cleft palate involves an appropriate method of feeding, followed by the surgical closure of the palate. Feeding reminders:

1. We recommend use of a standard, singlehole nipple that has been cross cut. Do not use nipples with multiple holes or one single large hole in the center, or an oversized one like a lamb's nipple.

2. The infant should be fed in the sitting position to reduce nasal regurgitation. If nasal regurgitation occurs during feeding in the sitting position, the cross cut on the nipple is too large.

3. Burp the infant after the intake of every 0.5 ounce of formula to get rid of the ingested air and forestall the sense of fullness and colic.

4. After the feeding, the infant should be placed in the prone position to avoid aspiration of regurgitated formula.

An obturator as a feeding appliance is used in some centers. This, however, has proved to be ineffective.

Congenital heart disease, which is noted to be present in about 7% of patients with cleft palate, should be treated by a cardiologist, and subacute bacterial endocarditis precautions should be taken at the time of palate surgery.

Primary surgical palate repair is usually done between 6 and 18 months of age. Some surgeons prefer to leave the hard palate open, in the belief that less interference with maxillary growth will occur. This approach, however, is controversial. Secondary palate surgery to close a functional oronasal fistula or pharyngoplasty to treat persistent palatal incompetence is recommended only when indicated.

Speech therapy following surgical closure of the cleft palate is indicated if a residual speech problem is diagnosed after surgery.

Orthodontic treatment is indicated in patients with clefting of the alveolar ridge. Cases of complete bilateral cleft of the lip and palate usually require the most extensive and long-term orthodontics management, and, in some cases, additional reconstructive surgery is needed to correct the maxillary hypoplasia.

Adenoidectomy should be avoided in a child with a repaired cleft palate or a submucous cleft palate. The hypertrophied adenoids help occlude the posterior pharynx and reduce mild forms of velopharyngeal incompetency that can cause hypernasal speech.

Submucous cleft of the palate is diagnosed by the presence of a bifid uvula, a thin blue line in the middle of the soft palate, and notching of the posterior border of the hard palate. Although the majority of patients with a submucous cleft palate are asymptomatic, a small percentage will show clinical manifestations similar to patients with overt clefts, such as serous otitis media, nasal regurgitation during feeding, and hypernasal speech. Surgical correction without adenoidectomy is required.

The Robin Sequence. The Robin sequence is associated with a moderate-to-severe degree of micrognathia, glossoptosis, and, in 80 per cent of patients, a U-shaped cleft of the palate leading to feeding and respiratory problems in the neonatal period. The majority of these patients show appropriate catch-up growth of the mandible by late childhood and do not require corrective surgery of the mandible. Congenital heart disease is associated in 13.6 per cent of cases and requires appropriate management.

Medical management in the immediate newborn period involves treating the upper airway respiratory obstruction, the feeding difficulties, and, if it develops, cor pulmonale.

The upper airway obstruction caused by the glossoptotic tongue is managed by keeping the infant in the prone position at all times. Frequent suctioning may be necessary if oral secretions seem to accumulate. Respiration should be monitored closely and an apnea monitor should be used if respiratory difficulty is moderate to severe. A plastic oral airway should be kept taped to the crib and used immediately if airway obstruction occurs. (Prior to insertion of the oral airway, make sure the tongue is not caught in the cleft of the palate.) Administration of oxygen should be based on the results of arterial blood gas determinations. If these simple measures do not relieve the airway obstruction, the infant should be intubated with an endotracheal tube to insure an adequate airway. (The airway may be kept patent with an endotracheal tube for 2 to 4 weeks.) We feel that a tracheostomy should be considered only if absolutely necessary.

Surgical management of glossoptosis and airway obstruction is used only if medical management is inadequate. Available procedures are tongue-lip adhesion, Kirschner wire fixation of tongue to mandible, and, as mentioned, tracheostomy, which is used only when all other treatment modalities are inadequate.

The infant is fed in the prone position. The use of a standard, single-hole nipple that has been cross cut is recommended. If the infant is unable to suck, feeding by gavage is resorted to. Formulas of increased calories should be considered if total daily intake is small. If these methods fail, gastrostomy should be considered.

If and when cor pulmonale develops, it should be handled by relieving the upper airway obstruction as delineated above. Surgical repair of the primary palate is usually performed at from 9 to 18 months of age, but only after all problems with glossoptosis and airway obstruction have resolved. Some surgeons prefer to leave the hard palate open, believing that there will be less interference with maxillary growth.

Secondary palate surgery, such as closure of oronasal fistula or pharyngoplasty to treat persistent palate incompetence, should be considered only when indicated.

Prognosis in these patients is good only if airway and feeding problems are handled aggressively from the start. Mental retardation and central nervous system damage occur secondary to anoxia and upper airway obstruction in the newborn period.

Unusual Clefts. Clefts other than the more common unilateral and bilateral cleft lip and/or palate are quite rare. They often extend into other areas of the face and can involve the base of the skull. Their severity cannot always be fully appreciated at birth and their total management is usually complicated.

Median Cleft Lip with Hypotelorism. The congenital anomalies in this syndrome are in the area of the primitive forebrain and frontonasal processes. This syndrome always includes hypoplasia of the nose and was once thought always to be associated with severe forebrain deformities inconsistent with life beyond a few months. Recent reports, however, have shown that occasionally the forebrain deformities are not as severe as the facial appearance might indicate and are, in rare cases, even absent. Computed tomographic scanning of the brain is helpful in determining the extent of forebrain involvement. If the prognosis is reasonable, median cleft lip repair can be carried out. Because of the marked upper lip deficiency, tissue from elsewhere often is required. The best donor site is the lower lip. Nasal correction should be done much later, during preadolescence or beyond.

Median Cleft with Hypertelorism. This syndrome involves the central portion of the face and can be thought of as persistence of the paired medial frontonasal processes rather than their normal fusion. The upper lip is cleft in the middle, the nose is bifid, and the orbits abnormally widely spaced. The brain is not involved, and intelligence and neuromuscular development are usually normal. Lip repair and partial correction of the bifid nose are usually possible during the first year of life. Correction of the hypertelorism and telecanthus and definitive nasal correction should be delayed until a later time, although the surgical techniques of craniofacial surgery are being applied to younger and younger individuals. This may prove to be of some benefit in reducing the incidence and severity of amblyopia and allowing binocular vision to develop.

Oro-Orbital Clefts (Tessier Cleft 4 or 5). As the name implies, this cleft extends from the upper lip into the orbit. The underlying maxillary bone and ipsilateral half of the nose are involved and at times the globe is small and sightless. Surgical correction can be carried out at a relatively early age, using a form of "Z"-plasty to the lip and cheek and a standard coloboma procedure to correct the lower eyelid cleft. Correction of the foreshortened and hypoplastic ipsilateral nose is more difficult and may require the use of a regional flap or free grafted tissue.

Lateral Facial Cleft (Tessier Cleft 7). This cleft extends from the commissure of the mouth laterally toward the ear in the line of the primitive junction between the maxillary and mandibular processes of the first branchial arch. The underlying bony structures, as well as the ear, can be involved and, if so, are hypoplastic. The cleft itself may not be complete but represented by a macrostomia appearance and a contracted scarlike band running toward the ear. Surgical repair of the lateral cleft can be carried out during the first year of life by correcting the macrostomia appearance and performing a series of Z–plasties along the cheek cleft or its scarlike representation. Mandibular bony and ear reconstruction are delayed for a few years and are more difficult to accomplish.

Median Cleft of Lower Lip. This cleft can be associated with a bifid tongue and mandible, but is not commonly associated with other facial anomalies. Surgical repair at an early age is possible.

Macrostomia. This condition can be thought of as a lateral cleft of the mouth in which the commissure of the involved side is placed more widely than normal. The distance from the center of the upper lip to the commissure is increased. It is often part of the first and second branchial arch syndrome in which hemifacial hypoplasia and ear deformities exist. Repair of the macrostomia, including the orbicularis oris muscle, can be carried out during infancy.

Lip Pits. Lower lip pits may be found as an isolated anomaly or with a cleft lip and/or palate. These pits may have a fistulous tract that leads to imbedded mucous glands and a watery mucous discharge that can be embarrassing to the individual. Treatment is by surgical excision, making sure all the glandular tissue is removed.

TONGUE AND FLOOR OF MOUTH

Ankyloglossia (Tongue-Tie). Most forms of tongue-tie require no treatment. If the tongue tip can be protruded from the mouth and touch the roof of the mouth, no anterior articulation defect will occur. More severe forms of tongue-tie should be released. Often the ankyloglossia is caused by an avascular web, which can simply be divided. More substantial forms with vascularity require a surgical procedure with Z-plasty lengthening of the web.

Bifid Tongue. The only problem associated with this deformity is cosmetic unless it is a manifestation of the orofacialdigital syndrome (see next paragraph). The defect is amenable to surgical correction.

Microglossia (Hypoglossia). This deformity presents as part of the orofacialdigital syndrome, in which there is hypoplasia of the tongue and mandible, as well as a small oral opening, and limb anomalies. Surgical mobilization of the tongue may aid the articulation speech problems that usually accompany this defect.

Macroglossia. Enlargement of the tongue may be an idiopathic generalized hypertrophy or may be secondary to hemangioma, lymphangioma, or neurofibroma, which can involve the tongue and floor of the mouth and can extend to contiguous structures in the neck and oral area.

The idiopathic form of macroglossia is often associated with Down syndrome or other forms of mental retardation, although it can occasionally occur alone. Early surgical treatment should be avoided, for sometimes, with facial growth, the tongue is accepted within the mouth. If by the age of 4 or 5 years the macroglossia continues to present problems with malocclusion, open bite, drooling, and social acceptance, surgical reduction can be carried out. This usually means marginal wedge excision, sometimes accompanied by anterior wedge excision. It should be understood, especially in those with any degree of mental retardation, that surgical reduction of the tongue may not correct the open mouth look and drooling pattern.

Hemangiomas in this area may show some spontaneous improvement with time, usually 4 or 5 years. Lymphangioma, the more common tumorous enlargement of the tongue, will usually show no improvement. Neurofibroma causes the most severe involvement. Biopsy of the tongue can be used to confirm the clinical impression. Some improvement is often possible by surgical excision, although complete removal is often not possible, and significant deformity can persist. Multiple surgical procedures are often required.

Dermoid Cysts. Benign congenital tumors, dermoid cysts are found on the undersurface of the tongue and the floor of the mouth. Surgical excision is definitive treatment.

Lingual Thyroid. This abnormally placed thyroid tissue presents as a tumor in the region of the foramen cecum. Radioactive iodine scan should be performed to determine whether cervical thyroid tissue is present. If surgical excision is carried out and no cervical thyroid is present, thyroid hormone replacement will be necessary to prevent hypothyroidism.

Ranula. Although this term can be applied to any cystic swelling in the floor of the mouth, it more specifically refers to a cystic dilatation of a blocked sublingual salivary gland duct. This condition will occasionally resolve spontaneously, but if no improvement is seen within a few months, surgical excision or marsupialization is indicated.

Drooling. Drooling during infancy and the toddler period is common. Assuming normal motor and sensory function in the oral region, it usually clears spontaneously with neuromuscular development and learning. In some individuals with cerebral palsy or other congenital and acquired brain damage syndromes, drooling persists and can present hygienic and social problems. An operation to decrease the amount of saliva present in the anterior portion of the oral cavity can lessen the severity of the drooling in many of these patients. Both submaxillary salivary glands are removed from an external approach, and both parotid (Stensen) ducts are diverted to the pharyngeal region through an intraoral operation. This surgery is usually performed after the age of 5 years, when it is clear that the problem is persistent.

DEFORMITIES OF THE LOWER JAW

Micrognathia (Retrusion of the the Lower Jaw). This condition may be congenital or acquired and in both cases may be unilateral, leading to asymmetry of the face, or bilateral. If congenital, it is usually present at birth; if severe, it may cause feeding and respiratory problems (see preceding section on Robin sequence). In most cases of Robin sequence, a certain degree of catch-up growth occurs, and most patients do not require extensive surgical correction. In some familial cases of isolated congenital bilateral micrognathia and in cases of the Treacher Collins syndrome, there is no evidence of catch-up growth, and the patient develops a "birdlike" profile.

Unilateral congenital micrognathia is associated with the first and second branchial arch syndromes and facioauriculovertebral anomaly syndromes. These patients show an asymmetric growth pattern of the mandible. Acquired micrognathia is caused by traumatic damage to the condylar head, resulting in temporomandibular ankylosis. When the damage sustained is bilateral, a fairly symmetric atresia of the mandible results. When the damage sustained is unilateral, shortening of the ramus and body of the mandible is limited to one side only; the patient's chin is deviated toward the affected side, and the body of the mandible on the unaffected side is flattened.

Relief of the temporomandibular ankylosis should be provided as early as possible by temporomandibular arthroplasty in order to restore mandibular movement and permit mastication. Correction of the micrognathic deformity, either unilateral or bilateral, is done by elongation osteotomy in conjunction with bone grafting. The procedure of the elongation osteotomy is limited to those patients whose second dentition has erupted. Milder firms of micrognathia may be treated orthodontically.

Mandibular Protrusion (Prognathism). This deformity is not apparent until the child reaches 5 to 6 years of age. It is important to distinguish whether the protrusion is skeletal or alveolar. The diagnosis, evaluation, and treatment of these pa-

tients require a team of orthodontist, oral surgeon, and plastic surgeon. Base-line cephalometric x-ray films and impressions of the jaws documenting the degree of class III type of malocclusion are necessary before treatment is started. Numerous surgical procedures involving osteotomy and wiring of the fragments of the mandible have been described for the patient with skeletal prognathism.

In alveolar prognathism, the alveolar process is pushed forward along a normal or somewhat too short mandibular base. The diagnosis of this condition is readily made from the cephalogram, and treatment is with osteotomy and retropositioning of the anterior alveolar process.

Mandibular Asymmetry. Mandibular asymmetry may be due to asymmetric prognathism or true condylar hyperplasia. The former condition is caused by unilateral hyperactivity of the condylar growth center. The mandible in these cases is displaced to the opposite side, causing the mandibular dentition to appear horizontally displaced, but not inclined. Lengthening of the condylar neck is noted by radiograph. Correction is by unilateral or bilateral sagittal splitting of the ramus, but this should be done only when no further changes in occlusion are noted and growth stops.

In the second type of asymmetry (true condylar hyperplasia), there is true enlargement of the mandibular condyle and lengthening of the condylar neck and ramus. This leads to an increase in height of the affected side of the body and relative shortness of the opposite side. Treatment in these cases is a combination of partial condylectomy and sagittal splitting of the ramus, followed by supplementary orthodontic treatment.

Trauma. Injuries in the oral region are quite common. Fortunately, most are minor and can be managed on an outpatient basis, using local anesthesia (lidocaine, 1 per cent, with epinephrine, 1:100,000). In very young and uncooperative patients, mild sedation and restraint are helpful. Morphine sulfate, 0.1 mg/kg (if older than 6 months), or a combination of meperidine hydrochloride, 25 mg/ml; promethazine hydrochloride, 8 mg/ml; and chlorpromazine hydrochloride, 5 mg/ml, in a dosage of 1 ml/25 lb to a maximum of 2 ml, is a safe and effective sedative. After administration, these sedatives are not effective until 30 to 45 minutes have elapsed. General anesthesia is necessary when the injury is more extensive and complicated or with intraoral involvement.

Wound preparation need not be elaborate, but should involve cleansing of the skin surfaces with a bland, nondetergent soap, irrigation of the wound with normal saline, and removal of devitalized tissue and foreign bodies.

The use of prophylactic antibiotics should be individualized. If used, they should be discontinued after a few days.

External sutures should be removed within 3 to

5 days; intraoral sutures, if not absorbable, within 7 to 14 days.

Lacerations. Lip lacerations should be repaired in layers—skin, muscle, mucosa. If the vermilion cutaneous junction ("white-roll") is involved, careful restoration of this important anatomic and aesthetic landmark must be accomplished if deformity is to be minimized. Muscle, when involved, should be repaired with an absorbable suture (catgut or polyglycolic acid) to avoid the lumpy feel to the long-term scar tissue around a permanent suture.

Intraoral lacerations can be repaired with either an absorbable or a permanent (silk) suture material. Silk sutures are soft and cause little reaction but must be removed, which is often a disadvantage in the very young and uncooperative child. Small lacerations involving only the mucosa often require no treatment, but deeper lacerations of the tongue and soft palate require repair if proper function and appearance are to be maintained, especially if the free border of these structures is involved.

Avulsions. Dogbites in the oral area often result in actual tissue loss (avulsion). Immediate reconstruction is usually possible and in most cases is indicated. "V" excision with direct closure is the procedure of choice in small avulsions of lip tissue. In larger avulsions, flap tissue and, occasionally, free grafts are required. Appropriate tetanus and rabies precautions must be undertaken and antibiotic prophylaxis is usually necessary. Close observation and followup are required.

Electrical Burns. This injury is the result of the intense heat developed as an electrical current arcs through the saliva at the oral opening in a child who inadvertently places a live extension plug into the mouth or chews through a "hot"cord. It is not truly an electrical injury, but rather a thermal one. Almost always full-thickness lip or cheek tissue is involved. Often the lateral oral commissure is destroyed.

This injury is best managed by allowing the necrotic tissue to slough spontaneously and the wound to heal secondarily. Reconstruction is then carried out later. This allows salvage of the greatest amount of tissue and necessitates the fewest surgical procedures.

During the early phases of this injury (5 to 10 days) hemorrhage from the labial artery might occur as the necrotic slough separates. Digital pressure can control this, and the hemorrhage will usually stop spontaneously. Occasionally, suture ligature is required to stop the bleeding. Antibiotics and liquid diet should be instituted during the acute phase of this injury.

Dental Avulsion. Permanent teeth that have been totally avulsed often can be salvaged by early (within a few hours) reimplantation. Some form of fixation is required; for this, a dental specialist should be consulted.

Jaw Fractures. These fractures are uncommon, due to the relative underdevelopment of the facial bones compared with the cranium. Because of this, the facial bones are more protected than in the adult. The principles of treatment include accurate reduction and thorough immobilization for a 3- to 4-week period. Intermaxillary fixation provides an accurate means of reduction and firm immobilization. Occasionally, open reduction and internal interosseous fixation are necessary.

Salivary Gland Tumors

IRVING M. POLAYES, M.D., D.D.S.

The major salivary glands—parotid, submandibular, and sublingual—and the minor salivary glands within the submucosal tissues of lip, cheek, and palate may give rise to solid tumors in the neonate, infant, preschool, preadolescent, and adolescent patient.

Hemangiomatous masses of the salivary glands should be allowed to plateau in their growth and expansion before any treatment plan is decided. Conservative treatment is the first approach. A large number of these lesions will involute and require nothing more than watchful waiting.

For patients in whom the mass has produced marked distortion of the external ear with recurrent episodes of external otitis, and in whom the increased size of the mass interferes with local function and destroys normal anatomic structures, a course of oral prednisone, 20 to 40 mg on alternate days for 3 to 4 weeks, may prove effective in promoting involution. If satisfactory progress has been made following a 2-week trial of prednisone, continue the same regimen for a third week and taper off all steroids during the fourth week. Injections of sclerosing agents, radiation, and carbon dioxide freezing are all ill-advised. Whether eventual use of the laser may solve the problem of this type of hemangioma remains to be seen.

If spontaneous involution of the hemangioma following a course of prednisone is not evident and symptoms indicate resection of the hemangiomatous mass, a careful parotidectomy by an experienced surgeon *with preservation of the facial nerve* by identifying its trunk and all branches is the treatment of choice. Because of the subcutaneous position of the facial nerve due to incomplete development of the mastoid process in the young child, there is a certain degree of risk to the facial nerve in any parotid surgical procedure. However, with careful technique and meticulous control of hemostasis, the risk can be minimized. Failure of a hemangioma to resolve after observation for 2 years is reason enough in the presence of symptomatology to surgically explore and remove the large vascular mass. In every case, the facial nerve must be meticulously dissected and preserved. Hemangiomas that appear later in childhood are likely to be cavernous and usually require surgical excision since most will not resolve on their own.

Pleomorphic adenomas present as solid masses with occasional cystic components. These tumors should be removed by segmental parotidectomy, which would include the majority of the lesions located in the lateral parotid segment. Those lesions that lie in the retromandibular protions of the parotid gland and may involve the deep parotid segment are less common in children, but when present require total parotidectomy. The benign mixed tumor must never be "shelled out" from its "capsule"; recurrence would be guaranteed since part of the tumor would then be left behind. It is always best to remove the attached glandular segment without exposing the tumor capsule at any point. Therefore, since the majority of mixed tumors are in the lateral parotid segment or exposed retromandibular and tail segment, a superficial or lateral parotidectomy containing the entire tumor mass with preservation of the facial nerve is the treatment of choice. It must be emphasized that with each recurrence of a mixed tumor, there is increased chance for malignant change in the tumor cell.

Warthin's tumor, on the other hand, is a tumor of lymphatic tissues, a benign mass that demonstrates technetium uptake on scanning. Little or no known malignant potential is attached to a Warthin's tumor except that it can expand to large proportions and compress adjacent tissues. Segmental or lateral parotidectomy is the treatment of choice, with preservation of the facial nerve.

The treatment in general for all tumor masses of the parotid is surgical. In each case, the facial nerve should be preserved and a segmental parotidectomy performed to include the specimen for diagnosis. Both the submandibular and sublingual glands drain through the same terminal duct system, and a tumor mass involving either of these glands carries a much higher incidence of malignancy than a tumor mass of the parotid. By removing both glands and the submandibular duct, the floor of the mouth is cleared, and adjacent submandibular nodes can be included in the specimen for diagnostic purposes.

The low-grade malignant tumors of the parotid, such as the mucoepidermoid carcinoma and acinic cell carcinoma, are best treated by parotidectomy with preservation of the facial nerve. It is probably a wise choice to perform a total parotidectomy in these cases to eliminate any possibility of secondary lesions remaining in the deep segment of the remaining parotid gland. A neck dissection is indicated if suspicious cervical nodes are palpable in the involved area of lymphatic drainage. One can include those nodes that are in continuity with the parotidectomy for examination as part of the specimen. Parotidectomy with preservation of the facial nerve without neck node dissection is more often than not adequate treatment for these tumors.

Care must be taken not to violate any portions of the acinic cell carcinoma in the site of parotidectomy. If the tumor mass involves facial nerve segments, these segments must be sacrificed. Immediate reconstruction of facial nerve segments in the child is indicated using microneuroanastomoses of available autogenous nerve graft, such as the greater auricular or greater occipital nerves.

Whether a neck node dissection is indicated for the low-grade malignant parotid tumor is decided by the findings of suspected adenopathy. In children, cervical adenopathy is not uncommon in both the submandibular group of nodes and the anterior cervical chain. Low-grade mucoepidermoid carcinomas have a very low incidence of metastatic spread to the cervical chain. Therefore, parotidectomy is adequate treatment for this lesion. However, it is always wise to dissect the nodes of the submandibular triangle and the parotid nodes in continuity with the specimen removed. If these nodes are negative on frozen section, there is no need for further neck node dissection. Follow-up must be maintained for several years, and any suspicious cervical adenopathy, especially in the ipsilateral neck, should be treated by elective neck node dissection.

Tumor masses involving the hard or soft palate are best treated by wide local resection for diagnosis and cure. Reconstruction of the defect can be effected by use of local flaps, skin grafts, or distant flaps to restore function and coverage of resected palatal areas. This treatment is adequate for low-grade mucoepidermoid and pleomorphic adenomas involving the minor salivary glands of the palate.

The treatment of tumors of salivary gland tissue is primarily surgical. Radiation and chemotherapy are poor secondary and tertiary choices. In the growing child, it is probably best to avoid radiation as a modality of treatment because growth and development of body parts are adversely affected to a much greater extent than they are by the surgical extirpative procedure alone.

Recurrent Acute Parotitis

EDWARD J. O'CONNELL, M.D., *and* JOHN T. TWIGGS, M.D.

Recurrent acute parotitis is an unusual and troublesome condition affecting persons from infancy to adulthood. The highest incidence is in 5- to 10-year olds. Treatment of the acute episode consists of symptomatic relief, re-establishment of salivary flow, and antibiotic therapy. Analgesia with aspirin or acetaminophen and heat to the affected gland are of benefit. The affected gland should be milked to encourage salivary flow. In some cases, probing the Stensen duct may be necessary to remove inspissated mucopus. The parents should be instructed in parotid massage and encouraged to use sialagogues, such as chewing gum.

Antibiotic therapy, though not proved to be of definite value, seems appropriate. Treatment with penicillin V (125 mg four times a day for children up to 6 years of age and 250 mg four times a day for children 6 years of age or older) should be begun after material for culture and sensitivity tests has been obtained from the Stensen duct. Typical oral flora (*Streptococcus viridans, Staphylococcus aureus,* and pneumococcus) usually grow on cultures, although anaerobic bacteria grew on cultures in two recent cases. If the patient is sensitive to penicillin, erythromycin (30 to 50 mg/kg every 6 hours to a maximum of 500 mg every 6 hours for 10 days) should be used. If inflammation has progressed after the first 24 hours of antibiotic therapy, the addition of therapy with a coagulase-resistant anti-staphylococcal drug (dicloxacillin, 25 mg/kg/24 hr in four divided doses) should be strongly considered.

The usual episode lasts from 4 to 6 days. A follow-up examination 4 to 6 weeks after the first attack is recommended. At this time, the parotid gland should be carefully examined bimanually to rule out small, partially obstructing lesions.

Preventing further attacks is much less rewarding than treating an acute attack. Prophylactic antibiotics, autogenous vaccines, and steroids have been of no benefit. Maintaining salivary flow by use of sialagogues, such as chewing gum, and, in some cases, preprandial parotid massage has appeared to be of some benefit. If recurrences continue, sialography should be done to rule out stenosis, stones, and obstruction. This procedure has also been reported to be of therapeutic value in some cases.

Because most children with recurrent parotitis have little trouble after adolescence, surgical therapy is seldom necessary. However, patients in late adolescence or older who have had many recurrences despite optimal medical management and have proximal ductal dilatation or cyst formation may benefit from surgical intervention.

Thyroglossal Duct Cysts

BURTON H. HARRIS, M.D.

A thyroglossal duct cyst is a remnant of the embryonic thyroglossal duct, a structure which at one time connected the foramen caecum of the tongue to the isthmus of the thyroid gland. Although failure of portions of this duct to obliterate can result in cyst formation anywhere along its course, thyroglossal duct cysts are almost always midline structures at or just inferior to the hyoid bone, distinctly above the "Adam's apple" (thyroid cartilage). When not infected, thyroglossal duct cysts are smooth, round, regular, and raised. Most appear after the second year of life.

The persistent connection with the oral cavity makes infection inevitable. Infection with mouth flora produces a red, swollen, tender, central cervical mass. Frequent warm compresses should be applied and antibiotic therapy with ampicillin or a cephalosporin begun. If the signs of inflammation do not begin to resolve promptly and convincingly within 24 hours, drainage becomes necessary. Aspiration with a 16 gauge needle should be attempted first. The infection will usually subside if sufficient pus and gelatinous material can be removed. In rare instances adequate drainage can be accomplished only by surgical incision. The child becomes a candidate for elective removal of the cyst about 6–8 weeks later, after all physical evidence of infection has disappeared.

Treatment is elective surgical removal. The operation is necessary to make a histologic diagnosis and to prevent infection. It should be done soon after the mass is noted, and should be preceded by a thyroid scan when the mass feels solid rather than cystic, or is associated with a lingual thyroid or uncertainty about the presence or location of other functioning thyroid tissue.

The goal is the prevention of recurrence by total excision of the cyst and the proximal vestige of the thyroglossal duct. The duct runs through the hyoid bone, so complete removal requires en bloc dissection of the cyst, the central one third of the hyoid bone, and the thyroglossal duct to its origin in the base of the tongue (the Sistrunk operation). The procedure is done with general anesthesia through a transverse skin crease incision. Although the operation is technically demanding, recovery is usually prompt, and most patients are discharged on the first or second postoperative day. The scar from an uninfected incision should be quite acceptable. The incidence of recurrent thyroglossal remnants is less than 5%.

Branchial Arch Cysts and Sinuses

BURTON H. HARRIS, M.D.

Branchial arch cysts and sinuses are caused by imperfect maturation of one of the four pairs of normal embryonic arches. Cell rests can persist anywhere along the arch, and appear later as a mass (cyst) or a skin opening (sinus), or both. The arch of origin can be determined from the location of the lesion, making its behavior and deep connections more predictable.

First branchial arch vestiges appear in front of the external ear or in the submaxillary triangle. They take an ascending path in close relation to branches of the facial nerve, and end by joining the middle third of the external auditory canal. Remnants of the second branchial arch, the most common, are found along the anterior border of the upper two thirds of the sternomastoid muscle. A complete tract would run upward through the neck, involve the structures of the carotid sheath and the hypoglossal and glossopharyngeal nerves, and terminate in the pharynx at the tonsillar fossa. The rare third arch lesions occur along the anterior border of the lowest part of the sternomastoid, with a tract that passes deep to the carotid arteries and above the laryngeal nerve, ending at the piriform sinus.

Treatment, after recognition of the congenital nature of the lesion, is complete surgical removal. The initial finding is either a mass or a small opening in the skin. Sinuses may drain mucoid, salivary-like fluid from the oropharynx or the epithelial cells lining the sinus. Flow often increases or becomes mucopurulent with respiratory infections. Cysts appear as asymptomatic deep cervical masses or as acute infections with cellulitis or an abscess. Warm compresses and penicillin or a cephalosporin are usually effective treatment.

Elective operation should be undertaken at a time of minimal or no drainage. If a sinus is present, insertion of a tear duct probe or injection with dilute methylene blue solution may be helpful. An elliptical incision around the skin opening is made, the tract is identified, and then an anatomic dissection of the tract from the surrounding structures is performed. Sometimes a parallel, "step ladder" incision higher in the neck becomes necessary as the tract is mobilized. Suture ligation at the point of origin completes the total removal.

Antibiotics and drains may be useful in cases of recent or continuing infection. Uninfected incisions heal nicely, and recurrence is rare.

Disorders of the Esophagus

K. C. PRINGLE, M. B., CH.B., F.R.A.C.S., *and* ROBERT T. SOPER, M.D.

Congenital disorders of the esophagus are, in general, more common and more serious than acquired lesions. Congenital lesions present at or soon after birth, whereas acquired lesions usually surface after the age of 6 months. All neonates with major congenital esophageal anomalies should be managed in high risk neonatal intensive care units staffed by pediatric surgeons, neonatologists, and pediatric radiologists. All investigations should be carried out in the center where the definitive treatment is performed.

Esophageal Atresia. Polyhydramnios is the usual prenatal sign of esophageal atresia. In the first few hours of life, the baby exhibits difficulty swallowing saliva, produces a frothy mucus from both nose and mouth, and has some respiratory distress. A 10 or 12 F catheter passed through the nose or mouth will be arrested within 9 or 10 cm of the alveolar ridges. X-ray reveals the atretic portion of the esophagus with the catheter in place and gas in the stomach and small bowel, heralding the presence of a fistula from the trachea to the distal esophagus. Associated anomalies are common.

Treatment begins by passing a sump tube into the upper pouch for continuous low pressure suction. The baby is nursed either upright in an infant seat or prone and slightly head down. The Waterston classification of these babies guides further treatment. Waterston's Group A babies (over 2.5 kg in birth weight without aspiration pneumonitis or other anomalies) can be primarily repaired via right thoracotomy (extrapleural approach) in the first day of life. Waterston's Group B babies (either 1.8 to 2.5 kg in birth weight and well, or larger babies with a moderate pneumonia or moderate associated congenital anomaly) can be staged with gastrostomy suction and a 2–3 day period to search for other anomalies, or for intensive physiotherapy to improve the lungs. Waterston's Group C babies (less than 1.8 kg in birth weight, or babies of any birth weight with either severe aspiration pneumonia or life-threatening associated anomaly) are best managed by staged repair: gastrostomy, ligation of the tracheoesophageal fistula, and placement of a feeding catheter. Delayed repair is undertaken after stabilization and satisfactory weight gain, perhaps weeks later.

A long gap between the proximal esophagus and the tracheoesophageal fistula occasionally prevents primary anastomosis. We divide the fistula and tack the distal esophagus as high in the mediastinum as possible at the first operation; later, an attempt is made to mobilize the upper pouch down to the fixed distal pouch, if necessary employing one or more circular myotomies in the upper pouch. We avoid cervical esophagostomy, since this commits the baby to a colon or gastric tube bypass. Although esophageal peristalsis is not normal after repair of an atresia, we feel that the esophagus functions better than either a colon or gastric tube bypass.

Babies with esophageal atresia and a gasless abdomen have no distal tracheoesophageal fistula. They are initially managed by suction of the proximal pouch and placement of a gastrostomy tube for feeding. Some time is spent elongating both proximal and distal esophageal pouches. Gastrostomy feeds are given by bolus to distend the stomach and the distal esophagus, and mercury-weighted bougies are used to stretch the upper pouch. After satisfactory weight gain, and when fluoroscopic examination with a bougie in the upper pouch and a Bakes' dilator in the lower pouch reveal that the two esophageal ends are close to each other, primary extrapleural repair is attempted. A long gap between the two esophageal pouches may require one or more circular myotomies to allow anastomosis.

POSTOPERATIVE COMPLICATIONS. Anastomotic leak occurs in 20–30% of babies postoperatively, heralded by spit or feedings draining from the chest tube. If the original repair was performed extrapleurally, this complication is a mild nuisance rather than the serious empyema that occurs with transpleural repair. Contrast swallow confirms the leak, and the baby is nourished by enteral feedings until the leak heals. A leak predisposes to anastomotic stricture, treated by retrograde Tucker dilatations over a silk suture.

Another major problem after successful repair is gastroesophageal reflux, which also may produce a troublesome anastomotic stricture. Most babies with an esophageal anastomosis will require one dilatation at some time in the postoperative period; if more than three dilatations are required, gastroesophageal reflux should be investigated. We treat gastroesophageal reflux by Nissen fundoplication. Occasionally, a leak will result in a recurrence of the tracheoesophageal fistula. This can be very difficult to diagnose but once confirmed, repeat operation (usually by a right transpleural approach) is required. The fistula is divided and both ends closed. A patch of pleura or pericardium must be sutured between the two suture lines.

"H Type" Tracheoesophageal Fistula. These patients usually present some weeks or months after birth with coughing and choking during feeds or with aspiration pneumonia. Diagnosis is usually confirmed by contrast esophagogram but may require sophisticated studies such as combined esophagoscopy and bronchoscopy. A fine catheter placed across the fistula facilitates surgical excision. About 85% of these fistulas can be repaired by a cervical approach; the remainder require thoracotomy. Both esophageal and tracheal ends of the fistula are closed and a flap of muscle is moved between the two suture lines.

Congenital Esophageal Web. These babies usually present with dysphagia, the web being recognized by its characteristic appearance on upper GI contrast swallow. The webs usually respond to one or more dilatations, but may require endoscopic resection or even open operative resection for definitive care.

Esophageal Duplications. Although these babies usually present with dysphagia, occasionally duplications are discovered as a mediastinal mass on routine chest x-ray. The simple duplication cyst usually can be excised via thoracotomy. Sometimes its anatomical location requires a more cautious approach, removing only the mucosa of the cyst through an incision in the muscularis; the muscle is then closed over the site of the repair. Occasionally, these foregut duplications have a fine connection with the esophageal lumen, which brings them into a spectrum of extralobar pulmonary sequestration. These lesions may have a significant sytemic blood supply that needs to be identified and ligated before the sequestration is removed; rarely they are associated with posterolateral diaphragmatic hernia.

Vascular Rings. These babies usually present with either respiratory distress in the first few months of life or dysphagia when weaned. Upper GI contrast reveals characteristic indentation of the proximal esophagus, angiography clearly defining the anatomy of the lesion. The site where the ring is divided depends on the anatomy. An anomalous right subclavian artery arising from the distal portion of the aortic arch may pass posterior to the esophagus. This is treated by simple ligation and division of the artery, usually through a left thoracotomy.

Achalasia. This anomalous motility problem is rare in children. Dysphagia, regurgitation of undigested food, aspiration pneumonia, and weight loss are the predominant complaints. The diagnosis is confirmed by upper GI contrast study and esophageal manometry. The best treatment is an anterior Heller myotomy. If the myotomy does not extend onto the stomach, an antireflux procedure is usually not required. However, if the myotomy extends onto the stomach, then it is best protected by a Thal or Dor-Nissen fundoplication.

Caustic Ingestion. Severe esophageal burns from ingestion of caustics have dramatically diminished in frequency and severity since the arrival on the market of the new "improved" Drano and Liquid Plummer, with the concentration of caustic in these two commercial preparations reduced from 30 to 10% and marketed in a bottle with a child-proof cap. The ideal first aid for caustic ingestion is to have the child drink a glass of milk immediately; the milk has a protective effect if swallowed within the first minute or two after injury. Emetics or gastric lavage are contraindicated.

Careful inspection will usually show some burns of oral mucosa. However, even in the absence of mouth burns, the full length of the esophagus should be assessed with careful endoscopy performed within 12–24 hours of the caustic ingestion. If endoscopy shows the characteristic whitish patches of full-thickness mucosal burn circumferentially at any point, a Silastic stent may be passed, as described by Reyes et al. A 3-week course of systemic steroids will then result in a much lower incidence of severe strictures. However, this treatment has significant morbidity. We prefer to manage children with significant noncircumferential full-thickness burns with a 3-week course of systemic steroids and antibiotics, closely observing for the development of strictures. We dilate caustic strictures repeatedly and have had some success with injecting them on a regular basis for 3 or 4 months with small amounts of triamcinolone. With the more mild caustics now available, esophageal replacement for caustic ingestion is rarely required. There may, however, be an increased risk of esophageal carcinoma in long term follow-up of patients with old caustic esophageal burns.

Peptic Esophagitis. This is most commonly due to gastroesophageal reflux, which is almost physiologic in the first year of life. This subject is dealt with in more detail in a following section.

Esophageal Foreign Bodies. Small children who habitually crawl around the floor putting foreign objects in their mouths occasionally have these objects lodged in the esophagus. The larger foreign bodies tend to get caught at the level of the cricopharyngeus or the aortic arch; when a foreign body hangs up at the level of the gastroesophageal junction, the child should be investigated for a peptic stricture. Blunt or rounded objects can usually be removed under fluoroscopic control by passing a Foley or Fogarty catheter beyond the object and inflating the balloon; the baby is then turned prone and head down, and the catheter is gently withdrawn under fluoroscopic control. Sharp foreign bodies such as open safety pins must be removed endoscopically. When possible, safety pins are closed and withdrawn into the endoscope. If this is not possible, the sharp end of the pin should be maneuvered into the endoscope and the endoscope and foreign body withdrawn together. Impacted food stuffs may lodge in the normal esophagus. Meaty foreign bodies may be softened by small quantities of papain, 5 ml every 30 minutes for 4 to 6 hours; if successful, this will allow the foreign body to pass into the stomach. Follow-up examination of the esophagus is necessary to exclude a stricture.

Gastroesophageal Reflux and Hiatal Hernia

HARVEY L. SHARP, M.D.

Until recently, the lower esophageal sphincter (LES) has been the focus of gastroesophageal reflux (GER) physiologic alteration and treatment. An increasing appreciation of a more diffuse motility disorder may lead to more successful treatment in the future. Everyone refluxes occasionally for short intervals of time. GER can range from normal to abnormal with variations in regards to frequency, length of time, and extent. Immature motility and low LES pressure are common in the newborn and "matures," usually by 10 months of age. Hiatal hernia occurs as frequently in normal individuals as in GER patients. Therefore, while hiatal hernia is a contributing physiologic factor, it is usually inconsequential otherwise. In the not so final analysis, GER may resolve without therapy when noted during infancy, or may initially respond 95% of the time to either medical or surgical therapy. The final analysis awaits better definition of the syndrome and long-term follow-up of the present treatment regimens.

Recent literature reflects a multiplicity of invasive diagnostic procedures for symptoms of GER. Faced with this, the family physician may opt to take a cost-effective humane approach to infants early in course of this disorder, avoiding most, and in "spitters" all, diagnostic procedures. The approach to treatment varies according to whether the patient is a) an infant with only GER, b) a GER plus other medical problems, or c) an older child. A large long-term physiologic and psychologic follow-up of medical or surgical therapy in GER has not been published. The long-term published results of previously reported short-term successes that are available for both medical and surgical approaches in children and adults have been disappointing. In addition, no controlled studies have been applied to diet or positioning, which have been the main elements of GER medical therapy. Short-term controlled studies evaluating motility altering medications in GER are encouraging.

DIETARY MANAGEMENT

Radiologists have illustrated that if the stomach is not overfilled with liquid or gas, refluxing may not occur. Therefore, the infant should be fed slowly, removing the nipple after every estimated ounce or two of milk to allow him to burp. Always feed in an upright position. Ad libitum feedings should be switched to 6 to 8 small-volume feedings per day. Formulas may be thickened with 1 tablespoon of cereal per ounce of liquid for the antral, nutritional, volume, and thickened ketchup effects. Older children eat six small-volume meals per day, avoiding foods that elicit chest pain. Fasting is instituted after 6 P.M. Weight gain is the earliest parameter of success, apparent within 7 days; in difficult cases this requires continuous drip feedings.

POSITIONAL MANAGEMENT

Parents can inform you about the various positions that cause regurgitant symptoms in their child. Many authorities advocate 24 hours in an upright position of at least 60° in infants. No follow-up studies are available to indicate whether being tied in this position is harmful to the infant. The child can object by increasing his intra-abdominal pressure, causing positional therapy to be counterproductive. In early cases, holding the baby upright in the mother's arms or in an infant seat for an hour after feeding is all that is required. Infant seats are wonderful as long as the child does not slump over. Otherwise the prone position is to be encouraged, since the esophagogastric junction is at the most superior part of the stomach. Special boards have been designed to maintain a prone position at the desired angle but are not commercially available. An 8-inch elevation of the head of the crib or bed is worthwhile only if the child will sleep and not migrate to a head-down position.

MEDICAL THERAPY

Irritability and abnormal head movements (Sandifer syndrome) in the infant and upper abdominal pain or "heartburn" in the older child are reflections of pain from esophagitis and occasionally gastritis. Although antacids seemingly would be utilized routinely for these symptoms of GER, which can result in dysmotility and stricture formation in the esophagus, they have not been administered properly in many published regimens. Because of the strong buffer effects of Milanta II, 5 to 20 ml can be administered 1 hour after feeding. Less costly antacids appear to be as effective as cimetidine in this inflammatory lesion as in others. In some instances bile reflux has been documented and cholestyramine advocated as a treatment. Long-term use has not been proven to be efficacious. In small, controlled studies, two motility altering medications (bethanechol and metoclopramide) have been demonstrated to be beneficial. Neither medication has been approved for GER in children. The incidence of side effects from long-term effective dosage remains to be documented in children. Other conditions, particularly respiratory or CNS, may respond adversely to these medications. Thus, unfortunately, these medications cannot be advocated for general use in GER at the present time. However, these or similar motility altering medications may play a more prominent role in the treatment of GER in the future.

SURGICAL THERAPY

Of the various procedures attempted in the past, the Nissen fundoplication is the current favorite. This involves an abdominal approach in which the fundus is wrapped around the esophagus to mechanically bar reflux of gastric contents into the esophagus. Immediate success rates have been as high as 95% in uncomplicated cases and 85% in those with other conditions that may contribute to continuing symptoms of vomiting, respiratory difficulty, or weight gain. Complication rates have been

stated to be as low as 0.6%; however, clearly this figure is too low if one includes all long-term and short-term complications. Otherwise, there would not continue to be as many variations of the Nissen procedure as there are other surgical approaches to this problem. Unique to this procedure are "tight Nissen," "slipped Nissen," "obstructed Nissen," and "herniated Nissen." Complications include dysphagia secondary to aperistalsis or peptic stricture. Other symptoms may arise from gastric ulceration, "gas bloat" syndrome when wrapped too tight to burp or regurgitate under normal circumstances, and recently the "dumping syndrome" is being documented more frequently. Dilatation is obviously indicated in patients with stricture. Indications for operation in GER include respiratory problems ranging from apnea to pneumonia, poor nutrition, esophagitis and stricture, and intractable vomiting. Surgical intervention has been most successful in stopping vomiting. No surgeon has advocated surgery until a "medical" regimen has failed and most surgeons with GER seek medical relief for years before submitting to a surgical procedure themselves.

THE PRESENT ROLE OF THERAPY

Initially, a carefully explained medical regimen should be attempted. The intensity of the therapeutic approach regarding diet, positioning, and antacids reflects a practical consideration of both the severity of the case and the family circumstances. If symptoms and signs of GER do not improve on this regimen, a 7 to 10 day hospitalization is required, during which the initial therapeutic approach is initially followed, then, if failure persists after 2 to 3 days of observation, advancing to the intensive medical regimen. Success with drip feedings, 24 hour positioning, and antacids should be evident by weight gain in 7 days. Only infants with other medical problems usually fail this regimen. Unless life-threatening complications continue to occur or other medical problems contraindicate, treatment failure should be evaluated on motility medications. Surgical intervention is indicated in those cases in which strictures are present, esophagitis will not resolve, or respiratory symptoms remain life threatening. Surgery is rarely necessary in the first year of life because of the natural course of the disease. Other medical problems may indicate earlier surgical intervention, but nutrition should be optimized before the procedure is attempted. The respiratory symptoms may persist after surgery in over 40% of cases because GER is not the cause. Malnutrition may remain a problem if GER is not the cause. While surgery usually stops the vomiting, it may accentuate an associated GER motility disorder. Long-term follow-up is required in GER treated medically in older children or surgically at any age.

Nausea and Vomiting

HARLAND S. WINTER, M.D.

Nausea and vomiting are symptoms that can be caused by many factors. Although nausea is an ill-defined sensation, it is accompanied by the physiologic changes of gastric hypoactivity and dilation. In contrast, vomiting is an active process in which the first portion of the duodenum contracts, causing reversal of flow through a relaxed pyloric sphincter. The stomach then contracts and its contents are forcibly expelled through the lower esophageal sphincter. Regurgitation, unlike vomiting, is an effortless explusion of gastric contents. Most causes of vomiting are self-limited and require supportive care only. If the child has lost more than 10% of his/her previous body weight, parenteral rehydration may be required. Early appropriate oral intervention may avoid such therapy. Sucking rather than chewing is often more easily tolerated and lollipops with a sweet aroma and taste may decrease the urge to vomit. Ice, popsicles, and decarbonated beverages such as Pedialyte, Lytren, and Gatorade are often successful because they can be swallowed without chewing. As even the sight of large volumes of fluid may cause nausea, beginning with 1 teaspoon of a clear liquid every 10 minutes and advancing to 1 tablespoon every 20 minutes, and then to 1 ounce every 30 minutes is often successful. After the acute episode and during recovery, soft pureed foods such as cereals, soups, and puddings that are low in fat are most easily tolerated. A search for a cause should precede any therapeutic intervention, as supportive therapy ultimately will not be successful if there is an underlying chronic problem.

CAUSES AND THERAPY

Anatomic. Vomiting from an anatomic problem may be caused by a congenital or an acquired lesion. Bile stained vomitus suggests an obstruction distal to the ampulla of Vater, as in Hirschsprung's disease, intussusception, malrotation, or duodenal obstruction; curdled and sour emesis suggests either an incompetent lower esophageal sphincter or a gastric/pyloric lesion such as antral web, pyloric stenosis, antral spasm, gastric ulcer, or pyloric channel ulcer; undigested food suggests esophageal obstruction, which may be caused by an esophageal stricture, diverticulum, or achalasia. If a newborn vomits blood, the mother's breasts should be checked for excoriation or infection. A nasogastric tube should be placed in the infant's stomach, and if blood is present, an APT test will distinguish fetal from maternal hemoglobin. If maternal hemoglobin is present, gastric lavage frequently resolves the symptoms. If fetal hemoglobin is present in the gastric aspirate, sepsis or a coagulopathy must be considered. Even if no obvious site of hemorrhage into the breast milk is identified, a guaiac of the milk from each breast is necessary. While awaiting the results of laboratory data, vitamin K, 1.0 mg IM, may be given prophylactically. Therapy of anatomic lesions often requires surgical intervention, but antacids and cimetidine may be useful in treating peptic lesions of the stomach, duodenum, and esophagus. These specific topics are covered elsewhere in the text. Nifedipine, an antianginal drug that is a calcium channel blocker, has been used in vasospastic angina and recently has been shown to decrease lower esophageal sphincter pressure. Because of this, it has been used in adults who have achalasia. Although this condition is rare in children and frequently requires a Heller myotomy, temporary relief may be obtained medically.

Metabolic. There are many metabolic abnormalities associated with nausea and vomiting: urea cycle abnormalities with hyperammonemia, familial protein intolerance, renal tubular acidosis, adrenal insufficiency, diabetic ketoacidosis, and renal failure. Successful treatment of the nausea and vomiting depends on correction of the metabolic abnormality; pharmacologic agents are of little value in controlling the vomiting. Supportive care as outlined above may provide some symptomatic relief.

Central Nervous System. Individuals with increased intracranial pressure, migraine, diencephalic syndrome, or seizure disorder may have recurrent episodes of vomiting. Frequently the vomiting is not preceded by periods of nausea. In the neonate who has had a difficult birth, vomiting may result from cerebral ischemia, cerebral edema, or intracranial hemorrhage. Vomiting from these causes is relatively refractory to medical control until the underlying problem is treated. Lead poisoning deserves special mention because of the possibility for chelation therapy.

Drug/Toxin. Oncology patients having radiation therapy or chemotherapy frequently experience some nausea and vomiting. Phenothiazines are most commonly used to control these symptoms because they act on the chemoreceptor trigger zone (CTZ) and the vomiting center. Thiethylperazine (Torecan), which comes as 10 mg tablets and suppositories, is used in older children, although the proper dose has not been definitely established. Perphenazine (Trilafon) also acts on the central nervous system, particularly the hypothalamus. As with other phenothiazines, its site and mechanism of action are not known. The appropriate dose for children has not been established, but 2, 4, 8, and 16 mg tablets are available. The major side effects of the phenothiazine compounds are extrapyramidal reactions that include trismus, torticollis, oculogyric crisis, hyperreflexia, dystonia, dysphagia, slurred speech, dyskinesia, and ataxia. Because of these side effects many physicians who regularly treat oncology patients with this class of antiemetics prophylactically administer diphenhydramine hydrochloride (Benadryl). Other untoward effects of the phenothiazine compounds are autonomic dysfunction, idiosyncratic or hypersensitivity reactions, and agranulocytosis.

Other classes of compounds also may be beneficial in treating the emesis associated with chemotherapy. Benzquinamide hydrochloride (Emete-Con) is a benzoquinolizine derivative that is unrelated chemically to phenothiazine compounds or other antiemetics. It can be given intramuscularly or intravenously. The mechanism of action is unknown, but antiemetic activity begins to occur within 15 minutes following injection. Although the proper dose has not been established in children, it is being used in controlled clinical situations. The most common adverse reaction is drowsiness, but allergic reactions and hypertensive episodes have occurred after administration. The recommended intramuscular dose is 0.5–1.0 mg/kg, with a maximum of 50 mg. The intravenous dose is 0.2–0.4 mg/kg with a maximum of 25 mg.

Other medications that have been used for chemotherapeutically induced nausea and vomiting include metoclopramide (0.3–0.5 mg/kg IV). This drug acts centrally on the chemoreceptor trigger zone as well as the gastric and esophageal smooth muscle. It potentiates gastric emptying by stimulating antral motility as well as increasing lower esophageal sphincter pressure and esophageal contractions. Its side effects include the drowsiness and extrapyramidal symptoms found with the phenothiazines. Because of this overlap, these two drugs should not be used concomitantly. Another investigational drug, domperidone (1.0 mg/kg IV) acts like metoclopramide but is reported to have fewer side effects. In preliminary studies, the active constituent of marijuana, delta-9-tetrahydrocannabinol, has also been shown to be effective in emesis related to chemotherapy. The antipsychotic tranquilizers, such as haloperidol, also may be associated with extrapyramidal reactions, but are reported to be of benefit in chemotherapeutic and radiation induced emesis.

Theophylline toxicity may present with headache, seizures, nausea, or vomiting. Approximately 90% of theophylline is metabolized by the hepatic P-450 microsomal enzyme system to four major metabolites. These metabolites plus the unmetabolized theophylline are excreted by the kidneys. A decreased clearance of theophylline has been reported in heart failure, cirrhosis, during therapy with erythromycin, and with influenza A or B infection. The mechanism in viral infection remains unclear but it is hypothesized that interferon, which is induced, may alter clearance by affecting the hepatic P-450 microsomal enzymes. For this reason children taking theophylline who develop a viral illness should be observed for theophylline toxicity, manifested by nausea and vomiting.

Toxins in food may cause self-limited episodes of vomiting. A reported outbreak of ciguatera fish poisoning was manifested by vomiting and diarrhea and resulted from fish contaminated with the dinoflagellate, *Gambierdiscus toxicus.*

Infection. Many acute infections, both viral and bacterial, are associated with nausea and vomiting. Rotavirus, which most frequently occurs during the winter months, commonly presents with vomiting as its first symptom but is also associated with diarrhea and upper respiratory tract symptoms. Approximately one fourth of gastroenteritis in neonates is caused by rotavirus. Although it is uncommon in the first 6 months of life, by 2 years of age over 60% of infants will have had an infection. Breast feeding or maternal antibodies do not seem to be entirely protective. Other viruses such as calicivirus may also cause acute vomiting episodes. Trimethobenzamide hydrochloride (Tigan) is frequently prescribed for nausea associated with gastroenteritis. A study with placebo as control showed that this antiemetic agent, which is supplied as 100 mg or 200 mg rectal suppositories, is not effective in controlling the vomiting of acute gastroenteritis. It may be beneficial in controlling the nausea.

Vomiting and nausea may also be caused by urinary tract infections, upper respiratory tract infections, hepatitis, pancreatitis, otitis media, or inflammatory bowel disease. Identification of the underlying problem will avoid unsuccessful symptomatic treatment.

Allergy. Allergies in infants may present with nausea and vomiting. These may be related to sinusitis with postnasal drip. Infants with cow's milk or soy protein intolerance may vomit when fed the offending antigen. Many of these children have an antritis that may delay gastric emptying and predispose to vomiting. Appropriate elimination diets may be beneficial but unnecessary restrictions need not be initiated if there is no clinical evidence to support this diagnosis. The vast majority of food intolerances resolve by 3 years of age, and persistence of symptoms should alert the physician to look for another etiology.

Pregnancy. "Morning sickness," or hyperemesis gravidarum may be quite debilitating in the early part of pregnancy. Pyridoxine (vitamin B_6), which is contained in the antiemetic Bendectin, may be of benefit. Although Bendectin has a long history of use during pregnancy, possible teratogenic effects are being investigated. To date, no conclusive evidence to support teratogenic effects has been reported.

Labyrinthine Abnormalities. Motion sickness or Meniere-like disorders are associated with nausea and vomiting. The presence of dizziness may alert the physician to one of these abnormalities. Antihistamines are the most commonly prescribed medications for motion sickness. The associated side effect, drowsiness, may improve the nausea by causing the child to lie down and relax.

Psychosocial. In the infant, a strained maternal-child or paternal-child interaction may result in stressful feeding situations and emesis. Overfeeding or a failure to pause during feeding may also cause intermittent vomiting. In children under 8 years of age, the pediatrician must be careful not to attribute recurrent vomiting to merely psychosocial issues. Children with gastroesophageal acid reflux and esophagitis may have secondary anxieties that manifest themselves as the major issue. In these situations medications merely obscure the underlying problems. The most successful outcome occurs when supportive attention is focused on understanding the nature of the stress.

Nausea and vomiting are symptoms that need explanation. Therapy depends upon the cause and although most children require limited symptomatic care, those whose symptoms fail to respond will require further investigation. In evaluating an infant or young child with vomiting, the clinician should always consider serious illnesses such as Reyes syndrome or meningitis, which can present with vomiting alone. In these illnesses, medication for control of emesis may be detrimental.

Constipation and Encopresis

MELVIN D. LEVINE, M.D.

Children are said to be constipated when defecation is inordinately difficult or when the event occurs too infrequently. Commonly the stools are hard and may be difficult to pass. While occasional periods of infrequent or difficult elimination are normal occurrences in childhood, *chronic* constipation can be a source of discomfort, inconvenience, and anguish. Longstanding retention of stool can lead to encopresis, in which a functional megacolon or megarectum develops secondary to obstipation, with resultant loss of control or fecal incontinence, commonly encountered in school children.

Most children with chronic constipation have no other organic pathology. However, in rare instances chronic constipation can be a sign of an anatomic, neurologic, or metabolic disorder. Possible are various forms of imperforate anus in the newborn, sometimes accompanied by vulvar or perineal fistulas. Atopic anus also can impair defecation. Myelomeningocele and other spinal cord defects commonly are associated with this disorder.

Although relatively rare, Hirschsprung's disease (aganglionic megacolon) is probably the most widely publicized neurogenic cause of constipation. It is particularly unusual to diagnose Hirschsprung's disease in a school-age child. Metabolic causes include hypocalcemia and hypothyroidism. Certain medications can cause infrequent bowel movements or hard stools. One example is methylphenidate (Ritalin), commonly used to treat attention deficits.

If all of the above organic causes of constipation are ruled out, it is inappropriate to assume that the problem is "psychogenic." Most cases represent neither organic nor psychiatric illness, but rather, a dysfunction, a bad habit, or a constitutional tendency toward sluggish bowel performance. Dietary factors may aggravate the process, but are seldom the sole cause.

MANAGEMENT

Newborn and Infancy. It is during the early months of life that the clinician must be most vigilant to possible anatomical causes of constipation that may require surgical intervention. In particular, Hirschsprung's disease may present at this time, often with symptoms of intestinal obstruction or necrotizing enterocolitis. The treatment of choice following appropriate diagnostic work-up generally is a colostomy followed by a pull-through operation late in the first year of life.

The newborn and infancy period also is a common time for symptoms of constitutional constipation to emerge. Treatment should be as noninvasive as possible, in order to prevent the induction of an "anal stamp," a permanent psychological scar associated with the later development of encopresis. The physician should emphasize to parents that the condition is benign, making every effort to minimize their anxiety. Frequent anal manipulations, such as digital disimpaction and the use of suppositories, should be discouraged. In mild cases, parents should be reassured and no therapy instituted. However, if the infant is uncomfortable and is producing consistently hard stools, one can add dark Karo syrup to feedings. Approximately 1–2 teaspooons per feeding generally is adequate. As the baby's diet becomes increasingly diversified, the need for such intervention diminishes. In rare cases, a mild laxative, such as milk of magnesia,may be needed. If so, use as little as possible (starting with ½ tsp a day).

Some infants have considerable discomfort on defecation. A mother may note that her baby constantly strains to have a bowel movement. In some instances, the infant is actually struggling *not to have one!* Such early evidence of voluntary withholding should be noted. Typically, the affected infant hyperextends his legs and clenches his fists while defecating. This may result from discomfort during bowel movements. The physician should ascertain that there are no problems in the perianal area causing painful defecation. The most common offender is chronic diaper dermatitis. Appropriate management of any such condition therefore is important in preventing habitual voluntary withholding.

The Toddler and Preschool Child. Training is the most critical event related to bowel function during this period. Some toddlers develop an aversion to defecation because of coercive or compulsively executed training. Improper training methods can result in constipation. For example, some children have difficulty defecating with their feet suspended in air. They can benefit from the use of telephone books or some other kinds of support while learning to use a toilet. Constipation related to training sometimes must be managed by postponing or modifying the training routine. Some toddlers and preschool children acquire an irrational fear of the toilet. Apprehension may center on the possibility of falling in or encountering "fish monsters" lurking in the bowl.

This can also be a time during which the manifestations of constitutional constipation seem to worsen. Treatment should remain nonaggressive, avoiding especially therapies that entail anal manipulation. Dietary alterations introducing high bulk foods (fruits, vegetables, bran-containing items) may be helpful. If this is ineffective, stool softeners should be given in small doses. Maltsupex is a palatable example. If this fails, small amounts of a mild laxative (such as Senokot granules, ½ tsp a day) can be instituted.

The School Years. There are many reasons why schoolchildren manifest chronic constipation. The phenomenon may be part of a continuing history of stool retention and poor bowel function that began in infancy or the toddler years. Or school itself may be an etiologic or at least aggravating factor. Some youngsters are reluctant to use school bathrooms because they lack privacy. They postpone defecation until safe, in the privacy of home. Some youngsters seem unable to "afford" to do this. That is, although they decline to use the bathrooms at school, they lose the urge when they get home. Over time, these children become constipated, and many develop a functional megacolon. Other schoolchildren acquire constipation because of a frenetic lifestyle. They race to meet the school bus each morning and are tightly scheduled all day. Homework, play, and alluring television shows occupy them until bedtime, leaving little time for something as trivial and uninteresting as defecation. Such children make relatively few trips to the bathroom and when they do their defecation is partial or incomplete because of their haste. Other

youngsters have significant attention deficits. These children are overactive, distractible, impulsive, and impersistent at tasks. They seldom finish anything they start, including defecation. They too ultimately develop chronic constipation.

An understanding of the pathophysiology of the schoolchild's bowel disorder can aid in counseling and management. Alterations in life style, provisions for more privacy of bathroom use in school, and various forms of behavior modification may be critical. In treating schoolchildren with chronic constipation, one should distinguish between those with the complication of incontinence (i.e., encopresis) and those who are fully continent.

SIMPLE CONSTIPATION (WITHOUT INCONTINENCE). Schoolchildren with uncomplicated constipation can be subdivided into those with overt symptoms and those with "occult stool retention." The latter group can be insidious and difficult to diagnose. Occult stool retention is one of the most common causes of recurrent abdominal pain. The diagnosis is often missed, since there may be no history of infrequent or hard stools. A plain supine x-ray of the abdomen in such instances reveals abundant retained feces, the removal of which often is associated with pain relief.

Most cases of uncomplicated chronic constipation can be alleviated by educating the child to use the toilet regularly and to remain in the bathroom long enough to achieve complete emptying. Laxatives such as senna (Senokot, 1 tablet a day) or danthron (Modane, 1 tablet a day) often are helpful. Treatment should be continued for 3–4 weeks. If symptoms persist, the child may benefit from the ongoing use of light mineral oil (1–2 tablespoons twice a day). In more severe or protracted cases, treatment may need to be more vigorous and long lasting. The regimen suggested for encopresis is recommended under these circumstances.

Encopresis. It is not unusual for schoolchildren with chronic constipation to develop encopresis. Varying degrees of severity are encountered, ranging from multiple large accidents per day to occasional bouts of incontinence or steady but slight leakage. Virtually all children with encopresis have at least intermittent constipation. Although emotional factors may complicate the picture, in most instances encopresis (like enuresis) is not caused by emotional factors. However, children who have suffered from this condition over a long period may become secondarily depressed, anxious, and socially withdrawn. Peer interactions, family harmony, self-esteem, and school performance can deteriorate as a result.

Most cases of encopresis ultimately resolve spontaneously; however, medical treatment can accelerate the cure and thereby diminish the suffering and psychological toll. Management of this condition can be divided into its component steps. The treatment is summarized in Table 1. The following is an elaboration on the steps involved:

1. DEMYSTIFICATION. The first step in treatment is education of the child and parents. The physician should explain normal colonic function, using drawings or diagrams. There can be discussion of the ways in which intestinal musculature propels stool; with consideration of the role of nerves within that musculature in providing signals indicating the need to defecate. It should be explained that some children go through a period when they do not completely empty their bowels. This results in the progressive accumulation of stool with the consequent chronic stretching of intestinal musculature and the loss of tone and strength. It also should be pointed out that the stretching results in diminished feedback from nerves, so that children fail to experience the urge or sensation of needing to move their bowels. A plain film of the child's abdomen can then be reviewed with the patient and parents. The physician

Table 1.

Treatment Phase		Treatment Program	Comments
Initial Counseling		1. Education and "demystification" 2. Removal of blame 3. Establishment and explanation of treatment plan	Include drawings, review of colonic function, joint observation of x-rays
Initial Catharsis	Inpatient	1. High normal saline enemas (750 cc bid) 3–7 days 2. Biscodyl (Dulcolax) suppositories bid 3–7 days 3. Use of bathroom for 15 minutes after each meal	Patient admitted when: 1) retention is very severe 2) home compliance likely to be poor 3) parents prefer admission 4) parental administration of enemas is inadvisable psychologically
	At home	1. In moderate to severe retention, 3–4 cycles as follows: a. Day 1–hypophosphate enemas (Fleet's Adult) twice b. Day 2–biscodyl (Dulcolax) suppositories twice c. Day 3–biscodyl (Dulcolax) tablet once 2. In mild retention, senna or danthron, one tablet daily for one to two weeks	1) Dosages or frequency may need alteration if child experiences excessive discomfort 2) Admission should be considered if there is inadequate yield
		Follow-up abdominal x-ray to confirm adequate catharsis	
Maintenance		1. Child sits on toilet twice a day at same times each day for 10 minutes each time 2. Light mineral oil (at least 2 tablespoons) twice a day for at least 6 months 3. Multiple vitamins, 2 a day, between mineral oil doses 4. High roughage diet 5. Use of an oral laxative (e.g., Senokot) for 1–2 mo daily in moderate or severe cases	1) A kitchen timer may be helpful 2) A chart with stars for sitting may be good for children under eight 3) Bathroom reading encouraged 4) Mineral oil may be put in juice or Coke or any other medium 5) Vitamins to compensate for alleged problems with absorption secondary to mineral oil 6) Diet should be applied, but not to the point of coercion
Follow-up		1. Visits every 4–10 weeks, depending on severity, need for support, compliance, and associated symptoms 2. Telephone availability to adjust doses when needed 3. In case of relapse: a. check compliance b. trial of oral laxative (e.g., Senokot) for 1–2 weeks c. adjust dosage of mineral oil 4. Counseling and/or referral for associated psychosocial and developmental issues	1) Duration of treatment program may be as long as 2–3 years or as short as 6 months 2) Signs of relapse: a) excessive oil leakage b) large caliber stools c) abdominal pain d) decreased frequency of defecation e) soiling 3) Physician should spend time alone with child 4) In cases slow to respond, physician should sustain optimism: persistence cures almost all cases eventually

All dosages and frequencies are calculated for an average-sized 7-year-old child. Appropriate adjustments should be made for smaller or larger patients.

can point out the accumulation of "rocks." It then is explained that the good thing about muscles is that they can be restored when they become weak. The treatment strategy is presented. It is pointed out that it is critical to begin treatment by establishing an entirely empty colon. After this, the goal will be to keep it as empty as possible over a period of months, so that the stretching can stop and the bowel can gradually return to its normal caliber, with restoration of muscle tone and feeling. It is important to point out that many other youngsters have this problem. A unique aspect of encopresis is that it is rare for any child who has it to have heard of any other who is similarly afflicted. Much anxiety can be relieved through demystification and the revelation that this is not an unusual condition. It also is helpful to emphasize that the problem is nobody's fault and that having it does not mean that a child is crazy, lazy, or immoral.

2. INITIAL CATHARSIS. A complete clean out is critically important at the beginning of treatment. In most instances this can be performed on an outpatient basis. In severe cases or when there is a very disturbed parent-child relationship, an inpatient program can be instituted. The components of these are summarized in Table 1. Following the initial catharsis the child should have a follow-up plain x-ray of the abdomen to establish that a good cleanout has been achieved. If this shows little or no improvement, the initial catharsis may need to be prolonged. If one begins a maintenance program following an incomplete cleanout, exacerbations are much more likely to occur.

3. MAINTENANCE. After the initial catharsis the youngster should be put on a laxative (Senokot, 1–2 tablets per day) or danthrone (Modane, 1–2 tablets per day). A stool softener should also be used. Most common and effective is light mineral oil. An average dose is about 2 tablespoons twice a day (for an average 7–8 year old). The flavor can be disguised with juice or soft drink. Light mineral oil should never be used when the bowel is impacted, since the lubricant itself is likely to leak around blockages, with the subsequent passage of a gold-colored liquid, which can be disconcerting as it streams down the legs of a schoolchild. In fact, if at any point during treatment excessive leakage of mineral oil is reported, one can assume that the youngster is again becoming retentive. In most cases after about a month of maintenance therapy, the laxative can be tapered off or discontinued. The stool softener should be continued for at least 6 months.

4. RETRAINING. A critical part of the treatment is retraining and toilet utilization. The child should be told to visit the bathroom twice a day at the same times eacy day, preferably after breakfast and supper. A minimum of 10 minutes should be spent therein. The youngster is told that he can read or listen to the radio, but he should try to empty out his bowel completely each time. In children under eight, it sometimes is helpful to set up a system of rewards, using a star chart, suitably embellished for each visit (with extra credit given for success).

It should be emphasized to parents that it is inappropriate to punish a child for having an accident. However, refusal to take medication or resistance to sitting on the toilet should constitute offenses. The child is not to blame for messing, but is to blame for not trying to do something about it. Following an accident a child should be required to clean himself. Underwear should be disposed of properly, although the child should not be expected to wash it, which could be interpreted as punitive.

For the child who soils himself in school, some arrangements may need to be made to provide a change of clothing in the nurse's office. Some youngsters may require a third visit to the bathroom, one that takes place in school. A sufficiently private setting for this should be sought. Most children feel strongly that they do not want school personnel to know about their problem, but most are agreeable to having one schoolperson aware of it. Their greatest fear is that peers will discover this most important secret. Therefore, every effort must be made to sustain their privacy.

5. FOLLOW-UP AND MONITORING. Encopresis is a chronic condition. The pediatrician should establish a strong alliance with the youngster and see him regularly (the frequency depending upon the severity and chronicity of the problem). During return visits, the physician should examine the child's abdomen and talk about management while alone with the youngster. There then can be joint discussions with parents. Medication needs to be "titrated." When exacerbations occur, laxative therapy should be increased or resumed. It is important that parents and the pediatrician be aware that in many cases several years are required for restoration of normal bowel function. Although this can be frustrating, persistence has its rewards. In severe treatment-resistant cases, the physician should periodically review the condition and consider the possibility of complicating psychosocial factors. Referral for a psychological or psychiatric evaluation may help, especially when the child seems to be noncompliant and unable to discuss the problem, or when there is evidence that serious family problems are interfering with management. Surgical consultation should be sought in treatment-resistant cases in which aganglionic megacolon is suspected. However, the latter is extremely rare among schoolchildren, whereas slowly responsive encopresis is a common condition.

Acute and Chronic Nonspecific Diarrhea Syndromes

PEARAY L. OGRA, M.D.

Diarrhea as defined by an increased number or decreased consistency of stools is one of the most frequently encountered symptoms in infancy and childhood. The mechanisms underlying the expression of diarrhea are diverse, and some of these are summarized in Table 1.

ACUTE NONSPECIFIC DIARRHEA

Acute Nonspecific Gastroenteritis. This usually benign and self-limiting disorder occurs typically in the winter months in localized outbreaks. It is most commonly due to acute infections with rotaviruses; less frequently to the Norwalk agent and other small, round viruses. Therefore, a more appropriate term would be acute viral gastroenteritis.

Most symptomatic infections with rotaviruses occur in children between 1–12 months of age and the diarrhea usually lasts for 2–6 days. Therefore, it is most important to determine whether the child is dehydrated and suffering fluid and electrolyte imbalance. Replacement of water and lost electrolytes is the mainstay of therapy. Oral administration of fluid and electrolytes has been highly effective in correcting the losses, even in continuing diarrhea. Replacement should be encouraged during the initial phase of the disease to correct mild to moderate dehydration, unless vomiting precludes fluid replacement by such a route.

The following guidelines have been suggested by many scientific groups for the use of oral electrolyte-glucose solution. It is recommended to initiate oral therapy in patients with dehydration and hypovolemia (regardless of the cause or the level of serum sodium) with the *World Health Organization (WHO) oral rehydration solution,* containing 90 mmol/L sodium, 20 mmol/L potassium, plus base and glucose at 111 mmol/L (approximately 2%). The amount of oral fluids administered to each infant must be based on clinical estimate of fluid and electrolyte deficits. Maintenance of hydration may be accomplished by supplementary oral rehydration solution with ad lib breast feeding, by one part of plain (or flavored) water for two parts of WHO solution or with potassium-containing juices.

It has also been suggested that, if possible, a separate maintenance and prevention solution may be used which contains carbohydrates as glucose (111 mmol/L), sodium (50–60 mmol/L), potassium (20–30 mmol/L), chloride anions (30–50 mmol/L), and a base content of bicarbonate or citrate at 30 mmol/L. In general, it is prudent to limit the intake of daily volume of such solution to about 150 ml/kg. Additional fluid may be given as plain water.

If vomiting is a major component of gastroenteritis, it is recommended that any oral intake be withheld for a few hours and the child be observed closely. Subsequently, oral fluids may be attempted, initially with small amounts of syrup of Coca-Cola and later with electrolyte solutions such as Pedialyte, or decarbonated soft drinks. Once vomiting has subsided, more liberal amounts of fluid in increasing frequency, followed by solids such as soup, applesauce, strained carrots, banana, or gelatin can be offered.

Transient monosaccharide intolerance is not uncommon during acute viral gastroenteritis. Therefore, it is advisable to monitor the infant's feces for reducing substances. If carbohydrate intolerance is suspected, sugar should be eliminated from the diet or reduced to less than 3% for a few days. Lactase should be introduced after 5–7 days after the disappearance of diarrhea.

Antiemetics should be discouraged, since they may render the assessment of clinical deterioration or dehydration difficult. Antidiarrheal agents such as diphenoxylate with atropine sulfate (Lomotil), paregoric, or other anticholenergic drugs have no place in the management of acute viral gastroenteritis, and may, in fact, be potentially harmful. These agents should not be used in most patients with acute viral enteritis.

Although most cases of acute gastroenteritis will resolve with the conservative management outlined above, some patients will require hospitalization for intensive management of dehydration and fluid and electrolyte imbalance. These patients should be rehydrated with appropriate IV electrolyte solutions. Subcutaneous administration of fluids is strongly discouraged. Oral or parenteral antibiotic therapy must be avoided unless specific indications for their use are clearly documented.

Nonspecific Enterocolitis. Although a number of disease entities listed in Table 1 may result in intractable diarrhea in infancy, it is not uncommon in pediatric practice to be faced with a child whose diarrhea is not attributable to any recognizable cause. Such cases of intractable diarrhea have also been referred to as nonspecific enterocolitis. The syndrome manifests in infants under 3 months of age as protracted, severe diarrhea. The infants are often admitted to the hospital with the body weight below the weight at birth, are severely dehydrated, and are malnourished, often to the point of cachexia. Evaluation and clinical management is often frustrating. Severe malnutrition at this age has a profound impact on subsequent growth and development; thus the management of these patients must be very aggressive.

Following initial evaluation, extensive examinations should be avoided. Severe dehydration is often associated with fluid and electrolyte imbalances and is sometimes complicated by sepsis as a termi-

Table 1. POSSIBLE MECHANISMS OF DIARRHEA AND REPRESENTATIVE
EXAMPLES OF THE ASSOCIATED CLINICAL SYNDROMES

Increased Fluid and Electrolyte Transport	Decreased Absorption	Changes in Functional Surface Area	Osmotic Factors	Other Factors
Infections	Celiac disease	Short bowel syndrome	Overfeeding	Irritable colon syndrome
Bacterial				
Viral	Ileal resection	Malnutrition	Intake of nonabsorbable solutes	
Antibiotic associated				Toxins
Parasitic infestations	Pancreatic and hepatic disorders	Scleroderma		
Fungal				
		Endocrinopathies		
Immune deficiency disorders	Fistula	Hirschprung's disease		
Carcinoid and other neoplasms	Blind loop syndrome			
Inflammatory bowel disease	Malrotation			
Regional enteritis				
Ulcerative colitis	Malabsorption syndromes			
Necrotizing enterocolitis				
Nonspecific enterocolitis				
Whipple's disease				
? Food allergy				

nal event. Therefore, the first management goals are to restore blood volume and correct electrolyte abnormalities and acidosis. After the infant has been somewhat stabilized, a few of the most helpful diagnostic procedures should be done, such as blood and stool cultures, determination of reducing substances in the feces, and qualitative determinations of stool fat and fecal pH.

The principal goal of subsequent therapy should be to support the infant through a relatively long period (usually 3–6 weeks) of nutritional replacement. Although some physicians prefer to rest the bowel for a short period, it is recommended to undertake a trial of oral alimentation, especially in patients whose clinical condition seems to improve rapidly after initial correction of metabolic and electrolyte abnormalities. Oral rehydration solutions, described earlier, given every 2–3 hours with gradually increasing amounts would be appropriate during the first 48 hours. If no increase in fecal frequency has occurred after 72–96 hours of dextrose and water feeding, the diet may be changed to a readily absorbable formula from which milk proteins and lactose have been eliminated. Pregestimil or Cho-free should be tried at a 10 KCal/oz concentration in small volumes of 1–2 oz every 3–4 hours. During oral alimentation, supplemental fluid and electrolytes should be given intravenously to maintain physiologic fluid and acid-base balance. If tolerance to oral feeding is good, increasing quantities and concentrations of the formula can now be given.

During oral alimentation, the infant should be watched very closely. This is because many infants may exhibit early improvement, only to relapse with diarrhea and dehydration as the concentration and

frequency or oral feeding is advanced. In such situations, it is recommended to return to small amounts of original well tolerated oral formula, and to supplement it with peripheral alimentation. This can be accomplished by infusion of 10% dextrose, 5% crystalline amino acid solution (Travasol), to provide a daily intake of 65 cal/kg of body weight at a rate of about 120 ml/kg per day.

Persistence of diarrhea, failure to gain weight, development of hypoalbuminemia, and reappearance of metabolic abnormalities are indications for the institution of total parenteral nutrition and elimination of all oral intake. A variety of regimens of total parenteral alimentation have been proposed and are discussed in more detail elsewhere in this book. In general, preparations providing 120–125 cal/kg/24 hr in 150 ml/kg/24 hr of volume have been found to be satisfactory for nutritional replacement in these infants. Usually 3 to 4 weeks of parenteral therapy will be required before the host can replace lost nutritional reserves and restore damaged intestinal mucosa. This will be clinically evidenced by significant weight gain and improvement in symptoms. At this point, oral alimentation should be reattempted for 4 to 6 days, as described previously, before parenteral alimentation is discontinued. In view of the high risk of potentially life-threatening infections often associated with central venous catheters, it is recommended to provide parenteral alimentation largely via peripheral veins. Central catheters should be introduced only as a last resort when peripheral veins are no longer available, or in critically ill infants.

The use of antibiotics, cholestyramine, or corticosteroids is not indicated and in general is not helpful in influencing the course of the disease.

CHRONIC NONSPECIFIC DIARRHEA

Chronic nonspecific diarrhea, or irritable colon syndrome, is a benign symptom complex that may manifest as colic in the neonate or increased fecal frequency in a toddler or older child with or without recurrent abdominal pain. These children are otherwise normal and exhibit normal growth and development, with no evidence of dehydration, malabsorption, or metabolic alterations. The syndrome can be a life-long condition and may manifest at any age. Most patients are between 8 months and 4 years of age, and have 4–8 loose stools per day. Most are in the second year of life and not yet toilet trained. The feces are loose, often foul smelling and mucoid. Stools will often contain undigested food particles. While some children may suffer a transient episode lasting a week or several months, others will continue to have loose stools intermittently or continuously for years. However, most patients appear to become asymptomatic after 3½ to 4 years of age.

No specific therapy is available. Counseling and reassurance of the parents based on repeated demonstration of normal growth and development during follow-up visits are usually adequate to allay their anxiety.

Assumption of upright position after feeding, introduction of chilled foods or low fiber diets, and bouts of infection or stress may aggravate the diarrhea. As a result, it may be appropriate to avoid chilled and hyperosmotic diets. However, dietary manipulations should be *carefully monitored* in order to avoid potential compromise of the child's nutrition.

Encouragement of early toilet training in young symptomatic subjects may also be quite helpful. Evidence suggests that the mouth to anus transit time for the ingested foods is increased in patients with irritable colon syndrome. Intake of high fiber, high residue diet and limiting oral stimulation by curtailing between-meal snacks in older children may be of considerable help in reducing the frequency and correcting the consistency of stools. Some patients with refractory and troublesome clinical manifestations have shown marked improvement with the oral use of cholestyramine.

Intractable Diarrhea of Infancy

THOMAS M. ROSSI, M.D.

Diarrhea in early life may be life-threatening if not promptly and properly managed. In addition to the immediate consequences of dehydration, acidosis, and electrolyte imbalance, less than adequate therapy may lead to a self-perpetuating and protracted state in which malabsorption of nutrients compromises the infant's nutritional status.

The syndrome of intractable diarrhea of infancy (IDI) has been arbitrarily defined as diarrhea, irrespective of its etiology, occurring in the first 3 months of life and persisting longer than 2 weeks. The mortality rate in the past has been high (45%) and "heroic" measures such as colectomy, ileostomy, and use of corticosteroids were of no benefit. Although older infants may suffer a similar syndrome, the definition emphasizes that young infants are more prone to the devastating effects of chronic diarrhea. The small-intestinal mucosa in young infants is more susceptible to injury and takes longer to recover from injury than in older children and adults. This may partially explain the greater susceptibility of infants to protracted diarrhea.

Typically, infants suffering from IDI present with similar histories and findings on physical examination. The diarrhea occurs shortly after birth. After several days of diarrhea, consultation with a physician is obtained. The infant is then gradually advanced from an oral electrolyte solution to dilute and hypocaloric formula and finally to a full strength (20 cal/oz) formula. This process may take several days to a week to complete. The practice has evolved, in part, from the finding of transient disaccharide malabsorption following acute infectious enteritis. In most infants, the diarrhea abates. However, in some this practice fails; the refeeding process is then repeated with a different formula. At times the infant is hospitalized and refed. Thus, insufficient calories may be provided for extended periods, weight gain ceases, and a gradual deterioration in nutritional status ensues.

On physical examination, nonspecific and variable degrees of marasmus are noted. The loss of subcutaneous tissue is striking. The ribs and vertebral column are prominent. Wasting of the extremities and buttock region is noted. Weight on admission approximates birth weight. Despite chronic malnutrition, the infant is most often biochemically well adapted to his condition. However, anemia, hypoalbuminemia, and abnormalities in serum electrolytes may occur. Stool cultures generally fail to reveal pathogens. The presence of reducing substances and an acidic pH confirm disaccharidase deficiency and carbohydrate malabsorption.

As IDI is a syndrome and not a disease, many entities are capable of initiating it. However, most act through the common pathophysiologic mechanism of injury to the small intestinal epithelial brush border area, resulting in disaccharidase, dipeptidase deficiency and impairment of transport mechanisms. Following injury to the epithelium, irrespective of the initial result, the same pathophysiologic chain of events follows. The subsequent malabsorption of nutrients leads to energy insufficiency, which impairs mucosal regeneration, ultimately adversely affecting pancreatic function and allowing bacterial overgrowth. A vicious cycle of self-perpetuating diarrhea is established.

The initial evaluation of an infant with diarrhea must therefore take into consideration the following: 1) the limited caloric reserves of young infants and their propensity for developing chronic diarrhea and malnutrition; 2) their need for adequate nutrition for growth and development; and 3) the fact that small intestinal mucosal injury and disaccharidase deficiency underlies most cases.

Keeping in mind the above considerations, our approach to an infant with diarrhea will depend on the stage in the progression to malnutrition that the infant exhibits. If the diarrhea is of a few days' duration and weight loss is not evident, a trial of dilute formula may be tolerated. Since small-intestinal mucosal injury underlies most cases, functional as well as anatomical disruption of the brush border occurs. Formulas consisting of complex carbohydrates, fats, and proteins require mature epithelial cells with intact digestive and transport systems for digestion and absorption. Not surprisingly, reintroduction of formula fails in some infants. If the diarrhea continues or malnutrition is evident, a semielemental diet such as Pregestimil should be used. Such formulas require minimal intraluminal and mucosal surface digestion, as they contain short polypeptides, short polymers of glucose, and a mixture of medium-chain and long-chain fatty acids. They are ideally suited for infants with small-intestinal mucosal injury.

To be deplored is the practice in which infants with intractable diarrhea undergo multiple attempts feedings at formulas containing similar complex carbohydrates, fats, and protein. Such multiple interchanges lengthen the course of the illness. During repeated trials with dilute (hypocaloric) formula, the infant may receive insufficient calories for extended periods. We therefore feel that Pregestimil should be used early in the course of diarrhea in young infants.

Infants who fail to show adequate weight gain or resolution of diarrhea while receiving adequate caloric intake in the form of a semielemental diet, should receive parenteral nutrition. The time period that one should observe the infant before instituting parenteral nutrition (PN) will vary according to the severity of the diarrhea and the state of nutritional debilitation. Careful, close monitoring is necessary. The clinical status of the infant, daily weights, fluid balance, serum electrolytes and acid base status, and also estimations of stool volume, pH, and reducing substances are necessary to help in the decision for the use of PN. The nutritional state of these obviously malnourished infants should not be allowed to deteriorate.

PN should be instituted without hesitation. Alimentation via central vein is most successful in restoring the nutritional status of the infant. Infants tolerate well a total fluid volume of 190–200 ml/kg/day. A dextrose solution of 20% containing 2.5–3.0 gm/kg/day of amino acids with added vitamins and trace minerals is the ideal solution. A 10 or 20% lipid solution is also available to provide calories in a concentrated form and also essential fatty acids. This is usually given in the amount of 1–2 gm/kg/day.

PN is generally continued until the patient's weight is restored to a value proportional to his height as recorded on the standard growth curves. While receiving PN, the patient should also receive small amounts, i.e., 1 oz, of Pregestimil 3 to 4 times a day. This should maintain the patient's interest in feeding and provide possible trophic factors through physiologic stimuli for mucosal regeneration associated with feedings. As the patient approaches ideal body weight, the volume and concentration of the semielemental diet can be gradually increased, with a concomitant proportionate decrease in the hyperalimentation rate. During the period of PN one can complete the diagnostic evaluation in search for the etiology of the diarrhea. A continuation of diarrhea while the patient is receiving PN should make one consider secretory diarrhea. The finding of a stool chloride concentration of > 90 mEq/L would confirm this suspicion. Causes of secretory state include bacterial toxins, tumors, and primary bile acid malabsorption. In the absence of a state of secretory diarrhea, one should pursue the long list of anatomic, metabolic, and pancreatic insufficiency entities that are capable of initiating the syndrome. In individual cases, small-intestinal biopsy, culture of duodenal fluid, and assessment of pancreatic enzymes may help.

If PN by the central route is not available, infants with IDI have been helped with peripheral alimentation using a 12% dextrose solution. One also has the option to add calories by giving Pregestimil via continuous nasogastric infusion.

As infants with IDI may show delayed healing of the small-intestinal epithelium, the semielemental formula should be continued exclusively for a period of 2–4 months. Thereafter, gradual advancement to a soy protein formula containing glucose polymers can be attempted.

Since the advent and use of elemental diets and PN by an approach such as outlined above mortality rate has been drastically reduced from the 45% stated previously to <5% in most reports. Follow-up studies indicate that when nutritional supportive measures are instituted early in the course, the weight and height velocities of affected infants can be expected to excel.

Irritable Colon Syndrome

MURRAY DAVIDSON, M.D.

The irritable colon syndrome remains imprecisely defined. For this discussion it is assumed to be a lifelong condition manifesting itself differently at different ages. In adults any one of three distinct patterns predominates in a particular individual: recurring constipation and severe abdominal pain, painless diarrhea, or alternating constipation and diarrhea. In children each of these three symptom complexes is most frequent in a specific age group, although there is some overlap. Painless diarrhea is usual between 6 months and 3 years of age. Recurrent abdominal pain most often presents between 3 years of age and adolescence. Alternating constipation and diarrhea are common in the adolescent but, as in adults, any of the three patterns may be experienced. Appropriate treatment for each age group is described here.

Nonspecific Diarrhea. Although not a serious disease, manifestation of the irritable colon as the nonspecific diarrhea syndrome requires appropriate management in the young child. The loose stools are *not* associated with food intolerances or malabsorption. Management should be with a full diet. In recent years it has been stressed that increasing the fat in the diet may be useful. Although this is certainly indicated in patients who are on low fat diets, it is not necessary to feed an increased amount of fat to children who are taking complete, balanced diets.

It is important that the mechanism of the diarrhea be explained and that parents be reassured that the condition is benign and self-limited. Exacerbations are related to episodes of physical stress such as teething, respiratory infections, and reactions to immunizations. The condition is associated more with an underlying tendency to constipation than with diarrhea. The loose stools do not pose the danger of dehydration or failure to thrive if a full diet is taken. There is no place for drug therapy in this condition, except for that directed against a concomitant infection, which may represent the inciting cause of the loose stools. Diodoquin, formerly prescribed in children and adults with the condition, has been demonstrated to be toxic to the eye and is contraindicated. Some suggest that psyllium seed, agar, or bran preparations may be helpful but additional data, acquired in controlled fashion, are necessary.

Abdominal Pain Group. Chronic recurrent abdominal pain (RAP), represents part of the continuum of symptoms in the irritable colon syndrome. The pain usually is restricted to the periumbilical area but sometimes may occupy either lower quadrant of the hypogastrium. It may be crampy and be present for much of the time, or it may occur as intermittent, griping spasms lasting for minutes to hours. The pain is sometimes difficult to distinguish from the pain of inflammatory bowel disease, which is more likely to be associated with weight loss, occurrence during the night, and changes in the blood count and erythrocyte sedimentation rate. These symptoms are usually absent in the irritable colon patient.

Management follows three broad principles. Foremost is reassurance of the patient and parents that the condition is not organic. It is extremely important that parents be reassured that the physician is not being casual. A careful history is taken, the patient is examined thoroughly, and the formulation and need for minimal work-up are explained deliberately and with sensitivity. However, excessive unnecessary and invasive studies beyond a routine urinalysis, blood count, screening chemistries, and erythrocyte sedimentation rate often cause the patient and family to fix on the possible organic origin of the symptoms and may make subsequent treatment more difficult.

A second aspect of management concerns discovery of possible upsetting features. The controversy about the relative importance of exciting factors vs the patient and his receptor organ is long standing. Some insist that the nature and degree of the irritating stimulant are of prime importance in the genesis of symptoms. Proponents of this view argue that virtually any individual may develop the clinical picture of the irritable colon syndrome if exposed to enough disappointment, anxiety, stress, or other exciting factors. Others hold that only certain individuals who are predestined congenitally or by conditioning may suffer these symptoms. They believe that, just as emotionally upsetting situations are not causative in inflammatory bowel disease, upsetting stimuli do not lead to the irritable colon syndrome. Nevertheless, aggravating environmental factors do exacerbate symptoms and produce dysmotility once an organic intestinal condition is present. They also do so in individuals with a predisposition to the irritable colon syndrome.

The physician must be sensitive to possible relationships between exciting factors and symptoms in the patient. It is important to evaluate the home situation, school situation, and relationships with friends and siblings. We find it useful to interview the mother and patient separately from one another at the initial visit. One may uncover possible areas of difficulty that each is reluctant to discuss in the presence of the other. Sensitive handling, support, and suggestions for relief of exacerbating factors follow from understanding by the doctor.

A third area of importance lies in attempting to limit the degree of rectal spasm and gaseous distention. It is best to do so via training to a regular daily bowel habit, a maneuver that may be difficult to accomplish. In patients with an underlying tendency to constipation, it may be necessary to employ a variety of adjuvants.

The child is instructed to attempt a regular 15 minute session on the commode following breakfast each day. If the patient is unable to evacuate with this maneuver despite attempts and willingness to do so, the bulk and softness of the stool are increased. Methylcellulose or psyllium seed preparations such as Metamucil are prescribed in the usual dosage before bedtime. Bran muffins or wafers containing added fiber may be substituted or added. Where this maneuver to increase bulk does not meet with success after a number of weeks, 1 or 2 ounces of plain mineral oil are added at bedtime to further ease passage of the morning stool. In very resistant cases a rectal suppository may be inserted each morning to stimulate regularity.

The treatment is continued with the addition of as many of these agents as are necessary for regular success over a period of a number of months. Stress is placed on achieving the complete evacuation each morning with only rare necessity for additional bowel movements during the day. Once this pattern has been achieved, the adjuvants are individually removed over a period of 3 to 6 months. If the treatment has been successful, the child should be able to continue to evacuate spontaneously each morning without artificial stimuli other than simple dietary modifications to increase bulk. This development of regularity is frequently important to prevent return of symptoms of RAP.

Acute bouts of pain are managed during all phases of the treatment by applications of a heating pad to the abdomen or immersion in a tepid bath. In some instances it may be necessary to relieve rectal spasm more directly by insertion of a suppository or rectal tube.

Alternating Constipation and Diarrhea. The adolescent most often suffers this pattern. Abdominal pain usually occurs during episodes of constipation and is located in the hypogastrium, as opposed to the periumbilical site complained of more by younger children. Intake of food or cold liquids frequently aggravates the pain; a bowel movement or the passage of flatus usually relieves it. In the alternate episodes of diarrhea, stools are semiliquid and contain considerable mucus, and sometimes consist almost entirely of mucus. Passage of stools is frequently an early morning phenemonon, and a number of disturbing periods of urgency may be experienced before and after breakfast. There may also be bowel movements in the early evening. The frequency and duration of the constipation and diarrhea episodes is variable.

Work-up is slightly different from that described for younger children. The older adolescent might require and tolerate more diagnostic studies. Anoscopy or sigmoidoscopy can be performed without preparation in patients with diarrhea in order to culture the adherent mucus and stool and to examine for possible amebae. Additional stool specimens should be cultured and examined for bacterial pathogens and amebae. Barium enema is usually not necessary but may prove useful if questions arise from equivocal findings in the sigmoid studies, blood counts, chemical screens, and/or erythrocyte sedimentation rates. A small-bowel series may be necessary to rule out Crohn's disease in the face of significant weight loss or other suggestive symptomatology. Lactose tolerance tests are also indicated in adolescents who have had bloating and diarrhea following ingestion of milk or milk products.

A major management feature consists of not allowing the adolescent to believe, at this critical stage of awakening self-identification, that the physician is disinterested. Reassurance of the parent is most important, but the adolescent is much more vulnerable if not personally reassured of the lack of organic bases for symptoms. Many adolescents take life very seriously, are often pessimistic and preoccupied with their symptomatology, and do not easily accept what they perceive to be unfounded reassurances. They are particularly suspicious of physicians who appear not to believe in the existence of their symptoms and who may imply that the youngsters are overly "nervous" without really being sick. This is viewed as rejection and is a patient turnoff. On the other hand, most adolescents welcome straightforward reassurance that they do not have serious, life-threatening disease from an individual who, from appropriate attention to the problem, has established his sensitivity, credibility, and a caring attitude. In some instances the environment may need to be altered to avoid stress, but this is usually not possible. Establishment of a supporting relationship with the physician with continued opportunities to ventilate may help the patient appreciate that relief of tensions in sports and other appropriate enjoyable avocations is helpful. A limited number of patients may be so seriously neurotic that psychiatric referrals are necessary.

Symptomatic relief may result from removal of some foods known to cause excessive distention and flatus, e.g., onions, carrots, beans, and cabbage. Lactose-containing foods may need to be withheld if a positive lactose tolerance test has been obtained. Food intolerances reported by patients should be tested for with repeated controlled feedings and withdrawals and these foods should be restricted when the relationship of symptoms with such empiric tests appears to be positive. Cold liquids should be avoided at times of severe symptoms. Application of heating pads and warm baths at times of pain may give prompt relief.

The measures described above for the development of a regular bowel habit should be carried out. In adolescents it may be possible to incorporate regular use of the psyllium seed preparations or bran in the diet to improve the general digestion. However, individual requirements for bran are variable and sufficient doses may be difficult to achieve in the patient with the irritable colon syndrome. Only doses large enough to ensure adequate bowel movement are useful. Small amounts often produce bloating and increased flatus, and are therefore frequently worse than none at all.

Recurrent Abdominal Pain

JAY A. PERMAN, M.D.,
and MELVIN B. HEYMAN, M.D.

Treatment of abdominal pain recurring at least monthly over a period of 3 or more months requires an organized and often time-consuming approach. The inconsistent and vague nature of the child's pain, which can be severe enough to interfere with daily activities, may lead to extensive and frequently unrewarding diagnostic investigations. Management must therefore begin with a carefully considered diagnostic evaluation. A thorough history, including home and social interactions, and physical examination are essential. It is estimated that only 10–15% of patients have a diagnosable organic cause of the symptoms, but this percentage may increase as diagnostic modalities improve. Thus, consultation with a pediatric gastroenterologist may be helpful if specialized testing is indicated.

Once a specific organic etiology is excluded, the goal of therapy is to return the child to a normal life by relieving symptoms and alleviating their effects on daily activities. Cessation of symptoms is the primary challenge. A review of the history, physical examination, and supporting laboratory data forms the basis for educating the entire family, including the patient, that while the pain is *real*, there is no associated physical abnormality. In particular, reassurance must be given that certain entities that the family and patient may fear, such as cancer or ulcers, do not account for the pain.

The process of educating and reassuring the patient and family usually evokes trust and confidence in the physician, permitting a change in the focus of the problem from the perceived pain to underlying emotional issues. Reduction of outside pressures and stress on the child is an important aim of the therapy. Opening lines of communication among family members is all that is needed in some cases of short duration. Psychological intervention is occasionally indicated, particularly when patients have associated behavior disorders or abnormal thought processes, and when parents have difficulty with discipline or their marriage.

Follow-up evaluations and family conferences to reinforce the initial treatment plan are very important. A physical examination during an episode of pain is especially significant in the reassuring process.

Medications have *no* role in the treatment of chronic recurrent abdominal pain of children.

Hospitalization is seldom required but may be useful to separate the patient from the family and environment. A brief hospitalization may also be helpful to observe the patient and perform specialized tests, if indicated, to exclude organic conditions.

Treatment requires diligence to exclude treatable disorders and persistence in dealing with patients and families. The benefit of treatment is supported by studies suggesting fewer relapses, shorter duration of each episode, and improved prognosis into adulthood when comparing treated versus untreated children with chronic recurrent abdominal pain.

Preoperative and Postoperative Care of Patients Undergoing Gastrointestinal Surgery

STEPHEN L. GANS, M.D.,
and EDWARD AUSTIN, M.D.

PREOPERATIVE CARE

In all instances, general preparation for gastrointestinal surgery includes correction of any depletions, such as fluid and electrolytes, blood components and coagulation factors, vitamins, and nutritives.

Preparation of the bowel itself depends on the site of the lesion (proximal or distal) and the presence or absence of an acute inflammatory process or obstruction. In the patient undergoing gastric or upper intestinal surgery who is without inflammation or obstruction, simply withholding feedings for 8 hours (in the neonate, 4 hours) is adequate. A nasogastric tube is placed in the stomach before induction of anesthesia.

When acute inflammation is present, peristalsis is diminished or has ceased, and fluid and air collect in the bowel—much as when a true mechanical obstruction exists. Under these circumstances the bowel should be decompressed by passing a nasogastric tube into the stomach as soon as the condition is known. This is best accomplished by using as large a tube (well lubricated and with several holes near its end) as will pass through the nares a measured distance into the stomach. The tube should be connected to intermittent suction and should be irrigated every 2 hours with a measured amount of normal saline (10 ml in the neonate, 15 or 20 ml in the older child) to ensure patency, and its position adjusted if the irrigating fluid is not returned. A tube that is not working is more harmful than no tube at all. It should not be plugged while the patient is being transported for x-rays or to the operating room. Small infant feeding tubes are not adequate for gastric decompression.

Before elective lower intestinal surgery the patient should be placed on a liquid diet for 3 days. Fecal residue in the colon is removed by warm normal saline enemas at this time. This should be the responsibility of experienced personnel. Retained stool makes surgery more difficult and more dangerous. The addition of antibiotics, either directly to the bowel preparation or systemically, is helpful. A solution of 0.1% neomycin in normal saline should be given as an enema or stomal irrigation 3 times within the 24-hour period before surgery. A broad spectrum antibiotic, such as cephalothin or erythromycin, may be given IV for 3 to 5 days postoperatively as the degree of contamination indicates. Cultures of the stool before surgery and of the bowel lumen intraoperatively may help if postoperative infection occurs.

When an indwelling bladder catheter is necessary it is best introduced in the operating room where sterile conditions are more secure.

POSTOPERATIVE CARE

Only aspects of postoperative care pertaining to the gastrointestinal tract are discussed here; other features of general supportive treatment are covered elsewhere.

All tubes, drains, and postoperative enemas should be managed under the direction of a member of the operating team who knows the details of the operation and who is in a position to assess the condition of the bowel and the security of any suture line.

The first basic need is effective decompression of the stomach and intestines until normal peristalsis is present and an anastomosis is patent. The use of a nasogastric tube in the manner described under Preoperative Preparation is satisfactory in most instances of short duration. Suction or gravity drainage should continue until good peristalsis is audible and flatus is passed, or, when there is an anastomosis, for at least 3 days. When long-term decompression is anticipated and critical, gastrostomy should be considered at the time of surgery. This procedure and its management are discussed elsewhere.

Feedings may be started when decompression is discontinued. Progress is made from clear liquids to low residue diet to full diet for age as quickly as is tolerated by the patient.

In the absence of mechanical or neostomal obstruction, failure of the gastrointestinal tract to move gas in normal fashion within 72 hours postoperatively suggests adynamic ileus. Treatment consists of prolongation of decompression by the previously described methods, attention to possible deficiencies in fluids, electrolytes, blood or its components, and treatment of infection, respiratory problems, and any other complications. If there are signs of sepsis, compromise of intestinal viability, leakage or abscess, prompt surgical intervention is indicated.

Finally, in catastrophic problems involving the bowel, when it will not function properly over a considerable period of time, much benefit can be derived by the use of total IV nutrition while permitting the intestines to recover.

Differences of opinion exist as to either the value or possible complications of routine use of antibiotics following gastrointestinal surgery. Believing that the greatest harm comes from going to either extreme, we suggest the following. Cultures should be made at surgery from free peritoneal fluid and from any open intestinal lumen. Antibiotics should not be used routinely for most gastric and upper intestinal surgery, but should be more commonly considered for lower bowel surgery. When suppuration is present in the peritoneum, when excessive contamination complicates the procedure, when questionably viable bowel remains in the peritoneal cavity, or when a suture line is considered insecure, antibiotics should be used.

ILEOSTOMY

Ileostomy is commonly used in the treatment of ulcerative colitis, but it is also sometimes used in the neonate for such conditions as necrotizing enterocolitis, meconium ileus, atresia of the ileum, or Hirschsprung's disease involving the entire colon. A small plastic collecting bag is placed over the stoma at the conclusion of surgery. This not only assists in measuring the output, which at times is copious, but also protects the surrounding skin from the irritating effects of ileostomy drainage. If properly fitted and applied, the bag will adhere to the abdomen for at least 24 hours with no damage to the skin or stoma and will be accident-proof during that time.

Skin irritation, an ever-present threat, occurs in varying degrees of severity. There are many ways to cope with this problem, but all depend upon the degree of meticulousness with which the patient is treated. Before applying the collecting bag, the surrounding skin should be thoroughly cleaned with a mild soap and warm water or a commercial skin cleaner. A disc of Stomahesive is fashioned to fit closely around the stoma. Small spaces between the disk and the stoma should be filled in with Orabase or karaya paste to provide a watertight seal. Any cracks, wrinkles, or dimples in the skin are sealed to prevent leakage of the appliance. Protecting the skin this way from contact with the ileostomy drainage will prevent most skin problems.

Persistent raw areas or shallow ulcers are more difficult, because an appliance will not adhere properly to this type of skin. Anti-inflammatory ointments such as triomcinolone (Kenalog) are useful in such situations. Nystatin (Mycostatin) powder and triamcinolone with neomycin, gramicidin, and nystatin (Mycolog) cream are usefulantimonilial agents. A neglected ileostomy may be tortuous. It is necessary sometimes to place the patient in the prone position on a Bradford frame so that all discharges from the intestine flow directly into a pan underneath until healing is accomplished.

Although most children with ileostomies can eat a normal diet, some may have difficulties with certain foods. In general, low residue diets are tolerated the best: lean meats, liver, hard-boiled eggs, cottage cheese, rice, gelatin, simple sugars, cooked cereals, orange juice, clear soups, and some cooked vegetables. Avoid or use great care with cabbage, turnips, corn on the cob or whole kernel corn, onions, nuts, raisins, coconut, berries with seeds, highly spiced or seasoned foods, and large amounts of candy or sweets, especially chocolate.

Complications are better avoided than treated. Fistulas are usually the result of faulty application or fitting of the bag. Most strictures occur at skin level and respond to gentle daily dilatation with the finger. Minor degrees of prolapse or herniation may be controlled by the wearing of an elastic girdle over the appliance. More severe strictures, prolapse, or herniation may require surgical revision. Obstruction may be due to edema or may result from eating large amounts of high residue foods. Irrigation with warm normal saline using a soft rubber bulb syringe or Foley catheter will bring relief.

Accustoming a child to the presence of ileostomy and its care requires patience and forbearance. However, in most instances children respond in a manner that most adults would do well to emulate. Local ileostomy clubs are source of great technical aid and psychologic encouragement.

COLOSTOMY

Colostomy is used as a temporary bowel-decompressing or stool-diverting arrangement in infants or children with aganglionic megacolon, ectopic or imperforate anus or other anorectal anomalies, atresia or stenosis of the colon, or severe injuries to the anus or lower bowel. There are many different types of colostomies and the site and type will depend on the location and nature of the lesion being treated as well as on the definitive or reconstructive procedures planned for the future.

Many surgeons recommend waiting 24 or more hours before opening the colostomy, but we have had no complications, particularly in the newborn with relatively sterile stool, from making this opening immediately at the time of surgery. A plastic collecting bag and a suitable skin protector are applied, as in ileostomy care. Gas may collect in the bag and can be released by piercing the bag with a small pin. This transparent bag permits one to measure fluid or blood loss and to observe viability of the colostomy and onset of function without having to change dressings. It also seals fecal drainage from a nearby incision and helps prevent skin irritation.

The plastic bag may be discarded and replaced every day or when full. When the incision is healed and the stools are becoming formed, the plastic bag can be replaced by a strip of petrolatum gauze over the bowel end and covered with an ordinary diaper. Some parents prefer to use adherent plastic bags more or less permanently, as with ileostomy. Others simply handle the colostomy as an "abdominal anus" by using the usual cleansing and diapering techniques.

Care of Bowel and Colostomy Stoma

Satisfactory results may be brought about by widely differing methods. In many infants, no special handling is necessary, particularly if the colostomy is to be present for a short time only. In others, the skin quickly becomes irritated or breaks down unless meticulous care is given. This can be controlled through diet, irrigations, or local skin therapy, singly or in combination. Constipating or low residue diets, depending on age, will prevent constant soiling with its resulting irritation. Irrigation of the bowel thoroughly once daily or every other day, combined with the above mentioned diet, may result in no intervening spontaneous stools, thus allowing the skin to heal. The best local therapy is cleanliness. Acid soaps and a very dilute vinegar solution are better than alkaline soaps and tap water. Zinc oxide ointment should be applied for minor irritation; antimonilial (Vioform), antibacterial (neomycin), or anti-inflammatory (hydrocortisone) preparations should be used when indicated.

Occasionally the skin becomes inflamed because of bag adhesives or adhesive solvents, or by traumatic adhesive bag removal. Under such circumstances this method should be discarded, or at least the cement or solvent changed.

Tincture of benzoin painted over the area regularly will toughen the skin. A drying lotion (calamine) will help relieve itching. Bleeding from the stoma or mucocutaneous junction is common and can be easily controlled by applying a layer of petrolatum over the bleeding surface. More serious bleeding may require cauterization or electrocoagulation.

Stricture usually occurs at the skin level. This is not ordinarily a problem in the infant with soft stools and a temporary colostomy. In others, gentle daily dilatations will open the aperture to a satisfactory size. If it does not, surgical removal of a circle of skin and resuture of the mucosal margins is an easily accomplished maneuver.

Pylorospasm

HAROLD MEYER, M.D.

Pylorospasm should be considered when vomiting occurs in the young infant. In the management of this problem, historical data obtained should include maternal attitude, feeding technique, amount taken by the infant, and the amount vomited. Although the maternal-infant relationship must be thoroughly investigated, at no point during information gathering should the mother be made to feel guilty.

Relief of parental anxiety is of primary importance in bringing about a resolution of the problem. The parents should be reassured that the vomiting is self-limited and that the symptom can be controlled. Assurance should also be given that the infant's nutritional status will be carefully monitored by the physician. Unless milk allergy is strongly suspected, formula changes should not be suggested. Maintaining the infant upright after feeding has not been found to be beneficial.

Infants have been shown to respond to anticholinergic drugs, such as Bentyl syrup (dicyclomine hydrochloride)—5 mg before each feeding or every other feeding may be helpful—and Donnatal elixir (each 5 ml contains phenobarbital, 16 mg; hyoscyamine sulfate, 0.1037 mg; atropine sulfate, 0.0194 mg; and hyoscine hydrobromine, 0.0065 mg). The dosage of Donnatal for a 10-pound infant is 0.5 ml before every other feeding. As this preparation is an elixir, it should be diluted before administration.

Side effects of the drugs should be looked for most carefully, e.g., flushing of the skin and fever. The combination of parental support and anticholinergic drugs should bring about enough improvement to enable discontinuance of medication after 3 to 4 weeks of therapy.

Pyloric Stenosis

ROBERT T. SOPER, M.D.,
and KEVIN C. PRINGLE, M.B.,Ch.B.,F.R.A.C.S.

Pyloric stenosis is the most common surgically correctible cause for vomiting in babies between 3 and 12 weeks of age. Pyloromyotomy, its corrective operation of choice, is perhaps the most successful and trouble-free operation that surgeons perform. Therefore, although pyloric stenosis may be a self-limited disease, its nonsurgical treatment by lengthy hospitalization for nasogastric suction and parenteral fluids and nutrition is hardly ever justified.

The duration of symptoms prior to diagnosis usually dictates preoperative therapy. When diagnosis is established early after only a few days of occasional vomiting, the infant's metabolic status is normal and operation can be undertaken without delay or special preparation. However, in most cases there is significant dehydration with hypochloremic, hypokalemic alkalosis, which requires correction before operation can be safely undertaken. In the extreme, neglected case, hepatic exhaustion of glycogen makes hypoglycemia a threat; several days of preoperative parenteral nutritional and fluid and electrolyte support may be required.

Once diagnosis is established, the first order of treatment is to empty the stomach of its curdled milk or contrast material. The pyloric stenosis itself never completely obstructs the pyloric channel; rather, it significantly narrows the channel so that it is easily plugged by curds and barium particles. If the latter are removed by gavage, then gastric juices and even ingested clear fluids pass out of the stomach in a relatively normal fashion.

Gastric gavage can sometimes be satisfactorily achieved with saline irrigations and aspiration gently carried out through the largest size nasogastric tube that will fit through the nose. However, more often than not these relatively small sized tubes become plugged so easily as to defeat effective gavage. It is best to place the baby in a prone position (to prevent aspiration) and then to pass a 14 or 16 F Robinson catheter through the mouth and into the stomach, through which warm normal saline can be irrigated for effective gavage; all residual barium and particulate matter are removed from the stomach. Once a clear saline return is achieved, the tube is removed and the baby made NPO until either operation or nasogastric suction is instituted.

With the stomach empty, it is possible to correct the baby's metabolic problems by oral feedings of 5% glucose in 0.5 N saline with KCl added. This is offered every 3 hours, with the infant placed in the right lateral decubitus position for the first half hour after each feeding (to facilitate gastric emptying). Although effective in preparing a baby for operation, this technique usually requires an additional day or two in hospital to achieve a normal metabolic status.

In most hospitals, metabolic correction is achieved intravenously. We usually rehydrate the patient with normal saline given at a rate of 200–250 ml/kg per 24 hours. Ten mEq KCl/500 ml are added as soon as an adequate urine output is achieved. Two to three gm of glucose can be added to each 100 ml of fluid, but 5% dextrose should not be used for fear of producing hyperglycemia and an osmotic diuresis. When half of the baby's calculated deficit has been replaced, the fluid is switched to 0.5N saline in 5% dextrose with 10 mEq KCl/500 ml and the rate decreased to 150–180 ml/kg per 24 hours. In the average case, 12–24 hours is sufficient to restore the electrolytes and pH to normal and allow safe operation. In the severely depleted patient, this preparation period may reach 24–48 hours, perhaps with the addition of 10% glucose or plasmanate to help repair the nutritional deficits.

Operation is not scheduled until the baby is clinically rehydrated and metabolically normal. The classic Fredet-Ramstedt pyloromyotomy is the operation of choice. Although feasible to perform under local anesthesia, pyloromyotomy is technically much simpler with general anesthesia, provided that anesthesiologists skilled in anesthetizing young infants are available. The operation is carried out with the stomach empty and with appropriate temperature and other monitoring devices in place.

Postoperatively, the patient is maintained NPO for four hours and a graduated feeding program is started: Offer 1 ounce 5% glucose q 2 h times 4; then offer 2 ounces 5% glucose q 2 h times 4; then offer 2 ounces ½-strength formula q 2 h times 4; then offer 2 ounces full strength formula q 2 h times 4; and then offer ad lib formula feedings q 4 h.

After the ad lib feedings have been well tolerated for 12 hours, the patient is ready for discharge, usually about 48 hours after operation. All babies will vomit some, which should not be cause for alarm. However, if vomiting persists, the feedings are withheld for 12 hours before resuming the feeding schedule. If the mother is breast-feeding, expressed breast milk is substituted for the formula; the baby is taken to the breast when the ad lib feedings are begun. We believe that the intravenous fluids should be discontinued when the feeding program is begun, to allow easier handling of the baby and better burping techniques.

Postoperative wound infections are rare and wound dehiscences are almost unheard of. Morbidity and mortality following pyloromyotomy are well below 1%. However, there are two operative complications that would cause the physician to vary the postoperative routine. If the surgeon perforates the mucosa while performing pyloromyotomy, he will close the perforation by sutures. Postoperatively these babies should have effective nasogastric suction for 24 hours before the above feeding routine is begun. Should the pyloric muscle not have been completely divided, persistent vomiting may recur postoperatively, not unlike that seen before operation. Under these circumstances, nasogastric suction and parenteral fluids and nutrition should be continued and reoperation delayed for at least 7 days, by which time the symptoms have usually abated. Reoperation for incomplete pyloromyotomy has not been required in our large university hospital for at least 30 years.

Peptic Ulcers

PETER K. KOTTMEIER, M.D.

The present confusion concerning both operative and nonoperative treatment of gastroduodenal ulcers in infants and children is partially related to the assumption that all these ulcers are "peptic ulcers." A correct classification of gastroduodenal ulcers in children is important not only to identify the cause—if possible—but also to select the appropriate therapy. True "peptic ulcers" in childhood are similar to adult peptic ulcers. Another group of children have gastroduodenal ulcers that appear to be neither secondary to stress nor compatible with peptic ulcers. These are loosely grouped together as "acute primary ulcers."

Acute Primary Ulcers. In patients with mild to moderate bleeding, gastric lavage with saline and buffering with antacids or milk will suffice to stop bleeding in most instances. In infants, care should be taken not to induce hypothermia with iced gastric lavage. In acidotic infants, the gastric lavage solution should be either isotonic lactate or isotonic half saline and half bicarbonate to reduce, or at least not to increase, a metabolic acidosis. The administration of isotonic crystalloid solutions, blood, or colloid depends on the amount of blood loss. If the blood loss is significant, either whole blood or packed cells and volume expanders can be used as replacement. In most instances an over-replacement should be avoided, since this may reinitiate gastric bleeding that may have stopped prior to the overadministration of blood.

If the blood loss within 24 hours exceeds the patient's blood volume, or if massive recurrent bleeding occurs, surgery is usually indicated. Since there is no recurrence of the ulcer formation after successful therapy, the most conservative operative procedure necessary to stop the hemorrhage should be used, such as the simple oversewing of isolated ulcers or suture ligation of bleeders. In an occasional infant with diffuse gastric ulcerations, a resection may be necessary, however. The perforation in a patient with a primary acute ulcer is also usually treated successfully by simple closure with or without the use of an omental patch.

A unique type of neonatal ulcer leading to gastric perforations within several days after birth has also been called an acute primary ulcer. Aspiration of the intraperitoneal air will improve diaphragmatic excursion and therefore respiration. The isotonic hypovolemia should be corrected with an initial push of isotonic solutions. The peritonitis, although predominantly chemical at onset, should be covered with broad-spectrum antibiotics. The operative procedure consists of closure of the perforation. If the patient recovers uneventfully, oral feedings can usually be resumed after 5 to 7 days; there is no need for postoperative antacids or other medications.

Chronic Primary or Peptic Ulcers. These usually begin at school age and increase during the teenage years. They represent the childhood equivalent of the adult peptic ulcer. The primary therapy, usually successful, consists of antacids between meals and at bedtime. Either magnesium or aluminum hydroxide can be used. Magnesium hydroxide appears to be a more powerful buffer, but serum hypermagnesemia has been reported not only in patients with renal failure but also in neonates, with resulting cardiorespiratory depression. While this is a rare complication, its possibility should be kept in mind with prolonged administration. Sodium bicarbonate, even though a powerful buffer, is contraindicated in view of the resultant alkalosis. Cimetidine appears to be as effective in children as in adults. There is no proof that special bland diets are of any help; gastric irritants should be avoided, however, including alcohol, aspirin, coffee, tea, and cola-containing drinks. Psychologic assistance in children with overlying anxiety problems may be useful. Diazepam (Valium) has been used successfully in children with psychogenic problems and in children with stress ulcers who have underlying or associated anxiety problems.

As in the adult, there is no unanimity as to the "ideal" operative procedure for peptic ulcers in children. Many investigators emphasize that the natural course of the childhood peptic ulcer is more benign than that of the adult. They report the response to medical therapy to be prompt in most instances. If surgery is necessary, limited operations, such as vagotomy and pyloroplasty, are supposed to suffice. Other series, however, show equally convincingly that childhood peptic ulcers often extend into adulthood and are more difficult to treat in the child than in the adult. Based on increased experience in the adult with selective or highly selective vagotomy, with or without drainage procedure or limited resection, the present trend toward truncal vagotomy plus pyloroplasty in children may change.

The indications for surgery in children with peptic ulcers consist of massive or repeated hemorrhage, perforation, obstruction, and the difficult to define "intractability."

Secondary or Stress Ulcers. In certain groups of patients, such as children with burns or CNS lesions, prophylactic therapy has been shown to decrease significantly the incidence of stress ulcers. The early use of milk feedings, immediately after stabilization of burn patients, can reduce gastric acidity and provide needed calories. Oral or nasogastric tube feedings of milk are given at 100 to 200 ml/kg body weight for 24 hr in divided hourly doses. The stomach is emptied prior to the

nasogastric tube feeding to prevent aspiration. Diazepam (Valium), given orally at 6-hour intervals in burn patients, is thought not only to decrease anxiety in burned children, but also to reduce gastric acidity through a direct effect on the hypothalamus. The nonoperative therapy of stress ulcers is otherwise similar to that described in patients with acute erosive gastritis. In contrast to patients with AEG, in patients with bleeding ulcers arterial embolization can serve as either a temporizing or definitive procedure when the general condition prohibits even a limited operative intervention. Stress ulcers can occur in either stomach or duodenum or both areas simultaneously. The majority of bleeding or perforating stress ulcers requiring operative intervention, however, are located in the duodenum. Since there is no recurrence of the ulcer once the underlying stress has ceased, the most conservative operative procedure able to control either hemorrhage or perforation is preferred.

Zollinger-Ellison Syndrome. This syndrome, responsible for multiple duodenal or jejunal ulcers, does occur occasionally in childhood. Non-beta pancreatic islet cells are responsible for the increased gastrin output, leading to a high gastric acidity. The treatment is identical to that in adults: total gastrectomy with esophagojejunostomy.

Gastritis

PETER K. KOTTMEIER, M.D.

Infectious gastritis, viral or bacterial, is uncommon even in children with "gastroenteritis." Bacterial gastritis can occur, however, in children with massive sepsis, such as, for instance, in emphysematous gastritis, where the therapy is directed toward the underlying etiology. Chronic granulomatous disease also occasionally can involve duodenum and stomach. Therapy is supportive, with appropriate antibiotics. Surgery is rarely indicated.

Acute gastritis is most commonly seen after the ingestion of medication or other chemicals. The therapy for acute gastritis after aspirin ingestion consists of the correction of a possible associated coagulopathy, restriction or appropriate selection of oral intake, and the temporary use of gastric antacids. Alcohol-induced gastritis is also self-limiting, after the discontinuation of alcoholic intake and symptomatic treatment. Gastritis due to the ingestion of corrosive agents is almost entirely limited to the ingestion of acid solution, such as hydrochloric acid. The attempt of buffering the ingested acid with alkaline solution is useless, since the corrosive effect of the acid is almost instantaneous. The stomach should be put at rest with nasogastric suction after careful insertion of a nasogastric tube to avoid perforation. Diffuse necrosis with perforation is the most likely complication, requiring prompt operative intervention. Gastritis due to lye or alkali ingestion is extremely rare. If it occurs, it is usually associated with esophageal burns and should be treated accordingly: proof of the burn via endoscopy, followed by the administration of steroids and antibiotics for approximately 3 weeks with re-examination.

Chronic gastritis can occur as a protein-losing, benign, hypertrophic gastropathy similar to Ménétrier's syndrome in the adult. It is occasionally associated with cyclic vomiting, viral infections, or eosinophilia, suggestive of a hypersensitivity reaction. Hypoproteinemia and anemia are present in most patients. Therapy consists of the correction of hypoproteinemia, either by infusion of protein or a high protein and low fat oral intake. In contrast to the adult Ménétrier's gastritis, it is usually self-limiting in children, responding promptly to supportive therapy. Bile gastritis, sometimes seen in adults after gastric operations, is rare in children. It can occur after gastrointestinal surgery such as bypass operations or duodenal obstruction. The gastritis due to the exposure of gastric mucosa to bile salts may respond to therapy with cholestyramine, antacids such as aluminum hydroxide, or bethanechol chloride (Urecholine) to stimulate gastric emptying, which is usually delayed. If this fails, a duodenogastric diversional operation is usually indicated to eliminate gastric bile stasis.

Acute Erosive Gastritis (AEG). Although the etiology of AEG is similar to that of stress ulcers, pathologic changes, therapy, and prognosis vary considerably. Stress ulcers are often confined to a single, predominantly duodenal site. Even multiple ulcers are limited to localized areas without the complete and diffuse gastric involvement seen in AEG. Since AEG often occurs in patients undergoing recognizable or anticipated stress, as in postoperative patients or patients with burns or CNS lesions, the therapy should be prophylactic in many instances. Although gastric acidity in children under stress is not necessarily increased, the breakdown of apical mucosal integrity allows back-perfusion of even normal acid, with subsequent gastritis and ulcerations. The breakdown of the mucosal integrity may be related to the diminution of energy source in the stressed patient; part of the therapy consists, therefore, of restoration or maintenance of an anabolic state in the stressed patient, if necessary through parenteral hyperalimentation. To prevent back-perfusion of gastric acid, buffers, such as antacids, or histamine receptor blockers, such as cimetidine, are used individually or together.

In patients in whom AEG has occurred, often leading to life-endangering bleeding, the following therapeutic approaches can be used: nasogastric tube suction with intermittent iced saline irrigation until the stomach is cleared of blood clots, followed by the instillation of antacids on an hourly basis. An attempt should be made to keep the gastric pH at or over 4. This can be supported or accomplished by the use of cimetidine. Cimetidine, a histamine receptor blocker, reduces basal and stimulated gastric acid output. It is also assumed to protect mucosal blood flow during hypotension. There is some evidence to suggest that a continuous intravenous infusion of cimetidine is preferable to a bolus infusion or oral administration in patients with AEG. Again, an attempt should be made to keep the gastric pH at or over 4. If the pH cannot be stabilized, uncontrollable sepsis or multiple organ failure is usually present or developing, with an extremely poor prognosis.

Other attempts to control bleeding from AEG consist of the systemic or localized arterial infusion of vasopressors. Arterial embolization, occasionally effective in children with localized duodenal bleeding, is usually not indicated with AEG in view of the diffuse gastric involvement.

Failure of nonoperative therapy requires operative intervention. As in adults, there is no uniformity of opinion as to what operative procedure is the most suitable. In contrast to patients with localized stress ulcers, in whom the most conservative procedure is usually recommended, substantial gastric resection with truncal vagotomy may be necessary for children with massive AEG, not only to control bleeding but also to prevent a rebleeding.

Fortunately, the prophylactic use of either antacids or cimetidine to control the gastric pH has reduced markedly the number of patients requiring operative intervention.

Malformations of the Intestine

E. THOMAS BOLES, JR., M.D.

Most congenital malformations of the intestines become symptomatic because of intestinal obstruction; therefore, relief of the obstruction is the primary goal of therapy. A few result in bleeding or inflammation, and some are asymptomatic.

DUODENAL ATRESIA AND STENOSIS

The newborn with congenital duodenal obstruction requires appropriate preoperative correction of any fluid and electrolyte abnormalities that may have developed. Evident dehydration with or without electrolyte disturbances requires adequate replacement and correction preoperatively. One method is to administer an intravenous bolus of 10 ml/kg of isotonic fluid (e.g., Ringer's lactate) and follow this by fluid calculated at a rate of 125 mg/kg/24 hr of a hypotonic solution (e.g., 0.45 normal saline with addition of 30 mEq. of KCl/L).

The response of the infant is essential in guiding fluid management with attention to urine output, urine osmolality or specific gravity, hematocrit, and physical examination, including vital signs, presence or absence of pulmonary rales, and peripheral edema. A more detailed review of appropriate intravenous replacement and maintenance therapy is found in the article on that subject. The stomach and duodenum should be emptied of fluid and air and decompression maintained. For a full-term infant a 10 F catheter may be passed into the stomach via the nose, the stomach aspirated, and the catheter attached to a source of low suction. Five small holes should be cut in the distal 5 cm of this catheter, and the most proximal hole should be above the diaphragm. Exact positioning of the catheter is important and may require an x-ray. Antibiotic therapy is unnecessary for the uncomplicated case.

The operation is most easily and safely performed under general endotracheal anesthesia with appropriate monitoring of pulse, heart sounds, blood pressure, and core temperature. Placement of the baby on a warming blanket, plastic drapes around the trunk, wrapping the extremities with sheet wadding, a cloth cap over the head, and the use of radiant heat lamps all are helpful in preventing hypothermia during the operation; the ambient temperature of the operating room should be at 75 to 80°F. Of course, intravenous fluid administration should be continued during the procedure.

A right upper quadrant transverse incision just above the umbilicus provides excellent exposure. It is not necessary and is undesirable to eviscerate the intestines. The right colon is mobilized and displaced to the left to expose the duodenum, and a Kocher maneuver is performed. This permits precise identification of the atretic or stenotic area. Gastrointestinal continuity is restored by duodenoduodenostomy. A very satisfactory technique is to make a transverse incision through the proximal duodenum and a vertical incision of the same length through the duodenum just distal to the obstruction, and to fashion the anastomosis with a single layer of interrupted 5–0 silk sutures. The possibility of a mucosal web originating proximal to the terminal end of the dilated proximal duodenum should be kept in mind. If such a web is missed and the anastomosis is done distal to its origin, obviously the obstruction will not be relieved. After the incision through the end of the proximal duodenum has been made, a hemostat can be passed through this opening into the stomach and out through a gastrotomy on the anterior wall of the stomach. Free passage ensures that a web is not present. If a web is present, it will reject passage of the hemostat. A gastrostomy tube is placed into the stomach and led out through a stab wound in the left epigastrium after the anastomosis has been completed.

Postoperatively the infant is returned to an isolette with appropriate humidity and temperature control. Intravenous water and electrolyte replacement is maintained. The nasogastric tube is removed the day following operation and the gastrostomy tube connected to a straight drain. Usually after 2 or 3 days the gastrostomy tube may be elevated and gastric residuals measured at 8-hour intervals. Usually the anastomosis opens up satisfactorily within 4 or 5 days and oral fluids may be started. The oral feedings are slowly progressed to an amount sufficient for maintenance of adequate hydration, and then progressively changed to a low-curd formula. Occasionally the anastomosis fails to open sufficiently within a week, and under these circumstances total parenteral nutrition should be started and maintained until full enteral feedings are tolerated.

Relief of the duodenal obstruction is excellent, and mortality and morbidity are low in uncomplicated patients. However, associated anomalies including Down's syndrome, cardiac defects, esophageal atresia, and imperforate anus are common and often multiple; so that the overall mortality of these babies is high.

MALROTATION AND VOLVULUS

Malrotation in an infant with intestinal obstruction is a surgical emergency because of the strong likelihood of associated volvulus. Often the diagnosis is made in the first few days of life, but in some the condition may not become apparent until later in infancy or in childhood.

Preoperative preparation depends on the status of the child. In the infant without peritoneal signs or indications of sepsis or hypovolemia, the preparation is similar to that for an infant with duodenal atresia except that antibiotics should be started preoperatively. Ampicillin and gentamicin are recommended. If the infant shows clinical or radiologic signs of volvulus, fluid resuscitation should be more vigorous and started with a "push" of 20 ml/kg. Metabolic acidosis is often present, and the addition of sodium bicarbonate in dosage appropriate to the intravenous regimen is required. In any event, resuscitation should be done promptly and vigorously, so that the infant can be brought to the operating room within an hour or two in satisfactory hemodynamic status.

Under general endotracheal anesthesia the abdomen is opened through a transverse incision as with duodenal atresia, except that the incision should be extended to the left with division of both rectus muscles. Volvulus is readily apparent, since only loops of small intestine are initially apparent and the colon cannot be seen. It is essential to eviscerate the small intestine. This will disclose the base of the mesentery and the volvulus itself. Reduction of the volvulus requires counterclockwise rotation of the small intestine one to three complete turns. After the volvulus has been corrected, and in the absence of devitalized gut, the usual anatomy found is an unattached right colon with a narrow mesenteric pedicle of the midgut. The ascending colon and the distal duodenum will be fused on their antimesenteric surfaces by a peritoneal band. This band is divided, and the ascending colon with its mesentery and the distal duodenum (often with some proximal jejunum) and its mesentery are carefully separated in a fashion analogous to opening the pages of a book. This results in displacement of the distal duodenum and proximal jejunum to the right and the proximal colon to the left. A catheter should be passed down the length of the duodenum to exclude a possible intrinsic mucosal web obstruction. This can be done by manipulating the nasogastric tube distally, or alternatively can be done through a gastrotomy. An incidental appendectomy is usually performed but a gastrostomy is unnecessary. Postoperatively, intestinal function returns to normal within 2 or 3 days. Antibiotics are discontinued 24 hours postoperatively if there is no evidence of intestinal vascular compromise.

If the intestine shows evidence of significant vascular compromise, management is more complex. It is helpful in the interim between detorsion of the volvulus and determining viability to return the midgut to the peritoneal cavity. If it is clear after an appropriate period of observation that a relatively short segment of intestine is devitalized, it should be resected. Depending on the status of the remainder of the gut and of the baby itself, either primary anastomosis or exteriorization with later anastomosis can be done. If a long segment or virtually all of the small intestines involved in the volvulus appear severely compromised, the abdomen is closed and a "second look" laparotomy performed 24 hours later. In some instances, at the second operation bowel that previously appeared gangrenous will be viable, and a limited resection will be possible that will permit the infant to have sufficient gut for normal function. Postoperatively these infants require close management of fluid, electrolyte, and blood volume status.

Results depend primarily on intestinal viability. In children without volvulus or with volvulus but no gangrenous intestine, the prognosis is excellent. In the few with devitalization of the entire midgut, resection is not advisable and the outcome is uniformly fatal. In those in whom a limited resection can be done, results are good in terms of mortality but may involve considerable morbidity if a short-gut syndrome ensues.

JEJUNOILEAL ATRESIAS AND STENOSES

The basic principles of preoperative management have been previously outlined; and achievement of normal fluid and electrolyte status,

nasogastric decompression, and maintenance of normal body temperature again deserve emphasis. Antibiotic therapy ordinarily is not necessary.

Laparotomy is performed through a transverse incision in the upper abdomen, and the exact anatomic situation is determined. The primary obstruction is easily found because of the marked discrepancy of intestinal caliber above and below the obstruction. The two ends may be separated, or may be in continuity with a diaphragm type atresia. Although most obstructions are solitary, occasionally multiple levels of obstruction are noted (15%). These are obvious when the intestinal segments are separated but not when distal diaphragmatic atresias occur. Therefore, the potency of the distal gut should be determined by injecting saline into the intestine just distal to the primary atresia and following this fluid down to the cecum.

The gut proximal to the atresia ordinarily ends in a bulbous dilatation. With high jejunal atresias this proximal bowel should be resected back to the ligament of Treitz. A short segment of intestine distal to the atresia is removed as well. Continuity is restored by a primary end-to-end anastomosis. A gastrostomy is routinely performed. When the atresia is in the distal ileum, the distal bulbous segment proximal to the atresia is resected and an end-to-side ileocecostomy constructed. Gastrostomy is not required in infants with distal obstructions.

For atresias in the midportion of the small gut there are two techniques, both of which work well in uncomplicated cases. An end-to-end anastomosis may be done after resection of the bulbous proximal segment and resection of a short segment of the distal gut. Alternatively, a Bishop-Koop technique may be used. Again, the bulbous proximal segment is resected and the end of the proximal segment is anastomosed to the side of the distal gut 3 or 4 cm distal to the proximal end. This proximal end is then opened and exteriorized as a vent. At a subsequent operation, this short span of distal gut is resected and closed.

The important points in postoperative management have been discussed previously. If function returns to the gut within a week and oral feedings can be initiated, there are usually few problems. If functional obstruction persists beyond this time, total parenteral alimentation should be started and continued until full enteral alimentation has been achieved.

In the past 25 years the success rate in infants with jejunoileal atresias has increased to over 90%. Such success is due to significant improvements in the techniques of surgical management and to the development of total parenteral nutrition.

COLONIC ATRESIA

Preoperative management parallels that for more proximal atresias. At laparotomy the dilated proximal colon is simply exteriorized as an end colostomy. This is easily managed postoperatively, and intestinal function permitting adequate oral feedings returns in a few days. A colostomy bag simplifies care of the colostomy, and the parents are instructed in the management of this appliance. Weeks or months later, when the baby is thriving, continuity is restored by an appropriate anastomosis, either a colocolostomy or an ileocolostomy. Mortality in such infants is close to zero, and morbidity is minimal.

Colonic atresia is occasionally associated with gastroschisis. In such an instance the blind proximal end is exteriorized and the gastroschisis managed either by primary closure or with the "silo" technique. Delayed anastomosis is done as with the uncomplicated case. Jejunoileal atresias occur very uncommonly with gastroschisis and are also managed with initial exteriorization. The prognosis of babies with the combination of gastroschisis and an atresia is nonetheless excellent.

MECONIUM ILEUS

This condition, invariably associated with cystic fibrosis, may be either uncomplicated or complicated, depending in all likelihood on whether an intrauterine segmental volvulus of small intestine has occurred. In the uncomplicated instance, the obstruction is an obturation type caused by inspissated meconium. The obstruction can often be cleared by a Gastrografin enema. Prior to such a procedure the infant should be managed as though a laparotomy were to be done; i.e., by correction of fluid and electrolyte abnormalities and nasogastric decompression plus systemic antibiotic administration. The enema procedure requires great care and should be done under fluoroscopic control with a surgeon in attendance. Because the enema fluid is hyperosmolar, the infant requires hypotonic fluid administration and careful monitoring during the procedure. When the Gastrografin reaches the dilated, air-containing small intestine, the procedure is discontinued. The loosened meconium usually begins to pass within 12 hours, with progressive relief of the obstruction. Complications occur rarely, particularly intestinal perforations, and, hence, the baby must be closely watched for such a possibility and follow-up x-rays taken.

If meconium does not begin to pass within 6 to 12 hours post enema, laparotomy should be done. Resection of the hugely dilated loop of small intestines is followed by a Bishop-Koop reconstruction. The distal segment can then be cleared of the obstructing concretions of meconium by instilling a dilute solution of pancreatic enzymes through the enterostomy vent. With either a successful enema procedure or a laparotomy, the preoperative measures are continued until relief of the obstruction is complete. Furthermore these babies, who are very vulnerable to respiratory infections, are nursed in isolettes using careful isolation techniques, and the appropriate prophylactic measures for cystic fibrosis are begun.

The complicated cases present with volvulus (sometimes complicated by perforation and meconium peritonitis), ileal or jejunal atresia, giant cystic meconium peritonitis, or a combination of these. Operation is required in all such infants, and the same preoperative measures as noted above are in order. At laparotomy the procedure is dictated by the pathology. If an atresia is found, the Bishop-Koop procedure as described in uncomplicated atresias works very well. With volvulus, resection of the devitalized segment and a double-barrel ostomy is advisable. Meconium peritonitis complicates the operation and may contribute to significant blood loss. Some type of ostomy, using either a double-barrel technique or the Bishop-Koop procedure, is safer than a primary anastomosis. Postoperatively these infants require particularly close attention to the problems of proper fluid and electrolyte balance, nutrition, and prevention of nosocomial infection.

DUPLICATIONS

Management of this very diverse group of lesions depends on their size and shape, and on the secondary problems resulting from their presence. The rare duodenal duplications are usually cystic. When proximally located, they often result in obstruction, with findings mimicking pyloric stenosis. At times they can be removed by stripping them away from the contiguous duodenal wall. If they are more distally located in the duodenum, the bile and pancreatic ducts may be immediately adjacent, and anastomosis of the common wall between duplication and duodenum is preferred.

Duplications in the small intestines may be either cystic or tubular, are located between the leaves of the mesentery, and share a common wall with the adjacent gut. The uncomplicated cystic and short tubular forms are resected along with the contiguous bowel, and continuity is restored with a primary anastomosis. If the duplication is complicated by volvulus or intussusception, resection is again done, but a double-barrel enterostomy may be wiser than primary anastomosis. Delayed secondary anastomosis is, of course, then necessary. In long tubular duplications, removal of the duplication with the contiguous intestine could result in the short-gut syndrome. In these, the mucosa of the duplication is removed by stripping it from its attachments to the muscularis. This can be done through a series of incisions through the seromuscular coat of the duplication, avoiding the mesenteric vessels. Complete mucosal stripping is important, since some or all of this mucosa may be gastric and hence responsible for intestinal bleeding. Leaving the seromuscular coat of these long duplications in situ does not appear to result in complications.

The rare hindgut duplication may involve the entire colon and rectum and the distal ileum. The mucosa of the duplication invariably is the same as that of the adjacent gut. These patients may be asymptomatic, with no obstruction or bleeding. In some the duplicated colons end in some form of imperforate anus (rectal atresia) malformation with obstruction. In others, the outer colon may end in a normal anus and the inner colon end in a rectovaginal or rectourethral fistula. In the former patients, a colostomy is required initially. In the latter, the two colons can be joined above the peritoneal reflection, and the mucosa leading to the rectovaginal or rectourethral fistula can be stripped out.

MECKEL'S DIVERTICULUM

This remnant of the omphalomesenteric duct usually is totally asymptomatic and requires no treatment, but may be responsible for profuse intestinal bleeding, intestinal obstruction, or discharge of intestinal contents from an umbilical sinus.

When symptomatic, rectal bleeding is most common. The bleeding may be profuse with resulting shock. The mucosa of the diverticulum in these cases is gastric, and a resulting ulcer in adjacent ileal mucosa produces the hemorrhage. At laparotomy the problem is usually obvious, but occasionally the diverticulum may be folded against the adjacent mesentery and be missed at first glance. In most instances, the diverticulum can be simply excised at its base on the antimesenteric surface of the ileum. If the base is quite wide or there is marked inflammation and induration, resection of a short segment of ileum with the diverticulum and a primary anastomosis may be necessary.

Occasionally a Meckel's diverticulum acts as the leading point in an ileoileal or, more commonly, an ileocolic intussusception. This will become apparent at laparotomy when the intussusception is reduced, and under such circumstances the diverticulum should be removed. This may be done primarily in many. However, if the involved gut shows marked induration and congestion, it is wiser to do this at a later laparotomy.

If the omphalomesenteric duct remains attached to the umbilicus, with or without patency, it may be responsible for a volvulus. This will be apparent at laparotomy, and the duct should be removed in its entirety after the volvulus is properly managed.

Rarely the omphalomesenteric duct remains patent throughout its length and results in the discharge of small intestinal contents from the umbilical opening. At laparotomy the duct is resected and the openings in the gut and at the umbilicus closed.

Very rarely a Meckel's diverticulum becomes inflamed, resulting in a clinical situation indistinguishable from acute appendicitis. At laparotomy, invariably with the wrong preoperative diagnosis, the inflamed diverticulum is identified as the culprit and is removed.

Foreign Bodies in the Gastrointestinal Tract

E. THOMAS BOLES, JR., M.D.

A swallowed foreign body that fails to pass uneventfully through the alimentary tract is most likely to become arrested somewhere along the course of the esophagus. If the foreign body reaches the stomach, and this is usually the case, the odds of it becoming arrested in its further passage down the gastrointestinal tract are exceedingly small, probably less than one time in 20. Accordingly, in most instances periodic observation of the patient, who is usually an infant or toddler, is all that is required.

The type and particularly the shape of the ingested object are important determinants of the possibility of its becoming arrested. Because most of these foreign bodies are visible radiographically, abdominal x-rays should be taken routinely. If the object is not radiopaque, it may be outlined by a small barium meal, although rarely a foreign body such as a toothpick may be ingested without symptoms and without knowledge of the parents, only to cause an inflammatory intra-abdominal lesion later as a consequence of ulceration or perforation through the intestinal tract.

If the object is rounded and smooth (marbles, coins, small plastic toys, etc.) the child may be followed on an outpatient basis, since the foreign body will almost certainly pass through safely. Usually this occurs within 2 days, and the parents should be asked to check the stools of the child to ensure passage and rejoice in this event. Even open safety pins almost always negotiate the gastrointestinal tract uneventfully.

It is possible for long, thin, pointed foreign bodies to become impacted at the pylorus, C-loop of the duodenum, duodenojejunal junction, or terminal ileum. Straight pins, bobby pins, and segments of pencils fall into this category. Hat pins are particularly dangerous. Children who have swallowed objects of this type should be observed in the hospital, and the progress of the foreign body documented by abdominal x-rays at 12 hour intervals. If there is failure of progression over a period of 2 to 3 days or if worrisome symptoms develop, the object should be removed. In the stomach and duodenum extraction can sometimes be performed successfully with the use of a flexible fiberoptic gastroduodenoscope. Otherwise, laparotomy with gastrotomy or enterotomy is required. Another type of foreign body of recent concern is the small alkaline battery, which is potentially harmful because the casing is not biologically sealed and may release corrosive fluid. Management is similar to that for long, pointed foreign bodies. If the foreign body does become arrested, it may erode the mucosa and produce bleeding or it may perforate through the intestinal wall. In the latter event a localized, walled off inflammatory process usually results. When either of these events occurs, the foreign body should be removed.

Rarely a foreign body gains access to the intestinal tract through the rectum. In infants, most often this is a glass thermometer that escapes upward or is broken off. These require prompt removal, which may be possible by digital manipulation alone. If this is not easily accomplished, proctoscopy under general anesthesia should be performed. In older children, a bizarre assortment of foreign objects will at times be inserted into the rectum. Often these pass without incident, but if they are large or fragile (e.g., light bulb), their extraction may prove to be a challenging exercise. Proctoscopy under anesthesia is ordinarily required.

Bezoars are masses of hair or vegetable fibers that form a cast in the stomach, sometimes extending down into the duodenum or even the upper jejunum. These are usually trichobezoars (hair balls) and occur most commonly in girls. Typically there is no history of eating hair, but clearly this is the mechanism. These patients are often asymptomatic, but symptoms that may develop include loss of appetite, intolerance of solid foods, vomiting, and abdominal pain. The child may show evidence of malnutrition and is often somewhat withdrawn or disturbed. The breath is characteristically fetid. A large, firm, movable mass is palpable in the upper abdomen. A barium swallow with fluoroscopy confirms the diagnosis by outlining the intragastric mass. Treatment is by gastrotomy, with removal of the bezoar, which forms a cast of the stomach. The small intestine should be traced down to the cecum to determine whether or not portions of the bezoar have separated from the main mass and have lodged downstream.

Intussusception

HARRY C. BISHOP, M. D.

Intussusception, the telescoping of bowel into itself, is a leading cause of acute intestinal obstruction in infants and is most common between the ages of 3 and 12 months. Ileocolic intussusception is the most common type and in over 90% of the cases it occurs without known cause. It usually occurs in a well infant, although there may be a preceding viral illness with gastrointestinal symptoms. It can occur in association with Henoch-Schönlein purpura, where a presumed hematoma of the bowel wall has acted as a lead point. In children over 2 years of age an inverted Meckel's diverticulum, a small intramural duplication, a polyp, or, very rarely, a lymphosarcoma of the ileum may be a lead point.

Characteristically, the patient has severe intermittent abdominal pain that recurs every 15 to 30 minutes. Between episodes of pain the infant or child is completely comfortable and may sleep. Occasionally, a small infant will present with lethargy and pallor rather than the more typical spasmodic pain, crying and flexing the legs or the abdomen. Vomiting usually occurs. Since the bowel mesentery is compressed between the intussusceptum (invaginated segment of bowel) and the intussuscipiens, venous obstruction occurs while the arteries are still pumping and this leads to edema and intraluminal bleeding and the typical currant jelly stool. As the intestine becomes more tightly incarcerated, the arterial supply is occluded, leading to less rectal bleeding and inevitably gangrene with associated signs of toxemia and complete intestinal obstruction. To avoid this potentially fatal result, early suspicion and confirmation of the diagnosis and reduction of the intussusception are essential. Examination of the abdomen will usually show soft distention and mild generalized tenderness. There may be a palpable "sausage-shaped" mass, most frequently along the transverse colon. Peristalsis is hyperactive initially and absent in the later stages of the disease. The intussusception may be felt on rectal exam if it has gone the full route through the colon. Rectal exam may produce a currant jelly stool appearing for the first time.

MANAGEMENT

All infants and children suspected of having intussusception should be hospitalized and under the care of a surgeon. Nasogastric suction is begun, as is intravenous replacement of fluid and electrolyte losses, blood is crossmatched, and the operating room is alerted for a possible emergency operation. With the surgeon attending, the patient is moved to Radiology, where a barium enema confirms the diagnosis and hydrostatic reduction will be attempted. If the patient is septic, has signs of perforation with peritonitis, or is considered critically ill, he or she may be taken directly to surgery rather than attempting hydrostatic reduction.

Barium Enema Reduction. Hydrostatic reduction is safe if properly performed. Most radiologists use a Foley catheter with the inflated balloon pulled down against the internal sphincter and the buttocks strapped tightly together. Thin barium is allowed to flow by gravity into the rectum, with the reservoir no higher than 3 feet above the table top. Manual manipulation through the intact abdomen is avoided. Steady hydrostatic pressure is exerted on the intussuscipiens, which is outlined by the barium column. Several attempts might be made, evacuating the barium between attempts. Intussusception usually reduces easily back to the cecal area but the last reduction through the ileocecal valve may be delayed. Some radiologists use glucagon or morphine, in an attempt to relax the bowel and the patient. It is vitally important for the reduction to be complete. Only if there is a free flow of barium into two or three loops of ileum can reduction be confirmed. If an intussusception has been reduced hydrostatically, the patient should remain in the hospital. He should be free of abdominal pain, his abdomen should be soft and free of a palpable mass, and he should pass stool and flatus in the early postreduction period. Careful observation is important to ensure complete reduction and rule out recurrence.

Unfortunately, the condition can start as an ileo-ileal intussusception, and then this whole mass prolapses through the ileocecal valve, producing a so-called ileoileocolic intussusception. This treacherous variation must be considered and the possibility eliminated only by a free flow of barium high into the ileum, guaranteeing a reduction of the ileoileal segment as well. If there is any doubt about the completeness of the reduction, the child should be taken to surgery and explored. Since the entrapped bowel is in danger of becoming gangrenous, early surgery is mandatory.

Indications for operation are 1) incomplete reduction of a known intussusception; 2) suspicion of a jejunojejunal or ileoileal intussusception with intestinal obstruction; and 3) perforation during the barium enema, which is rare if the proper safeguards are taken.

If operation is scheduled, antibiotics should be given preoperatively, assuming that the bowel has been damaged. Most surgeons use a right lower quadrant McBurney type incision, which can be enlarged if necessary. An intussusception should be milked out from the distal end proximally, with great care to avoid splitting the bowel wall. At no time should the bowel be pulled from the opposite end. Frequently the appendix will have invaginated into the intussusception and may be traumatized. Ileal mesenteric lymph nodes are frequently enlarged, and it is difficult to know whether these were there primarily or occurred as a result of the intussusception. If the bowel can be completely reduced, there is always edema of the lead point and the Peyer's patches may seem hypertrophied. The cyanotic bowel frequently will improve once the reduction has been accomplished, especially if covered with warm gauze sponges. Care is taken to look for a lesion leading to the intussusception, as mentioned above. Most surgeons feel appendectomy can be safely accomplished, and often it is wise to include an appendectomy, since the appendix has been damaged. If the intussusception is gangrenous or cannot be reduced manually, the bowel is resected and ordinarily a primary anastomosis is done. The bowel would be resected if perforation occurs during the attempted reduction, but a careful effort should be made to avoid this complication. Postoperatively these patients are continued on nasogastric suction, intravenous replacement and support, and antibiotics. They frequently have a low-grade fever that might last for 2 or 3 days, presumably from damage of the intestinal wall.

Recurrent Intussusception. If the symptoms of intussusception occur following hydrostatic reduction, one must suspect that the original reduction was incomplete or that an etiological lead point lesion is present. Therefore, surgical exploration is indicated for any recurrence. A rare patient will repeatedly intussuscept and require resection of the ileocecal area or suturing of the terminal ileum up along the ascending colon. A very rare individual might have a chronic intussusception without the acute symptoms, which may be discovered while investigating mild abdominal complaints. These patients should be explored.

Postoperative Intussusception. Jejunojejunal or ileoileal intussusception can occur during the early postoperative period following other unrelated operative procedures. It is frequently confused with paralytic ileus or obstruction due to adhesions and cannot be diagnosed by barium enema. Early surgical exploration is therefore indicated when this diagnosis is suspected.

Hirschsprung's Disease

MARC I. ROWE, M.D.,
and DAVID A. LLOYD, M.D.

Hirschsprung's disease is due to congenital absence of ganglion cells in the submucosal and intermuscular neural plexuses of the intestinal wall. The disease always affects the distal rectum and extends proximally for varying distances. The result is functional obstruction of the colon. The diagnosis is confirmed by demonstrating absence of ganglion cells on rectal biopsy.

Three clinical groups are identified.

1. The Neonate Who Fails to Pass Meconium and Becomes Distended. Proper management depends on an accurate diagnosis, since ileal atresia and meconium ileus may require laparotomy, and meconium plug syndrome and small left colon syndrome can be dealt with by rectal washouts. The diagnosis is suspected on barium enema but requires rectal biopsy for confirmation. Suction biopsy has greatly facilitated prompt diagnosis. The recommended treatment is initial diverting colostomy in ganglionic bowel, followed later by definitive surgery.

2. Acute Enterocolitis. This usually occurs in infants who present with an acute severe illness, abdominal distention, fulminating diarrhea, and hypovolemia. Less commonly, the presentation is milder, with chronic diarrhea and failure to thrive. Hirschsprung's disease should be suspected in a child with severe diarrhea associated with abdominal distention. The diagnosis is suggested by marked colonic distention on plain radiographs. Improper treatment of this serious condition may be fatal. Initial management consists of correcting fluid and electrolyte deficits, care being taken to avoid rapid correction of hypertonic dehydration if present. Urgent colostomy is performed; where possible the diagnosis is first confirmed by urgent rectal biopsy.

3. Chronic Constipation. Hirschsprung's disease may present in older children with chronic constipation, abdominal distention, and failure to thrive. The diagnosis may be made by barium enema and is confirmed by rectal biopsy. In most patients, preliminary colostomy is required to decompress the distended bowel and allow adequate washouts, followed later by definitive surgery. Occasionally, when distention is not severe, colonic washouts are followed by definitive surgery.

A particularly troublesome form of Hirschsprung's diseases is *total colonic aganglionosis.* Here the entire colon and variable lengths of ileum, and rarely the entire intestine, are involved. Patients usually present as newborns with low small bowel obstruction. The barium enema is suggestive but seldom diagnostic. The diagnosis of aganglionosis is made by rectal biopsy, but at operation the typical transitional zone cannot be found in the colon, necessitating multiple biopsies to identify ganglionic bowel. Ileostomy is required.

Three different procedures are in common use for the definitive treatment of Hirschsprung's disease, and all yield satisfactory results. The Swensen procedure involves resecting the aganglionic colon to a level just above the anus. The ganglionic bowel is anastomosed to the low rectal cuff. The Duhamel procedure involves resection of the aganglionic bowel down to the lower rectum. The rectal stump is closed and the ganglionic bowel is drawn down behind the rectal stump and sutured side-to-side, forming a pouch with an anterior wall composed of aganglionic rectum and a posterior wall consisting of ganglionic bowel. In the endorectal pull-through operation (Soave), the aganglionic bowel is resected down to the rectum. The mucosa is stripped from the aganglionic rectal stump, leaving a muscular tunnel through which ganglionic bowel is drawn and anastomosed at the level of the anus. Long-segment Hirschsprung's disease is usually treated by the Duhamel procedure, with or without the Lester Martin modification.

Ulcerative Colitis and Crohn's Disease

MARVIN L. DIXON, M.D.,
and W. ALLAN WALKER, M.D.

The major chronic inflammatory diseases of the bowel, ulcerative colitis (UC) and Crohn's disease or regional enteritis, share similar clinical features and treatment methods. However, in recent years, clinical manifestations of the two have become more distinct and differences are emerging in their responses to therapy.

Regional enteritis may involve the entire alimentary tract, but the ileocolic region or small bowel is involved in about 80% of affected individuals. About 20% with Crohn's may have colonic disease alone, making its differentiation from UC difficult at times. Crohn's disease often is insidious in onset and is characterized by crampy abdominal pain, low grade fever, anemia, diarrhea (usually unaccompanied by gross blood), and weight loss. Growth retardation is seen in up to 20% of affected children and adolescents. Radiographically, there may be asymmetrically involved "skip" areas with transmural ulcerations and rectal sparing. The tendency to develop fistulas, intra-abdominal abscesses, and strictures increases with duration of disease, often making multiple surgical resections necessary. Arthralgias, arthritis, erythema nodosum, uveitis, pericholangitis, and nephrolithiasis are the more commonly seen extraintestinal manifestations of regional enteritis and may actually predate gastrointestinal symptoms.

In contrast, ulcerative colitis is limited to the large intestine, except for occasional "backwash" ileitis. In children, UC involves the entire colon more frequently than in adults and also seems to be less responsive to medical therapy. Children with ulcerative colitis often complain of diarrhea, hematochezia, tenesmus, and rectal urgency more than abdominal pain. Weight loss may be seen but growth retardation occurs less frequently than in Crohn's disease. The risk of malignancy increases with the extent and duration of the disease, such that after the first decade of disease, 20% of affected children per decade will develop cancer. Colectomy, if done before a malignancy develops, is curative. At endoscopy one finds mucosal friability and inflammation, most marked distally. Extraintestinal manifestations are similar in frequency to Crohn's disease, with less liver disease and nephrolithiasis being reported.

Therapeutic goals for ulcerative colitis and regional enteritis are similar—mainly to suppress inflammation and induce a remission so that normal growth and development can ensue. Similar agents and modalities are used with varying results. Therapy must be individualized, based on an affected child's symptoms, extent of disease, and response to treatment.

Anti-Inflammatory Agents

Corticosteroids have been the mainstay of therapy for UC and regional enteritis; they are definitely beneficial in acute attacks and exacerbations of UC and Crohn's disease, but have no long-term benefit in preventing exacerbations. The initial attack of UC or Crohn's disease is usually the most responsive to steroids, and the same patient may respond differently during subsequent attacks of illness. In addition, steroids seem to be less effective in the same patient as time progresses.

Depending on the severity of illness, prednisone or its parenteral equivalent prednisolone should be started at 1 to 2 mg/kg/day up to 40 to 60 mg/day in 2 to 3 divided doses. Those with severe attacks of ulcerative colitis or proctitis characterized by dehydration, fever, anemia, and frequent stools (more than 10 per day) often benefit from topical steroids in addition to parenteral steroids. Hydrocortisone suppositories (15 and 25 mg), enemas (100 mg in 60 ml of tap water or normal saline), or foam (10% hydrocortisone giving 80 mg/dose or 40 mg methylprednisolone/unit enema) may be used twice daily initially and tapered to once daily in 2 to 3 weeks. Every-other-day use should be attempted after 2 to 3 weeks of daily use, discontinuing the topical steroids after 6 to 8 weeks if symptoms permit. During severe attacks of UC, topical steroids should be administered cautiously. They are tolerated poorly by young children and, hence, used infrequently. Their effects are maximal if they are retained for longer than an hour, and there is variable systemic absorption of from 30 to 65% of the administered dose. Finally, one may begin therapy with topical steroids, along with sulfasalazine, in children newly diagnosed with UC who have moderate disease; this may avert a course of systemic steroids.

In Crohn's disease, the initial steroid dose is generally continued for 2 to 4 weeks, after which an attempt to taper it should be made based on clinical symptoms and laboratory data. Following the sedimentation rate can be especially helpful if it was previously elevated. The drug should be tapered by 5 to 10 mg every 1 to 2 weeks. An every-other-day dosage regimen may be tried in an attempt to lower the incidence of steroid side effects. However, this often does not lead to the same amount of disease

suppression as daily steroids. Should a decrease in steroid dosage be met by increased disease activity, the amount being given should be increased to or above the previous level at which disease suppression occurred. After 3 to 6 weeks of higher steroid dosage, an attempt should again be made to slowly reduce the dose.

Acute attacks of UC seem to respond to steroids more rapidly than do acute attacks of Crohn's disease. The reduction in steroid dosage is often begun within 1 to 2 weeks after starting steroids and is completed within 4 to 8 weeks. There is no evidence that "maintenance" steroids prolong disease-free intervals or decrease the frequency of attacks; thus steroids should be discontinued once remission is achieved.

ACTH (1–1.5 U/kg/day IM, SQ, or IV over 8 hrs) has also been used for acute attacks of Crohn's disease and UC. It is felt that response is better than with systemic steroids, particularly when increasing doses of steroids seem to be ineffective. The use of ACTH, however, should be discouraged because it depends on adrenal responsiveness, enhances unwanted mineralocorticoid effects, may cause hyperpigmentation, and, most important, does not allow for precise dose regulation.

Extensive small bowel disease may interfere with absorption of oral steroids, but this may be bypassed by giving the drug parenterally. Finally, if one is concerned about in vivo conversion of prednisone to its active form after oral ingestion, prednisolone can be used.

Although corticosteroids are important in the therapy of inflammatory bowel disease, they are not without untoward effects, among the most significant being their potential to interfere with growth in children and adolescents whose underlying disease may already have affected their somatic development. In addition to growth suppression, corticosteroids increase susceptibility to infection and predispose to hypertension, hyperglycemia, subcapsular cataracts, and osteoporosis. Electrolytes must be followed closely in those with diarrhea because steroids potentiate calcium and potassium losses. The alterations in physical appearance that high dose steroids cause may worry some children and their parents. All should be reassured that the physical changes will go away when the steroids are stopped. Finally, the use of steroids is contraindicated in the presence of intestinal perforation or peritonitis.

Sulfasalazine

Unlike steroids, sulfasalazine has been found to decrease the likelihood of exacerbations in UC. Colonic bacteria degrade sulfasalazine into its active moiety, 5-aminoasalicylic acid and sulfapyridine. The drug seems to have no effect on the small intestinal disease of regional enteritis but may have some effect on the colonic disease. Therapy of mild to moderate attacks of UC should be begun with sulfasalazine (40–60 mg/kg/day in three divided doses or 2 gm/day for those less than 25 kg and 3 gm for those greater than 25 kg, up to 4 gm/day). No convincing data exist to show that sulfasalazine is useful during severe attacks of UC, and it is usually begun within 10 to 14 days of onset of an acute episode. Eighty percent of those with mild attacks will be better within a month of starting sulfasalazine. Recurrences have been prevented with 2 gm/day in adults or 30 mg/kg/day in children.

Side effects of sulfasalazine may occasionally interfere with its use. Headache, nausea, vomiting, anorexia, and rash are commonly experienced and are considered minor side effects. Allergic reactions, hepatoxicity, hemolysis, and myelosuppression also occur and are of more concern. Minor side effects can be lessened by not taking the drug on an empty stomach. Also, if introduction of the drug is met by minor side effects, the drug dosage should be decreased and subsequently increased slowly over several days. The enteric coated preparation may lead to fewer side effects but can, on occasion, pass undigested in the stool. When treating sexually active teens, one should remember that azospermia and sperm motility problems have been reported. There has been one report of sulfasalazine induced exacerbation of UC. Finally, sulfasalazine is known to interfere with folic acid metabolism, so folate levels and the CBC should be monitored, particularly in those on the drug chronically, and supplemental folate given if needed.

Other Agents

Azathioprine has not been effective in controlling active Crohn's disease or in preventing recurrences but it may be useful in those unable to wean from steroids. Hampering the more widespread use of azathioprine is the lack of convincing data of its efficacy as well as its serious side effects and complications, including pancreatitis, renal failure, and leukopenia. The drug is used at 1 to 2 mg/kg/day.

The active metabolite of azathioprine, 6-mercaptopurine, has been reported to be effective in Crohn's disease in conjunction with steroids by allowing the steroid dosage to be decreased, by promoting fistula closure, and by lessening disease symptoms. In one trial evaluating the efficacy of 6-mercaptopurine in adults, one third of the study participants took longer than 3 months to respond. In addition, reversible side effects (nausea, leukopenia, pancreatitis) occurred in about 10%. Studies on the effectiveness of azathioprine and 6-mercaptopurine in children are nonexistent, and hazards of their use may obviate potential benefits.

Recently, promising data have emerged on the use of metronidazole* in patients with regional enteritis. It seems particularly helpful in perirectal disease and promotes healing of perianal lesions at 800 mg/day in adults. It has been suggested that metronidazole may be more effective than sulfasalazine for colonic disease accompanying Crohn's.** Children should get 20 to 40 mg/kg/day in 2 or 3 divided doses for 3 to 4 months. Drawbacks are reports of teratogenicity in animals and side effects in humans that include anorexia, vomiting, a metallic taste, paresthesias and neutropenia.

Nutritional and Diet Aids

Total parenteral nutrition (TPN) and elemental diets are a useful adjunct in the therapy of inflammatory bowel disease. TPN has been used to treat malnutrition felt to be contributing to growth failure, to improve nutritional status preoperatively, to meet nutritional needs while a patient is NPO, to decrease disease activity, and to allow adaptation of a short bowel after large intestinal resections. Temporary remissions have been induced in up to 80% of patients with regional enteritis and up to 33% of patients with UC by using TPN. Parenteral nutrition has been found to cause improvement in Crohn's disease and should be considered for those who have not responded to medical intervention. It has enabled several patients with persistent steroid requirements to be successfully cared for at home. And finally, it has been shown to effect up to 75% closure rate of enteric fistulas. Unfortunately, fistula closure, except for fistulas occurring postoperatively, is not permanent and most fistulas require eventual surgical resection.

Results from the use of elemental diets have been equally encouraging. Although the effects were short-lived, brief periods of elemental alimentation temporarily re-established growth in children with protracted growth arrest and regional enteritis. Continuously infused elemental diets administered for 3 weeks at the time of diagnosis of Crohn's disease led to remission without additional therapy. A soft silicone nasogastric tube can be used for infusion. The diets should be advanced in volume and concentration while monitoring urine sugar and serum electrolytes, calcium, and glucose.

Maintaining adequate nutrition in children with inflammatory bowel disease is of paramount concern. Even in those with few symptoms, the daily caloric intake is about 80% of that expected based on size. This decreased intake may be related to anorexia, often seen in those with chronic disease. Also, affected children may consciously limit their

---

*Safety and efficacy of metronidazole in children have not been established.

**This use of metronidazole is not listed by the manufacturer.

intake to avoid episodes of abdominal pain. One should encourage a well-balanced, nutritious diet of sufficient calories, estimated to be about 140% of the ideal caloric intake in children with inflammatory bowel disease, to promote growth.

Dietary restrictions should be avoided, as specific foodstuffs have not been found to correlate with disease exacerbations. High roughage foods may irritate the intestine during attacks marked by moderate diarrhea and bleeding, and it is prudent to avoid these at those times. An empiric trial of a milk-free diet has been advocated soon after diagnosis because milk ingestion often leads to more severe diarrhea.

There may be fat malabsorption with widespread disease involvement of the small intestine or following surgical resection. Luminal bile salts can be decreased from an interrupted enterohepatic circulation or bacterial overgrowth. Medium chain triglycerides may be substituted for long chain fats in the presence of steatorrhea. Terminal ileal disease may interfere with vitamin B_{12} or zinc absorption. If the Schilling test is abnormal, then vitamin B_{12} should be given (100–200 μg SQ q 2 wks). Supplemental folate may be needed (1–3 mg/day) in the presence of sulfasalazine. Supplemental calcium and vitamin D may be needed for those on chronic corticosteroids because of the steroids' ostoepenic effects. Foods high in potassium should be encouraged for those with hypokalemia secondary to chronic steroid use.

In general, there should be few restrictions while attempting to prevent deficiencies by the judicious use of supplements.

Symptomatic Therapy

The abdominal pain and diarrhea seen in regional enteritis and UC are unfortunate indicators of disease activity. Suppressing the underlying inflammation will ameliorate these symptoms. Unabsorbed bile salts may pass to the colon, be deconjugated, and inhibit sodium and H_2O reabsorption, and a trial of cholestyramine may help diminish diarrhea.

Symptomatic improvement in the diarrhea can often be achieved by using opium derivatives (codeine, paregoric, deodorized tincture of opium) and seem more effective than diphenoxylate (5 mg qid) in controlling diarrhea. During acute attacks, or in the presence of toxic megacolon, these agents should be used cautiously, as they may cause colonic dilatation or worsen it if it is already present. In addition, in children antidiarrheal agents may hamper accurate assessment of fluid losses secondary to intraluminal pooling. Occasionally, these agents cause intestinal spasm and aggregate symptoms. The belladonna alkaloids have been used for their antispasmodic effects but the response is often poor. Codeine often works well for pain, but with

persistent or unusually severe pain consider the possibility of intestinal perforation, intra-abdominal abscess or an extraintestinal source such as biliary or renal colic.

Surgery

The need for surgery is clear in IBD when dealing with an intestinal perforation, intra-abdominal abscess, persistent stricture, disease unresponsive to bowel rest and anti-inflammatory agents, fistulas, and "uncontrollable" hemorrhage. Growth retardation has responded to surgical intervention in 20 to 50% of affected children, with the best results seen in 12- to 16-year-olds. The optimal time to operate when medical therapy has not led to improvement is not clear, but surgery performed for growth failure should be done before epiphyseal closure. A decision to operate is complicated by the high rate of disease recurrence (10–50%) seen in regional enteritis, especially in the presence of ileocolic disease. The reluctance of physicians to recommend surgery in Crohn's disease is understandable but there is often an unduly long wait before surgical intervention in UC. Concerns about surgical morbidity and the undesirableness of a colostomy in a child or adolescent are valid, but a prolonged bout of diarrhea and bleeding should not be tolerated. Colectomy should be considered for all those with UC who continue to be symptomatic after a good trial of topical and systemic corticosteroids and TPN, remembering that colectomy will be curative and abate the risk of malignant degeneration. Severe unremitting extraintestinal symptoms will also improve after surgical resection.

Emotional Care

The onset of UC and its exacerbations frequently seem to occur at times of anxiety, stress, and emotional upset, but there are no good data for a psychogenic basis for the disorder. Consequently, routine psychotherapy or psychiatric evaluations are not indicated. These children and their parents need an empathic, supportive caretaker. Uncertainty regarding disease course and prognosis engenders much anxiety, often unexpressed among these children and their families. Questions and concerns should be addressed honestly and in understandable terms. Adolescents may find upsetting the changes in appearance secondary to steroid use. Knowledge that the steroids cause these changes may encourage many youngsters to be noncompliant in their use, and reassurance that the changes are temporary must be reiterated. One must attempt to involve the adolescent patient in sharing the responsibility for his or her care.

Finally, some parents may benefit from meetings with groups consisting of parents of similarly affected children. Adolescents with this problem often find similar group contacts useful as well.

Necrotizing Enterocolitis

FRANK R. SINATRA, M.D.

Early recognition and prompt institution of therapy have dramatically decreased the mortality and necessity for surgical intervention in neonatal necrotizing enterocolitis (NEC). Since many of the signs and symptoms of NEC are often nonspecific (thermal instability, apnea, decreased activity) an extremely high index of suspicion must be maintained when caring for premature neonates. This is particularly important if there is a history of perinatal hypoxia, shock, low Apgar scores, exchange transfusion, patent ductus arteriosus, hypothermia, or hyperviscosity. If there is any clinical suspicion of NEC medical therapy should be instituted immediately.

Medical Therapy. Once the diagnosis is suspected all enteral feedings should be immediately discontinued. Continuous nasogastric suction is instituted using a Replogle tube or similar sump-type catheter. This allows continuous decompression with minimal gastric mucosal trauma. Supine, upright, and decubitus abdominal radiographs are immediately obtained and examined for intestinal distention, pneumatosis intestinalis, portal venous gas, and free intraperitoneal air. If distention alone is noted and the infant appears well and is without clinical or laboratory evidence of septicemia, nasogastric suction and supportive intravenous fluid therapy are continued. The infant's clinical status must be frequently re-evaluated and repeat abdominal radiographs should be obtained every 6–8 hours. Serum electrolytes, pH, complete blood count, platelet count, and blood gases should be closely monitored. Stool should be evaluated for white blood cells and occult blood. Cultures of blood, stool, urine, and CSF should be obtained. If no evidence of pneumatosis intestinalis develops and all clinical and laboratory findings remain normal, nasogastric suction can be discontinued in 5–7 days and cautious reinstitution of oral feedings can be slowly started after 7–10 days.

Infants in whom pneumatosis intestinalis or portal venous gas is noted radiographically or in whom clinical or laboratory findings of sepsis (temperature instability, apnea, lethargy, acidosis, leukocytosis, leukopenia, thrombocytopenia) are present should immediately be started on parenteral antibiotics. Although culture results may subsequently alter antimicrobial therapy, initial treatment should be directed against the wide spectrum of aerobic and anaerobic organisms that may be present in cases of enteric sepsis. Our initial antibiotic therapy consists of the following: ampicillin, first week of life, 50–100 mg/kg/day (q 12 H), 1–4 weeks of age, 100–150 mg/kg/day (q 8 H); gentamicin, first week of life, 5 mg/kg/day (q 12 H), 1–4 weeks of age, 7.5 mg/kg/day (q 8 H); and clindamycin, 25 mg/kg/day (q 6 H).

Many neonatal intensive care centers add oral gentamicin or colistin at doses of 10–15 mg/kg/day. Nasogastric instillation of one sixth of the total dose is given at 4 hour intervals, following which the nasogastric suction tube is clamped for 1 hour. We do not routinely add oral antibiotics in uncomplicated cases but have instituted oral therapy in cases of recurrent NEC.

In addition to nasogastric suction and antibiotic therapy, meticulous care must be given to all aspects of neonatal supportive care. Fluid and electrolyte balance and a thermoneutral environment must be carefully maintained. Adequate blood volume, peripheral perfusion, and oxygenation are mandatory in the prevention of further mucosal damage. Particular attention must be directed toward nutritional support. Once blood volume and fluid and electrolyte status has been stabilized, 10% dextrose and 2% amino acid solutions can be provided via a peripheral vein. In infants older than 1 week and in whom there is no significant hyperbilirubinemia, lipid emulsions can be started, beginning with 1 gm/kg/day over 24 hours. Infants with confirmed NEC should be kept on nothing by mouth for approximately 14–21 days. If peripheral vein access cannot be maintained, a central venous, Broviac-type catheter should be inserted. This technique has the advantage of being able to provide a higher caloric intake but may be associated with an increased incidence of infectious and mechanical complications.

Feedings may be slowly restarted after 14–21 days, using small volumes of dilute formula. Formula concentration and volume are slowly increased as the infant is gradually weaned from parenteral nutritional support. During this time the infant is carefully monitored for any signs of recurrent NEC, such as abdominal distention, increasing gastric residuals, or abnormal stooling.

Surgical Therapy. Surgery is reserved for the infant with radiographic evidence of perforation or the infant in whom medical therapy has been unsuccessful. Situations in which medical therapy should be considered unsuccessful include 1) persistent hypotension, metabolic acidosis and/or coagulopathy; 2) progressive abdominal wall edema, induration, or erythema; and 3) radiographic evidence of a fixed, unresolved area of involvement.

The surgeon should attempt to resect all grossly necrotic bowel and leave behind any potentially viable bowel. A "second-look" procedure can be performed if a questionably viable segment of bowel is left. All reasonable attempts should be made to avoid creating a short-bowel syndrome. In patients with a single, localized area of involvement, it is sometimes possible to perform a primary anastomosis; however, in most cases an ileostomy and a separate mucous fistula should be created. Reanastomosis should be postponed for several weeks until nutritional status is improved and radiographic studies have been performed to identify areas of obstruction in the diverted segment. Stricture formation is common in severe NEC. Fluid and electrolyte losses from the ileostomy may require fluid, sodium, and bicarbonate supplementation. This is especially important in very small premature infants.

Following reanastomosis, infants who have undergone significant terminal ileal resection may develop chronic diarrhea due to bile acid malabsorption. In some infants cholestyramine,*a bile-acid-binding resin, may be necessary to prevent chronic diarrhea.**In small infants it is important to uuse an initially small dose (250 mg q.i.d.) in order to avoid hyperchloremic acidosis and/or intestinal obstruction. Parenteral vitamin B_{12} may also be required on a monthly basis owing to loss of B_{12} absorption sites.

Peritonitis

MELVIN I. MARKS, M.D.

Primary Peritonitis. The treatment of peritonitis depends on both host factors and infectious etiologies (Table 1). Paracentesis by percutaneous needle aspiration is the essential diagnostic test, since the Gram stain provides a rapid and major guideline to initial therapy.

Primary disease in normal hosts is easiest to treat,

Table 1. PERITONITIS

Type	Most Common Infectious Agent
Primary	*Streptococcus pneumoniae, S. pyogenes*
Bowel perforation	*Escherichia coli, Bacteroides fragilis,* group D streptococci
Peritoneal dialysis	*Staphylococcus epidermidis, S. aureus,* gram-negatives, yeasts
Nephrotic syndrome	*Streptococcus pneumoniae, E. coli*
Other	
V-P shunt	*S. aureus, S. epidermidis,* gram-negatives
Septicemia	Variable
Tuberculosis	
Pelvic inflammatory disease	*Neisseria gonorrheae, Ureaplasma urealyticum, Chlamydia trachomatis,* anaerobic bacteria, *Actinomyces* (with intrauterine device)

*Dosage of cholestyramine has not been established for infants and children.

**This use of cholestryramine is not listed by the manufacturer.

since the usual causes (*Streptococcus pneumoniae* and *S. pyogenes*) are highly sensitive to penicillin and host immune responses are normal. In such cases, parenteral or oral penicillin should be administered in doses of approximately 100,000 units/kg/day and continued for one week. Most antimicrobials (amphotericin B may be an exception) diffuse well into peritoneal fluid, so direct instillation is rarely necessary. However, this route may be useful when an intraperitoneal catheter is in place, as in patients undergoing peritoneal dialysis (see below). The route of systemic antimicrobials is not critical, although some patients with peritonitis may be vomiting, and a few have paralytic ileus, and may be unable to take drugs orally.

When peritonitis is part of a generalized sepsis syndrome, management must be more aggressive and includes cardiovascular support, hydration, and nutrition. Cultures of blood, peritoneal fluid, and urine should be obtained before starting antibiotic therapy.

Peritonitis may also be a component of pelvic inflammatory disease. Here, gonococci, gram-negative aerobes, anaerobes, and chlamydia may be responsible. Cefoxitin, 150 mg/kg/day, divided q 6 h (maximum 12 gm), plus gentamicin, 7 mg/kg/day, divided q 8 h, is a useful initial regimen. Subsequent gentamicin doses and frequency should then be determined by measuring peak and trough serum concentrations of the drug until steady state is achieved.

Bowel Perforation. Peritonitis associated with intestinal gangrene and bowel perforation is often due to enteric gram-negative bacteria (e.g., *Escherichia coli*), anaerobes (e.g., *Bacteroides fragilis*), and gram-positive cocci (e.g., group D *streptococci*). Antibiotic combinations are often useful in initiating therapy for such patients. Ampicillin (200 mg/kg/day), plus gentamicin (7 mg/kg/day), plus clindamycin (25 mg/kg/day) are recommended. Other appropriate initial programs include combinations of beta-lactam (penicillins or cephalosporins) and aminoglycoside drugs. As mentioned, the aminoglycoside dose and frequency should be adjusted by means of serum drug assays. Of course, if examination of the peritoneal fluid reveals yeasts, acid-fast bacilli, or other causes, then specific alterations in therapy are indicated. Insertion of drains and peritoneal lavage are not necessary if surgical repair of the perforation, drainage of abscesses, and surgical debridement of necrotic tissue are carried out. In fact, intraperitoneal aminoglycosides and povidone-iodine may add to the morbidity by increasing peritoneal inflammation or by toxic effects after systemic absorption.

Dehydration is common, and adequate fluids and electrolyte management are indicated. Diagnosis and treatment of shock may also be needed.

Nephrotic Syndrome. The common causes of peritonitis in patients with ascites, hypogammaglobulinemia, edema, and other manifestations of nephrotic syndrome are *S. pneumoniae,* other streptococci, and occasionally *Haemophilus* or *E. coli.* The initial Gram stain is very important. If the patient is not too ill, one can usually initiate therapy with penicillin (100,000 units/kg/day) or ampicillin (200 mg/kg/day) directed at the pneumococci. Subsequent adjustments may be necessary, depending on culture results. The younger the infant, the more likely it is that *Haemophilus* may be present. In more debilitated hosts, *E. coli* or other enteric bacilli are more likely. If the patient is extremely toxic and appears septic, ampicillin, 200 mg/kg/day, and gentamicin, 7 mg/kg/day, may be useful initially.

Peritoneal Dialysis. Patients with indwelling peritoneal catheters who develop peritonitis present special problems. Since staphylococci are the most common causes, early diagnosis by demonstrating neutrophils and/or bacteria in the peritoneal fluid, should be followed by antistaphylococcal therapy. If the patient is not vomiting and is only mildly ill, dicloxacillin 50–75 mg/kg/day (divided q 6 h) will usually be effective.* The efficacy of this therapy should be documented by serial examinations and cultures of the peritoneal fluid obtained via the catheter. Such therapy should be continued for 10–14 days, if the catheter is not removed, or approximately 5 days after removal. In many cases, catheter removal may not be necessary if peritonitis is diagnosed and treated early.

The causative agents in patients receiving peritoneal dialysis are extremely diverse. Hence, early examination of the peritoneal fluid for yeasts, gram-negative bacteria, anaerobes, and, occasionally, atypical mycobacteria should be carried out. Each requires specific therapies.

Another way to treat peritonitis in these patients is to include antibiotics in the peritoneal dialysate. If bacterial peritonitis is suspected, cephalothin, cephapirin, or other cephalosporins may be mixed in the dialysate. Generally, final concentrations of 5–10 μg/ml should be aimed for. Since, with the exception of penicillin, these are usually stable in dialysate fluid for 24 hours, these fluids can be prepared in advance.

When yeasts are the cause of the peritonitis, the therapy is more complicated. Although continuous peritoneal lavage has resulted in successful treatment in some cases, this is not usually recommended. Oral 5-fluorocytosine, ketoconazole, or parenteral miconazole can be tried initially. If the patient fails to respond within 48–72 hours, intraperitoneal antifungal therapy should be added.

Miconazole or amphotericin B can be added to the dialysate directly (a final concentration of 2–5 μg/ml should be adequate). In vitro susceptibilities can be useful for guiding therapy for 5-fluorocytosine, although it is less useful for amphotericin B and some of the other antifungal agents. Intraperitoneal amphotericin B may be extremely painful and may limit this type of treatment. Treatment should be continued for at least 2 weeks and, if the catheter is left in place, 6 weeks may be more prudent.

Other Causes of Peritonitis. Treatment of other causes of peritonitis depends on the specific pathogenesis or cause. For example, rarely, a ventriculoperitoneal shunt may erode the bowel wall and lead to bowel perforation. In this circumstance, surgical repair of the perforation and adjustment or replacement of the peritoneal end of the shunt is necessary. The specific causes of granulomatous peritonitis might be defined by peritoneal biopsy and/or culture and examination of peritoneal fluid. When diagnosed, tuberculosis should be treated with isoniazid and rifampin (or other appropriate antituberculous combinations) for 9–12 months. Histoplasma peritonitis should be treated with amphotericin B for at least 6 weeks. The use of ketoconazole for treatment of fungal peritonitis is still experimental.

Aggressive diagnostic approaches should be used in all cases of peritonitis; this includes examination and culture of the peritoneal fluid and blood cultures. Most antimicrobials diffuse well into the peritoneal cavity, thus intraperitoneal instillation is rarely needed. In some cases, however, this is the most practical way of giving antimicrobials and, as in patients receiving peritoneal dialysis, may be the most effective and well-tolerated method for treatment of mild early peritonitis. Patients with signs of severe peritonitis should be hospitalized, receive a paracentesis and cultures of blood and urine, and be treated with parenteral antimicrobials and other supportive therapies. If bowel perforation is suspected, surgery should be done as soon as possible. With these approaches, the feared complications of peritonitis can be averted in most cases. The role of surgical drainage should not be underestimated in patients whose peritonitis is secondary to intra-abdominal abscess formation.

Hyperbilirubinemia Due to Metabolic Disturbances

AUDREY K. BROWN, M.D.

Conditions associated with hyperbilirubinemia related to metabolic disorders in bilirubin metabolism are listed in Table 1. In two of these disorders, neonatal hyperbilirubinemia and Crigler-Najjar

---

*This dose may exceed that recommended by the manufacturer.

Table 1. METABOLIC DISORDERS OF BILIRUBIN METABOLISM

Unconjugated Hyperbilirubinemias
  Neonatal hyperbilirubinemia
    in preterm infants
    in term infants

  Familial non-hemolytic unconjugated hyperbilirubinemia
    Gilbert disease
    Crigler-Najjar syndrome

  Familial Conjugated Hyperbilirubinemias
    Dubin-Johnson syndrome
    Rotor syndrome

disease, the aim of therapy is to prevent kernicterus. In other disorders of bilirubin metabolism, Gilbert, Dubin-Johnson, and Rotor syndromes, the role of the physician is to identify and diagnose the disorders and thus spare the patient unnecessary intervention, for these disorders do not require specific treatment.

Unconjugated Hyperbilirubinemia

Neonatal Hyperbilirubinemia. Effective management of neonatal hyperbilirubinemia requires that we first define and distinguish it from "physiologic" neonatal bilirubinemia, which can be expected in the majority of newborn infants.

Since most infants exhibit some neonatal jaundice, the limits, nature, and pattern of its appearance and disappearance are well recognized. Hyperbilirubinemia is a departure from this pattern, including 1) jaundice on the first day of life; 2) a rise in serum bilirubin in excess of 5 mg/dl/day; 3) persistence of bilirubin levels greater than 3 mg/dl beyond the first week of life (full term infants); 4) the presence of direct reacting serum bilirubin concentration greater than 1 mg/dl at any time; and 5) a serum indirect bilirubin concentration of 10 mg/dl at any time. In all of these situations every effort should be made to determine whether an underlying cause or clinical circumstances require addressing. For example, early jaundice or levels of bilirubin greater than 10 mg/dl in the first 24 hours of life are almost universally associated with a hemolytic process or enclosed hemorrhage. An increased concentration of direct reacting bilirubin in the serum is a common sign of neonatal infection such as pyelonephritis or sepsis or a sign of hepatic disease.

Preterm Infants (Less than 2000 Gram Birthweight). The degree of hyperbilirubinemia to be anticipated is directly related to the degree of immaturity of the neonate. The mean peak serum bilirubin in infants of birthweight less than 2000 grams is about 9 mg/dl, and 62% will have serum bilirubin levels greater than 10 mg/dl. In 3 to 8% of autopsied infants weighing less than 1500 grams,

kernicterus, i.e., yellow staining of the gray matter of the basal ganglia, can be found even when serum bilirubin levels have been less than 10 to 15 mg/dl; this occurs chiefly in sick infants with acidosis and/or hypoxia.

These considerations have led to recommendation that in infants weighing less than 2000 grams or in sick infants less than 2500 grams hyperbilirubinemia be prevented as soon as possible through the early use of phototherapy.

Phototherapy instituted early (at 24 ± 12 hours of age) and continued for 96 hours in very small infants has been found to prevent or at least limit neonatal hyperbilirubinemia. In a recent trial, only 23% of infants receiving such treatment developed bilirubin levels greater than 10 mg/dl and no kernicterus was found in infants treated this way.

If one attempts to use exchange transfusions alone rather than phototherapy to control hyperbilirubinemia in low birthweight infants, about one fourth of all infants of birthweight less than 2000 grams would have to receive or exchange transfusion in order to limit indirect bilirubin to levels that have been recommended as "safe," i.e., 10 mg/dl in infants weighing < 1000 grams or 15 mg/dl in high risk infants weighting < 1500 grams.

Even these relatively low levels of bilirubin have in rare instances been associated with the finding of kernicterus at autopsy. Present information does not permit selection of limits of serum bilirubin that will ensure against kernicterus. Nevertheless, since phototherapy appears to be a safe, noninvasive means of preventing and limiting hyperbilirubinemia, its early use in very low birthweight infants is recommended.

In infants of birthweight > 2000 grams, phototherapy instituted at a serum bilirubin of 10 mg/dl will usually prevent a rise to 15 mg/dl unless there is significant hemolysis. The daily decrease in serum bilirubin that occurs with phototherapy does not usually exceed 2 mg/24 hours when white light is employed. This degree of response is seen in the first day or two of phototherapy and lessens as the therapy continues. This apparent decrease in effectiveness is probably due to the reabsorption of the bilirubin that enters the intestine during light phototherapy, since photobilirubin formed by the action of light is unstable and reverts to the unconjugated natural bilirubin in the intestine. In this form it can be reabsorbed and enters the enterohepatic circulation. This phenomenon probably also accounts for the slight "rebound" in serum bilirubin level following cessation of phototherapy.

Full Term Infants (≥2500 grams). Less than 20% of all full term infants will have serum bilirubin levels greater than 10 mg/dl and only 6% will have levels over 12 mg/dl. Any infant with levels in this range should be investigated for the cause of this degree of hyperbilirubinemia, since it may be the clue to an otherwise unrecognized infection, hemolytic disease, metabolic disorder, hepatic disease, etc. The underlying disorder may also need treatment.

Overt clinical or pathologic evidence of kernicterus is rarely found in full term infants in the absence of hemolytic disease, such as that attributable to isoimmunization or G6PD deficiency. Bilirubin levels in excess of 20 mg/dl are rarely seen in this group in the absence of increased red cell degradation but can occur in inherited Crigler-Najjar syndrome. Any infant with serum bilirubin concentration $\geq$ 20 mg should receive an exchange transfusion. In the presence of hemolysis, one may anticipate a rise to this level if the bilirubin is 10 mg/dl at 24 hrs or 14 mg/dl at 48 hrs; early exchange transfusion is often indicated in such cases since phototherapy usually does not control such a rapid rise in bilirubin.

The degree to which bilirubin encephalopathy or impaired neurologic development occurs when serum bilirubin levels are in excess of 15 mg/dl is uncertain. Poor motor development has been attributed to sustained serum bilirubin levels in excess of 15 mg/dl even in infants of this birthweight.

When attempting to control hyperbilirubinemia with phototherapy it is important to realize that the daily bilirubin decrement associated with phototherapy is limited; phototherapy instituted at a level of 10 mg/dl has been shown to be more effective in preventing a further rise in serum bilirubin than if it is instituted at serum bilirubin 13 or 15 mg/dl.

Phototherapy and Hemolytic Disease

The rate of bilirubin clearance by phototherapy (i.e., 2 mg/24 hrs) is usually not sufficient to control hyperbilirubinemia associated with hemolytic processes and such clearance may not be reflected by a decrease in serum bilirubin. However, phototherapy, even in cases of hemolysis, may be a useful adjunct to exchange transfusion while waiting for blood to arrive or following the use of exchange transfusion. It should be recognized that the underlying process of hemolysis will continue despite phototherapy. If phototherapy alone is used in mild ABO hemolytic disease to control hyperbilirubinemia, sensitized red blood cells will continue to be destroyed and correction of resultant anemia by simple transfusion may be necessary before the end of the first week or later in the month. Hematocrit and reticulocyte counts must therefore be performed frequently in any hemolytic disorder in the first few weeks of life, even though hyperbilirubinemia has been controlled.

In any situation in which phototherapy is used, the bilirubin should be below 10 mg/dl before it is discontinued. Serum bilirubin must be re-evaluated at 12 and 24 hours after cessation of therapy to be sure that the hyperbilirubinemia has been controlled. Only a minimal "rebound" of about 1 mg/dl should be attributed to the cessation of therapy.

Breast-Feeding and Neonatal Jaundice

Two types of neonatal jaundice have been ascribed to breast-feeding: 1) that which is seen in the first week of life, accounting for slightly higher concentrations of bilirubin than seen in bottle-fed infants, and 2) that which begins in the second week of life and continues for several weeks while the infant continues breast-feeding.

Breast-"Feeding" Jaundice—First Week. This may be related more to the pattern and adequacy of breast-feeding than to factors in breast milk itself. Many pediatricians contend that serum bilirubin concentrations are slightly higher in breast-fed than in bottle-fed infants and that the incidence of hyperbilirubinemia is increased in such infants. Not many prospective studies have borne this out, though recent studies have supported such an association at 4 to 6 days of life. It should be remembered that in some studies adequacy of fluid intake is controlled. Further, it is usual for mothers enrolled in studies to receive instruction and encouragement regarding breast-feeding. These factors could easily reduce the trend toward increased bilirubin levels in infants under study. It is possible that in ordinary clinical settings some breast-fed infants may receive inadequate fluid volume; such infants are more likely to become jaundiced.

Starvation enhances bilirubin absorption from the intestine and promotes bilirubin formation through stimulation of heme oxygenase.

Management of hyperbilirubinemia in the first week of life in the breast-fed infant should include encouragement of the mother's efforts to breast-feed, since poor lactation with restriction of oral intake probably promotes bilirubin formation and retention, as does starvation.

Breast "Milk" Jaundice—Beyond the First Week. Jaundice persisting beyond the first week of life in some breast-fed infants may be related to factors in the milk rather than to the pattern or adequacy of feeding. The extent to which such factors contribute to bilirubin retention before the second or third week of life is not known. In about 2% of lactating mothers, breast milk contains substances that may inhibit bilirubin conjugation as well as promote its reabsorption from the intestine. This breast milk jaundice can be associated with significant elevation of serum indirect reacting bilirubin in the range of 10 to 20 mg/dl and can persist for several weeks. While no case of bilirubin encephalopathy has been reported secondary to this type of hyperbilirubinemia, there is no reason to believe that it could not occur. The "protective" factors may be that the infants are usually full term and beyond the first week of life. If additional adverse events occur (such as intercurrent infection), such "protection" against toxic effects of bilirubin may not suffice.

The diagnostic as well as therapeutic test of "breast milk jaundice" is interruption of breast milk feeding for 36 to 48 hours, after which a significant decrease in serum bilirubin occurs. Following this may be a rise to a lower plateau if breast-feeding is resumed. It is usually safe to continue breast-feeding, but the mother should be aware that the jaundice may not clear completely for several weeks. She must inform the physician of any intercurrent infection or change in the infant's feeding pattern and activity.

Other Notable Causes of Neonatal Hyperbilirubinemia

Galactosemia and hypothyroidism must be considered in any case of prolonged jaundice in the newborn. Galactosemia may rapidly produce hepatic damage and may lead to accumulation of direct as well as indirect reacting bilirubin. Specific management of both of these disorders is directed at the underlying metabolic defects.

Familial Nonhemolytic Unconjugated Hyperbilirubinemia. Gilbert Syndrome. Beyond the neonatal period serum bilirubin levels are usually at or below 0.8 mg/dl in the normal population. When hemolysis and/or liver disease are excluded there remains a small proportion, about 5% of the population, who have elevated levels of serum bilirubin attributable to familial disorders of bilirubin metabolism. The commonest form of familial unconjugated, nonhemolytic hyperbilirubinemia is the Gilbert syndrome. It affects 2 to 5% of the population and is probably inherited as an autosomal dominant. Jaundice is mild and intermittent; it may deepen during an intercurrent infection and is associated with malaise, nausea, and some discomfort over the liver. The serum bilirubin level rarely exceeds 3 mg/dl. Other liver function tests are normal. There is no bilirubin in the urine. Histology of the liver is normal but bilirubin glucuronyl transferase is less than normal. There is a mild impairment of BSP clearance. The serum bilirubin increases during fasting, and in doubtful cases the increase in serum unconjugated bilirubin following a 400 calorie diet for 24 hours may be used diagnostically, since the bilirubin rises on fasting.

Phenobarbital (3 to 5 mg/kg/day) is effective in reducing the serum bilirubin but is probably unnecessary, since the bilirubin levels are not dangerous and prognosis is excellent.

Crigler-Najjar Syndromes, Types I and II. An extreme form of familial nonhemolytic jaundice, associated with very high serum unconjugated bilirubin levels, is Crigler-Najjar syndrome. Two types have been described. In type I, no bilirubin glucuronyl transferase is found in the liver and there is no conjugated bilirubin in the bile. In the past, patients usually died in the first year. Those who survived were severely retarded. In type I there is no response to phenobarbital. In type II, although glucuroynl transferase is absent, patients do respond to phenobarbital, and bilirubin can be maintained at 3 to 10 mg/dl while they receive phenobarbital in doses of 10 mg/kg/day.

In both types, bilirubin levels must be kept under control throughout life, for the patient may develop kernicterus suddenly during viral infections or other illness. Serum bilirubin levels may rise above 20 mg/dl in the first week of life, and the levels must be reduced through the use of repeated exchange transfusions and/or phototherapy to prevent bilirubin encephalopathy.

Both types of Crigler-Najjar syndrome respond to phototherapy, and since type I cannot be controlled with phenobarbital, these patients are managed throughout life with phototherapy. Success has been reported with the use of blue fluorescent light from 10 high-intensity 20 watt T-12 special blue lamps (Westinghouse). Patients require phototherapy for 8 to 12 hours nightly.

Recently it has been suggested that the concomitant use of cholestyramine in doses of 4 to 8 gm daily increases the efficacy of phototherapy. As indicated earlier, during phototherapy, unstable photobilirubin composed of geometric isomers of bilirubin is cleared by the liver without requiring glucuronidation. In the bile, these forms of bilirubin revert to the more stable "natural" unconjugated bilirubin, which can be absorbed and, through enterohepatic circulation, again contribute to the bilirubin load imposed on the liver. Such reabsorption can be reduced by cholestyramine.

Familial Conjugated Hyperbilirubinemia

This rare disorder is associated with a chronic benign intermittent jaundice with conjugated hyperbilirubinemia and bilirubinemia.

Macroscopically the liver is greenish-black, hence the name black-liver jaundice. On section, the liver cells show a brown pigment that is neither iron nor bile. The pigment gives the staining reaction of lipofuscin.

Pruritus is absent; serum alkaline phosphatase and bile acid levels are normal. There is poor excretion of the contrast media used in intravenous cholangiography.

Pregnancy and the use of oral contraceptives reduce hepatic excretory function, and jaundice in these patients may be exacerbated. There is no specific treatment, but prognosis is excellent. The role of the physician is to be aware that this entity may mimic other disorders of obstructive biliary disease.

Rotor Syndrome. This form of chronic familial hyperbilirubinemia resembles Dubin-Johnson syndrome but no brown pigment is found in the liver cells. Further, the gallbladder opacifies on cholecystography and there is no secondary rise in the BSP test. While there is BSP retention, it appears to be related to a defect in hepatic uptake rather than to excretion. There is no treatment for this benign condition.

Cirrhosis

JOEL M. ANDRES, M.D.

Cirrhosis is an irreversible end-stage liver disease characterized by widespread fibrosis that interferes with hepatocellular nutrition and alters hepatic hemodynamics. Prevention of cirrhosis is the optimal treatment goal since medical and surgical therapy do not reverse this slowly progressive process. For the most part, treatment is supportive or directed toward the complications of cirrhosis.

Nutritional. Anorexia and poor nutrition are frequently observed in children with cirrhosis. Inadequate bile acid excretion (cholestasis) leads to steatorrhea, which may improve with a low-fat diet supplemented with medium-chain triglycerides. In the absence of liver failure, a diet high in protein (2 gm/kg/24 hr) and carbohydrate should be encouraged. The fat-soluble vitamins A, D, E, and K are given in twice the usual daily requirements. Patients with hypoprothrombinemia usually respond to daily oral vitamin K (2.5 to 5.0 mg) but may require parenteral therapy. The daily requirement of vitamin D increases to at least 2000 IU in the child with liver disease; oral $1,25 (OH)_2$-cholecalciferol is usually effective in treating rickets at doses greater than 0.1 μg/kg/24 hr.

Hematologic. Nutritional anemia is unusual in patients with cirrhosis, but hypochromic anemia secondary to blood loss and the anemia of splenic hemolysis may be severe enough to require blood transfusion. In advanced cirrhosis, thrombocytopenia is usually the first indicator of hypersplenism, and leukopenia can lead to infection, but impaired coagulation is the major hematologic manifestation of cirrhosis. Coagulation factors are proteins synthesized in the liver and include fibrinogen (factor I), prothrombin (factor II), and factors V, VII, IX, and X; factors II, VII, IX, and X are vitamin K–dependent factors. Decreased activity of these coagulation factors and thrombocytopenia are a serious problem for the poorly compensated child with cirrhosis; intramuscular vitamin K (5 to 10 mg/dose), fresh frozen plasma (10 ml/kg/dose), and platelet concentrates can be administered to decrease the potential for bleeding.

Hemodynamic. A life-threatening complication, such as bleeding esophageal varices, requires accurate diagnosis and aggressive management. Supportive treatment, however, is probably the most important aspect of therapy and includes administration of fresh whole blood to re-establish adequate intravascular volume, correction of electrolyte abnormalities such as hypokalemia, and prevention of hyperammonemia secondary to bacterial degradation of intestinal blood. Intravenous infusion of vasopressin* (10 to 20 units diluted with 20 ml of saline in the older child) over 10 to 15 minutes may cause cessation of bleeding from varices. Two to three repeat doses are sometimes necessary, and control of bleeding is monitored by intermittent gastric aspiration. Selective intraarterial vasopressin is less often utilized in children but provides an effective means of controlling variceal and nonvariceal bleeding lesions, especially in the older patient. Rarely, esophageal balloon tamponade with a pediatric Sengstaken-Blakemore tube is needed when bleeding continues despite conservative and vasopressin therapy, and only in preparation for portal decompression surgery.

Ascites. Initial treatment efforts are directed at dietary salt restriction; ascites will often diminish or not progress with the patient on a low-sodium intake (less than 1 to 2 gm/24 hr). Pharmacologic diuresis can be followed by rapid reaccumulation of ascites and precarious "effective" blood volume. Therefore, the smallest dose of diuretic is needed for adequate diuresis. Spironolactone is one of the safest agents because of its potassium-sparing effect and is known to inhibit aldosterone at the distal renal tubule in a starting dose of 3 mg/kg/24 hr. Urine electrolytes must be carefully checked during therapy; if urine sodium continues to be low (less than 15 meq/1) after 72 to 96 hours, the dose is doubled and may subsequently be increased to 10 mg/kg/24 hr.** Chlorothiazide (20 to 30 mg/kg/24 hr) is added if spironolactone is not effective. The more potent diuretics, furosemide and ethacrynic acid, are considered for use if the ascites continues to be refractory. It should be emphasized that excessive diuresis reduces "effective" plasma volume, and a weight loss of no more than 800 to 1000 gm/24 hr is reasonable in the edematous patient with ascites and from 200 to 300 gm/24 hr in the child with cirrhosis but without peripheral edema.

Other complications of diuretic therapy include hyponatremia, hypokalemia, and encephalopathy; obviously, serum electrolytes and acid-base balance must be carefully monitored. Paracentesis is hazardous but may be necessary to provide symptomatic relief from dyspnea and abdominal distress

---

*This use of vasopressin is not listed in the manufacturer's official directive.

**Ten mg/kg/24 hr may exceed dosage recommended in the manufacturer's official directive.

such as esophageal reflux. The potential for bacterial contamination of ascitic fluid is significant and the most common organism is *Diplococcus pneumoniae*. Salt-poor albumin (1 gm/kg/dose) may be given during this procedure, and should be infused prior to parenteral diuretic therapy if the blood volume is suspected to be low, especially in the hypoalbuminemic patient. Decompressive portal shunts or continuous peritoneovenous shunting of ascitic fluid (LeVeen) are reserved for patients with intractable ascites.

Encephalopathy. Portal-systemic encephalopathy is a frequent complication in advanced cirrhosis. Therapy should focus on identification and treatment of precipitating causes of hepatic coma, such as gastrointestinal bleeding; electrolyte abnormalities, especially hypokalemia; excessive dietary protein; infection; and the use of drugs, such as sedatives, analgesic agents, and diuretics. Gastrointestinal blood should be evacuated, using aspiration and cleansing enema techniques. Neomycin retention enemas and oral neomycin (100 mg/kg/24 hr) suppress the growth of colonic bacteria that produce proteolytic enzymes, such as urease. Lactulose (10 to 30 gm tid) will also decrease blood ammonia by increasing intraluminal acidity via bacterial degradation of this synthetic disaccharide; this is followed by retention of ammonium ion in the gut lumen, and the pH gradient favors movement of ammonia from blood to intestine. Theoretically, lactulose and neomycin are mutually exclusive. Also, general supportive measures are essential, including correction of electrolyte abnormalities; discontinuance of all dietary protein and drugs, especially sedatives and diuretics; treatment of infection; and maintenance of normal serum glucose and osmolality. Exchange transfusion and hemodialysis have not been therapeutically effective, but development of extracorporeal artificial support systems offers hope for the future. Some patients with end-stage chronic liver disease may be candidates for liver transplantation.

Tumors of the Liver

R. PETER ALTMAN, M.D.

Mass lesions arising from the liver can be benign or malignant. Included among the former are cystic and solid tumors. Cystic tumors are often congenital. When solitary, the cyst can often be excised or removed by wedge resection. Alternatively, large cysts require internal drainage to the intestine or marsupialization to the peritoneal cavity.

Benign hepatic adenomas may rupture spontaneously. The intraperitoneal hemorrhage represents an acute abdominal crisis, and emergency surgical resection is life-saving.

Hemangioma and hemangioendothelioma present as mass lesions, or with signs and symptoms of cardiac failure as a result of massive shunting through the tumor. Circumscribed, solitary lesions can be resected, but massive tumors have been treated by hepatic artery ligation or radiologic embolization. Involution of the tumor may be hastened by radiation therapy or the administration of steroids. Extensive hepatic resections are justified if conservative measures fail to control symptoms.

Mesenchymal hamartoma, a tumor of uncertain origin, frequently has cystic and solid components. Surgical excision is recommended.

Focal nodular hyperplasia is benign but can be confused with malignant hepatic tumors angiographically. Surgery is recommended if the tumor is localized, but extensive radical resections are not justified.

Malignant tumors include hepatoblastoma, hepatocellular carcinoma, and rhabdomyosarcoma. None of these has a favorable outlook. The clinical presentation is that of a painless abdominal mass, often of massive proportions. Elevated levels of alpha-fetoprotein in the serum are suggestive of hepatoblastoma, but the test is not specific for this tumor.

Hepatocellular carcinoma is seen in older children. There is a predilection for this malignancy to develop in patients with chronic liver diseases, including cirrhosis, resulting from metabolic disorders (alpha$_1$-antitrypsin deficiency), glycogen storage disease, or chronic active hepatitis.

Rhabdomyosarcoma arises from the bile ducts, and children with this tumor are often jaundiced.

The treatment for all malignant liver tumors is radical surgical excision. These operations should be undertaken only after thorough diagnostic evaluation, including angiography, has been performed in order to delineate the extent and anatomy of the tumor. Occasionally, preoperative chemotherapy will reduce the bulk of the tumor-making resection tenable. Even the largest of liver malignancies can usually be removed by anatomic resection of major portions of the liver.

Survival depends upon complete surgical excision. At present, the results of adjunctive chemotherapy and radiation have been disappointing.

Portal Hypertension

SHEILA SHERLOCK, D.B.E., M.D.

Portal hypertension is nearly always due to obstruction to blood flow in the portal venous system. It can be divided into two main categories: presinusoidal, and sinusoidal or postsinusoidal. It is important to make the distinction. In the presinusoidal type of portal hypertension, hepatocellular function is intact, whereas in the second form it is defective, and liver cell failure is liable to be precipitated by hemorrhage. Treatment depends upon accurate localization of the site of obstruction and, if possible, knowledge of the cause.

Management Before and Between Hemorrhages. Apart from any treatment necessary for underlying cirrhosis, the child should be allowed to lead as normal a life as possible and attend ordinary school. Provided the spleen is not too large, games and physical education may be allowed. Particularly vigorous sports, such as football, must be forbidden. The child should not be allowed to become overly tired. The school principal should be informed of the situation, and the parents should not press the child to be too competitive in either work or play.

Note should be taken of fecal color and the parents told to report if it becomes black. Hemoglobin estimations should be done if the child appears anemic or passes black stools. Oral iron treatment is given as required. The cirrhotic child requires occasional estimations of the prothrombin time, and intramuscular vitamin K_1(5 mg) may be useful from time to time.

Hemorrhage commonly follows an upper respiratory tract infection, and this should be avoided if possible and all necessary inoculations given. If infection develops, it should be taken seriously and broad-spectrum antibiotics given from the start. Drugs containing acetylsalicylic acid must be avoided. Cimetidine is given at the first indication of bleeding.

Undue attention should not be paid to the platelet and leukocyte counts. Although both may be low, the effects on the patient are not definite. Multiple infections are unusual. Low values should not indicate splenectomy.

Management of Hemorrhage. Endoscopy should be done, using a pediatric endoscope. If the technique has not been performed previously, an emergency percutaneous splenic venogram is performed.

If the patient is cirrhotic, hepatic precoma and coma may be precipitated by the hemorrhage. This should be anticipated by giving no protein by mouth, keeping the bowels moving freely, giving an enema if necessary, and prescribing oral neomycin, 15 mg/kg 4 times a day for 3 days. All types of sedation should be avoided. If the child has extrahepatic portal venous obstruction and normal hepatic function, there is virtually no danger of the development of hepatic precoma. The precoma regimen is therefore unnecessary, and sedation can be given as required. It is unusual for these patients to bleed before the age of 4 years.

Blood transfusion is usually necessary. In patients with extrahepatic portal obstruction, hemorrhages are likely to be multiple over years. The greatest possible care must be taken to preserve peripheral veins for further transfusions and to give absolutely compatible blood.

If liver cell function is adequate, the bleeding usually ceases spontaneously. If liver cell function is deficient and if the bleeding continues, I prefer to use vasopressin* (Pitressin) IV, although this route is not recommended by the manufacturer. This drug lowers portal venous pressure by constriction of the splanchnic arterial bed, causing an increase in resistance to the inflow of blood to the gut. It controls hemorrhage from esophageal varices by lowering portal venous pressure. A large dose, 1 unit per 3 kg of body weight, is given well diluted in 5 per cent dextrose intravenously in 10 minutes. Mean arterial pressure increases transiently, and portal pressure decreases for 45 minutes to 1 hour. Control of hemorrhage is shown by the disappearance of blood from gastric aspirates and by serial pulse and blood pressure readings. Abdominal colicky discomfort and evacuation of the bowels, together with facial pallor, are usual during the infusion. If these are absent, it may be questioned whether the vasopressin is pharmacologically active. Inert material is the most common cause of failure. Regular vasopressin injections may be repeated in 4 hours if bleeding recurs, but efficacy decreases with continual use. The ultimate failure of vasopressin to control terminal hemorrhage reflects hepatocellular failure rather than improper method of treatment.

The value of vasopressin is its simplicity of use. In an emergency it can even be used in the home. Special nursing and medical care are not essential. The short duration is obviously unsatisfactory, and the side effects are unpleasant even if short-lived. However, this dosage is necessary to achieve an adequate reduction in portal pressure.

If vasopressin fails to produce the desired effect, the Sengstaken trilumen esophageal compression tube is used. A special small-sized tube is available for pediatric use. A rubber tube is inflated in the esophagus at a pressure of 20 to 30 mm Hg, slightly greater than that expected in the portal vein. Another balloon is inflated in the fundus of the stomach. The third lumen communicates with the stomach. The tube is passed relatively easily if the pharynx is well anesthetized. When the tube is in position, traction has to be exerted, and this causes difficulty. Too little traction means that the gastric balloon falls back into the stomach. Too much traction causes discomfort, with retching, and potentiates gastroesophageal ulceration.

The compression tubes are very successful in controlling bleeding from esophageal varices. They

---

*This use of vasopressin is not listed in the manufacturer's directive; 1 unit/3 kg may exceed manufacturer's recommended dosage.

do, however, have many complications. They should not be left inflated longer than 24 hours. Their use should be part of a plan of management culminating either in surgery or in withdrawal of the tube and conservative treatment if the patient's condition is too poor. Complications include obstruction of the pharynx with consequent asphyxia, aspiration pneumonia, and ulceration of pharynx, esophagus, and fundus of the stomach. The tube is not well tolerated by the patient. Skilled nursing is required for supervision of the patient while the tube is in position.

Emergency surgery is rarely necessary. If bleeding does not cease or if it recurs and active intervention becomes essential, the best surgical method is probably transhepatic sclerosis of the portal and splenic vein tributaries feeding the varices. In patients having normal liver function, and in whom the splenic venogram or mesenteric angiogram has shown a portal or superior mesenteric vein of adequate caliber, a portacaval or mesocaval shunt may be performed. Emergency shunt surgery has a high mortality rate if the patient has cirrhosis and, if possible, should be avoided in this circumstance. Esophageal transection or direct ligation of varices is occasionally necessary in children with extrahepatic portal vein destruction and exsanguinating bleeding.

Elective Surgery. Prophylactic surgery is not indicated. The patient must have bled from varices before operation can be considered. The choice of procedure depends largely upon the state of the portal venous system as revealed by splenic venography or selective splanchnic angiography. If the portal vein is patent and of adequate caliber, end-to-side portacaval anastomosis is the most satisfactory procedure. In experienced hands this operation carries a low mortality rate of less than 5 per cent. Because of vein size, the operation can rarely be undertaken before the age of 10 years. It carries a small risk of shunt encephalopathy. In children this is particularly small, and in the presence of a normal liver, e.g., obstruction to the portal vein at the hilus of the liver, the changes are almost nonexistent. In the presence of cirrhosis, the possibility varies with the degree of underlying damage to the liver. The operation should not be performed in the presence of jaundice, ascites, or a past history of hepatic coma.

Splenorenal anastomosis may be considered in portal venous occlusion if the splenic vein is of adequate size. It is less efficient than a portacaval anastomosis, because the shunt is small and often occludes. The danger of post-shunt encephalopathy, however, is very small.

Superior mesenteric vein–inferior vena caval shunt is used to treat portal hypertension in patients who have occlusion of the portal and splenic veins, making neither available for anastomosis.

The vena cava is transected just proximal to the junction of the two iliac veins, and the distal segment is ligated. The proximal segment is then anastomosed to the side of the intact superior mesenteric vein. Sometimes an intervening Dacron graft is used and the superior mesenteric vein and inferior vena cava so anastomosed side-to-side. Failures may be due to superior mesenteric vein thrombosis, and the mortality rate is about 10 per cent.

Direct attacks on the varices and on various dangerous collaterals are numerous and rarely of long-lasting benefit. They include splenectomy, transection of the esophagus, partial and total gastrectomy, and partial esophagectomy. In general, they are not to be recommended. Patients with extrahepatic portal venous obstruction rarely die of exsanguinating hemorrhage. Conservative management usually helps them over the acute episode. Bleeding becomes more infrequent as time allows for the opening of collateral vessels to the renal and lumbar veins. Ultimately, portal pressure may decrease. This possibility may be lessened with repeated operations and removal or transection of such benign collaterals. The operative and postoperative mortality rate of the local operations on varices in a cirrhotic patient with borderline liver function is high, and the ultimate benefit doubtful.

Chronic Active Hepatitis

SHEILA SHERLOCK, D.B.E., M.D.

Chronic active hepatitis is diagnosed by the continuation for longer than 6 months of fluctuant hepatocellular jaundice with increased transaminase and gamma globulin levels.

If specific causes, such as Wilson disease, can be excluded, then immunosuppressive therapy, usually with prednisolone, must be considered. The indications for such treatment are not clear-cut, but if the serum transaminase levels are increased five times and gamma globulin levels are more than twice elevated, steroid therapy should be given. Liver biopsy findings of piecemeal necrosis with inflammation and bridging necrosis between portal zones and central areas are also indications. The initial dose is 0.4 mg/kg of prednisolone for 2 weeks. This is then reduced to a maintenance dose of 0.2 mg/kg.

Twenty per cent of patients fail to respond, deteriorate, develop hepatocellular failure, and die. In such patients a trial of higher doses of prednisolone (0.8 mg/kg) is worth considering. Prednisolone usually must be used for at least 6 months. Attempts are made to withdraw therapy when serum bilirubin, transaminase, and, if possible, gamma globulin levels are normal. Relapses follow discontinuation of treatment in about half of the patients, usually within 6 months of stopping, and necessitate reinstitution of the drug. Children who are hepatitis B antigen–positive respond less well to prednisolone than do those who are negative. In this group, if clinical and biochemical improvement has not followed 6 months' therapy, it should be stopped. Antiviral therapy must be considered but, at present, no satisfactory agent is available.

Retardation of growth may be a problem in those less than 10 years old. In these children, alternate-day therapy with prednisolone, 0.4 mg/kg every other day, must be considered. This may minimize the effects of corticosteroids on growth. Alternatively, if complications such as facial mooning, obesity, growth retardation, or diabetes are a problem, then prednisolone (0.15 mg/kg) may be combined with azathioprine (1 mg/kg). Azathioprine alone gives less satisfactory results than when prednisolone is used.*Corticosteroid therapy is of particular value in preventing deaths during the first 2 years after diagnosis, when the disease is most active. Although most patients end with cirrhosis, a lesion which is irreversible, there are many examples in which the disease has become inactive and the patients have survived 10 to 20 years.

Disorders of the Hepatobiliary Tree

JOYCE D. GRYBOSKI, M.D.

Biliary Atresia. Biliary atresia is a significant disorder in the neonate, its incidence being reported as between 1 in 8000 and 1 in 20,000 live births. It is responsible for one third of all cases of neonatal jaundice.

Only 10–12% of affected infants have correctible atresia. Here the lesion is either a distal atresia with patent proximal hepatic ducts or a cystic dilatation of the ducts adjacent to the hilus of the liver. In most instances there is a patent gallbladder. Correction is accomplished by anastomosis of the patent extrahepatic bile duct or the gallbladder to a Roux-en-Y jejunostomy.

The more common and *noncorrectible form* of biliary atresia consists of a nonpatent extrahepatic biliary tree and an absent or nonfunctioning gallbladder. The Kasai operation has considerably altered the near-uniform fatal prognosis. In this procedure, the nonfunctioning extrahepatic ducts are removed and the jejunum is anastomosed to the hilus of the liver. The procedure requires patent intrahepatic bile ducts, greater than 150 μ in diameter, for flow to occur in all patients. Successful flow

may be established in 86% of those with ducts less than 150 μ and in only 12% of those with no demonstrable ducts. Success rates of 80 to 90% are reported if surgery is performed before 2 months of age. Overall, the surgical success rate is directly related to the timing of operation, for it falls to 60% in those operated between 2 and 3 months, and to 20% in those operated after 3 months of age. This is largely due to progression of the disease. A 5 year survival rate reported in the Japanese literature is 36%. Although early results in the United States have been poor, more recent studies report up to 50% of patients alive and 25% free of jaundice 1 to 6 years after operation.

Complications are related to progression of the underlying disease and to the surgical procedure. Modification of the Kasai operation to include wide dissection at the base of the fibrous remnant and incorporation of a cutaneous stoma to divert or decompress the biliary drainage has significantly improved the earlier results.

Bile flow may never be established because of severe liver disease and paucity of intrahepatic ducts. Ten to 15% of infants in whom bile flow has been established may show a decrease in or cessation of flow. If this occurs within 2 months of surgery, reoperation with further excision of the liver hilus and reanastomosis of the jejunum will establish flow in half. Some recommend a course of systemic steroids (methylprednisolone or hydrocortisone) 3 to 5 mg/kg/24 hr) for 2 to 3 days. Flow that decreases after 3 months is less amenable to surgery and represents progression of liver disease. Closure of the external conduit is performed after 1 or more years when bile flow has remained adequate, liver function and histology are improved, and there is no evidence of cholangitis.

Postoperative and recurrent cholangitis is a major problem, occurring in more than half of successful portoenterostomies. Stasis is implicated. Cholangitis is less common in those who had correctible lesions and the gallbladder or external ducts anastomosed to the jejunum. This complication is signaled by fever, leukocytosis, right upper quadrant tenderness, deteriorating liver function, decreased bile flow, and jaundice. The incidence decreases markedly between 6 and 12 months. Second or third generation aminoglycosides are the antibiotics of choice, for these attain the highest biliary levels. Tobramycin, 6 to 7.5 mg/kg/24 hr,*with the frequent addition of carbenicillin, 500 mg/kg/24 hr for 7 to 10 days, is recommended. In our experience intravenous cefamandole, 50 to 100 mg/kg/24 hours, has been highly effective. Continued maintenance therapy with oral trimethoprim/sulfamethoxazole, 10 mg/kg/24 hr in four divided

---

*This use of azathioprine is not mentioned in the manufacturer's directions.

*This dose may exceed that recommended by the manufacturer. Serum levels should be monitored.

doses, or cephradine, 25 to 50 mg/kg/24 hr in three or four divided doses, during the first year, may suppress recurrent infection.

Cholangitis that develops after 12 months usually indicates obstruction, and the patient should be evaluated and treated surgically.

Nutritional deficiencies may present early and continue even after successful establishment of bile flow. The unavailability of bile acids or of levels less than those necessary for micellarization of lipids results in malabsorption of fats and fat-soluble vitamins. Supplementation with water-soluble vitamins is necessary for years after operation and should be in dosages two to four times the recommended daily requirements. Vitamin A as Aquasol A should be given in a dosage of 1500 to 25,000 IU per day, and vitamin A levels should be monitored to avoid toxic levels. Vitamin D is administered as D_2 in a dosage of 5000 IU per day or as 1,25, $(OH)_2D_3$, 0.1 μg/kg/day. 25-hydroxycholecalciferol is used for treatment of those with rickets. Vitamin K, 0.1 to 5 mg/kg/day, is given orally, but if bleeding is evident and the prothrombin fails to correct, vitamin K must be administered intramuscularly. Vitamin E requirements are 100 to 400 IU, provided by Aquasol E.

Mineral deficiencies exist as well. Since steatorrhea impairs calcium absorption, calcium intake should be increased to provide 50 to 200 mg of elemental calcium/kg/day with 25 to 50 mg/kg/day of elemental phosphorus. Zinc deficiency has been reported, and supplements of at least 10 mg/day are recommended.

Overall nutritional support consists of a diet high in proteins and low in fats. Formula, such as Pregestimil, which contains medium chain triglycerides, is now readily available. In older children medium chain triglyceride oil may be used.

Pruritus and xanthomas are complications of longstanding disease. Phenobarbital, 5 to 10 mg/kg/day to attain serum levels of 10 to 20 μg per ml, may have a choleretic effect. The clinical response, however, must be titrated against the sedative effect of the drug. Cholestyramine,* which binds intraluminal bile acids, should be used only in children with some evidence of bile flow. The usual dosage is ½ to 1 packet given four times daily to a maximum of 8 gm (each packet contains 2 gm). In addition to its being gritty and rather unpalatable, reported complications from its administration have been intestinal obstruction, hyperchloremic acidosis, and increased steatorrhea.

Portal hypertension complicated by splenomegaly, hypersplenism, ascites, and bleeding from esophageal varices develops in infants with established or progressive liver disease and cirrhosis. Ascites is treated with salt restriction to approximately 500 mg/day. Diuretics such as spironolactone, 3 to 5 mg/kg/day in divided doses, or furosemide, 1 to 2 mg/kg/dose, may be used if diet does not control the ascites. Serum electrolytes must be monitored carefully. Paracentesis should be avoided unless there is severe respiratory distress.

Bleeding esophageal varices are treated medically with intravenous vasopressin (Pitressin)* in dosage of 2 to 4 milliunits/kg/min in 5% dextrose over a 20 to 30 minute period every 4 hours for 24 hours. The Sengstaken-Blakemore tube may be placed in the esophagus to control bleeding if the above treatment fails. A chest film must determine the accuracy of placement of the balloon in the distal esophagus, and the balloon itself should be deflated every 6 hours to prevent pressure necrosis of the esophagus. It should not be left inflated for more than 24 hours. Excellent results are now reported with endoscopic sclerosis of varices using sodium morrhuate injection. However, the child must be big enough to tolerate endoscope and sclerosing equipment. Prospective studies are under way in adults, using propranolol, a beta-blocker, in prevention of esophageal bleeds, but there is no information available on its use in children.

The long-term results of shunting procedures in this age group are not promising and, since there is often spontaneous improvement with the development of collateral circulation, these operations are not indicated.

Liver transplantation is now a viable alternative to the Kasai procedure, but is limited because of the few centers in which it is performed and the few donor livers available for infants. Results have improved dramatically with the use of Cyclosporin A, an investigational immunosuppressive agent, in combination with low-dose steroid therapy.

Choledochal Cyst. This uncommon form of ductal cholestasis is estimated to occur in 1 : 13,000 to 1 : 15,000 live births, and affects females 3 to 4 times more often than males. Associated lesions are frequent and must be evaluated before or during surgery. The most common malformation is dilatation of the cystic duct, and often of the hepatic ducts. Biliary atresia is associated in 12% and common duct diverticulum in 10 per cent. A few patients have a choledochocele. Others have extrahepatic cysts, stenoses, and anomalous junction of the pancreaticobiliary system. Complete excision of the cyst followed by choledochojejunostomy is the treatment of choice. Simple aspiration of the cyst is unacceptable, and with choledochocystojejunostomy there occurs a high

---

*Dosage of cholestyramine in children has not been established.

*This use of vapopressin is not listed by the manufacturer.

incidence of cholangitis. Further support for complete cyst excision lies in an increased carcinoma risk, with a recent survey from the American Academy of Pediatrics reporting a 4.7% incidence.

The complications of untreated choledochal cyst are cholangitis, calculus formation, and biliary cirrhosis with portal hypertension.

Despite adequate surgical correction of the extrahepatic lesion, patients may have recurrent disease from intrahepatic lesions such as intrahepatic cysts or primary biliary atresia. Cholangitis and complications of portal hypertension are treated as described under Biliary Atresia.

Caroli's Disease. Also known as congenital segmental dilatation of the intrahepatic biliary tree, this disease occurs in the simple form known as Caroli's disease or in association with congenital hepatic fibrosis. Cystic spongiosis of the renal medulla and cystic disease of the pancreas are associated diseases.

The large intrahepatic ducts are involved, and cystic dilatations reach 10 to 45 mm in diameter. Cholangitis secondary to biliary stasis is the most frequent form of presentation, and recurrent episodes of cholangitis plague affected patients. The medical treatment is similar to that described under Biliary Atresia, with children requiring long-term maintenance antibiotic therapy. Since periods of infection are associated with bacterial deconjugation of bile acids, rendering them ineffective in lipid micellarization, attention to nutritional needs and vitamin and mineral supplementation is indicated.

Rarely, the cystic dilatations are confined to one lobe of the liver, and in such instances hepatic lobectomy may be indicated. A new technique of transhepatic drainage of the biliary tree has provided drainage in some patients.

If infection can be controlled, those with the simple form of the disease survive well into adult life. Those with congenital hepatic fibrosis will develop portal hypertension and all of its complications.

Sclerosing Cholangitis. This is seen in patients with inflammatory bowel disease, usually ulcerative colitis. It may involve the external biliary tree, the region of ductal bifurcation, and even the intrahepatic bile ducts. The only available therapy is that to relieve biliary obstruction and to treat cholangitis. T-tube external drainage or cholecystoduodenostomy, cholecystojejunostomy, and even hepaticojejunostomy have been employed to relieve obstruction. Corticosteroids have been beneficial in a few patients but their action is temporary. Colectomy does not affect the course of sclerosing cholangitis. Cholangitis progresses to biliary cirrhosis and portal hypertension, and carries an increased incidence of biliary tract carcinoma.

Intrahepatic Cholestatic Syndromes. Familial cholestatic syndromes vary from the relatively benign recurrent intrahepatic cholestasis to Byler's syndrome, which leads to death in childhood or early adolescence from cirrhosis. In the intermediate forms lymphedema, atypical facies, and peripheral pulmonary stenosis (Alagille syndrome) may also occur. Regardless of type, nutritional, vitamin, and mineral deficiencies must be addressed as described under Biliary Atresia.

Diseases of the Gallbladder. Until recently, *Cholelithiasis* was considered rare during childhood, and usually occurred in the postpubertal child. Disease was usually associated with a history of underlying hemolysis or infection. Recently, asymptomatic stones are being reported in 7- to 10-year-old children with a history of mild neonatal jaundice and in infants of several months whose postpartum course was complicated by prematurity, necrotizing enterocolitis, ileal resection, or sepsis. Increased incidence has been reported in children who have received long-term parenteral hyperalimentation, many of whom had ileal resection or disease.

Ileal resection or malfunction predisposes to the formation of cholesterol gallstones. It has also been suggested that in the presence of cholesterol saturated bile, some unstable bilirubin is converted to an insoluble form.

In view of this evidence, it may be possible to avert cholelithiasis by feeding small increments of fat in order to stimulate bile flow during long periods of hyperalimentation. Certainly the development of cholecystitis is an indication for intravenous antibiotic therapy and cholecystectomy. Most calculi are large and asymptomatic and may be watched with caution until the patients are of a size to warrent their removal. Multiple small calculi are more likely to produce complications within the common duct or the pancreatic duct and should be removed.

Medical therapy using chenodeoxycholic acid has resulted in dissolution of stones and lessened bile saturation in some adults, but it must be considered in view of years of administration. It has not been used in children.

Hydrops of the gallbladder may occur in the absence of biliary tract infection or stones. With the use of ultrasonography, it is being recognized with greater frequency. Originally associated with upper respiratory infection, salmonella, streptococcal, and pseudomonas infections or sepsis, it is now seen as a manifestation of Kawasaki's disease, and in prematures and neonates. In infants, hydrops of the gallbladder has been attributed to poor peristalsis and stasis, and often resolves spontaneously after initiation of oral feeding.

Infection, if identified, must be treated vigorously. Serial ultrasonography will determine increase or decrease in gallbladder size. If there is no increase in size and the patient is not toxic, watchful waiting is appropriate. If the size continues to increase, perforation may be imminent and cholecystectomy should be performed, and the biliary tree should be examined for abnormalities such as stenosis, atresia, or torsion.

Acute cholecystitis unassociated with stones is extremely rare but has been reported with typhoid fever, typhus, diphtheria, scarlet fever, shigellosis, viral gastroenteritis, and respiratory tract infection. Rarely it has been caused by infestation by *Giardia lamblia* or *Ascaris lumbricoides*. Malformations of the biliary tree, spasm of the sphincter of Oddi, and gastric heterotopia in the gallbladder are other associated causes. Specific treatment with second or third generation aminoglycosides for 48 hours and cholecystectomy is curative.

Spontaneous perforation of extrahepatic bile ducts occurs during the first days of life and should be considered in a previously well infant who becomes irritable, anorectic, febrile, and jaundiced and has increasing abdominal girth. Cholangiography will show extravasation of dye into a saclike structure, and ^{131}I rose bengal or other isotopes will show normal liver uptake but, 24 hours later, isotope concentrated under the diaphragm or free in the peritoneal cavity. Medical therapy is unsuccessful and surgical therapy consists of immediate drainage of the area of perforation. Exploration should not be attempted and the gallbladder is left in place. Spontaneous closure will occur after several weeks, during which the infant is fed parenterally.

Trauma or *battering* may result in traumatic hemobilia, avulsion of the bile ducts, or late biliary stricture. Traumatic hemobilia results from formation of intrahepatic pseudocysts which suddenly empty into the biliary tree. Surgical removal of the edges of the cystic cavity with drainage of the lesion is the only therapy. Treatment for avulsion of the bile ducts consists of drainage and repair of the tear.

Benign *tumors of the biliary tree*, such as papilloma, adenoma, and fibroma, are more common than malignant ones and are treated by simple excision. The most common malignant tumor is sarcoma botryoides; less frequent ones are rhabdomyosarcoma and cholangiosarcoma. These are treated by excision followed by radiotherapy but the prognosis for long-term survival is poor.

Pancreatic Diseases

KENNETH L. COX, M.D.

ACUTE PANCREATITIS

The general principles of treatment of acute pancreatitis are (1) to treat hypovolemia and electrolyte abnormalities, (2) to relieve pain, (3) to reduce pancreatic secretions, and (4) to remove the precipitating cause.

Correction of hypovolemia should begin imme-diately, utilizing a large-bore central venous catheter for fluid replacement and to monitor central venous pressure. Hypotension and low central venous pressure should be corrected as rapidly as possible with plasma, dextran, albumin, or whole blood. Shock is the main cause of death in acute pancreatitis. Shock is primarily a result of exudation of plasma into the retroperitoneal space and peripheral vasodilatation caused by increased kinin activity.

After hypovolemia has been corrected, the rate of intravenous infusions should be reduced so as to provide maintenance plus replacement of ongoing losses from nasogastric suctioning and exudation into the peritoneal and retroperitoneal spaces. Monitoring urine output and central venous pressure are mechanisms for assessing the adequacy of the fluid replacement. Major complications of treatment of severe acute pancreatitis are pulmonary edema and congestive heart failure; these usually occur 3 to 7 days after the onset of pancreatitis. Though in many cases the cause is unknown, in some cases fluid overload has occurred because of excessive fluid replacement. Thus, the amount of fluid replacement must be adjusted frequently for changes in intravascular volume.

Serum electrolytes, including calcium and magnesium, serum creatinine, and blood urea nitrogen determinations, will aid in selecting the appropriate electrolyte composition of intravenous solutions. Since between 2 and 17 per cent of patients with acute pancreatitis have renal failure, potassium should not be added to IV solutions until stable urine output has been established. In addition to maintenance sodium chloride and potassium chloride of 3 mEq/kg/24 hr and 2 mEq/kg/24 hr, respectively, losses from nasogastric suctioning should be replaced. Though 5 per cent dextrose solutions should be initiated, hyperglycemia and hypoglycemia occasionally seen in severe pancreatitis warrant careful monitoring of urinary reducing substances and blood glucose concentrations and changing the concentration of dextrose in the IV solution appropriately. Symptomatic hypocalcemia, i.e., tetany and seizures, should be treated with IV calcium gluconate, 0.1 to 0.2 gm/kg/dose (not over 2 gm) as a 10 per cent solution administered slowly and stopped for bradycardia. For asymptomatic hypocalcemia, replacement may be accomplished by adding 10 ml or more of 10 per cent calcium gluconate to each 500 ml of IV solution. In severe pancreatitis, serum electrolytes, including calcium, should be measured at least daily so that adjustments in the electrolyte composition of IV solutions can be made if necessary.

Pancreatic exocrine secretions are reduced by fasting the patient. Usually feeding should not be reinstituted until abdominal pain and ileus have resolved and serum amylase, urinary diastase, and the amylase-creatinine clearance ratio have returned to normal. If oral alimentation cannot be taken within 5 days, then parenteral nutrition should be given. Since carbohydrate is less of a stimulant to pancreatic exocrine secretion than are protein and fat, the initial diet should consist of carbohydrates only. If the carbohydrate diet is tolerated without worsening or exacerbating symptoms, then a low-fat and protein diet may be given. Again, the diet should be discontinued if symptoms should recur.

Nasogastric suctioning should be used to relieve nausea, vomiting, and abdominal pain. Since there is no evidence that gastric suctioning alters the clinical course of pancreatitis, it is not required in the treatment of mild-to-moderate pancreatitis. However, in severe pancreatitis or marked ileus, nasogastric suctioning should be used.

Relief of the severe abdominal pain associated with pancreatitis not only is important for patient comfort but also may reduce the cephalic phase of pancreatic secretion. Morphine sulfate should be avoided because it may worsen pancreatitis by causing sphincter of Oddi spasm. Meperidine hydrochloride (Demerol) may be administered IV or IM at 1 to 2 mg/kg every 3 to 4 hours for severe abdominal pain. If this does not reduce pain sufficiently, then the effect of Demerol can be potentiated by administering chlorpromazine (Thorazine) at 1 mg/kg IM simultaneously.

Other therapies for acute pancreatitis remain controversial. Prophylactic antibiotics have not been shown to be beneficial. Secondary infection of the pancreas, usually by streptococci, coliforms, or staphylococci, occurs in 2 to 5 percent of cases of pancreatitis. Identification of the infective organism(s) and the antibiotic sensitivities will allow selection of the appropriate antibiotics. If pancreatic abscess forms, surgical drainage is usually necessary. There is insufficient clinical evidence that suppressors of pancreatic exocrine secretion, such as anticholinergic drugs, glucagon, somatostatin, calcitonin, and tranquilizers, and inhibitors of pancreatic enzymes, such as aprotinin (Trasylol)*and epsilon-amino-caproic acid (EACA), are useful in the management of acute pancreatitis.

Persistence of abdominal pain and of elevation of serum amylase levels for 2 or more weeks after the onset of acute pancreatitis suggests the formation of a pseudocyst. Ultrasonography is an effective method of identifying pseudocysts, differentiating pseudocysts from inflammatory masses, and monitoring the size of pseudocysts. Many pseudocysts spontaneously resolve in 4 to 12 weeks. If the pseudocyst persists for 6 or more weeks or is en-

larging, surgical internal drainage of the cyst into the stomach or upper small intestine has been the treatment of choice. More recently, ultrasonography has been used to guide percutaneous needle aspiration of the cysts and to place catheters for external drainage. This technique may be particulary useful in patients who are poor operative candidates.

Pancreatic fistulas most often occur following pancreatic trauma or drainage of pseudocysts. Most fistulas will spontaneously close. Those that have a high output or interfere with providing adequate oral alimentation often require prolonged periods of fasting and total parenteral nutrition. Intravenous lipids can be given as a part of TPN therapy since they do not appear to stimulate pancreatic secretion. Rarely, surgical closure of the fistula is necessary.

Chronic and recurrent acute pancreatitis are rarely seen in children. Continued exposure to the precipitating cause, i.e., alcohol, cholelithiasis, child abuse, and so on, or familial pancreatitis must be considered. Hereditary pancreatitis is transmitted autosomal dominantly and is associated with lysinuria and cystinuria in some cases. Most cases of hereditary pancreatitis require total pancreatectomy for control of symptoms. Endoscopic retrograde cholangiopancreatography (ERCP) should be performed if etiology is unknown, since congenital papillary stenosis may be identified and treated by endoscopic papillotomy. ERCP may identify other obstructive abnormalities such as gallstones choledochal cysts, or duplication cysts that can be surgically corrected. Malabsorption due to pancreatic exocrine insufficiency and, rarely, diabetes mellitus requiring insulin therapy are sequelae of chronic pancreatitis. Malabsorption should be treated with oral pancreatic enzyme replacement therapy. Severe chronic abdominal pain may require prolonged fasting, using home parenteral nutrition or pancreatectomy.

PANCREATIC EXOCRINE INSUFFICIENCY

Cystic fibrosis, Shwachman-Diamond syndrome (pancreatic insufficiency and bone marrow hypoplasia), and chronic pancreatitis are main causes of pancreatic exocrine insufficiency in children.

Oral pancreatic enzyme extracts are the primary treatment, independent of the cause. The dose of pancreatic enzymes extract to be administered with meals depends upon the severity of pancreatic exocrine insufficiency, the patient's age, the fat content of the diet, and the type of enzyme preparation. In general, dietary fat restriction is not necessary, and approximately 8000 lipase NF units (one Cotazym capsule or one Viokase tablet) should digest at least 15 gm of dietary fat. Higher doses of enzymes may not improve digestion and may result in hyperuri-

---

*Aprotinin is an investigational drug and may not be available in the United States.

cemia. Ineffectiveness of oral pancreatic enzymes to completely correct malabsorption is in part due to the suboptimal pH of the stomach for enzyme activity. Reduction of gastric acidity with antacids or cimetidine or protection of preparations with enteric coating (Pancrease or Cotazyms) has been reported to improve enzyme activity. However, clinical studies have not consistently shown improvements in fat and protein absorption or nutritional state of the patients when cimetidine, antacids, or enteric-coated preparations were used.

Deficiency of fat-soluble vitamins D, A, K, and E may occur with severe malabsorption. Clinical manifestations from vitamin deficiencies are rarely seen. Occasionally, bleeding diathesis due to hypoprothrombinemia from vitamin K deficiency and hemolytic anemia from vitamin E deficiency will occur. Prevention of vitamin deficiencies is usually accomplished by reducing malabsorption with oral pancreatic enzymes and by administering a multiple vitamin preparation at twice the minimal daily requirements. Additional supplementation with water-miscible vitamin E, 50 to 100 U daily, and with vitamin K, 0.5 to 5 mg daily, should be given to those who have severe malabsorption or laboratory evidence of deficiency in these vitamins.

Advising patients and families of the appropriate diet for age and dose of oral pancreatic enzymes will usually allow normal growth and development without significant malabsorptive symptoms. Occasionally, additional calories in the form of dietary supplements will be desired, or limited fat restrictions in the diet, i.e., a 15 to 20 per cent fat diet, will be necessary to control steatorrhea. Because elemental dietary supplements like medium-chain triglycerides and predigested protein are unpalatable, children will often refuse to take these preparations, especially for long periods of time. In these cases, nonelemental dietary supplements, such as Ensure, Sustacal, and Meritene, given with enzymes may be more acceptable.

ISOLATED PANCREATIC ENZYME DEFICIENCIES

Isolated pancreatic enzyme deficiencies are extremely rare. Diagnosis is made by pancreatic secretory studies revealing normal concentrations of pancreatic enzymes in duodenal aspirates except for the absence of a single enzyme.

Isolated lipase deficiency is an autosomal recessive disease that presents shortly after birth with oily diarrhea. Standard oral pancreatic enzyme preparations, as are used in cystic fibrosis, will correct the malabsorption.

Isolated amylase deficiency usually presents after 1 year of age. As starch becomes a larger part of the diet, watery diarrhea occurs. Analysis of the stool will reveal reducing substances (Clinitest positive at more than ¼ per cent) and an acid pH of less than

6.0. The diagnosis can be confirmed with a starch loading test, i.e., failure of blood glucose to rise following ingestion of 50 gm of starch per square meter of body surface area. Treatment consists of starch elimination and supplementation with disaccharides.

Isolated trypsin or trypsinogen deficiency presents shortly after birth with diarrhea, anemia, hypoproteinemia, edema, and severe failure to thrive. Absence of trypsin or trypsinogen results in lack of proteolytic enzyme activity in duodenal secretions. Treatment consists of standard oral pancreatic enzyme preparations.

Isolated enterokinase deficiency is an autosomal recessive disease that will also present in the neonatal period with severe watery diarrhea, failure to thrive, anemia, hypoproteinemia, and edema. Enterokinase is produced in the brush border of the proximal small intestine. Since this enzyme is necessary for the activation of trypsin, duodenal aspirates lack proteolytic enzyme activity, which can be activated by adding enterokinase to the aspirate. Enterokinase can be assayed in the small intestinal biopsies. Standard oral pancreatic enzyme preparations are the required treatment.

CONGENITAL MALFORMATIONS

Annular pancreas is a ring of pancreatic tissue encircling the descending portion of the duodenum. Surgical intervention consists of a duodenoduodenostomy or duodenojejunostomy. The pancreas is left undivided so as to avoid formation of pancreatic fistulas. Pancreatic function is normal in these patients.

Approximately 2 per cent of the population have ectopic pancreatic tissue. Ninety per cent of these occur in the stomach, duodenum, or jejunum. Occasionally, the ectopic pancreas will produce abdominal pain, gastrointestinal obstruction, bleeding, or intussusception. When these complications occur, the ectopic pancreatic tissue should be excised.

PANCREATIC TUMORS

Pancreatic tumors in children are very rare. Most are endocrine-secreting tumors, e.g., insulinoma, gastrinoma, VIPoma, and so on.

Ninety per cent of insulinomas are solitary tumors. Severe hypoglycemia often results in irreversible neurologic sequelae. Diazoxide, from 5 mg/kg/24 hr up to 20 mg/kg/24 hr, will usually prevent hypoglycemia. Most children who have insulinomas during the first year of life will have remission before 5 to 6 years of age. Thus, surgical resection is not usually necessary in these younger children if hypoglycemia is prevented by diazoxide. Earlier surgery is indicated in children with localized tumors seen after 1 year of age or who have hypoglycemia that is poorly controlled by diazoxide. Blind resections are often unsuccessful.

Twenty per cent of gastrinomas are solitary and benign. Gastrin secreted by the tumor stimulates gastric acid secretion, resulting in multiple gastric and duodenal ulcers and often diarrhea. Fasting serum gastrin levels may be only marginally elevated, but will be markedly elevated (> 400 pg/ml) following IV secretin injection or calcium infusion. In adults, cimetidine, an H_2-receptor antagonist, has been shown to be an effective drug for controlling symptoms caused by the gastric hyperacidity. Those whose symptoms are not controlled by cimetidine usually require a total gastrectomy. Since the tumors are usually multiple and difficult to localize, surgical resection is often impossible.

Fortunately, carcinoma of the pancreas rarely occurs in children. However, recent reports from Japan indicate an increasing incidence in pancreatic carcinomas in children. Since clinical manifestations usually do not appear until extensive metastasis has occurred, prognosis of pancreatic carcinoma is poor, with a mean survival of 6 to 9 months after diagnosis in adults. Pancreaticoduodenectomy is recommended for the rare patient who has a small, localized lesion. In those with inoperable disease, supportive therapy consists of providing adequate nutrition and analgesia.

Cystic Fibrosis

JOHN J. HERBST, M.D.

Cystic fibrosis is the most common severe inherited disease in North America. Successful treatment of this chronic progressive disease requires awareness of its many manifestations. A team approach is the best way to coordinate patient care. Improvements in care have markedly enhanced the quality as well as the length of life (present projected mean age of survival in excess of 19 years).

Pulmonary complications including infection, bronchiectasis, atelectasis, hematemesis, pneumothorax, cyanosis, hypercapnia, and cor pulmonale account for most of the morbidity and mortality. In the immediate newborn period, intestinal obstruction due to inspissated meconium is a major problem, and severe malabsorption due to absence of pancreatic enzymes is usually present. The challenge in management of the malabsorption problems in patients who have decreased appetite due to chronic pulmonary infections is to arrange for sufficient intake to allow for body maintenance and growth, as well as the extra caloric requirements related to chronic infection and malabsorption. The average life span has doubled in the last 14 years, and many of these people are entering into an active late adolescence and adult life. This has created pressing needs for help and counseling services in the area of education, jobs, marriage, parenthood, and obtaining financing for increasingly sophisticated and expensive medical care.

Since many patients may go for decades without hospitalization, it is obvious that most care is administered at home. Thus, at the time of diagnosis it is important that both patient and parents be extensively educated in the nature of the disease, the specifics of home care, and its genetic implications. This includes instruction in performing postural drainage, use and cleaning of inhalation equipment, if needed, nutrition, and instructions on administration of vitamins, pancreatic supplements, and antibiotics. The education process is often facilitated by a short period of hospitalization.

Following initial evaluation and institution of care, the patient should be seen several times at 2 to 4 week intervals to document improvement, adjust therapy to the patient, give remedial instruction on care to parents or patient, and answer questions. Thereafter, intervals can be cautiously lengthened. Usually patients should be seen at least every 2 to 3 months. At return visits a careful interval history is obtained and an examination is performed. Emphasis is placed on eliciting changes in history of cough, sputum production, exercise tolerance, and rates of increase in height and weight. Careful inquiry into appetite, food intake, and changes in stooling patterns is important. A stable or slight decrease in weight, a poor appetite, or decreasing activity can be early clues of increasing pulmonary infection. Routine chest films and pulmonary function studies obtained at least once a year can be useful to document progression of disease. Sputum culture or a deep throat culture after an induced cough is invaluable in guiding antibiotic therapy. In patients old enough to cooperate, use of a simple screening pulmonary function test such as a peak flow or FEV_1 can give the first clue to increasing pulmonary disease.

Changes in clinical status, especially pulmonary symptoms, may be rapid, but the usual course is one of slow progression. If the progression of pulmonary disease or the patient's general condition is not improved after aggressive outpatient therapy, hospitalization is indicated, usually for at least two weeks, with emphasis on pulmonary toilet, antibiotics as indicated by cultures, and nutritional support.

Prevention of complicating diseases is important. Routine immunizations are essential and should be administered even if a cough is present, so long as the patient is not actually ill. Yearly immunizations against influenza are strongly recommended.

PULMONARY THERAPY

The severity of pulmonary problems varies greatly among patients, and decisions on the modalitites to be used and for how long are based on the patient's response. Much of the therapy is empiric and symptomatic, and the effectiveness of many specific aspects are unproved. The effect of each part of the care program may be quite small by itself, but they are often additive. Because of the variability of the disease and diversity among individuals, some modalities may greatly benefit some patients but be of little or no value to others. Close supervision and continuity of care are especially important. The concept of a team approach with aggressive therapy of the chronic pulmonary complications has almost doubled the expected life span of cystic fibrosis patients in the last 15 years.

Aerosol Therapy. This is used to deliver fluid to the lower respiratory tract to help thin the thick mucoid secretions. It can also be used to deliver medication to the lower respiratory tract (usually bronchodilators, antibiotics, and mucolytics).

Small compressor-driven nebulizers can be utilized to deliver the mist; ultrasonic units are more expensive but more quiet and deliver a greater volume of fluid. All units should be carefully cleaned each day and allowed to air dry after each use. Mist is usually delivered for 15–20 minutes prior to postural treatment but may also be used after postural therapy. If medication is added it is usually administered in a volume of about 4 ml.

Decongestants and bronchodilators are often used. ⅛% phenylephrine in 10% propylene glycol is a common mixture. If patients have clinical evidence of bronchospasm or if it is documented on pulmonary function testing, bronchodilators are especially indicated. Mucolytic agents (usually N-acetylcysteine) may be added to the mist treatment. We employ 2 to 4 ml of 10 to 20% N-acetylcysteine for 10 minutes. This substance can be irritating and may induce bronchospasm. For this reason it is usually used for only short periods and usually in association with bronchodilators.

Antibiotic aerosol therapy is not effective and one runs the risk of sensitization to a drug or of encouraging bacterial resistance. If used, it should be as an adjunct to vigorous systemic antibiotic therapy. Drugs often used are 1 gm methicillin or carbenicillin, 750 mg ticarcillin, and 20 mg of colistimethate, gentamicin, or tobramycin per treatment 4 times a day.

Physical Therapy. This is utilized to help remove thick mucopurulent material from the lungs. It is generally felt to be extremely useful, especially if it induces sputum production. Often it is preceded by inhalation therapy. We routinely teach the postural drainage technique at the time of diagnosis, even if there is no evidence of pulmonary disease. If there is a cough, postural drainage should be initiated at least once a day, twice daily if there is sputum production. In school children it is usually difficult to arrange more than 2 episodes per day, but some patients with severe bronchiectasis will benefit markedly from 3 or 4 treatments a day. We teach parents the various positions and recommend that the session last at least 20 minutes. Patients are encouraged to cough forcefully as they change positions. In older, cooperative patients, exhalation assisted by manual vibration and compression of the ribs is performed at the completion of each position. When properly performed, vigorous percussion with cupped hands is not uncomfortable.

Infants and children can be positioned most effectively on the therapist's lap. Use of the tilt board, pillows, or a folding therapy table is helpful in positioning older patients. Older patients are taught to perform postural therapy on themselves. We are not convinced that mechanical percussors are more effective than manual clapping. If the patient is large and strong enough (usually about age 14) a percussor with vertical movement can be helpful in areas they cannot reach and can be a great aid in independent living.

Antibiotic Therapy. In most patients with cystic fibrosis, chronic and recurrent pulmonary infections are the major cause of illness, leading to progressive pulmonary disease and eventual death. Antibiotic therapy is a most important aspect of care. Its goal is to reduce the severity and delay the progression of infection as much as possible, but there is little agreement as to specifics. Several studies have shown that aggressive treatment of acute infections with appropriate antibiotics, including intensive outpatient treatment of staphylococci and inpatient treatment of *Pseudomonas aeruginosa,* improves pulmonary function and weight gain. Frequent cultures are necessary for intelligent selection of antibiotic therapy. In older patients sputum culture is most useful, especially if the specimen is stained to be certain there are few squamous epithelial cells, indicating that the specimen came from the lung. In smaller children, nasotracheal cultures are useful, and deep throat culture at the time of induced coughing is a reasonable alternative, especially for outpatient care. Early in the course, patients are likely to be infected with *Streptococcus pneumoniae* and *Hemophilus* species. Staphylococci and *Proteus mirabilis* are also common pathogens. Eventually most patients became infected with *Pseudomonas aeruginosa.* Choice of antibiotic therapy is made difficult by the fact that infection is usually low grade, and it is difficult to differentiate between colonization and infection with organisms. Patients may also have exacerbation of pulmonary symptoms due to viral or mycobacteria infections. Signs of acute infections such as high fever, pleuritis, or tachypnea are often absent. In addition to deteriorating chest findings or radiographic changes, more subtle findings such as increasing cough, especially paroxysmal night cough, increased irritability, decreased activity, anorexia, poor weight gain, or weight loss should be sought. Frequent use of screening pulmonary function tests such as peak flow, FEV_1, or MMEF is useful in detecting increases in pulmonary disease. Because the severity of pulmonary disease is so variable, antibiotic therapy will vary from a short course of a single antibiotic to continuous treatment with several antibiotics. Prolonged use of low-dosage antibiotic therapy is to be avoided, since it encourages growth of resistant organisms.

Most exacerbations of pulmonary infections are treated at home. More intensive use of inhalation therapy and postural drainage is always advised. Except in special circumstances, the choice is limited to orally administered antibiotics. The choice should be guided by frequent cultures. Tetracycline should not be used in children under 9 years of age to prevent staining of teeth. Most often one is treating *Staphylococcus* and/or *Hemophilus*. Dicloxacillin and cephalexin are very useful antistaphylococcal antibiotics, and ampicillin, amoxicillin, sulfonamides, and tetracyclines are usually effective against staphylococci and hemophilus. Occasionally *Pseudomonas* species, especially cepacia, are sensitive to chloramphenicol or trimethoprim-sulfa. Antibiotic therapy should be continued at least 2 weeks. More severely involved patients often require 4 to 6 weeks of therapy. Continuous therapy is sometimes indicated, especially if cessation of antibiotics is regularly followed by increasing cough, auscultatory findings in the lung, or other symptoms.

If aggressive outpatient treatment of pulmonary infection with mist, postural drainage, and optimal oral antibiotics is unsuccessful, the patient is hospitalized for IV antibiotic therapy, more intensive inhalation therapy, and postural drainage. It is most convenient to use small scalp vein needles or indwelling cannulas with attachments for intermittent use. This allows the patient to be free between infusions. We do not change them on a schedule and a single cannula may be maintained for up to 7 days. If the parent or patient is trained, this technique may also be used to finish up a course of antibiotic therapy at home. Occasionally, when peripheral veins are difficult to cannulate and quickly thrombose, insertion of a subclavian catheter or other central line dramatically decreases stress and discomfort associated with intravenous antibiotic therapy. We seldom use the intramuscular route, since the muscle mass is usually small and injections quickly become very painful.

Most patients notice significant improvement in 3 to 5 days. In-hospital therapy is continued for at least 14 days to ensure optimal improvement in lung function.

Because *Pseudomonas, Staphylococcus,* and *Hemophilus* are commonly cultured, usually 2 or even 3 antibiotics are used in combination. Cystic fibrosis patients often metabolize antibiotics differently, and it is advisable to monitor drug levels. For example, these patients excrete aminoglycosides much more rapidly than normal, and doses above the usual manfacturer's recommendations are routinely used. We usually initiate treatment with gentamicin or tobramycin at a dose of 8 to 9 mg/kg/24 hours. After monitoring blood levels, it is often necessary to increase the dose by as much as 50% and administer it every 6 instead of 8 hours. Choice of antibiotics is usually guided by culture and sensitivity reports, but occasionally empirical changes should be made if the patient is not improving. Therapy for *Staphylococcus* should usually be included even if it is not cultured. It may not have been cultured because of sampling error or overgrowth of *Pseudomonas* if the specimen was not plated immediately after expectoration.

Allergies and Reactive Airway Disease

Cystic fibrosis patients have allergies at least as often as the general population. Symptoms may not be severe or may be difficult to distinguish from those of cystic fibrosis. Allergic rhinitis is commonly seen. Antihistamines and decongestants may not thicken lower respiratory secretions as much as feared, and often provide symptomatic relief. Bronchospasm, often not related to a particular allergen, can be detected by use of pulmonary function tests before and after bronchodilation. Sputum and nasal smears for eosinophils, peripheral blood counts, serum immunoglobin E levels, and careful history taking are important aids. Oral theophylline in the range of 15 to 20 mg/kg/24 hours is often dramatically helpful. Nausea and other gastrointestinal side effects may preclude attainment of full therapeutic blood levels, but addition of metaproterenol is often useful. Occasionally aerosolized bronchodilators or steroids in the form of beclomethasone, systemic steroids, and immunotherapy are indicated to control associated atopic disease.

Bronchoscopy and Lavage. Indications for the use of these procedures are unclear. Techniques have varied from lavage of large volumes of fluids to use of small volumes to irrigate the trachea or main bronchus only. Our experience has not been encouraging. Tracheostomy does not help in the long-term care of these patients, since it interferes with effective coughing and clearance of sputum.

Expectorants. No systemic drug has been proven to help in clearance of secretions from the lungs. Prolonged use of iodides is associated with goiters. Beyond assurance of patient hydration, we do not recommend use of expectorants.

PULMONARY COMPLICATIONS

Atelectasis. Lobar atelectasis, even if discovered on a routine chest roetgenogram, should be aggressively treated wth antibiotics. The usefulness of blow bottles or intermittent positive pressure breathing is debated, and there is risk of iatrogenic pneumothorax with intermittent positive pressure breathing.

If there is no improvement within a week, bronchoscopy and lavage of the bronchus to remove a mucous plug or other secretions is indicated. We prefer a rigid endoscope in order to have a large channel for irrigation, suctioning, and adequate oxygenation. The procedure may be repeated if necessary. If the patient is otherwise well, treatment at home with vigorous postural therapy to the affected area is continued, since resolution may occur in the ensuing weeks and months. Occasionally resolution does not occur, and atelectasis may cause infection, fever, chronic cough, and large amounts of purulent sputum if the lobe or segment does not become fibrosed. In such cases, lobectomy or segmental resection of the chronically infected, nonfunctioning lung may be indicated.

Hemoptysis. Small amounts of blood-tinged sputum are common in cystic fibrosis patients with extensive bronchiectasis. It is wise to reculture the patient and review antibiotic therapy. If mild hemoptysis (less than 30 ml) continues, aggressive inpatient antibiotic treatment is indicated. Patients with continuing or massive hemoptysis should be admitted for intensive antibiotic therapy. Blood should be available if there is evidence of blood pressure changes or significant decrease in the hematocrit. Postural drainage is stopped until bleeding ceases for 18 to 24 hours and then restarted gently with gradual advancement to vigorous clapping. Investigation for clotting abnormalities, especially vitamin K deficiencies, is mandatory. The patients are very apprehensive as well as dyspneic, and constant assurance and nasal oxygen are very helpful.

If hemoptysis continues, one may localize the site of bleeding with bronchoscopy. Percutaneous catheterization and angiography of the bronchial arteries may also identify the source of bleeding and allow embolization of the bleeding vessel. Lobectomy of functioning lung tissue should be avoided if possible.

Pneumothorax. This complication is being recognized more frequently in older patients. Treatment principles are the same as for noncystic fibrosis patients. If the pneumothorax is stable and less than 10%, the patient can be observed. If it is larger than 10% or under tension, immediate closed thoracotomy with insertion of a pleural catheter is mandatory. Unfortunately, there is a high rate of recurrence. Chemical pleurodesis using tetracycline inserted into the chest tube has been advocated, but open pleurodesis with oversewing of blebs and basal pleural abrasion with stripping of the apical pleura is much more likely to provide a permanent solution.

Aspergillosis. Allergic aspergillosis is usually self-limited. Intensive bronchodilator therapy with systemic and aerosolized bronchodilators is indicated, and steroids may be used if needed. The organisms should be assessed for sensitivity to the available antifungal agents, but systemic treatment with amphotericin or other agents is rarely necessary.

Acute Respiratory Failure. A severe infection can lead to acute respiratory failure in patients with extensive but stable disease. With intensive care, including oxygen and respirator care, these patients can usually return to their previous state of health. Postural therapy is even more important at this time, but it may have to be administered for a longer period. If a respirator is required, careful attention should be given to frequent suction of pulmonary secretions from the endotracheal tube.

Chronic Respiratory Failure. As survival is prolonged, many patients develop chronic respiratory failure. Watchful care of pulmonary toilet and attention to all details of care can maximize remaining lung function. If there is acute deterioration of lung function, these patients will not benefit from continuous ventilatory assistance. Although no conclusive studies demonstrate the effectiveness of low-flow nasal oxygen, the data on improvement in longevity and quality of life in adults with chronic obstructive pulmonary disease are very encouraging. Most patients improve somewhat with antibiotic treatment. We routinely use outpatient low-flow nasal oxygen starting at 24 minutes in patients with arterial P_{O_2} in room air under 50 to 55 torr. There is usually a prompt improvement in chronic fatigue, dyspnea, and headache. Patients are more mobile and some have been able to work in sedentary occupations.

Cor Pulmonale. Cor pulmonale carries an ominous prognosis. Aggressive treatment of pulmonary infections is indicated, as is use of supplemental oxygen to maintain an arterial P_{O_2} of at least 50 torr if it can be done without depressing the respiratory drive with hypercapnia. Diuretic therapy is important, especially acutely. Furosemide, 1 mg/kg, should be given immediately and may be repeated every 12 hours as needed. Salt restriction is usually indicated, and carbenicillin and ticarcillin should be used with caution because of the relatively high sodium content. The value of digitalis is questioned, and the nausea and headaches associated with use of tolazoline, as well as its marginal effectiveness, discourage its use.

GASTROINTESTINAL THERAPY

Pancreatic Deficiency. Most cystic fibrosis patients will have pancreatic insufficiency. This causes massive steatorrhea and can be detected by a simple Sudan stain of the stool. We see no need for routine quantification of steatorrhea with 72-hour stool collections. Pancreatic enzymes should be given with meals, or just prior to or following the meal. The dose is variable; enough enzymes are given to improve stool odor and consistency and to allow growth. Inactivation of the enzymes by gastric acid is a major difficulty in using exogenous pancreatic enzymes. The introduction of enteric coated enzymes (Pancrease and more recently Cotazym-B) has greatly facilitated care. The usual dose in older children is 1 to 3 capsules with each meal plus smaller amounts taken with snacks. In infants, a half capsule is usually sufficient. In small children, a capsule can be opened and mixed with cereal, apple sauce, etc. Children should be cautioned not to chew the enteric coated spheres, since this will negate the effect of the enteric coating. As the child grows, the amount of enzymes needed also increases. Symptoms of bloating, diarrhea, and abdominal distention often decrease during the teenage years. In rare patients an unusual mouse-like odor is associated with use of the enteric coated products, and in a few cases the spheres have been noted intact in the stools. In these cases, and for those infants who will not swallow the microspheres, nonenteric coated tablets and capsules are available. The efficiency of these products can be increased by depressing acid secretion with cimetidine, but considerations of costs and the risks of using such a drug over a lifetime make us reluctant to do this on a routine basis.

Most children are maintained on a regular diet, with the main goal being normal increases in height and weight. Many tolerate a normal amount of dietary fat, which is an excellent source of calories. Only if a normal diet is not tolerated are fats restricted. Normal absorption is seldom obtained, and usually 1.5 to 2 times normal intake of calories are required to allow for malabsorption, the caloric expenditure of chronic lung infection, body maintenance, and growth. Poor growth is usually associated with anorexia related to chronic pulmonary infections. It is often impossible to overcome this anorexia consciously, and excessive demands by parents or physicians to consume more food can cause unnecessary stress. In our experience, extensive efforts to routinely add medium-chain triglycerides to the food of older children are not worth the effort. All patients are given supplemental vitamins, including vitamin E.

Special formulas are often indicated during infancy. Many of these children are severely malnourished, and many have anasarca and hypoproteinemia. Formulas with hydralized proteins or medium-chain triglycerides (Pregestimil, Portagen, Nutramigen) can greatly accelerate nutritional rehabilitation in these children. We usually continue these formulas until the child has attained normal height and weight for age. Exogenous enzymes must be administered with these formulas,

since lipase is necessary for optimal absorption of medium-chain as well as long-chain triglycerides.

Meconium Ileus. Meconium ileus occurs in approximately 10% of patients and is the most common cause of neonatal intestinal obstruction. Gastrografin enemas with flushing of contrast media above the area of obstruction will often draw water into the bowel and flush out the inspissated meconium. Gastrografin is hypertonic, and careful attention to fluid balance, with an intravenous infusion during the procedure, is indicated to prevent dehydration and shock. In approximately one half of these patients, there will be associated volvulus, atresia, or meconium ileus, and in all surgical intervention is necessary. Once the obstruction is relieved, special attention to nutrition is required; if enteral feedings cannot be instituted within a day or so, parenteral nutrition should be employed. Only rarely is meconium ileus not caused by cystic fibrosis; patients should be treated as having cystic fibrosis until the diagnosis is proved by quantitative determination of sweat chlorides with pilocarpine iontopheresis.

Meconium Ileus Equivalent. In 15% of patients there are episodic accumulations of obstructing mucoid bowel contents in the distal ileum. There are usually severe cramps and a decrease in bowel movements. The patient often mistakenly interprets this as an indication that enzyme dosage should be decreased. Actually, the pancreatic enzyme dosage should be increased, and in fact tripled for a few days. Laxatives such as mineral oil, Colace, or Dulcolax should be added. Large saline enemas often will give relief. Acutely, N-acetylcysteine (Mucomyst), 1 tbsp of 20% solution 2 to 3 times a day by mouth, can help relieve the obstruction. If these efforts are unsuccessful, therapeutic enemas with water soluble contrast material under fluoroscopic control, and use of a long intestinal tube for proximal decompression are needed. If attacks are recurrent, careful attention to adequate intake of pancreatic enzymes, use of Colace or mineral oil, and judicious early use of N-acetylcysteine can prevent severe symptoms.

Intussusception. There is an increased incidence of intussusception in patients with cystic fibrosis. It may occur at any age and is usually ileocolic. It frequently follows a 1 or 2 day history of "constipation," and the cramps and other symptoms may simulate a severe episode of the much more common meconium ileus equivalent. If intussusception is suspected, a barium enema should be administered to the cecal area. If the problem is severe meconium ileus equivalent, the barium may be drained and Gastrografin used to flush out the obstruction. This approach reserves the expensive, hypertonic, irritating contrast material for situations where it is needed, and any interfering feces in the colon will have been flushed out by the less irritating barium suspension. If an intussusception is reduced, the patient should be carefully observed for signs of intestinal necrosis caused by compromised blood flow.

LIVER DISEASE

An occasional infant has transient cholestatic jaundice due to inspissated bile, which requires no specific therapy. The most common liver disorder is nutritional fatty liver, which is best treated by enzyme therapy and careful attention to diet. Focal biliary cirrhosis is found in 25% of postmortem examinations and is pathognomonic of cystic fibrosis. One fifth of these patients (or 5% of all people with cystic fibrosis) will progress to a multinodular cirrhosis with development of portal hypertension. There is no specific therapy; the main problems are related ascites, hypersplenism, and bleeding varices. As with adult forms of biliary cirrhosis, hepatic function usually remains adequate until late in the course.

The principles of management are the same as for other liver diseases. The mainstay of treatment of ascites is institution of a low-sodium diet. If necessary, diuretics (usually hypochlorthiazide and a potassium-sparing diuretic such as spironolactone) are used; more aggressive measures are rarely needed.

Variceal bleeding can be a fatal complication. Vitamin K should be administered if the prothrombin time is prolonged. Acutely, nasogastric intubation, saline lavage, and infusions of vasopressin(Pitressin, 0.15 to 0.5 U/m^2/min)*can help control bleeding. If the bleed is significant, upper gastrointestinal endoscopy is indicated to identify the site of bleeding, since experience with portal hypertension in adults indicates that over half of all bleeds are not from ruptured varices. If variceal bleeding is severe and persistent, a Sengstaken-Blakemore tube can be of use. A portacaval anastomosis can decrease portal vein pressure and prevent subsequent bleeding. If there is severe hypersplenism and splenectomy is indicated, a splenorenal anastomosis can give good results. If there is severe pulmonary disease and the patient is a poor surgical risk, endoscopic sclerosis of the varices or use of propranolol to lessen portal venous pressure should be considered. Any patient with portal hypertension should be cautioned to avoid salicylates, since their effect on platelet function can greatly increase the likelihood of bleeding. Prophylactic shunts to prevent an initial variceal bleed are not indicated.

In autopsy series, up to 10% of older patients will have gallstones or other evidence of biliary tree obstruction. Usually these abnormalities are asymptomatic but if the patient has stones and has colic or pain typical of cholelithiasis, surgical correction is indicated.

Pancreatitis. Fifteen per cent of cystic fibrosis patients will have normal pancreatic function and may develop acute or recurrent pancreatis. It is often difficult to separate symptoms of cholelithiasis, pancreatitis, and nonspecific bloating and pain associated with cystic fibrosis. Acutely, nasogastric drainage, intravenous fluids, and meperidine for pain are the most important factors in care.

Rectal Prolapse. This is especially common in newly diagnosed patients with poor weight gain, and usually occurs at defecation. Often it will reduce spontaneously if the patient lies on his abdomen. If not, the rectal mucosa can be replaced manually. If the prolapse is huge and the bowel edematous, placing the patient in the knee-chest position and continuously but gently compressing the bowel is usually successful. Often, as the steatorrhea is controlled, the prolapse ceases. If prolapse continues to occur, most children can be taught to self-reduce it by placing a piece of toilet tissue over it and applying finger pressure. Usually by the time the patient is 6 or 7 years old the prolapse ceases. We have not found it necessary to perform surgical precedures on these children.

MISCELLANEOUS PROBLEMS

Salt Depletion. Especially in hot climates, salt losses can be high. Parents should liberally salt the food of younger patients, and older patients may require 500 mg salt supplementation 2 to 3 times a day, especially in the summer. In recent years, salt depletion, along with potassium depletion and alkalosis, is being recognized much more frequently, since all added salt has been removed from infant foods, thereby decreasing salt intake by up to 60%. Infants, especially those being breast fed, frequently require supplementation of 2–3 mEq/kg of potassium and sodium.

Hyperglycemia. An altered carbohydrate tolerance caused by pancreatic fibrosis with some destruction of the islets occurs in most older patients. If there is no polyuria or significant glucosuria, no therapy is required. Approximately 3% will eventually develop overt diabetes and require insulin. Severe diabetic acidosis is rare in these patients.

Nasal Polyps and Sinusitis. Nasal polyps are a recurrent problem in about 15% of cystic fibrosis patients. Attempts to prevent recurrence or to decrease the size of the polyps using beclomethasone nasal spray are reasonable; if the polyps completely obstruct one or both nasal passages, they should be removed.

Opacification of the sinuses on radiographs is almost a universal finding. If patients have chronic sinusitis with pain, fever, and a septic course, surgical drainage can be very useful.

---

*This use of vapopressin is not listed by the manufacturer.

Reproductive Problems. Many cystic fibrosis patients have delayed sexual maturation and short stature. Boys are almost always sterile because of azospermia related to obstruction in the vas deferens. Only about 2% will be capable of fathering children. Many pregnancies have occurred in cystic fibrosis women, and anyone with regular menses should be regarded as being fertile. Patients should be informed of these factors and counseled regarding the increased risks of pregnancy in patients with severe chronic lung disease.

Surgery. Many patients have relatively normal pulmonary function and the main adjustment to routine care will be careful attention to pulmonary toilet just before and after surgery. In more severe patients, every effort should be used to employ local anesthesia if surgery is needed. Often 1 to 2 weeks are employed in maximizing pulmonary therapy prior to required surgery, and anesthesia time is kept to a minimum. Endotracheal intubation should be done in all patients and careful endotracheal suction to aid in removal of pulmonary secretions is important. After surgery, intensive postural drainage is initiated as soon as feasible.

Malabsorption Syndromes and Chronic Diarrhea

EMANUEL LEBENTHAL, M.D.,
and MYRON SIEGEL, M.D.

In this country the major causes of malabsorption in infancy and childhood are cystic fibrosis (pancreatic insufficiency) and celiac disease (small intestinal mucosal injury). In addition, many congenital digestive enzyme deficiencies and intestinal transport abnormalities can result in malabsorption because of reduced digestive or absorptive capacity. Hirschsprung's disease, gastroschisis, ileal atresia, or short bowel syndrome due to small bowel resection can also result in malabsorption.

Infants early in life who suffer from protracted diarrhea will have prolonged small intestinal mucosal injury and a prolonged period of malabsorption. Chronic diarrhea due to secretory diarrhea caused by hormones elaborated by tumors is rare in infants and children. The main problem during early infancy is prolonged diarrhea associated with small intestinal villus atrophy and secondary malabsorption.

The mucosal injury, loss of the polarity of the mature epithelial cells, and disorganization of the brush border area of the absorptive surface of the mature epithelial cells can cause malabsorption of nutrients, vitamins, and minerals, including trace elements.

Depending on the extent of the changes, there may be loss of enzymes responsible for hydrolysis of short polymers of glucose and disaccharides as well as hydrolysis of short polypeptides, tripeptides, and dipeptides. When the injury progresses the active and facilitated transport of elemental nutrients such as glucose, galactose, and fructose or amino acids are also diminished. As a consequence, the severity of the malabsorption can reach an extreme that at times can be resolved only by excluding food per os and institution of total parenteral nutrition. However, if only the hydrolytic enzymes are affected, but the active and facilitated transport of glucose and amino acids remain intact, an elemental diet per os might suffice. Thus, assessment of mucosal changes and enzymatic activities can help determine the appropriate method of nutritional rehabilitation of the malabsorptive state.

A state of partial malabsorption occurs in early infancy with partial maldigestion of fats and starches owing to the absence of pancreatic amylase and the low pancreatic lipase and bile acid concentrations in the duodenal fluid. Also, in prematures there is reduced lactase activity due to immaturity of the small intestine. This can result in lactose malabsorption. Thus, in our recommendations for support in malabsorptive states in early infancy, we must consider not only organic disease but also "physiologic" malabsorption secondary to immaturity.

"PHYSIOLOGIC" (EARLY INFANCY) MALABSORPTION

Available data indicate that in early infancy (up to 6 months of age) there is an impaired ability to digest and absorb fat, as well as limited capacity to hydrolyze and absorb starches. However, studies on the digestibility and absorption of nutrients, minerals, and vitamins in premature, full-term, and compromised infants are scarce.

Neonates can digest and absorb an adequate quantity of dietary protein, although their digestive capacities are limited. Ten-day-old infants can completely digest and absorb 1.3% protein in cow's milk (about 1.95 gm/kg/day) but not 1.5% (about 2.25 gm/kg/day). Similarly, 4- to 6-month-old infants can completely digest and absorb 2.5% protein in cows' milk (about 3.75 gm/kg/day) but not 2.7% (about 4.05 gm/kg/day). Younger infants therefore have a relatively lesser capacity to digest protein than older infants. An important issue regarding the protein content of the diet is its relationship to caloric intake. The calculated values of dietary nitrogen requirements, based on growth measurements from the second to the tenth month of life, show a decline from 600 mg/100 kcal at 2 months of age to 250 mg/100 kcal at 10 months of age, suggesting a decrease in the relative protein requirement with age and caloric intake. A natural decrease in protein content is found in human milk as lactation progresses. Although the lower limit of protein requirement per kilocalorie is not known, most studies suggest that 1.6 gm/100 kcal during the first 3 months and 1.4 gm/100 kcal from 4 to 6 months of age are adequate. Infant formulas normally contain 2.2 to 2.3 gm/100 kcal, substantially higher than the level of protein shown to be adequate in clinical trials. Formulas for premature infants contain even higher levels (2.7 to 3 gm/100 kcal). The absorption of native protein depends on the nature of the protein and the age of the individual. There is, however, ample evidence of macromolecular absorption in humans. It is more marked in the premature than in the mature infant. Circumstantial evidence in infants shows that antigen absorption decreases progressively with age. Adverse reactions to cow's milk protein become progressively less common during the first year of life. These are reasons for restricting infants to human milk, which presents little antigenic load.

Neonates, particularly premature ones and those small for gestational age, relatively inefficiently digest and absorb lipids. Neonates have low levels of lipase in the duodenum. In addition neonates, particularly premature ones, have an intraluminal concentration of bile acid (1 to 2 mmole/L) below the critical micellar concentration (2 mmole/L) and therefore insufficient to solubilize lipids and their hydrolytic products. Physiologically, intragastric lipolysis by lingual lipase may be important in view of inefficient duodenal lipid digestion. The composition of dietary lipid has been shown to greatly influence the level of absorption and retention. Term and preterm infants digest and absorb fats from human milk better than fats from cow's milk or formula, in part because of the presence of two human milk lipases. Other contributing factors are the source of triglycerides and their fatty acid composition. Vegetable fats are absorbed better than animal fats. Triglycerides with saturated fatty acids are not utilized as well as those with unsaturated fatty acids. In neonates, portal transport appears to be operative and lymphatic transport partially deficient. Thus short- and medium-chain fatty acids, which are absorbed directly into the portal system, are absorbed and transported more readily than long-chain fatty acids. Excess Ca^{++} in cow's milk causes a high excretion of fatty acids, especially the saturated variety. In neonates, a high intake of Ca^{++} may hinder lipid retention. Conversely, high lipid intake has been found to lower Ca^{++} absorption and may lead to hypocalcemia. Estimation of the coefficient of lipid absorption in premature babies may vary from 58.3 to 88.7%, and in full-term infants from 71.7 to 95.3%. The wide ranges in part depend on the type and amount of fats ingested. The structural interaction of fat with other dietary constituents is also important. Lipids in milk exist as fat droplets with surfaces covered by thin films of phospholipid and protein, which impede the action of pancreatic lipases in vitro.

Carbohydrate intake in infancy makes up 35 to 55% of the total calories in the diet. The period from infancy to childhood has three phases, each with a different major source of dietary carbohydrate. In the initial phase the main carbohydrates, lactose and sucrose, are derived from human milk or formula in the absence of solids. A transitional phase follows the introduction of solid food; various polysaccharides, mainly starches, are added. In the final phase the shift to solid food is complete and polysaccharides predominate. The optimal amounts of disaccharides that can be hydrolyzed in vitro by the whole small intestine at various gestational ages have been calculated. By 26 to 34 weeks, sucrase and maltase activities approach 70% and lactase activity only 30% in full-term infants. These findings suggest that infants born during the sixth to eighth months of gestation can utilize maltose, sucrose, and isomaltose pretty well but not lactose. Thus, premature babies may not tolerate milk-based formulas as well as full-term infants. It may be advisable to include sugars other than lactose in formulas designed for premature babies if greater carbohydrate absorption is required or if lactose is poorly tolerated. Most studies show that pancreatic amylase activity in the duodenal fluids of infants up to age 4 months is low or absent. In premature infants of 32 to 34 weeks gestation, virtually no pancreatic amylase can be detected in the duodenum during the first month of life, and the capacity to hydrolyze long polymers of glucose is limited.

CARBOHYDRATE MALABSORPTION

The hydrolysis and absorption of individual carbohydrates may be impaired by a variety of diseases. In those associated with moderate to severe injury to the small intestinal mucosa, all the disaccharidase activities are depressed. Lactase activity seems to be the most sensitive to injury, for it is the first disaccharidase activity to decrease and the slowest to recover. Infants and children with severe architectural disarray of the intestinal villus and changes in the brush border membrane may also suffer impairment of monosaccharide transport. The acquired monosaccharide intolerance usually indicates severe changes in the intestinal mucosa. However, the discussion of secondary carbohydrate malabsorption as well as secondary protein and fat malabsorption will be included in the section on small intestinal mucosal injury.

The main congenital and inborn errors of specific carbohydrate malabsorption are presented in Table 1.

Glucose-Galactose Malabsorption. This is a rare autosomal recessive disorder of glucose and galactose transport from the intestinal lumen to the

Table 1. CARBOHYDRATE MALABSORPTION

Congenital

Glucose–galactose malabsorption
Fructose malabsorption
Sorbitol and mannitol malabsorption
Sucrase–isomaltase deficiency
Lactase deficiency
    a. congenital
    b. adult type
Trehalase deficiency
Pancreatic insufficiency with amylase deficiency

Developmental

Lactase deficiency in prematures
Pancreatic amylase deficiency in early infancy

Secondary

Acquired monosaccharide malabsorption (glucose, fructose, and galactose)
Disaccharide malabsorption (lactose, sucrose, maltose, and alpha limit dextrins)
Pancreatic insufficiency (pancreatic amylase deficiency) due to pancreatitis, malnutrition, etc.

---

enterocyte. Patients present with watery diarrhea with the initiation of enteral feedings, usually in the first week of life. Diarrhea resolves when feedings are withdrawn and resumes when feedings are reintroduced. Some villous atrophy may be noted in an intestinal biopsy performed when the patient has severe diarrhea and malnutrition, but a biopsy obtained from a patient under proper treatment will show normal histology and disaccharidase activities. Patients have flat glucose and galactose tolerance tests; such tests should be performed only on patients in good clinical condition. Stools of undiagnosed patients are acidic and contain large amounts of carbohydrates. Fructose absorption is an unrelated facilitated transport mechanism; therefore, treatment consists of feeding a synthetic formula containing 4 to 8% fructose. Absorption does not improve with age but as patients get older they may be able to eat small amounts of carbohydrate other than fructose with few or no symptoms.

Fructose Malabsorption. Fructose is an increasingly important commercial sweetener. Some children complain of abdominal symptoms after ingesting fructose-containing foods. Incomplete absorption is associated with abdominal cramps or diarrhea. Patients with these symptoms after ingestion of large amounts of fructose should have their intake restricted. Recently, the development of an inexpensive conversion of glucose derived from corn syrup into fructose has resulted in increased use of fructose, especially in soft drinks. The major natural source of fructose is dried figs, dates, prunes, and grapes.

Sorbitol and Mannitol Intolerance. Absorption of the sorbitol and mannitol used in dietetic candies and gum is slow in all individuals, and overinges-

tion can lead to an osmotic diarrhea. Restriction of the appropriate foods should lead to resolution of symptoms.

Congenital Disaccharidase Deficiencies. These inherited disorders are associated with normal intestinal mucosa. Specific enzymes are absent from the intestinal brush border.

Sucrase-Isomaltase Deficiency. This is inherited as an autosomal recessive disorder. Sucrase is responsible for sucrose hydrolysis, and isomaltase hydrolyzes the 1,6 branch chain linkages of alpha limit dextrins hydrolyzed from amylopectin starch. Patients generally develop watery diarrhea with the introduction of sucrose or starches, although some will develop mild chronic diarrhea. Especially in more subtle presentations, the clinical picture may simulate celiac disease, as the onset of symptoms may coincide with the introduction of cereals.

Patients generally have acidic stools (pH < 5.5). Sucrose is not a reducing sugar, so reducing substances will be detected only after acid hydrolysis. This can be tested by adding 10 drops of 1.0N HCl to 5 drops of liquid stool and boiling for a few seconds. A Clinitest tablet is then added.

A small bowel biopsy with measurement of disaccharidase activities will reveal normal or mildly abnormal villous histology with complete absence of sucrase and isomaltase activity. Typically, maltase activity is reduced but still present.

Elimination of sucrose and starch from the diet will eliminate symptoms. Corn and rice starches, which have fewer 1,6 bonds, may be tolerated to a limited degree in some patients. Meats, fish, poultry, and dairy products are well tolerated. Liquid medications, which generally contain sucrose, must be avoided. Table 2 provides guidelines for a sucrose restricted diet.

Congenital Lactase Deficiency. This is extremely rare in infancy. Patients present with diarrhea with the introduction of feeds and have acidic stools containing reducing substances. A small bowel biopsy will reveal absence of lactase with normal histology. Other disaccharidases should be normal.

Infants do well with soy-based, lactose-free feedings. In older children, small amounts of lactose may be tolerated and adding Lact-Aid to milk to predigest most of the lactose might be successful. In patients intolerant of any lactose, adequate calcium and vitamin intake must be insured. Table 3 provides guidelines for a lactose-free diet.

Congenital Lactose Intolerance. Congenital lactase deficiency must be distinguished from congenital lactose intolerance. In this disorder, diarrhea is minimal and patients have severe systemic symptoms including vomiting, failure to thrive, dehydration, lactosuria, aminoaciduria, renal tubular acidosis, liver dysfunction, and bleeding. No specific defect has been identified and these patients

Table 2. SUCROSE RESTRICTED DIET

Foods Allowed	Foods Avoided
Milk, unsweetened evaporated milk and cream	Sweetened condensed milk and formulas containing sucrose
Asparagus, broccoli, Brussels sprouts, cabbage, cauliflower, celery, chard, chicory, cucumber, lettuce, mushrooms, spinach, tomatoes, bamboo shoots, radishes, potatoes (0.3 gm/100 gm)	Peas, dried beans, lentils, turnips, parsnips, other vegetables not listed in foods to include or those not tolerated
Grapes, fresh cherries, dried Kadota figs, blackberries, cranberries, currants (red and white), lemon, loganberries, medium ripe strawberries (0.3 gm/100 gm)	Those not on the list of fruits to include or those not tolerated
Fried, hard cooked, soft cooked, poached eggs	
Fresh meat, fish, ham	Check all commercially prepared meats and fish
All cheeses	
Bread (homemade), spaghetti, macaroni (without sugar)	Breakfast cereals, wheat germ, rice, bran
Butter, margarine, cooking oil, lard, salad dressing (oil and vinegar)	Mayonnaise, salad dressing (French, Roquefort, Thousand Island, Russian)
Cocoa (unsweetened), coffee, tea, vegetable juice, "special" eggnog (see recipes)	Malted milk, milk shake, Kool-Aid, pop
Salt, pepper, gravy, spices, herbs, vinegar	Olives, pimiento, pickles (sweet and sour)
Chicken and beef broth, boullion, consomme	
Glucose (dextrose) and artificial sweeteners	Sugar (cane, beet, granulated, powdered, brown), jam, honey, jelly, candy, molasses, maple syrup, frosting
Homemade cake, cookies, ice cream using glucose (see recipes), gelatin tapioca, diabetic chocolate	Commercially prepared pies, cookies, cakes, diabetic products (unless mentioned elsewhere), ice cream, sherbet, any food prepared with sugar
	Salad dressing, pickles, chutney, medicines made up in syrup

do have small intestinal lactase activity. Treatment consists of a milk-free diet. Patients may be able to tolerate lactose by 6 to 18 months of age.

Late Onset Lactase Deficiency. Late onset lactase deficiency is common in populations other than those of northern European ancestry. Low lactase levels can be found in the otherwise normal small bowel biopsies of children as young as age 5, although often onset is later. The association of vague symptoms of abdominal pain with adult onset lactase deficiency has been reported, although in most of these cases the abdominal pain does not appear to be caused by the lactase deficiency. When diarrhea is clearly associated with lactose ingestion, a lactose restriction is reasonable. Many patients will tolerate small volumes. In some patients who would like to drink milk, Lact-Aid will improve tolerance. Patients who need a milk-restricted diet should have adequate calcium intake assured by eating green leafy vegetables or taking calcium supplements.

Congenital Trehalase Deficiency. Trehalase is a sugar found in mushrooms. Two families have been reported with clinical signs of trehalase intolerance. Absence of the small intestinal enzyme trehalase was demonstrated. Treatment of the disorder involves removal of mushrooms from the diet.

FAT MALABSORPTION

"Physiologic" fat malabsorption and secondary fat malabsorption due to small intestinal mucosal injury and pancreatic insufficiency are the main issues in infancy. However, there are very rare congenital and inborn errors of fat malabsorption (Table 4) that will be discussed.

Lipase Deficiency. Isolated pancreatic lipase deficiency is extremely rare. It has been described in only two families. Patients develop steatorrhea soon after birth. Diagnosis is based on an absence of lipase in duodenal fluid. Treatment consists of using pancreatic enzyme supplements.

Abetalipoproteinemia. This is a rare autosomal recessive disease in which patients are unable to synthesize apoprotein B in the intestinal mucosa. As a result, they cannot form chylomicrons or the

Table 3. LACTOSE-FREE DIET

Foods Allowed	Foods Avoided
Lactose-free formulas, fruit juices, carbonated beverages, Kool-Aid, cocoa without added milk solids, nondairy cream or milk substitutes, coffee, tea	Milk (fresh, evaporated, condensed, dried, butter), frappes, ice cream soda, "Great Shakes," Instant Breakfast
French, Italian, or Vienna bread. Homemade fresh toast without added milk. Unkneaded biscuits, saltines, graham, oyster, soda crackers, Triscuits	Breads, rolls, biscuits, muffins made with or enriched with milk solids (hamburger and frankfurter buns), pancakes, waffles, doughnuts, pop-tarts
All types of cereals	Check all commercial breakfast and baby cereals
Jell-O, water ice, popsicles, fruit pie (pie crust made without butter or regular margarine), tapioca, homemade cornstarch pudding, or junket made with fruit juice or milk substitute	Cakes, cream pie, cookies made with milk, ice cream, ice milk, sherbet, custard, commercial pudding mixes
Milk-free cookies such as fig bars, gingersnaps, lemonsnaps	
Kosher margarine, lard, vegetable oil, cream substitutes such as Coffee Rich or Coffee Mate	Butter, margarine, sour cream, whipped cream, salad dressing made with milk, mayonnaise
All types of fruits	
All types of meat, fish, and poultry	Creamed meats, gravies, processed or canned meats such as luncheon meat, sausage, hash, frankfurters unless 100% pure meat, commercial hamburgers
Eggs	All kinds of cheeses
All potatoes or substitutes (macaroni, rice, spaghetti)	Potatoes mashed with milk or butter
Clear soups, broth	Creamed soups
Limit amount of sweets for good dental hygiene: sugar, jam, jellies, syrups, honey, candies such as gum drops, Canada mints, Planter's Jumbo Block, Good n' Fruity, Dots, Necco Wafers, Mason's Black Crows	Candies made with milk chocolate, butter, or cream, butterscotch
All kinds of vegetables	Vegetables in butter or creamed sauce
Mustard, relish, catsup, salt, pepper, spices, peanut butter, gravy without added milk or cream, potato chips, pretzels, pickles, olives	Yogurt

Table 4. FAT MALABSORPTION

Congenital and inborn errors of metabolism
  Lipase deficiency
  Abetalipoproteinemia
  Hypobetalipoproteinemia
  Chylomicron retention disease
  Wolman's disease
  Intestinal lymphangiectasia
  Defective intestinal bile acid reabsorption

Developmental
  Low pancreatic lipase in prematures and early infancy
  Low bile acid pool and critical micellar formation in intestinal fluids in prematures and early infancy

Secondary
  Decreased pancreatic lipase and colipase due to pancreatitis, malabsorption, pancreozymin deficiency
  Decreased conjugated bile acids due to bacterial growth
  Diminished monoglyceride absorption due to severe mucosal injury

very low density lipoproteins that are eventually converted to low density lipoproteins.

Patients present in the first year of life with diarrhea, abdominal distention, steatorrhea, and failure to thrive. Frequently, the initial clinical picture may be indistinguishable from that of other causes of steatorrhea, such as celiac disease or cystic fibrosis. As patients get older, gastrointestinal symptoms may improve but ataxia, muscle weakness, nystagmus, and retinitis pigmentosa develop. Milder forms of the disease exist in which patients have hypolipoproteinemia.

Characteristic laboratory findings include decreased plasma cholesterol and triglyceride levels and acanthocytes on hematologic smear. Vitamin A, vitamin E, and carotene levels are very low. Lipoprotein electrophoresis shows absent or very decreased beta-lipoproteins, and small bowel biopsy shows enterocytes engorged with fat droplets.

High doses of vitamin A and vitamin E may delay the development of neurologic and retinal lesions. Recommended doses are 100 IU/kg/day vitamin E and 7500 to 25,000 IU/day vitamin A. Nutrition is enhanced through the use of medium chain triglyceride (MCT) oil, which does not require chylomicrons for absorption. A low fat diet will reduce steatorrhea.

Chylomicron Retention Disease. Patients have recently been described with findings similar to these patients with abetalipoproteinemia but who have apoprotein B. These patients develop steatorrhea in infancy and have low levels of carotene, vitamin A, and vitamin E as well as hypoprothrombinemia. On light microscopy, their small bowel biopsies are indistinguishable from those of patients with abetalipoproteinemia. Electron microscopy suggests a defect of chylomicron secretion. Some of these patients have developed neurologic and ophthalmic findings similar to those of patients with abetalipoproteinemia.

Suggested treatment is a low fat diet supplemented with medium chain triglycerides; vitamin A, 15,000 IU/m²/day; vitamin E, 100 IU/kg/day;* and vitamin K, 5 mg/day.

Wolman's Disease. In this rare autosomal recessively inherited lipid storage disease secondary to lysosomal acid esterase deficiency, cholesterol esters and triglycerides accumulate in all organs. Patients develop diarrhea, hepatomegaly, and failure to thrive.

Abdominal x-rays may show adrenal calcifications, and the bone marrow shows lipid-filled macrophages. There is no treatment, and patients generally die before 1 year of age.

Lymphangiectasia of the Small Intestine. This refers to dilatation of the lymphatics in the small bowel. Families with multiple affected siblings have been described in the congenital type, although the precise inheritance has not been defined. Intestinal lymphangiectasia has been described in association with Turner's syndrome and Noonan's syndrome. Patients with inherited forms may have associated lymphatic anomalies such as lymphedema of an extremity. Secondary lymphatic dilatation can occur as a result of inflammatory obstruction of lymphatics or back pressure due to heart failure. Leakage of lymph can lead to substantial protein and fat losses. Patients can present at any age, although those with the congenital form frequently present in infancy with steatorrhea, abdominal protuberance, failure to thrive, chylous effusions, hypoproteinemia, and deficiencies of fat soluble vitamins. Lymphopenia is often present. A small bowel biopsy is diagnostic.

In cases of secondary lymphatic dilatation, relief of the primary cause is the preferred therapy. Rarely, a congenital lesion will be resectable, as determined by mesenteric lymphography. If surgical resection is not possible, a diet containing 5 grams or less of fat will reduce lymphatic drainage and may help induce remissions. Medium-chain triglycerides bypass the lymphatics and are a useful nutritional supplement. Fat soluble vitamin supplements are also necessary. In severe cases, parenteral nutrition and bowel rest may help induce remission.

Bile Salt Depletion. Intraluminal bile salt deficiency can result from abnormalities at any point in the enterohepatic circulation. Parenchymal liver disease such as neonatal hepatitis or bile duct obstruction from biliary atresia will prevent bile salt excretion into the intestinal lumen. Bile salt deconjugation from bacterial contamination (discussed below) will make bile salts unavailable for micellar formation. Ileal dysfunction due to severe ileitis in Crohn's disease or due to surgical resection of the ileum will impair the reabsorption of bile salts by active transport. Recently, two patients have been described with an apparently congenital defect of this active transport mechanism, as determined by in vitro analysis of ileal transport of taurocholic acid.

Relatively mild cases of ileal dysfunction can cause enough bile salt malabsorption to induce a secretory diarrhea in the colon, but not enough to result in intraluminal bile salt depletion. In these cases, the reserve capacity of bile salt production will compensate for the increased losses of salts in the stools. Binding of intraluminal bile salts with cholestyramine,* 250 to 500 mg/kg/day, given as 2 to 4 doses to a maximum of 4 gm (1 packet) 4 times per day, may be effective in some cases. The drug itself may produce steatorrhea by further depleting intraluminal bile salts and has also been associated with intestinal obstruction and metabolic acidosis. Failure of cholestyramine to treat the diarrhea in many cases may be due to metabolism of unabsorbed fatty acids to long chain hydroxy acids, which can act as cathartics. Cholestyramine may also be used as a choleretic in the treatment of cholestasis in the same doses.

Some cases of bile salt depletion can be corrected by appropriate therapy. Patients with extrahepatic biliary atresia can often have bile flow restored surgically (usually by a portojejunostomy [Kasai] procedure). Crohn's ileitis may respond to prednisone. Most cases of neonatal hepatitis will resolve following appropriate supportive therapy.

Similar principles apply to the management of all causes of intraluminal bile salt depletion. Diets

---

*Dosage of cholestyramine has not been established for infants and children.

must be altered to provide adequate nutrition and adequate amounts of fat soluble vitamins. MCTs are well absorbed without a critical micellar bile salt concentration, and use of an infant formula containing MCT oil, such as Portagen, can improve nutrition in infancy. In older patients, cooking with MCT oil or using it in foods such as salad dressing may be beneficial. Supplementation with fat soluble vitamins A, D, E, and K is necessary. Water soluble preparations of A, E, and K are available. Aquasol A, 5000 IU/day; Aquasol E, 50 IU/day; and water soluble vitamin K, 5 mg twice a week, are generally effective but doses may be varied for individual patients. In all patients with bile salt depletion, intestinal absorption of vitamin D will be affected. Patients with parenchymal liver disease may also have impaired ability to perform the 25-hydroxylation step in the liver. The proper vitamin D dose can be best evaluated by monitoring serum 25 (OH) D levels. Both standard vitamin D and 25 (OH) D preparations are available. Doses in excess of 5000 IU/day of vitamin D may be necessary. Three to five μg/kg/day is a suggested starting dose for 25 (OH) D.

Patients with cholestatic disease may benefit from phenobarbital, 5 mg/kg/day, to lower serum bilirubin and bile salt levels. Cholestyramine may also be useful as described above.

PROTEIN MALABSORPTION

The main diseases related to protein malabsorption are secondary protein intolerances, protein-losing enteropathies, and acquired amino acid and polypeptide malabsorption due to severe mucosal injury. A number of rare inherited disorders of amino acid transport have been identified (Table 5). We will discuss only defects associated with diarrhea or malnutrition.

Lysinuric Protein Intolerance. These patients have a defect of the basolateral membranes of the intestine and the kidney, resulting in malabsorption of the dibasic amino acids lysine and arginine and increased urinary excretion of these acids. Patients have low plasma levels of arginine, ornithine, and lysine. The lack of ornithine interferes with the urea cycle, resulting in hyperammonemia with the ingestion of a large protein load. Formula-fed infants develop diarrhea and vomiting at birth. Breast-fed infants tend to develop symptoms after weaning, as the low protein in breast milk offers some protection. Other features are aversion to protein, growth retardation, hepatosplenomegaly, muscular weakness, and fragile hair. Some patients develop seizures and coma after ingesting large amounts of protein.

The most effective therapy is a diet containing citrulline, 2 to 3 mg/day, and a diet of 1 to 2 gm/kg of protein/day. This diet appears to prevent hyper-

Table 5. PROTEIN MALABSORPTION

Congenital and inborn errors of metabolism
  Neutral amino acid malabsorption
  Basic amino acid malabsorption
  Amino acid-glycine malabsorption
  Enterokinase deficiency
  Trypsinogen deficiency
  Pancreatic insufficiency (with endo- and exopeptidase deficiency)

Secondary
  Acquired amino acid malabsorption in severe small intestinal mucosal injury
  Polypeptide and dipeptide malabsorption
  Pancreatic insufficiency (with endo- and exopeptidase deficiency) due to pancreatitis, malnutrition, etc.
  Secondary protein intolerance
  Protein-losing enteropathies
    Intestinal lymphangiectasia
    Menetrier's disease
    Severe mucosal injury
    Crohn's ileocolitis
    Ulcerative colitis

ammonemia and improve protein nutrition.

Methionine Malabsorption. Patients with selective methionine malabsorption have defects of branch chain amino acid and serine absorption. Symptoms include sporadic diarrhea, mental retardation, convulsions, and tachypnea. Patients have blue eyes and white hair.

A low methionine diet will improve the diarrhea and neurologic symptoms and color the hair.

Trypsinogen and Enterokinase Deficiencies. In addition to selected transport deficiencies, protein malabsorption can result from inherited enzyme deficiencies. Absence of pancreatic trypsinogen and absence of enterokinase (an intestinal enzyme) have been described as isolated enzyme deficiencies. Enterokinase converts trypsinogen into trypsin and trypsin activates trypsinogen as well as other pancreatic proteases. Trypsinogen deficiency is diagnosed by absence of trypsin activity in duodenal fluid, and enterokinase deficiency by absence of activity in a small intestinal biopsy. Growth failure, diarrhea, hypoproteinemia, and edema can be found in both cases. Pancreatic enzyme replacement is appropriate therapy in both instances.

Protein Intolerances. Protein intolerance, particularly milk protein sensitivity, is overdiagnosed in many infants and children. This is due to the absence of a reliable test to establish the diagnosis and the tendency to blame vague complaints such as fatigue, restlessness, or frequent colds on food allergies. In addition, it is possible to confuse protein intolerance with intolerance secondary to an inability to digest the associated carbohydrate. This confusion is particularly apt to occur in patients intolerant to cow's milk with a secondary lactase deficiency due to intestinal mucosal injury. Confusion may also arise in older children or adults with a genetically determined lactase deficiency. Patients with gastrointestinal symptoms secondary to protein sensitivity generally have vomiting and diarrhea of varying severity. Microscopic blood in the stool is frequently reported. The most commonly implicated proteins are milk, soybean, fish, shellfish, eggs, nuts, and wheat.

Clinical response to the double blind administration of protein isolates in capsules is the best method of diagnosis but this is not generally available. Resolution of symptoms with removal of the offending food, appearance of symptoms within 48 hours of ingesting small amounts of the food, and disappearance again when the food is stopped will ascertain the diagnosis in severe cases. More subtle symptoms may require multiple challenges. Particularly with cow's milk, an assessment of lactose tolerance by small bowel biopsy, hydrogen breath test, or lactose tolerance test may also be necessary.

Treatment is removal of the offending protein from the diet. In infancy, substitution of a soy protein formula may be successful, although soy protein sensitivity may occur.

Patients with intestinal mucosal injury (discussed below) appear more inclined to develop multiple protein sensitivities, as larger peptides may cross the damaged mucosa, provoking an immune response that causes gastrointestinal or systemic symptoms. In cases of cow's milk and soy sensitivity, a casein hydrolysate formula such as Nutramigen may be necessary. The shorter peptide chains of protein hydrolysates generally do not produce protein sensitivity. Infants with sucrose intolerance, as well as protein sensitivity due to mucosal injury, may require Pregestimil, which also contains casein hydrolysate but has short-chain glucose polymers instead of the sucrose in Nutramigen.

When they are 2 years old, infants who had relatively mild symptoms can be rechallenged with the offending food, starting with small amounts to see if restriction is still necessary. Parents of children with protein sensitivity should be advised to read food labels carefully to avoid inadvertent exposure to the offending protein.

SMALL INTESTINAL MUCOSAL INJURY

General Considerations. Diseases that injure small bowel mucosa cause villous atrophy and an associated loss of membrane bound hydrolases, including disaccharidases and dipeptidases. More extensive mucosal injury can result in loss of the capacity to absorb the main essential nutrients such as glucose, amino acids, and fatty acids. Many diseases are associated with mucosal injury (Table 6), including celiac disease, tropical sprue, intractable diarrhea of infancy, acute infectious gastroenteritis,

Table 6. DIARRHEA DUE TO MUCOSAL INJURY

Intractable diarrhea of infancy
Celiac disease
Small bowel contamination
Pathogenic *Escherichia coli*
Giardiasis
Tropical sprue
Viral gastroenteritis
Congenital crypt hypoplasia
Immunodeficiency syndromes
Dermatitis herpetiformis
Hirschsprung's enterocolitis
Secondary disaccharidase deficiencies
Secondary monosaccharide malabsorption
Protein sensitivity

and parasitoses such as giardiasis. Neomycin, kanamycin, methotrexate, colchicine, and other drugs can cause mucosal injury. Protein-calorie malnutrition can cause significant villous atrophy.

Intolerance to lactose can occur with relative mild injury, with sucrose intolerance generally limited to more severe cases. In the most serious atrophy, the loss of surface area can result in monosaccharide intolerance (fructose, glucose, and galactose). Patients with monosaccharide intolerance cannot tolerate carbohydrates. However, the short-chain glucose polymers found in corn syrup sugars are generally well tolerated by patients with significant intestinal mucosal injury, including those under 6 months of age who do not produce significant amounts of pancreatic amylase. This may be due to an alternate pathway of digestion provided by intestinal glucoamylase. This enzyme has a high affinity for glucose polymers with 5 to 9 glucose units. Although this enzyme is membrane bound, it appears to adequately digest short-chain glucose polymers even in many cases of severe intestinal mucosal damage. These polymers provide a lower osmotic load than monosaccharides and, as high osmotic feedings can themselves result in diarrhea, glucose polymers are recommended for patients with significant intestinal mucosal injury.

In addition to carbohydrate intolerance, intestinal mucosal injury results in the absorption of relatively long peptide chains. As a result, some patients will develop protein sensitivity if given casein and whey or soy based formulas. Casein hydrolysates seem to be less capable of inducing protein sensitivity.

Severe mucosal injury may produce steatorrhea secondary to the loss of surface area for absorption. MCT oil, which can be partially absorbed without digestion, may help in the nutrition of these patients.

These considerations can be applied to the treatment of a variety of clinical conditions where the end result is severe small intestinal mucosal injury.

Pregestimil, containing corn syrup sugars, casein hydrolysate, and 40% of the fat as MCT oil, has been used successfully in many infants with significant mucosal injury.

Intractable diarrhea, a significant cause of diarrhea due to mucosal injury in early infancy, is covered in another chapter.

Celiac Disease. Celiac disease results from severe villous atrophy due to the gluten-containing grains wheat, rye, barley, and oats. There is a wide variability in presentation. Patients under 2 tend to have more obvious gastrointestinal complaints while older children and adults have more subtle symptoms. The infant with celiac disease classically has frequent loose, bulky, pale, oily, foul-smelling stools after a 3 to 6 month period of exposure to gluten. Such patients also have a distended abdomen and wasted buttocks, and are quite irritable. At times stools are bulky but not loose, and some infants are even described as constipated. Growth failure is frequently seen in infants, but the diagnosis has been made in patients without growth failure.

Diarrhea is frequently less apparent in the older patient. These patients can present with a wide variety of symptoms including growth failure, abdominal pain, weight loss, and rickets or bleeding disorders secondary to an inability to absorb fat soluble vitamins. Other findings are iron-, folate-, or rarely B_{12}-deficiency anemias and edema due to protein-losing enteropathy.

Untreated patients with celiac disease have an increased incidence of lymphoma and carcinoma of the small bowel, as was emphasized in a recent report of over 250 adults with celiac disease and malignancy. Therefore, a proper diagnosis is mandatory to correctly identify patients who need lifelong gluten restriction. Unfortunately, the proper diagnosis of celiac disease remains cumbersome. A small intestinal biopsy with findings of villous atrophy, loss of nuclear polarity and pseudostratification of epithelial cells, elongated crypts with an increased mitotic index, and increased plasma cells in the lamina propria suggests celiac disease, but unfortunately these findings can be seen with other causes of villous atrophy. Therefore, it is necessary to demonstrate a normal mucosa on a gluten-free diet and return of abnormal histology after a gluten challenge. Clinical response to a gluten-free diet is not a satisfactory means of diagnosis, since it will result in an unnecessarily restrictive diet in patients without celiac disease. Clinical tolerance to the reintroduction of gluten unfortunately does not exclude celiac disease and may expose these patients to an increased risk of malignancy along with subtle symptoms such as vague abdominal pain and growth failure.

At the time of presentation, severe villous atrophy can result in low lactase and sucrase activity, and lactose and sucrose restrictions may be necessary. These should be temporary, as healing occurs with a gluten-free diet. In patients requiring carbohydrate restriction, cautious relaxation of the restrictions can be attempted after the first month, starting with sucrose.

Fat soluble vitamin supplementation is worthwhile early in therapy owing to the frequent malabsorption of fat soluble vitamins. Parenteral vitamin K will be necessary in patients with prolonged clotting studies. Anemias due to malabsorption of iron, folate, or B_{12} should be treated appropriately. Patients with severe vomiting, diarrhea, dehydration, and shock consistent with celiac crisis need prompt intravenous corticosteroids, 2 mg/kg/day of methylprednisolone.

The basic treatment is a gluten-free diet. This same diet is necessary for patients placed on a gluten-free diet as part of the diagnostic evaluation for celiac disease. Strict avoidance of wheat, rye, barley, and oats is necessary. In some families better compliance may be achieved by placing the entire family on the diet. A sample guide for patients and parents is shown in Table 7. Gluten-free recipe books will encourage tolerance.

Available books include:

1. Celiac Disease—Recipes for Parents and Patients. Hospital for Sick Children, Toronto, Canada, 1968
2. Good Food, Gluten Free. Keats Publishing, Inc., New Canaan, Connecticut, 1976
3. Gluten-Free Cooking. By Pat Murphy Gurst, M. Stevens Agency, P.O. Box 3004, Frankfort, KY 40603, 4th Printing, 1982.

Hospital dietitians may be aware of parent groups who also have recipe ideas. To insure that healing is complete, it is generally worthwhile to wait until about 1 year off the gluten before performing the small bowel biopsy. This will avoid unnecessary biopsies. If the patient is asymptomatic on gluten challenge, it is wise to wait another year before performing a challenge biopsy, as in some patients a prolonged challenge is necessary before histologic abnormalities appear on the biopsy.

Tropical Sprue. This condition, of unknown etiology, can present in a manner similar to celiac disease but is limited to patients who live in or have visited the tropics. Other causes of malabsorption, including parasitic or bacterial infection and celiac disease, need to be ruled out. Villous atrophy is usually seen in the small bowel biopsy, although the diagnosis has been made in patients with normal histology but malabsorption of two unrelated substances such as fat and B_{12}.

Patients may be deficient in a variety of nutrients. Megaloblastic anemia is often seen as a result of malabsorption of folate and/or B_{12}. Other observed deficiencies are iron, calcium, and vitamins A, D, and K. Steatorrhea is common and hypoproteinemia is seen frequently. Treatment should

Table 7. FOODS TO ALLOW AND FOODS TO AVOID ON A GLUTEN-FREE DIET

Food Groups	Allow	Avoid
Beverage	Carbonated beverages, artificially flavored fruit drinks; coffee, tea, decaffeinated coffee, pure instant coffee*	Cereal beverage. coffee beverages containing cereal grains, root beer**
Meat	Pure meat, fish, fowl, and eggs, guaranteed pure meat cold cuts,* sausage*; aged cheese, cottage cheese, cream cheese; peanut butter; soybeans; peanuts	Commercially prepared meat and egg products**; breaded meats, meat loaf, and meat patties; processed cheese,** cheese foods and dips**; texturized or hydrolyzed vegetable protein products**
Fat	Butter, margarine, cream, vegetable oil, shortening, nuts, olives, mayonnaise, gravies and sauces made with allowed thickening agents	Nondairy cream substitutes**; commercial salad dressing**; commercially prepared gravies and sauces
Milk	Milk, yogurt	Commercial chocolate milk, malted milk, instant milk drinks,** hot cocoa mixes**
Starch	Specially prepared bread and other baked products made with the following flours: corn, rice, potato, soybean, gluten-free wheat starch	Any homemade or commercially prepared baked goods or mixes containing wheat (except wheat starch), oats, rye, graham, or barley; buckwheat; pancakes**; bran or wheat germ; commercially prepared corn muffins**; gluten bread
	Corn and rice cereals	Cereals containing wheat, oats, rye, barley, bran, wheat germ, graham, bulgur, or millet
	Potatoes, rice, hominy grits	Commercial rice mixes, pasta, noodle, spaghetti, and macaroni products
	Thickening agents: corn flour, cornstarch, cornmeal, potato flour, potato starch, gluten-free wheat starch, soybean starch, arrowroot starch, tapioca, gelatin	All others
Vegetable	All except those in "Avoid" column	Any commercially prepared with cheese sauce or cream sauce, canned baked beans
Fruit	All except those in "Avoid" column	Commercially prepared pie fillings**; thickened fruit.
Soup	Homemade broth; vegetable or cream soups thickened with allowed flours and starches	Commercially prepared soup,** soup mixes**; bouillon** and broth**; any containing barley, pasta, or noodles
Dessert	Gelatin; meringues; custard; cornstarch, rice, and tapioca puddings; specially prepared desserts made of allowed flours and cereal-free baking powder, junket	Commercially prepared desserts and mixes**; cookies, cakes, pie, piecrust, pastries, pudding, ice cream,** sherbet, ice cream cones
Sweets	Sugar, honey, jelly, jam, molasses, corn syrup, pure maple syrup, pure baking chocolate, pure cocoa, coconut	Flavored syrups**; chocolate and other commercial candies
Miscellaneous	Salt, pepper, other spices and herbs, dry yeast, food coloring, and extracts	Prepared catsup**; mustard;** horseradish; bottled meat sauces,** soy sauce,** pickles; seasoning mixes;** cake yeast;** chewing gum;** baking powder**
	Wine, rum, brandy, vermouth, cognac	Beer, ale, alcoholic beverages distilled from cereal grains
Food Labeling	The patient should be advised to read product labels carefully and avoid sources of gluten: wheat, oats, rye, barley, bran, wheat germ, bulgur, millet, graham, durham, and malt. Possible sources of gluten in processed foods include stabilizers, emulsifiers, cereal additives, and vegetable protein. If there is any doubt, the product should be avoided until absence of gluten is verified by the manufacturer or by a brand name list prepared by the research unit of a hospital or university.	

*Check label carefully to be sure gluten is not an ingredient.
**Avoid unless absence of gluten is verified by the manufacturer or by special brand name product lists.
(Adapted from Pemberton CM, Gastineau CF (eds): *Mayo Clinic Diet Manual*. Philadelphia, W. B. Saunders, 1981.)

be directed at correcting these nutritional deficiencies. B_{12} should be given parenterally because of the frequency of malabsorption. In many patients administration of B_{12} and folate not only corrects the nutritional deficiencies but also improves the sense of well-being. Correction of these deficiencies may play a part in healing the intestinal mucosa. Tetracycline, 50 mg/kg/day maximum 1 gm/day for a few weeks, is successful in many cases.*Sulfonamides may be tried as an alternative. In patients who relapse, long term tetracycline therapy, for 6 months, is indicated. In cases of secondary carbohydrate deficiency due to intestinal mucosal injury, temporary exclusion of the appropriate carbohydrate may be worthwhile.

Contaminated Small Bowel Syndrome. Small bowel contamination can have a variety of causes. In most cases there is stasis of small intestinal contents allowing bacterial overgrowth. Examples include anatomic abnormalities such as strictures resulting from Crohn's disease and motility disorders such as intestinal pseudo-obstruction, abnormal motility due to gastroschisis, or postoperative areas of stasis such as intestinal blind loops. Other abnormalities that make conditions favorable for bacterial overgrowth are immune deficiency states, resection of the ileocecal valve, and malnutrition, particularly in the tropics where malnourished children ingest large numbers of bacteria owing to their unsanitary living conditions. As described below, bacterial overgrowth in immune deficiency states generally is not severe enough to demonstrate a clear association between bacterial overgrowth and malabsorption.

Normally the luminal contents of the upper small intestine contain less than 10^4 bacteria per ml. Concentrations of greater than 10^7 bacteria per ml are clearly abnormal. Steatorrhea results from bacterial deconjugation of bile salts. Deconjugated bile salts cannot form micelles, and depletion of conjugated bile salts below the critical micellar concentration results in fat malabsorption. B_{12} malabsorption is caused by bacterial utilization or conversion to inactive metabolites. Carbohydrate and protein malabsorption are also due in part to bacterial consumption, but the mechanisms are not completely understood. Serum folic acid may be increased, apparently as a result of synthesis of folic-acid–like compounds by the bacterial contaminants. Not all findings are present in all patients with bacterial overgrowth. Only about one third of B_{12} deficiency patients have steatorrhea.

The best treatment is definitive correction of a surgically correctable lesion. If this is not possible, antibiotic therapy can reduce bacterial overgrowth. There are no rules about the best method of therapy. Because of the mixed flora usually seen, culture and sensitivity may not provide a definitive choice of antibiotic. Tetracycline has been successful, as has lincomycin, which is a good drug to treat anaerobic overgrowth. Both continuous therapy and intermittent therapy, such as 2 weeks out of each month, have been successful.

Recently, 10 infants with persistent diarrhea were treated with oral gentamicin for 3 days and a combination of metronidazole and cholestyramine for 5 days. (S. Afr. Med. J. 58:241, 1980). All 10 patients improved with this therapy. Small bowel contamination was not documented, although the authors assumed this to be a factor in the persistent diarrhea of these patients. Further experience may determine if this therapy has a role in the care of young infants with persistent diarrhea due to small bowel contamination.

Nutritional support of patients with a contaminated small bowel should include B_{12} injections. When steatorrhea is present, medium chain triglycerides and fat soluble vitamin supplements are necessary. If antibiotic therapy is successful, less intensive nutritional support will be necessary.

Giardiasis. Giardiasis is a parasitic infection that can present with symptoms ranging from short term, self-limited illness to severe chronic malabsorption and growth failure. Areas of endemic infection have been noted but sporadic cases occur as well. Contaminated water supplies as well as person to person contact have been responsible for disease transmission.

Patients with hypogammaglobulinemia are particularly susceptible. Small bowel histology has revealed lymphoid nodular hyperplasia and absence of plasma cells in the lamina propria of many of these patients.

Diagnosis can be made by examining stool specimens for giardia cysts. Examination of 3 specimens will improve the yield. Examination of a small bowel biopsy or duodenal fluid may be diagnostic in patients with no evidence of giardia in the stool.

Quinicrine (Atabrine), 6 mg/kg/day (maximum of 300 mg/day) in 3 divided doses for 10 days, is the treatment of choice, although intolerance due to nausea and vomiting may occur. Metronidazole (Flagyl) has been used successfully but, because of findings of carcinogenesis and mutagenesis in animals, this drug is not recommended. Despite this caution, the successful use of combined quinicrine and metronidazole has been reported in an adult patient whose infection was unresponsive to either drug alone. Furazolidone (Furoxone) can be used in patients who do not tolerate quinicrine. A recent study found furazolidone, 8 mg/kg/day in 3–4 divided doses, better tolerated, particularly in young patients. Because of this improved tolerance,

---

*The use of tetracycline during the period of tooth development (fourth month of fetal development through the eighth year of life) may cause permanent discoloration and inadequate calcification of teeth.

furazolidone was also more effective. The maximum dose is 200 mg/kg/day. The greater expense of furazolidone makes quinicrine a reasonable first choice, although furazolidone has the advantage of being available in a liquid form, 50 mg/15 ml. Furazolidone is contraindicated in patients under 1 month, owing to the risk of hemolysis. In hypogammaglobulinemia patients longer periods of treatment may be necessary. Investigation of contacts, particularly family members, may reveal a source of infection. Failure to treat an asymptomatic carrier can result in reinfection.

Table 8. OTHER CAUSES OF CHRONIC DIARRHEA

Anatomic abnormalities
  Short bowel syndrome
  Intestinal lymphangiectasia

Pancreatic insufficiency
  Cystic fibrosis
  Shwachman-Diamond syndrome
  Malnutrition
  Johanssen-Blizzard syndrome

Bile salt insufficiency
  Cholestatic liver disease
  Small bowel contamination
  Defects of ileal bile salt reabsorption
    Ileal resection
    Ileitis, i.e., Crohn's disease
    Congenital deficiency of bile salt reabsorption

Metabolic and endocrine abnormalities
  Acrodermatitis enteropathica
  Abetalipoproteinemia
  Wolman's disease
  Adrenal insufficiency
  Hypoparathyroidism
  Hyperthyroidism

Malabsorption in developing countries
  Malnutrition
  Contaminated small bowel syndrome
  Tropical sprue

Miscellaneous
  Nonspecific diarrhea of infancy

Immune Deficiencies. Giardiasis is often seen in patients with hypogammaglobulinemia. Although it has been reported in other immune deficiency states, it is not clear whether the incidence is above that of the general population.

Selective IgA deficiency has been associated with diarrhea and steatorrhea. Some patients have responded to a gluten-free diet, although the absence of IgA-secreting plasma cells makes their small bowel biopsy picture different from that of typical celiac disease. A patient with selective IgA deficiency has been reported who required parenteral feeding and later an elemental diet because of an apparent hypersensitivity to food proteins.

Bacterial overgrowth has been found in immune deficiency patients but a correlation with diarrhea and malabsorption has not been established, nor has an association between treatment of patients with bacterial overgrowth and immune deficiency and improvement of malabsorption.

MISCELLANEOUS

Acrodermatitis Enteropathica. Acrodermatitis enteropathica is a cause of chronic diarrhea associated with zinc deficiency. Patients have an abnormality of zinc transport in the intestine, possibly resulting from an absence or abnormality of zinc binding ligands within the intestine. Human milk gives some protection because zinc binding ligands are present in it. Formula-fed infants present early in life and breast-fed infants after weaning. Patients develop moist or scaling erythematous eruptions about the mouth, anus, and interdigital areas. Alopecia, dystrophic nails, photophobia, conjunctivitis, and glossitis may also be present. The rash may occur before or with the onset of diarrhea. Loss of taste sensation, anoxeria, irritability, lethargy, and depression are associated symptoms. Diarrhea tends to be intermittent, and usually there is steatorrhea. A deficiency of essential fatty acids in the serum has been described, and addition of Intralipid intravenously can help.

Diagnosis is based on a low plasma zinc (< 65 to 70 μg/dl) in association with typical clinical findings. Blood samples should be collected appropriately, as contamination can occur from glassware or rubber stoppers, raising the measured zinc level. Some patients with typical findings have been reported to have normal serum zinc levels, and some of these have responded to oral zinc therapy.

Oral therapy with zinc sulfate or zinc acetate to provide 10 to 45 mg/day of elemental zinc should maintain normal zinc levels. Zinc acetate causes less gastric irritation. A liquid preparation of zinc acetate providing 1 mg Zn/ml given 2 to 3 times a day 1 hour before meals has been used successfully.

Zinc deficiency can also be secondary to other diseases causing malabsorption, including Crohn's disease and celiac disease. Secondary zinc deficiencies will also respond to appropriate zinc replacement. Doses should be individualized and serum levels monitored.

Endocrine Abnormalities. Diarrhea may be a presenting finding in patients with adrenal insufficiency, hypoparathyroidism, and hyperthyroidism. Treatment of these conditions is discussed elsewhere in this text.

Nonspecific Diarrhea of Infancy. This diagnosis describes a group of patients generally between 8 months and 3 years of age who have persistent loose stools but who otherwise are in apparent good health. Growth and weight gain are normal. The physician must be confident that these patients have no significant abnormality before making this diagnosis. The extent of investigation must be individualized. Some patients, with a history of reduced fat intake, have responded to a 50 gm fat diet. Reassurance of parents and good follow-up to insure that the patient continues to thrive despite loose stools are necessary.

SURGICAL ASSOCIATED ENTITIES

Short Bowel Syndrome. After extensive small bowel resection, malabsorption occurs as a result of a loss of mucosal surface area, loss of mucosal enzymes, and reduced transit time in the small bowel. Malnutrition and decrease in enteric hormones may impair exocrine pancreatic function, leading to further malabsorption. A reduction of duodenal pH secondary to gastric hypersecretion may also impair pancreatic enzyme function. Loss of ileum results in loss of functions specific to that region, particularly the active uptake of B_{12} and conjugated bile acids. Thus, loss of substantial amounts of jejunum may be better tolerated than loss of a large portion of ileum. When the ileocecal valve is resected, a further decrease in transit time as well as small bowel contamination may contribute to malabsorption. Parenteral alimentation has allowed long term survival in patients intolerant to enteral feedings. Infants with greater than 40 cm of small bowel beyond the ligament of Treitz and an intact ileocecal valve usually tolerate enteral feeds well, and patients with only 25 cm of small bowel and an intact ileocecal valve have tolerated feeds. If the ileocecal valve is resected, greater than 40 cm of small bowel beyond the ligament of Treitz is generally needed for tolerance of enteral feedings. Patients with extensive ileal resection will need parenteral B_{12} therapy. The dose must be individualized but the long half-life of B_{12} should allow relatively infrequent injections. Unabsorbed bile salts can produce a secretory diarrhea, and if losses are enough to significantly deplete intraluminal bile salt concentrations, patients will develop steatorrhea. While cholestyramine therapy can be tried to treat the secretory diarrhea (250–500 mg/kg/day divided 2–4 times a day up to 4 gm [1 packet] 4 times a day),*this is usually unsuccessful. This appears to be due to bacterial metabolism of fatty acids to long-chain hydroxy acids, which can be potent cathartics. A low fat diet with MCT oil, which does not require a critical micellar concentration of bile salts for absorption, may have more success than cholestyramine use. Patients with steatorrhea but without secretory diarrhea should also benefit from a low fat diet supplemented with MCT oil used in cooking and in foods such as salad dressing.

Continuous drip enteral feedings may be successful in patients otherwise intolerant of enteral feedings. Elemental feeds that include monosaccharides, amino acids, and essential fatty acids may be successful, but some patients may be intolerant of the high osmotic load. Patients with adequate absorptive function may tolerate drip feeds of semielemental, lower osmotic feedings. Osmolyte contains short chain glucose polymers as well as casein hydrolysate. Fifty percent of the fat is MCT oil. The caloric density is 1.06 kcal/ml. In young infants Pregestimil, which has a similar composition, may be successful. Pregestimil is a complete infant formula, unlike Osmolyte, and contains 0.67 kcal/ml. These patients will require supplements of fat soluble vitamins A, D, E, and K in doses individualized for each patient (see discussion on bile salt insufficiency). Small bowel contamination should be treated as discussed above.

Anticholinergic agents and opiates are generally contraindicated. They tend to produce abdominal distention and may exacerbate small bowel contamination.

Patients intolerant to enteral feeds can be maintained on home parenteral nutrition.

Hirschsprung's Disease and Enterocolitis. Hirschsprung's disease, aganglionic megacolon, is commonly associated with constipation. Some patients develop overflow diarrhea leaking around a bolus of hard stool. There will be absence of the normal internal sphincter relaxation reflex on rectal manometry and frequently a dilated colon proximal to the affected area on unprepared barium enema. Definitive diagnosis is made by full-thickness rectal biopsy showing absence of ganglia, and treatment consists of removal of the aganglionic segment and a pull-through procedure.

Hirschsprung's enterocolitis is a serious complication that can occur before or after surgery for removal of the aganglionic segment. Patients develop severe diarrhea, apparently from small intestinal mucosal injury, and carbohydrate and other nutrient intolerances. Parenteral alimentation may be necessary until the small intestine is sufficiently recovered. In mild cases, Pregestimil may be a successful alternative to parenteral nutrition, as in other patients with intestinal mucosal injury. It also appears to be the feeding of choice in infants being weaned from parenteral nutrition.

Recurrent episodes of enterocolitis require repeated periods of nutritional support.

PANCREATIC INSUFFICIENCY

Exocrine pancreatic insufficiency in childhood is due to cystic fibrosis in over 90% of cases. The second most common cause is Shwachman-Diamond syndrome, consisting primarily of pancreatic insufficiency, bone marrow dysfunction (most commonly neutropenia), and growth retardation. Associated features are metaphyseal dysosto-

---

*The dosage of cholestyramine in infants and children has not been established.

sis, eczema, elevated fetal hemoglobin, and rarely, diabetes mellitus, Hirschsprung's disease, and testicular fibrosis. Exocrine pancreatic function can be impaired temporarily in patients with protein calorie malnutrition (see below) but is usually restored with return of adequate nutrition.

Permanent pancreatic insufficiency requires pancreatic supplementation, dietary therapy, and vitamin supplements. The optimal method of administering pancreatic supplementation is controversial. If standard supplements are given, enzyme activity will be lost if the intragastric pH falls below 4. Aluminum hydroxide and sodium bicarbonate have reduced steatorrhea in these patients, although with sodium bicarbonate, the risk of metabolic alkalosis is real. Antacids containing calcium or magnesium appear to impair fat absorption perhaps by forming soaps or by interfering with glycine-bile salt conjugates. Inconsistent results have been obtained with the use of cimetidine with pancreatic supplements.

An alternative approach is use of pH-sensitive enteric coated tablets such as Pancrease. As long as the gastric pH stays below 6, the enteric coating will remain intact. If the pH rises above 6 and subsequently drops below 4 with the enzymes still in the stomach, activity will be lost.

A recent study demonstrated no significant difference in effectiveness between pH-sensitive capsules and conventional pancreatic enzyme preparations without antacid supplements in adults with pancreatic insufficiency secondary to chronic alcoholic pancreatitis (Gastroenterology 84:476, 1983). Further studies are needed, but if there is indeed no significant difference between enteric coated and standard preparations such as Cotazyme or Viokase, the standard preparation would be more cost effective.

Doses of pancreatic supplements must be individualized. Guidelines include a decrease in steatorrhea and appropriate weight gain with appropriate or moderately increased caloric intake. Preparations should be given before each meal. A reasonable dose for a 2-year-old is usually about 1 Pancrease capsule, 2 Cotazyme capsules, or a teaspoon of Viokase powder. The presence of erythema on the buttocks suggests irritation from an excessive amount of enzymes. Very high doses also carry the risk of uric acid renal stones caused by the purines present in the supplements.

These patients should avoid greasy or fatty foods. Medium chain triglycerides are absorbed more efficiently than long chain triglycerides. Malnourished patients may benefit from supplemental MCT oil, but generally this is not necessary with appropriate supplements. Fat soluble vitamin supplements will avoid vitamin deficiencies due to malabsorption. With appropriate enzyme supplements, maintenance doses of these vitamins should be adequate.

MALNUTRITION

It is frequently difficult to determine whether severe malnutrition induces diarrhea or chronic diarrhea induces malnutrition. Chronic diarrhea and malnutrition worldwide make up one of the most significant problems in pediatrics. Generally patients in underdeveloped countries live in poverty in places of poor sanitation. Breast-feeding can be valuable in prevention by reducing exposure to contaminated water supplies. Children suffering malnutrition and diarrhea generally have intestinal mucosal injury and will benefit from semielemental feedings such as Pregestimil. Parenteral nutrition is often necessary; unfortunately, facilities for this therapy are frequently unavailable. Small bowel bacterial contamination (previously described) and parasitic infestation must also be treated. Feeding tolerance may be impaired owing to a deficiency of pancreatic enzymes. Pancreatic insufficiency generally resolves with proper nutrition.

NEW THERAPEUTIC MODALITIES—HOME PARENTERAL NUTRITION

Patients with severely impaired small bowel function require parenteral alimentation. Candidates include patients with short bowel syndrome, intractable diarrhea, severe Crohn's disease, or intestinal pseudo-obstruction. Patients with chronic debilitating illness such as cystic fibrosis may benefit from the nutritional support.

Catheters that can be clamped safely, such as the Broviac or Hickman catheters, allow intermittent infusion of solutions, which allows patients to be independent during the day and to receive parenteral nutrition at night. This mode of therapy has been used successfully in infants, children, and adults, and can be done at home with proper training.

The use of large vessels for these infusions allows the use of hypertonic solutions. Infants under age 2 generally tolerate between 150 and 180 ml/kg/day. Older patients can be given 3000 ml/M^2/day, to a maximum of 4000 ml/day. Patients need to adapt to increasing glucose loads. Generally patients will tolerate 12.5% dextrose initially and can be advanced 2.5% a day to a maximum of 20%. Patients may tolerate up to 25% dextrose if the extra calories are necessary. Two to three gm/kg of protein in the form of a crystalline amino acid solution is generally used. Patients with significant protein losses have been given 4 gm/kg/day. Lipid preparations can be given separately through a Y-connector into the central venous catheter. These solutions are available in concentrations of 10 and 20%. Available 10% solutions provide between 0.9 and 1.1 kcal/ml and therefore can provide an excellent source of calories. Doses of 3 gm/kg/day are generally well tolerated, although some patients will develop turbid serum and elevated triglycerides requiring a lower dose. Two to four gm/kg twice a week should provide enough essential fatty acids to prevent essential fatty acid deficiency. When a lipid preparation is used, fluid from the glucose and protein source should be reduced by a volume equal to that of lipid given. At least 24 nonprotein calories should be provided per gram of protein infused to insure that amino acids will be incorporated into protein rather than being utilized as an energy source.

Suggested values for minerals and electrolytes are shown in Table 9. B_{12} and folate can be added to the bottle once a week. The dose of B_{12} is 2 to 5 μg/day. For folic acid, 50 μg/day can be given to infants less than 1 year old and 100 to 400 μg/day can be given to older children. Vitamin K, 1 to 5 mg, should be given intramuscularly biweekly to infants. Adolescents can receive 10 mg biweekly. One to three ml of a multivitamin preparation should be added daily.

Table 9. SUGGESTED ELECTROLYTE AND MINERAL COMPOSITION OF PARENTERAL NUTRITION

Sodium (as chloride)	3–4 mEq
Potassium (as phosphate and chloride)*	2–4 mEq
Calcium (as gluconate)	1–4 mEq
Magnesium (as sulfate)	0.25 mEq
Phorphorus as potassium phosphate)*	1.36 mmole
Zinc (as sulfate)	150–300 μg
Copper (as sulfate)	20–40 μg

*Potassium, as phosphate, should be limited to 2 mEq/kg/day; additional potassium should be provided as the chloride salt.

(Adapted from Lebenthal E (ed): Textbook of Gastroenterology and Nutrition in Infancy. New York, Raven Press, 1981.)

Further experience will no doubt lead to new recommendations. For instance, biotin deficiency associated with alopecia and a crusting exfoliative rash around the eyes, nose, mouth, and perianal region has been described in patients receiving prolonged parenteral nutrition. One hundred μg/day of biotin is probably adequate.

Patients to receive home parenteral nutrition will need to adapt to the shorter infusion period. Once the patient is tolerating his full amount of parenteral nutrition, infusion time can be reduced by 2 hours/day so that the total fluid is given over a period of 10 to 14 hours. To avoid hypoglycemia, the rate should be reduced gradually over the last hour. This is usually done by reducing the rate by half over the first 30 minutes and by half again over the second 30 minutes before stopping the infusion completely.

Careful instruction of patient, parents, and health care personnel in the proper care of the cen-

tral venous catheter is essential for successful use of total parenteral nutrition. Use of sterile technique in changing dressings and tubing will prevent sepsis, which is the major complication of parenteral nutrition. Monitoring of the metabolic parameters, as suggested in Table 10, will alert the physician to significant abnormalities in nutrition, electrolyte, and glucose parameters along with abnormalities of liver function, which can be seen frequently with prolonged parenteral alimentation. As indicated before, serum should be inspected periodically (daily when lipids are first begun) for turbidity. Initially, serum triglycerides should be monitored once or twice a week, as significant triglyceride elevations can occur without visual evidence of serum turbidity.

Table 10. SUGGESTED MONITORING SCHEDULE DURING TPN

Variable to Be Monitored	Suggested Frequency (per week)*	
	Initial Period	Later Period
Growth variable		
Weight	7	7
Length	1	1
Head circumference	1	1
Metabolic variable		
Blood or plasma		
Na, K, Cl	3–4	1
Ca, Mg, P	2	1
Acid-base status	3–4	1
Urea nitrogen	2	1
Albumin	1	1
Liver function studies	1	1
Lipids**		
Hemoglobin	2	2
Urinary glucose	2–6/day	2/day
Prevention and detection of infection		
Clinical observations (activity, temperature, etc.)	Daily	Daily
WBC and differential	As indicated	As indicated
Cultures	As indicated	As indicated

*Initial period is the time during which a full caloric intake is being achieved. Later period implies that the patient has achieved a metabolic steady state. In the presence of metabolic instability, the more intensive monitoring outlined under the initial period should be followed.

**See text.

(Reprinted from Lebenthal E (ed): Textbook of Gastroenterology and Nutrition in Infancy. New York, Raven Press, 1981.)

With proper patient monitoring and a well organized, dedicated health care team, home parenteral nutrition can be a safe and effective means of long term nutritional support.

Disorders of the Anus and Rectum

MARC I. ROWE, M.D.,
and DAVID A. LLOYD, M.D.

Anal Fissure. Fissure-in-ano is a superficial longitudinal tear of the anoderm, usually in the anterior or posterior midline, caused by passage of a large, hard fecal mass. The resulting pain and anal spasm lead to retention of stool, constipation, and eventual passage of another hard stool with further trauma. If this cycle is not broken, a chronic lesion results. Fissures typically occur during infancy and early childhood and are the most common cause of rectal bleeding in infancy. The presenting symptoms are painful defecation with bleeding, the blood being on the surface of the stool rather than mixed with fecal matter. The diagnosis can be made by gently spreading the buttocks and inspecting the everted anus. Passage of a test tube or anoscope is painful and seldom helpful. Treatment consists of initial softening of the stool by oral mineral oil, followed by daily bulk laxatives (e.g., Metamucil). Warm sitz baths after each bowel movement will ease pain and spasm. Persistent symptoms suggest a chronic fissure and require an examination under anesthesia. If a relatively acute and superficial lesion is found, this can be successfully treated by gently but firmly stretching the anus to relieve sphincter spasm. A chronic deep fissure will necessitate complete excision.

Perianal Abscess and Fistula-in-ano. A perianal abscess originates in the anal crypts and spreads to the perianal subcutaneous tissues where it presents as an acute painful swelling. Initial treatment consists of warm sitz baths and local drainage. This may suffice, but persistent drainage or recurrent infection suggests a perianal fistula, which has an internal opening at the infected crypt and extends either superficial to or through the external anal sphincter to open on the perianal skin. Under general anesthetic, the fistula is defined and either laid open or completely excised, and allowed to heal by secondary intention. Recurrent fistulae, particularly in older children, require investigation to exclude chronic inflammatory disease, notably Crohn's disease.

Injuries to the Anus and Rectum. Injuries usually result from ingestion or insertion of foreign bodies, careless use of thermometers or enemas, traumatic endoscopy, or from accidents or child abuse. The injuries encompass superficial anal tears, disruption of the sphincter mechanism, and perforation of the rectum above or below the peritoneal reflection. Contamination of the peritoneal cavity leads to peritonitis. The extent of the lesion cannot be determined by superficial examination, and careful evaluation under general anesthetic, usually with endoscopy, is required.

Superficial lacerations may be left open or sutured, depending on severity. Injuries to the sphincter muscles must be repaired, and if the damage is extensive, a temporary diverting colostomy ensures good healing. Broad-spectrum antimicrobials are required for all major lesions. Perforation above the peritoneal reflection necessitates immediate laparotomy with closure of the perforation and a diverting colostomy. Perforation below the peritoneal reflection usually can be managed with broad-spectrum antibiotics and careful observation. The need for colostomy depends on the extent of the injury and the degree of contamination.

Foreign bodies are removed by endoscopy. Large foreign bodies lying transversely across the rectum, particularly those with sharp ends, are best handled by dividing the object in two and removing the pieces separately.

Rectal Prolapse. Prolapse of the rectum is the circumferential descent of one or more layers of the rectal wall through the anus. Mucosal prolapse involves the mucosa only; prolapse of all the layers of the rectal wall is known as procidentia. Prolapse is fairly common during the first two years of life and extremely uncommon thereafter. The relative mobility and lack of fixation of the rectum in the young child and the loose attachment of the rectal mucosa to the muscularis are thought to be the reasons for the high incidence in early childhood. Conditions that may initiate prolapse are those producing sudden increases in intra-abdominal pressure or leading to excessive straining at stool. These include chronic respiratory infections, constipation, diarrhea, polyps, and worms. Specific disorders associated with prolapse of the rectum are neurologic abnormalities such as meningomyeloceles, sacral agenesis, exstrophy of the bladder, and cystic fibrosis. Toddlers undergoing bowel training usually have no specific defect.

A careful search is made for specific etiologic factors, which are then treated. Prolapse usually is self-limiting. Management includes prompt reduction and strapping the buttocks together to hold in the rectum. Persistent prolapse requires admission to hospital and either injection of 30% saline solution perirectally in front of the coccyx or placement of a nylon or an absorbable Thiersch suture around the anus.

Imperforate Anus Anomalies. The various forms of imperforate anus can usually be diagnosed, and treatment planned, by simple inspection of the perineum. Since continence is dependent on the rectum being surrounded by the levator ani muscular sling, a major differentiating point is whether the rectum terminates above or below the sling.

In girls, there are usually three forms of this anomaly. If only one orifice is noted, the probable diagnosis is a persistent cloaca. In this form of imperforate anus, there has been failure of separation of the hind gut from the urogenital system, resulting in the upper vagina, the hind gut, and the urethra opening into a single orifice. This is a complex anomaly with the rectum ending well above the levator ani sling. Temporary colostomy is required followed by later reconstructive surgery.

If two openings, one urethral and one vaginal, are identified, this suggests that the rectum communicates with the vagina as a rectovaginal fistula. The communication may be either high in the vagina or low, ending just above the hymenal ring. High lesions terminate above the levator ani sling and are best treated by temporary diverting colostomy and later definitive operation. Lower lesions may terminate below the levator ani sling and can be treated via a perineal approach, usually by transposing the anal opening to a posterior position on the perineum.

The presence of three openings signifies an ectopic anus. This is a definite low lesion, since the rectum has passed through the puborectalis sling. This lesion, however, is frequently misdiagnosed and called a rectovaginal fistula because the ectopic anal opening is in very close proximity to the hymen and must be carefully searched for. Treatment of this low lesion is either a cutback anoplasty or transposition of the anal opening to a more posterior location. In either case, results are excellent and perfect continence is the rule.

In the male, the high lesion is usually a result of failure of the urogenital system to separate from the hind gut. The rectal opening communicates with the posterior urethra above the levator ani musculature. The diagnosis can usually be made by observing the passage of meconium-stained urine. A diverting colostomy is necessary, followed later by a pull-through operation at 9 to 12 months of age.

There are two forms of low lesion in the male. The ectopic anus or perineal fistula presents as an opening anterior to the normal position of the anus. The external sphincter muscle can usually be identified posterior to this opening. A cutback anoplasty is adequate. A covered anus is a normally situated anus that is either partially or completely covered by a membrane or a ridge of skin. Often this ridge is well defined and is termed a "bucket handle." Occasionally a track leads up over the scrotum and may contain drops of meconium. Simple excision of this skin cap suffices. Dilatations may be necessary to prevent stricture.

A major contribution to the understanding of imperforate anus was made by Stephens, who recognized that the levator ani musculature was essential for continence, and devised an operation to assure proper placement of the rectum within this musculature. The Stephens operation, which became the procedure of choice, entailed identification of the levator ani sling, through which the rectum was passed under direct vision. This was done by either a sacroperineal or a sacroperineoabdominal approach. Although continence was better after Stephens' operation, compared with older abdominoperineal operations, the results were not always satisfactory. Recently Pena and DeVries have described a procedure emphasizing the importance of not only the levator ani musculature but the entire muscular complex including the muscles frequently described as the external anal sphincters. Their operation consists of a posterior midline incision extending from the sacrum through the anal area. The entire musculature is divided in the midline, and the rectum is carefully placed between the halves of the muscles, which are sewn around the anus and rectum. The initial results of this procedure have been encouraging.

_7_

Blood

Anemia of Iron Deficiency, Blood Loss, Renal Disease, and Chronic Infection

JOHN N. LUKENS, M.D.

IRON DEFICIENCY ANEMIA

The treatment of iron deficiency requires replenishment of body iron and correction of the factor or factors responsible for the deficiency state. Patients compromised because of severe anemia may require blood transfusion to rapidly correct cardiac decompensation. Iron supplements are indicated for groups at high risk for developing nutritional iron deficiency.

Iron Replacement. Iron can be given orally, intramuscularly, or intravenously. *Oral iron* is the safest, least expensive form of treatment, and is as effective as parenterally administered iron. There is no indication for the intravenous infusion of iron in children.

The treatment of choice for iron replenishment is ferrous sulfate. Ferrous gluconate and ferrous fumarate, while as effective, are more expensive. Numerous other iron salts, with and without adjuvants, are marketed with claims of improved palatability, enhanced absorption, or fewer side effects. Most of these preparations are therapeutically inferior to ferrous sulfate and all are more expensive. Ascorbic acid is a popular additive because of its known potential to increase iron absorption. However, the amount of ascorbic acid added to most iron preparations is much less than that needed to significantly influence absorption. In addition, ascorbate potentiates the undesirable side effects of oral iron. Thus, an increase in the dose of iron achieves the same result at a lower cost. Enteric coated tablets and sustained release capsules should be avoided, as they ensure transit of iron beyond the site of maximal absorption.

Ferrous sulfate is marketed in a variety of concentrations and forms for use in children of different ages. A concentrated solution containing 15 mg elemental iron per 0.6 ml is administered by calibrated dropper to infants and small children. An elixir, intended for toddlers, contains 30 mg elemental iron per 5 ml. Tablets and capsules contain 60 mg. elemental iron.

The elemental iron content of the ferrous salt is used for dosage calculation. For ferrous sulfate, the elemental iron content is 20% by weight. An optimal therapeutic response is obtained with 5 mg elemental iron/kg/day (ferrous sulfate, 25 mg/kg/day). The usual adult dose of 180 mg elemental iron/day should not be exceeded. Larger doses are more likely to produce gastrointestinal disburbances without effecting a more rapid recovery. The daily dose is divided into three portions and given with meals. While meals interfere somewhat with iron absorption, the reduction in absorption is more than offset by better tolerance and patient compliance. If there are apparent side effects despite this precaution, the dose of iron should be decreased by 50%. Speed in the repair of iron deficiency is rarely important.

Subjective improvement may be noted within a day or two after starting iron therapy: irritability is less prominent, spontaneous activity increases, pica is corrected, and appetite returns. A reticulocytosis, inversely proportional to the initial hemoglobin concentration, is noted within 3 to 5 days. Reticulocytes are maximal (5–10%) at 5–10 days. The rate of hemoglobin rise is a function of the magnitude of anemia. The more severe the anemia, the greater is the daily increment in hemoglobin concentration. Approximately 18 days after initiation of therapy, the hemoglobin reaches a level midway between the initial value and that which is normal. Irrespective of the severity of anemia, approximately 2 months are required to achieve a normal hemoglobin concentration. Full doses of iron are continued for 2 months after correction of anemia in order to provide iron reserves. Suboptimal response to iron most commonly reflects failure of iron administration, inadequate dosage, or use of an iron preparation that is poorly absorbed. Less frequently, a coexistent infection compromises marrow response to iron or ongoing blood losses obscure an appropriate marrow response. Rarely, treatment failure is due to iron malabsorption.

Side effects of oral iron therapy are more frequently encountered in adults than in infants and children. Adverse symptoms potentially related to medicinal iron include constipation, diarrhea, heartburn, and abdominal cramps. Temporary staining of teeth by liquid preparations can be avoided by using a straw or by placing the iron directly on the back of the tongue with a dropper.

Iron tablets should be dispensed in bottles equipped with safety caps. Parents are instructed to ensure inaccessibility of the tablets to small children. Because of their relatively low iron concentration, liquid preparations pose little or no risk of accidental iron poisoning.

Parenteral iron therapy is painful, expensive (relative to oral therapy), and attended by a slight but measurable risk of hypersensitivity reaction. The rate of hemoglobin rise is no greater than with iron given by mouth. Nevertheless, the intramuscular injection of iron is indicated in the face of steadfast noncompliance, for situations in which ongoing iron losses exceed that which can be absorbed by the oral route, and for states of iron malabsorption. Most iron deficient patients with peptic ulcer disease and inflammatory bowel disease do not require parenteral iron.

The parenteral iron preparation with which there is greatest experience is iron dextran (Imferon). This is a complex ferric hydroxide with high molecular weight dextrans in a colloidal solution containing 50 mg elemental iron/ml. The total required dose is calculated as follows: dose (mg Fe) = weight (kg) × desired increment Hgb (gm/dl) × 2.5.

An additional 10 mg iron/kg is given in order to ensure replenishment of stores. The calculated dose is given over several days so as not to exceed 2 ml/day. Care is taken to deliver the preparation deep into the upper outer quadrant of the buttock. The skin and subcutaneous tissue are retracted laterally prior to insertion of the needle in order to avoid staining the skin.

Blood Transfusion. Because the response to iron is prompt and predictable, blood transfusion is rarely indicated. It is reserved for children whose anemia is of such severity as to produce frank or impending cardiac decompensation. In this setting, sedimented red blood cells are given as a modified exchange transfusion. Patient blood is replaced with packed red cells in 10 to 20 ml increments. The volume of the exchange need not exceed 20 ml/kg.

Correction of Predisposing Factors. It is very important to identify and correct the factors responsible for the deficiency. Iron deficiency is properly viewed as the expression of a primary disturbance rather than as a complete diagnosis in itself. Curtailment of milk consumption is required for infants whose deficiency is nutritional. Substitution of an evaporated milk preparation or a non-milk-based formula for cow's milk is necessary to arrest the occult blood loss of milk-induced enteropathy. Nutritional counseling is provided for those of high school and college age. Search for occult disease is necessary when dealing with unexplained iron deficiency.

Preventive Measures. The risk of iron deficiency in the first years of life can be minimized by adoption of simple feeding practices. These include encouragement of breast feeding, avoidance of unmodified whole cow's milk during the first year, inclusion of foods that promote iron absorption (fruit and fruit juices, meat, poultry), and avoidance of excessive weight gain. Iron supplements are required during the first year if the recommended daily requirement (2 mg iron/kg) is to be met. For infants receiving cow's milk formulas, this is conveniently provided by using an iron-fortified formula. A medicinal iron supplement (2 mg/kg/day) is indicated for infants receiving milk formulas not fortified with iron. Twice this amount is required by small preterm infants after 3 months of age. Breast-fed infants, also, require an iron supplement between 6 and 12 months of age despite the high bioavailability of iron in human milk. The negative iron balance of breast-fed infants after 3 to 6 months of age is due in part to a progressive decline in the iron content of breast milk and in part to a decrease in breast milk consumption that follows introduction of solid foods.

BLOOD LOSS ANEMIA

The management of blood loss anemia is dictated by the volume and chronicity of bleeding. The needs of patients who have sustained massive acute hemorrhages are different from those of individuals who have experienced chronic or remote bleeding.

Acute Blood Loss. Not until 20% or more of the blood volume is lost do disturbances in circulatory dynamics occur. Consequently, no therapy is required for blood losses unattended by alterations in vital signs unless recurrence of bleeding is anticipated. With losses of 30 to 40%, all the symptoms and signs of shock are observed: peripheral perfusion is poor, the skin is moist and cool, the blood pressure and central venous pressure are low, and the heart rate is accelerated. These physical findings are of far greater value than is the hemoglobin concentration in assessing the need for therapy. Since several hours are required for plasma volume expansion, the magnitude of acute blood loss is not revealed by alterations in hemoglobin concentration just after the event.

The immediate need is expansion of the blood volume, best accomplished with the transfusion of whole blood. If the urgency of the situation obviates the delay inherent in obtaining properly cross-matched blood, plasma or a plasma protein solution may be infused until blood is available. Approximately 20 ml/kg of the most readily available product is given by rapid intravenous infusion. The need for subsequent infusions can best be assessed by monitoring the central venous pressure. The initial transfusion is followed by repeat infusions of 10 ml/kg until a measurable central venous pressure is obtained and peripheral circulation is restored.

If massive volumes of blood are lost, the infused blood must be fresh in order to prevent a "washout" of platelets and factor VIII. In general, coagulopathy resulting from massive blood transfusion is encountered only if more than the estimated blood volume of the recipient is replaced in a 24 hour period.

Chronic or Remote Blood Loss. The signs and symptoms of chronic or remote blood loss are those of anemia rather than hypovolemia. Because blood loss imposes a drain on iron, the anemia characteristically has all the morphologic and biochemical hallmarks of iron deficiency.

Anemia is usually well compensated. Because volume overload is a potential problem, blood is not given unless there is cardiac decompensation. This is best managed with a small exchange transfusion (20 ml/kg). The use of sedimented red cells instead of whole blood facilitates rapid correction of anemia and permits creation of a volume deficit. Correction of the iron deficiency that almost always accompanies chronic blood loss follows the principles described in the section dealing with iron deficiency anemia.

ANEMIA OF RENAL DISEASE

The anemia associated with severe renal failure has multiple contributing factors. Red blood cell production is limited, in part because of decreased erythropoietin production by the kidneys and in part because of decreased stem cell responsiveness to erythropoietin; red cell survival is shortened; blood is lost into dialysis equipment; and folate availability may be limited by poor dietary intake and by loss to dialysis baths. Contaminants in hemodialysis fluids (copper, nitrates, chloramines) may also trigger hemolytic episodes. The most significant of these contributing factors is deficient erythropoietin production. Since erythropoietin is not available for clinical trials, treatment of the anemia is symptomatic rather than substantive.

The cornerstone of therapy is blood transfusion. The indication for transfusion is based on symptoms rather than on an arbitrary level of hemoglobin concentration. Most active children with renal disease tolerate moderately severe anemia remarkably well. This is due at least in part to enhancement of oxygen unloading secondary to increased red cell 2,3-diphosphoglycerate. Symptoms attributable to anemia are infrequently experienced until the hemoglobin drops below 7 to 8 gm/dl. Many children tolerate 5 gm/dl. with impunity. When dictated by symptoms, blood is given as sedimented red cells (approximately 10 ml/kg). If symptoms are alleviated, transfusions are repeated when symptoms recur. In the absence of symptoms, the hemoglobin concentration is allowed to fall until it stabilizes at approximately 5 gm/dl.

Patients on chronic hemodialysis programs are at risk for iron deficiency because of loss of blood into the dialysis apparatus. Therapeutic amounts of iron are indicated for such individuals unless the iron requirement is satisfied by blood transfusions. Since folate is dialyzable, reserves of this essential nutrient are also readily exhausted. Folate-limited erythropoiesis is easily prevented by giving 1 mg folic acid (pteroylglutamic acid) daily.

ANEMIA OF CHRONIC INFECTION

A wide variety of chronic infectious, inflammatory, and malignant states are associated with a mild anemia having well defined morphologic, kinetic, and biochemical features. The anemia is mild and nonprogressive. Rarely is the hemoglobin concentration less than 8 to 10 gm/dl. The significance of the anemia is its disclosure of a primary disease. Therapeutic efforts should be focused on the underlying disease rather than on the anemia. If anemia is so severe as to justify blood transfusion, additonal pathogenetic mechanisms should be sought. Coexistent iron deficiency is particularly common. Chronic gastrointestinal blood loss associated with inflammatory bowel disease or salicylate therapy given for rheumatoid arthritis regularly compounds the anemia of chronic disease. The contribution of iron deficiency is best determined by the extent to which anemia is corrected by a 6 to 8 week trial of therapeutic iron.

Aplastic Anemia

PHILIP LANZKOWSKY, M.D.,
and ROBERT FESTA, M.D.

Aplastic anemia may be acquired or constitutional.

Acquired Aplastic Anemia. The treatment of severe acquired aplastic anemia consists of bone marrow transplantation, transfusion therapy, general supportive care, hormonal therapy, and immunosuppressive therapy.

BONE MARROW TRANSPLANTATION. Approximately 40 per cent of patients with acquired aplastic anemia have histocompatible siblings with identical HLA matching and D-locus compatibility. The latter determines antigens responsible for graft rejection and graft-versus-host disease and can be tested by mixed lymphocyte culture. In patients with severe aplasia, bone marrow transplantation should be the initial treatment modality. The decision to perform bone marrow transplantation should be made early in the course of the disease, before the patient has been exposed to platelet or granulocyte antigens or has developed an infection. Early transplantation maximizes survival in severe aplastic anemia. The overall survival rate of transplanted patients is 50 to 60 per cent, which is better than the 10 to 20 per cent survival in untransplanted patients.

HLA typing should be done immediately on the patient and all siblings. It is mandatory that no family member be a donor for any blood products, since this greatly enhances the probability of rejection if a transplant is to be performed.

The two major obstacles to successful transplant and prolonged survival are (1) failure of engraftment, and (2) graft-versus-host (GVH) disease. Failure of engraftment occurs in 30 to 40 per cent of patients with aplastic anemia and in most cases is due to sensitization to minor transplantation antigens, which are inherited independently of the major HLA complex or due to prior transfusions. The immune system of the patient must be suppressed for the foreign marrow graft to be accepted. Several preparatory immunosuppressive regimens are currently in use, including high-dose intravenous cyclophosphamide, alone or combined with other agents such as procarbazine and antithymocyte globulin, with or without total body irradiation (TBI). Patients sensitized by blood transfusions require more aggressive preparation in an attempt to decrease graft rejection.

With complete engraftment, GVH disease becomes the next major problem, occurring in about 50 to 70 per cent of successfully transplanted patients. Early GVH following transplant is treated with a variety of agents, including high-dose corticosteroids, L-asparaginase,* and antithymocyte globulin (ATG).† Prophylactic treatment with methotrexate* does not prevent GVH, but cyclosporin A† may be more effective. Unfortunately, many patients who survive early acute GVH progress to a chronic GVH phase that carries a high risk of fatal interstitial pneumonia. The use of methotrexate, corticosteroids, ATG, and melphalan has not met with great success in ameliorating the chronic phase of GVH.

Finally, severe infection is the most common complication of bone marrow transplantation and ultimately accounts for the majority of deaths. During the first 30 days, when neutropenia is most severe, bacterial and fungal infections are common. Specimens for culture must be obtained during febrile episodes, and broad-spectrum antibiotics to cover both gram-positive and gram-negative organisms are indicated after appropriate cultures have been obtained. A reasonable regimen includes ticarcillin 200 mg/kg/24 hr in four divided doses and amikacin, 15 mg/kg/24 hr in three divided doses. However, different antibiotic regimens may be utilized, depending on the microbial flora and the sensitivities of the organisms at the particular institution. Systemic fungal infections present a severe problem, and, if suspected, intravenous amphotericin should be used with an initial daily dose of 0.25 mg/kg. The amount is increased daily until a dose of 1 to 1.5 mg/kg is reached. Another agent, miconazole,* may be useful for treating systemic fungal infections. The recommended dosage is 20 to 40 mg/kg in 3 divided doses. The new agent acycloguanosine is proving extremely effective in controlling varicella-zoster and herpes virus infections.

Interstitial pneumonitis is a late complication. It may occur in 60 per cent of patients and be responsible for death in 25 per cent of transplanted patients. It may be due to cytomegalovirus or *Pneumocystis carinii,* but the cause of most cases is not known. If *Pneumocystis carinii* is documented by lung biopsy, trimethoprim, 20 mg/kg/24 hr, and sulfamethoxazole, 100 mg/kg/24 hr in 4 divided doses, are used. The incidence of interstitial pneumonia is greater in patients with severe GVH disease.

TRANSFUSION THERAPY. In patients with aplastic anemia in whom bone marrow transplantation is not possible because a histocompatible donor is not available, transfusion therapy plays a major role in support.

Complete red cell typing is done on all patients to identify minor blood groups and avoid the development of red cell antibodies. Leukocyte-depleted washed red cells or frozen packed red cells should be used since they reduce the incidence of febrile reactions and sensitization. The hemoglobin level should be kept at a level—9 to 10 gm/dl—that keeps the patient free of symptoms due to anemia.

---

*This use is not listed in the manufacturer's official directive.
†Investigational drug.

*Safety and efficacy of miconazole for use in children under one year of age have not been established.

In patients in whom a drug-induced or spontaneous recovery does not occur, an outpatient program utilizing subcutaneous desferrioxamine may be used to prevent or delay the complications of transfusional hemosiderosis.

Long-term platelet support poses certain problems. Platelet transfusions are indicated for overt bleeding episodes and for preparation for surgery. Six units of platelets/m^2 will raise the platelet count approximately 50,000/mm^3. The use of prophylactic platelet transfusion to maintain platelets above 20,000/mm^3 is controversial and increases the risk of antibodies against platelet antigens. Such antibodies diminish the effectiveness of platelet transfusion, and we prefer to use platelets only if signs of bleeding develop. The risk of sensitization is reduced by using HLA-matched platelets or single-donor platelets, and this makes long-term platelet support more manageable.

Granulocyte transfusions are indicated in neutropenic patients (granulocytes <500/mm^3) with culture-proven bacterial septicemia, for those with bacterial infection localized to organs, e.g., pneumonia and cellulitis, and for those patients in whom clinical signs and symptoms point to a serious bacterial infection prior to culture results. White cell transfusions can cause fever, chills, and blood pressure changes, and the use of meperidine (Demerol), diphenhydramine (Benadryl), and acetaminophen (Tylenol) can lessen these side effects. In addition, the allosensitized patient can sequester granulocytes in organs such as the lung, resulting in major organ dysfunction. Granulocyte transfusions should be given for a minimum of 5 days if maximal effect is to be achieved and should be irradiated prior to administration.

In regard to transfusion therapy, it is of the utmost importance that family members not be used as donors as long as the possibility of bone marrow transplantation exists.

GENERAL SUPPORTIVE CARE. Infection remains the main cause of death in patients with aplastic anemia. Febrile episodes in the neutropenic patient require the use of broad-spectrum antibiotics after appropriate culture specimens are obtained. The skin should be swabbed with povidone-iodine (Betadine) prior to any blood drawing or fingerstick, to lessen the risk of iatrogenic infection. Although the use of prophylactic antibiotics is not recommended, there is increasing evidence that prophylactic trimethoprim-sulfamethoxazole may reduce the incidence of gram-negative sepsis in neutropenic patients.

HORMONAL THERAPY. In severe cases of aplastic anemia, androgens probably do not improve the extent of recovery or survival. However, in patients who lack a compatible donor, a trial of androgens is indicated. No one androgenic preparation appears to be more advantageous over another but oxymetholone is most frequently used. The initial dose is 4 to 6 mg/kg and the drug should be given for several months since responses, when they do occur, are often delayed. If a therapeutic effect is obtained, the drug is tapered to the lowest effective dose. The side effects of androgen therapy include liver dysfunction (cholestatic jaundice, hepatomegaly, peliosis hepatis), hepatocellular carcinoma, growth retardation due to premature closure of the epiphyseal plate, and virilization. In addition to androgens, prednisone in a dose of 0.5 to 1.0 mg/kg has also been employed in aplastic anemia. Corticosteroids have no role in hematologic recovery, but small doses counterbalance the growth retardant effects of androgens by delaying the closure of the epiphyseal plate. In addition, steroids may decrease the bleeding tendency in thrombocytopenic patients.

Androgens have been reported to be of benefit in patients with mild-to-moderate aplasia. However, since these patients may require little in terms of supportive care, we prefer to observe them closely rather than subject them to the side effects of virilization, growth retardation, and possible induction of hepatoma.

IMMUNOSUPPRESSIVE THERAPY. Investigations in aplastic anemia have recently centered on the concept of an immune-mediated failure of hematopoiesis in some patients. Reports by several groups have appeared describing recovery in aplastic anemia following immunosuppressive therapy with agents such as Cytoxan, antilymphocyte globulin (ALG), and antithymocyte globulin (ATG). ATG, while still considered investigational, should be recommended as primary therapy in patients who do not have a histocompatible donor.

Constitutional Aplastic Anemia. The management of these patients is similar to that of patients with acquired aplastic anemia. Evaluation of the nature of the associated congenital anomalies and their correction where possible is of great importance. developing aplastic anemia at a later date.

Although improvement in survival with drug therapy has occurred, prolonged survival has uncovered an increased risk of myeloblastic or myelomonocytic leukemia and hepatocellular carcinoma (probably secondary to androgen therapy) in these patients.

PURE RED CELL APLASIA

Pure red cell aplasia may be congenital or acquired. The distinction is important since the treatment for each is quite different.

Congenital. Patients with the congenital form, commonly known as Diamond-Blackfan syndrome, usually show anemia within the first year of life.

Treatment consists of prednisone at a daily dose of 2 mg/kg as soon as the diagnosis is established, since early initiation of therapy improves the response to steroids. In the responsive patient, evidence of bone marrow and peripheral blood improvement should occur in 1 to 3 weeks. If no response occurs, a dose of 3 mg/kg may be tried. Erythroid hyperplasia in the bone marrow, accompanied by an increased hemoglobin level and reticulocyte count, portends a favorable response. Once a satisfactory hemoglobin level has been attained ($\geq$ 10 gm/dl), the dose should be tapered to the lowest level to maintain an acceptable hemoglobin level. Alternate-day maintenance therapy is desirable since this lessens growth retardation and other steroid-related side effects. Occasionally, a rare patient may be weaned off prednisone completely.

In the patient who does not respond to steroids after 3 to 4 weeks, therapy should be tapered and discontinued and a transfusion program initiated. Another trial of steroids may be tried at a later date. A long-term transfusion program will result in transfusional hemosiderosis, and chelation with subcutaneous desferrioxamine should be instituted to delay the complications of iron overload.

The long-term prognosis for these patients is generally good, and spontaneous remission occasionally occurs as late as 10 years of age. There have been some reports of the development of leukemia in older patients.

Acquired. The most common disorders associated with acquired erythroid hypoplasia in the pediatric age group are idiopathic transitory erythroblastopenia; transitory anemia caused by infections, drugs, chemicals, and toxins; and transitory erythroid hypoplasia in hemolytic anemias.

Idiopathic transitory erythroblastopenia generally requires no therapy except for observation. The natural course of this illness is complete recovery in several weeks. The hemoglobin level should be carefully observed and transfusions used if symptoms develop or if the hemoglobin falls below 5 gm/dl. Steroid therapy is not indicated unless resolution fails to occur in a reasonable amount of time, such as 8 weeks. In such unusual cases, a trial of prednisone may be given. In contrast to the congenital form, prolonged steroid therapy is not required.

Acquired red cell aplasia secondary to drugs, toxins, and so on is treated by removal of the offending agent and supportive transfusion, if necessary, until recovery occurs.

Transitory hypoplastic crises can occur in patients with a number of hemolytic conditions—hereditary spherocytosis, sickle cell anemia, G-6-PD deficiency, and so on. Factors that lead to the development of such crises are infection and folic acid deficiency. Often such hypoplastic crises can be the presenting feature of an underlying hemolytic anemia. The aplasia is generally self-limited, with recovery beginning in 10 to 14 days. Therapeutic measures include treatment of any underlying infections and institution of folic acid and supportive transfusion, if necessary. Once recovery has occurred, an investigation for the possibility of a congenital hemolytic anemia should be undertaken.

Megaloblastic and Macrocytic Anemias

BARTON A. KAMEN, M.D., Ph.D.

Regardless of etiology, all megaloblastic and macrocytic anemias appear morphologically identical. Once the correct diagnosis of a folate or cobalamin deficiency is made, a therapeutic trial of folate or cobalamin can be initiated according to guidelines to be outlined. Since a deficiency may be secondary to a malabsorption syndrome, in addition to simple replacement therapy, treatment should be designed to ameliorate the underlying etiology (for example, a gluten-free diet in celiac disease). Another important consideration during treatment of a deficiency of folate or cobalamin is knowing that a failure of an appropriate response to oral therapy may be secondary to compliance or such a severe malabsorption syndrome that there is inadequate absorption. Therefore, a trial of parenteral treatment may be indicated. In cases of a functional deficiency of folate or cobalamin such as occur in an inborn error of metabolism or transport, only massive doses of vitamin may be helpful. These cases will only be diagnosed by appropriate biochemical tests, often on cultured fibroblasts obtained by skin biopsy. Inborn errors are rare and patients often show mental deficiency, aminoacidemia, and growth failure rather than simple cases of anemia.

A simple dietary deficiency of folate (such as "goats' milk anemia") could be treated with as little as 50 to 100 μg of folic acid daily; however, it has become standard practice to treat with 250 to 1000 μg daily to insure adequate absorption and because of the availability of commercial preparations. In cases of dietary malabsorption, as much as 5000 μg (5 mg) can be given daily to ensure adequate replenishment of folate stores. Adequate replacement will be marked by a brisk reticulocytosis within 48 to 96 hours, which peaks in 4 to 7 days. This is often preceded by a fall in serum iron as effective erythropoiesis resumes. A normal hemoglobin is achieved in 2 to 6 weeks. The duration of replacement therapy depends on the etiology of the deficiency. If a dietary deficiency is corrected, then supplemental folate treatment for as little as 4 weeks is satisfactory. In cases of malabsorption, several months' or chronic treatment may be indicated. After discontinuing therapy, followup should include checks at 4 to 6 weeks of serum folate and the morphology of both leukocytes and erythrocytes for 4 to 6 months. In cases of congenital malabsorption or inborn errors, up to 5 mg of folic acid or leucovorin (5-formyltetrahydrofolate) may be given daily to insure adequate supply.

A cobalamin deficiency secondary to a malabsorption syndrome, surgery, or pernicious anemia should be treated only with parenteral medication. Responses can be seen with as little as 25 μg daily; however, it has become standard to treat adults with 1000 μg monthly because of the body's ability to store cobalamin. An exact requirement for children has not been established. Doses of 200 to 1000 μg monthly have been satisfactory.

A deficiency of transcobalamin II (transport protein) should be treated with 1000 μg (1 mg) 2 to 3 times weekly to insure adequate cobalamin uptake. Similarly, patients with inborn errors (e.g., some cases of methylmalonic acidemia) also will benefit only from massive doses (1 to 2 mg) administered daily.

A hematologic response to adequate cobalamin therapy is generally 1 to 2 days behind a response to folate. Reticulocytosis occurs on days 3 to 4, peaks at days 6 to 8, and returns to normal at about 3 weeks.

Rarer metabolic causes of a macrocytic anemia, that is, thiamine deficiency, have occurred in products of consanguineous marriages who have presented neurologic abnormalities. The anemia was responsive to 25 mg of thiamine daily. Inborn errors of pyrimidine and purine metabolism (e.g., orotic aciduria and Lesch-Nyhan syndrome) can be treated with uridine and adenine, respectively. These conditions are unresponsive to folate and cobalamin.

In megaloblastic anemia caused by anticancer therapy, treatment with leucovorin is not indicated unless there are other stigmata of a folate deficiency, such as stomatitis or gastrointestinal disturbance.

Since megaloblastic anemias are not acute events, the need for blood transfusion, which is rarely necessary, should be based only on a symptomatic anemia (e.g., cardiac failure).

Hemolytic Anemia

JAMES A. STOCKMAN III, M.D.

Hemolytic anemias may be congenital or acquired. Such anemias are the result of some defect within the internal environment of the red cell, at the red cell membrane, or extrinsic to the red cell. Thus, the hemolytic anemias can be broadly classified in the following manner:

Intrinsic defects: red cell enzyme deficiencies (examples include the disorders of the Embden-Meyerhof pathway, principally hexokinase deficiency and pyruvate kinase deficiency, and of the pentose phosphate shunt, principally glucose-6-phosphate dehydrogenase deficiency; hemoglobinopathies (will be discussed elsewhere); and red cell membrane abnormalities, principally hereditary spherocytosis and hereditary elliptocytosis. *Extrinsic defects:* autoimmune hemolytic anemia and microangiopathic hemolytic anemia.

The major difficulties observed with the hemolytic anemias depend on the degree of anemia present and the fact that aplastic crises are potential.

Transfusion therapy is generally employed in the chronic hemolytic anemias only if the cardiac vascular status is significantly compromised by the magnitude of the anemia. Most children can tolerate levels of chronic anemia as low as 5 to 6 gm/dl of hemoglobin with relatively little difficulty. In some children, even with no evidence of cardiovascular compromise, transfusion therapy may be justified if growth retardation occurs. In either case, chronic transfusion therapy may be necessary, and the principles of management outlined in the article on the thalassemias should be followed. In many instances chronic transfusion therapy need only be employed in the first few years of life, after which splenectomy can be safely performed. Transfusion therapy may be sporadically necessary in the management of aplastic crises. Even transient suppressions of red cell production, usually initiated by infection, can result in dramatic and rapid declines in the hemoglobin level. The specific details of transfusion therapy will be discussed in each section that follows.

Splenectomy is the treatment of choice for certain of the hemolytic anemias, such as hereditary spherocytosis or drug-refractory autoimmune hemolytic anemia. Splenectomy should be delayed if at all possible until the patient is at least 4 years of age, to reduce the risk of postsplenectomy infection. Administration of the multivalent pneumococcal vaccine should precede splenectomy. The antibody response to this vaccine is limited prior to 2 years of age, so splenectomy prior to this carries an even greater risk. Prophylactic penicillin administration postsplenectomy has been advocated to diminish the postsplenectomy infection rate but is still of unproved benefit. Any child who develops a febrile illness postsplenectomy must be considered to be at high risk of having a septicemia with an encapsulated organism, such as the pneumococcus or *Hemophilus influenzae*. Such children should be examined and a cultured specimen obtained, and then treated with therapeutic doses of penicillin or ampicillin pending the culture reports.

Folic acid should be administered to all patients with chronic hemolysis since such patients have an increased nucleic acid turnover and a greater requirement for folate. Folate deficiency is usually first detected by a rise in the red cell mean corpuscular volume. Folate deficiency should be prevented by the administration of folic acid, 1 mg, given daily. Except for those forms of hemolytic anemia associated with red cell intravascular fragmentation, there is no increased requirement for iron. In fact, most children with hemolytic anemias absorb excessive dietary iron which, together with the iron deposited from transfusions, may ultimately result in hemosiderosis. For this reason, the use of medicinal iron is not only not indicated but in fact may be dangerous.

RED CELL ENZYME DEFICIENCIES

Defects of the Embden-Meyerhof Pathway—Hexokinase (HK) Deficiency and Pyruvate (PK) Deficiency. Both these disorders present with varying severities. The newborn period may be the only time of life that any specific complications may occur. The rate of hemolysis may be such that hyperbilirubinemia is of sufficient magnitude to require exchange transfusion therapy. Also, at 1 to 2 months of age, at the time of the so-called physiologic anemia that most infants experience, patients with HK and PK deficiency may have a transient, exaggerated degree of anemia, requiring a period of transfusional support. In later life, transfusional support may be occasionally necessary. As with any chronic hemolytic anemia, folic acid should be administered. At any given level of hemoglobin, subjects with PK deficiency seem to have a better exercise tolerance than do subjects with HK deficiency. This is true because the metabolic block at the PK step on the Embden-Meyerhof pathway results in an elevated red cell 2,3-diphosphoglycerate concentration, which facilitates oxygen delivery.

Splenectomy is indicated in patients with PK deficiency when transfusion dependency is present or when the degree of anemia appears to produce a functional impairment with respect to either exercise tolerance or growth. The results of splenectomy are unpredictable, unlike hereditary spherocytosis. In most cases, the anemia is significantly improved but not totally eliminated. No currently available technique predicts favorable or unfavorable responses to splenectomy. Since splenectomy is not completely ameliorative of the anemia in PK deficiency, its use should be carefully tailored to the needs of the patient. This also applies to HK deficiency. Splenectomy would be expected to abolish transfusion requirements and improve the degree of anemia.

Since the major metabolic consequence of defects of the Embden-Meyerhof pathway is diminished production of red cell adenosine triphosphate, approaches are being evaluated using agents such as inosine to circumvent the enzyme block. This is still experimental.

Defects of the Pentose Phosphate Shunt. Glucose-6-phosphate dehydrogenase (G6PD) deficiency is probably the most common inherited defect in the world. Over 100 variants are known to exist. The most common occur in people whose origins are around the Mediterranean basin (G6PD Mediterranean) and in blacks (G6PD A$^-$ variant). G6PD deficiency may be associated with sporadic or chronic hemolysis, with the latter variants constituting what are known as the chronic nonspherocytic hemolytic anemias.

In those variants of G6PD deficiency not associated with chronic hemolysis, no treatment is necessary unless a hemolytic episode occurs. Such episodes are occasioned by the ingestion of oxidant medicinals, chemicals, or food substances such as fava beans. Inhalation of vapors of oxidant agents, such as mothballs, may also result in hemolysis. Substances known to trigger hemolysis:

Antipyretics and analgesics	*Sulfones*
Acetanilide	Sulfoxone (Diasone)
Acetophenetidin	Thiazolsulfone
(phenacetin)	(Promizole)
Antipyrine*	Diaminodiphenyl
Aminopyrine*	sulfone (DDS)
Antimalarials	*Infections*
Chloroquine†	Infectious
Quinine*	mononucleosis
Primaquine	Bacterial pneumonias
Pamaquine	Viral respiratory
Quinocide	diseases
Plasmoquine	Infectious hepatitis
Sulfonamides	*Diabetic Acidosis*
Sulfacetamide	*Miscellaneous*
(Sulamyd)	Dimercaprol (BAL)
Sulfanilamide	Methylene blue
Sulfapyridine	Naphthalene
Salicyazosulfapyridine	Phenylhydrazine
(Azulfidine)	Acetylphenhydrazine
N$_2$-Acetylsulfanilamide	Probenecid (Benemid)
	Quinidine*
Nitrofurans	Fava beans*
Nitrofurantoin	Nalidixic acid
(Furadantin)	(Neg-Gram)
Furaltadone (Altafur)	Orinase
Furazolidine	p-Aminosalicylic acid
(Furoxone)	Trinitrotoluene*
Nitrofurazone (Furacin)	Neosalvarsan

*Produces hemolysis in Caucasians only.
†Produces mild hemolysis in G6PD-deficient Blacks if given in large doses.

Occasionally, for reasons not well understood, infections or severe systemic metabolic derangements may initiate hemolysis in G6PD-deficient individuals.

In subjects with the G6PD A⁻ variant (most deficient blacks), the hemolysis is self-limited and the degree of anemia only mild or moderate, rarely severe. This appears to be the result of a longer red cell enzyme half-life in the G6PD A⁻ variant, compared with the G6PD Mediterranean variant. Generally in these patients, an offending drug can be continued if necessary without further worsening the anemia. Individuals with the G6PD A⁻ variant usually do not require transfusional support at the times of hemolysis, while the Mediterranean variant can be associated with so severe an anemia as to result in death. In such instances, transfusion support is lifesaving. When transfusions must be given but the offending drug, infection, or metabolic derangement cannot be eliminated, transfused units of blood are best screened for G6PD deficiency.

G6PD deficiency occasionally causes hyperbilirubinemia in the newborn period. In some instances this results from maternal ingestion of the causative agents but it may result from their direct administration to the infant. The hyperbilirubinemia may be severe enough to require exchange transfusion.

In the G6PD deficiency variants associated with congenital nonspherocytic hemolytic anemia, a low-grade hemolysis is usually continuously present and patients are at the same risks as the others. The likelihood of neonatal jaundice is greater, as is the need for transfusion in the newborn period. Aplastic crises may occur, and folic acid administration is recommended. Splenectomy is not recommended for patients with these variants.

Studies have indicated that high-dose alpha-tocopherol (vitamin E) may reduce the degree of hemolysis that occurs in subjects with congenital nonspherocytic hemolytic anemia associated with G6PD deficiency. Vitamin E is a natural antioxidant, which may protect the red cell from damage from nondetoxified free radicals in G6PD deficiency. The dose required appears to be between 1200 and 1600 units daily.

Glutathione reductase deficiency is a relatively uncommon defect of the pentose phosphate pathway. It is generally unassociated with any significant problem and requires no treatment.

DEFECTS OF THE RED BLOOD CELL MEMBRANE

The most common inherited defects of the red cell membrane are hereditary spherocytosis (HS), hereditary elliptocytosis (HE), hereditary stomatocytosis, and hereditary pyropoikilocytosis.

Hereditary spherocytosis most probably represents more than one disorder of the red cell membrane. For this reason, the clinical expression of the disease may be variable. The anemia may be mild or severe. The management of HS involves prevention of its complications and potentially splenectomy.

Aplastic crises may occur in HS. Sometimes several family members are affected at one time. Megaloblastic anemia may occur if folic acid supplementation is not given. This is most frequently observed during pregnancy or recovery from an aplastic crisis when the folate requirement is greatest. Gallbladder disease is quite common in HS. By the age of 10 years, 5 per cent of children will have gallstones. By the second to fifth decade, this rises to 50 per cent. Complications can be prevented or improved by splenectomy.

One of the truisms of medicine is that subjects with true hereditary spherocytosis are improved by splenectomy. Whether the benefits of splenectomy justify the subsequent risk of infections in all patients remains controversial. Certainly splenectomy is justified in anyone with anemia, significant hemolysis, or a family history of gallbladder disease. Such individuals probably have a greater risk of aplastic crisis and certainly have a high probability of developing cholelithiasis and cholecystitis. Splenectomy will correct the anemia and eliminate hemolysis but does not improve the red cell morphology, which generally appears worse because of the increased numbers of circulating spherocytes. As cautioned previously, splenectomy should be deferred till age 4 to 6 years and should be preceded by the administration of the pneumococcal vaccine.

Occasionally, following an improvement postsplenectomy, hemolysis will return. This invariably indicates the presence of an accessory spleen verifiable by the loss of Howell-Jolly bodies from the red cells on peripheral smear and by splenic scan. Patients who have not had a splenectomy who have cholecystitis should probably have their spleens removed to prevent the occurrence of common duct stones. This is best done at a second operation to minimize the risk of infection at the time of the cholecystectomy.

Some neonates with HS will develop hyperbilirubinemia requiring exchange transfusion. Occasionally, transfusion therapy is necessary in the management of HS, especially in the first few months of life.

Hereditary elliptocytosis and *hereditary stomatocytosis* are generally very mild disorders requiring no treatment. In more severe cases, the complications are potentially those of HS and the management would be the same.

Hereditary pyropoikilocytosis is a rare disease presenting in infancy or childhood. It is a severe, often transfusion-dependent hemolytic anemia, characterized by extreme poikilocytosis with budding red cells, fragments, spherocytes, elliptocytes, and other bizarre poikilocytes. Heating increases the fragmentation. Splenectomy will improve but not completely cure individuals with hereditary pyropoikilocytosis.

EXTRACORPUSCULAR DEFECTS

Disorders exclusive of the red cell that may result in hemolysis include the immune hemolytic anemias and the effects of toxins, venoms, thermal injury, and mechanical injury.

Immunohemolytic Anemia. The management of immune-mediated hemolysis depends on an identification of the etiology of the immune disturbance. Immune-mediated hemolysis may be secondary to drug administration, infections, connective tissue diseases, cancers, and inherited or acquired immune deficiency states. When no cause can be found, which is the usual case in children, the disturbance is known as autoimmune hemolytic anemia (AIHA).

In drug-induced immune mediated hemolytic anemia, antibodies formed against the drugs may be IgG or IgM. Although several mechanisms of interactions between the red cell, the antibody, and the offending drug are possible, withdrawal of the drug and its in vivo catabolism usually results in termination of the hemolysis, and no further management is necessary. Occasionally, hemolysis will continue for a period even upon withdrawal of the drug. An example of this is α-methyldopa–induced hemolytic anemia. In this circumstance the management would be the same as that of autoimmune hemolytic anemia.

Infections may result in IgG- or IgM-mediated hemolytic anemia, the latter most often representing a cold agglutinin. Such antibodies are common in mycoplasma infections and are of little or no consequence. They may also occur with infectious mononucleosis and cytomegalovirus infection. If cold agglutinins are associated with hemolysis, this is usually mild and transient. Treatment should consist of providing a warm environment. Transfusions are rarely required but, if needed, the blood should be carefully warmed to 37°C using a commercially available blood warmer. The use of a water bath or warm water basin should be avoided because of the risk of inadvertent thermal hemolysis of the transfused blood.

In the immune hemolytic anemias associated with connective tissue disorders and cancers, the antibody is most frequently an IgG and the process may deposit complement on the red cell. The hemolytic anemia is best managed by aggressive treatment of the underlying disease. Steroid and immunosuppressive therapy are usually beneficial, as discussed below in reference to AIHA.

Unusual antibodies resulting in immunohemolytic anemia frequently occur in association with congenital and acquired defects of the immune system. The treatment is the same as for AIHA.

AIHA is a fairly uncommon occurrence in children. Management of this disorder, which is usually IgG-mediated, involves exclusion of any primary underlying disease. If no cause can be found, then therapy should begin.

Systemic corticosteroids are the initial agents of choice in the management of AIHA. The starting dosage of prednisone is 2 mg/kg/24 hr. Divided doses are preferable since controlled studies analyzing single dose administration have not been performed. Occasionally, patients will initially respond only to extraordinarily high doses of corticosteroids (prednisone, 6 mg/kg/24 hr). Such doses can safely be administered only for relatively brief periods.

The mechanism of action of steroids is probably multifold, involving decreased immune clearance, dissociation of antigen and antibody, and finally reduction in antibody synthesis. The first two of these actions usually result in a rapid rise in hemoglobin within just a few days. If a satisfactory rise in hemoblogin is observed, the dosage of corticosteroids can be reduced after about 2 to 4 weeks. It is wise to make all steroid adjustments slowly. For example, after 2 weeks at 2 mg/kg/24 hr, the dose may be reduced to 1 mg/kg/24 hr over the next 2 to 3 weeks. Subsequent tapers should be even more gradual. Some patients may require incredibly small doses of steroids (even below physiologic levels) to maintain a normal hemoglobin concentration. Alternate-day therapy may be attempted but, as with most hematologic disorders, controlled trials of this method of administration have not been performed. If corticosteroid therapy is ineffective in the management of AIHA or if the steroid side effects are unacceptable, other therapies should be initiated.

Immunosuppressive therapy is indicated when steroid therapy has failed. In most instances, it is begun only if in addition to steroid nonresponsiveness the patient has not improved with splenectomy. No specific immunosuppressive combinations have been shown to be most effective. Cyclophosphamide* may be begun at a daily dosage of 2 mg/kg and advanced as tolerated to 5 mg/kg, depending on its hematologic toxicity with respect to thrombocytopenia and neutropenia. The neutrophil count should be maintained above 1000 cells/μl. Cyclophosphamide requires a constant state of hydration to prevent bladder irritation. Azathioprine* is another immunosuppressive that may be utilized. Both these agents may be given in conjunction with corticosteroids. The duration of immunosuppressive therapy must be tailored to the patient's response. Other forms of immunosup-

---

*This use of these drugs is not listed by the manufacturer.

pressive therapy in the management of AIHA are experimental. There are now several reports of management of adults with immune-mediated hemolysis with chronic plasmapheresis. Its use in children is made difficult because of technical considerations.

Splenectomy should be considered in steroid-refractory patients. Since up to 70 per cent of children will respond to splenectomy, this form of therapy is usually recommended before alternative immunosuppressive therapies. There is no absolute, predictable way to determine the effectiveness of splenectomy before the procedure is performed. A careful search for accessory spleens must be made at surgery, and all the precautions previously listed must be observed.

Transfusions should be reserved unless they are truly needed, since in many instances it will not be possible to find completely compatible units. Transfusions should be begun slowly in order to observe any early transfusion reaction. Despite the greater risks than normal involved with the transfusions of blood in AIHA, the procedure can usually be accomplished successfully without untoward reactions.

Thermal Injury. Blood exposed to high temperatures, either in vivo (burns) or in vitro (blood warming), may hemolyze. This is a self-limited problem but may require appropriate transfusion support.

Mechanical Red Cell Injury. Causes of mechanical red cell injury include malfunctioning heart valves, intravascular prostheses, abnormal vasculatures (hemangiomas or areas of vasculitis), intravascular fibrin deposition (disseminated intravascular hemolysis), and crush injury or excessive marching. Treatment of mechanical red cell injury is directed at the underlying cause. Transfusion therapy is usually only of very transient benefit. If the underlying cause cannot be corrected or if the correction itself is riskier than the anemia (as in some cases of cardiac surgery), then the only management possible is prevention of iron deficiency. Chronic intravascular hemolysis results in large urinary iron losses as hemosiderin in shed tubular cells. Ferrous sulfate in a dosage of 5 mg/kg/24 hr is usually sufficient to maintain iron stores. If the iron losses are extremely rapid, periodic intravenous iron administration may be necessary.

Thalassemia

CAROL B. HYMAN, M.D.

SPECIFIC TREATMENT

No specific treatment of the thalassemias is available. Bone marrow transplantation, primarily for young infants, is being tried. However, even if the transplant procedure is successful, it must be con-

sidered investigational, as the long term risks from preparatory chemotherapy and/or radiation are not known. We do know that under present day management, most patients can expect to live to at least the third or fourth decade. Also, it can be anticipated that in the future drugs to increase hemoglobin synthesis and/or genetic engineering procedures will be effective in treating the basic abnormality.

SUPPORTIVE CARE

Transfusion Therapy. Patients who cannot maintain a hemoglobin level of approximately 7 gm/dl should be on a regular transfusion program to prevent chronic hypoxemia and suppress ineffective erythropoiesis. A transfusion program to maintain the hemoglobin level at 10.5 gm/dl or greater will enable patients to feel well and carry out most age-appropriate activities. Young adults, especially those who are active, may feel better with a pretransfusion hemoglobin level of 12 to 13 gm/dl. This transfusion program will diminish or prevent development of the bony abnormalities usually associated with the thalassemias, decrease spleen size and, to a lesser extent, improve growth and development. Dietary iron absorption is also decreased. It should be noted that once patients have become accustomed to a high hemoglobin level, symptoms may occur if the level is allowed to drop. For this reason, and because fluctuation in hemoglobin level is not physiologic, our patients are transfused at 2- to 3-week intervals. In fact, some patients require less blood on a biweekly than a triweekly schedule. Frozen red cells or washed red cells less than a week old should be used, as unwashed cells may result in febrile reactions. Neocytes, the most recently produced red cells from a unit of blood, are being used at some centers. Given with partial exchange transfusion, the intertransfusion interval can be increased and total red cell requirement decreased by as much as one third. However, these procedures are costly and wasteful of blood, since only part of each unit is used. Caution should be observed with the rate of infusion of blood or other fluids in iron loaded patients to prevent fluid overload or heart failure. The older the patient, the less tolerant he or she will be of fluctuations in blood volume. Our patients receive each unit over 3 to 4 hours and wait at least 2 to 4 hours between units. Adults may require 12 to 24 hours between units.

Splenectomy. Splenectomy should be considered for correction of hypersplenism with a red cell transfusion requirement above expected (greater than 250 ml/kg/year), for leukopenia or thrombocytopenia, and for massive splenomegaly. Prior to determining whether the procedure should be done, the degree of hypersplenism and the risks of rupture from trauma or discomfort from spleen size should be weighed against the benefits of leaving the spleen in situ. The spleen's protective effect against severe overwhelming infection, especially from pneumococcus and *Hemophilus influenzae,* are well known. The role of the spleen as an innocuous storage site for excess iron is not well understood. The author feels it may offer a greater protective effect for the heart and other organs than has been previously appreciated, and this may be enough to counteract some of the risks of the higher transfusion requirement.

If splenectomy is necessary, consideration should be given to performing a partial splenectomy. At this time, partial splenectomy is not "standard procedure" for thalassemia, as data on its effectiveness are not available. If partial or complete splenectomy is planned, Pneumovax, a vaccine that provides partial immunity to some strains of pneumococci, should be given at least 2 weeks prior to the procedure. Patients and their parents should be educated to the risks of postsplenectomy infection, and this education should be reinforced repeatedly over the following years and for the lifetime of the patient. This education is more valuable than prophylactic antibiotics. However, prophylactic penicillin, 250 mg b i d, should be prescribed and patients instructed to call WITHOUT DELAY if they develop fever of 101.5°F or above. Patients who live a distance from the medical center may be given a supply of ampicillin if they can be depended upon to call the physician and complete a course of therapy if needed.

Management of Chronic Iron Overload. Deferoxamine (DF), is the best iron chelating agent available for clinical use. Its effectiveness depends on dose, time in blood stream, total body iron, and the chelatable iron pool. DF is expensive and 20 mg/kg per day is the most cost effective dose, but higher doses increase iron excretion. DF must be given parenterally, as oral absorption is minimal. Daily intramuscular (IM) DF removes only one third of iron intake by transfusion, and subcutaneous (SQ) DF is inadequate to prevent continued iron accumulation. Therefore, we use a combined SQ-IV treatment program. SQ DF, 40 mg/kg over 8 to 10 hours, for 5 to 6 days per week is recommended. For SQ therapy, each 500 mg vial of DF is dissolved in 1.2 ml distilled water without preservative and the total volume increased to 7 ml with normal saline in a 10 ml syringe attached to a 25 G or a 27 G long tube butterfly needle. The needle is inserted in the thigh or lower abdominal wall, and the drug is administered by continuous infusion, using a mechanical pump (Auto-syringe, Farmington, Vermont). The maximum IV dose, 15 mg/kg per hour, is infused at the time of transfusion and, if possible, for as many hours as practical thereafter, as it has been found that there is greater iron excretion after than during transfusion. If this is not possible, IV pulse therapy for approximately 48 hours at regular intervals should be considered to prevent continued iron accumulation, or in older patients to lower the total body iron load. For in-

fants and young children too small to use the pump, IM DF can be used. Although there is no consensus of opinion, the author believes that chelation therapy should begin when the patient is as young as possible to prevent the chelatable iron from being transported to the heart or other parenchymal organs. With DF, iron is excreted in the urine, coloring it orange-red, and in the stool in variable amounts. Toxicity is minimal, and side effects include abdominal discomfort, mild diarrhea, itching at the injection site and, with rapid IV infusions, possible lowering of the blood pressure. Cataracts may occur but are very rare. Therefore, the patient should be seen by an ophthalmologist at 6-month intervals. To ensure the availability of chelatable iron, ascorbic acid, 50 mg, should be given after the daily dose of DF is started. Vitamin C without DF or in large doses is contraindicated, as it can increase iron toxicity, especially to the heart and, if given with meals, can increase food iron absorption.

Diet. Patients should be advised to avoid citrus and other high vitamin C containing foods with meals. Tea and cocoa are excellent mealtime beverages, as they interfere with dietary iron absorption. Vitamin E supplements are necessary to counteract the oxidant effects of iron. Infants should receive 100 units, young children 200 units, and older children and adults 400 units per day. Folic acid, 1 mg per day, should be given to all patients.

COMPLICATIONS OF THALASSEMIA AND CHRONIC IRON OVERLOAD

Cardiac. The primary cause of death in thalassemia is cardiac disorders. Congestive heart failure, arrhythmias and pericarditis should be aggressively treated, preferably by a cardiologist familiar with cardiac problems due to chronic iron overload.

Diabetes and Other Endocrine Abnormalities. These should be managed as indicated. Patients who do not go through puberty or develop secondary sex characteristics should be given replacement therapy.

Magnesium Depletion. Magnesium depletion is a frequent problem and may manifest with increased neuromuscular irritability with cardiac arrhythmias, eyelid twitching, generalized muscle aches, neck pain, and changes in affect. Hypomagnesemia must be corrected, as it may significantly increase cardiac arrhythmias from chronic iron overload. The serum magnesium level should be observed at regular intervals beginning in early childhood and, if low, oral magnesium supplements given. If oral magnesium supplements are insufficient to maintain the serum magnesium level, intravenous infusions of magnesium sulfate may be required.

THALASSEMIA INTERMEDIA

This clinical term includes those patients with beta thalassemia who can maintain a hemoglobin level of 6 to 7 gm/dl or greater without regular transfusions. Each patient should be individually evaluated to determine if transfusion therapy and/ or splenectomy is indicated, as symptoms may be severe and crippling. The long term risks of chronic hypoxemia and erythroid hyperplasia with osteoporosis, bony deformities, energy wastage, retardation of growth and development, and marked splenomegaly must be weighed against the problems associated with a chronic transfusion program. Severe hemosiderosis, from increased oral iron absorption, can be a significant problem and requires diet modification, including folic acid and vitamin E supplements as outlined above, and sometimes chelation therapy. After considering the factors discussed above, splenectomy or partial splenectomy may be necessary.

THALASSEMIA TRAIT

The diagnosis of beta thalassemia trait (thalassemia minor) is important for three reasons: 1) to differentiate it from iron deficiency anemia and avoid the chronic use of hemotinics. The exception is during pregnancy, when folic acid may prevent the hemoglobin from falling as low as would otherwise occur. 2) To reassure the affected individual that this is not a disease and will not cause illness or affect longevity. 3) For genetic counseling. Screening of family members who are potential parents should be carried out.

HEMOGLOBIN H DISEASE

This is a moderately severe form of alpha thalassemia and manifests as thalassemia intermedia, with a hemoglobin level of approximately 7 to 10 gm/dl. Symptoms are usually less severe than those of beta thalassemia intermedia, as ineffective erythropoiesis is less marked. Although these patients do not require regular transfusions, sporadic transfusions may be necessary. The red cells are susceptible to oxidant stress, so drugs such as sulfonamides, antimalarials, and high doses of salicylates should be avoided. Cholelithiasis, hypersplenism, and hemosiderosis from increased absorption of dietary iron may be problems. Splenectomy or partial splenectomy should be considered (as discussed above) for correction of severe hypersplenism. Diet modification and vitamin E supplements as outlined are advisable.

Adverse Reactions to Blood Transfusion

DENNIS GOLDFINGER, M.D.

The transfusion of blood components carries with it many potential risks. Patients may experience adverse reactions to the cellular or noncellular constituents of blood; many such reactions are im-munologically mediated. Many diseases can be transmitted from the donor to the recipient. Infection also may be transmitted to the recipient by contamination of the blood during collection or storage. The anticoagulants and preservatives, as well as the accumulated products of cellular metabolism and breakdown, can cause undesired effects. Whenever the decision is made to transfuse a blood component, the relative hazards of the transfusion should be balanced against the possible benefits to the recipient. Only when the patient is clearly in need of transfusion, and the potential value outweighs the risk, should the component be transfused.

Transfusion reactions often are totally avoidable; therefore, the key to safe transfusion therapy is prevention of reactions rather than treatment. When transfusion is necessary, the likelihood of adverse effects can be minimized by careful selection of the proper blood component. Close clinical monitoring of patients receiving transfusions can result in early detection of adverse reactions and prevention of serious complications, should such reactions ensue. By discontinuing transfusion at the onset of a reaction, thereby limiting the quantity of blood transfused, serious complications often can be avoided.

REACTIONS TO RED BLOOD CELLS

Acute Hemolytic Transfusion Reactions. Red blood cells may be transfused to treat either acute or chronic anemia and may be administered as packed, washed, or frozen red blood cells, or as whole blood. The most feared complication of such transfusion is the acute hemolytic transfusion reaction. This reaction may result when the patient possesses antibodies directed against the transfused red blood cells. Usually, the most severe reactions are caused by ABO incompatibility, although equally dangerous reactions may result from antibodies to other (minor) red blood cell antigens. The most common cause for ABO-incompatible transfusion is clerical error (i.e., the patient is given the wrong unit of blood).

Acute hemolytic transfusion reactions must be prevented rather than treated. Sophisticated serologic techniques have been developed for the detection of abnormal red blood cell antibodies that may be directed against one or more of the minor red blood cell antigens. Therefore, the danger of acute hemolytic transfusion reactions in alloimmunized recipients has been reduced significantly. Reactions due to ABO incompatibility can be avoided effectively by paying meticulous attention to positive identification of the unit of blood to be infused and the intended recipient. The process that ensures that errors in identification will not occur begins with proper collection of the pre-transfusion blood specimen for typing and cross-matching, extends to careful handling of the patient blood sample and units of blood in the blood bank, and ends with positive identification of the patient and the unit of donor blood prior to the start of transfusion.

If a patient receives incompatible red blood cells and develops an acute hemolytic transfusion reaction, two significant complications may ensue—acute renal failure and disseminated intravascular coagulation (DIC). Appropriately, treatment is directed toward preventing these complications. The most important therapeutic consideration is to minimize the volume of incompatible red blood cells transfused. Therefore, as soon as a transfusion reaction is suspected, the infusion of red blood cells should be stopped. Usually, if only a small volume of red blood cells has been transfused, specific therapy will be unnecessary (the designation of a "small" volume of red blood cells depends on the size of the recipient, but might be defined as an amount less than 5 to 10 per cent of the patient's blood volume). Additional red blood cell transfusion should be avoided until the cause for the hemolytic reaction has been identified and compatible blood can be provided safely.

Patients who receive relatively large volumes of incompatible red blood cells may develop hypotension, shock, and DIC. These complications, in turn, may lead to acute renal failure. It is now clear that renal failure is not caused by the action of hemoglobin on the kidney. Free hemoglobin is neither directly toxic to renal tubular epithelium nor does it precipitate in the tubules, causing blockage of urine excretion. Instead, renal failure, if it occurs, appears to be due to ischemic damage to the tubules, resulting from decreased renal cortical blood flow. The widely held belief, therefore, that prevention of acute renal failure can be achieved by the use of diuretics to "flush out" the kidneys makes little sense. Instead, treatment should be aimed at restoration of normal blood circulation. Blood pressure should be maintained by the infusion of fluids (either colloids or crystalloids) and by the use of appropriate drugs. Those drugs that help restore systemic blood pressure, as well as improve renal cortical blood flow, probably are most useful. Dopamine would seem to be the most logical pharmacologic agent for achieving these objectives. However, this drug has not been used extensively in the specific treatment of acute hemolytic transfusion reactions, so its value cannot be stated with certainty.

The development of DIC is a significant risk for patients who receive large quantities of incompatible red blood cells. Early institution of anticoagulation with heparin might be of benefit in preventing this complication and should be considered on an individual basis (the potential benefits of heparinization must be weighed against the possible risks). While "prophylactic" heparinization has never been evaluated as a treatment modality in patients suffering acute hemolytic transfusion reactions, it is a logical therapeutic intervention for preventing the often fatal complication of DIC, provided that it is instituted before significant activation of the clotting system has occurred. If prophylactic heparinization is deemed appropriate, fully anticoagulating doses should be used, unless relative contraindications exist. In this case, minidoses must suffice. Anticoagulation probably need be maintained only so long as the stimulus for DIC exists (perhaps 6 to 24 hours). This short course of therapy also serves to minimize the likelihood of hemorrhagic complications from heparin.

Delayed Hemolytic Transfusion Reactions. Patients receiving transfusions may become alloimmunized to red blood cell antigens. Months or years later, the concentrations of these antibodies present in the patient's plasma may decline to such low levels that they are undetectable by routine pretransfusion tests. If, under these circumstances, the patient again is transfused with red blood cells that possess an antigen to which sensitization has occurred previously, the patient may develop an anamnestic response, generating large quantities of antibody within approximately 1 to 5 days after transfusion. This may result in a delayed hemolytic transfusion reaction, with rapid destruction of the transfused red blood cells. The patient's hematocrit may fall and jaundice may develop. Although renal failure may be precipitated by a delayed hemolytic transfusion reaction, this is an extremely rare occurrence. Therefore, specific therapy usually is not indicated for patients suffering such reactions. Instead, the most important factors are to recognize that a delayed hemolytic transfusion reaction has occurred and to avoid transfusion of additional incompatible red blood cells. As soon as the identity of the offending antibody can be determined, it usually will be possible to provide safe, compatible blood for further transfusion.

REACTIONS TO LEUKOCYTES OR PLATELETS

Febrile, Nonhemolytic Transfusion Reactions. Fever and chills are the most frequent adverse effects encountered in recipients of blood transfusions. While such signs and symptoms may result from the transfusion of incompatible red blood cells, their most common cause is from a reaction to transfused leukocytes. If fever or chills develop, the transfusion should be stopped immediately and an investigation begun to determine whether a hemolytic transfusion reaction has occurred. If there is no evidence of a hemolytic reaction, it can be assumed that fever has resulted from a reaction to leukocytes. No specific therapy is indicated for the fever, although antipyretics (e.g., acetaminophen) may be administered.

Patients who have suffered febrile, nonhemolytic transfusion reactions usually can be transfused safely with leukocyte-poor red blood cells. Further transfusion, therefore, should be accomplished with either buffy coat–poor, saline-washed, or frozen red blood cells—all of which are leukocyte-poor.

Alloimmunization to Leukocyte and Platelet Antigens. Transfusions of whole blood or packed red blood cells expose the recipient to large numbers of leukocytes and platelets. This could result in alloimmunization to leukocyte and platelet antigens. If it is desirable to prevent such sensitization, because of possible compromise of future granulocyte or platelet transfusions or because the patient may be a candidate for an organ transplant, red blood cell transfusions may be accomplished with leukocyte-poor blood components. Such products are less likely to sensitize the patient, owing to their reduced content of leukocytes and platelets.

Graft-Versus-Host Disease. Many blood components contain significant numbers of viable lymphocytes. If such immunocompetent lymphocytes are transfused to immunodeficient patients, the cells may survive, replicate, and initiate a reaction to the foreign tissues of the recipient. This could result in the syndrome of graft-versus-host disease, a complication that is frequently fatal. Treatment of this reaction may be ineffective, so prevention is most important. Severely immunoincompetent patients may be transfused safely with irradiated blood products. The administration of 1500 to 3000 rads of radiation to lymphocyte-containing blood components (whole blood, red blood cells, platelet concentrates, granulocyte concentrates) renders the lymphocytes incapable of replication and prevents graft-versus-host disease.

Post-Traumatic Pulmonary Insufficiency. During the storage of units of blood, large numbers of microaggregates form, consisting of degenerated leukocytes and platelets and possibly fibrin. These particles may be small enough to pass through the standard 170-micron filter used for blood administration. Therefore, large amounts of particulate debris, ranging in size from approximately 20 to 150 microns, may be transfused to the patient. Since the first capillary bed encountered by the blood following intravenous infusion is in the lungs, the microaggregates become trapped at that point. It has been suggested that occlusion of the pulmonary microcirculation by transfused particulate debris may contribute to the development of post-traumatic pulmonary insufficiency, or "shock-lung." The possible dangers of microaggregates in stored blood are greatest for patients receiving massive transfusion. Avoidance of infusion of microaggregates to patients receiving large amounts of blood can be achieved by transfusion of relatively fresh blood (less than 7 days old), by the use of special microaggregate filters, or by washing stored blood prior to transfusion. Saline-washed red blood cells have an additional advantage for patients receiving massive transfusion, in that the undesirable products of red blood cell metabolism, which accumulate in stored blood, also are eliminated during the washing procedure (see below).

REACTIONS TO SUBSTANCES CONTAINED IN PLASMA

Urticarial Transfusion Reactions. The development of hives during or shortly after transfusion is the second most frequently encountered transfusion reaction. These reactions are not dangerous and need not be investigated as possible hemolytic reactions, unless other signs and symptoms suggestive of possible hemolytic reaction (e.g., chills or fever) also occur. Urticarial transfusion reactions can be treated with antihistamines (e.g., diphenhydramine [Benadryl]). Patients who have experienced repeated urticarial transfusion reactions should be treated with an antihistamine 30 minutes prior to transfusions or should receive washed or frozen red blood cells that are nearly devoid of plasma.

Anaphylactic Transfusion Reactions. Patients who are totally deficient in immunoglobulin A (IgA) proteins may develop severe anaphylactic reactions to transfusions of blood components containing IgA. These reactions can be prevented by transfusing washed or frozen red blood cells that are devoid of most plasma (and devoid of IgA proteins). If transfusions of platelet concentrates or fresh frozen plasma are required, these components must be collected from IgA-deficient blood donors. Registries of IgA-deficient blood donors are maintained by the American Red Cross and by several other blood banking institutions.

If a patient should develop an anaphylactic transfusion reaction, treatment should be similar to that used for other forms of anaphylaxis. Treatment is aimed at combating respiratory distress and circulatory collapse. Epinephrine probably is the most useful drug to be used in this situation, as it is in other forms of anaphylactic shock.

Circulatory Overload. Patients who receive too much blood too quickly may develop acute volume overload. This can be an extremely severe, possibly lethal, complication that could result in acute pulmonary edema or sudden death. In the case of red blood cell transfusion, circulatory overload is entirely preventable by following two simple rules: nonbleeding, anemic patients should be transfused with packed red blood cells rather than whole blood; and they should receive no more than two units of packed red blood cells daily. Even severely anemic patients who are not bleeding seldom require immediate elevation of their hemoglobin concentration by more than 2 to 3 gm/dl.

The only time that volume overload should be risked is in the management of patients with coagulation factor deficiencies. For those deficiencies in which concentrates of the required coagulation factor are not available, it is necessary to administer the missing factor by transfusions of fresh frozen plasma. Relatively large amounts of fresh frozen plasma may be required, in order to raise the concentration of a particular coagulation factor to hemostatic levels. Under these circumstances, diuretics can be administered in an effort to reduce circulatory overload. Patients who show signs of cardiac failure from excessive transfusion should be treated in the same manner used to treat heart failure from other causes (e.g., diuretics, morphine, phlebotomy, and so on).

Transfusion of Antibodies to Red Blood Cells. Patients who receive plasma containing antibodies that react with their own red blood cells may develop hemolytic transfusion reactions. The most common cause for these reactions is the administration of ABO-incompatible plasma. This could result from transfusion of ABO-incompatible platelet concentrates (since each unit of platelets contain approximately 50 ml of plasma). The patient may develop a positive direct Coombs test and evidence of mild hemolysis. Very rarely does a more severe, acute hemolytic transfusion reaction occur. This complication should be prevented by avoiding transfusion of excessive quantities of ABO-incompatible plasma.

Citrate Toxicity. Patients who receive large quantities of blood components may develop signs and symptoms of hypocalcemia, resulting from the infusion of citrate anticoagulant. This is rarely a significant problem, except for patients receiving massive amounts of blood (as in the case of exchange transfusion). To prevent or combat this complication, such patients may be given supplemental calcium solutions intravenously. However, care must be taken not to give too much calcium, because iatrogenic hypercalcemia probably is a greater hazard than citrate-induced hypocalcemia.

Transfusion of Blood Cell Metabolites. During storage of blood components, there may be accumulation of large quantities of lactic acid and ammonia from the metabolic activity of the various cellular constituents. In addition, significant amounts of potassium may leach out of the blood cells, resulting in concentrations of potassium as high as 75 mEq/l in the supernatant plasma. Complications from the infusion of these substances are likely to be a problem only in patients receiving massive transfusions or exchange transfusions. The risk of complications from these substances can be avoided best by transfusing relatively fresh blood products (less than 7 days old) to patients receiving massive transfusions. If relatively fresh blood is unavailable, saline-washed red blood cells may be substituted for packed red blood cells, since the washing procedure rids the red blood cells of unwanted contaminants.

INFECTIOUS COMPLICATIONS

Post-transfusion Hepatitis. Hepatitis remains the most frequent serious complication of blood transfusion. Current estimates suggest that as many as 20 per cent of transfused patients acquire hepatitis, and many such patients develop severe, chronic liver disease. The only means available for preventing post-transfusion hepatitis is by avoiding transfusions wherever possible. In addition, products prepared from pooled plasma (e.g., lyophilized Factor VIII and Factor IX concentrates) should be avoided, if single donor blood components can be substituted safely. Frozen or saline-washed red blood cells may have a reduced risk of transmitting hepatitis compared with packed red blood cells, although proof of their relative safety is lacking. Finally, it has been suggested that administration of immune serum globulin to recipients of transfusions may prevent some cases of hepatitis, but studies of the efficacy of such prophylaxis are inconclusive, and routine administration of immune serum globulin to transfusion recipients currently is not recommended.

Cytomegalovirus Infection. There is increasing evidence that cytomegalovirus infection may be transmitted by blood transfusion. The risk appears to be greatest for relatively immunodeficient patients, especially neonates. Prevention may be possible by selecting blood from donors with low levels of anticytomegalovirus antibodies (such donors are less likely to be cytomegalovirus carriers), or by transfusing leukocyte-poor blood components (since the cytomegalovirus appears to be carried in peripheral blood leukocytes). Leukocyte-poor red blood cells may be supplied most efficiently by transfusing saline-washed red blood cells, since this product also may avoid many of the other hazards of red blood cell transfusion therapy.

Malaria. Transfusion-transmitted malaria is a known hazard of red blood cell transfusion, although its occurrence is extremely uncommon. Prevention is by excluding blood donors who are likely to be carriers of malarial parasites. Consideration of the rare complication of transfusion-transmitted malaria should be given to transfused patients who subsequently develop unexplained fever.

Transfusion of Contaminated Blood. Transfusion of blood that has been contaminated in vitro with bacteria can result in an extremely severe reaction, manifested by chills, fever and circulatory collapse. The risk of blood contamination has been reduced to minimal levels by the development of blood collection systems which utilize sterile, disposable plastic bags. In the event that heavily contaminated blood is transfused, the patient will develop severe septic shock, and this must be treated with circulatory support and antibiotics.

Autologous Blood. One final consideration in the prevention of transfusion reaction is the use of autologous blood for transfusion. The technique of autologous blood transfusion is most valuable for patients scheduled for elective surgical procedures. Patients may donate blood prior to surgery, and the blood can be stored either in the liquid or frozen state for subsequent reinfusion during surgery or postoperatively. Even relatively small children can donate blood safely, simply by removing a small volume of blood (e.g., one-half pint instead of a full pint) at each donation. These small volume collections can be pooled into volumes of approximately one pint and stored in the frozen state until the time of surgery. Autologous transfusion eliminates almost all of the hazards of blood transfusion therapy, especially the risk of post-transfusion hepatitis.

Sickle Cell Disease

ROLAND B. SCOTT, M.D.

Rational therapy of this disease is based upon recognition that the syndrome consists of a number of clinical hemoglobinopathies of variable occurrence and morbidity. The most frequently encountered types in the United States are homozygous sickle cell disease (sickle cell anemia), sickle cell-hemoglobin C disease, and the sickle cell-beta-thalassemia syndromes. The course of the disease is usually characterized by periods of remission (steady state) and exacerbation (crises). The approach to treatment is generally based upon the nature of the crises and the presence of complications.

PERIOD OF REMISSION

Anemia is usually not present at birth; however, it characteristically appears 4 to 6 months postnatally and is variably persistent for the remainder of life. In the absence of infections and complications, patients tend to compensate reasonably well for the anemia during the steady state, and blood transfusions are not necessary when the patient is active and comfortable. In the periods between crises, one should determine and record the patient's physical and hematologic status. This is also a good time to perform elective surgical and dental procedures. Folic acid, 1.0 mg daily, is recommended to supply the need created by the hyperplasia and increased activity of the bone marrow in this disease.

Neonatal detection of sickle cell disease by hemoglobin electrophoresis on cord blood samples taken in the delivery room now offers an opportunity to place sickle cell infants under parental and medical supervision and surveillance for the pre-

vention and early detection of life threatening infections such as sepsis, pneumonia, and meningitis. Inasmuch as *Streptococcus pneumoniae* is a common and virulent offender, some clinicians now employ a preventive regimen of prophylactic penicillin administered orally daily or intramuscularly at monthly intervals during infancy. Pneumococcal vaccine (Pneumovac, Merck, Sharpe and Dohme, or PnuImmune, Lederle) is recommended for infants and children at ages 1–2 years or older.

ACUTE CRISES

Vaso-occlusive or Pain Crisis. Vaso-occlusive crises are the most frequently observed. They vary considerably in frequency, duration, and degree of intensity. Analgesics and adequate hydration are the two most dependable agents for control of acute pain. Mild forms with bearable pain and lassitude can often be treated in the home with bed rest and water or other fluids orally (20 ml per kg of body weight per 24 hours) divided into 4 or more portions. Acetaminophen (Tempra or Tylenol) is recommended in single doses of 60 mg for infants under one year and for other ages the following: children 1–4 yrs, 60 to 120 mg; 4–8 yrs, 120 to 240 mg; 8–12 yrs, 240 mg.

If persistent pain is not relieved by the above drugs, then codeine phosphate alone or combined with Empirin or Tylenol may be used. The dose of codeine for children 12 years and younger is about 3 mg/kg/24 hours, divided into six doses. The elixir of Tylenol with codeine (12 mg codeine phosphate per teaspoonful) is convenient for small children. In patients 12 years or older, the following agents will often relieve moderate to severe pain associated with vaso-occlusive crises:

Codeine phosphate, 15–30 mg, often prescribed orally in such compounds as Tylenol or Empirin.

Meperidine, usually administered intramuscularly in doses of 30 to 70 mg every 3 or 4 hours. The main adverse effect is respiratory depression. This drug should be used with caution because long term administration can be associated with drug/psychic dependence.

Papaverine hydrochloride,*usually given orally (tablets) in dosage of 30 to 60 mg three to five times daily for local pain associated with vascular spasm.

Pentazocine hydrochloride (Talwin),**oral dose: 25–50 mg repeated in 3 or 4 hours; intramuscular: 15–30 mg every 3 or 4 hours.

Talwin compound—supplied in caplets, each containing pentazocine hydrochloride 12.5 mg equivalent and aspirin 325 mg. Dose for older

---

*The safety and efficacy of papaverine in children have not been established.

**The safety and efficacy of pentazocine in children under 12 years of age have not been established.

child is 1 caplet three or four times daily.

Morphine sulfate—reserved for treatment of severe pain. Administer subcutaneously or intramuscularly in single dose of 0.1–0.2 mg/kg and repeat every 3 to 5 hours until pain is controlled.

Indomethacin (Indocin) has been useful for short-term (2 weeks or less) administration in adolescents when pain is combined with local tenderness and swelling of soft tissues, especially in joints and extremities, in dosages of 1 mg/kg body wt orally every 6 to 8 hours. (This drug has not been officially approved for use in persons under 14 years of age).

For pain of moderate to severe intensity in children, codeine is often effective and perhaps should be the drug of first choice, as it has a long duration of action (4–5 hours), oral medication is effective in pain control, and the hazard of dependency is less common than for the other narcotics in common use. Morphine is a more effective analgesic and sedative; however, it must be given parenterally to achieve maximum efficacy and repeated use has a higher addiction risk; therefore, its use in children should be reserved for control of severe painful episodes. Meperidine has a relatively short duration of action (2 to 4 hours) and patients who frequently receive this agent often exhibit physical drug dependency. Also, seizures have been reported after its administration. Adjuvant agents such as hydroxyzine and phenergan are popular with the staff of many hospitals; however, their value as potentiators of narcotic analgesics is questionable, but they may have some value as sedatives. Vaso-occlusive crises in children usually last 4 to 14 days with a mean of about 5 or 6 days followed by an asymptomatic steady state of variable duration.

Occasionally, when analgesics and parenterally administered fluids cannot control severe pain in hospitalized patients, partial exchange blood transfusions may bring relief by reducing the mass of sickled cells in the circulation. The goal of this method is to reduce the Hb S-containing cells to less than 45%. Once this objective has been achieved, small transfusions of packed red blood cells can be administered every 3 to 4 weeks to keep the Hb S less than 45% in patients when vaso-occlusive crises are refractory to conservative medical management. The chief hazards of prolonged or frequently repeated blood transfusions are alloimmunization, hepatitis, and iron overload. Supplemental oxygen is recommended for hypoxic patients with low PO_2.

Painful crises in children are often associated with anorexia, febrile illness, and other conditions that contribute to dehydration; hence parenteral administration of fluid is important. I recommend 5% dextrose in ¼ strength saline infused at the rate of 2000 to 2500 ml/M^2 per day. Sodium bicarbon-

ate should be reserved for patients with documented acidosis. Intravenous fluids should be carefully monitored to avoid overloading the circulatory system in these children, who often exhibit cardiomegaly associated with varying degrees of anemia. Children should be encouraged to take fluids orally when feasible. Conditions that have frequently been associated with the onset of pain crises should be avoided. In children and adolescents, infections, dehydration, physical exertion, emotional stress, trauma, exposure to chilling, and inclement weather have been identified as precipitating agents.

Children with sickle cell disease may also exhibit pain associated with hand-foot syndrome, joint effusions (arthropathy), osteomyelitis, ankle ulcers, acute chest syndrome, gallbladder disease, biliary tract obstruction, hepatic infarcts, priapism, avascular necrosis of bone especially involving the femur or humerus, cardiovascular manifestation, musculoskeletal crises, and abdominal distention with transient adynamic ileus. Appropriate therapeutic measures should be individualized for the particular patient.

HEMATOLOGIC CRISES

The aplastic crisis is the most frequently observed hematologic crisis in the United States. The transient depression of hematopoiesis is often associated with acute infections, particularly of the viral type. The degree of anemia is variable and on occasion is sufficiently severe to warrant a transfusion of packed red blood cells. Recovery is usually prompt and is heralded by a significant increase in the reticulocyte count.

The so-called hyperhemolytic crisis is uncommon in my experience and is associated with an increase in bilirubin and a reticulocytosis. It can be confused with G6PD deficiency in a patient with sickle cell anemia, especially during a febrile illness when antipyretic agents are being administered. Transfusion of packed red blood cells is indicated for significant anemia (Hb < 5 gm).

Megaloblastic crisis may occur in sickle cell disease due to folic acid deficiency. This type is more frequently observed in African inhabitants, especially during pregnancy. It can be prevented by folic acid prophylaxis but if the anemia is severe, blood transfusion should be administered, with due care to avoid cardiopulmonary overload.

The sequestration crisis involving the collection of large pools of blood in viscera, especially the spleen, can be life threatening. This crisis is most commonly observed during infancy and early childhood. Sudden death may occur from hypovolemic shock. Treatment is by administration of whole blood and saline solution to restore circulatory volume; however, overloading of the cardiopulmonary circulation is to be avoided. Splenectomy may be necessary in selected cases to prevent repetitive crises. This type of crisis should not confused, however, with splenomegaly due to chronic and long-standing splenic infarction.

INFECTIONS

Many sickle cell anemia patients exhibit an immunodeficiency that makes them particularly susceptible to a number of infectious agents. Infants and young children are quite vulnerable, particularly to *Streptococcus pneumoniae* and *Haemophilus influenzae,* which are frequently identified with sepsis, bacteremia, meningitis, and pneumonia. In view of the occurrence of sudden death in patients with sickle cell anemia due to these two pathogens, initial therapy for suspected septicemia in children should be ampicillin. When ampicillin resistant *H. influenzae* infection is encountered, chloramphenicol or an antibiotic such as cefamandole may be a suitable alternative. *Salmonella* and *Staphylococcus aureus* can cause osteomyelitis in these patients, which requires both vigorous antibiotic therapy and orthopedic consultation. Pneumonia caused by mycoplasma often presents a protracted course with delayed resolution. Erythromycin is recommended. In general antibiotic therapy should be given parenterally without delay at the onset of febrile illness, particularly in children with homozygous sickle cell disease.

TRANSFUSION THERAPY

Blood transfusions are of value in treating certain complications of sickle cell disease. However the risk/benefit ratio should be carefully evaluated whenever the decision is made to use this therapy. The common risks are iron overload, hepatitis, alloimmunization, and the induction of hyperviscosity. Currently transfusions are used to prepare patients with sickle cell disease for anesthesia and surgery. For elective surgery, packed erythrocytes in dosage of 10 ml per kg body weight can be given to maintain the hemoglobin at 12 gm/dl. It may be advantageous to space the transfusions over several days prior to surgery. When simple transfusions are employed in preparing patients for elective surgery it is important to keep the hematocrit below 35% in order to avoid hyperviscosity. Partial exchange transfusion is recommended for major operations and emergency surgery in order to provide a hematocrit of 30 to 35% and sickle hemoglobin less than 25%. Following transfusion, the preoperative administration of intravenous fluids prevents dehydration due to an increase in blood viscosity. Following surgery, oxygen should be administered until the effects of anesthesia and sedatives have abated.

Partial exchange transfusions have been used in some medical centers for a variety of clinical conditions including the following: 1) prevention of recurrence of cerebrovascular accidents; 2) prevention of crises and complications in pregnancy; 3) prevention of severe and frequently recurring vaso-occlusive crises; 4) treatment of chronic nonhealing leg ulcers; 5) treatment of protracted priapism. Usually an attempt is made to keep the level of sickle hemoglobin below 40 to 50%. Once a patient has been brought to an acceptable level of hematocrit and percentage of sickle hemoglobin, maintenance at these levels can be achieved by simple transfusions of packed erythrocytes given every 3 to 4 weeks. This will suppress the patient's own erythropoiesis. Chronic transfusion regimens predispose patients to iron overload and hemochromatosis, which may warrant the use of chelation therapy. Selective transfusion with young erythrocytes (neocytes), which theoretically have a longer life span than do regular donor red cells, could decrease transfusion frequency and hopefully reduce iron deposits in patients who require chronic transfusion therapy. However, the use of expensive cell separators is required for this procedure.

The frequent use of blood transfusions for the management of patients with sickle cell disease is resulting in an increasing incidence of alloimmunization reactions. This has been attributed in part to the Caucasian origin of much of the donor blood, which results in sickle cell anemia patients becoming isoimmunized to blood antigens such as the Duffy system, which is largely absent in people of African descent. Other offending blood group antibodies include the Rh, Kell, and Kidd systems. Some patients with sickle cell disease have become isoimmunized to so many antigens or to such common blood groups that transfusion becomes almost impossible. Therefore, complete genotyping before transfusion has been suggested for patients who will be on a transfusion program for long periods of time, because the typing will be difficult to obtain if they prove to be immunologic responders later. An alternative management plan to prevent transfusion reactions is the use of autologous blood for transfusion. For example, patients who are scheduled for elective surgery may donate blood prior to the surgical operation for cryopreservation and storage for subsequent reinfusion during or after surgery. This eliminates most of the hazards of blood transfusion including isoimmunization and hepatitis.

Polycythemia

SHELLY C. BERNSTEIN, M.D., Ph.D.,
and DAVID G. NATHAN, M.D.

During the first week of life, hemoglobin values above 22.0 gm/dl or hematocrit values of more than 65% should be considered evidence of polycythemia. In childhood and adolescence, hemoglobin values above 17.0 gm/dl or hematocrit values of more than 50% are significant. The diagnosis should be verified by venipuncture; capillary blood samples should not be used. Hemoconcentration due to dehydration must be excluded as a cause.

NEONATAL POLYCYTHEMIA

Polycythemia in the neonate may be due to twin-to-twin transfusion, maternal-fetal transfusion, delayed cord clamping, placental insufficiency, congenital adrenal hyperplasia, maternal diabetes mellitus, Down's syndrome, or Beckwith's syndrome. The signs and symptoms may consist of lethargy, plethora, cyanosis, jaundice, respiratory distress, congestive heart failure, seizures, priapism, thrombocytopenia, renal vein thrombosis, necrotizing enterocolitis, hypoglycemia, and hypocalcemia. Many infants with polycythemia are, however, asymptomatic. Prophylactic treatment is not recommended. However, all infants with polycythemia should be monitored carefully, and at the first sign of symptoms, treatment should be instituted. Treatment should be designed to reduce the venous hematocrit value to approximately 60%, accomplished by partial exchange transfusion, using fresh frozen plasma to reduce the hematocrit value while maintaining the blood volume. The volume of exchange may be estimated from the following formula:

Volume of exchange (ml) =

$$\frac{\text{Blood volume} \times (\text{Observed Hct} - \text{Desired Hct})}{\text{Observed Hct}}$$

The infant's blood should be removed in volumes of 10 ml for full-term (and smaller volumes for low-birth weight) infants and replaced with an equal volume of fresh frozen plasma. A blood volume of 80 ml/kg may be estimated for newborn infants. The procedure is usually performed through an umbilical venous line. Simple phlebotomy should not be performed unless the infant is hypervolemic.

CHILDHOOD POLYCYTHEMIA

Primary Polycythemia. POLYCYTHEMIA VERA. This disorder consists of an increase in red cell mass of unknown etiology, often accompanied by thrombocytosis, and is rarely seen in childhood. The Polycythemia Vera Study Group recommends phlebotomy for patients under the age of 40 years. Erythropheresis with isovolemic exchange of fresh frozen plasma or Ringer's lactate, rather than simple phlebotomy, should be performed to maintain the hematocrit between 40 and 45%. Patients with complications (such as symptomatic splenomegaly, vascular obstruction, or symptoms associated with hypermetabolism) or with extreme thrombocytosis (platelet counts greater than $1.0 \times 10^{12}1/1$) should be treated with myelosuppressive agents. Hydroxyurea* at a dose of 30 mg/kg, orally, in three divided doses per day is given until the platelet count falls to $1.0 \times 10^{11}/1$. At that time, busulfan at a dose of 0.12 mg/kg (maximum dose of 6 mg) orally per day for 7 days is given. This dose may be repeated for another 7 days if significant myelosuppression does not occur. Periodic pulses of busulfan may be required to control thrombocytosis and may need to be performed on a regular basis. Repeated erythropheresis will lead to iron deficiency, causing an increase in whole blood viscosity related to decreased erythrocyte deformability, as well as thrombocytosis. Therefore, iron deficiency should be avoided by oral iron supplementation.

BENIGN FAMILIAL POLYCYTHEMIA. This term is used to describe familial cases with increased red cell mass that are otherwise normal, with no other recognizable etiology. Therapy is not required unless the patient is symptomatic due to hyperviscosity. Erythropheresis or phlebotomy may then afford symptomatic relief.

Secondary Polycythemia. These conditions refer to an increase in red cell mass secondary to a recognizable cause and may result from tissue hypoxia, leading to a compensatory response of erythropoietin, or from increased production of erythropoietin despite normal tissue oxygenation.

CYANOTIC CONGENITAL HEART DISEASE. Children with cyanotic congenital heart disease with a right-to-left shunt develop polycythemia in response to chronic systemic arterial desaturation. Symptoms are headaches, irritability, anorexia, and dyspnea. In addition, polycythemia, when accompanied by iron deficiency, may be associated with an increased incidence of intravascular thrombosis and a consumptive coagulopathy. Arterial saturation should be surgically corrected, if possible. If the patient is symptomatic, reduction of hematocrit values should be attempted cautiously by partial exchange transfusion or erythropheresis. Since acute phlebotomy in these patients may result in vascular collapse, cyanotic spells, cerebrovascular accidents, or seizures, sudden hemodynamic alterations should be avoided. Erythropheresis should be performed, removing aliquots of blood (5 ml for infants and 30 ml for older children) and infusing equal volumes of fresh frozen plasma, estimating the total exchange volume from the above formula. The hematocrit should be reduced to 60 to 65% over 30 to 60 minutes. Strict adherence to critical blood volume maintenance must be made. Because of the complications associated with iron deficiency and polycythemia, iron deficiency should always be corrected. These measures have led to reduced

---

*Dosage not established for children in manufacturer's directive. This use of hydroxyurea is not listed by the manufacturer.

coagulation abnormalities, decreased operative mortality, and symptomatic improvement in polycythemic patients with cyanotic congenital heart disease.

ABNORMAL HEMOGLOBINS. A number of hemoglobin variants have been described with a marked increase in oxygen affinity and compensatory polycythemia via increased production of erythropoietin. Other than erythrocytosis, affected individuals have minimal clinical manifestations, with the exception of one reported family with Hb Malmö, the children of which were reported to have cardiovascular symptoms. Hematocrit values rarely are high enough to necessitate treatment.

Congenital methemoglobinemia due to NADH-diaphorase I deficiency and acquired methemoglobinemia due to the exposure to various agents capable of oxidizing heme iron to the ferric state may produce cyanosis and polycythemia. Treatment of methemoglobinemia, regardless of the etiology, is dictated by the severity of the hypoxia. Most patients with hereditary disease require no therapy. Severe methemoglobinemia can be treated initially by methylene blue in a dose of 1 to 2 mg/kg administered intravenously as a 1% solution. Further treatment is accomplished with daily oral doses of methylene blue, 1 to 2 mg/kg.

INAPPROPRIATE ERYTHROCYTOSIS. Polycythemia has been associated with a number of tumors in which erythropoietin secretion is elevated, such as Wilms' tumor, hepatoma, cerebellar hemangioblastoma, and benign lesions of the kidney such as cysts and hydronephrosis. Endocrine disorders such as pheochromocytomas, aldosterone-producing adenomas, Cushing's syndrome, as well as exogenous administration of testosterone or growth hormone may also cause increased red cell mass. Correction of the underlying condition results in elimination of the polycythemia.

Leukopenia, Neutropenia, and Agranulocytosis

A. KIM RITCHEY, M.D.

The total leukocyte count is the sum of five specific types of leukocytes: neutrophils, monocytes, eosinophils, basophils, and lymphocytes. Leukopenia is defined as a total leukocyte count of less than 4000/mm³ in the white population and 3000/mm³ in the black population. The lower counts in blacks are due to an absolute reduction of neutrophils. Leukopenia is most commonly associated with infectious illnesses, is usually mild, and is managed by treating the underlying infection.

We will discuss the management of the patient with the abnormally low neutrophil count, or neu-

tropenia. Agranulocytosis has come to mean a severe degree of neutropenia, although in the strictest sense it is a deficiency of all granulocytes, including eosinophils and basophils. Neutropenia in the white population is defined as a neutrophil count of less than 1500/mm³. The same criteria cannot be used in black people, however, since studies have demonstrated a lower mean neutrophil count in healthy black adults and children. Therefore, neutropenia in black people may be defined as a neutrophil count of less than 1000/mm³. However, in a study of healthy black children between ages 1 and 5 years the range of normal neutrophil counts included values as low as 388/mm³. In all infants between the ages of 2 weeks and 6 months the lower limit of normal is 1000 neutrophils/mm³.

There are three situations in which neutropenia may be seen in clinical practice: 1) in infectious illness, 2) in blood dyscrasia, malignancy, or the treatment thereof, and 3) as an isolated finding without apparent cause. Infections are the most common cause in children, with viral infections being most frequent. The neutropenia is usually mild to moderate and resolves within a week or two. Management is directed at treatment of this underlying infection. Neutropenia in blood dyscrasia and malignancy is frequently severe, prolonged, and associated with high morbidity and mortality. Finally, isolated neutropenia without apparent cause frequently is a diagnostic and therapeutic dilemma and will be considered next.

Isolated neutropenia can be discovered at any time of life, although it is uncommon. It is often accompanied by a compensatory monocytosis, but red cells and platelets are normal. Neutropenias have been divided into those due to decreased production, those due to increased destruction, or a combination of the two. Productive neutropenias include those due to drugs (mainly cytotoxic agents, but also the semisynthetic penicillins), Kostman's infantile genetic agranulocytosis, Schwachman's syndrome of pancreatic insufficiency and bone marrow dysfunction, cyclic neutropenia, copper deficiency, and anorexia nervosa. Destructive neutropenias include isoimmune neutropenia, neutropenia with immunoglobulin deficiency, autoimmune neutropenia, hypersplenism, and neutropenia secondary to drugs. In some familial forms of neutropenia and in the chronic benign form the pathogenesis is not well delineated.

The work-up of a patient with isolated neutropenia depends somewhat on the presenting age and clinical features. It is most important to perform at least weekly, and preferably twice weekly, CBC's for 6 to 8 weeks. These will confirm the neutropenia and establish the pattern as cyclic or chronic. Documentation of neutrophil counts at the time of infection is helpful in prognosticating the risk of infection. A bone marrow aspiration should be performed to rule out the rare occult malignancy and to document the myeloid status of the marrow. The hydrocortisone and epinephrine stimulation tests are used to assess the marrow reserve and marginating pool of neutrophils, respectively. These tests, although of interest, are generally not helpful in classification or management. Immunologic evaluation should include antineutrophil antibodies, quantitative immunoglobulins, ANA, C_3, C_4, and possibly T & B cell studies. Miscellaneous studies include those for exocrine pancreatic function, liver function tests, serum copper, vitamin B_{12}, folates, and urine metabolic screen.

Since isolated neutropenia is associated with a markedly variable risk of infectious complications, management is individualized. For example, the patient with chronic benign neutropenia usually has little difficulty with infections, while Kostman's infantile genetic agranulocytosis is lethal. Only careful observation will differentiate the low-risk from the high-risk patient, classification notwithstanding. In general, the neutropenic patient is able to lead a normal life under the watchful eye of parents and physician. Promptly diagnosed infections will usually respond to routine antibiotic therapy, especially if the neutrophil count is known to rise in response to infection. A trial of prophylactic antibiotics (such as trimethoprim-sulfamethoxazole) is indicated in patients with frequent episodes of bacterial infection. An obviously ill or hyperpyrexic child should be handled in the same manner as the neutropenic patient with cancer (see below).

A few patients with isolated neutropenia may benefit from specific treatment. The patient known to be taking a drug associated with neutropenia should have therapy stopped or an alternative nontoxic drug substituted if possible. Corticosteroids increase the neutrophil count in 50% of patients with autoimmune neutropenia. A trial of prednisone (1–2 mg/kg/day) for 2 to 3 weeks is indicated in patients with neutrophil autoantibodies, but its long-term use must be weighed against the risks of steroid toxicity. Corticosteroids have not been helpful in other patients with neutropenia and their use may increase the risk of infection. Splenectomy is not of sufficient benefit to warrant the risk of postsplenectomy sepsis. Finally, Kostman's infantile genetic granulocytosis is highly lethal and appears to be due to a defective myeloid stem cell. A recent report of bone marrow transplantation with resolution of the neutropenia in a patient with this disorder warrants serious consideration of this potentially life-saving procedure.

The risk of serious infection is highest in neutropenic patients with blood dyscrasias, such as aplastic anemia, or patients undergoing myelosuppressive chemotherapy or radiation therapy for cancer. The degree of risk is directly related to the absolute neutrophil count. With a neutrophil count between 1500 and 1000/mm^3 there is no increased risk, between 1000 and 500/mm^3 the risk increases slightly, but below 500/mm^3 the risk rises exponentially. A febrile patient with a neutrophil count of less than 100/mm^3 has a greater than 70% chance of being infected. If the period of neutropenia is prolonged, the risk of infection increases and treatment is less likely to be successful. The immunosuppression that accompanies most cancer chemotherapy renders these patients susceptible to opportunistic infections with fungi, viruses, and protozoa, especially *Pneumocystis carinii*.

Neutropenia per se is not an indication for hospitalization. Indeed, home management of the afebrile patient is preferred in order to decrease exposure to hospital organisms. Since Hughes et al.* initially demonstrated the efficacy of chronic trimethoprim-sulfamethoxazole in preventing *Pneumocystis carinii* pneumonia, numerous reports have indicated the added benefit of decreased bacterial infections in neutropenic patients taking this drug. Trimethoprim (5 mg/kg/day)-sulfamethoxazole (25 mg/kg/day) in two divided doses should be administered on a chronic basis to all cancer patients at high risk of infection. (Ironically, a potentially significant side effect of this drug is neutropenia.) Another aspect of home management includes avoiding obviously infected individuals. Although every attempt should be made to advocate a normal life-style for these patients, including attending school, restrictions on group activities may be necessary, especially during periods of severe neutropenia. Parents should be taught to take oral or axillary temperatures, since rectal temperatures may seed the blood stream with fecal flora. Finally, parents should be told to notify their physicians of all temperatures greater than 101°F (38.5°C). The febrile neutropenic patient should *not* be managed at home.

A febrile patient with a granulocyte count of less than 1000/mm^3 needs to be evaluated and treated. A thorough physical exam usually will not help to identify a source of infection due to a poor inflammatory response secondary to the neutropenia. Nonetheless, careful attention should be directed to all potential infection sites, remembering to inspect and palpate for tenderness in the perianal region. Bacterial and fungal cultures of blood (at two different times), oropharynx, urine, perianal region (not rectal), and any suspicious skin lesions are routine. Lumbar puncture with CSF examination and bacterial and fungal cultures is mandatory in any patient with central nervous system (CNS) or

---

*Hughes, W. T., Kuhn, S., Chaudhary, S. et al.: Successful chemophophyloxis for *Pneumocystis carinii* pneumonitis. N. Engl. J. Med. 297:1419,1977.

meningeal symptoms or signs, but is not performed on all febrile neutropenic patients, since the incidence of CNS infection is surprisingly low.

Empiric antibiotics are essential in the febrile patient and should be started immediately after cultures have been obtained. The bacteria most frequently isolated in neutropenic cancer patients are *Staphylococcus aureus, Escherichia coli, Pseudomonas aeruginosa,* and *Klebsiella pneumoniae.* The relative distribution and antibiotic sensitivity of these organisms will vary between institutions and must be kept in mind when selecting antibiotics. Intravenous antibiotic therapy should include an aminoglycoside (gentamicin, tobramycin, or amikacin) and an anti-*Pseudomonas* penicillin (carbenicillin or ticarcillin). Some institutions add a cephalosporin or a penicillinase-resistant penicillin, especially if aminoglycoside resistance of *S. aureus* is a problem.

If an infection is identified, either by culture or subsequent physical findings, specific therapy for that infection should be instituted. Although treatment will depend on the organism and site, as a general rule a bactericidal antibiotic should be part of the regimen, since bacteriostatic drugs alone are inadequate in neutropenic patients. The "routine" duration of therapy may have to be extended if granulocytopenia persists.

In the neutropenic cancer patient with pneumonia additional drug treatment is necessary, because of the risk of other treatable opportunistic infections. Besides the bacterial pathogens, treatment for *Pneumocystis carinii* and *Legionella pneumophila* must be considered. The infiltrate pattern may be of help since *P. carinii* is the most likely cause of interstitial pneumonia, though it has been associated with focal pneumonias. As such, trimethoprim-sulfamethoxazole (20 mg/kg/day as trimethoprim in 4 divided doses) either orally or intravenously is begun along with the empiric antibiotics noted above in neutropenic patients with pneumonia. If the disease progresses within 3 days open lung biopsy should be done to rule out trimethoprim-sulfamethoxazole-resistant *P. carinii, L. pneumophila,* fungi, and viruses.

The duration of empiric antibiotic therapy has not been well defined for the patient without a specific focus of infection. In general, the patient who becomes afebrile, who develops no sign of localized infection, whose cultures remain negative, and whose granulocytopenia has resolved may have his antibiotics discontinued after 3 to 4 days. A similar patient whose granulocytopenia persists in the severe range should probably have antibiotics continued for at least 7 days, although there is some evidence that treatment should continue until the granulocyte count is greater than 500/mm³. The patient who remains febrile and neutropenic for 7 days should be scrutinized for occult infection, and empiric antifungal therapy should be considered.

Granulocyte transfusions are indicated in patients with documented gram-negative septicemia not responding to antibiotic therapy after 24 to 48 hours, since this patient subgroup has a clear improvement in survival with this therapy. The initial course consists of daily granulocytes for 4 days, after which the need for granulocytes is reassessed, based on the patient's clinical status, surveillance cultures, and persistence of neutropenia. Non-septicemic, febrile patients given granulocytes have not shown a clear-cut survival advantage over comparable patients not receiving granulocytes. Also, although prophylactic granulocytes were associated with a decreased number of infections in bone marrow transplant recipients, no difference in survival compared to those not receiving granulocytes was noted. Therefore, granulocyte transfusions should not be routinely used other than in patients with septicemia not responding to antibiotics.

Finally, general measures for the care of the hospitalized patient with neutropenia include the following. Laminar airflow rooms decrease the incidence of infection in the compromised host and should be utilized whenever possible. In hospitals not equipped with such a specialized environment, the patient should be in a private room, and handwashing should be strictly enforced for anyone entering the room. Gowns, gloves, and masks are of no further benefit. Obviously infected individuals should not be allowed in the patient's room. Instrumentation should be avoided and prior to venipunctures and fingersticks the skin should be carefully cleansed with betadine and alcohol. Only butterfly needles should be used for intravenous therapy, and the IV site should be changed every 3 days.

Hemorrhagic Disorders

GERALD S. GILCHRIST, M.B., B.Ch.

PLASMA COAGULATION FACTOR DEFICIENCIES

Inherited Disorders

General Principles of Management. The hemophilias and other inherited disorders of blood coagulation are characterized by an inherited inability to produce one of the plasma factors needed for normal hemostasis or by the inheritance of an abnormal molecule with reduced procoagulant activity. The tendency to "spontaneous" bleeding into joints and muscles, particularly in those with severe deficiencies (< 1% of normal), produces serious physical, economic, and psychosocial problems. Thus the treatment of patients with hemophilia requires a multidisciplinary team approach of which only one component is the replacement of the missing factor by transfusion of material harvested from normal human plasma. The replacement therapy itself can produce serious complications, such as hepatitis, and contribute to the development of circulating inhibitors to the missing factor and to development of immune-complex disease related to the repeated infusion of plasma proteins from large pools of blood donors. Repeated exposure to blood products may also contribute to susceptibility to acquired immune deficiency syndrome (AIDS).

Even patients with mild to moderately severe hemophilia can encounter musculoskeletal hemorrhage and are sometimes more seriously affected by many of the psychosocial complications that result from restrictions placed on a young child's participation in peer-related activities, particularly contact sports.

The interdisciplinary approach to the management of patients with hemophilia and other inherited disorders of blood coagulation has resulted in the designation of Comprehensive Hemophilia Diagnostic and Treatment Centers at institutions around the United States and in Canada. These have the resources and expertise to provide a complete range of services to the affected patient and the family. In larger metropolitan areas, patients may receive their primary and ongoing care at the Centers, but in rural and less densely populated areas, it is essential that primary care physicians outside the Center participate actively in the development and execution of appropriate management programs designed to meet individual needs. We recommend periodic in depth evaluations at a Center to monitor the appropriateness of the replacement therapy program, to detect significant complications of the disease or its treatment, and to ensure that the patient is given every opportunity to participate appropriately in the mainstream of society. At these sessions, patients are evaluated by a pediatric hematologist, orthopedic surgeon, specialist in physical medicine, dental surgeon, geneticist, and social service consultant. The plasma is screened for an inhibitor and for evidence of liver and kidney disease.

After this multidisciplinary evaluation, the program for the upcoming year is reviewed with the patient, and, if necessary, appropriate modifications are made. This includes a replacement therapy plan, exercise programs to maintain or restore joint function, and communication with primary physicians, schools, employers, and appropriate community, regional, and state agencies. Plans are also developed for surgical or medical consultation or treatment of other problems identified during the evaluation. More frequent evaluations may be necessary. Between visits to the Center patients are expected to submit monthly reports documenting the site and frequency of bleeds and the nature and response to replacement therapy. This is of particular importance for patients on home treatment programs. These records are reviewed by the Center personnel and appropriate contacts made with the patient, family, and primary physician regarding any recommended changes in treatment. This type of contact is greatly facilitated by hemophilia nurse specialists and social workers experienced in dealing with hemophilia patients and their problems.

Participation in most normal peer-group activities should be encouraged, and this often requires contacting school personnel to emphasize this. From both a physical and psychologic viewpoint, we prefer to have children participate in routine physical education programs to the extent they are able. Contact sports should be avoided. As an alternative, we recommend early entry in a competitive swimming program, for swimming provides an excellent physical and psychologic outlet for the patient. Attempting to isolate or overprotect the hemophiliac from all types of potentially dangerous activity can produce psychologic problems that ultimately may prove more devastating than the physical crippling. The physician has the ultimate responsibility of advising appropriate restrictions for individual patients, taking all these factors into consideration.

Replacement Therapy. The prevention and treatment of hemorrhage and musculoskeletal deformities rank high in the list of priorities for the patient with hemophilia. At present, material for replacement therapy must be extracted from normal human plasma, although animal products have been developed and used with some success, particularly in Europe. However, the problem of species differences and the rapid development of antibodies to these animal products have limited their usefulness.

Ideally, providing adequate levels of the missing factor on a continuing basis would allow the hemophilia patient to live a completely normal life. Unfortunately, the shortage of human plasma, the short half-life of the missing factors, and the cost and various complications of treatment preclude the routine prophylactic use of replacement therapy. Therefore, treatment for most patients must be directed at controlling hemorrhage rather than attempting to prevent it.

Factor VIII and Factor IX, the two factors most commonly lacking in inherited disorders, can be concentrated into relatively small volumes, and this helps to overcome the volume limitation that precludes the use of whole human plasma to produce hemostatic levels of the missing factor. As an example, 1 ml of average normal fresh frozen plasma contains approximately 0.7 unit of Factor VIII coagulant activity, and, in order to elevate the circulating level by 50 per cent in a 10-kg child, one

Table 1. PRODUCTS FOR COAGULATION FACTOR REPLACEMENT

Product	Fibrinogen	II, VII, X	VIII:C*	VIIIR:VWF†	IX	XI	V	VIII	XIII
Fresh-frozen plasma	+	+	+	+	+	+	+	+	+
Cryoprecipitate	+	0	+	+	0	0	0	0	0
Factor VIII concentrates	0 or ±	0	+	0	0	0	0	0	0
Prothrombin complex concentrates	0	+	± ‡	0	+	0	0	0	0

* Factor VIII coagulant activity.
† Ristocetin-Willebrand factor activity.
‡ Contain small amounts of Factor VIII, which can result in stimulation of inhibitor production.

would have to infuse approximately 350 ml of fresh frozen plasma. If cryoprecipitate or one of the commercially produced concentrates is used, the same amount of Factor VIII can be infused in as little as 10 to 30 ml, depending on the potency of the particular concentrate.

Cryoprecipitate and fresh frozen plasma are extracted from single donor units of blood in most blood banks, but the more potent lyophilized concentrates are made from pools of plasma obtained from hundreds or even thousands of donors. The use of material from large pools increases the risk of hepatitis and, possibly, other complications in the recipient, so their *routine* use in all factor-deficient patients cannot be recommended. This applies particularly to the mildly affected patient in whom one might anticipate a relatively low life-time exposure to blood and blood products. As with all forms of therapy, the clinician must carefully weigh the potential risk of a particular blood product against its potential benefits. Although one might prefer to use a single donor product to treat minor hemorrhagic episodes, this approach would fail in the face of an intracranial bleed in a patient with Factor IX deficiency for whom no single donor concentrates are available and in whom the volumes of fresh frozen plasma needed to control hemorrhage would seriously overload the cardiovascular system.

In developing a rational replacement therapy program, one must have a knowledge of the potency of the various therapeutic products available for replacement therapy, an awareness of the levels of the missing factor needed for hemostasis in the particular clinical situation, and the approximate infusion half-life of the missing factor.

Table 1 lists the various products available for the treatment of coagulation deficiencies. In the United States, five pharmaceutical companies produce Factor VIII concentrates, and there are two commercially produced prothrombin complex concentrates. The potency of the concentrates varies considerably, but each vial has the number of units of activity listed on the product label. Table 2 lists the equivalent volumes of products containing Factor VIII or Factor IX that contain 100 Factor VIII or Factor IX units, respectively. Table 3 lists the approximate half-disappearance times of various coagulation factors following infusion. The decay patterns are complex, but for practical purposes these figures reflect the approximate time for the initial peak levels to decrease by 50 per cent.

The in vivo recovery of the missing factor depends on its molecular weight and whether or not it is evenly distributed within the intra- and ex-

Table 2. EQUIVALENT VOLUME CONTAINING 100 u* OF ACTIVITY

Product (ml)	Factor	
	II, VII, IX, X	VIII
Reference plasma	100	100
Fresh-frozen plasma	125	140
Cryoprecipitate†	—	15–25
Factor VIII concentrate	—	2–5
Prothrombin complex concentrate	4	—

*u is defined as the amount of coagulant activity present in 1 ml of plasma having 100 per cent activity.
†The factor VIII content of individual bags is variable. The average bag of cryoprecipitate contains 100 Factor VIII units with a range of 50–200 u.

Table 3. APPROXIMATE BIOLOGIC HALF-LIFE OF COAGULATION FACTORS AFTER INFUSION

VII	4–6 hours	XI	48 hours
VIII	12 hours	Fibrinogen	72 hours
V	20 hours	II	72 hours
IX	24 hours	XIII	10+ days
X	36 hours		

travascular spaces. For example, after infusion of a given quantity of Factor VIII, almost all of it is measurable in the circulation, and approximately 1 unit of factor VIII/kg of body weight will elevate the in vivo factor VIII level by approximately 2%. On the other hand, when compared with factor VIII, factor IX is a smaller molecule, and, since it is distributed extravascularly, will only produce 25 to 50% of the increment after infusion. These figures are approximations but are of practical value in day-to-day patient management.

FACTOR VIII DEFICIENCY (HEMOPHILIA A, CLASSIC HEMOPHILIA). One Factor VIII unit/kg will elevate the plasma level by 2 per cent. To achieve a 50 per cent level in a 20-kg child, 500 VIII units are given by rapid infusion. This would require approximately five bags of cryoprecipitate, ± 700 ml of plasma or 10 to 20 ml of concentrate. After ± 12 hours the level will have dropped to 25%, and, in order to maintain levels above 25% over a period of time, infusions will have to be repeated every 12 hours using a dose calculated to produce a 25% increment in plasma VIII level. The potency, in vivo recovery, and half-disappearance time are quite variable so that levels of VIII may have to be monitored by specific assay. This is not usually necessary in the treatment of isolated joint or muscle hemorrhage but is critical in the management of intracranial hemorrhage or in patients undergoing major surgery. This information allows the dose to be adjusted when it is essential that minimum plasma levels be maintained.

FACTOR IX DEFICIENCY (HEMOPHILIA B, CHRISTMAS DISEASE). The in vivo recovery of Factor IX is lower than that of Factor VIII. One Factor IX unit/kg elevates the circulating plasma level by only about 1%. Thus, in order to achieve a peak postinfusion increment of 50%, 50 u/kg would have to be administered. A 20-kg child would require 1000 to 1200 ml if fresh frozen plasma is used. Concentrates contain ± 500 IX units in 20 ml so that the 1000 units of activity can be administered in a volume of 40 ml. Because of the longer biologic half-life of Factor IX, the infusions can be given less frequently. However, it should be appreciated that the first phase of Factor IX disappearance is rapid, and if high hemostatic levels are needed over a prolonged period of time the frequency of infusions may approach that used in Factor VIII replacement. In potentially life-threatening situations or to cover surgical procedures, laboratory monitoring of plasma factor levels is critical.

Although we have the impression that lower levels of Factor IX may be adequate to produce hemostasis in various clinical situations, we use the same general guidelines as are used for Factor VIII-deficient patients. This means that most severely affected hemophilia B patients will have to be treated routinely using concentrates. With milder deficiencies we attempt to control minor bleeding with fresh frozen plasma, but major trauma or surgery usually necessitates the use of concentrates, with their increased attendant risk of hepatitis transmission.

VON WILLEBRAND DISEASE (VWD). VWD is characterized by a deficiency of a plasma factor that is necessary for the promotion of normal platelet adhesiveness and the synthesis of Factor VIII coagulant activity. Both sexes are equally affected. Bleeding tends to be mucosal and cutaneous, although hemarthroses can occur in patients with extremely low Factor VIII levels. Epistaxis is common in childhood and is often aggravated by local lesions in the nose and, during the winter months, by reduced humidity. Thrombin-soaked nasal packs and cauterization are sometimes needed and may require replacement therapy coverage. Menorrhagia can be severe but can usually be controlled with cyclic oral contraceptive therapy.

Infusion of normal (and even hemophilic) plasma stimulates exaggerated in vivo production of coagulant Factor VIII activity, which may be sustained at hemostatic levels for 72 hours or longer. The secondary rise in circulating Factor VIII occurs over a 10- to 24-hour period. Thus, to prepare a patient for elective surgery an infusion of plasma (10 to 15 ml/kg) or cryoprecipitate (1 bag/10 kg) is given 8 to 24 hours earlier. In an emergency, enough cryoprecipitate should be given to produce an immediate rise in Factor VIII coagulant activity to 50%. This will provide adequate coverage during the period of in vivo synthesis. The decision to provide further therapy is determined by monitoring the plasma Factor VIII level. We aim to maintain the circulating Factor VIII above 50% for 10 days after a major operation.

The bleeding time is often shortened 2 to 4 hours after infusion, but rarely to normal levels. In our experience, hemostasis has been satisfactory in spite of failure to correct the bleeding time or in vitro platelet adhesiveness.

FACTOR XI DEFICENCY (HEMOPHILIA C, PTA DEFICIENCY.) Very little Factor XI enters the extravascular space so that one can apply the same dosage calculations as for Factor VIII. No concentrates are available, but satisfactory hemostasis can be maintained because the biologic half-life is from 40 to 48 hours. A series of three plasma transfusions in a dose of 10 ml/kg every 6 to 8 hours will produce a peak rise in Factor XI of about 50%, and levels above 25% can be maintained easily with daily transfusions of 10 ml/kg or less. In an emergency, partial exchange transfusion may be necessary if circulatory overload is a concern.

FACTOR XII DEFICIENCY (HAGEMAN DISEASE.) Deficiency of Factor XII is not associated with abnormal hemostasis. No particular precautions or replacement therapy is needed in spite of the markedly prolonged in vitro coagulation times.

FACTOR XIII DEFICIENCY. Deficiency of fibrin-stabilizing factor is easily treated. A single monthly infusion of 2 to 3 ml of plasma/kg is sufficient to maintain normal hemostasis and correct the abnormal in vitro clot solubility. To reduce exposure to plasma from multiple donors, a single, healthy compatible donor can be identified for periodic plasmapheresis, since most patients will require 250 ml of plasma or less every 4 weeks.

CONGENITAL AFIBRINOGENEMIA, HYPOFIBRINOGENEMIA, AND DYSFIBRINOGENEMIA. Normal hemostasis requires plasma levels of 60 to 80 mg/dl and can be readily achieved with single donor cryoprecipitate, which contains about 250 mg per bag. After infusion, fibrinogen enters the extravascular space. Two to four bags of cryoprecipitate per 10 kg body weight will elevate plasma fibrinogen by 50 to 100 mg/dl. This can be administered over an 8- to 12-hour period to minimize volume overload, depending on the volume of cryoprecipitate in each bag. Adequate circulating levels can be maintained by daily infusion of 0.6 to 1 bag of cryoprecipitate per 10 kg body weight.

DEFICIENCIES OF FACTORS II, VII, OR X. These rare inherited disorders do not respond to vitamin K therapy. Their in vivo recovery is similar to that of Factor IX although their biologic half-lives vary. The same principles for the use of plasma or prothrombin complex concentrates apply. A rare condition, characterized by congenital deficiency of all the vitamin K-dependent clotting factors, is partly corrected by oral vitamin K, suggesting that there is a defect in vitamin K metabolism.

FACTOR V DEFICIENCY. Factor V is extremely labile, and only fresh or fresh-frozen plasma should be used for replacement therapy. The in vivo recovery and biologic half-life are similar to those of Factor IX, and the same general principles apply. Factor V is not a vitamin K-dependent factor and is not present in cryoprecipitate or other concentrates.

Special Treatment Situations. MUSCULOSKELETAL HEMORRHAGE. We stress prompt recognition and treatment of hemarthrosis or intramuscular bleeds, particularly those involving the gastrocnemius muscle or if nerve compression is suspected. All patients or parents should be made aware of the early signs and symptoms of hemarthrosis and the need for early treatment, which should be made readily available on an outpatient basis if the patient is not on a home treatment program. If treatment is given in an emergency room, clinic, or doctor's office, an outline of the patient's treatment program should be kept on file as an ongoing prescription for replacement therapy. Physician evaluation is not necessary for patients who are known to the facility and have demonstrated a working knowledge of hemophilia and its treatment. Naturally, if the well-informed patient or parent requests it, intervention by a physician is certainly indicated.

A smooth-flowing system is essential to the success of an outpatient treatment program. Traditionally, when the need for replacement therapy had to be evaluated with each bleed, treatment was inevitably delayed because the average physician in an emergency room is usually less well-informed about hemophilia than the patient.

Our procedure is to have the patient's treatment program on record in the emergency room, blood bank, or any other treatment facility, but, in addition, we advise the patient to carry a copy of the program at all times. At the earliest sign of bleeding into an area that would require replacement therapy, a phone call is made to the treatment facility with a request that the appropriate number of vials or bags of material be prepared for infusion at the time the patient anticipates arriving there. Occasionally, less responsible patients fail to keep these appointments, to the chagrin of the hospital personnel, but this is a rare occurrence in our experience and should alert one to re-evaluate whether that particular patient's treatment program is appropriate. Table 4 lists the principles for outpatient or home therapy for the treatment of musculoskeletal bleeding. Joint aspiration is rarely indicated and then only to relieve pressure symptoms in a markedly swollen joint.

Table 4. GUIDELINES FOR REPLACEMENT THERAPY OF JOINT OR MUSCLE HEMORRHAGE

Treat at *earliest* sign of hemarthrosis or intramuscular bleed.

Increase Factor VIII or IX level to 40 to 60 percent of normal.*

Repeat dose at 24 hours if no response.

Physician evaluation if still symptomatic at 40 hours.

Maintain mobility unless pain or swelling is severe.

*It is often possible to produce hemostasis with lower levels if the treatment is instituted very early.

Specific factor assays are not needed to monitor treatment unless the clincal response is considered unsatisfactory. If assay is indicated and the increment in factor level is not consistent with the dose infused, the possibility of an inhibitor or some deterioration in the potency of the infusion material has to be considered.

The presence of synovitis with hypervascular friable synovium should be suspected in patients who have repeated bleeds into a single joint with documented satisfactory increments in plasma procoagulant levels. The inflamed synovium sets the stage for recurrent hemorrhage. In order to break this vicious cycle we initially prescribe short 4 to 5 day courses of prednisone (40 mg/m²/day in three divided doses) to be administered in conjunction with replacement therapy. If this fails to have the desired effect after 6 to 8 weeks of observation, a longer course of prednisone (3 to 4 weeks) is considered. Alternatively, a prophylactic infusion program aimed at maintaining factor VIII or IX levels above 5% can be effective in this situation. In selected instances, synovectomy should be considered in a joint that is the site of recurrent hemorrhage with synovial thickening but before radiographic evidence of hemophilic arthropathy has developed. In older patients, joint replacement has successfully eliminated painful, crippling deformities in weight-bearing joints.

DENTAL MANAGEMENT. Preventive dental care should be part of the hemophiliac's overall treatment plan. Most routine dental procedures can often be performed without replacement therapy, particularly if regional anesthesia is avoided. We advise local infiltration of the affected tooth if local anesthesia is needed. Loss of deciduous teeth is not usually associated with significant bleeding, but, if persistent, oozing can usually be controlled with thrombin-soaked gauze. Extraction of permanent teeth requires appropriate replacement therapy, with the aim of achieving a 50% level of the missing factor immediately prior to the procedure. Epsilon-aminocaproic acid (EACA, Amicar) is given orally or intravenously to inhibit fibrinolytic activity in the oral cavity. This prevents the fibrin clot in the tooth socket from dissolving. Clot formation is also enhanced by packing the socket with thrombin-soaked oxidized cellulose.* The dose of EACA is 100 mg/kg body weight every 6 hours, and treatment is continued for 7 to 10 days. It is most easily administered as a 25 per cent syrup, which contains 1.25 grams in each 5 ml, but is also available in tablet form. The drug should not be used in the presence of hematuria or if there is evidence of active intravascular coagulation. With a single infusion of replacement therapy and adequate consolidation of the clot, no further replacement therapy is usually necessary unless the clot is dislodged from the tooth socket.

EPISTAXIS AND INTRAORAL HEMORRHAGE. Epistaxis is more common in patients with VWD than in those with hemophilia. Packing with thrombin-soaked oxidized cellulose (see Dental Management, just discussed) is helpful if other local measures fail. Replacement therapy may be necessary, particularly if the oozing is generalized without an identifiable bleeding point to cauterize.

The toddler with hemophilia tends to have problems with intraoral bleeding as a result of trauma to the tongue, lips, frenum, or oral mucosa. Because

it is impossible to "immobilize" these areas, the clot is easily dislodged, leading to recurrent bleeding and the need for repeated doses of replacement therapy. This series of events can be modified by prompt replacement therapy aimed at elevating factor levels to 50%, local application of thrombin-soaked oxidized cellulose, and oral EACA as recommended for dental procedures.

PAIN CONTROL. One of the goals of early control of bleeding is to reduce the need for analgesia. Particularly in older patients with established hemophilic arthropathy, drug abuse and addiction can be serious problems. In addition, aspirin and aspirin-containing drugs should not be used because of their action on platelet function and their ability to aggravate the pre-existing hemostatic defect. A list of aspirin-containing drugs is available from the National Hemophilia Foundation. Although other nonsteroidal anti-inflammatory drugs such as ibuprofen (Motrin) or indomethacin affect platelet function, the effect is rapidly reversed when treatment is discontinued. In contrast, the effect of aspirin persists for the life span of the exposed platelet. Thus nonsteroidal anti-inflammatory drugs deserve a trial in patients with symptoms suggestive of arthritis in joints which have been the site of recurrent hemorrhage in the past. Recently we have begun using nonacetylated salicylates (Trilisate [choline magnesium trisalicylate] or Disalcid [salicylsalicylic acid], 500–1000 mg b i d), which do not affect platelet function but do have an anti-inflammatory effect. Although their effects on platelet function are less well defined, phenylbutazone, phenothiazides, and phenacetin should be avoided in patients with bleeding disorders.

HEMATURIA. Hematuria is often unresponsive to replacement therapy in spite of hemostatic blood levels being attained. Bed rest for 24 to 48 hours seems to be advantageous in some patients. Prednisone, 40 to 60 mg/m^2/24 hr in divided doses, usually causes the hematuria to subside in 48 hours, after which time the dose should be tapered and stopped over the next 3 days. EACA is contraindicated in the management of hematuria and can produce thrombosis in the urinary tract under these circumstances.

INHIBITORS. Approximately 10% of severely affected hemophiliacs develop inhibitors that are capable of neutralizing infused Factor VIII or Factor IX. Some patients have low titers of inhibitor and do not have an anamnestic rise in inhibitor level after an infusion. These inhibitors can often be overcome by treating with larger and more frequent doses of the missing factor. In patients with more potent inhibitors, a number of therapeutic approaches have been tried. Some investigators have recommended withholding replacement therapy, hoping that the inhibitor titer will drop, but in our experience this rarely happens and usu-

---

*Oxycel or Surgicel saturated with a solution of powdered thrombin dissolved in 0.5% sodium bicarbonate.

ally leads to increasing disability resulting from untreated musculoskeletal hemorrhages. Various trials of immunosuppressive therapy have not met with success in hemophiliacs with inhibitors. In life-threatening situations, exchange transfusion utilizing the continuous-flow centrifuge has been effective in replacing the patient's inhibitor-containing plasma with normal plasma. The beneficial effect is temporary since the antigenic stimulus invariably produces an anamnestic antibody response and even higher levels of inhibitor within 5 to 7 days.

The most recent approach to producing hemostasis in Factor VIII-deficient patients with high inhibitor levels ($\geq$ 5 Bethesda units) utilizes "activated prothrombin complex concentrates" that bypass the need for Factor VIII in the hemostatic "cascade." Both of the commercially produced concentrates in the United States—Konyne (Cutter) and Proplex (Hyland)—have produced satisfactory hemostasis in doses of 25 to 50 Factor IX units/kg body weight. Recently, however, the degree of activation has been much more variable from one production lot to another, and therapeutic effect is less predictable. Autoplex (Hyland), an activated prothrombin complex concentrate specifically developed for the purpose of treating patients with inhibitors, is now available. A dose of 50 "Factor VIII correctional" units/kg has been found to control hemarthrosis. Up to 100 u/kg every 6 to 24 hours may be needed to control more serious hemorrhage. Unfortunately, no satisfactory laboratory test has proved useful in monitoring therapy. Cost and supply may limit the availability of Autoplex and it should not be used in conjunction with fibrinolytic inhibitors or in the presence of active intravascular coagulation.

HEAD INJURY. Any significant injury to the head in a patient with an inherited disorder of blood coagulation deserves immediate replacement therapy prior to proceeding with careful neurologic evaluation. Similarly, a patient with hemophilia should receive replacement therapy if a headache lasts for more than 6 to 8 hours. We instruct patients to immediately infuse sufficient material to elevate the factor level to 100%. Surgical evacuation of intracranial accumulations of blood ideally should be undertaken in Hemophilia Centers, where facilities are available for careful monitoring of blood levels.

NERVE COMPRESSION. Compression of peripheral nerves can occur whenever bleeding is into a closed fibromuscular compartment. Hemorrhage into the iliopsoas sheath can lead to permanent femoral nerve palsy. Early recognition and prompt replacement therapy are essential. On occasions surgical decompression is necessary if there is danger of permanent loss of neuromuscular function.

MAJOR SURGERY. Elective surgical procedures should be undertaken only in hospitals with facilities to monitor coagulation factor levels and only after it has been established that the patient has no evidence of an inhibitor. Factor levels above 30% have to be maintained for 7 to 10 days after major procedures.

Emergency surgical procedures should be performed after administering enough of the missing factor to produce a blood level of 100%. If specific factor assays cannot be done, normalization of the partial thromboplastin time can be accepted as reasonable indirect evidence of satisfactory response, but the patient should be transferred to a Hemophilia Center as soon as possible if such transfer is considered safe on clinical grounds.

Home Infusion Therapy. Home therapy should be considered only if the patient requires reasonably frequent transfusions and after careful psychosocial evaluation of the patient and the family. Formal training in infusion procedures and intravenous technique is mandatory, and it is the responsibility of the supervising physician to ensure that the patient and family are completely familiar with the indications for treatment and the signs and symptoms that would mandate physician evaluation.

Home treatment has obvious psychologic and economic advantages for both the patient and the family. In addition to making early treatment more available, home therapy also means that, for the first time, many of the patients have some control over their lives and the management of their disease. Home infusion is not without hazards, however. These include lack of medical supervision, increased danger of hepatitis in relatives, poor intravenous technique, overutilization of material, product deterioration, and illegal use of intravenous equipment. Although many people have expressed concern about poor intravenous technique at home, we have not encountered any serious problems. We insist that the patient and family keep detailed records, and, as with the outpatient treatment program, they are advised to check with the physician if more than two successive daily infusions are needed for control of a single bleeding episode. Furthermore, each patient on the home infusion program must return at least once a year for evaluation of the total management program. A number of studies have shown that there is increased use of replacement therapy initially but this eventually levels off. However, even if replacement therapy utilization remains high, this is usually balanced by the reduced cost to the patient and the improvement in school and work attendance. To guard against product deterioration, it is essential that the patient have adequate instructions and facilities for storage. To ensure that patients who are traveling in other areas receive prompt and appropriate replacement therapy, each patient is provided with a card outlining the diagnosis and the dose of replacement therapy. This is also useful in protecting patients who have to account to law enforcement authorities for the venipuncture marks and the possession of venipuncture equipment.

The institution dispensing the infusion material has an obligation to guard against abuse and sale of venipuncture equipment through illegal channels. To monitor this, we insist that all materials be returned to the Clinic after their use, and spot checks are made to ensure that used syringes, needles, and other equipment are returned. Patients are encouraged to restock their supply when they have enough material left for only one infusion. Ordinarily we supply enough for four infusions at a time, and this can be done through the mail. The patient is required to periodically mail in treatment records to ensure that the treatment program is appropriate.

Prophylactic Replacement Therapy. Although it is now possible to provide satisfactory prophylaxis, it is not a practical consideration for most patients. However, it may be indicated in selected situations as, for example, in patients who have had repeated CNS hemorrhage or for the control of repeated hemarthrosis into a single joint (see above). Prophylaxis is also required during periods of intensive physical therapy.

Dose schedules have to be individualized. For Factor VIII we generally advise infusions every 2 to 3 days, with doses calculated to raise the VIII level to 40 to 50 per cent. Lower doses and less frequent treatment often can produce the desired effect by maintaining Factor VIII levels above 2 to 3% of normal.

Educational Resources. A wide variety of educational materials is available from the National Hemophilia Foundation, 25 West 39th Street, New York, New York 10018. These include informative brochures suitable for patients, physicians, teachers, nurses, and other individuals who deal with the hemophilic patient and family. The brochures cover subjects such as pain control, physical therapy, financial counseling, teaching home therapy, and so on. In addition, the Foundation publishes a directory of Hemophilia Treatment Centers and descriptions of state and federal programs for assisting the hemophiliac and the family. The World Federation of Hemophilia, 1170 Peel Street, Room 1126, Montreal, Quebec, Canada H3B 2T4 publishes a "Guide for Traveling Hemophiliacs," which lists Hemophilia Centers located in over 40 countries.

Acquired Disorders

Vitamin K Deficiency

HEMORRHAGIC DISEASE OF THE NEWBORN

Prevention. In healthy full-term infants, the problem of hemorrhagic disease of the newborn has been virtually eliminated by the administration of vitamin K at or soon after delivery. The naturally occurring compound—vitamin K_1 oxide (phytonadione)—is the preferred form because synthetic vitamin K analogues can produce hemolysis. Neonatal hemolysis and the risk of kernicterus are a particular problem in the presence of a deficiency of red cell glucose-6-phosphate dehydrogenase. It has been well established that as a little as 0.025 mg of vitamin K_1 can prevent deficiencies of the vitamin K-dependent factors in a neonate with reasonably mature liver function. Thus the recommended dose of 0.5 to 1.0 mg intramuscularly or subcutaneously or 1 to 2 mg orally is already far in excess of the neonate's physiologic needs, and higher doses have no added beneficial effect. Particularly with the water-soluble analogues, higher doses increase the risk of kernicterus. Infants of mothers being treated with phenytoin (Dilantin) or phenobarbital are occasionally found immediately after birth to have hemorrhage secondary to depletion of vitamin K–dependent factors. This is in contrast to the usual case of hemorrhagic disease of the newborn in whom the various clotting factors are transferred transplacentally and symptoms become manifest only beyond the first 24 hours of age. Some recommend the administration of vitamin K during labor to the mother who is on anticonvulsant therapy, to prevent bleeding secondary to the trauma of delivery.

Treatment. Premature infants, particularly those with complications such as hypoxia, acidosis, or infection, do not respond to the administration of vitamin K as well as healthy term infants. When hemorrhagic manifestations are proved to be due exclusively or in large part to a deficiency of vitamin K–dependent factors, the clinician has to resort to the use of replacement therapy with fresh or fresh-frozen plasma if the patient is not responsive to vitamin K. The amount of procoagulant that can be safely administered to the newborn in this fashion is limited by the relatively low concentrations of procoagulants in whole plasma. On an average, plasma contains 1 unit of procoagulant activity in each ml, and an infusion of 10 ml/kg will produce an elevation of only about 10 per cent in the circulating level of Factor IX and the other vitamin K–dependent factors. Because of concern for volume overload, central venous pressure should be constantly monitored, particularly if an umbilical vein catheter is already in place for other reasons. As a practical approach, 10 ml of fresh-frozen plasma/kg body weight can be administered every 12 hours, and this should provide hemostatic levels of the missing factors, although the levels of each procoagulant will vary because of variations in in vivo recovery and intravascular biologic half-life. For example, Factor VII, although stable in stored plasma, has a short in vivo disappearance time of 4 to 6 hours. In contrast, 50% of infused prothrombin (Factor II) is still present 72 hours later.

Prothrombin complex concentrates are commercially available. In these concentrates the vitamin K–dependent factors are concentrated in approximately 1/25 the volume, compared with plasma. However, because of the increased risk of hepatitis, these concentrates should not be used unless it has been impossible to provide satisfactory hemostatic levels with single-donor plasma.

High-risk neonates should continue to receive supplemental parenteral or oral vitamin K, particularly if they are receiving broad-spectrum antibiotics or total parenteral nutrition.

IMPAIRED INTESTINAL ABSORPTION. Vitamin K deficiency can develop as a result of fat malabsorption and after prolonged administration of broad-spectrum antibiotics. Thus patients with conditions in which vitamin K deficiency might be anticipated should receive the water-soluble form of the vitamin prophylactically. For treatment of bleeding in these situations, intramuscular or intravenous vitamin K_1 should be given. Replacement therapy with blood products is rarely necessary.

LIVER DISEASE. In advanced liver disease, there is defective synthesis of the vitamin K–dependent clotting factors, and treatment with vitamin K is often ineffective. If there is overt bleeding or if the patient is being prepared for surgery, plasma infusions may be necessary. If possible, prothrombin complex concentrates should be avoided because of the added risk of hepatitis in the face of pre-existing liver dysfunction. Thrombosis is another recognized complication of treatment with prothrombin-complex concentrates, and this hazard may be increased in the patient with liver disease who is unable to clear activated coagulation factors from the circulation.

COUMARIN ANTICOAGULANTS. The coumarin anticoagulants are rarely used therapeutically in pediatric practice but they can cross the placenta, producing neonatal bleeding. More commonly, accidental ingestion of medication or rat poison can produce severe depletion of vitamin K–dependent factors. Intravenous administration of 50 mg of vitamin K_1 will normalize the prothrombin time within 6 to 12 hours, regardless of how much dicumarol is taken. The synthetic water-soluble analogues are less effective than the naturally occurring compound.

Circulating Anticoagulants. Circulating inhibitors of coagulation can develop in children without pre-existing coagulation factor deficiency. They may be directed against specific coagulation factors but are usually nonspecific and appear to be directed against the prothrombinase complex. They are rarely associated with abnormal hemostasis, in spite of significant in vitro abnormalities. Treatment is directed at the underlying disease as, for example, in systemic lupus erythematosus. We have not encountered problems at renal biopsy, even when significant in vitro inhibition is present. Many of these inhibitors, particularly those detected during "preoperative screening," seem to be related to viral infections and gradually disappear over weeks or months without specific therapy.

PLATELET DISORDERS

Thrombocytopenia

Treatment varies with the severity of the thrombocytopenia and the pathophysiologic basis for the reduction in platelet count. In general, patients with levels of normally functioning platelets above 50,000/mm³ have normal hemostasis. In the presence of platelet dysfunction, however, hemostasis is defective in spite of normal levels of circulating platelets. At the other end of the spectrum, children with conditions such as immunologic or so-called idiopathic thrombocytopenic purpura (ITP), characterized by shortened platelet survival and maximal compensatory production of platelets, may have reasonably normal hemostasis and normal bleeding times even with platelet counts as low as 10,000/mm³.

Impaired Platelet Production (Leukemia, Aplastic Anemia). Reduced production of platelets is usually the underlying mechanism for the thrombocytopenia complicating *aplastic anemia, acute leukemia,* and other conditions characterized by *bone marrow failure.* However, intravascular coagulation and fibrinolysis precipitated by complicating infection or by the disease process itself can aggravate the degree of thrombocytopenia. Platelet transfusions may be needed in acute leukemia during the period of induction of remission, at times of drug-induced pancytopenia, or at relapse. Because of the increase in the use of bone marrow transplantation, platelet transfusions should be used sparingly because exposure to foreign lymphocytes in platelet concentrates may enhance graft rejection at the time of bone marrow transplantation, particularly in patients with aplastic anemia. The use of "prophylactic platelet transfusions," particularly from family members, appears to be contraindicated in any patient who may be a candidate for bone marrow transplantation in the near or distant future. Children with documented immune deficiency or those who are to receive intensive immunosuppressive therapy are at risk to develop graft-versus-host disease (GVD) related to the infusion of viable donor lymphocytes. This problem is obviated by irradiating all blood products prior to administration.

Obviously, in the presence of active or potentially life-threatening hemorrhage, platelet replacement using random unrelated donors should not be withheld. Ultimately, however, restoration of normal platelet count can be expected only when the underlying disease process is brought under control.

Immune Thrombocytopenia (ITP). In so-called *idiopathic thrombocytopenic purpura* (ITP), one of the commonest causes of thrombocytopenia in children, the reduced platelet count results from the production of autoantibodies directed against the patient's platelets, usually following a relatively mild viral infection. Splenic sequestration of antibody-coated platelets is enhanced, and the degree of thrombocytopenia depends on the ability of the bone marrow to compensate for varying degrees of shortened platelet survival. Underlying disorders, such as *systemic lupus erythematosus* or *lymphoma,* must be sought and, if present, treated appropriately.

The treatment of ITP has been the subject of controversy for many years. A number of studies have demonstrated that corticosteroid therapy shortens the time from diagnosis to *normalization* of platelet count. However, the natural history of the disease is such that hemorrhagic manifestations usually clear within a week or two of onset whether or not corticosteroids are given and in spite of persistently low platelet counts. It is during this period that normalization of the bleeding time can be documented in the absence of an increase in platelet count. Thus *clinical* improvement does not necessarily depend on a rise or normalization of the platelet count. In addition, the use of corticosteroids has not reduced the incidence of chronic cases.

One of the major concerns of clinicians caring for these patients is the risk of intracranial hemorrhage, but this is a very rare complication and usually occurs within the first few days of illness, often before treatment can be instituted or expected to exert a therapeutic effect. Thus in the presence of mild clinical bleeding confined to the skin or mucous membranes, it is our policy to hospitalize the patient for a few days of observation. Within 3 to 7 days the hemorrhagic manifestations have subsided and the patient is discharged to home care, where the parents are advised to take reasonable precautions against significant trauma. We advise against bicycle riding, tree climbing, skating, sledding, and contact sports, but in older children who can take reasonable precautions, there is no contraindication to returning to a normal classroom situation. If after approximately 6 months the platelet count has not risen above 50,000/mm^3, a trial of corticosteroid therapy is indicated. Prednisone, 40 to 60 mg/m^2/24 hr in three divided doses, is administered for 4 weeks. Whether or not there has been a response, the dose should be tapered over 4 to 6 weeks. By monitoring the platelet count during drug withdrawal, it is possible to define a minimal dose level at which an adequate platelet level might be maintained.

In patients who respond initially but relapse after discontinuing prednisone therapy, it seems reasonable to attempt reinduction with a more gradual taper. This alternative is often unacceptable to teenagers who become very concerned about the cosmetic effects of corticosteroids even for these relatively short treatment periods. Under these circumstances, and where platelet counts above 50,000 cannot be maintained without treatment, splenectomy should be considered. Permanent benefit can be anticipated in well over half the patients subjected to splenectomy. In patients who have previously had a response to prednisone therapy, the drug should be administered for a week prior to surgery in order to achieve and maintain hemostatic platelet levels. However, it should be stressed that even with severe thrombocytopenia it is rare to encounter excessive bleeding at splenectomy in these patients.

We usually have platelet concentrates available in the blood bank to be administered only if the surgeon encounters excessive oozing during the operative procedure. To my recollection we have never had to administer platelets under these circumstances and, in any event, their effect would be short-lived since infused platelets are rapidly cleared from the circulation as they become coated with antibody. Even in patients who have not previously responded to therapy, corticosteroid coverage is essential during the perioperative period to protect against the effects of adrenal insufficiency.

Relapse after splenectomy-induced remission should alert the clinician to search for an accessory spleen by ^{99m}Tc scanning. If present, removal of the accessory spleen usually results in a second remission. In many cases these relapses are transient and, like the initial episode, are often provoked by a minor viral infection. These patients are considered to have a "compensated thrombolytic state," and relapse is precipitated either by an increase in the rate of platelet destruction or decreased platelet production. They usually recover within a week or two but are often given corticosteroids, which in my experience does not alter the natural history of the condition in this rare but troublesome group of patients.

Even in the absence of proven long-term benefits from corticosteroid therapy, it seems prudent to treat patients with fulminating hemorrhage or intracranial bleeding at the time of diagnosis. Although platelet transfusions are not considered appropriate as routine therapy in patients with ITP, transient hemostasis may be achieved that could be critical in a life-threatening situation.

Approximately 5% of patients will fail to achieve remission after an appropriate period of observation followed by an adequate trial of prednisone and splenectomy. In these cases, immunosuppressive therapy with cyclophosphamide or azathioprine has been used with variable success. Vincristine sulfate, which has some immunosuppressive qualities and has a positive effect on platelet production, has produced remissions in adults with ITP. Vinblastine-treated random donor platelets have been transfused to adults with ITP with the intent of delivering a "cytotoxic" agent to the areas of platelet sequestration. High dose intravenous gamma globulin has been reported effective in a small number of children with chronic or intermittent ITP. At present, all these immunotherapeutic approaches must be considered investigational. Their use should only be considered after the risks of such therapy have been carefully weighed against the hazards of chronic thrombocytopenia in a particular patient.

Neonatal Thrombocytopenia. Thrombocytopenia in the high-risk neonate is most commonly related to intrauterine or postnatal infection. Treatment is usually directed against the underlying disease process. Less frequently, neonatal thrombocytopenic purpura develops as a result of transplacental passage of platelet antibodies from either a mother with active or "compensated" autoimmune thrombocytopenia or one who is isoimmunized by her infant's platelets. Isoimmunization occurs when the mother lacks antigens present on the infant's platelets, and the mother becomes immunized against fetal platelets in much the same way as the erythrocytes are affected in hemolytic disease of the newborn. There is then passive transfer of material antibodies across the placenta, which react with antigens on the fetal platelets. The PLA-1 antigen has been most frequently incriminated in isoimmune neonatal thrombocytopenia.

In symptomatic newborn infants with platelet counts below 20,000 to 30,000/mm^3, prompt therapy is indicated. The ideal form of therapy in isoimmune thrombocytopenia is the transfusion of platelets that lack the antigen against which the antibody is directed. These nonreactive platelets can be obtained from the mother and washed free of antibody before transfusing the infant. If previous infants have been affected, maternal platelets can be harvested by plateletpheresis prior to delivery so that they can be available for transfusion soon after birth if the infant is affected. Alternatively, if the offending antigen has been identified with a previously affected infant, an unrelated donor lacking the antigen could be used as a source of platelet concentrate for the affected infant. If compatible platelets are not available, as is true in most cases of maternal autoimmune thrombocytopenia, we recommend proceeding with exchange transfusion using freshly drawn whole blood (< 24 hours from donation) from a random donor. This will have the effect of removing circulating antibody from the infant's circulation while providing at least temporary correction of the thrombocytopenia with donor platelets. Subsequent platelet transfusions may be necessary if the platelet count is not sustained at hemostatic levels. Although they are frequently rec-

ommended, corticosteroids have not been proved to be of benefit in neonatal thrombocytopenia. Without specific therapy, recovery can be anticipated in 4 to 6 weeks, by which time most of the maternal antibody would have been cleared from the fetal circulation.

One preliminary study has produced evidence to suggest that administration of corticosteroids to mothers prior to labor can elevate the fetal platelet count. Some have recommended that subsequent infants born to the mothers of infants with neonatal thrombocytopenia be delivered by cesarean section. We only make this recommendation if a prolonged or difficult labor is anticipated and to date have not experienced problems with major hemorrhagic manifestations in neonates delivered vaginally. The rationale for advising cesarean section is to avoid trauma to the delivering head during vaginal delivery. An alternative to this approach is to measure platelet counts in the presenting fetal scalp prior to deciding on the need for cesarean section.

Cyanotic Congenital Heart Disease. In cyanotic congenital heart disease, the degree of thrombocytopenia is related inversely to the height of the hematocrit, which in turn contributes to increasing blood viscosity. Although thrombocytopenia is rarely severe enough to produce hemorrhagic symptoms, the risk of postoperative hemorrhage is increased, and it is important to attempt to correct thrombocytopenia either before or after open heart surgery. In patients with platelet counts of less than 100,000/mm^3 who are scheduled for bypass procedures, arrangements should be made to have platelets available for transfusion after extracorporeal circulation is discontinued. Another approach is a modified exchange transfusion, with removal of red cells and replacement by normal plasma or 5% human albumin before operation with the aim of reducing the hematocrit reading to about 60%. The dramatic rise in platelet count observed after this procedure suggests that redistribution of platelets within the circulation may play a role in the pathogenesis of thrombocytopenia.

Disorders of Platelet Function

An increasing number of congenital and acquired disorders are now recognized and should be suspected in any patient having a normal platelet count with a prolonged bleeding time.

Inherited Disorders. GLANZMANN THROMBASTHENIA, BERNARD-SOULIER SYNDROME, "STORAGE POOL DISEASE." For the increasing number of inherited disorders of platelet function now recognized, no specific therapy is usually available to correct the basic platelet defect so that transfusion of normal platelets is required to cover serious bleeding episodes or major surgical procedures. Since these patients are not on any form of immunosuppressive therapy, there is a strong likelihood that they will develop antibodies directed against donor platelets. This problem can be circumvented by identifying donors who are compatible with respect to HLA antigens. This reduces the possibility of developing resistance to future transfusions, and transfusions from these donors are often effective when the patient has become resistant to transfusion from random donors.

Congenital afibrinogenemia is associated with platelet dysfunction presumably due to the lack of fibrinogen on the platelet surface. Transfusion of plasma or cryoprecipitate corrects both the prolonged bleeding time and the in vitro platelet abnormalities.

Patients with *type 1 glycogen storage* disease have abnormalities of platelet function, but the hemorrhagic tendency is mild although it does tend to become more severe with advancing age. Correction of the underlying metabolic disturbances results in correction of the platelet abnormalities, but this often takes up to a week so that careful preparation is needed prior to major surgical procedures in this group of patients.

Acquired Disorders. UREMIA. Abnormal bleeding in patients with chronic uremia is often associated with abnormal platelet function, related in part to elevated levels of serum guanidinosuccinic acid. Hemodialysis or successful renal transplant corrects both the bleeding time and the in vitro abnormalities of platelet function. More recently, the administration of cryoprecipitate has been shown to correct the platelet abnormalities in this group of patients although the mechanism by which it exerts this effect is not clear. The chronically uremic patient with a bleeding diathesis that can be ascribed to abnormal platelet function can be treated initially with cryoprecipitate. If this fails to accomplish the desired therapeutic effect, hemodialysis should be undertaken.

DRUG-INDUCED PLATELET DYSFUNCTION. A number of commonly used drugs have been shown to produce abnormal platelet function. Aspirin is the most widely used of these agents, but antihistamines, antidepressants, tranquilizers, alpha-adrenergic blocking agents, local anesthetics, and nonaspirin analgesics like phenylbutazone and indomethacin may have similar effects. In general, few of these agents produce symptomatic bleeding unless there is an underlying hemostatic defect. Discontinuing the particular medication will result in a return to normal of platelet function; the in vitro abnormalities may persist for up to a week after aspirin administration but the effect is more transient after exposure to other nonsteroidal anti-inflammatory drugs.

Platelet Transfusions

To minimize the hazard of volume overload in the pediatric patient and to improve utilization of blood components in general, platelets are usually administered in the form of platelet concentrates. Although there is significant risk of spontaneous and life-threatening hemorrhage at platelet counts below $10,000/mm^3$, many patients are able to maintain adequate hemostasis under resting conditions so that the platelet count should not be used as the sole indication for transfusion. This is particularly true in patients who have thrombocytopenia characterized by increased platelet turnover. Platelet transfusions should, however, be considered in the severely thrombocytopenic patient with leukemia or marrow aplasia with evidence of active hemorrhage, even if only in the form of spontaneous petechial eruptions. Patients with platelet counts between 10- and $50,000/mm^3$ are at risk from hemorrhage related to varying degrees of trauma; platelet transfusions aimed at raising and maintaining the platelet count above $50,000/mm^3$ would be necessary to cover minor or major surgical procedures. Patients with platelet counts above $50,000/mm^3$ are usually able to maintain normal hemostasis if platelet function is normal and there is no associated coagulation defect.

Although most blood banks can now provide sufficient quantities of platelet concentrate to meet the needs of the thrombocytopenic patient, current routine blood bank procedures do not evaluate the compatibility of platelets for transfusion. Thus, there is significant risk of developing platelet antibodies after transfusion of platelets from random donors, resulting in unresponsiveness to future platelet transfusions. This is a particular concern in patients with aplastic anemia since immunosuppressive therapy is usually not part of their treatment program. Thus, in embarking on a platelet transfusion program for an individual patient, the risk of hemorrhage at the time of transfusion has to be carefully weighed against the future needs of the patient, the likelihood of antibody production, and the potential for marrow graft rejection due to transfusion of foreign lymphocytes.

Patients with qualitative platelet disorders or those with aplastic anemia who are not candidates for bone marrow transplantation and in whom long-term platelet transfusion programs are anticipated should be typed with respect to the HLA antigens, since these seem to relate closely to platelet antigens. If HLA-compatible donors can be identified, transfusion from these donors has proved very effective for long periods of time in patients who have developed resistance to transfusion of platelets from random donors.

The dose of platelet concentrate can be calculated based on observations that platelets derived from 1 unit of whole blood produce an average increment in platelet count of $13,000/mm^3/m^2$ body surface. The administration of 6 units of platelet concentrate/m^2 will produce an increment in platelet count of $50,000/mm^3$ or above in the majority of recipients. If hemorrhage continues in spite of an adequate increment in platelet count, a search should be made for a local lesion to account for the continued bleeding. Febrile patients with or without to platelet transfusions, as measured by increment in platelet count, but even with a less than satisfactory rise in the platelet count, hemostasis can often be achieved and maintained. To evaluate response to a platelet transfusion, the platelet count should be obtained prior to the transfusion. 1 hour after its completion, and again the next morning. On an average, 50 per cent of the infused platelets will have disappeared from the circulation after 24 hours, so that it is often necessary to repeat the transfusion every 2 to 3 days.

Fresh platelet concentrates have a limited shelf life. To maintain adequate inventories of blood components, it is extremely helpful to the blood bank for the clinician to attempt to anticipate the patient's platelet transfusion requirements as far in advance as possible. Methods for long-term platelet cryopreservation are being actively explored. When the techniques are perfected and become more generally available, it will be possible to stockpile platelet concentrates from selected donors, or from the patients themselves while in remission, for use at some future time.

Acute Leukemia

LUCIUS F. SINKS, M.D.

ACUTE LYMPHOBLASTIC LEUKEMIA (ALL)

Acute lymphoblastic leukemia is a curable disease in a significant number of cases. Therapy is based on the concept that multiagent chemotherapy will effectively control the disease for a prolonged period of time after which, and upon the cessation of the therapy, the disease will not recur. The therapy conceptually involves the following phases: (1) induction, (2) sanctuary treatment, (3) maintenance therapy, and (4) cessation of therapy.

Furthermore, since we can now identify various subclasses of ALL that have different anticipated outcomes, the therapy should be modified to reflect these differences. However, the eventual therapy for these subgroups still remains in the area of clinical research, so that, at the present time, there does not exist unanimous agreement as to the optimal treatment.

Acute Lymphoblastic Leukemia—Standard Risk. Children between the ages of 2 and 9 years at the time of diagnosis and with white cell counts of 20,000 or less per mm^3 are considered standard risk or good risk patients, assuming they do not have positive T-cell markers.

The induction therapy varies somewhat from study to study but basically incorporates the use of vincristine, given at a dose of 2 mg/m^2 once weekly IV, and prednisone, 40 mg/m^2 daily given p o. This is followed by L-asparaginase, at 1000 units/kg IV daily for 10 days. (There are other schedules currently in use according to the study design.) Ninety to ninety-five per cent of such children will go into complete remission. The sanctuary therapy phase is designed to decrease the incidence of leukemic infiltration in the central nervous system, gonads, liver, and spleen, but special emphasis has been placed on preventing so-called meningeal leukemia, as otherwise 50% of the children will develop this life-threatening complication. Recent studies show that this group of ALL patients do very well in terms of complete disease control if they receive three courses of intermediate dose methotrexate, 500 mg/m^2 IV for 24 hours. One third is given as push and two thirds is dripped in over the remaining 24 hours. At 48 hours they receive 12 mg/m^2 of leukovorin IV or IM. Each course is repeated every 3 weeks. At the same time 12 mg/m^2 of methotrexate are given intrathecally (IT). The IT methotrexate is initiated at day 15 during induction and given weekly for three doses and then with each dose of IV methotrexate. Upon completion of the sanctuary phase of therapy, patients are placed on maintenance therapy consisting of 6-mercaptopurine, 75 mg/m^2 po daily, and methotrexate, 15 mg/m^2 po once weekly. Pulse doses of vincristine, one IV dose every month, are given with 7 days of prednisone po. This is repeated monthly for six months, then given every twelve weeks. One expects that 70% of these patients will remain disease free at 3 years.

Upon completion of 4 years of such therapy with no evidence of recurrent disease, therapy is discontinued and the patient observed.

Clinical research continues to address the question of central nervous system prophylaxis, principally refining the role of cranial irradiation. Maintenance programs in this group of patients have been quite successful, but the vexing question of the optimal time to discontinue therapy remains to be answered to everyone's satisfaction.

Acute Lymphoblastic Leukemia—High Risk (Non-T-cell). These children usually respond quite well to the induction regimen described above, but the proportion going into remission is usually 85 to 90%. Cranial irradiation remains the standard therapy for the sanctuary phase of this group of patients, in combination with intrathecal methotrexate. The dose of radiation is somewhat in question as to whether 1800 or 2400 rads is the optimal dose, considering effectiveness and long-range toxicity. There has been concern during recent years that radiation can cause impairment of intellectual capacities, especially in younger children, as well as give rise later to life-threatening leukoencephalopathy. Maintenance therapy is usually the same as previously described, but efforts in clinical research studies are focusing on improvement, as one expects less than 50% of these high risk patients to remain in complete remission for three years.

The proper time to discontinue therapy within this group also is an unresolved question. One fears, particularly in males, that early cessation of therapy will lead to testicular relapse. This rate of relapse is undoubtedly related to the effectiveness of systemic therapy. We have seen that patients receiving intermediate dose methotrexate have far better control of testicular relapse than those who do not. We now recommend 4 years of systemic therapy before discontinuing maintenance, and then follow patients carefully.

The 10 to 15% of children with ALL who have T-cell markers on their lymphoblasts tend to be teenage males with high white blood cell counts and mediastinal masses, who unfortuantely have a very poor prognosis despite the fact that many will go into remission with current induction treatment. Currently, these patients are the subjects of newer and more intensive approaches in terms of chemotherapy. Since there is no accepted standard therapy for this group of patients, it is recommended that they be referred to a center where a research program is being conducted.

Relapsed Patients. Patients who relapse while on treatment have a very poor prognosis; those who relapse after cessation of therapy have a slightly better prognosis. Although these patients often can be induced into remission, the duration of the second remission is short. At this time the option of bone marrow transplant should be considered, and if there is a suitable donor, there exists a viable alternative. As high as 40% of relapsed patients with identical twin donors have had prolonged remissions. Obviously, this represents a small proportion of patients.

If marrow transplant is not possible, other regimens of maintenance chemotherapy must be utilized. Such schedules are highly dependent on the previous chemotherapy utilized, as well as prior central nervous system prophylaxis.

ACUTE MYELOBLASTIC LEUKEMIA

The therapy of acute myeloblastic leukemia (AML) and related forms, such as myelomonocytic and promyelocytic, has lagged behind the effective development described for ALL. It is only recently that one can expect greater than 70% of such children to go into remission and, furthermore, to expect that a good proportion of them will remain in remission at 2 years.

The combination of cytosine arabinoside and one of the anthracycline drugs, daunorubicin (DNR) or Adriamycin (ADR), has led to the improved induction rates. Usually either a 7-day course of cytosine arabinoside at 100 mg/m² daily is given with a 3-day course of DNR or ADR. DNR is given at a dose of 45 mg/m² IV × 3 and ADR at

a dose of 30 mg/m² × 3. The use of ADR has led to a high incidence of necrotizing enterocolitis and death in some patients, so there appears to be less toxicity with DNR.

Although the induction rates have increased recently, there still exists a real problem with maintenance schedules. The schedules to date have not been impressive, and there is now a real interest in aggressive consolidation therapy following induction and then *no* subsequent maintenance. One of the most promising approaches involves consolidation with very high doses of cytosine arabinoside, 3 gm/m² every 12 hours for 3 days. There are increased problems with toxicity, such as chemical conjunctivitis, cerebellar signs, dystonia (temporary), and prolonged hematologic depression. However, this current approach projects 40% of patients in remission at 4 years. This is in contrast with the usual figure of 20% of patients at 3 to 4 years.

Another viable option that exists if there is a suitable matched donor is bone marrow transplantation following induction. In this select population, 50% of the patients are in complete remission at 3 to 4 years.

The entire management of these patients requires far more supportive measures and clinical skill than does the current management of children with ALL. Infection, bleeding, necrotizing colitis, and prolonged hematopoietic depression all require trained and skilled professionals. Therapy should be undertaken only where such personnel are available.

Family Support. The medical therapy of acute leukemia in children brings with it an obligation to support not only the patient but also the family. This support must be made available by utilizing various members of a team, as it is far too great an emotional load to place on the physician alone to perform this task.

After the initial shock of the diagnosis of such disorders, many man hours must be spent educating and supporting the family. Soon after going into remission, the children and adolescents are encouraged to enter school. This often formidable challenge requires a special effort and program to effectively have the child re-enter the normal social environment.

Neuroblastoma

F. ANN HAYES, M.D.,
ALEXANDER A. GREEN, M.D.,
and ALVIN M. MAUER, M.D.

Neuroblastoma, a malignancy of neural crest origin, is one of the most common neoplasms in children. At presentation, one half of the affected patients will be under 2 years of age and 70% already will have metastatic spread of the tumor. The most important prognostic factor at diagnosis is the extent of disease (stage). Infants less than 1 year of age at diagnosis have a better prognosis compared with older children but, even in this more favorable group, the prognosis is related to stage of disease.

The staging system for neuroblastoma, which has proved effective from our studies, is shown in Table 1.

Table 1. STAGING SYSTEM FOR NEUROBLASTOMA

Stage I	Localized tumor completely resected
Stage IIA	Localized tumor grossly resected but with microscopic residual disease through capsule
IIB	Localized tumor unresectable without invasion of regional nodes
Stage III	Metastatic disease
IIIA	Regional or systemic spread without bone or marrow disease
IIIB	A single bone lesion without generalized bone or marrow disease
IIIC	Generalized bone and/or bone marrow disease

Surgery. Surgery may have three roles in the initial phase of treatment of the child with neuroblastoma: biopsy for diagnosis, staging of clinically localized disease, and curative resection for Stages I and IIA disease. Extensive attempts at initial surgical resection with the potential for compromise of normal structures are contraindicated. Most children with locally unresectable tumors can be cured with chemotherapy and a "second look" surgical approach. Children with metastatic disease have no improvement in prognosis or response to other therapeutic modalities by surgical attempts to remove tumor volume (debulking procedures).

Proper surgical staging requires regional node biopsies; if the tumor is present in the abdomen, a liver biopsy is essential because only microscopic evidence of tumor frequently is found.

Radiation Therapy. The role of radiation therapy in neuroblastoma is currently controversial. Children with Stages I and IIA disease, regardless of age, have essentially a 100 per cent cure rate with only surgical resection and should not be exposed to the long-term hazards of radiation therapy. All infants under 1 year of age and over 75 per cent of older children with Stage IIB disease can be cured with current chemotherapy programs. For the child with metastatic disease, there has been no evidence that radiation therapy, including total body irradiation, has improved the clinical outcome.

Currently, we administer radiation therapy to those children whose tumors have been demonstrated to be resistant to chemotherapy or for palliation of painful lesions uncontrolled by chemotherapy.

Chemotherapy. More than 85% of children with neuroblastoma will have surgically unresectable tumor at presentation; therefore, effective chemotherapy is essential for control of their disease. The most effective single agents are cyclophosphamide, Adriamycin, cisplatin, and the epipodophyllotoxin VM-26.* Less effective agents also used commonly include vincristine and dacarbazine (DTIC).

In our experience, cyclophosphamide is best combined with Adriamycin in the following schedule; cyclophosphamide, 150 mg/m^2 IV for 7 days followed by doxorubicin, 35 mg/m^2 once on day 8. This cycle is repeated every 3 weeks with subsequent courses of cyclophosphamide being given by mouth. When followed by second look surgery and resection of residual primary tumor, where necessary and possible, this program results in long-term disease-free survival in essentially all infants under 1 year of age and more than 75% of older patients with Stage IIB disease. The same treatment course is curative for about 60% of infants with Stage III disease, including those with bone metastasis. This treatment program will induce a complete clinical response in 50% of children over 1 year of age with Stage III disease. However, most of these children will subsequently relapse and die of tumor.

Another effective combination has been the use of cisplatin in a dose of 90 mg/m^2 IV, followed in 48 hours by VM-26* IV in a dose of 100 mg/m^2. This schedule has resulted in complete clinical responses in about 30% of children over 1 year of age with previously treated tumor.

In our current treatment program, all four of these drugs are used in the combinations and schedules described above for the treatment of children over 1 year of age with Stage III disease.

The immediate side effects of these agents include nausea; vomiting; bone marrow suppression with anemia, leukopenia, and thrombocytopenia; and alopecia. Additionally, there are special drug-related toxicities, such as the cardiomyopathy of doxorubicin, the hemorrhagic cystitis of cyclophosphamide, and the renal and otic toxicity of platinum. Side effects can be minimized by close follow-up, dose limitation where necessary, and a full awareness of the potential complications.

In spite of the improving complete clinical response rates for the older child with disseminated disease, the long-term survival for these children remains poor. Since this group of children comprises 60% of the patients with neuroblastoma, clinical and laboratory research efforts must center on this group with such an unfavorable prognosis.

It is essential that children with neuroblastoma be referred to pediatric cancer centers upon diagnosis so that proper staging can be cone. Treat-

---

*Investigational drug.

ment programs must be designed so that those children with potentially curable disease will survive with the fewest possible short- and long-term consequences. In this setting, those children whose clinical presentation is associated with poor prognosis can receive the benefits of the most current therapy, giving them the best quality and duration of survival possible. Considerable clinical experience with these treatment programs is necessary to get maximal benefit with minimal complications. It is important for the family physician to be aware of the child's therapy and potential complications, because programs are designed to allow the patient to spend as much time as possible at home. The family physician must be closely involved with the cancer center physicians in providing continued care.

8

Spleen and Lymphatic System

The Postsplenectomy Syndrome

A. KIM RITCHEY, M.D.

Since the original description by King and Schumacher of five infants with fatal infections following splenectomy, the syndrome of postsplenectomy sepsis has received considerable attention. The dramatic, rapidly progressive course of this disorder with a mortality rate of 50 to 75% warrants this special consideration. Following splenectomy, the immunologic and filtering functions of the spleen are lost, exposing the patient to an increased risk of sepsis and meningitis, primarily due to encapsulated bacteria. The pneumococcus is the most frequent causative organism followed by *Hemophilus influenzae* type B and the meningococcus. The clinical syndrome is characterized by rapid progression from malaise and fever to death, often within 12 to 24 hours, due to failure to clear these encapsulated organisms. The risk of postsplenectomy sepsis depends on the age of the patient and the nature of the underlying disorder. Children under the age of 2 are at the greatest risk, with a decreasing risk thereafter. Although statistically the 4 years following splenectomy are when most episodes of overwhelming infection occur, the risk in the splenectomized patient at any age or at any time after surgery never is as low as the general population. When splenectomy is performed for hereditary spherocytosis, idiopathic thrombocytopenia, or ruptured spleen, the degree of risk is quite low, while it is much greater in Hodgkin's disease, thalassemia and congestive splenomegaly. The highest risk occurs in disorders with a concomitant immunologic defect, such as Wiskott-Aldrich syndrome.

Management of the postsplenectomy syndrome can be divided in two areas: preventive measures and acute management.

Prevention. A laudable goal for the "management" of the postsplenectomy syndrome is prevention. Steps to help accomplish this are as follows:

1. *Avoid splenectomy* when possible; for example, by nonoperative management or partial splenectomy in the patient with a ruptured spleen. Splenectomy should no longer be considered routine.

2. *Postpone elective splenectomy* until after the period of highest risk for postsplenectomy sepsis, i.e., about 5 years of age.

3. *Administer pneumococcal vaccine* at least 1 to 2 weeks prior to elective splenectomy and as soon postoperatively as possible in patients requiring emergency splenectomy. If the vaccine is given before the age of 2, it should be repeated again after the second birthday. In all other patients, booster immunization is not recommended at the present time.

4. *Prophylactic antibiotics* have a role in the management of the patient whose spleen has been removed, but clear-cut guidelines are not universally accepted. Prophylactic penicillin effectively decreases mortality from pneumococcal infection in splenectomized rats, but a well controlled human study has not been reported. Anecdotal data on the use of prophylactic penicillin in splenectomized patients with Wiskott-Aldrich syndrome, however, support the use of this regimen in preventing the postsplenectomy syndrome. Disadvantages of prophylactic antibiotics include emergence of resistant organisms, problems of compliance, and a false sense of security leading to delays in seeking medical attention with febrile illnesses.

Although some physicians recommend prophylactic antibiotics for all patients, we treat only patients at high risk of postsplenectomy sepsis, including children under the age of 5 and patients of any age with an underlying high risk disease (e.g., Wiskott-Aldrich). Penicillin or amoxicillin in doses of 125 or 250 mg twice a day is recommended. Therapy should be at least to age 5 in young children and lifelong in high risk patients. Use of prophylactic antibiotics *in no way* affects the management of acute, febrile illnesses.

5. *Education* of both patient and parents regarding the signs, symptoms, and management of postsplenectomy synrome are crucial to preventing morbidity and mortality. Education should begin prior to splenectomy.

Acute Management. Patients and parents should be told to seek medical attention for illness with fever greater than 101°F (38.5°C). This somewhat arbitrary temperature guideline encompasses most cases of postsplenectomy syndrome. Parents should be further advised that nonfebrile illnesses accompanied by vomiting, headache, or lethargy also require medical attention. If the patient looks well and no clearcut, nonbacterial cause of the illness is discovered, a blood culture and complete blood count are obtained and a dose of ampicillin (20 mg/kg) is administered parenterally. If the patient continues to look well after a few hours of observation, he may be sent home on oral amoxicillin therapy at weight adjusted doses until the blood culture is negative (usually 48–72 hours). The patient should return immediately if any clinical deterioration occurs.

If the patient looks very ill and/or is hyperpyrexic (temperature >104°F [40°C]), he should be presumed septic and admitted to the hospital for prompt diagnostic work-up and treatment. Cultures of blood, spinal fluid, and nasopharynx should be obtained, as should a chest x-ray. Therapy should be initiated with intravenous penicillin (300,000 u/kg/day divided q4h) and chloramphenicol (100 mg/kg/day divided q6h). Treatment duration and modification will depend on the results of CSF cell count, Gram stain, and culture results. Gram stain of the peripheral blood buffy coat occasionally reveals the causative organism in a bacteremic patient. Vigilance for the development of shock and disseminated intravascular coagulation is paramount, and maximum supportive care should be readily available.

If splenectomized patients know they will be in situations where medical care is not available, they should carry a supply of amoxicillin in case of illness. At the first sign of fever they should take a double dose (age adjusted) and continue regular doses every 6 hours until medical attention can be obtained.

Finally, children with sickle cell disease who have lost splenic function and children with congenital asplenia (Ivemark syndrome) are at high risk for developing the postsplenectomy syndrome and should be managed in the same fashion as patients who have lost their spleen at surgery.

Disorders of the Spleen

A. KIM RITCHEY, M.D.

Although the spleen was long considered a nonessential vestige by the ancients, we are now aware of a number of crucial functions performed by this reticuloendothelial organ: 1) clearance of particulate antigens and senescent or damaged red cells from the blood; 2) production of antibodies and opsonins, especially in response to intravenous particulate antigen; 3) removal of red cell inclusions, such as Howell-Jolly bodies, Heinz bodies, and surface vesicles ("pocks") without damaging the cell; and 4) storage of platelets and Factor VIII. Splenic activity can be assessed by the traditional liver-spleen radionuclide scan or a relatively new semiquantitative method involving enumeration of red cells containing pocks, using interference phase microscopy with Nomarski optics. Normals have less than 1% "pocked" red cells while asplenic individuals have greater than 12%.

The spleen is rarely the site of primary disease, yet reflects a variety of other disease processes, usually as splenomegaly. Functional activity is not lost when splenomegaly ensues. Indeed, enlargement of the spleen may be associated with *hypersplenism,* a condition characterized by accelerated destruction or "pooling" of red cells, platelets, and neutrophils —alone or in combination—resulting in peripheral cytopenias. Platelet and neutrophil counts are usually only moderately depressed and infrequently produce clinical symptoms. Red cell destruction may lead to an increased transfusion requirement. Although splenectomy will cure hypersplenism, it is rarely indicated and must be weighed against the risk of aggravating the underlying disease and the risk of postsplenectomy sepsis.

SPLENOMEGALY

The number of conditions associated with splenomegaly are legion. Some of the commonly associated diseases are listed below:
1. Infectious: Infectious mononucleosis; congenital infections ("TORCH"); subacute bacterial endocarditis; typhoid fever; sepsis; tuberculosis; histoplasmosis; malaria; schistosomiasis.
2. Hematologic: Sickle cell disease and its variants; β-thalassemia; hereditary spherocytosis; autoimmune hemolytic anemia.
3. Oncologic: Leukemia; lymphoma.
4. Storage: Gaucher's disease; Niemann-Pick disease.
5. Collagen vascular: Rheumatoid arthritis; systemic lupus erythematosus.

6. Miscellaneous: Cysts; histiocytosis; congestive splenomegaly (secondary to cirrhosis of the liver or obstruction of portal or splenic veins).

Management of splenomegaly in all cases is by medical treatment of the underlying disorder, where such treatment exists. Although splenectomy for selected conditions has been considered routine in the past, our understanding of the risk of post-splenectomy infection has changed this approach. However, it may still play an important role in the management of the selected patient with splenomegaly and is considered below.

SPLENECTOMY

Surgical excision of the spleen must be considered with regard to the effect on the underlying disease process and to the subsequent risk of infection. In hereditary spherocytosis, for example, splenectomy is "curative," while in certain cases of congestive splenomegaly it may worsen the clinical situation. Similarly, the risk of postsplenectomy sepsis following removal for traumatic rupture is quite low, while it is extremely high in splenectomized infants with Wiskott-Aldrich syndrome. General guidelines for managing the prospective splenectomy candidate are as follows:

1. The risk of postsplenectomy sepsis is higher in infants and young children; thus splenectomy should be postponed until the child is over 5 years of age, if possible.
2. Pneumococcal vaccine is less effective in patients without spleens, so it should be administered at least 1 or 2 weeks prior to splenectomy.
3. Patient and parent education regarding the risks and management of postsplenectomy infection should begin before splenectomy.

Selected disorders in which splenectomy may play a role in management of the underlying diseases are considered below.

HEREDITARY SPHEROCYTOSIS (HS). There is no question that splenectomy will prevent the premature destruction of red cells in this disorder. However, HS is a clinically heterogeneous disorder and indication for splenectomy must be individualized. The patient with a mild course may not need splenectomy, while the child with severe hemolysis and growth failure may require it at an early age. In most instances, however, the child can be managed medically until the age of 5 or older.

AUTOIMMUNE HEMOLYTIC ANEMIA (AIHA.) This disorder in childhood, unlike in adults, is usually self-limited and splenectomy is not often necessary. In the patient with acute AIHA unresponsive to steroids and transfusions, splenectomy is appropriate, though the results are unpredictable. Splenectomy is also indicated in the patient with chronic AIHA who requires large doses of steroids to maintain the hemoglobin and is at risk for the complications of steroid therapy.

IDIOPATHIC THROMBOCYTOPENIC PURPURA (ITP). Like AIHA, ITP is self-limited in 85 to 90% of children. In the acute phase of the illness splenectomy has no role except in rare patients with life-threatening bleeding, such as central nervous system hemorrhage. Splenectomy for the few children who develop chronic ITP must be individualized. Criteria for selection include severity of thrombocytopenia, the sedentary nature of the child, and the emotional effect of restriction of activity. Splenectomy in chronic ITP is usually curative, though complete remission or freedom from relapse cannot be guaranteed.

GAUCHER'S DISEASE. Splenectomy may be indicated in patients with Gaucher's disease whose spleens become so large as to cause physical symptoms. Splenectomy may in some instances exacerbate the bony involvement of this disorder.

SPLENIC CYSTS. Cysts of the spleen may be congenital or may follow trauma. Although splenectomy has been considered the treatment of choice in the past, partial splenectomy to preserve some splenic function should be considered if surgically feasible.

CONGESTIVE SPLENOMEGALY (BANTI'S SYNDROME.) This disorder, characterized by splenomegaly and hypersplenism, is due to obstruction of the splenic or portal veins or to cirrhosis of the liver. The symptoms are those of an enlarged spleen, hypersplenism, and the underlying condition. If portal hypertension is a major component, bleeding from esophageal varices is a frequent initial manifestation. Before splenectomy is considered, the site of obstruction must be determined, usually by angiography and portal pressure determinations. If only splenic vein obstruction is identified, splenectomy is curative. However, splenectomy alone in the face of cirrhosis or portal vein obstruction is contraindicated. Portacaval shunting with or without splenectomy may be indicated in the patient with recurrent bleeding from esophageal varices.

RUPTURE OF THE SPLEEN

Rupture of the spleen should be suspected in patients with left upper quadrant pain with or without splenomegaly following serious trauma to the left side, such as in motor vehicle accidents or contact sports. Enlargement of the spleen predisposes to traumatic rupture. Management of splenic trauma is in flux at the present time, with more attempts at nonoperative management or partial splenectomy. Preliminary data indicate that splenic preservation is safe in patients who are hemodynamically stable and closely monitored in the hospital. These newer techniques have the advantage of preventing the postsplenectomy syndrome.

Children who undergo splenectomy for trauma have a 50% incidence of *splenosis* (heterotopic autotransplantation of splenic tissue within the peritoneal cavity). This partial activity may help to explain the relatively low incidence of overwhelming infection in patients splenectomized for traumatic rupture. By periodically measuring the percentage of pocked red cells, development of splenosis can be documented. Since splenosis can become evident years after splenectomy, it is reasonable to enumerate pocked red cells every 6 months for 2 to 3 years. Although splenosis is felt to protect against postsplenectomy sepsis to a variable degree, documented cases of overwhelming sepsis have been reported in patients with splenosis. Therefore, the same cautious management of febrile episodes in patients splenectomized for ruptured spleen is indicated whether or not splenosis has been documented.

Lymphangitis

MAX L. RAMENOFSKY, M.D.

Lymphangitis is an inflammation of the lymphatic channels due to a local spreading distal infection. This was referred to in the past as "blood poisoning." Clinically lymphangitis is manifested as painful red streaks starting distally and moving proximally from the site of an infection. Regional lymph nodes are also usually affected.

In children, erysipelas is the most common cause, although deep puncture wounds are often incriminated. The most common organism is the streptococcus, and consequently any bacterial therapy is directed at eradicating this organism. Other occasionally involved organisms are staphylococcus and the gram-negative organisms.

Treatment. The infection at the site of entry must be cleaned, cultured, drained (if indicated), and appropriately dressed. Initial antimicrobial therapy is penicillin, and the route of administration is dictated by the severity of the illness. Usually, oral penicillin V, 250 mg every 6 hours, is adequate for the child under 10 years of age. For the older child, 500 mg every 6 hours is a reasonable dosage. The child who is septic and toxic and whose disease process is rapidly progressing should receive parenteral penicillin G, 100,000 u/kg/day. Should the child be sensitive to penicillin, erythromycin, 50 mg/kg/day in four divided doses is effective therapy. Antibiotics should be continued for 10 days and the physician should be alert for complications of streptococcal infection. Should staphylococcus be the offending organism, dicloxacillin, 50 mg/kg/day in four divided doses orally, or methicillin, 100 mg/kg/day IV, for severe infections should be used.

Puncture wounds deserve special attention when they result in lymphangitis. The puncture may have resulted in the inoculation of *Clostridium tetani*, which in the unimmunized child may be cata-

strophic. The puncture should be opened in a sterile fashion, irrigated, and dressed. If tetanus prophylaxis is not adequate, tetanus toxoid, 0.5 ml, or tetanus immune globulin, 250 units IM, should be given.

Patients at special risk for the development of lymphangitis as well as lymphadenitis are those in whom there is an abnormality of the lymphatic drainage system, such as lymphedema. The streptococcus is a common offending organism in this situation, although gram-negative organisms are more frequently cultured than in patients who do not have lymphedema. The appropriate antimicrobial drug should be started depending on the results of the culture. Oral penicillin V at doses described previously should be the drug of choice until the cultures return.

Lymph Node Infections

(Lymphadenitis)

MAX L. RAMENOFSKY, M.D.

Lymph node enlargement is common in childhood and adolescence but quite rare in the newborn. The most common cause of a mass in the neck during childhood is an enlarged lymph node, and it must be differentiated from other congenital cystic cervical masses such as branchial cleft cyst, thyroglossal duct cyst, and cystic hygroma. Infectious causes should be differentiated from noninfectious causes such as hyperplasia or neoplasia. Lymph node infections are either acute, developing over a period of 2 to 3 days, or chronic, developing over weeks to months.

Lymph nodes anywhere in the body provide drainage from other more peripheral areas. The location of the node(s) will give one an indication of where to look for the primary infection. The most common inflamatory lesion of a cervical lymph node is suppurative lymphadenitis, which is generally an acute process. The most common chronic cervical lymph node infections are atypical mycobacterial lymphadenitis, tuberculous lymphadenitis, and cat-scratch disease.

ACUTE SUPPURATIVE CERVICAL LYMPHADENITIS

Acute suppurative lymphadenitis is generally thought to be secondary to bacterial entry at some distal site. In the child it is most common from the first to the eighth year. Prior to the penicillin era, the most common offending organism was group A beta-hemolytic streptococcus. At present, the most common organism is *Staphylococcus aureus,* with streptococcus occupying the second position, and gram-negative organisms and anaerobes being found with increasing frequency.

There is a sudden onset of a rapidly growing, painful, red swelling in the neck, 2 to 3 days after an upper respiratory infection. The patient may be febrile and appear toxic. A leukocytosis is usual, with a left shift. At this point, unless the mass is fluctuant, needle aspiration or drainage is not recommended. A diligent search for the primary organ of entry should be done. In cervical lymphadenitis, sites to be carefully examined are the ears, the pharynx for tonsillitis or pharyngitis, and the oral cavity, particularly for dental caries and dental abscess. Therapy is started with an antistaphylococcal drug such as dicloxacillin sodium, 25 mg/kg/day orally, or methicillin, 100 mg/kg/day IV in four divided doses for 10 days. At these dosages both staphylococci and streptococci are adequately covered. The use of the antibiotics for greater than the prescribed interval is to be discouraged, as prolonged use often results in a chronic granulomatous lymphadenitis that will neither resolve nor fluctuate.

The lesions should be followed at frequent intervals and the antibiotics continued for 10 days. If, however, the lesion softens and becomes fluctuant, incision and drainage are mandatory and should be carried out following the principles of adequate drainage with optimal cosmesis. The incision should be along Langer's lines in the neck, with insertion of a soft rubber drain and a collecting dressing. At the time of drainage an adequate culture and Gram stain should be done to identify the offending organism. Anaerobic cultures should be included in the examination. The antibiotic may be discontinued twenty-four hours after a lesion has been drained unless there is evidence of a spreading cellulitis. The drain should be removed when there is adequate saucerization of the wound.

On occasion organisms other than staphylococci and streptococci have been identified. Of particular note is the plague-causing organism *Yersinia pestis*. Tularemia is another cause of cervical lymphadenitis but is usually associated with an eye infection or skin ulceration. The treatment for *Yersinia pestis* is streptomycin, 30 mg/kg/day, or chloramphenicol sodium succinate, 50 mg/kg/day IV, in four divided doses for 10 days if the child is less than 8 years of age. For older children, tetracycline, 25 to 50 mg/kg/day in four divided doses, is effective therapy. Occasionally the involved nodes from plague or tularemia require incision and drainage but these nodes should not be drained until after 24 hours of antibiotic therapy.

CHRONIC LYMPHADENITIS

Most patients with chronic lymphadenitis have enlarged, nontender, asymptomatic cervical masses.

Mycobacterial Lymphadenitis. Most cases of mycobacterial cervical lymphadenitis are no longer due to *Mycobacterium tuberculosis* but to atypical mycobacteria (MOTT, mycobacteria other than tuberculosis). Cervical lymphadenitis due to *M. tuberculosis* is usually an extension of a primary pulmonary infection and thus involves the supraclavicular nodes. Cervical lymphadenitis due to atypical mycobacteria is thought to be a primary infection gaining entrance through the pharynx or tonsils and thus involves higher cervical nodes such as the submandibular group.

The nodes of the child with tuberculous lymphadenitis are generally large, matted, and asymptomatic. Evidence of pulmonary tuberculosis is frequently found when the cervical lymphadenopathy is encountered but progress of the disease from lymphadenitis to pulmonary tuberculosis is rare. Central necrolysis of the involved nodes with the development of sinus tracts is uncommon but may occur if the nodes have not been aspirated or were incompletely excised at biopsy.

MOTT infection occurs in high cervical lymph nodes, generally the submandibular group. Very rarely will there be extranodal involvement and then only in the child who is immunosuppressed either primarily or secondarily. The involved nodes are usually large, matted, fixed, and nontender. The nodes of MOTT are likely to break down spontaneously and drain externally with the development of sinus tracts.

Diagnosis. The diagnosis of *M. tuberculosis* can be aided by identification of pulmonary tuberculosis on chest films. Skin testing will identify most children with mycobacterial infections. Most of these children have a positive skin test to PPD-S, first strength. In children having atypical mycobacterial lymphadenitis this is not so. Use of first strength PPD-S in MOTT infections will yield negative or questionable results in over half of children tested. Second strength PPD-S may confirm infection due to MOTT.

Treatment. The treatment of tuberculous lymphadenitis is antituberculous chemotherapy. Regardless of how the diagnosis is made, antituberculous chemotherapy should be instituted and continued for 2 years. Complete resolution of the disease is to be expected, including cutaneous sinus tracts. Chemotherapeutic agents for tuberculous lymphadenitis are isoniazid, 10 to 20 mg/kg/day up to 300 mg daily, and rifampin, 10 to 20 mg/kg/day up to 600 mg daily.

The treatment of lymphadenopathy due to atypical mycobacteria is complete excision of the involved nodes including culture. Antituberculous chemotherapy is neither indicated nor necessary. The vast majority of these children are cured, if all the involved nodes are removed.

CAT-SCRATCH DISEASE

Although the etiology of cat-scratch disease has never been proven, the infectious agent is thought to be a member of the Chlamydia genus, other members of which cause Lymphogranuloma venereum and psittacosis. Cat-scratch disease is the most common cause of chronic, nonbacterial lymphadenopathy.

The disease is generally transmitted by the scratch of a kitten, but monkeys and dogs as well as a thorny plant have been implicated in transmission. The animal carrier is not affected by the disease nor does it react with the antigen of cat-scratch disease.

Patients, when closely questioned, give a history of a minor scratch by a kitten 2 to 4 weeks before the onset of the lymphadenopathy. The inoculation site generally reveals a papule or blister. The most common sites of lymphadenopathy, corresponding to a distal inoculation site, are, in order of decreasing frequency, axillary, cervical, preauricular, submandibular, and epitrochlear.

Diagnosis. The diagnosis can be confirmed by a positive reaction to a skin test antigen prepared from the purulent aspirate of an involved node. As the antigen is not commercially available and difficult to obtain, the appropriate history with the findings of a chronic lymphadenitis allows a presumptive diagnosis of cat-scratch disease.

Treatment. There is no chemotherapy available for this disease. Excision of the involved node is generally curative, but on occasion aspiration will allow the node to heal. Culture and histologic evaluation of the aspirated or excised material will exclude other causes of chronic lymphadenopathy. Supportive care for such symptoms as headache, malaise, fever, and vomiting is indicated.

Cat-scratch disease is self-limited, and complete resolution is to be expected.

Lymphedema

BRIGID G. LEVENTHAL, M.D.,
and CHARLES S. TURNER, M.D.

Lymphedema may occur secondary to a traumatic, infectious, or surgical event. Lymphedema of the arm, for example, is a rather common complication of treatment for breast cancer; however, in the pediatric age group lymphedema is usually primary.

Attempts at medical management should be made in all patients. The patient's daily schedule should be altered to avoid prolonged standing and allow opportunities to elevate the extremity once or twice daily. In the early phase, it is vital to make every effort to control the swelling and prevent massive increase in extremity diameter. To assist this the patient should wear a firm elastic support at all times. Measurements for stockings should be made after a period of bed rest. Meticulous skin

care is important to avoid infection. Diuretics can be beneficial, particularly in the early course of management, and general weight loss may assist mechanical drainage of lower extremity lesions. Impairment of function, unsightly appearance, and fatigue related to the size and weight of the extremity are common symptoms. In addition, considerable morbidity and occasional death can occur in patients with lymphedema due to recurring episodes of cellulitis. These should be treated vigorously with antibiotics.

Indications for surgery are usually the huge size of the extremity or recurring cellulitis that in time becomes truly disfiguring. Surgery reduces the size of the extremity, but does not affect the basic lymphatic defect, so it should not be considered early in the course of the disease. Many surgical procedures have been proposed for lymphedema, which generally have two theoretical bases: excision of affected tissue or attempted physiologic restoration of lymphatic drainage. Physiologically designed procedures have not been uniformly successful in reconstructing lymphatic flow, and most recent reviews recommend excision of the skin and subcutaneous tissue with a thick split-thickness skin graft. Complications of these operations consist primarily of wound infections, hematomas, and necrosis of skin flaps. Patients who have already suffered recurrent cellulitis and lymphangitis are most likely to have a poor result after surgery, with cellulitis and lymphangitis continuing unabated after the operation. All patients must have adequate supportive care after surgery, with continued attention to limb elevation and elastic stockings.

Lymphangioma

BRIGID G. LEVENTHAL, M.D.,
and CHARLES S. TURNER, M.D.

Lymphangiomas are benign tumors thought to represent a developmental malformation arising as a result of sequestration of embryonic lymphatic vessels.

Simple lymphangiomas should be resected for cosmetic or functional reasons but complete excision is often difficult because of the multiple finger-like extensions of these tumors, which may render excision impractical because it results in excessive sacrifice of normal tissue. Complete excision is considered the treatment of choice for cystic hygroma and should be performed as soon as possible. Fluid will continue to reaccumulate as long as the endothelial cells are intact, so drainage of the lesions will not result in permanent control. However, the excision of a large cervical lesion in a very small infant may be a formidable procedure, and in a high-risk infant it may be advisable to delay surgery until an acceptable size and weight are achieved. This may require some measure of local control, such as intermittent incision and drainage of the tumor. Another reason to delay surgery may be the existence of active infection within the cystic tumor, but this delay should last only until the infection is controlled. Leaving the tumor in situ will only result in possible increased risk of secondary infection and hemorrhage, as well as tumor growth with extension into vital structures and increasing deformity.

Radiotherapy is generally not accepted as therapy for these benign and somewhat radioresistant lesions, and injection of sclerosing materials usually leads to no permanent improvement, but merely thickening of the cyst wall with increase in the difficulty of later definitive surgery. In some patients with lesions in the lining of the gastrointestinal tract, resection is being achieved with a diathermy snare.

Prior to surgery there should be a definition of the extent of the tumor by the most adequate technique, usually a computed tomography (CT) scan for neck lesions or lymphangiogram for extremity lesions. These tumors are often more extensive than is appreciated on external examination. About 10% of cervical tumors, for example, show extension into the mediastinum. Axillary and cervical lesions may interconnect.

The peri- and postoperative mortality in patients with cystic hygroma is 2 to 3%, with most reported operative deaths being related to tension pneumothorax or bronchopneumonia. An additional 1 to 2% of patients may die of nonoperative causes, such as associated congenital anomalies.

Complete excision is curative in over 75% of patients. Partial excision is curative in only 15 to 25% but the tumor may be reduced in size so that no further surgery is required. In some patients, however, multiple operations are required, particularly in patients in whom the vital structures of the oral cavity and neck are involved, which renders resection difficult and which may require reconstructive procedures in addition to resection. In one series, the average number of operations was 1.2 in patients whose tumor could be completely resected, and 5.2 in those whose tumor could not.

Malignant Lymphoma

LUCIUS F. SINKS, M.D.

The lymphomas represent several different disorders having in common a neoplastic process involving lymph nodes. Included in this group are Hodgkin's disease, non-Hodgkin's lymphoma, and Burkitt's lymphoma.

Table 1. ANN ARBOR STAGING FOR HODGKIN'S LYMPHOMA

Stage I:	Involvement of single lymph node regions (I) or single extralymphatic sites (I^e).
Stage II:	Involvement of two or more lymph node regions on one side of the diaphragm (II), or localized involvement of extralymphatic organs or sites and one or more nodal regions on the same side of the diaphragm (IIe).
Stage III:	Involvement of lymph node regions on both sides of the diaphragm, which also may be accompanied by localized involvement of extralymphatic organs or sites (IIIe) or, for example, spleen (III^s) or both (III^{s,e}).
Stage IV:	Diffuse or disseminated involvement of one or more extralymphatic organs or tissues, with or without lymph node involvement.

Each stage is subclassified into A or B according to the presence or absence of constitutional symptoms. These are unexplained fever of 38° C or more, night sweats, and unexplained weight loss of more than 10% body weight. Superscripts, after laparotomy, are applied to indicate sites of involvement, e.g., liver, spleen, lung, bone marrow, pleura, bone, and skin, respectively.

HODGKIN'S DISEASE

This disease is very effectively treated and cured. In early stage disease (Stage 1) (see Table 1), over 90% of the patients are expected to be cured. The therapy is radiotherapy alone or in conjunction with combination chemotherapy. Even though the therapy is effective, a number of clinical research trials are underway to refine it to ensure minimal long-range side effects. When dealing with children and adolescents with this disease, long-range side effects are of prime consideration. Such effects include secondary oncogenesis, growth impairment, breast atrophy, immune suppression, and sterility.

Stage I and II Disease. Early stage disease is usually treated by radiotherapy alone, with so-called extended fields to a dose of 3500 rads, based on the fact that the patient undergoes a staging laparotomy with splenectomy and that one is confident that no occult disease is located beneath the diaphragm. Such surgical staging procedures are avoided in children under the age of 5 because of the fear of life-threatening sepsis.

There currently exists a rational concept of radiation to *involved* fields only in combination with multiple drug chemotherapy in stage II disease. This has the advantage that the patient can be staged by nonsurgical means and offers the advantage of reduced size of the radiation field. This is particularly important in avoiding breast tissue atrophy in the prepubescent female. The administration of systemic chemotherapy thus ensures that occult disease below the diaphragm that has escaped detection by nonsurgical techniques will be adequately treated. This approach is comparable to extended field radiation; however, it will be several years before we can appreciate the relative long-range toxicities of the two different approaches.

Stage III and IV. In the patient with defined stage III disease, the current therapy best utilized in this age group is multiple drug chemotherapy followed by radiotherapy at 3500 rads directed to bulky disease only. Such therapy is very effective in controlling disease for prolonged periods of time. Fortunately, a smaller proportion of young children and adolescents present with advanced stage disease.

Staging. The surgical staging technique is less desirable in situations where systemic chemotherapy is utilized; however, when performed, it involves a splenectomy, periaortic lymph node biopsy, liver biopsy, bone marrow biopsy, and if radiation to the pelvic area is anticipated, an attempt at oophoropexy is made to remove the ovaries from the intended field.

Nonsurgical staging is undergoing technologic improvement as CT scans mature and replace older methods of radiologic procedures, such as lymphangiograms, which are extremely difficult to perform in young children and should only be attempted by skilled personnel.

Combination Chemotherapy. The original successful multiple drug chemotherapy of nitrogen mustard, prednisone, procarbazine and vincristine (MOPP) has paved the way for a number of other equally successful and, in some cases, less toxic combinations. One such is CVPP, which includes lomustine (CCNU), Velban, prednisone, and procarbazine. This combination has been equally effective and is less toxic. It also avoids the potential carcinogen nitrogen mustard. This has become of increasing concern as a number of adults who have been re-treated for relapsing Hodgkin's disease with MOPP and radiotherapy have developed acute leukemia.

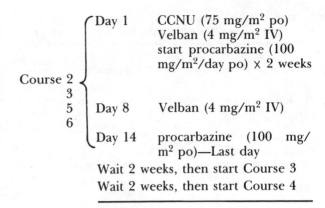

Wait 2 weeks, then start Course 3

Wait 2 weeks, then start Course 4

NON-HODGKIN'S LYMPHOMA

This disease in children and adolescents is usually a diffuse histiocytic or lymphocytic process involving lymph nodes; rarely is there a focal histologic pattern. In this age group the disorder is much more rapidly progressive than in older people and has a great tendency to involve the bone marrow, thus producing a leukemia-like picture.

The progressive and systemic nature of this disease dictates that the evaluation and staging of the patient be swift and that systemic therapy be administered.

Staging is controversial and does not influence the choice of therapy as it does in Hodgkin's disease. Radiation therapy plays a lesser role than it does in Hodgkin's and is usually limited to radiating bulky disease.

A number of combination chemotherapy schedules have been tested. The LSA$_2$–L$_2$ combination described by Wollner and associates at the Memorial Hospital for Cancer and Allied Diseases, New York, has gained wide acceptance, and although difficult to administer, has been successful. The most recent review demonstrates an 80% disease-free survival curve for such children, with a median of 7½ years. This includes all stages of disease (Table 2).

LSA$_2$–L$_2$ Schema with Drug Doses

INDUCTION PHASE. On the first day 1200 mg/m^2 cyclophosphamide are given in a single push injection to reduce the bulk of the tumor. Radiation therapy to the major site of primary disease is started either on the same day or within the next 3 days. On day 3 or 4, a 28-day course is started. This consists of daily oral prednisone, 60 mg/m^2; weekly intravenous injections of vincristine, 1.5–2.25 mg/m^2; intrathecal methotrexate, 6.25 mg/m^2, between the first and second vincristine injections, and two consecutive doses of intravenous daunomycin, 60 mg/m^2 each, between the second and third vincristine injections.

Dose and Schedule
CVPP Schedule

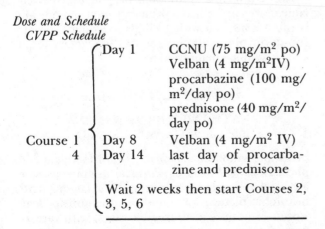

Nodal	Stage	Extranodal
One area.	I	One single site
Two or more areas either above *or* below diaphragm	II	One site + regional node. Two sites + regional nodes either above *or* below diaphragm
Two or more areas above *and* below diaphragm	III	Two or more sites above *and* below diaphragm
All extensive intrathoracic		All extensive intrathoracic
All extensive intraabdominal		All extensive intraabdominal
Central nervous system and/or bone marrow involvement	IV	Central nervous system and/or bone marrow involvement

*Memorial Hospital Staging System

After completion of this 28-day course and while the prednisone dose is being tapered, two more intrathecal injections of methotrexate are given, 2 to 3 days apart.

CONSOLIDATION PHASE. This phase starts within 1 week from the last dose of intrathecal methotrexate and consists of a combination of 15 doses of cytosine arabinoside, 150 mg/m², intravenously daily (Monday through Friday) and thioguanine given orally, 75 mg/m², 8 to 12 hours after the injection of cytosine arabinoside. If the white blood count remains adequate on the fifth day of cytosine arabinoside, the patient continues to receive the same dosage of thioguanine over the weekend. However, both drugs are discontinued temporarily if there is bone marrow depression; this usually occurs after the initial seventh to tenth doses of the combination and ordinarily recovers within 7 to 10 days. Hence, the patient may receive more than 15 doses of thioguanine orally but may receive only 15 doses of intravenous cytosine arabinoside. This first phase of the consolidation averages 30 to 35 days.

The second consolidation phase starts immediately after completion of the 15 doses of cytosine arabinoside and entails the administration of L-asparaginase intravenously, 6,000 u/m² daily for a total of 12 injections. Within 2 to 3 days after the last injection of L-asparaginase, two more intrathecal injections of methotrexate are given. These are followed within a few days by an intravenous injection of 1,3-bis(2-chloroethyl)-1-nitrosourea (BCNU), 60 mg/m², which completes the consolidation. The average duration of induction and consolidation is 125 to 132 days.

MAINTENANCE PHASE. Maintenance starts 1 to 2 weeks after the end of consolidation and comprises 5 cycles of 5 days each, with intervals of 7 to 10 days between cycles.

The first cycle starts with oral thioguanine, 300 mg/m², for 4 days, followed by intravenous cyclo-

phosphamide, 600 mg/m² on the fifth day. The second cycle consists of oral hydroxyurea, 2400 mg/m²/day for 4 days, followed on the fifth day by daunomycin, 45 mg/m² intravenously. In the third cycle, oral methotrexate, 10 mg/m²/day, is given for 4 days, followed on the fifth day by intravenous BCNU, 60 mg/m². The fourth cycle consists of daily injections of cytosine arabinoside, 150 mg/m² for 4 days, followed by the intravenous injection of vincristine, 1.5 mg/m² on Day 5. The fifth cycle consists only of two intrathecal injections of methotrexate, 6.25 mg/m² 2 to 3 days apart. The sequence of cycles, beginning with thioguanine, is restarted after a 7- to 10-day rest period. Each of these five-cycle courses of therapy usually takes from 55 to 65 days.

The initial therapy of non-Hodgkin's lymphoma requires very careful clinical observation, to avoid life-threatening complications secondary to acute tumor lysis, such as uric acid stones and hyperkalemia, and other problems, such as sepsis and bleeding. In these patients allopurinol should be started at the time of diagnosis and the serum potassium levels should be carefully monitored to avoid sudden cardiac arrest.

The incidence of central nervous system (CNS) involvement in this disorder is quite high in patients with bone marrow involvement and a leukemia-like picture. Under these conditions, the treatment may be modified to utilize prophylactic CNS measures such as cranial radiation. If CNS disease is detected during treatment by demonstration of blast cells in the cerebrospinal fluid, then effective therapy such as cranial radiation and intrathecal methotrexate must be used.

Non-Hodgkin's lymphoma involving the bowel, usually the terminal ileum, is one of the few instances where surgery plays an important role. These tumors and usually a segment of bowel should be resected and then the patient treated with chemotherapy. Radiation is sometimes necessary if bulky disease is left and is nonresectable.

Non-Hodgkin's lymphoma may in unusual circumstances present as a primary tumor of bone and is often confused with Ewing's sarcoma. Therapy should involve radiotherapy to the primary lesion with systemic chemotherapy.

Burkitt Lymphoma

NATHANIEL BROWN, M.D.,
and GEORGE MILLER, M.D.

Burkitt lymphoma is an acute non-Hodgkin lymphoma characterized by (1) focal tumor masses in a typical anatomic distribution; (2) a characteristic histologic picture; (3) rapid progression to death within 3 months in untreated cases, with rare reported cases of spontaneous remission; and (4) a high rate of initial response to chemotherapeutic agents.

Treatment of Burkitt lymphoma should begin as soon as the diagnosis is established. Since prognosis can be correlated with the extent of tumor "burden," it is customary in most centers to complete a quick (1-day) set of staging studies. All patients should have a bone marrow aspiration and lumbar puncture, and cytocentrifuged cerebrospinal fluid should be examined for the presence of tumor cells, which occasionally are noted at the time of initial presentation. In addition, a chest radiograph, intravenous pyelogram, bone films, [67]gallium citrate scan, complete blood count, serum electrolytes, and assessment of renal function are recommended.

Therapy begins with the concept that Burkitt lymphoma is generally a multisystemic disease at the time of clinical presentation. Usually, after the initial workup and staging procedures, multiple foci of tumor have been demonstrated, and all patients can be presumed to have diffuse "microscopic" disease. Hence, systemic chemotherapy is the chief mode of treatment, with surgery and radiotherapy confined to adjunctive roles.

Soon after Burkitt's description of the disease, it became evident that this cancer is particularly susceptible to cytotoxic agents. While effective therapy can produce survival statistics that nearly rival those of acute lymphocytic leukemia, the treatment strategies for these two lymphoid malignancies are quite different. The principles of therapy of Burkitt lymphoma have been most extensively articulated by Ziegler and associates at the National Cancer Institute (U.S.A.) and include (1) use of three to six semicontinuous cycles of cytotoxic agents to induce complete remission; (2) careful clinical monitoring (including bone marrow and CSF) for evidence of tumor relapse; and (3) aggressive treatment of CNS relapse or relapse at other sites, with type of treatment depending on site and time of relapse. Ziegler has noted that relapse in the first 3 months often includes the original tumor site and may consist of cells resistant to the agents used for remission induction, while relapse occurring later often involves distant body sites and may respond to renewed use of the induction protocol.

In general, regimens employing cyclophosphamide in high, single doses (at least 40 mg/kg, or 1000 mg/m^2, IV) have been most successful, with complete remission being induced in 80 to 95 per cent of presenting cases. Most current protocols also employ other drugs, with the hope that remission will be prolonged and the chance for survival enhanced. At the National Cancer Institute (U.S.A.), these other agents include vincristine, methotrexate, and prednisolone. Depending on the extent of disease at the time of presentation, three to six cycles of induction therapy are given at close intervals, allowing time only for recovery of the peripheral blood granulocyte count to 1500/mm^3 (generally about 2 weeks).

Unlike acute lymphocytic leukemias, maintenance chemotherapy has not proved important in Burkitt lymphoma to date. Similarly, while current protocols often routinely employ intrathecal therapy with methotrexate or cytosine arabinoside, prospective studies have failed to demonstrate the effectiveness of these agents, or craniospinal irradiation, for CNS prophylaxis. Intrathecal methotrexate or cytosine arabinoside is often effective in treating demonstrated CNS disease, however.

The use of other treatment modalities in Burkitt lymphoma is currently controversial. Surgery is felt by some authorities to be indicated for resection of abdominal tumors. In such instances, when the primary tumor bulk is often large, resection may prolong survival by reduction of tumor bulk and, in some cases, by allowing for improved renal function, if this has been compromised by the tumor.

It has been found that patients with less tumor bulk and normal renal function fare much better on the intense induction therapy regimen that Burkitt lymphoma demands. Patients with extensive disease or with renal compromise are particularly prone to succumbing in the first week of therapy to the so-called acute tumor lysis syndrome, a metabolic complication of rapid tumor-cell breakdown that results in metabolic acidosis with hyperuricemia, hyperphosphaturia (and hyperphosphatemia if renal function is compromised), hyperproteinemia, and hyperkalemia. Affected patients present severe management problems and may die suddenly from cardiac arrhythmia. To avoid this complication, the syndrome should be anticipated in every case of Burkitt lymphoma; hence, it is crucial that uricosuric agents (e.g., allopurinol) be used before and during chemotherapeutic efforts. When severe hyperuricemia is present, hemodialysis or peritoneal dialysis may be necessary.

Ideally, all patients presenting with Burkitt lymphoma should be treated by experienced oncologists, preferably at a center where this disorder is studied in a prospective, controlled fashion. With optimal treatment on current protocols, it appears that 40 to 50% of new patients will enjoy long-term survival. Current basic research continues to focus on the cause of the disease. The Epstein-Barr virus induces certain neoplastic changes in normal B-lymphocytes in vitro, including the ability to proliferate continuously in culture. Using recombinant DNA techniques, defined fragments of the EBV genome have been cloned in bacteria, and the function of these viral genes is being studied. It seems likely that detailed knowledge of the virus-induced changes in cellular proliferative capacity will afford important information on the regulation of growth in normal and neoplastic human cells and may ultimately prove directly beneficial in our treatment of Burkitt lymphoma.

9

Endocrine System

Hypopituitarism

BORIS SENIOR, M.D.

At the present time, treatment of growth hormone deficiency remains limited to the use of growth hormone extracted from human pituitary glands obtained at autopsy, one gland yielding approximately 8 units of growth hormone. The growth hormone is made available by the National Pituitary Agency and is restricted to children with clear-cut evidence of growth hormone deficiency who are participants in an approved research study and who would be expected to benefit from the therapy. Growth hormone is also now available from two commercial sources and is also restricted to children with unequivocal evidence of deficiency. The National Pituitary Agency provides growth hormone at no charge; the cost of a year's supply from the commercial sources is between $5,000 and $10,000. Efforts are also being made to produce human growth hormone using recombinant DNA technology.

It is important to explain to the parents and to a child who is old enough to understand what response may be expected to the therapy. Frequently, expectations are unrealistic, sometimes excessively so. Disappointment could lead to treatment being abandoned. Growth of approximately 7 to 11 cm may be seen during the first year of treatment, but the response is far from uniform. Thereafter, the rate of growth tends to slow and follow the curve parallel to the normal growth track. The younger the patient and the taller the parents, the better the response is likely to be.

Failure to respond adequately may be due to (1) Incorrect diagnosis—the need to be sure of the diagnosis before treatment is begun has been stressed; (2) An inadequate dose—increases in the amount of growth hormone are needed with time; (3) Failure to administer the growth hormone—no one enjoys injections, and children can easily develop an avoidance pattern; (4) Deficiency of thyroid hormone—a significant number of patients who are euthyroid when tested initially become mildly hypothyroid months or years later. Failure to detect and treat hypothyroidism will result in poor growth; and (5) Antibodies—improved extraction procedures provide a growth hormone that is not as prone to produce antibodies as earlier extracts were. Nevertheless, antibodies may occur. Even if present, antibodies need not necessarily inhibit the growth-promoting effect of growth hormone, but they may do so.

The human growth hormone can be administered by the parents or by the patient after instruction in the technique. It is given as an intramuscular injection three times weekly. Other than the trauma of the injection, no local or systemic ill effects occur. Depending on the age of the patient, the dose is between 0.5 and 4 units per injection; an average dose is 6 units/m²/week. Treatment is continued as long as the patient is able to and does respond or attains a height of 162.5 cm.

THYROID-STIMULATING HORMONE (TSH)

A deficiency of TSH may be present when the diagnosis of hypopituitarism is first made or may develop months or years later. Accordingly, even if thyroid function appears normal at first, one must continue to test at regular intervals, particularly as the clinical manifestations of secondary hypothyroidism tend to be subtler and milder than in primary hypothyroidism. If hypothyroidism is present, therapy consists of L-thyroxine. The dose is approximately 0.004 mg/kg once daily. In younger children, the per kilogram dose is higher and in older children the per kilogram dose is lower, with a range of 0.008 mg/kg down to 0.002 mg/kg. The adequacy of the dose is monitored by the clinical findings and by measurement of the concentrations of T_4 and T_3 in the blood.

ADRENOCORTICOTROPIC HORMONE (ACTH)

ACTH deficiency will result in diminished secretion of cortisol, but aldosterone secretion will remain adequate so that the concentrations of electrolytes in the blood remain normal. A deficiency of cortisol may lead to fasting hypoglycemia in the newborn period, but, in older subjects, clinical signs of the deficiency may only manifest with the stress of an infection or surgical procedure. Because of this, many withhold maintenance therapy except during periods of stress. We find that children who are deficient in cortisol may have little in the way of specific complaints but frequently comment that they feel stronger and more vigorous once maintenance treatment is introduced. Accordingly, we administer cortisone acetate, 0.6 mg/kg/24 hr in two doses, two thirds in the morning and one third at night. Because excess cortisone impairs growth and inhibits the growth-promoting effect of human growth hormone, care is needed so that no more cortisone is given than is necessary.

The patients are instructed to double the dose with any illness. If a patient is subjected to major stress, such as a surgical procedure, therapy consists of intramuscular cortisone acetate, 5 to 10 mg/kg for 24 hours before the procedure and daily thereafter as needed. Hydrocortisone hemisuccinate, 50 to 100 mg, is also kept available at all times for additional emergency intramuscular or intravenous use.

GONADOTROPINS

Puberty is frequently delayed in patients with isolated deficiency of growth hormone. Thus, absence of secondary sex characteristics in either sex at the usual ages need not necessarily imply that gonadotropins are lacking. As with diagnosis of deficiencies of the other tropic hormones, careful clinical observation, together with assays of luteinizing hormone and follicle-stimulating hormone, is needed.

Boys. Human chorionic gonadotropin, 1000 international units IM three times weekly, will stimulate the Leydig cells to produce testosterone. However, testosterone cypionate, 100 to 200 mg IM every 2 weeks, will be as effective in inducing secondary sex characteristics, at less cost and with far fewer injections. Later, when fertility is desired, treatment with menopausal gonadotropins is used to produce sperm.

Girls. We use cyclical therapy to induce secondary sex changes and menstruation. Premarin, 0.625 mg daily, is given continuously for 3 months and thereafter for the first 21 days of each calendar month. At this stage, Provera, 5 mg, is given in addition to the Premarin on days 14 through 21 of the calendar month.

DIABETES INSIPIDUS

This may be present as an isolated disorder or associated with deficiencies of anterior pituitary hormones. Again, it is important to be aware that a space-occupying lesion may be responsible and that continued careful surveillance is necessary.

Pitressin tannate in oil now has been supplanted by DDAVP (1-desaminocysteine-[8-D-arginine]-vasopressin acetate) as the therapy of choice. This synthetic analog of vasopressin contains 0.1 mg of DDAVP/ml. The dose varies from 10 μg once daily to 20 μg twice daily. Owing to its long duration of action, a single evening dose may suffice. It is administered intranasally through a soft, graduated plastic tube.

Tall Stature

EDGAR J. SCHOEN, M.D.

Large doses of sex steroids administered to tall children will shorten their ultimate height. But why treat a normal condition with potent agents? Tall stature is generally considered a social advantage, and sex steroids have potential risks. The indications for limiting height are psychosocial and cultural. Thus, the decision to treat a tall child must be carefully considered and must be based on informed agreement between the physician, the child, and the parents.

WHOM TO TREAT?

We do not treat tall stature unless the predicted mature height is over 183 cm (72 inches) in girls and over 198 cm (78 inches) in boys. There must be a strong desire for treatment in both parents and child. Typically, the patient is healthy and tall, is accompanied by very tall parents, and has a family history of tall ancestors. Only rare diseases cause increased height; among these are Marfan's syndrome, cerebral gigantism, hyperpituitarism, thyrotoxicosis, the feminizing testis syndrome, homocystinurea, and Klinefelter's syndrome. All candidates for estrogen or androgen treatment should, before considering therapy, receive a thorough examination to rule out the above conditions.

Mature height in normal tall children can be accurately predicted from age 9 years by assessing bone age according to the Gruelich and Pyle *Atlas* and using the tables of Bayley and Pinneau found in the back of the *Atlas*. Alternative systems using the Tanner-Whitehouse 2 (TW2) or the Roche-Wainer-Thissen (RWT) methods give comparable results. Height prediction should be based on accurate measurements, and bone age roentgenograms should be read by experienced observers.

Before treatment, it should be established that the child's ultimate height exceeds the limits mentioned, and that the child and parents understand the short-term and potential risks of treatment and feel that the psychosocial benefit of a modest shortening of height (an average of 5 cm (2 inches) in most series) outweighs these risks. After explaining these factors to the child and the parents separately, on at least two visits, we document the discussions in the record and ask the parents to sign a consent form.

HOW TO TREAT?

Girls. Treatment is started when the bone age is between 11 and 13 years and there is evidence of spontaneous puberty. In some instances, postmenarchal girls have been treated, but results seem better with earlier therapy. We use 10 mg conjugated estrogens (Premarin)* daily, adding 10 mg medroxyprogesterone acetate (Provera) for the last 7 days of each month. Others, believing that estradiol is a more natural estrogen, prescribe 0.3 mg ethinyl estradiol (Brevicon) daily, adding 10 mg norethindrone (Norlutin) daily for the last 7 days of each cycle. We currently use continuous rather than intermittent therapy.

Monthly menstruation usually begins 1 to 2 days after stopping the progestin and generally continues for a few days. Treatment is continued until bone age is 15 to 16 years, and the average duration of therapy is 1.5 to 2 years.

The patient is seen monthly during the first 90 days of therapy and every 3 months thereafter until growth has ceased. Bone age is determined every 6 months to assess acceleration of development.

Boys. Therapy is begun when the bone age is 12 to 14 years. We use testosterone cypionate (Depo-testosterone)† if necessary, a long-acting ester, 400 mg intramuscularly every 3 weeks. Treatment is continued until bone age reaches 17 to 18 years, a period usually lasting 1.5 to 2 years. Follow-up routine is similar to that described for girls.

SIDE EFFECTS (SHORT-TERM) AND RISKS (LONG-TERM) OF THERAPY

Girls. Secondary sexual characteristics progress rapidly, and the patient and family should be prepared for the physical and psychological changes of puberty. Morning nausea may occur during the first week of therapy. There is often hyperpigmentation of the nipples and areolae and a tendency toward increased weight gain. A few girls develop painful breast lumps, which usually disappear in a few weeks; breast fibroadenoma and intraductal papilloma have been reported, as has ovarian cystadenoma. Occasional mild, transitory hypertension is seen. Thromboembolic phenomena, a feared complication of estrogen administration, have not been reported in the vigorous, healthy young girls selected for therapy of tall stature. High-risk factors such as diabetes mellitus, varicose veins, marked obesity, and hyperlipidemia should preclude estrogen treatment.

Menses usually begin spontaneously within 8 weeks of completing treatment. Future fertility does not appear to be impaired in girls who have had high-dosage estrogen treatment for tall stature; many are now raising normal families.

The principal long-term side effect of high-dosage estrogen treatment is anxiety that therapy predisposes to future cancer, a fear not supported by any evidence to date.

Boys. Rapid pubertal changes should be anticipated, as in girls. There often is improved self-image and confidence. Acne, if present, may become worse and require local treatment. There is often increased weight gain. The testes decrease in size while on therapy but gradually increase to normal adult size within 1 to 2 years after cessation of treatment.

Thyroid Disease

DELBERT A. FISHER, M.D.

The spectrum of thyroid disease in pediatric patients is broad, and the therapeutic decisions often controversial. precise diagnosis highly sophisticated in vitro and in vivo procedures are available. Treatment in the pediatric setting, however, is less precise, and rarely emergency oriented. Long-term considerations thus become important: concerns such as the early thyroid hormone dependency of the central nervous system, thyroid hormone requirements for normal somatic growth, the radiation sensitivity of the child's thyroid gland, and the long life expectancy of children.

NEWBORN GOITER

In areas of the world without endemic goiter, thyroid enlargement in the newborn indicates either compromised capacity to synthesize thyroid hormones or neonatal hyperthyroidism. Therapy must be directed to possible local obstructive effects of the goiter as well as the associated thyroid dysfunction. Maternal ingestion of iodides for treatment of asthma or thyroid disease, or maternal antithyroid drug treatment for hyperthyroidism may

---

*This use is not listed in the manufacturer's instructions for Premarin, Provera, Brevicon, Norlutin.

†This use is not listed in the manufacturer's instructions for Depo-testosterone.

result in fetal goiter. On occasion the goiter can be very large, especially that due to iodine. If the airway is obstructed in the newborn with goiter, careful positioning with neck extension is appropriate with or without intubation. In severe cases, tracheostomy and/or subtotal thyroidectomy may be necessary.

Iodide-induced goiter in the newborn of a mother without hyperthyroidism or Graves' disease will spontaneously disappear within a period of 2 to 3 months. Remission can be hastened by administration of exogenous Na-1-thyroxine in a dose of 8 to 12 μg/kg/day for 3 months. It is important to document thyroid status in such infants by objective laboratory tests (serum thyroxine [T_4], free T_4 index, and TSH concentrations) before therapy and 1 month after discontinuing thyroid medication to exclude the possibility of permanent hypothyroidism.

NEONATAL GRAVES' DISEASE

If a mother has Graves' disease or a history of Graves' disease, neonatal thyrotoxicosis is a possible diagnosis. Such infants may or may not have a goiter at birth but usually have some enlargement of the thyroid gland. Because of transplacental passage of maternal antithyroid drugs and because the fetus converts T_4 predominantly to the inactive metabolite reverse T_3, the newborn with Graves' disease will usually appear euthyroid at birth. Thyroid function tests and careful follow-up of all newborns of mothers with Graves' disease or a history of Graves' disease is essential for early diagnosis. Therapy must be vigorous and includes sedatives and digitalization as necessary, and administration of a thionamide drug (propylthiouracil or methimazole) and/or iodides. The thionamides inhibit hormone synthesis; iodides potentiate this effect and, in addition, block thyroid hormone release. Adequate doses of both drugs are essential for most effective therapy. Propylthiouracil or methimazole* should be administered in doses of 5 to 10 mg/kg/day or 0.5 to 1.0 mg/kg/day, respectively, in divided doses at 8-hour intervals. Strong iodine solution (5 per cent iodine and 10 per cent potassium iodide, 126 mg of iodine per ml) is given in doses of 1 drop (about 8 mg iodine) every 8 hours. If a therapeutic response is not observed within 48 to 72 hours, the dose of both drugs (iodides and thionamide) can be increased 30 to 50 per cent.

Propranolol hydrochloride also is useful in controlling sympathetic overstimulation and can dramatically reduce cardiac rate; the recommended dose is 2 mg/kg/day divided into 2 or 3 portions. Finally, adrenal corticosteroids acutely inhibit thyroid hormone secretion in Graves' disease, and these drugs can be useful in unusually severe cases. Minimal effective doses have not been established, but the usual 2 mg/kg/day anti-inflammatory dose of prednisone would seem appropriate.

The need for careful follow-up cannot be overemphasized. In a significant proportion of infants prolonged or intermittent disease may ensue.

CONGENITAL HYPOTHYROIDISM

Congenital hypothyroidism is an important therapeutic problem in the newborn and small infant; diagnosis is difficult and delayed treatment can lead to irreversible mental retardation. The diagnosis may be suspected on the basis of results of newborn screening of blood T_4 and/or TSH levels or from clinical suspicion. The hypothyroidism may be *primary* due to thyroid dysgenesis, an inborn defect in thyroid hormone metabolism, or goitrogen exposure, or it may be *secondary* due to a hypothalamic-pituitary disorder.

Treatment of primary hypothyroidism is accomplished by administration of replacement thyroid hormone. Several preparations are available including synthetic Na-1-thyroxine (T_4), synthetic Na-1-triiodothyronine (T_3), combinations of synthetic thyroxine and triiodothyronine in a 4:1 ratio, thyroid USP, and thyroglobulin. Thyroid USP is a cleaned, dried, and powdered preparation of porcine or bovine thyroid gland previously deprived of connective tissue and fat. Thyroglobulin is the relatively purified porcine thyroid storage protein with a molecular weight approximating 700,000. Equivalent doses of the several preparations are Na-1-thyroxine, 100 μg (0.1 mg); Na-1-triiodothyronine, 25 μg (0.025 mg); $T_4 + T_3$, 50 to 60 μg and 12.5 to 15 μg, respectively; thyroid USP, 60 mg (1 gr); and thyroglobulin, 60 mg (1 gr).

Of these preparations Na-1-thyroxine is the drug of choice. It is more uniform in its potency and absorption; it is easily measured in serum and it provides physiologic serum T_3 levels since most of the circulating T_3 normally is derived from T_4 by monodeiodination in tissues. The dose of oral T_4 for infants is 8 to 12 μg/kg/day. The usual total daily dose during the first 6 months ranges from 30 to 50 μg (0.03 to 0.05 mg) (Table 1). Approximately 50 to 75% of the drug is absorbed so that the absorbed dose is less than the total dose.

In adults with hypothyroidism a rapid increase in metabolic rate may produce uncomfortable symptoms and cardiac decompensation if there is underlying cardiac disease. Therefore, treatment usually is begun with a small dose of hormone and the dose is increased gradually to optimal replacement levels. In infants, in contrast, it is important to achieve optimal replacement promptly in order to minimize the period of CNS thyroid hormone deficiency. The estimated total replacement dose is given orally

---

*This dosage may be somewhat higher than the manufacturer's recommendations.

Table 1. DOSE OF ORAL NA-1-THYROXINE FOR REPLACEMENT THERAPY OF HYPOTHYROIDISM IN INFANCY AND CHILDHOOD

Age	Usual Oral Dose of Na-1-Thyroxine	
	(μg/kg/day)	(Range of Dose μg)
1 to 6 months	7 to 12	30 to 50
6 to 12 months	6 to 8	50 to 100
1 to 5 years	4 to 6	75 to 150
5 to 10 years	3 to 5	100 to 200
10 to 20 years	2 to 3	100 to 250

from the first day of treatment. Some have advocated a relatively large intravenous priming dose of T_4 to achieve normal circulating levels more rapidly. Ten to 20 μg/kg of the IV preparation of Na-l-thyroxine can be injected intramuscularly daily for 2 days, after which oral medication can be substituted. Two to 4 weeks usually are required to observe the maximal effects from a constant dosage. In infants with severe hypothyroidism, this period may be more prolonged. In an occasional infant with a delayed diagnosis and severe disease associated with manifest or suspected cardiac disease a more gradual approach to optimal therapy over 4 to 6 weeks may be indicated. Overtreatment acutely produces tachycardia, excessive nervousness, disturbed sleep patterns, diarrhea and other findings suggesting thyrotoxicosis. Excessive dosage over a prolonged period may produce premature synostosis of the cranial sutures, undue advancement of bone age and osteoporosis.

Adequacy of therapy is judged, first, by clinical evidence of normal growth and development and lack of signs and symptoms of toxicity. Growth in length and weight should be plotted monthly during the first 3 months and at 2- to 3-month intervals thereafter during the first year. Bone age should be assessed at 3 months and at 6 to 12 months of treatment. Thereafter, 12- to 24-month evaluations will suffice. Measurements of circulating hormone concentrations are essential to assess adequacy of treatment. Measurements of T_4, TSH and, on occasion, T_3 are helpful. Serum T_4 levels should be adjusted to the upper two thirds of the normal range for age. At this time the serum TSH level should be normal or mildly increased, and the serum T_3 concentration within the normal range of age. Serum TSH concentrations tend to remain mildly elevated in the face of normal serum T_4 concentrations in infants with congenital hypothyroidism during T_4 treatment. This presumably is due to resetting of the T_4 negative feedback mechanism as a result of fetal hypothyroidism.

If the hypothyroidism is *secondary,* due to hypothalamic-pituitary dysfunction, treatment with adrenal corticosteroids and growth hormone (GH) is necessary if deficiencies of ACTH and GH are documented. Adrenal insufficiency may be manifest as failure to thrive and/or hypoglycemia in the neonatal period. GH deficiency also may contribute to hypoglycemia and may impair growth after 3 to 6 months.

HYPOTHYROIDISM IN CHILDHOOD AND ADOLESCENCE

Acquired hypothyroidism before 5 or 6 years most commonly results from delayed failure of the thyroid remnant in infants with thyroid dysgenesis, but inborn defects in thyroid hormone synthesis, ingested goitrogens, chronic thyroiditis or hypothalamic-pituitary disease may be involved. After 5 to 6 years the same spectrum of etiologies is involved, but hypothyroidism most commonly is due to chronic lymphocytic (Hashimoto's) thyroiditis. Surgery or radioiodine treatment also can result in hypothyroidism.

Irreversible brain damage is not a likely result of hypothyroidism acquired after 2 or 3 years of age. By this time CNS growth is largely complete. Delayed growth, however, may be marked, and most commonly is manifest as delayed tooth development and eruption, delayed skeletal growth and maturation, and linear growth retardation. Aberrations in pubertal development and menstrual irregularities are common. These manifestations are reversible with adequate replacement therapy. As in infants, the treatment of choice is oral Na-l-thyroxine. The replacement dose on a body weight basis decreases progressively with age (Table 1). The dosage should be adjusted at 2- to 4-week intervals to a level which maintains the serum T_4 concentration in the mid-range of normal together with normal T_3 and TSH concentrations. In contrast to adults, it is not necessary in most children with hypothyroidism to increase the dose of replacement T_4 gradually. Initial administration of the total daily estimated replacement dose will result in a gradual increase in serum T_4 concentrations over a 3- to 4-week period. If cardiac disease is suspected, more gradual replacement may be indicated.

Treatment of secondary hypothyroidism in childhood or adolescence may require stimultaneous replacement with adrenal corticosteroids, growth hormone and gonadal steroid(s).

SUPPURATIVE THYROID DISEASE

Acute suppurative thyroiditis is rare in childhood. Infected thyroglossal duct cysts or thyroglossal duct remnants are more common. Therapy is directed to the offending organism(s) as well as the underlying embryologic abnormality. Surgical drainage may be necessary acutely. Definitive surgery is delayed and is conducted on an elective basis after resolution of the acute infection.

ACUTE-SUBACUTE NONSUPPURATIVE THYROIDITIS

This entity usually is referred to as subacute thyroiditis because the course runs several weeks to several months. The disorder is self-limited and of uncertain cause, although it seems likely that most cases are of viral etiology. There are local and systemic manifestations of the inflammatory process as well as a transient hypermetabolism due to release of thyroid hormones from the damaged follicular cells. There is no specific therapy; antithyroid drugs are of little benefit. Symptomatic treatment (usually salicylates) for the local and/or systemic discomfort is helpful. Patients with marked painful goiter have been treated with adrenal corticosteroids, but such therapy usually is not warranted. When hyperthyroid manifestations are marked, propranolol may be useful.

HASHIMOTO'S THYROIDITIS

Hashimoto's thyroiditis, or chronic lymphocytic thyroiditis, is an autoimmune disease most frequently involving only the thyroid gland. Occasionally, however, Hashimoto's thyroiditis is associated with other endocrine gland autoimmunity and deficiencies. These include the pancreas and diabetes mellitus, the adrenal gland with adrenal insufficiency, the parathyroid glands with hypoparathyroidism and, on rare occasions, the gonads with hypogonadism. Autoimmune gastritis with pernicious anemia and cutaneous moniliasis sometimes are associated. Treatment of all the endocrine gland deficiencies may be necessary. Most frequently, however, the disease involves only the thyroid gland and presents as a mild to moderate euthyroid goiter. The disease remits spontaneously in about one third of children. The remainder gradually develop hypothyroidism. There is no specific therapy, but if the goiter is large, if the serum TSH concentration is elevated, or if the patient is clinically hypothyroid, replacement therapy with Na-l-thyroxine is indicated. Some physicians favor thyroxine treatment of all children with Hashimoto's thyroiditis to avoid mild, undiagnosed hypothyroidism.

NONTOXIC DIFFUSE COLLOID GOITER
(Simple Goiter; Colloid Goiter)

Simple colloid goiter refers to a smooth, symmetrical enlargement of the thyroid gland in a euthyroid patient without detectable abnormality in thyroid function tests or thyroid autoantibody titers. It is most common during adolescence in females and has been referred to as adolescent goiter. The goiter usually disappears spontaneously and requires no treatment. Some prefer to prescribe thyroid hormone replacement therapy, particularly if the goiter is large.

JUVENILE HYPERTHYROIDISM

Chronic hyperthyroidism in childhood usually is due to Graves' disease, but less commonly can be associated with Hashimoto's thyroiditis, hyperfunctioning thyroid nodule(s) or, rarely, TSH hypersecretion. Treatment is directed to the thyroid hormone hypersecretion and the cause of the hyperthyroid state when possible.

Treatment of the hyperthyroid state may be accomplished with antithyroid drugs, surgery or radioiodine. Radioiodine treatment is not considered the approach of first choice in children. There is a 10% incidence of permanent hypothyroidism during the first year after treatment and an additional 2 to 3% incidence yearly thereafter. Thus 10 to 20 years post-treatment about half of radioiodine treated patients will be hypothyroid. Projection of this figure suggests that hypothyroidism is nearly inevitable in children thus treated. Additionally, in contrast to adults, children after radioiodine therapy of thyrotoxicosis may have an increased incidence of thyroid malignancy, including both adenoma and carcinoma. The experience, however, is limited to date, both in terms of numbers of children treated and the duration of follow-up. Finally, the results are not uniformly good. About 10% of children treated with radioiodine have experienced relapse and about 5% have been operated upon subsequently.

Surgery has the disadvantages of a finite mortality, considerable morbidity, and a significant incidence of complications. These include recurrent laryngeal nerve damage with vocal cord paralysis and permanent hypoparathyroidism. The combined incidence of the latter problems has varied from 1 to 8% in several reports, and probably averages 2 to 3% in most clinics. In addition, there is a 25% incidence of permanent hypothyroidism after 15 to 20 years. For these reasons, surgery is not usually considered the therapy of first choice.

Medical therapy with antithyroid drugs is considered the treatment of choice by most pediatric endocrinologists. Both propylthiouracil (PTU) and methimazole (Tapazole) are effective. These are drugs of the thionamide class which act by inhibiting the organification of iodine and hormone synthesis by the thyroid gland. PTU also inhibits peripheral tissue conversion of thyroxine to triiodothyronine, but this action is of lesser importance in chronic therapy of thyrotoxicosis. Both drugs can produce skin rash, drug fever, agranulocytosis and rarely a collagen-vascular-like reaction. Drug fever and rashes occur in 3 to 5% of cases and disappear promptly on withdrawal of medication. Agranulocytosis occurs in 0.2 to 0.3% and usually is observed during the first 6 to 8 weeks of treatment. Agranulocytosis resolves upon drug withdrawal and administration of antibiotics.

Initial therapy is instituted with PTU, 5 to 7 mg/kg/day, or methimazole, 0.5 to 0.7 mg/kg/day*, in 3 divided doses at about 8-hour intervals. The dose is increased if improvement is not observed within 2 to 3 weeks. Nearly all patients will respond to PTU in doses of 10 to 15 mg/kg or methimazole in doses of 1 to 1.5 mg/kg/day. However, an occasional patient may require as much as 20 mg/kg/day* for control. Methimazole has a longer half-life than PTU, and some patients will maintain effective blockade of thyroid hormone synthesis with once-daily drug administration, particularly after remission has been induced. PTU often can be given in 2 daily doses.

In patients with severe disease or distressing cardiovascular symptoms, propranolol** is useful adjunctive therapy; 0.1 to 0.3 mg/kg IV followed by 2 mg/kg/day orally in divided doses, or oral therapy alone has been utilized. The dose of propranolol can be increased to 4 to 6 mg/kg/day.

Potassium iodide in large doses potentiates the action of thionamide drugs and inhibits thyroid hormone secretion. The effect, however, is transient. Therapeutic doses for hyperthyroidism range from 2 to 4 mg/kg/day, usually given as strong iodine solution or a saturated solution of potassium iodide. The inhibitory effect on hormone synthesis and/or release usually persists 10 to 40 days. Thus potassium iodide is most useful for short-term treatment of severe disease and for preoperative preparation of patients for surgery.

After the patient has become euthyroid, which usually takes 30 to 90 days, the daily dose of medication can be reduced to 3 to 4 mg of PTU/kg or 0.3 to 0.4 mg of methimazole/kg. Treatment must be monitored with measurements of serum T_4 concentrations to ensure an adequate drug effect and avoid hypothyroidism. Measurements of serum T_3 concentration often are useful when the clinical assessment and serum T_4 measurements are in disagreement; on occasion the antithyroid medication will be adequate to inhibit T_4 but not T_3 secretion, and the patient will appear euthyroid or even hyperthyroid, with low levels of serum T_4. Serum TSH measurements are helpful in assessing drug-induced hypothyroidism.

It is possible in follow-up either to adjust the antithyroid drug dosage to maintain normal thyroid hormone levels or to continue a blocking dose which produces hypothyroidism and maintain the

patient on exogenous Na-l-thyroxine in replacement doses. The duration of antithyroid drug treatment cannot be predicted and usually is considered long-term—1 year or more. The rationale is that Graves' disease, like other autoimmune disorders, usually remits spontaneously. Drug treatment only maintains a euthyroid state as we await such remission. The remission rate approximates 25% each 2 years. As a general rule, patients with continuing goiter not due to drug-induced hypothyroidism will experience exacerbation of hyperthyroidism if treatment is withdrawn. Also remission is not likely if the thyroid gland remains nonsuppressible.

At the end of 1 year, if the goiter has disappeared and the patient is euthyroid, treatment can be discontinued. Some physicians prefer to document suppressibility before drug withdrawal. Perhaps 30% of patients will remain in remission off treatment after 1 year, and some feel that 3 months of treatment is adequate to define this group. The majority require long treatment; perhaps 50% will require 4 or more years of treatment before remission occurs.

If drug toxicity ensues, the drug becomes ineffective for patient or pharmacologic reasons, or if the goiter is large and unresponsive to a reasonable drug treatment regimen, alternative treatment may be considered. If an experienced thyroid surgeon is available, thyroidectomy may be preferable. Radioiodine is a viable alternative in the adolescent. It should be emphasized, however, that the physician threshold for abandoning medical therapy should be kept relatively high. These patients require frequent follow-up, support and encouragement.

Graves' ophthalmopathy is common in juvenile patients, but usually is not severe. Lid retraction, lid lag, stare and mild to moderate proptosis are seen, but severe infiltrative changes, proptosis and eye muscle weakness are rare. Thus, specific treatment for ophthalmopathy is not usually necessary during childhood and adolescence. If periorbital edema should occur, the patient should sleep with the head of the bed elevated. Patients with diplopia should wear an alternating eye patch. If the eyelids fail to close properly a protective shield at school or while sleeping is useful. More severe disease requires consideration of adrenal corticosteroid treatment and/or surgery.

THYROID NODULES

Thyroid nodules in children are significant for three reasons: they may herald underlying thyroid disease, they may be hyperfunctioning nodules and produce hyperthyroidism, or they may represent carcinoma. In the first instance, the approach is to the basic disease, often Hashimoto's thyroiditis. Functioning nodules producing clinical and chemical thyrotoxicosis require treatment, and surgery is

---

*These doses may be higher than manufacturer's recommendations.

**Manufacturer's precaution: Data on use of propranolol in children are too limited to permit adequate directions for use.

the most frequently employed and reliable therapeutic modality. Partial thyroidectomy is conducted with minimal risk of recurrent nerve or parathyroid gland damage. Functioning nodules not resulting in hyperthyroidism have a very low incidence of malignancy and can be followed without treatment. Nonfunctioning or "cold" nodules—those which do not concentrate radioiodine—are considered potentially malignant. The likelihood of carcinoma in a cold nodule in an otherwise normal thyroid gland approaches 40% in children. Most of these are thyroid follicular cell neoplasms, but about 5% are medullary carcinomas secreting calcitonin and can be identified with a serum calcitonin measurement with or without stimulation.

It is difficult to differentiate malignant and nonmalignant masses in the remainder of cases. Surgery is indicated if there is a prior history of therapeutic radiation to the head or neck, if the nodule is hard, if there is evidence of tracheal invasion (dysphagia, hoarseness or cough) or vocal cord paralysis, if adjacent lymph nodes are involved, or if there are distant metastases. If none of these malignancy criteria is present thyroid suppression with 0.2 to 0.3 mg of Na-l-thyroxine daily can be employed. If over a period of 4 to 6 months the nodule grows, or if over a period of 12 months the nodule does not decrease in size, surgery is indicated. If the nodule decreases in size longer follow-up is in order. It is important to remember that thyroid follicular cell carcinomas in children are rather indolent neoplasms and do not require urgent treatment.

Parathyroid Disease: Hypoparathyroidism and Pseudohypoparathyroidism

JOSEPH I. WOLFSDORF, M.D.

The aim of treatment is to restore normal serum levels of calcium and phosphate while avoiding the deleterious effects of hypercalcemia. Three forms of treatment are available: large doses of vitamin D, dihydrotachysterol (DHT), and 1,25-dihydroxyvitamin D_3 (calcitriol). Large doses of vitamin D used to be the mainstay of treatment, but the other choices are safer and more convenient. Because vitamin D is slowly metabolized, its action tends to be cumulative; therefore after months of therapy hypercalcemia may develop, which may persist for many weeks despite stopping treatment.

1,25-Dihydroxyvitamin D_3, the natural, active form of vitamin D, is synthesized from 25-hydroxyvitamin D by 1-α-hydroxylase in the kidney. It has been widely used to treat hypoparathyroidism and pseudohypoparathyroidism, and is both safe and highly effective. The great advantage of 1,25-dihydroxyvitamin D_3 is its rapid onset of action (1 to 4 days) and short biologic half-life (less than 9 days); if hypercalcemia occurs, serum calcium levels return to normal within a few days of stopping the medication. I recommend 1,25-dihydroxyvitamin D_3 as the treatment of choice for hypoparathyroidism and pseudohypoparathyroidism; however, it is expensive.

If 1,25-dihydroxyvitamin D_3 cannot be used, DHT, an analog of vitamin D that does not require hydroxylation at the 1-carbon position, is equally effective in treating hypoparathyroidism. DHT and 1,25-dihydroxyvitamin D_3 have similar biologic effects; both stimulate intestinal absorption of calcium, mobilize calcium from bone in the absence of parathyroid hormone, and increase the renal excretion of phosphate. Hypercalcemia must be avoided, and the patient's serum calcium level should be measured frequently: twice weekly for the first few weeks after starting treatment, and thereafter at progressively less frequent intervals once stable levels have been achieved. To prevent deleterious effects of hypercalciuria on the kidney, it is advisable to measure calcium and creatinine in urine samples obtained at each visit. A ratio of calcium to creatinine in the urine that exceeds 0.4 indicates hypercalciuria, and is an indication to reduce the dose of medication even though the serum calcium level is not obviously above the normal range. Both 1,25-dihydroxyvitamin D_3 and DHT have a small margin between therapeutic and toxic doses; consequently the serum calcium level should be maintained in the lower range of normal—8.5 to 9.5 mg/dl. Attempts to keep the calcium closer to 10 mg/dl will result in more frequent episodes of hypercalcemia. If hypercalcemia does occur, stop the medication immediately and, after the serum calcium has returned to normal, restart at a lower dose.

The dose required for each patient must be established empirically, starting at the lower end of the recommended dose range.

1,25-Dihydroxyvitamin D_3 (calcitriol): The usual daily dose in children is 0.25 to 1.0 μg or approximately 0.015 to 0.025 μg/kg/24 hr.

Dihydrotachysterol: The usual daily dose in infants and young children is 0.1 to 0.5 mg; for older children and adults, 0.5 to 1.0 mg (0.01 to 0.02 mg/kg/24 hr).

Vitamin D_2 (ergocalciferol) is the cheapest available agent. The dose of vitamin D required to restore normal levels of serum calcium and phosphate in hypoparathyroidism far exceeds physiologic requirements. The maintenance dose averages 2000 I.U. (50mg) /kg/day, but sensitivity to vitamin D varies from individual to individual. The initial requirement of vitamin D is similar in pseudohypoparathyroidism; however, in this disorder the dose can often be reduced later.

Therapy is initiated with 2000 I.U./kg/day by mouth. The liquid form of vitamin D is preferred because it permits precise adjustment of dose. The liquid is administered directly into the patient's mouth from a tuberculin syringe. Unacceptable variation in the size of the dose can occur when the medication is given with a dropper.

In patients with symptomatic hypocalcemia, treatment with vitamin D can be started with a dose of 8000 I.U./kg/day. The serum calcium is measured daily, and as soon as the level reaches 9.0 mg/dl, the dose of vitamin D should be reduced to 2000 I.U./kg/day.

Most patients achieve normal serum calcium levels without the addition of calcium salts. The routine use of calcium salts in addition to either DHT or 1,25-dihydroxyvitamin D_3 is usually neither necessary nor desirable. Patients who do not respond satisfactorily to treatment with DHT or 1,25-dihydroxyvitamin D_3 may benefit from additional calcium, either as calcium lactate or gluconate, in a dose of 5 to 10 grams daily. The administration of aluminum gels to bind intestinal phosphate is usually not necessary.

Resistant mucocutaneous candida infections often occur in patients with hypoparathyroidism. Local and oral nystatin usually controls the infection but eradication of candida with presently available medications is seemingly impossible.

Tetany and Hypocalcemic Seizures. Tetany or seizures due to hypocalcemia are treated with calcium salts given intravenously. This involves the cautious administration of a 10% solution of calcium gluconate (9.4 mg of elemental calcium per ml) in a dose of 2 ml/kg of body weight. During the infusion of calcium, the heart rate should be monitored, preferably with an electrocardiogram. The appearance of bradycardia is an indication to halt the infusion. Too rapid an infusion of calcium may cause cardiac arrest. Maintenance administration of calcium gluconate in a dose of 500 mg/kg/24 hr should follow the acute treatment. During the acute phase, the serum calcium level should be determined daily or twice daily to assess the efficacy of therapy and prevent hypercalcemia.

HYPOPARATHYROIDISM REFRACTORY TO TREATMENT

Occasionally one encounters a patient who, after an initial favorable response, becomes resistant to treatment. There is not always a clear explanation for this phenomenon. Certain patients with autoimmune idiopathic hypoparathyroidism have intestinal malabsorption that impairs the absorption of orally administered fat-soluble steroids. Larger doses of DHT or 1,25-dihydroxyvitamin D_3, to-

gether with supplementary calcium salts, usually produce normal levels of serum calcium. In addition, the steatorrhea may improve, suggesting that hypocalcemia itself adversely affects intestinal absorption of fat.

Magnesium deficiency is another cause of resistance to treatment. It should be remembered that hypomagnesemia frequently accompanies hypocalcemia in patients with hypoparathyroidism. When the hypoparathyroidism is treated, the magnesium level rises, though usually less rapidly than does the calcium level. Certain patients, however, are resistant to vitamin D therapy and respond more favorably after magnesium has been given. Magnesium can be given intramuscularly as magnesium sulfate (0.2 ml/kg of 50 percent $MgSO_4 \cdot 12H_2O$). If renal function is normal, the serum magnesium concentration will fall to pretreatment levels in 4 to 6 hours, so that repeated injections are necessary to maintain normal concentrations. For chronic treatment, oral magnesium as magnesium chloride, citrate, or lactate, 2 to 4 mEq/kg/24 hr in divided doses, can be used.

HYPERCALCEMIA

Hypercalcemia is defined as a serum calcium concentration greater than 11 mg/dl.

The aims of treatment are to initially lower the serum calcium concentration quickly and then to eliminate the underlying cause of the hypercalcemia whenever possible. The rationale of treatment is to augment calcium excretion, diminish absorption of calcium from the gut, and decrease its resorption from bone.

The diet should be low in calcium and all sources of vitamin D eliminated. In addition, the patient should not be exposed to sunshine during the hypercalcemic phase.

The urinary excretion of calcium is increased by providing a high fluid intake. Isotonic saline at 2 to 4 times the maintenance rate, combined with furosemide, 1 mg/kg every 6 to 8 hours, produces natriuresis and calciuresis. Fluid and electrolyte intake and output must be monitored carefully to prevent dehydration and depletion of electrolytes.

Hypercalcemia unresponsive to these measures necessitates more aggressive treatment. Intravenous infusion of phosphate cannot be recommended because of the danger of metastatic calcification. Intravenous infusion of isotonic (0.12M) sodium sulfate may cause hypernatremia and is rarely used today. Oral phosphate (Neutra-Phos, a solution of sodium and potassium phosphate), although slower in its onset of action and less predictable in effect, does not carry the same risks as intravenous phosphate. One should provide 1 to 3 grams of phosphorus in divided doses each day. Each 300 ml of Neutra-Phos solution supplies 1 gram of phosphorus. Gastrointestinal discomfort and diarrhea are common side effects.

Although the beneficial effect may be delayed for several days, pharmacologic doses of glucocorticoids (prednisone, 1 to 2 mg/kg/24 hr) interfere with intestinal calcium transport and are effective in reducing the hypercalcemia of vitamin D intoxication, sarcoidosis, and adrenal insufficiency. Glucocorticoids have a mild calciuretic effect but are rarely effective in the hypercalcemia of hyperparathyroidism. On the other hand, in tumor-associated hypercalcemia, steroids may be valuable, primarily because of their direct antitumor action. In this situation, the hypercalcemia often takes several days to respond, and other measures are required in the interim.

Mithramycin, an antineoplastic antibiotic, is a patent calcium-lowering agent that directly inhibits bone resorption. It is given intravenously over 4 hours in a dose of 25 μg/kg. It is usually effective within 12 to 36 hours and the effect persists for 3 to 7 days. Thrombocytopenia is a potential side effect.

Calcitonin is another agent that may be used to treat resistant hypercalcemia. It inhibits mobilization of calcium from bone and to some extent reduces renal tubular reabsorption of calcium. The response occurs within 2 to 3 hours but is transitory; hence, calcitonin must be administered every 12 hours. Calcimar (salmon calcitonin) is given either as an intramuscular or subcutaneous injection. The recommended starting dose is 4 MRC units/kg. If within 24 to 48 hours the response has not been satisfactory, the dose can be increased to a maximum of 8 MRC units/kg, given every 6 hours. Its lack of toxicity makes calcitonin an attractive hypocalcemic agent.

If the measures described above fail, either peritoneal dialysis or hemodialysis against solutions low in calcium may be undertaken as a last resort. Dialysis can rapidly reduce a high level of serum calcium. Occasionally a patient with primary hyperparathyroidism does not respond to these measures and requires an emergency parathyroidectomy. Whatever the therapeutic approach, the treatment of a hypercalcemic crisis is a holding measure until the underlying disease can be tackled definitively.

PRIMARY HYPERPARATHYROIDISM

This disorder is extremely rare in children. The treatment of hyperparathyroidism is either subtotal or complete parathyroidectomy. Recently, a new strategy has been recommended, involving total parathyroidectomy and the transplantation of a portion of the excised parathyroid gland into the muscles of the patient's forearm. If the grafted tissue becomes hyperplastic, causing a recurrence of the hypercalcemia, it is easy to remove.

Disorders of the Adrenal Gland

MARIA I. NEW, M.D.,
LENORE S. LEVINE, M.D.,
and JEAN W. TEMECK, M.D.

It is prudent for every patient with adrenal insufficiency to wear a medic-alert bracelet, medallion, or card.

ADRENAL HYPERPLASIA DUE TO ENZYMATIC DEFICIENCY OF STEROIDOGENESIS

Classic (Congenital) (CAH). In the virilizing forms of this disorder (21-hydroxylase, 11β-hydroxylase deficiency, and 3β-hydroxysteroid dehydrogenase deficiency), females usually have clitoromegaly. If clitoromegaly is mild, the clitoris may become hidden by the labia majora as the child grows and is under treatment. However, most cases require surgery involving either removal (resection) of redundant erectile tissue with preservation of the sexually sensitive glans clitoris or clitoral recession. The procedure is usually done at the age of 1 year. A vaginoplasty may also be necessary and is generally performed during early adolescence.

Incomplete virilization occurs in males with cholesterol desmolase deficiency, 3β-hydroxysteroid dehydrogenase deficiency, and 17α-hydroxylase deficiency. The virilization may be so incomplete as to make the female sex assignment more appropriate. Surgery is performed to correct the genital abnormality to conform with the sex of assignment. Sex hormone replacement is necessary to induce and maintain secondary sex characteristics at puberty.

The glucocorticoid deficient forms of this disorder (21-hydroxylase, 11β-hydroxylase, 3β-hydroxysteroid dehydrogenase, 17α-hydroxylase, and cholesterol desmolase deficiency) require cortisol replacement. This not only corrects the deficiency but also suppresses ACTH oversecretion. Therefore, excessive stimulation of the androgen pathway, and consequently further virilization, is prevented, allowing normal growth and puberty. Of the various forms of steroid treatment available, we employ hydrocortisone. The dose varies widely depending on the patient, but the average requirement is 20 to 25 mg/m^2/day in two or three divided doses.

The mineralocorticoid deficient forms (salt-wasting 21-hydroxylase, 3β-hydroxysteroid dehydrogenase, cholesterol desmolase, 18-hydroxylase, and 18-dehydrogenase deficiency) require salt-retaining hormone replacement. Fludrocortisone (Florinef) is most commonly used and the usual dose is 0.05 to 0.1 mg/day. It is also helpful in patients with simple virilizing 21-hydroxylase deficiency with high plasma renin activity (PRA), where the addition of salt-retaining steroids to the treatment regimen suppresses renin and may permit a decrease in the glucocorticoid dose. Sodium chloride tablets may be used for infants in a dose of 3 to 5 mEq/kg/day. There is a 17 mEq Na^+/tablet which may be divided into two to four equal parts, crushed, and added to the infant's formula.

Therapy should be regulated by clinical and biochemical parameters. Clinically, it is important to monitor the child's growth and pubertal development. Biochemically, sensitive measurements of control are serum 17-hydroxyprogesterone and Δ4-androstenedione. In females and prepubertal males, serum testosterone is also useful but not in newborns and pubertal males.

PRA is a helpful index of therapeutic control in virilizers as well as salt-wasters. PRA is closely correlated with the ACTH level, and normalization of PRA may result in decrease in ACTH. Also, normalization of PRA allows for improved statural growth. Monitoring of PRA is also helpful in these forms of CAH with mineralocorticoid excess (11β-hydroxylase and 17α-hydroxylase deficiency). In the mineralocorticoid-deficient forms, PRA is increased in poor control, and in the mineralocorticoid-excess form, it is suppressed.

Follow-up visits should occur at 3 month intervals. In addition to monitoring the above parameters above, a bone age should be obtained yearly.

Nonclassic 21-Hydroxylase Deficiency

Symptomatic (Acquired or Late Onset) Deficiency. The nonclassic 21-hydroxylase deficiency form results from a milder defect in 21-hydroxylation than the congenital classic form. It may be symptomatic or asymptomatic.

Signs of excess androgen production in affected patients are not noted at birth, but at some time thereafter. Onset may not be until adulthood. Treatment consists of glucocorticoid replacement in the same doses as in the congenital form.

Asymptomatic (Cryptic) 21-Hydroxylase Deficiency. This is noted in family members of patients with classic CAH. In contrast to the patient with classic and nonclassic CAH, affected family members are asymptomatic. They may have one gene for a severe 21-hydroxylase deficiency and one gene for a mild deficiency, or two genes for the mild deficiency. No treatment is needed, as growth, puberty, and fertility are normal.

PRIMARY HYPERALDOSTERONISM

This condition is rarely seen in childhood. In children it is predominantly due to bilateral adrenal hyperplasia, as opposed to an aldosterone producing tumor. When a tumor is present, surgical removal, if feasible, is the treatment of choice. Response to surgery is less satisfactory in cases due to bilateral hyperplasia, and spironolactone is effective drug therapy. Spironolactone, an aldosterone antagonist, may also be used preoperatively in the surgical management of primary hyperaldosteronism due to a tumor. Amiloride (Midamor), a potassium-sparing diuretic, is also effective. These agents may be used alone or in combination with diuretics, β-blockers, and vasodilators to control the hypertension.

DEXAMETHASONE-SUPPRESSIBLE HYPERALDOSTERONISM

This familial disorder is similar to primary hyperaldosteronism except that in the former the aldosterone hypersecretion is completely and rapidly suppressed with dexamethasone. The hypertension always remits in children given glucocorticoid therapy, though it does not always do so in adults despite aldosterone suppression. Thus, early diagnosis and treatment are essential to cure this form of hypertension. Adequacy of the glucocorticoid treatment can be monitored not only by blood pressure measurement but also by measurement of PRA, which is suppressed in the untreated state and rises to normal with effective treatment.

ACUTE ADRENAL INSUFFICIENCY—EMERGENCY TREATMENT

This is a medical emergency that requires prompt recognition and treatment. It may be precipitated in the hypofunctional adrenal cortical conditions (e.g., CAH, Addison's disease) when patients are not yet diagnosed or are noncompliant with therapy or are stressed. It may also occur with trauma and bacteremia and during surgery in patients who are steroid dependent. There may be significant hyponatremia, hyperkalemia, hypoglycemia, and dehydration with shock. Therapy consists of volume expansion and steroid replacement:

Infuse normal saline in 5% dextrose at 1.5 to 2 times maintenance (i.e., 2250 to 3000 ml/m²/day). Use plasma or plasmanate at 10 to 20 ml/kg or normal saline at 20 ml/kg over 1 hour if patient is in shock.

Administer hydrocortisone sodium succinate (Solu-Cortef) in a stat dose of 2.0 mg/kg IV push or IM. One may estimate the emergency dose of hydrocortisone by IV bolus as follows: for an infant, give 25 mg; for a small child, 50 mg; a larger child or adolescent, 100–150 mg. After the emergency dose, use hydrocortisone at 100 mg/m²/day as a continuous IV infusion or every 6 hours IM.

Give deoxycorticosterone acetate (DOCA) stat at 2 mg IM. A repeat dose is usually not needed more than once daily, but this should be determined by the patient's electrolytes. It should be remembered that large doses of glucocorticoids (hydrocortisone) have some mineralocorticoid action which, coupled with normal saline infusion, may make the use of DOCA unnecessary in the acute situation.

To treat hyponatremia, calculate the patient's sodium deficit as follows: (normal serum Na$^+$ − observed serum Na$^+$) × body weight (kg) × 0.6. Administer half of the total sodium deficit in the first 8 to 12 hours with IV fluids, in addition to maintenance sodium.

Resistant hyperkalemia may require a kayexalate enema; rarely are other measures needed.

It is imperative not to overtreat the child. This may lead to sodium and fluid overload with resulting hypertension, hypernatremia, edema, congestive heart failure, and hypokalemia, with muscle weakness. Monitor the patient's clinical condition, weight, input/output, blood pressure, electocardiogram, and serum electrolytes very closely.

As the patient recovers and is able to tolerate liquids, IV fluids and medications may be tapered over a few days, and when a single AM dose is reached, they may be discontinued. If a short-acting glucocorticoid such as hydrocortisone was used for less than 3 days, therapy may be discontinued without tapering. It is essential to search carefully for the cause of the adrenal insufficiency. If the problem was acute, no further treatment is necessary. If the problem is one of chronic insufficiency, then maintenance steroid replacement is required. The oral dose of hydrocortisone may vary from 12.5 to 25 mg/m^2/day in two or three divided doses, and fludrocortisone from 0.05 to 0.15 mg/day.

When a patient with chronic adrenal insufficiency is stressed, e.g., during a febrile illness or surgery, the oral dose of hydrocortisone must be doubled or tripled, depending on the degree of stress and the condition of the patient. If oral therapy is not tolerated, the drug must be given parenterally. The stress dose of parenteral hydrocortisone is 40 to 60 mg/m^2/day in three or four divided doses. If the stress is a febrile illness, the increase should be continued for the duration of the illness and then maintenance therapy resumed. If the stress is surgery, administer either IV or IM hydrocortisone in the above dose 24 hours prior to surgery. Continue the same on the day of surgery, but divide the total dose into three equal portions: one on call to the operating room, one as a continuous infusion during surgery, and one in the immediate (same-day) postoperative period. Thereafter, depending on the procedure and the patient's condition, continue the same stress dose of hydrocortisone for 3 to 5 postoperative days, at which time the maintenance regimen may be resumed.

For emergency surgery, administer hydrocortisone 50 mg IV or IM on call to the operating room for a small child, and 100 mg IV or IM for a larger child or adolescent, and continue the management outlined above during the operative and postoperative period.

If a patient has received glucocorticoids in the past year, it is prudent to follow the above protocol in times of major stress such as surgery.

PRIMARY ADRENAL INSUFFICIENCY (ADDISON'S DISEASE OR BILATERAL ADRENALECTOMY)—MAINTENANCE TREATMENT

This disorder requires replacement with glucocorticoid and mineralocorticoid hormones. The usual maintenance dose of hydrocortisone ranges from 12 to 20 mg/m^2/day in two or three divided doses, and fludrocortisone 0.05 to 0.1 mg/day.

Important parameters to monitor treatment include growth, blood pressure, serum electrolytes, and PRA. It is also important to concomitantly treat infection (e.g., tuberculosis or histoplasmosis), if this is the underlying etiology.

SECONDARY ADRENAL INSUFFICIENCY (ACTH DEFICIENCY)

In contrast to primary adrenal insufficiency, secondary adrenal insufficiency is characterized by deficient glucocorticoids but normal mineralocorticoid function. This occurs in steroid treated or hypophysectomized or hypopituitary conditions. Glucocorticoid replacement is the same as that described for primary adrenal insufficiency.

ACTH UNRESPONSIVENESS

Therapy is the same as for secondary adrenal insufficiency.

CUSHING'S SYNDROME

Treatment depends on the etiology. It may be iatrogenic or secondary to an adrenal tumor or result from excess ACTH secretion from either the pituitary or a nonpituitary source.

If it is due to an adrenal tumor, surgical resection, if possible, is the treatment of choice. When an autonomously functional unilateral adrenal adenoma is removed, as is usually the case, the remaining adrenal is often atrophic. Therefore, these patients should be supplemented with glucocorticoid therapy before, during, and after surgery until the remaining adrenal gland returns to normal, which may take many months, depending on the duration of pituitary-adrenal suppression. If bilateral tumors were present, then total adrenalectomy is indicated, and the patient must take lifelong glucocorticoid and mineralocorticoid treatment in the doses outlined for primary adrenal insufficiency.

If the cause is a nonresectable adrenal carcinoma, the following agents may be tried: o,p'-DDD (mitotane [Lysodren]), an adrenocorticolytic drug; metyrapone, an 11-hydroxylase inhibitor of cortisol production; cyproheptadine hydrochloride, a serotonin antagonist that suppresses ACTH; and aminoglutethimide, which blocks conversion of cholesterol to Δ5-pregnenolone in the adrenal cortex. However, these agents are not without side effects; there has been limited experience with them in children; and results are disappointing.

When the syndrome is secondary to a nonpituitary source of ACTH, i.e., "the ectopic ACTH syndrome," treatment is that of the underlying disease.

Cushing's disease refers to bilateral adrenal hyperplasia resulting from excessive ACTH secretion by the pituitary. Several treatment options are available. Recent advances in surgical techniques include selective surgical removal of the pituitary microadenoma(s) via the transsphenoidal route. Postoperatively, the resulting pituitary insufficiency, primarily ACTH, is usually temporary, but replacement glucocorticoid therapy is needed until normal pituitary/adrenal function returns. Pituitary irradiation is another treatment option. Total bilateral adrenalectomy is outdated and has two major disadvantages: the need for lifelong steroid replacement therapy, and the postoperative risk of Nelson's syndrome.

VIRILIZING, FEMINIZING, AND NON-FUNCTIONAL ADRENOCORTICAL TUMORS

Treatment is surgical removal in resectable cases. If the tumor is also cortisol-producing, then the patient requires glucocorticoid replacement until the remaining adrenal gland returns to normal.

Additional modes of therapy include radiation, drugs, and chemotherapy. O,p'—DDD (mitatane) destroys both normal and cancerous adrenal tissue. Therefore, it is important to initiate glucocorticoid replacement therapy when a response occurs (usually in several weeks). Mineralocorticoid replacement may also be necessary. Among the chemotherapeutic agents that have been used, alone or in combination, are alkylating agents such as cyclophosphamide, doxorubicin, and fluorouracil. Many others have been tried, but in the cases reported in the literature, there has been only limited success with these agents.

PHEOCHROMOCYTOMA

Pheochromocytoma generally arises from the adrenal medulla, but it may be found anywhere along the sympathetic chain. Definitive treatment consists of surgical excision. In children it may be bilateral, in which case bilateral adrenalectomy is necessary, as well as subsequent lifelong glucocorticoid and mineralocorticoid therapy. Three major complications may occur during surgery: severe hypertension, tachyarrhythmias, and hypotension. The first two result from excessive discharge of catecholamines during manipulation of the tumor, and the latter from catecholamine withdrawal and hypovolemic shock. Appropriate preoperative and operative management of the patient is crucial in preventing these complications. Preparation usually begins 1 to 3 weeks before surgery. To control catecholamine release, the patient is placed on α-blockers with or without β-adrenegic blocking agents. The most commonly used α-blocker is phenoxybenzamine hydrochloride (Dibenzyline). It is administered orally and, because of its long half-life, is given on an every 12 hour basis. The usual starting dose is 5 mg every 12 hours. However, the dose must be adjusted to the individual patient and this should occur in the hospital.

Phentolamine (Regitine) is equally effective but less satisfactory for prolonged use because of its short half-life. It is particularly useful, however, when these patients develop acute hypertension, such as during a diagnostic radiographic procedure or during surgery. The emergency dose of phentolamine is 1 mg intravenously or intramuscularly.

Additional preoperative therapy with β-adrenergic blocking agents is appropriate when α-blockade alone is not satisfactorily controlling the catecholamine excess or when tachyarrhythmias develop. β-blockers are myocardial depressants, and in patients with hypertensive cardiomyopathy, may precipitate congestive heart failure. Propranolol (Inderal) is the most commonly used β-blocker. The usual dose is 5 to 10 mg orally every 6 to 8 hours, but again, the dose must be adjusted to the needs of the individual patient. The emergency dose for tachyarrhythmias is 1 mg administered IV over 1 minute.

Most recently, metyrosine (Demser) has been used in combination with adrenergic blockade when the latter alone is not sufficient treatment. Metyrosine is a tyrosine hydroxylase inhibitor that reduces the production of catecholamines. The usual starting dose is 5 to 10 mg/kg/day orally every 6 hours. Again, the dose must be adjusted to the needs of the individual patient.

There should be close intraoperative monitoring of these patients, including both central venous and arterial pressure. Also, during surgery it is essential to administer an adequate amount of intravenous fluid to prevent hypovolemic shock once the tumor is resected. Preoperative administration of phenoxybenzamine may also be helpful, as it permits intravascular volume expansion by its α-blocking capability.

Intraoperatively, hypertension can be controlled with either phentolamine or sodium nitroprusside IV. Supraventricular tachyarrhythmias can be treated with propranolol IV, and ventricular arrhythmias with lidocaine. It should be reiterated that hydrocortisone should be available, so that in cases of bilateral adrenalectomy a continuous IV infusion may be begun.

If hypertension persists for longer than 48 hours postsurgical removal, one must suspect a remaining tumor. In children, these tumors may be not only multiple but also extra-adrenal. This emphasizes the importance of complete abdominal exploration at surgery. It is important to document normal plasma and/or urinary catecholamines, as patients may be normotensive and asymptomatic postoperatively but still have residual tumor.

It is wise to follow these patients and their families for many years, because these tumors may recur, and because of their association with conditions such as multiple endocrine adenomatosis, neurofibromatosis, and von Hippel-Lindau disease.

PREMATURE ADRENARCHE

This is a benign condition of isolated sexual hair growth (pubic, with or without axillary hair) in boys less than 9 and girls less than 8 years of age. The source of androgens is most likely the adrenal gland.

No treatment is indicated, but close follow-up is necessary to assess the patient's growth velocity and note if additional signs of puberty appear. In this condition, the growth velocity is either normal or slightly accelerated. The bone age is usually slightly more advanced than the chronological age but compatible with the height age. On follow-up, these patients should show no other signs of virilization than the presence of sexual hair, and no other signs of puberty should appear. Baseline and follow-up serum androgens and 24-hour urinary 17-ketosteroids are elevated but remain in the early pubertal range. Serum 170HP, gonadotropins, and the response to LHRH stimulation are all at prepubertal levels.

Endocrine Disorders of the Testis

JOSEPH I. WOLFSDORF, M.D.

DISORDERS OF THE FETAL TESTIS

A variety of rare disorders can cause failure of the fetal testis to secrete normal amounts of testosterone. These include defects of testosterone biosynthesis, syndromes of testicular hypoplasia such as XY testicular dysgenesis, XO/XY mosaicism, Leydig cell agenesis, and deficiency of pituitary gonadotropins. A lack of testosterone results in incomplete differentiation of the external genitalia. At one end of the spectrum, the external genitalia may be indistinguishable from that of a phenotypic female, while at the other end, the child may be a normal-appearing male with a microphallus.

When the appearance of the genitalia dictates that a baby with a Y-cell line is to be raised as a girl, there is a high risk of a tumor developing in that child's gonadal elements. In general, the risk is low before the age of 10 years; nevertheless, removal of the gonads should be performed once the diagnosis has been made.

MICROPHALLUS

Growth of the microphallus in response to the administration of androgens has been most satisfactory in patients whose hypogonadism is due to gonadotropin deficiency.

Depot testosterone cypionate or enanthate, 25 to 50 mg intramuscularly (IM) monthly for 3 months, will stimulate growth of the penis (increased stretched length and corporal mass) provided that the child does not have androgen resistance. Lack of a response suggests a very limited growth potential and, in a child less than 18 months of age, raises the question of possible sex reassignment.

SEXUAL INFANTILISM

Puberty in boys normally commences at about 11 years of age. Because pubertal development cannot occur spontaneously in boys with primary or secondary hypogonadism, androgen therapy is indicated to induce puberty and to maintain virilization after sexual development is complete. Therapy should commence when the bone age has reached 11 years.

Because of their potency and the steady response obtained, I recommend a long-acting ester of testosterone, either testosterone cypionate or enanthate. Peak blood levels are attained within a few days and levels return to baseline by 3 or 4 weeks. Both preparations are administered IM and have similar pharmacokinetic properties. An advantage of using the natural androgen testosterone is that its blood level can be monitored to be maintained in the desirable range.

For the first year of treatment, to prevent unduly rapid growth and epiphyseal maturation, use 100 mg monthly. Thereafter, the dose is increased to 200 mg at 2 to 3 week intervals for 2 to 3 years or until full development is attained. A maintenance dose of either 200 mg every 2 weeks or 300 mg every 3 weeks produces serum testosterone concentrations that fluctuate within the normal adult range. This regimen also keeps serum LH and FSH concentrations in the normal range in patients with primary hypogonadism.

Orally active androgen preparations can be used if the patient is unwilling to receive injections, and if taken regularly, will produce androgenization. The oral agents, however, are not as potent as the long-acting testosterone esters. The response to oral androgens is said to be limited in patients with gonadotropin deficiency and cannot bring about complete sexual development. This does not appear to be the case in primary testicular failure.

Methyl testosterone (17-α-methyltesterone) is a 17-α-substituted alkyl derivative that retains its androgenic potency while still being active orally. Fluoxymesterone (the 9-α-fluoro-11-α-hydroxy derivative of 17-α-methyl testosterone) is a related orally active androgen. Both compounds are satisfactory for maintenance therapy. The usual maintenance dose of methyltestosterone is 10 to 40 mg daily. Fluoxymesterone has a longer half-life and the usual dose is 10 to 20 mg daily.

The 17-α-alkylated steroids, especially methyltestosterone, may cause alterations of liver function. Fluoxymesterone has a lesser effect on liver function. These steroids can cause nausea and intrahepatic cholestatic jaundice, which are rapidly reversible upon stopping the medication. The long-acting esters do not damage the liver. Patients receiving high doses of these steroids for prolonged periods, as in treatment of aplastic anemia, may develop hepatic adenomas, peliosis hepatis, and even hepatocellular carcinoma.

Sodium chloride and water retention are inherent properties of androgens and may cause edema in patients with a pre-existing tendency to retain fluid. All androgens can cause acne and gynecomastia. Within a few days of starting treatment with large doses in a eunuchoid individual, frequent erections may occur. This may be embarrassing and psychologically disturbing; this response subsides with continued treatment at the same dose.

KLINEFELTER'S SYNDROME

Klinefelter's syndrome is probably the most common cause of hypogonadism. Pubertal development usually commences at an average age and often progresses normally. Androgen replacement therapy is indicated only for patients whose testosterone production is inadequate.

Gynecomastia is not amenable to medical treatment. Indeed, high doses of testosterone may make the condition worse. Thus, when gynecomastia is severe and causes embarrassment, reduction mammoplasty is the only available treatment.

Infertility in Klinefelter's syndrome is irreversible.

CONGENITAL BILATERAL ANORCHIA ("VANISHING TESTES SYNDROME")

This is a rare disorder in which testicular degeneration occurs after male sexual differentiation has been completed. Silastic prosthetic testes are available in various sizes and should be implanted in the scrotum to give the child a normal appearance.

CONSTITUTIONAL DELAYED PUBERTY

Individuals whose somatic growth and osseous development are slow (constitutional slow growth) are apt to have delayed onset of puberty. Not infrequently, pressure from peers and family members contributes to rather severe psychological disturbances. Consequently, while remembering that this is not a disease but a variation of normal, treatment with androgens may be justified in instances where counseling and reassurance are to no avail.

A prerequisite for such treatment should be the attainment of at least age 14 years and a thorough evaluation to exclude an identifiable organic disease of the hypothalamus, pituitary, or testes. The aim of therapy is to promote growth and induce puberty, thereby reassuring the boy that he is not abnormal.

Before undertaking such therapy, the patient and his parents must be warned that testosterone may cause advancement of skeletal maturation at a rate that exceeds linear growth. This may compromise the attainment of the boy's genetically determined adult height. Furthermore, although no other deleterious effects of such treatment are known, little is known about the long-term outcome of this therapy.

I use a long-acting ester of testosterone, 100 mg IM monthly for 6 months; after this time there is usually some evidence of sexual maturation, which the boy and his family find reassuring. Treatment is then stopped for at least 6 months. During the off-phase, spontaneous progression of sexual development usually occurs. Occasionally, a second 6-month course of testosterone therapy is necessary.

PRECOCIOUS PUBERTY

In boys, an organic disorder causes true isosexual precocity in about 60% of cases. Whenever possible, the underlying disorder must be treated appropriately. Precocious puberty may precede the onset of detectable neurologic signs; thus, prolonged careful observation may be necessary to exclude a cerebral lesion before a diagnosis of idiopathic precocious puberty can be made safely. When precocity is idiopathic, the aim of therapy is to slow the rate of epiphyseal maturation, which, unchecked, compromises adult height, and to retard the progression of secondary sexual characteristics. This is done by inhibiting the secretion of gonadotropins by the pituitary. Currently, no ideal therapy is available.

If puberty has started only a year or two earlier than normal and its progression is not unduly rapid, treatment may be withheld.

At present, medroxyprogesterone acetate (Depo-Provera) is the only potentially effective medication available for this purpose in the U.S.A. It is given in a dose of 100 to 200 mg IM every 2 to 4 weeks, or orally in a dose of 10 mg b i d or q i d. One should use the lowest effective dose. The effects of therapy can be monitored by measuring levels of testosterone, measuring linear growth, and assessing the progression of bone age. If a beneficial effect is observed, therapy may have to be continued for several years. Unfortunately, medroxyprogesterone acetate is not invariably effective.

Several adverse effects have been reported. Because of its weak intrinsic glucocorticoid activity, prolonged administration can cause suppression of the hypothalamo-pituitary-adrenal axis. Very large doses can cause Cushing's syndrome. Alterations in chromosome structure and testicular histology have also been noted.

European endocrinologists have advocated cyproterone acetate as the drug of choice in treating precocious puberty. Unfortunately, this agent is not available for use in the U.S.A. It has both antigonadotropin and antiandrogenic activity. Given orally in a dose of 70-150 mg/m²/day, it uniformly stops progression of pubertal development and, when the bone age is less than 11 years, slows growth velocity and the rate of osseous maturation.

Preliminary clinical studies using highly potent analogs of LHRH to treat precocious puberty have produced promising results. This form of treatment is still in the investigational phase.

A major component of the management of precocious puberty is support and counseling for the child, his family, and others involved in the child's daily affairs. This entails simple sex education to the extent that the child is capable of comprehending. Serious adjustment problems may occur because the boy's mature appearance belies his ability to cope with the psychosocial adjustments that face him. Parents are frequently anxious and bewildered and need assistance in understanding the nature of their child's premature development. A simple explanation, indicating that a normal process has merely occurred earlier than usual, is reassuring. Families must also be helped to understand that their son's psychological development is concordant with his chronologic age. They should expect attitudes and behavior commensurate with his actual age and not his physical size and appearance.

Gynecomastia

NOEL K. MACLAREN, M.D.

NEONATAL GYNECOMASTIA

In almost all newborn infants, breast tissue is palpable soon after birth and increases by engorgement within the first few days of life. It is the result of maternal estrogens transmitted to the fetus, and it resolves spontaneously within weeks·or, exceptionally, months. No therapy is required other than normal infant skin hygiene. More pronounced gynecomastia with modest galactorrhea, or "witches milk," is occasionally encountered. Prolactin levels are not distinguishable from the normal neonatal hyperprolactinemia. Parents must not manipulate these breasts to get rid of the "witches milk," as this can cause inflammation and, in girls, permanent breast damage.

Prepubertal Gynecomastia

The rare finding of gynecomastia before puberty requires a vigorous search for a possible source of exogenous estrogens, and a careful history to exclude ingestion of contraceptive pills, application of estrogen-containing cosmetic creams or, more rarely, consumption of estrogen-fattened chicken meat. Should none of these be identified, and if the disorder is progressive or features of virilization are found, work-up for congenital adrenal hyperplasia (especially 11β hydroxylase deficiency), an estrogen-secreting adrenal tumor, testicular neoplasia, or trophoblastic (hCG secreting) tumor should be undertaken. For diagnosis and therapy of these problems, the reader is referred elsewhere. For patients with idiopathic prepubertal gynecomastia with negative findings in the above work-up, specific therapy is not required.

PUBERTAL GYNECOMASTIA

In almost all boys approaching mid-puberty, puffiness and hyperemia of the areolae together with a subareolar nodule of breast tissue, which may be tender, is to be expected. Introspective boys and their parents need strong reassurance that such changes are a normal accompaniment to increased levels of male hormone and to the ascent to manhood. Adolescent gynecomastia is seldom greater than 4 cm and can be expected to resolve spontaneously within 6 to 18 months as more adult levels of testosterone are encountered. Excessive gynecomastia, however, requires work-up to exclude estrogen-secreting tumors of the adrenals or testes (Leydig cell type), trophoblastic tumors, hyperthyroidism, or chronic liver disease. A careful history should exclude drug taking such as use of marijuana or phenothiazine. A history of galactorrhea warrants testing for prolactinomas. Adolescent testicular growth (more than 4 ml or 2.5 cm length) will exclude Klinefelter's syndrome. When the appropriateness of testicular volume for age and stage of sexual development is equivocal, gonadotropin levels should be determined.

Severe physiologic gynecomastia with more than 5 cm of breast tissue and marked areolar changes will seldom resolve completely. Such cases are occasionally familial, and modest increases in the ratios of plasma estradiol to testosterone levels are often seen. We discuss the probable outcome with the boy and his parents, and urge early mammoplasty if we feel the chance of spontaneous reversal in a reasonable time is unlikely. Black patients with a history of keloid scarring should be cautioned about the cosmetic risks involved with mammoplasty.

Testosterone therapy is *not* indicated in adolescent gynecomastia and will actually increase breast size. Whereas the use of testosterone is associated with increased virilization in patients with Klinefelter's syndrome, the gynecomastia usually persists.

Ambiguous Genitalia

BARBARA M. LIPPE, M.D.

Ambiguous genitalia should be classified as a medical emergency. Not only might there be immediate medical concerns such as a salt-losing crisis or shock but also there is the urgent psychologic need to assign a sex of rearing. Parents invariably ask "what is it?" even before they ask "how is it?" and the physician must minimize this anxiety. Thus, treatment begins with a rapid diagnostic test series to establish an etiology for the ambiguity.

MANAGEMENT OF THE FAMILY

(1) We establish a single physician who communicates most of the information to the family;

(2) We allow the family to examine the baby, and we name all structures, explaining, e.g., this may be a phallus that has not developed fully, or, this may be an overdeveloped clitoris that will shrink soon, or, we can tuck it up where it belongs.

(3) We explain that we may need to examine internal structures to clarify what the baby was *meant to be.* This is a major part of our approach. We explain that some babies have one genotype but are reared as the opposite; others have the potential to be either phenotype; no one factor, not even a chromosome, determines gender. It is sometimes appropriate to say, "The way this baby's hormones work and the insides have formed, it was meant to develop into a girl. Something caused it to overdevelop a bit, but we can correct this."

(4) We discourage hospital personnel from making the parents fill in a birth certificate until a name and sex are determined.

(5) We discourage the use of a neuter name; such a name would always carry the initial doubts. An unambiguous name reinforces the sex assignment.

(6) A multidisciplinary team assists with the diagnosis (endocrinologist, geneticist, radiologist, surgeon, etc.), led by the person with the most experience with this problem, usually a pediatric endocrinologist.

Definitive treatment cannot be instituted until the pathogenesis has been elucidated. It must be recognized that external genitalia develop in two stages: (1) by morphogenic events, identical in the male and female, occurring in the first 6 weeks of gestation, resulting in the genital tubercle, urogenital sinus, and anal canal; and (2) subsequent differentiating events mediated by the absence or presence of testosterone or dihydrotestosterone (DHT). Bladder exstrophy, penoscrotal transformation, and agenesis of the phallus occur as a result of the former, independent of gonadal or hormonal causes. Masculinization occurs if testosterone is secreted from a gonad, as in the normal male fetus or in the fetus with gonadal intersex where some testicular tissue is present. It also occurs if the testosterone is secreted by the fetal adrenal, as in the female fetus virilized by congenital adrenal hyperplasia (CAH) or maternal ingestion or secretion and transfer of androgen. Incomplete masculinization occurs when testosterone is not synthesized, as in enzyme defects of steroidogenesis, or is not converted by 5 alpha reductase to DHT, or the target organ is insensitive.

MANAGEMENT OF THE INFANT

Repeat physical examinations within the first few hours and days is mandatory: A gonad in the labioscrotal fold may not become palpable until later; a hernia may develop; an imperforate anus may be demonstrated. Dehydration or shock can occur in adrenal enzyme deficiencies, and weight gain fails to occur in patients with salt-losing CAH.

A vagina, cervix, uterus, and fallopian tube(s) may all be demonstrated with a single contrast study. Conversely, ultrasonography of the pelvis may demonstrate a cervix and uterus that did not communicate with the contrast-filled urethra. Ultrasonography can also identify gonads in the inguinal canal(s), although it is not useful for intra-abdominal gonads in the neonate.

Laboratory Studies. CHROMOSOMES. The karyotype may not indicate the gender or diagnosis (up to 80% of true hermaphrodites may have a 46,XX karyotype, and 10% may be XY and 10% mosaic), but it may confirm the sex when virilization of the female due to congenital adrenal hyperplasia (CAH) is diagnosed, while a mosaic karyotype indicates a gonadal intersex problem. A buccal smear usually does not show mosaicism and is often inaccurate in the newborn.

BLOOD FOR ADRENAL STEROIDS. Most forms of CAH can be diagnosed with assays for plasma steroids, eliminating the need for 24-hour urine collections. The most common adrenal enzyme deficiency that presents with virilization of the female is 21-hydroxylase deficiency. The most accurate and rapid method of diagnosis is the determination of plasma 17-alpha-hydroxyprogesterone. Abnormal values are usually 10 to 200 times higher than in normal neonates. This test is performed on plasma mailed to several reference laboratories widely available across the country. Similarly, 11-hydroxylase deficiency (form of CAH) can be diagnosed using a specific compound-S (deoxycortisol) plasma assay. 3-Beta-hydroxysteroid dehydrogenase deficiency (rare form of CAH), in which both adrenal and gonadal steroids cannot be synthesized, is less easily diagnosed by the plasma steroid profile; 24-hour urine steroid analyses may also be required.

BLOOD FOR ELECTROLYTES. In salt-losing CAH, serum sodium decreases in the first 10 days of life, either accompanied or followed by hyperkalemia. Thus, monitoring of electrolytes is mandatory.

BLOOD FOR GONADOTROPINS AND GONADAL STEROIDS. In some forms of ambiguity the gonads may be severely defective, effectively acting like "streaks" by the time of birth. In these cases, the hypothalamic-pituitary gonadal axis may increase the secretion of FSH and LH. If gonadal failure is due to lack of hypothalamic-pituitary function (male with hypopituitarism and a microphallus) the gonadotropins do not rise. The normal testis secretes documentable amounts of testosterone in the first weeks of life; thus measurement of testosterone can indicate presence or absence of a functioning testis.

STIMULATION TESTS. In complex patients whose contrast studies, plasma steroids, and karyotype do not provide a clear diagnostic profile, we perform an HCG or ACTH stimulation test.

EXPLORATORY SURGERY. Prior to definitive sex assignment, it is sometimes necessary to know precisely the gonadal histology and internal genital anatomy, in which case exploratory surgery must be performed in the first weeks of life. More often a sex of rearing has been already assigned and the surgery, designed to remove a gonad(s) and/or inappropriate genital organ(s), may be delayed and performed in conjunction with a stage of the external genital repair.

Definitive Treatment

Definitive treatment consists of three possible modalities: medical management, surgical reconstruction, and hormone replacement.

CAH requires cortisone therapy in quantities that will not only replace the deficiency but also suppress the enzymatically blocked adrenal from producing precursor hormones. After intensive treatment of the neonate, the dosage should be individualized according to growth, bone age, physical examination and steroid secretion pattern. Most patients are adequately controlled with 25 mg of cortisone per square meter given orally in divided doses. If salt loss is present, DOCA, 1 mg IM q 12 hours, is given for acute therapy, and fludrocortisone acetate (Florinef), 0.05-0.1 mg orally thereafter.

In cases of morphogenic anomalies or gonadal intersex, medical therapy in childhood is usually not indicated, but in both these and CAH patients, surgical reconstruction should be initiated early. There is good evidence that gender identity is established by the end of the second year. Thus, some repair of the externalia should be undertaken by 18 to 24 months of age so that phenotypic identity is preserved.

Recession and reduction of the clitoris is mandatory in children reared as females. We try to avoid total clitorectomy. Conversely, total reconstruction of the phallus is rarely possible, so that a male with agenesis of the phallus usually undergoes gonadectomy and the scrotal skin is preserved for later use in vaginal reconstruction.

We feel that if the internal structures (such as a gonad or mullerian remnant) need removal, this should be done in infancy. There is no good evidence that the gonads are necessary for normal prepubertal growth or psychosocial development. On the contrary, it has been our experience that parental anxiety about the possible effects of a heterosexual gonadal structure and the traumatic experience of laparotomy in a teenager makes early removal preferable.

At the expected time of puberty, hormonal replacement will be necessary in the gonadectomized child. If one gonad is intact, physical examination and measurement of plasma gonadotropins (follicle-stimulating hormone and luteinizing hormone) and plasma sex steroids may be used to assess its potential function and obviate the necessity of replacement therapy. If replacement is indicated in the female, we use small doses of estrogen (10–20 μg of ethinyl estradiol). Initially, even lower doses may be used to prevent too rapid epiphyseal fusion. The estrogen is given in a cyclic fashion whether a uterus is present or not. Similarly, progesterone is added during the last part of the artificial cycle so that a state of unopposed estrogen (potentially carcinogenic) is not created. We give the estrogen from days 1 to 23 of a calendar month, adding Provera, 2.5 to 10 mg on day 10 and continuing both until day 23, with no medication until day 1 of the next month.

In the male, androgen therapy may be initiated with oral methyltestosterone linguets (10 mg daily). As masculinization progresses, the dose can be increased, with an eventual shift to a parenteral depo preparation (100–200 mg of testosterone enanthate in oil every 2–3 weeks).

In rare cases a hypothalamic or pituitary lesion may have been responsible for failure of virilization in the male. If so, and if the gonads are intact, intramuscular administration of gonadotropins may bring on sexual development and fertility. In the future, the synthetic gonadotropin releasing hormone may be available.

Surgical therapy is usually staged: reconstruction of the phallus or recession of the clitoris is performed in early childhood, while vaginal reconstruction is delayed until hormone therapy has been instituted or the patient is in spontaneous puberty. When testes are absent, small testicular prostheses may be inserted prior to school age, to be followed by removal and replacement with larger ones during adolescence. Conversely, some males prefer to delay prosthesis placement until adolescence, so that only one surgery is necessary.

10

Metabolic Disorders

Infants Born to Diabetic Mothers

NAOMI D. NEUFELD, M.D.

Advances in the obstetrical care of the pregnant diabetic patient, coupled with a greater understanding of the etiology of specific fetal disorders, have led to a significant reduction in both neonatal morbidity and mortality rates in infants of diabetic mothers (IDM). Nonetheless, the rates of perinatal morbidity are still significantly greater than in normal preganancies; thus, the care of such infants is extremely critical. Care should begin in the prenatal period and, to be performed well, is best conducted in a tertiary medical center where the team approach of obstetrician, pediatrician, and specialist in diabetes is practiced.

The aims of prenatal care are (1) to strictly regulate diabetic control of the pregnant patient. Patients with poor diabetic control have a significantly higher incidence of fetal loss, and ketoacidosis in particular is associated with extremely high fetal losses. Better metabolic control has been shown to significantly reduce neonatal morbidity and mortality rates; and (2) to monitor continued viability and well-being of the fetus and allow prolongation of pregnancy to as near term as possible.

MATERNAL MANAGEMENT

Most authorities consider maternal hyperglycemia a major predisposing factor in the development of clinical complications in IDM. Since improvement of fetal outcome has been shown to occur with good metabolic control of maternal diabetes throughout pregnancy, diabetic patients should be seen on a weekly basis for supervision of dietary and insulin therapy. The aims are to maintain fasting blood glucose at 100 mg/dl and postprandial blood glucose at less than 140 mg/dl and

to prevent ketoacidosis. Insulin doses should be adjusted according to home urine test results for glucose and acetone, as well as the history of hypoglycemic episodes. Recent studies have suggested a role for home monitoring of blood glucose in pregnancy as an improvement in the care of these patients, leading to further reduction in perinatal morbidity rates. Rigorous diabetic management using a regimen of multiple insulin injections or continuous insulin infusion by portable pump has been shown to significantly reduce perinatal morbidity in diabetic pregnancy. It remains to be shown whether such management in the early stages of pregnancy would reduce the incidence of major congenital anomalies. Should diabetic control be difficult to achieve early in pregnancy, patients should be hospitalized for careful supervision.

FETAL WELL-BEING

Tests of fetal well-being in pregnancy should be performed routinely. Ultrasonography at 18 to 20 weeks will give a fairly accurate determination of fetal size, confirming the duration of pregnancy and ruling out the presence of gross fetal anomaly. Serial determinations may be performed to assess rate of fetal growth. Urinary estriol, protein, and creatinine determinations should be performed at least weekly after 30 weeks' gestation. After 33 weeks' gestation, pregnant patients should have nonstress testing or oxytocin challenge tests for assessment of fetal and placental function. Patients with falling urinary estriol values, abnormal stress or nonstress testing, pre-eclampsia, or poor diabetic control should be admitted to the hospital immediately for close supervision.

Patients with uncomplicated pregnancies should be hospitalized at 36 to 37 weeks' gestation for further management. Alterations in insulin and dietary therapy during the hospital stay are made in

304

accordance with the results of blood glucose determinations obtained two to four times daily. Prevention of hyperglycemia during the latter stage of pregnancy has been associated with a significant reduction in the incidence of fetal macrosomia and postnatal hypoglycemia. Use of techniques such as closed- or open-loop continuous insulin infusion devices during this period may further reduce the incidence of these problems. During that time, the daily urinary estriol determinations and weekly tests of fetal well-being mentioned above should be performed.

Prior to delivery, fetal lung maturation is assessed by amniocentesis, utilizing lecithin/sphingomyelin ratio (L/S) determinations or lung maturity profiles, which include measurement of phosphatidylglycerol and disaturated phosphatidylcholine. Since documented cases of the respiratory distress syndrome (RDS) have been shown to occur in IDM who have L/S ratios of 2:1, a ratio of 3.5:1 or greater may be necessary to assure good fetal outcome.

Timing of the delivery of the IDM should take into account the variables of maternal and fetal well-being described. Planning of the delivery should include the the pediatrician, who is informed about the expected fetal status and who will be present in the delivery room to initiate resuscitation therapy as needed, as well as to identify other specific problems. The need for elected caesarean section for predetermined fetal macrosomia should be considered in order to avoid birth injury.

GENERAL NEONATAL MANAGEMENT

If maternal blood glucose values are normalized during pregnancy as described above, such infants should appear to require very little attention since the incidence of perinatal morbidity is reduced to normal. On the other hand, if normal blood glucose values are not documented during diabetic pregnancies, such infants should be monitored as outlined herein. Following delivery, essential information, including Apgar score, weight, sex, and any obvious congenital anomalies, should be carefully recorded by the nursing staff. A specimen of cord blood should be sent to the laboratory for glucose and pH determinations at that time. Infants are transferred to the stabilization nursery, where they are warmed and more carefully examined. Assessment of gestational age by Dubowitz criteria is recorded. Detailed examination of the heart, lung, kidneys, and extremities and the presence of obvious congenital anomalies and birth injuries, including Erb palsy, fractured clavicle, phrenic nerve injury, or intracranial hemorrhage, should be noted. Blood studies for initial determinations of glucose (using Dextrostix or BG Chemstrips), calcium, hematocrit, and bilirubin should be obtained according to the following schedule:

Glucose: 1, 2, 4, 6, 8, 12, 24, 36, 48 hrs of age
Calcium: 6, 12, 24, 48 hrs of age
Hematocrit: 2, 24 hrs of age
Bilirubin (total and direct): 24, 48 hrs of age

The incidence and severity of the specific problems seen in IDM are related directly to the severity of the maternal diabetes, as judged by the White criteria, as well as to the degree of prematurity at birth. Near-term infants with gestational diabetes have a reported incidence of perinatal morbidity of 25% or less. Infants delivered prior to 37 weeks of mothers with severe, long-standing diabetes have morbidity rates at birth approaching 60%. These infants in particular have a significantly greater incidence of serious complications, including major congenital malformations and hypocalcemia.

SPECIFIC PROBLEMS OF THE IDM

Hypoglycemia is defined as blood glucose value of less than 30 mg/dl in infants of any gestational age. This is the most common metabolic complication, occurring in as many as 56 per cent of IDM. Most often it occurs between 1 and 1.5 hours of live. Oral feedings of glucose water should begin within 1 hour of life, and assessment of blood glucose should continue in association with feedings until stable. By 12 hours most infants are on formula with transfer to breast feedings as soon as possible, and supplemental feedings of glucose-water are given as necessary to prevent hypoglycemia.

For infants who are unable to feed well or whose hypoglycemia cannot be managed by oral feedings, treatment with intravenous glucose infusions at a rate of at least 6 mg/kg/min, or that rate which results in normal steady-state glucose levels, should be given. The use of hypertonic glucose in bolus doses should be avoided since, in the presence of persisting hyperinsulinemia, this may lead to rebound hypoglycemia. Treatment with glucagon, while recommended by some, is usually not necessary. In the usual case this is a transient phenomenon lasting no more than 24 to 48 hours. Persistance of hypoglycemia beyond 48 hours often necessitates glucocorticoid treatment. Persistence of hypoglycemia despite glucocorticoid therapy should prompt investigation for causes, such as beta-cell hyperplasia (nesidioblastosis) or islet cell tumor (see article on Hypoglycemia).

While the incidence of the *respiratory distress syndrome* has been reduced significantly because of a greater understanding of pathophysiology and improvement in prenatal care, this still remains a major form of neonatal morbidity in diabetic pregnancies. Treatment of RDS is discussed elsewhere in this book.

The peak incidence of *hypocalcemia* occurs within 48 hours of birth and is increased in the presence of other known causes of the disorder. Treatment is usually begun when calcium levels are less than 7 mg/dl. The treatment of choice is with calcium gluconate (10 per cent) given either orally or intravenously. Acute symptomatic hypocalcemia is treated with 2 ml/kg of intravenous calcium gluconate given slowly (1 ml/min or less), with the careful monitoring of heart rate. (*Note:* calcium should not be added to intravenous solutions containing sodium bicarbonate since an insoluble precipitate, $CaCO_3$, will form). Oral supplementation can be continued with the addition of diluted calcium salts to formula at a dose of 0.5 to 1.0 gm/kg/24 hr.

To prevent further aggravation of hypocalcemia (neonatal tetany), feedings with only those formulas with low-phosphate loads should be provided. Breast milk is ideal, and nursing is beneficial for both the infant and the diabetic mother. Other specially prepared low-phosphate formulas such as PM 60/40 (Ca^{++}, 400 mg/l, P, 200 mg/l) can be used. Treatment is usually necessary for 4 to 5 days: during this time calcium levels should be monitored every 12 to 24 hours and supplemental calcium provided accordingly.

Persistence of hypocalcemia or its resistance to treatment should lead to a search for other causes. Hypocalcemia may occur in the presence of renal insufficiency, defective Vitamin D metabolism, or hypomagnesemia. Treatment of these disorders is described elsewhere in this book.

Hyperbilirubinemia is another problem commonly observed in the IDM, occuring in as many as 37 per cent of infants in one series. The etiology of this disorder is unclear, although both polycythemia with increased hemolysis and hypoglycemia have been implicated. Treatment of the jaundiced infant is described elsewhere in this book.

POLYCYTHEMIA AND HYPERVISCOSITY SYNDROMES

The occurrence of elevated hematocrit (greater than 65 per cent for a venous sample obtained within 2 hours of birth) is very common in IDM, although the exact incidence is not known. A direct relationship between the viscosity and venous blood hematocrit has been defined. The clinical findings in such infants are due to the increased viscosity of blood flow in the venous bed and include respiratory distress, cyanosis, jitteriness, jaundice, thrombocytopenia, necrotizing enterocolitis, and gangrene. Treatment, which is aimed at lowering the hematocrit to between 50 to 60 per cent with exahdnge transfusion, is carefully detailed in the article on Hyperviscosity Syndromes.

Renal vein thrombosis, an unusual complication of polycythemia, is seen with a greater frequency than normal in IDM and is often associated with asphyxia and hypotension. Clinical manifestations include hematuria and renal enlargement. Treatment is conservative, based upon careful fluid and electrolyte management coupled with heparin therapy. These are temporizing measures that permit observation for spontaneous resolution of the disorder. In rare instances, surgical intervention may be required.

The major cause of death in IDM in several recent studies was that associated with fatal *congenital anomalies* of various types, including severe cardiovascular defects, skeletal malformation such as sacral agenesis, and anencephaly-meningomyelocele. Careful management of maternal diabetes in the early stages of pregnancy has been suggested as the best means of lowering the incidence of these anomalies, which occur now in as many as 6% of all diabetic pregnancies. Treatment is dictated by the nature and severity of the particular lesion.

Diabetes Mellitus

MARK A. SPERLING, M.D.

Diabetes mellitus is a disease of disturbed energy metabolism caused by deficiency of insulin secretion or insulin action at the cellular level, which results in altered fuel homeostasis involving carbohydrate, protein, and fat. It is the most common endocrine/metabolic disorder of childhood, with important consequences on physical and emotional development. It acutely affects the quality of life through the need for daily insulin injections and self-monitoring, and chronically it affects morbidity and mortality through the complications that affect small and large blood vessels resulting in retinopathy, nephropathy, neuropathy, ischemic heart disease, and obstruction of large vessels. This disease has an overall prevalence rate of approximately 1 in 500 children under age 20 years, with an annual incidence of 16 new cases per 100,000 children. The incidence and prevalence in American black people is one third to one half that in the Caucasian population.

TREATMENT

Prevention through education of the family, patient, and responsible physican to recognize and treat diabetes prior to ketoacidosis is the best form of therapy. The decline in incidence of ketoacidosis at initial presentation of diabetes bears witness to the success of this approach.

In treating an established case of diabetic ketoacidosis in childhood, the following principles should be employed:

1. Establish the diagnosis through determination of the blood concentration of glucose, ketones, acid-base status, and electrolytes. Obtain a blood culture, examine the urine for bacteria and white cells, and obtain an electrocardiogram to rapidly provide an index of hyperkalemia (if T-waves are peaked). The electrolyte and acid-

base status is re-examined every 2 to 4 hours until the pattern of return to normal is evident. Catheterization of the bladder is not indicated in children; if considered necessary, bag collection or condom drainage permits an assessment of urine output. Also, for each patient, a flow sheet is constructed detailing fluid input and output, timing and dose of insulin administration, electrolytes, and acid-base status.

2. Correct fluid and electrolyte disturbances.
3. Correct acidosis through the use of bicarbonate as indicated.
4. Provide adequate insulin to restore and maintain intermediary metabolism in a normal state.

Fluid and Electrolyte Therapy

Fluid and electrolyte therapy is the most important single factor in treating diabetic ketoacidosis. Typical losses of water and major electrolytes in children, and the composition and rate of replacement in a 30-kg child are depicted in Tables 1 and 2.

One may assume dehydration to be of the order of 10%. Based on response, adjustments can subsequently be made. The initial hydrating fluid should be normal saline; in children less than 10 years of age, the initial hydrating fluid may be 0.5 normal saline. It should be recalled that hyperosmolarity is virtually universal in diabetic ketoacidosis. Thus,

even normal (0.9%) saline is hypotonic relative to the patient's serum osmolality. A gradual decline in osmolality is desirable, as too rapid a decline in osmolality is a consistent factor identified as predisposing to cerebral edema, one of the major complications of therapy in children. For the same reason, the rate of fluid replacement is adjusted so as to provide only one half of the calculated deficit over the initial 8 hours, extending replacement of the remaining one half of fluid deficits over the next 20 to 30 hours, and to commence glucose replacement as a 5% solution when blood glucose approaches 300 mg/dl.

Potassium should be started early, as total body potassium is very depleted during acidosis, even if

Table 1. FLUID AND ELECTROLYTE MAINTENANCE AND LOSSES IN DIABETIC KETOACIDOSIS

	Maintenance Requirements*	Losses†
Water	2000 ml/m²	100 ml/kg (range 60–100 ml/kg)
Sodium	45 meq/m²	6 meq/kg (range 5–13 meq/kg)
Potassium	35 meq/m²	5 meq/kg (range 4–6 meq/kg)
Chloride	30 meq/m²	4 meq/kg (range 3–9 meq/kg)
Phosphate	10 meq/m²	3 meq/kg (range 2–5 meq/kg)

*Maintenance is expressed in surface area to permit uniformity because fluid requirements change as weight increases.

† Losses are expressed per unit of body weight since the losses remain relatively constant as a function of total body weight.

Table 2. FLUID AND ELECTROLYTE LOSSES AND REPLACEMENT IN A CHILD WEIGHING 30 KG (∼ 1m²) WITH DIABETIC KETOACIDOSIS

	Loss in 10% Dehydration	Maintenance Requirement *(36 hr)*	Working Total *(36 hr)*
Water (ml)	3000	2250	5500
Sodium (meq)	180	65	250
Potassium (meq)	150	50	200
Chloride (meq)	120	45	165
Phosphate (meq)	90	15	100

Replacement Procedure	Fluid	Sodium	Potassium	Chloride	Phosphate
Hour 1	500 ml of 0.9% NaCl (normal saline)	75	—	75	—
Hour 2	500 ml of 0.45% NaCl (0.5 normal saline) plus 20 meq of KCl	35	20	55	—
Hour 3 to 12 (200 ml/hr for 10 hours)	2000 ml of 0.45% saline with 30 meq/L of potassium phosphate	150	60	150	40
Sub total Initial 12 hours	3000 ml	260	80	280	40
Next 24 hours 100 ml/hr	0.2 normal saline in 5% glucose with 40 meq per liter of potassium as the phosphate	75	100	75	60
Total over 36 hours	5400 ml	335	180	355	100

serum potassium is normal or elevated. Also, whereas potassium moves from intra- to extracellular sites during acidosis, the reverse occurs with alkalosis, particularly during provision of insulin with existing endogenous hyperglycemia, or with provision of exogenous glucose. Thus, therapy results in a shift of potassium back to the intracellular compartment and may produce hypokalemia. In our experience and that of others, hypokalemia is more common than hyperkalemia. Hence, after the initial fluid replacement of approximately 20 ml/kg has been provided, potassium should be added to subsequent infusates; serum potassium concentrations should be monitored periodically. An electrocardiogram provides a rapid assessment of hyperkalemia (high-peaked T waves) or hypokalemia (low T waves with presence of U waves). Potassium should not be infused if the urinary output is impaired. Finally, the total potassium deficit cannot be replaced in the initial 24 hours of therapy, so potassium supplements should be continued for several days.

Provision of excess chloride is almost inevitable (see Table 2) and may aggravate acidosis. However, excess chloride can be reduced through use of phosphate that is significantly depleted in diabetic ketoacidosis. Moreover, phosphate together with glycolysis is essential for, and related to, the formation of 2,3-diphosphoglycerate (2,3-DPG), which governs the oxygen dissociation curve. Thus, with deficiency of 2,3-DPG, the oxygen dissociation curve shifts to the left, that is, more oxygen is retained by hemoglobin and less is available to tissues, thereby predisposing to lactic acidosis. Acidosis tends to shift the oxygen dissociation curve back to the right (Bohr effect), thereby "compensating" in part for 2,3-DPG deficiency. As acidosis due to the accumulation of ketoacids is corrected through the provision of insulin with or without provision of bicarbonate, the effects of 2,3-DPG deficiency may no longer be "compensated" and release of oxygen to tissues be impaired. Provision of phosphate thus promotes the formation of 2,3-DPG, permits the oxygen dissociation curve to shift to the right, and facilitates the release of oxygen to tissues and the correction of acidosis. Finally, hypophosphatemia is associated with resistance to insulin action.

Although the recovery of 2,3-DPG by phosphate therapy is accelerated, one must be aware of the potential for precipitating hypocalcemia through excessive use of phosphate solutions. Hence, we recommend the use of potassium chloride alernating with a balanced solution of potassium phosphate, as outlined in Table 2. In addition, we recommend that serum calcium be measured periodically; symptomatic hypocalcemia requires appropriate treatment with calcium gluconate.

The nitroprusside reaction that routinely measures "ketones" reacts only with acetoacetate but not with beta-hydroxybutyrate. The normal ratio of beta-hydroxybutyrate to acetoacetate is approximately 3:1, but is commonly 8:1 and occasionally higher in diabetic ketoacidosis. Since with correction of acidosis, beta-hydroxybutyrate dissociates to acetoacetate, there is often an impression of persistence of ketonemia and ketonuria despite clinical improvement in the patient. For this reason, ketone bodies, as routinely measured, are not always a reliable index of therapeutic response.

Use of Bicarbonate

With provision of fluid and electrolytes, as well as insulin, metabolic acidosis usually corrects spontaneously, owing to the interruption of ketogenesis, the metabolism of ketones to bicarbonate, and the generation of bicarbonate by the distal renal tubule. Concerns over the use of bicarbonate center on four issues. First, alkalosis shifts the oxygen dissociation curve to the left, thereby diminishing the release of oxygen to tissues and potentially providing a mechanism for developing lactic acidosis. Second, alkalosis accelerates the entry of potassium into the intracellular space, and hence may produce hypokalemia. Third, provision of bicarbonate according to the calculated base deficit overcorrects and may result in alkalosis. Fourth, and perhaps most important, bicarbonate may lead to worsening in cerebral acidosis, while the plasma pH is being restored to normal. This is because HCO_3^- combines with H^+ and dissociates to CO_2 and H_2O. Whereas bicarbonate passes the blood-brain barrier slowly, CO_2 diffuses freely, thereby exacerbating cerebral acidosis and possibly cerebral depression. On the other hand, severe acidosis, with a pH of 7.1 or less, diminishes respiratory minute volume, may produce hypotension with peripheral vasodilation, impairs myocardial function, and may be a factor in insulin resistance. For these reasons, our recommendation is to not use bicarbonate unless the pH is 7.2 or below. We recommend that at a pH of 7.1 to 7.2 and below a pH of 7.1, 40 meq of HCO_3^-1m^2 and 80 meq of HCO_3^-/m^2, respectively, should be infused over 2 hours, and acid-base status re-evaluated prior to further alkali therapy. Bicarbonate should not be given by bolus infusion, as it may precipitate cardiac arrhythmias.

These principles of fluid and electrolyte therapy and correction of acidosis are the basis of ketoacidosis treatment, and often result in clinical and biochemical improvement even before the initiation of insulin. However, insulin is essential to restore intermediary metabolism.

Insulin Therapy

The continuous low-dose infusion method using a priming dose of 0.1 unit/kg followed by 0.1 unit/kg/hr is described in Table 2. It is now clear that the constant low-dose insulin infusion method is a very effective, simple, and physiologically sound form of therapy that has gained wide acceptance as the preferred method for administering insulin during diabetic ketoacidosis. The principle of the method is based on the ability to provide a constant, steady insulin concentration in plasma that approximates the peak concentration attained in normal individuals during an oral glucose tolerance test. Presumably, the same steady concentration is perceived at the cellular level, permitting a steady metabolic response without the fluctuations imposed by fluctuating insulin concentrations as must occur with intermittent forms of insulin therapy. Indeed, it has been demonstrated that with continuous low-dose insulin infusion the rate of decline, that is, the slope of the line, is constant for a given patient, although the actual slope varies from patient to patient. Because of this linearity of the response, the time at which blood glucose will approximate 300 mg/dl can usually be predicted and hypoglycemia avoided since there will be no residual subcutaneous or intramuscular depots of insulin. Concern that the insulin may adhere to glass and tubing is unfounded, and effective delivery of insulin can be provided without the use of albumin or gelatin added to the infusate bottle. Moreover, the insulin infusion can be provided by gravity drip, without the use of a special pump, although such a pump is helpful. However, it has been our policy to infuse the insulin into a separate vein from that used for the fluid and electrolyte therapy. After calculating the amount of insulin required over the initial 6 to 8 hours, this amount is added to a 250- or 500-ml bottle of 0.5 normal saline. Some of this mixture is run through the tubing and discarded; this procedure "saturates" the insulin-binding sites in the tubing. The insulin infusion can then begin in the patient at the rate calculated to provide the required dose as in Table 2. When blood glucose concentration approaches 300 mg/dl, the electrolyte solution is made up in 5 per cent glucose, and the rate of insulin infusion is halved to 0.05 units/kg/hr. Alternatively, the insulin infusion may be discontinued, and insulin may be given subcutaneously at a dose of 0.25 to 0.5 unit/kg immediately and every 6 to 8 hours while maintaining the glucose infusion, until the child can fully tolerate food. Subsequent insulin therapy using a combination of intermediate- and short-acting insulin is as described below.

With this regimen, intermediate-acting insulin is usually begun within 24 to 36 hours after commencing therapy, but 3 to 5 days is the usual time required to stabilize the insulin dose. During this time, a recognizable precipitating cause, such as infection, is appropriately treated. In addition, for both new and recurrent episodes of ketoacidosis, the time required for stablization should be utilized to educate parents and patients in the management of the child's diabetes mellitus, including proper insulin dose, injection technique, nutritional requirements, exercise, and monitoring of urine or blood. This education should be carried out by a team consisting of physician, dietitian, and nurse with special training in diabetes.

MANAGEMENT OF THE CHILD WITH TYPE I DIABETES

Insulin Regimens

The pattern of insulin concentration in the serum of normal humans during the course of 1 day consists of a basal level on which several secretory episodes coinciding with food intake are superimposed. The rise in insulin levels is synchronous with and proportional to the rise in blood glucose. Moreover, insulin is secreted into the portal circulation, and its first target organ is the liver, the key organ governing the initial disposal of a glucose load. It is naive, therefore, to expect that a single injection of intermediate-acting insulin given subcutaneously can permit the normal pattern; periods of excessive insulin resulting in a tendency to hypoglycemia, or periods of inadequate insulin resulting in hyperglycemia, or both, are inevitable. Even with injections of regular fast-acting insulin prior to each meal, normalization of blood glucose is not entirely achieved, although the degree of control is clearly improved, as are the wide fluctuations of blood glucose. It is unrealistic, however, to expect children to permit thrice daily injections of insulin.

At the onset of diabetes, or following recovery from ketoacidosis, the total daily dose of insulin is of the order of 0.5 to 1.0 unit/kg. Long-acting insulins are not routinely used in children. In view of the slow onset of intermediate-acting insulin, some fast-acting regular insulin also is given. With the single daily dose regimen, about two thirds of the total dose is intermediate-acting (NPH, Lente, and so on) and the remainder is quick-acting given 30 minutes before breakfast. The two insulins should be drawn up in the same syringe and always in the same sequence, so that any residual insulin in the "dead space" remains constant and insures greater stability of the patient once a therapeutic dose is established. Disposable syringes with fine needles, minimal dead space, and easy-to-read calibration for use with U-100 insulin have become standard and easily available. For smaller children, syringes calibrated to a maximum of 50 units are available. Adjustments in the insulin dose can be made, depending on the pattern of blood glucose or urine glucose spill. For example, if the predominant glucose spill in the urine occurs from midmorning to noon, the quick-acting form of insulin is increased; if the predominant glucose spill occurs in the late afternoon or evening, the longer-acting insulin is increased. Each increase should be approximately 10% and, except for the stabilization period following initial diagnosis when changes may be made daily, subsequent changes should be made at 2- to 3-day intervals, depending on response.

Many children can be managed with a single daily insulin injection. The initial phase of recovery of metabolic equilibrium is characterized by a period of replenishment of body tissues depleted during the evolution of diabetes. Hence, insulin requirements for the first few days may exceed the guidelines outlined above. Similar considerations will apply to nutritional requirements as outlined below.

If there is persistent nocturia or significant fasting hyperglycemia with morning glucosuria, one should consider "splitting" the total daily insulin dose. We particularly recommend twice daily injections in children aged less than 5 to 6 years, and during the pubertal growth spurt. Of the daily total of insulin, two thirds is given before breakfast and one third before the evening meal; each injection consists of intermediate- and short-acting insulin in the proportion of 2:1 or 3:1. For example, in a 30-kg child, a typical regimen at 1 unit/kg would consist of 14 units of NPH and 6 units of regular insulin before breakfast, and 6 units of NPH plus 4 units of regular insulin before the evening meal. Individual adjustment should be made according to response. With explanation of the rationale for this recommendation, patients' and parents' acceptance of, and compliance with, this twice-daily regimen has been remarkably good. For infants and children less than 5 years old, twice daily injections have regularly resulted in smoother control of blood glucose, with fewer episodes of hypoglycemia. Also, during the pubertal growth spurt, a twice-daily regimen often permits better metabolic control. Our recommendation, however, is not intended to convey an attitude of rigidity, particularly as there is evidence that twice-daily injections may not result in better metabolic control than the once-daily injections except in selected patients. Therefore, with children who are hesitant about twice-daily injections, we comply with their wish for single daily injections so as not to foster guilt, and in order to maintain confidence in the patient-family-physician relationship.

The technique of insulin injection should be taught to parents and patient, using rotating sites on arms, thighs, buttocks, and abdomen. With this rotation and the availability of the purer, single-peak insulin, lipodystrophic changes, either atrophy or hypertrophy, are far less common—indeed, they are quite rare. The rotation also helps to ensure absorption and prevent fibrosis. Some children find the abdominal wall to be a painful injection site; in these children this site may be omitted. Depending on their physical and psy-

chologic maturity, children over the age of 10 to 12 years should be encouraged to administer their own insulin injections and to monitor their own response. The assumption of responsibility for self-monitoring may be gradual, requiring a transitonal period during which parents and child participate. Once the child has assumed total responsibility, the parents must resist overprotection.

Hypersensitivity to insulin is uncommon in children. Local skin reactions may sometimes occur; these are characterized by burning, itching, tenderness, erythema, or urticaria within hours of an injection. These reactions usually resolve spontaneously over a period of days. Antihistamines may be used if necessary. Generalized reactions with severe urticaria or angioneurotic edema are rare and may spontaneously resolve, but treatment usually involves a change in the insulin, for example, from a mixed beef-pork preparation to a pure pork preparation. Desensitization also may be necessary, as may a short course of steroids. Rarely, insulin resistance develops due to a local tissue enzyme that destroys injected insulin; these patients require expert care in specialized hospital units. After several months of insulin therapy, nearly all patients can be demonstrated to have antibodies to insulin. In most, these antibodies do not interfere with metabolic response, although they may promote instability by acting as a reservoir of insulin that may be released at unpredictable times. Rarely, children with antibodies develop true insulin resistance characterized by an insulin requirement in excess of 2 units/kg/24 hr. A change to a preparation of pure pork or pure beef insulin usually resolves the problem, but a course of steroids may be necessary. Antibodies causing allergy are usually of the IgE class; IgA and IgM antibodies may be responsible for resistance.

Diet

The word diet connotes restriction and denial and, therefore, imposes a source of anxiety and often rebellion on the part of parent and patient. We therefore recommend avoidance of the word diet and speak to our patients and parents about "nutritional requirements" and "meal plans." In this context, there is no special diet for the diabetic child; rather, there are nutritional requirements that must be met for optimal growth and development. In addition, the capacity to secrete insulin in response to a meal is negligible, and since the dose of insulin is predicated on caloric intake, regularity of the eating pattern for the chosen dose of insulin becomes paramount. In general, the nutritional requirements of diabetic children are similar to those of healthy nondiabetic children of similar age, sex, weight, and activity, eating the foods of their own cultural, social, and ethnic backgrounds. The guidelines to be listed are generally applicable, but the needs of each child must be separately and individually planned and adjusted.

Total caloric intake is based on size or surface area and can be obtained from standard tables; a general rule is 1000 calories plus 100 calories for each year of life. The composition of these calories should be approximately 55 per cent carbohydrate, 30 per cent fat, and 15 per cent protein. In general, we recommend that approximately 70% of the carbohydrate content be derived from complex carbohydrates such as starch and that intake of sucrose or other highly refined sugars be avoided. Complex carbohydrates require digestion and absorption so that the plasma glucose rises slowly, whereas freely available glucose as obtained from refined sugars, including carbonated beverages, is rapidly absorbed, causing marked hyperglycemia with wide swings in the degree of metabolic control. Carbonated beverages should therefore be of the sugar-free variety, and we encourage the use of saccharin despite the recent controversy surrounding its use. Although concern in children is centered on the potential effect of a cumulative dose, recent studies provide no evidence of an association between saccharin, in the moderate doses likely to be used, and bladder cancer. Sorbitol and xylitol should not be used as artificial sweeteners in diabetics as they are products of the polyol pathway implicated in some of the complications of diabetes. Fructose has antiketogenic effects and thus might serve as a useful substitute for glucose in diabetics. However, the caloric content of fructose is equal to that of glucose.

The fat intake is adjusted so that the polyunsaturated/saturated (P/S) ratio is increased to 1.2:1.0 from the usual American average of 0.3:1.0. To achieve this desirable ratio, fats derived from animal sources are reduced and substituted by polyunsaturated fats derived from vegetable sources. This can be achieved by substituting margarine for butter and vegetable oil for animal oils in cooking, and by substituting lean cuts of beef and increased amounts of veal, chicken, turkey, and fish for fatty meats such as ham, bacon, and fatty ground beef. In addition, cholesterol intake may be limited by these measures and by limiting the number of egg yolks consumed. There is ample evidence that these simple measures reduce serum LDL cholesterol, a predisposing factor to atherosclerotic disease.

The total daily caloric intake may be divided so as to provide two tenths at breakfast, two tenths at lunch, and three tenths at dinner, leaving one tenth each for midmorning, midafternoon, and evening snacks; in older children, the midmorning snack may be omitted and the extra one tenth of balanced calories taken with lunch. Various organizations, including the American Diabetes Association, have prepared simplified methods of providing balanced meals based on these principles. The American Diabetes Association's meal plans are based on food exchanges; within each exchange of carbohydrate, protein, and fat, a wide variety of foods can be substituted or exchanged.

Thus, for practical purposes, there are few if any restrictions, and each individual may select a diet based on personal taste or preference that may be translated into the exchanges or modified with the help of the physican or dietitian. Emphasis should be placed on regularity of food intake and on the constancy of carbohydrate intake; substitution within the carbohydrate exchanges is permissible so long as total carbohydrate intake is constant. Occasional excesses on special occasions such as birthdays, parties, and holidays not only are permissible but are encouraged so as not to foster rebellion and stealth in obtaining desired food. Similarly, cakes, doughnuts, and candies are permissible on occasions as long as the food exchange value and carbohydrate content are considered in that day's meal plan. Special adjustments in meal planning (and insulin) must be made during the adolescent growth spurt and with vigorous exercise. Above all, adjustments must be constantly made to meet the needs of each individual, and flexibility rather than rigidity is of the essence in children. Special brochures and pamphlets describing the exchanges and sample meal plans for children are usually available from regional diabetes groups; their use should be encouraged.

Exercise

Exercise is an integral part of growth and development. No form of exercise, including competitive sports, should be forbidden to the diabetic child, who should not be made to feel different or restricted. A major complication of exercise in diabetes is hypoglycemia reactions during or within hours after exercise. If hypoglycemia does not occur with exercise, adjustments in diet or insulin are not necessary and glucoregulation is likely to be improved through increased utilization of glucose by muscles. In diabetes, the major contributing factor to hypoglycemia with exercise is an increased rate of insulin absorption from its injection site consequent upon increased blood flow in the exercising limbs. Thus, one approach to minimize hypoglycemia is to choose an injection site least likely to be exercised. For example, if the exercise involves primarily leg muscles, the upper arms are used as the injection site and vice versa. The abdomen may be more suitable when both arms and legs will be used. However, from the practical point of view, exercise usually involves all limbs, with an increased blood flow throughout the body. One additional carbohydrate exchange may be taken before exercise, and readily available glucose in the form of orange juice, carbonated beverage, or candy should be available during and after exercise. With experience, as well as trial and error, each child and parent guided by the physician learns the optimal approach for the individual. Occasionally, when exercise is programmed at regular times and is frequently associated with hypoglycemia, the daily dose of insulin may need to be reduced by 10%. Exercise also improves glucoregulation by increasing insulin receptors, and lipid metabolism by raising HDL (high-density lipoprotein) cholesterol.

Monitoring

The education of each family and patient must stress the importance of self-monitoring via urinary glucose and ketone spill as guidelines for adjusting insulin dosage and nutritional needs. A carefully maintained record charting the urine glucose content before each major meal and the evening snack is desirable, but rarely accurately maintained by children. The tests are performed on second void specimens; that is, the bladder is emptied and the urine discarded; half an hour later a second specimen is obtained for testing, to more accurately reflect the metabolic situation at the time of testing. These records are notoriously unreliable, however, for several reasons. There may be self-delusion, reliance on memory with charting of records immediately prior to the visit with the physician, attempts to please the physician and avoid guilt or rebuke, and the cumbersome nature of the tests, involving 2 drops of urine, 10 drops of water, plus the tablet for glucose (Clinitest), and urine directly on the tablet for ketone measurement (acetest). The most frequently omitted test is at noon while at school; children object to the potential embarrassment. When reliable readings indicate 2% or more glucose in the urine for 48 hours, the insulin dose should be increased by 10%. Conversely, when urine is consistently negative for glucose for 48 hours, insulin may need to be reduced by 10% if hypoglycemia reactions ensue, or if blood glucose levels (determined via glucose oxidase strips) are 60 mg/dl or less. In the absence of symptomatic hypoglycemia and documented low blood glucose levels, absence of glucosuria does not warrant a reduction in insulin as these patients show desirable metabolic control. Consistent patterns of excessive urine glucose spill at fixed times in the morning or afternoon allow rational changes in the morning or evening dose and type of insulin.

Intelligent and honest individuals or families learn to adjust; they should be encouraged to avoid dependence on the physician. When in doubt, the physician may request a fractional 24-hour urine collection. The urine may be collected in three fractions: 8:00 A.M. to 2:00 P.M., 2:00 P.M. to 8:00 P.M., and 8:00 P.M. to 8:00 A.M. Assessment of volume and semiquantitative or quantitative glucose in each sample permits rational decision in regard to adjusting the type and dose of insulin.

In highly motivated young adults who have been intensely educated in diabetes, self-monitoring of blood glucose before and 2 hours after each meal, using glucose oxidase strips such as Dextrostix in conjunction with a reflectance meter, or Chemstrips, with appropriate insulin adjustment based on blood glucose level, has permitted an unprecedented degree of control. It remains to be seen whether this can be done in children, but the required discipline is likely to preclude this possibility. Pain may not be the limiting factor; a small portable device that automates capillary blood-letting in a relatively painless fashion is now commercially available (Autolet).

The physician also has available measurement of glycosylated hemoglobin (HbAlc) that can provide a long-term index of control. HbAlc represents hemoglobin to which glucose has been nonenzymatically attached. The reaction occurs in the blood stream after hemoglobin is synthesized in bone marrow. Because the reaction is slow, proportional to the prevailing blood glucose concentration, and continues irreversibly throughout the 120-day life span of the red blood cell, the level of glycosylated hemoglobin is a reflection of the integrated "time-averaged" blood glucose concentration over the preceding 2 to 3 months. The test procedure, when properly performed in the laboratory, is not confounded by an isolated episode of hyperglycemia nor is it subject to manipulation as are reported urine test results. In this regard, measurement of HbAlc is superior to urine testing and to random or fasting blood glucose measurements, which reflect an isolated instance in the continuum of metabolic change. Moreover, the stress of obtaining blood may be sufficient to raise blood glucose concentration upon which is based the assessment of control or the recommended changes in insulin dosage. Consequently, we do not perform occasional fasting blood glucose measurements in our patients, relying instead on HbAlc measurement as an objective index of compliance and long-term control. Periodic evaluation by HbAlc measurement may also help resolve questions relating the degree of control to the subsequent development of complications.

Hypoglycemic Reactions

All diabetic children experience a hypoglycemic reaction during the course of their disease. Hypoglycemia occurs suddenly or over minutes, in contrast to diabetic ketoacidosis, which develops over hours or days. The symptoms and signs are those due to an outpouring of catecholamines, including trembling, shaking, sweating, apprehension, and tachycardia, and those due to cerebral glucopenia, including hunger, drowsiness, mood or personality changes, mental confusion, seizures, and coma. There is now evidence that these symptoms may occur with a sudden drop in blood glucose to levels that would not meet the criteria for hypoglycemia (less than 60 mg/dl) in healthy subjects. The avoidance of severe hypoglycemic episodes should be a major treatment objective; they have been implicated in ultimately provoking epileptic seizures and there is an increased frequency of abnormal electroencephalographic findings.

The occurrence of hypoglycemia in a diabetic child indicates an inappropriate level of insulin effect for that individual's energy intake and expenditure. Common causes include the evolution of the honeymoon phase after initial diagnosis, errors in insulin dosage, inadequate caloric intake and exercise in the absence of increasing caloric intake. The most important factor in the treatment of hypoglycemia is education for patient and family to be familiar with the symptoms and signs and to avoid known precipitating factors outlined above. Acutely, a carbohydrate-containing snack, or a drink such as orange juice or sugar-containing carbonated beverage, or candy (each equivalent to 5 to 10 grams of glucose) should be taken. Patients, parents, and teachers should also be instructed in the use of glucagon; 0.5 mg given intramuscularly is particularly useful when the patient is losing consciousness or is vomiting. If exercise is the precipitating factor, the patient should be instructed to take additional calories prior to exercise and, if hypoglycemia persists, to reduce the morning dose of insulin by 10%.

The Somogyi Phenomenon and Brittle Diabetes

Hypoglycemic episodes that may be mild and manifest as late nocturnal or early morning sweating, night terrors, and headaches and that alternate rapidly within 4 to 6 hours with ketosis, hyperglycemia, ketonuria, and severe glucosuria should arouse suspicion of the Somogyi phenomenon. This has been aptly described as "hypoglycemia begetting hyperglycemia" and is believed to be due to an outpouring of counter-regulatory hormones in response to the insulin-induced hypoglycemia. The coexistence of this brittle form of diabetes with daily insulin doses of more than 2 units/kg suggests that the phenomenon is present and that the insulin dose should be reduced. Brittle diabetes implies that control of blood glucose fluctuates widely and rapidly, despite frequent upward adjustment of the insulin dose.

Although the Somogyi phenomenon may be the most common cause of the instability or brittleness in children, the early morning rise in blood glucose following nocturnal hypoglycemia appears to be primarily due to waning of biologically available insulin and not to counter-regulatory hormones. Therein lies the dilemma: increasing the insulin dose may exacerbate the nocturnal episodes without improving metabolic control. When this syndrome is clinically suspected, the insulin dose should be decreased by 10% and further reductions made at 3-day intervals; abrupt reduction of insulin may precipitate ketoacidosis. In other patients with brittle diabetes, better control is often achieved by a change from single to twice-daily insulin injections; by a change from beef-pork mixtures to pure pork or pure beef insulins, which may circumvent problems with antibodies that bind insulin and act as a reservoir of potentially releasable insulin; and by attention to psychologic problems that are the basis for manipulative and deliberate errors in insulin or nutritional intake or both.

Psychologic Aspects

Diabetes in a child affects the lifestyle and interpersonal relationship of the family unit. Anxiety and guilt are common in parents. Similar feelings, coupled with denial and rejection, are common in children, particularly during the rebellious teenage years. No specific personality disorder or psychopathology is characteristic of diabetes; similar feelings are observed in families that have members with other chronic disorders.

In diabetic patients, these feelings are expressed as nonadherence to instructions regarding nutrition and insulin therapy, or noncompliance with self-monitoring. Deliberate overdosing with insulin, resulting in hypoglycemia, and omission of insulin or excesses in nutrition, resulting in ketoacidosis, may be pleas for help, manipulative events to escape family surroundings perceived as undesirable or intolerable, or, occasionally, manifestations of suicidal intent. Over-protection by parents is frequent and often not in the best interest of the patient. Feelings of being different or of being alone are common, and not unjustified in view of the restrictions imposed by schedules requiring urine testing, insulin administration, and nutritional limitations. Furthermore, publicity regarding the likelihood of developing complications and of decreased life span in Type 1 diabetes must foster anxiety. In addition, misinformation abounds regarding the risk of developing diabetes in siblings or offspring, or the risk of pregnancy in young diabetic women. In turn, this information fosters further anxiety.

Many of these problems can be averted through knowledge, understanding, and patience and counseling based on correct information and the fostering of attitudes that do not perceive the patient as a cripple but rather as a productive and potentially reproductive member of society. Recognizing the impact of these problems, various local and regional associations have organized peer discussion groups; feelings of isolation and frustration improve with the sharing of common problems. Summer camps for children organized by various organizations, offer an excellent opportunity to learn and share under expert supervision. Reinforcement of education regarding diabetes, insulin dose and technique of administration, nutrition, and exercise and hypoglycemia reactions can be performed by medical and paramedical personnel. And the presence of peers with similar problems affords newer insights for the diabetic child.

Referral for psychologic help or for specialists' advice is sometimes clearly indicated. In managing diabetes in children and adolescents, pediatricians or family physicians should be aware of their pivotal role as counselors and advisors, as well as physicians, and of the possibility of recourse to expert advice when necessary.

Infections and Surgery

Infections. Systemic or local infections are no more common than in nondiabetic children. During intercurrent illnesses, including infection or trauma, diabetic children should take additional insulin: 10 to 20 per cent of total daily insulin should be administered as the regular (short-acting) form before each meal if glucosuria remains pronounced (5 per cent) and ketonuria is present so that the development of ketoacidosis is aborted.

Patients who are vomiting should nevertheless take some insulin: approximately 50 per cent of the daily dose is a general rule. If vomiting continues and the patient cannot tolerate clear liquids, admission to hospital and consideration of intravenous therapy with glucose and electrolytes are warranted.

Surgery. If surgery is elective, the patient should be admitted to the hospital 24 hours before, and the usual nutritional requirements and insulin provided. Supplemental regular insulin also may be given for more optimal control of blood glucose. On the morning of surgery, an infusion of 5 per cent glucose in 0.45 per cent saline plus 20 meq of potassium chloride/l is begun, and regular insulin is added to the infusate bottle so that 1 unit of insulin is provided for each 2 to 4 gm of administered glucose. The blood glucose concentration should be monitored at periodic intervals before, during, and after surgery so that glucose levels remain at approximately 120 to 150 mg/dl through appropriate changes in the dose of insulin and/or glucose delivered. This regimen may be continued during the operative and postoperative period and discontinued when the patient is awake and capable of oral food and fluid intake. The rate of infusion should provide maintenance fluid requirements plus estimated losses during surgery. During the interval between liquid and solid foods, insulin therapy should be given as the regular form at 0.25 unit/kg at 6-hour intervals, with appropriate adjustments based on blood glucose or urinary glucose spill. When solid food is tolerated, the insulin regimen used prior to surgery can be instituted. These metabolic aspects should be under the guidance of a physician experienced in diabetes, working in conjunction with the responsible surgeon.

If emergency surgery is needed, an intravenous line that provides 5 to 10% glucose in 0.45 per cent saline plus 20 meq of potassium chloride/l is begun and insulin added to the infusate to provide 1 unit for each 2 to 4 gm of glucose infused. Again, blood glucose concentration should be maintained at approximately 120 to 150 mg/dl. Where possible, rehydration and metabolic balance should precede surgery. Following surgery, the regimen described above can be instituted. Patients undergoing minor surgery under local anesthesia can have their usual insulin and food intake; losses through vomiting should be replaced through intravenous glucose.

The desirable objectives in managing a diabetic child who has surgery are to prevent hypoglycemia during anesthesia, severe fluid loss, or diabetic acidosis. The regimens described are generally applicable, but vigilance and individual adjustment for each patient are necessary to achieve these desirable goals.

NEUROVASCULAR AND OTHER COMPLICATIONS OF DIABETES IN CHILDREN: RELATION TO CONTROL

The increasing survival of the diabetic child as a result of the availability of insulin, fluid and electrolyte therapy, antibiotics, and modern anesthesia is associated with an increasing prevalence of complications that affect the microcirculation of the eye (retinopathy) and kidney (nephropathy), the nerves (neuropathy), as well as large vessel disease and cataracts. Statistics recently compiled by the Public Health Service, National Institute of Health, indicate that retinopathy is present in 45 to 60% of insulin-dependent diabetic patients after 20 years of known disease and in 20% after 10 years. The incidence of proliferative retinopathy increases progressively with increasing years of known disease; 40% of diagnosed patients are less than 19 years of age. Lens opacities are present in at least 5% of diabetics aged less than 19 years. Diabetic nephropathy is also common—up to 40% after 25 years of diabetes in children; renal disease may account for about half of the deaths in long-term insulin-dependent diabetics. The preponderance of clinical, experimental, and biochemical studies now strongly suggests an association between control and later development of complications. In addition, these studies implicate some possible biochemical pathways that might be responsible for these complications.

Clearly, genetic predisposition plays a part. Equally clearly, all debate relative to humans remains moot, because conventional treatment modes have resulted in varying degrees of imperfect metabolic control without restoration of the fine moment-to-moment regulation of normal physiologic events. Nevertheless, within the imperfection imposed by currently available treatment, there still appears to be a relationship between the degree of control and the development of complications. Consequently, as long as reduction of these late complications remains a possibility, physicians treating children with diabetes have an enormous responsibility of maintaining metabolism as near normal as is compatible with the physical and psychologic well-being of each child. Despite the potential for developing complications, survival for 40 years or more is feasible.

AUTOIMMUNE DISEASES ASSOCIATED WITH CHILDHOOD DIABETES

Chronic lymphocytic thyroiditis (Hashimoto thyroiditis) is frequently associated with Type I diabetes in children. The prevalence of thyroid cytoplasmic antibodies in the sera of patients with Type I diabetes is 2 to 20 times the rate found in control populations, and as many as 1 in 5 insulin-dependent diabetics may have thyroid antibodies in their serum. However, only a small proportion go on to develop clinical hypothyroidism and in these the interval between diagnosis of diabetes and thyroid disease is an average of 5 years. Therefore, we advocate routine palpation of the thyroid gland in all children with insulin-dependent diabetes. If the gland feels firm or enlarged, thyroid antibodies and serum thyroid-stimulating hormone (TSH) concentrations should be measured. A TSH level of greater than 10 μU/ml indicates existing or incipient failure of thyroid function, which warrants replacement with thyroid hormone. A slowing in the rate of growth may also indicate thyroid failure and suggests the need for measurements of serum thyroxine and TSH concentration. When two features such as diabetes and thyroid disease coexist, the possibility of adrenal insufficiency should be borne in mind. This may be heralded by decreasing insulin requirements due to an increasing frequency of hypoglycemia, increasing pigmentation of the skin and buccal mucosa, salt craving, weakness, asthenia, postural hypotension, or frank addisonian crisis indicating primary adrenal failure. This syndrome is unusual in the first decade of life but may become apparent in the second decade or later.

In addition to thyroid and adrenal disease, circulating antibodies to gastric parietal cells or to intrinsic factor are two to three times more common in patients with Type I diabetes than in normal subjects. There is a good correlation between the existence of gastric parietal cell antibodies and the presence of atrophic gastritis, and between circulating antibodies to intrinsic factor and malabsorption of vitamin B_{12}. Thus, the possibility of megaloblastic anemia should be considered in Type I diabetes, although its occurrence in children is rare.

TRANSIENT DIABETES OF THE NEONATE

Onset of persistent, insulin-dependent diabetes before age 6 months is most unusual. Transient diabetes mellitus in the neonate has its onset in the first week of life and is self-limited in duration, lasting only several weeks to months before spontaneous resolution. It occurs most invariably in infants who are small for gestational age and is characterized by hyperglycemia and pronounced glucosuria resulting in severe dehydration, but with only minimal or no ketonemia or ketonuria. Insulin response to glucose or tolbutamide is low to absent; basal insulin concentrations are normal. Following spontaneous recovery, the insulin responses to these same stimuli are brisk and normal. Occurrence of the syndrome in consecutive siblings has been reported. Permanent diabetes has not recurred in any affected infant who has recovered. Transient diabetes of the neonate should be distinguished from severe hyperglycemia occurring in diseases associated with abnormalities of the central nervous system and disturbances of electrolytes. These patients are usually older infants who respond promptly to rehydration with a minimal requirement for insulin.

Once the disease is recognized, insulin therapy is mandatory. One to 2 units/kg of an intermediate-acting insulin in divided doses brings dramatic improvement and accelerated growth and weight gain. Attempts to gradually withdraw the insulin therapy may be made as soon as recurrent hypoglycemia manifests or after 2 months of age. Parents should be reassured regarding the transient nature of the disease and excellent prognosis.

Hypoglycemia

NOEL KEITH MACLAREN M.D.,
and MARVIN CORNBLATH, M.D.

Clinical hypoglycemia is the association of an abnormally low blood sugar with a variety of signs and symptoms which are improved with glucose administration or food. The clinical state results from decreased glucose availability to the central nervous system and the induced catecholamine response. Weakness, apathy, irritability, hunger, bizarre behavior, mental confusion, apnea, cyanosis, hypothermia, convulsions, and coma, together with pallor, sweating, tremulousness, tachycardia, and shock may result.

The Dextrostix is a useful screening technique, but a reliable laboratory glucose determination of blood or cerebrospinal fluid must be done in every patient before therapy is initiated. In addition, a further blood sample should be obtained prior to treating the acute episode of hypoglycemia, since the underlying cause of the hypoglycemia can often be diagnosed on this *critical blood sample*. A minimum of 2 to 4 ml of serum or plasma should be frozen and saved for determination of insulin, growth hormone, and cortisol, as well as metabolites, such as alanine β-hydroxybutyrate, uric acid, and lactate. The first urine specimen after the episode should be analyzed for ketones and reducing sugars (Clinitest tablet).

In neonates with persistent or recurrent hypoglycemia, as well as in older infants and children, an abbreviated glucagon (0.05 mg/kg not to exceed 1 mg, given IM or IV) tolerance test (0, 10, 20 minutes) during a hypoglycemia episode should be performed to differentiate between hypoglycemia due to hyperinsulinism and that due to other etiologies. A brisk, significant hyperglycemic response to glucagon implicates hyperinsulinism. In instances of nonresponse to glucagon, the test should be terminated with IV glucose. The initial *critical blood sample* can still be diagnostic and should always be obtained.

NEONATAL HYPOGLYCEMIA

Hypoglycemia has been defined in the neonate as replicate whole blood glucose values of less than 20 mg/dl in the infant under 2500 gm, less than 30 mg/dl in full-size infants during the first 72 hours of life, and less than 40 mg/dl thereafter. Plasma or serum glucose values tend to be 15 to 20% higher than those of whole blood, depending on hematocrit. Most infants with hypoglycemia have clinical manifestations such as twitching, jitteriness, apathy, cyanotic spells, hypothermia, pallor, limpness or convulsions. Symptomatic infants should be treated if the Chemstrip reads 40 mg/dl or less while waiting for the diagnostic laboratory blood results.

Give 2 ml (0.5 gm) per kg of 25 per cent glucose IV at the rate of 1 ml/min, and continue the infusion with glucose in water to provide 6 to 10 mg/kg/min for at least 24 hours, or at increased rates until the blood sugar is stable in the normal range. Blood glucose levels should be carefully monitored and the rate of glucose infusion altered accordingly The total 24-hour fluid requirement determines the concentration of glucose to be used. If the total requirement is 65 to 85 ml/kg/day, use 15 to 20% glucose; if it is 115 to 145 ml/kg/day, use 10% glucose. After 12 to 24 hours, add 40 mEq/L NaCl (0.2N saline) to the glucose solution. If parenteral fluid therapy alone is required beyond 24 to 48 hours, add potassium (1 to 2 mEq/kg/day as KCl) and monitor serum potassium levels. Oral feedings should be introduced as soon as clinical manifestations subside. Therapy can be tapered off after blood sugar levels have remained over 30 to 40 mg/dl for 24 to 48 hours by changing to 5% glucose and then stopping.

Never discontinue hypertonic glucose abruptly, for a reactive hypoglycemia may ensure.

If symptoms persist beyond 2 to 4 hours despite a sustained elevation in blood sugar, the hypoglycemia may have been associated with one of a variety of underlying conditions, of which CNS hemorrhage, congenital defects, sepsis, respiratory distress syndrome, hypoplastic left heart syndrome, asphyxia or anoxia, and metabolic aberrations such as hypocalcemia are the most common. Thus it is necessary to diagnose and treat all associated disease as well.

If blood sugar levels remain under 30 mg/dl with adequate glucose therapy, start hydrocortisone (Solu-Cortef), 5 mg/kg/day every 8 hours, by the oral, IM, or IV route. Hydrocortisone can be tapered when the blood sugar has remained over 30 mg/dl for 48 hours, and stopped after 3 days. During treatment, blood sugar should be monitored at 2- to 6-hour intervals.

Glucagon, 0.05 mg/kg IM or IV (not to exceed 1 mg), can be used with effect in asymptomatic infants of diabetic mothers or initially in symptomatic infants while the IV infusions are being started. However, glucagon and epinephrine are not recommended for treating any other neonate with hypoglycemia.

Rarely, despite the above therapies, chronic or persistent hypoglycemia may occur, may be life-threatening, and may be responsible for permanent CNS damage. Thus, an aggressive diagnostic and therapeutic approach is indicated as noted below (see diazoxide and pancreatic surgery for hyperinsulinism).

HYPOGLYCEMIA OF INFANCY

Inborn Errors of Hepatic Carbohydrate Metabolism. Such disorders may result in hypoglycemic episodes from the neonatal period or from early infancy, and tend to ameliorate with age.

HEPATIC GLYCOGEN STORAGE DISEASES. *Type I* (glucose-6-phosphatase deficiency). A diet containing 60 to 70% of the caloric requirement as carbohydrate (glucose, maltose or starch and containing no or little fructose or galactose), 15% as protein and the remainder as fat, given at 3- to 4-hour intervals, plus a continuous nasogastric drip of glucose or Vivonex-HN (glucose, oligosaccharides, fat 0.8% and protein 18% during the night is indicated for older infants.

Type III (amylo-1,6-glucosidase or "debrancher" deficiency). Hypoglycemia is less frequent and usually follows episodes of caloric deprivation, intercurrent infections, or gastrointestinal upset. Since gluconeogenesis is intact, a high protein diet with regular meals and a bedtime snack is advised.

Types VI and IX (phosphorylase and phosphorylase-kinase deficiency). Hypoglycemic episodes are mild and infrequent. The measures for type III generally apply.

Type O (glycogen synthetase deficiency) probably is very rare, and severe hypoglycemia is reported within a few hours of fasting. Frequent feedings, high in carbohydrate and protein, should be the basic approach.

Type IV (brancher α-1,4 glucan: α-1,4 glucan 6-glyosyl transferase deficiency): Progressive early cardiac and hepatic failure is characteristic in this rare disease. High protein–low carbohydrate diets enriched with corn oil should be offered. Purified α-glucosidase from *Aspergillus niger* has been given with possible benefit. None of these therapies appears to improve the prognosis.

GALACTOSEMIA (galactose-1-phosphate uridyl transferase deficiency). Strict avoidance of lactose-containing milk, foods, and sweets is essential to prevent the associated postprandial hypoglycemia and other sequelae.

FRUCTOSE INTOLERANCE (fructose-1-phosphate aldolase deficiency). Postprandial hypoglycemia episodes date from the introduction of sucrose into the diet. Give a fructose-free diet, avoiding table sugars, sweets, and fruits, and substitute glucose as the dietary sugar.

FRUCTOSE-1,6-DIPHOSPHATASE DEFICIENCY. A special diet consisting of 56% utilizable carbohydrate (glucose, maltose or lactose), 12% protein and 32% fat has been reported to be effective; however, intercurrent illness may require alkali and glucose therapy.

Inborn Errors Resulting in Hypoglycemia

MAPLE SYRUP URINE DISEASE. Hypoglycemia is a common accompaniment of an oxidative decarboxylation defect of the ketoacids of valine, leucine, and isoleucine. The hypoglycemia may be due in part to hyperleucinemia (see under hyperinsulinism), and should be treated with IV glucose and protein withdrawal until the infant's condition is stable. A diet restricted in the above amino acids to ensure appropriate blood levels of them will usually prevent hypoglycemia. Intermittent forms may respond to thiamine administration.

METHYLMALONIC ACIDURIA (methylmalonyl CoA carbonylmutase deficiency). Hypoglycemia frequently accompanies episodes of infection or trauma resulting in metabolic organic acidosis. Treatment should be symptomatic. Some patients improve with vitamin B_{12} treatment.

TYROSINOSIS (para-hydroxyphenylpyruvic acid oxidase deficiency). Hypoglycemia in variable degree accompanies the picture of hepatic dysfunction. Distinction between tyrosinosis and neonatal hepatitis is difficult. Treatment of hypoglycemic episodes is by carbohydrate administration. Dietary restriction of tyrosine and methionine is often prescribed but with little effect.

Endocrine Disorders Associated with Hypoglycemia

HYPOPITUITARISM. A syndrome of congenital hypopituitarism has been described that may result in profound life-threatening hypoglycemia from the first hours of life. Associated findings are jaundice, hepatomegaly, midline abnormalities, edema, and often microphallus in the male. Multiple endocrine deficiencies usually are present, and therapy consists of glucose and steroids, followed by specific replacement therapy. Growth hormone deficiency may result in hypoglycemic episodes from early life; however, they become less frequent during the school years, owing perhaps to larger body size. Replacement therapy with human growth hormone at 1 to 2 units thrice weekly is indicated. In combined GH and corticotropin deficiency, a trial of GH therapy alone is justified if there is no mineralocorticoid deficiency, since glucocorticoid therapy retards the growth response from GH treatment. If hypoglycemia persists, cortisone acetate, 0.75 to 1.0 mg/kg/day (25 mg/m²/day) in divided doses (one half this dose if IM) is effective.

ADRENAL INSUFFICIENCY. Congenital hypoplasia of the adrenals, corticotropin unresponsiveness, and rarely congenital virilizing hyperplasia may be associated with hypoglycemia. Cortisone replacement therapy as above is indicated. During intercurrent illnesses, the dose should be doubled.

HYPERINSULINISM. Inappropriately high insulin secretion may occur in infancy, associated with the "infant giant," Beckwith-Wiedemann syndrome, or without physical stigmata. Histologically the pancreas may show beta cell hyperplasia, nesidioblastosis, or beta cell tumor. Surgery is often required in such cases and should not be delayed in infants refractory to adequate glucose, diazoxide, and/or glucocorticoid therapy. If a discrete tumor is not palpated at laparotomy, a subtotal pancreatectomy removing at least 80 to 90% of the pancreas should be carried out. Diazoxide may be used postoperatively if necessary, but considerable salt retention may occur in smaller infants (see below). Infants with hypoglycemia and elevated insulin values after oral leucine should be given leucine restricted diets. The diet must be adequate in leucine for growth, but divided into 3 or more meals to provide small amounts of leucine. Offer carbohydrate 30 minutes after feeds and before sleep. For infants, S-14 (Wyeth) is recommended, but SMA-26, Enfamil, Bremil, or Similac can be used. Diazoxide may induce striking improvement in those responding poorly to diet. Partial pancreatectomy may be necessary in leucine-sensitive patients with beta cell hyperplasia or adenoma.

Drug Therapy. For many infants, regular feeding schedules and avoidance of overnight fasting are adequate. For others, attacks become recurrent and further measures are necessary.

DIAZOXIDE. This drug is a thiazide derivative. It has a major action in inhibiting insulin secretion. Its side effects include hypertrichosis, hypotension, salt retention, hyperuricemia and low IgG levels. In the neonate, anorexia, vomiting, striking salt and water retention and even hypertension have been noted, especially with higher doses (>12 to 15 mg/kg/day). In practice, hirsutism (hypertrichiasis lanuginosa) is frequently encountered, and parents should be warned about this before its appearance.

Start with 6 mg/kg/day in 8- to 12-hour doses by mouth, and increase as necessary to maximum doses of 20 to 25 mg/kg/day. Doses near 10 mg/kg/day usually are effective. Diazoxide should *not* be discontinued *suddenly* after prolonged use.

STEROIDS. Oral cortisone acetate (5 mg/kg/day) or prednisone (1 to 2 mg/kg/day) in 2 to 3 divided doses is often effective. The steroid dosage should be reduced by about 20% weekly until the lowest dose compatible with freedom from hypoglycemia is reached. Steroids will retard growth and cause other problems, and should be withdrawn slowly after prolonged use.

ADRENERGIC DRUGS. These offer the theoretic advantages of inhibiting insulin release, mobilizing fat stores, and promoting hyperglycemia. Sus-Phrine or epinephrine, 0.3 ml subcutaneously, may be useful in treating an acute episode and can be given by parents in an emergency. Ephedrine may be used in long-term management, particularly in patients who fail to respond to hypoglycemia with increased catecholamine output.

GLUCAGON. In infants with hyperinsulinism, glucagon may produce a dramatic response. Give 0.05 mg/kg, not to exceed 1.0 mg total dose, IV or IM. If the infant responds to glucagon, parents should be taught to administer it at home in an emergency. Continuous infusions of glucagon at 15 mg/kg/min may be useful especially in concert with somatostatin infusions.

SOMATOSTATIN. Continuous IV infusions of somatostatin at 4–8 mg/kg/min are usually effective; however, the effect is short lived. This form of therapy should be offered only as an adjunct once definitive management, e.g., pancreatectomy, has been decided upon. This therapy should be considered experimental. Platelet count should be monitored.

HYPOGLYCEMIA IN LATE INFANCY AND CHILDHOOD

Any of the previously mentioned endocrinopathies may occur at this age. Hypoglycemia may occur in children with psychosocial growth retardation. These patients have a functional hypopituitarism with GH and ACTH deficiency. Placing of the child in an environment providing affection and concern produces dramatic improvement.

The frequency of *islet cell tumor* increases with age but it remains a rare cause of hypoglycemia at any age. Treatment is surgical. In patients who have persistent hypoglycemia after partial pancreatectomy, diazoxide may be effective. Streptozotocin, which selectively destroys the pancreatic beta cells in animals, has had restricted and limited use in humans with beta cell carcinoma. Curiously, the human beta cell may be relatively resistant to damage by this drug. For adults, 2 to 5 gm have been given IV at 1- to 4-week intervals for 2 to 3 doses. Nausea and vomiting are usual. This drug is experimental, highly unstable, and difficult to use and relatively ineffective.

Drug ingestion or the malicious administration of insulin should always be considered as a cause of hypoglycemia. Overdose of insulin or hypoglycemic drugs may respond to glucagon (0.5 to 1 mg by injection). Alcohol taken during fasting can cause serious hypoglycemia by inhibiting hepatic gluconeogenesis. In all cases of *alcohol ingestion,* the child should have his stomach washed out and be admitted to the hospital for monitoring blood sugar levels. If he is drowsy, IV glucose is given at a rate of 6 to 8 mg/kg/min. Hypoglycemia may complicate severe aspirin overdose. Glucose therapy as outlined previously is given for hypoglycemia occurring in Reye's syndrome, hypothermia, malnutrition states and diarrheal disorders.

Ketotic Hypoglycemia of Childhood. Ketotic hypoglycemia was the most common syndrome of hypoglycemia in childhood; however, for unknown reasons it became less frequently recognized. It rarely occurs before 1 year of age, and attacks seldom persist into puberty. Hypoglycemic episodes are widely spaced and can be largely prevented with frequent high-protein, high-carbohydrate, low-fat meals coupled with the routine testing for ketonuria at bedtime, on rising and at times of illness. If ketonuria is found, attacks may be prevented with sugar in the form of candy, carbonated drinks, or sweetened juices. This must be continued until the ketonuria clears. If vomiting, coma, or convulsions occur, give Instant Glucose* or Monojel or 0.5 to 1 gm of IV glucose per kg by push, followed by 0.5 gm/kg/hour until food can be taken. Glucagon is characteristically ineffective and the poor response is often diagnostic. Treatment with glucose is essential. Steroids prevent attacks but are seldom required since most children respond to dietary measures.

The clinical picture of ketotic hypoglycemia may be seen in children with isolated growth hormone deficiency, adrenal insufficiency, or panhypo-

---

*Tubes of Instant Glucose and absorbable gel are available from the Diabetes Association of Greater Cleveland, 10205 Carnegie Avenue, Cleveland, Ohio 44106.

pituitarism. The initial *critical plasma sample* (see above) should provide the information to lead one to suspect these diagnoses. Definitive testing and specific treatment are indicated for specific confirmed hormone deficiencies.

Hypoglycemia often constitutes a medical emergency, and glucose administration is required, although some patients will respond to glucagon or epinephrine. Rational therapy subsequently depends on identification of the cause.

Diabetes Insipidus

JOHN F. CRIGLER, JR., M.D.

There are essentially two types of diabetes insipidus (DI)—neurogenic and nephrogenic. The former is vasopressin-responsive, since it results from a deficiency of antidiuretic hormone production due to destruction of cells of the supraoptic and paraventricular nuclei of the hypothalamus. Symptoms of polydipsia and polyuria in these patients may vary considerably because the deficiency of vasopressin is incomplete or other hypothalamic-pituitary dysfunctions (deficiencies of ACTH, TSH, and growth hormone, disturbance in the recognition of water requirements, and so on) that influence water balance are present. Both these factors may have a role in defining therapeutic needs. Conversely, the polydipsia and polyuria of patients with nephrogenic DI, which is frequently familial and characteristically marked, is vasopressin-resistant, for the basic defect is in the response of the nephron to antidiuretic hormone. This fundamental difference in the pathophysiology of the two disorders determines the nature of treatment for each.

It is possible, however, at times to apply with advantage the therapeutic procedures used to treat patients with nephrogenic diabetes insipidus to patients with neurogenic DI when use of vasopressin preparations presents unacceptable risk for the benefit received. The latter condition may apply to infants in the first year or two of life when adequate calories characteristically carry with them water loads in excess of amounts that can be excreted under the continuous antidiuresis produced by the longer-acting vasopressin preparations. It may apply also to patients with loss of ability to recognize water requirements (hypo- or hyperdipsia inappropriate for their state of water balance) who have complete vasopressin deficiency or are unable to tolerate drugs that alter thirst and augment antidiuretic hormone activity. For this reason, treatment of nephrogenic diabetes is discussed first.

Nephrogenic DI (Vasopressin-Resistant). The approach to treatment of this disorder is limited at the moment to minimizing water required for obligatory solute excretion by the kidney. Healthy persons eating a normal diet excrete 500 to 600 mosm/m^2/24 hr of solute. At a urine concentration of 100 mosm/kg (specific gravity approximately 1.001), 5 to 6 l/m^2/24 hr of water are required to excrete this amount of solute, and additional water would be necessary to cover requirements for insensible loss, stool, and growth. Reduction of the osmolar load by a low-solute diet (fasting reduces solute excretion to approximately 375 mosm/m^2/24 hr and a minimum of 200 mosm/m^2/24 hr has been accomplished in persons taking only glucose 100 gm/m^2/24 hr) can significantly decrease water requirements. Such diets are of significant benefit if they are accepted by the patient to a degree that total caloric intake is not compromised. Under these conditions, a low-solute diet represents a therapy without significant risk.

Diuretics that promote sodium excretion have been found to be antidiuretic, especially when administered to patients on a low-solute diet. This paradoxic effect seems to result from increased isotonic reabsorption of filtered sodium in the proximal tubule so that little reaches the more distal portion of the nephron for hypertonic reabsorption of sodium with formation of a hypotonic urine. Thus some conservation of water is accomplished. A low-sodium diet, however, is necessary to obtain an optimal effect, and, therefore, potassium supplementation may be required. Chlorothiazide (1 gm/m^2/24 hr in three divided doses) or hydrochlorothiazide (0.1 gm/m^2/24 hr in three divided doses) in conjunction with a low-solute diet has been most widely used. Other investigators, however, have reported comparable benefit from spironolactone, ethacrynic acid, and furosemide. Close supervision of all patients receiving diuretics is required to avoid metabolic or serious toxic side effects that can occur with these drugs.

Neurogenic DI (Vasopressin-Responsive). It seems obvious from the fact that neurogenic DI results from a total or partial deficiency of vasopressin secretion that antidiuretic hormonal replacement therapy would be all that is required for successful treatment. The regulatory nature of the neurohypophyseal-renal system with its ability to rapidly adjust water excretion to environmental factors (diet, including especially water and solute intake; activity; fasting; and so on), the pathophysiologic variations of antidiuretic hormone deficiency in and between patients, and the pharmacologic properties of the vasopressin preparations available for therapeutic use, however, make it necessary to consider these factors individually in prescribing treatment, especially in infants and young children.

While there is an almost infinite upper limit of the normal kidney to excrete water (12 to 15 l/m^2/24 hr after a few months of age and about one third this amount below 3 months), which is seldom reached even by patients with DI who often do well on 3 to 4 $l/m^2/24$ hr, water requirements under full continuous antidiuretic hormonal effect are very restrictive (approximately 1.6 $l/m^2/24$ hr for infants with normal activity and diet; 1 $l/m^2/24$ hr for 3 years and up). Since normal infants on formula receive approximately 2.5 $l/m^2/24$ hr of water, it is evident that a period free of antidiuretic hormonal activity is required daily to prevent the occurrence of hypo-osmolality with symptoms of water intoxication. For this reason, long-acting (24 to 48 hours or longer) vasopressin preparations, such as Pitressin tannate in oil (PTO), should not be used and even 1-desamino-8-D-arginine vasopressin (DDAVP, desmopressin), the preferred therapeutic agent today, with an intermediate duration of action (8 to 20 hours), should be used with caution and probably only at night when its use would be followed by the minimum daily period of water intake. The latter suggestion is particularly important since the duration of antidiuretic activity of DDAVP varies in and between patients and, over the range of dosages usually given (2.5 to 20 μg per dose, 0.025 to 0.2 ml), does not appear to be dose-related. While lysine vasopressin (Diapid) is sufficiently short-acting to be used successfully in infants on a schedule of two to three times per day, it has the disadvantage of producing significant pressor effects and nasal irritation on occasion.

For these reasons, it is advisable initially to treat all infants (and particularly neonates) with frequent feedings (every 3 to 4 hours) of a relatively low-solute formula to determine whether water requirements are sufficiently great to necessitate the use of one of the shorter-acting vasopressin preparations. As long as a relatively normal feeding schedule for age with normal progress in growth and development can be maintained, vasopressin therapy is not indicated. When nocturnal water loss becomes great enough to interrupt sleep, a short intermediate-acting vasopressin preparation should be given at bedtime. When polydipsia disrupts daytime activities, a similar preparation can be begun during the day, keeping in mind that a short period free of vasopressin activity is required each day to prevent water intoxication in children up to 2 to 3 years of age.

In older children, adolescents, and adults, the analog of arginine vasopressin, DDAVP, has become the preparation of choice for treatment of patients with neurogenic diabetes insipidus. The two modifications of the arginine vasopressin molecule, deamination of the hemicysteine in position 1 and substitution of D-arginine for L-arginine in position 8, change the antidiuretic vasopressor activity from 1:1 to 2000:1 when the duration of biologic activity is considered, with a coincident decrease in oxytocic activity. It thus is the most specific antidiuretic hormone available for clinical use and has been used successfully now for prolonged periods in patients of all ages and during pregnancy, with minimal side effects.

Several points concerning its pharmacologic properties are worth emphasizing. Per cent absorption from the nasal mucosa decreases as the dosage is increased and appears to be slow, which may be a factor in explaining its prolonged action. Other factors possibly explaining its prolonged effect are resistance to enzymatic degradation, increased lipophilicity, which would alter its volume of distribution, and smaller steric size, which may facilitate its reabsorption by the renal tubules. Limited studies in patients, using a specific radioimmunoassay, show peak plasma levels occurring from 1 to 5 hours after intranasal administration, with plasma half-lives of from 0.4 to 4 hours and a duration of action of 8 to 20 hours.

Probably as a consequence of these pharmacokinetics, a wide range in dosage of DDAVP has been reported, although most patients respond to 10 to 40 μg daily given in two doses. Since the preparation is expensive and dosages variable but unrelated to age and body size, initial dosage of 2.5 to 5 μg (0.025 to 0.05 ml) before bed and on arising are recommended, with subsequent increases in 2.5 μg (0.025 ml) increments until nocturia and daytime polyuria are satisfactorily controlled. DDAVP is administered intranasally via a plastic catheter calibrated to deliver 0.05, 0.1, and 0.2 ml of the preparation (100 μg/ml). Very young children can be taught to deliver the medication intranasally by inserting the tip of the catheter into the nose and blowing swiftly on the opposite end. The rapid exhalation lifts the soft palate, which permits delivery into the nasal cavity without passage into the pharynx. This is a simple and effective way to administer intranasal medication without inducing undesirable coughing, aspiration, or loss of material into the pharynx.

Side effects with DDAVP have been very uncommon. Headaches have been reported and appear to be dose-related and probably due to a local nasal effect. At large dosages (40 μg), increases in blood pressure have been reported, but the high antidiuretic-to-pressor ratio of DDAVP gives a wide margin of safety with respect to this and other pressor or oxytocic side effects. In infants and in older patients with a disturbed mechanism for recognizing water requirements, too continuous use can be associated with water intoxication.

We have noticed and a number of other investigators have reported a change in the duration of response with duration of usage so that an increase in dose may be required. Indeed, significant variations in peak urinary osmolality and volume on a constant dose are often seen, and more rarely a patient will need larger and more frequent doses to obtain a satisfactory response (up to 20 μg X 4/24 hr). Various factors may cause this apparent tolerance, including variability of rate of absorption, change in urinary clearance which for arginine vasopressin has been shown to increase fivefold or more with rapid hydration, changes in the dynamics of binding at the nasal-cell membrane, or a variation in inactivation by peptidases. To date, however, no antibodies to DDAVP have been identified. In such patients, the use of an agent such as chlorpropamide,* clofibrate,† or carbamazepine in low doses capable of prolonging the action of DDAVP may be of value.

The pharmacologic properties of DDAVP and its ease of administration with essentially absent side effects have markedly reduced the use of other vasopressin preparations. Vasopressin tannate in oil (PTO), which previously was the preparation of choice in children over 3 years and adults, can still be effective for patients who require multiple daily doses of intranasal preparations, including DDAVP, and have a tolerance for intramuscular injections. Such repeated intranasal therapy not only may make treatment inconvenient but increases the cost significantly. When PTO is used, we recommend the administration of a full ampule (1 ml) at all ages when the use of such a long-acting preparation is physiologically sound (from 3 years up), since in our experience of over 25 years significant acute side effects have not been evident and its duration of action when used at this dose has been most prolonged and consistent.

Of the short-acting vasopressins, only lysine vasopressin (Diapid) is generally available. Its intranasal use is limited primarily to conditions in which a longer-acting preparation presents significant risk. These conditions, as mentioned, are present in infants and young children whose daily calories are taken with water loads greater than permitted with prolonged full ADH effect and in patients who have an inability to recognize water requirements. In these patients, a spray in each nostril (approximately 18 μg) at bedtime and perhaps once during the night if the patient wakes may have a significant effect on nocturia and water balance without running the risk of water intoxication. DDAVP, however, is preferable even in these patients, if a period of diuresis can be recognized easily and is always permitted between doses, since its pressor activity is so low.

Finally, there are the nonhormonal drugs, which can be taken orally and which have an antidiuretic effect if the vasopressin deficiency is not complete. The most widely used has been the sulfonylurea chlorpropamide, which appears to potentiate the vasopressin effect at the nephron by inhibiting the action of prostaglandin E_1. This mode of action appears to explain its insulin-dependent hypoglycemic effect as well as its less well-recognized effects on blood pressure, phosphorus excretion, and restoration of thirst in patients with hypodipsia. In this latter group of patients with DI, chlorpropamide* given in single daily doses of 150 mg/m^2 or less has been especially beneficial and, if the dose is kept minimal, hypoglycemia rarely has occurred in our experience, even in patients with anterior pituitary deficiencies. Chlorpropamide may also be of use in patients with a temporary partial vasopressin deficiency but normal thirst during convalescence from surgery, during radiation therapy, or to augment the effect of administered lysine vasopressin, or DDAVP. Other prostaglandin E_1 inhibitors, such as aminopyrine and acetaminophen, are less effective and, though less toxic, are seldom used.

Clofibrate and carbamazepine (Tegretol), which appear to stimulate vasopressin secretion by different mechanisms, have been used to a limited extent. Both drugs have significant side effects, especially carbamazepine, so their use for long-term treatment is not recommended. Clofibrate† in low dosages (0.5 gm) that are usually tolerated has been reported of value in prolonging the action of DDAVP.

Rickets

WILLIAM H. BERGSTROM, M.D.

Nutritional Needs. During an infant's first year, 50 mg/kg of calcium and 25 mg/kg of phosphorus per day will prevent or cure rickets when absorption is assured by vitamin D. Human milk is usually sufficient, but rickets is still seen occasionally in breast-fed infants, and supplementation (400 IU/24 hr) is advisable. Prematurity, parenteral alimentation, and food faddism (e.g., variants of the macrobiotic diet) are risk factors; calcium, phosphorus, and vitamin D intakes should be estimated and supplemented if necessary. The rapid proportionate growth rate of small premature infants approximately doubles calcium and phosphorus requirements; neither can be met by human milk. For reasons presently obscure, the vitamin D require-

---

*This use of chlorpropamide is not listed by the manufacturer.
†Safety and efficacy of clofibrate in children has not been established. This use is not listed by the manufacturer.

*This use of chlorpropamide is not listed by the manufacturer.
†Safety and efficacy of clofibrate in children has not been established. This use is not listed by the manufacturer.

ment is similarly increased by parenteral alimentation.

Anticonvulsant Rickets

Phenytoin and phenobarbital reduce calcium absorption and may cause rickets when vitamin D intake is at or below 400 IU/24 hr. If dietary calcium is adequate, bone lesions heal on 800 to 1000 IU/24 hr.

Hepatic Rickets

Either hepatitis or biliary atresia may cause rickets (and hypocalcemic tetany). Both malabsorption and inadequate hydroxylation of vitamin D may occur; it is difficult to tell which predominates, since both lead to low plasma 25-hydroxyvitamin D_3. Most patients respond to vitamin D either orally (3000 to 4000 IU/24 hr as Drisdol) or parenterally (125,000 IU IM once a month). 1,25-Dihydroxyvitamin D_3 (0.5 to 1.5 μg/24 hr) should be ideal but is not yet approved for this use. The osteoporosis of chronic liver disease does not respond to vitamin D or its metabolites.

Pseudodeficiency (Vitamin D-Dependent) Rickets

This hereditary defect in renal l-hydroxylase (usually recessive but rarely an irregularly penetrant dominant) can be treated with pharmacologic doses of vitamin D (up to 100,000 IU/24 hr) or physiologic doses (0.5 to 1.5 μg/24 hr) of 1,25-dihydroxyvitamin D_3 (Rocaltrol). As in hypophosphatemic rickets, treatment is lifelong.

Primary Hypophosphatemic Vitamin D-Resistant Rickets

This X-linked transport defect reduces both intestinal and renal tubular phosphate absorption; rickets is the result of hypophosphatemia. Oral phosphate (1.5 to 2.0 gm of phosphorus/24 hr in 4 to 5 doses as Neutra-Phos or sublaxative doses of Fleet Phospho-Soda [5 ml = 0.5 gm P]) partially restores serum phosphorus. Vitamin D (25,000 to 100,000 IU/24 hr), dihydrotachysterol (0.2 to 1.0 mg/24 hr) or 1,25-dihydroxyvitamin D_3 (0.5 to 1.5 μg/24 hr) is also necessary to prevent the hypocalcemic effect of oral phosphate and to enhance transmembrane phosphate transport. Vitamin D is economical and convenient; dihydrotachysterol's short half-life facilitates dose adjustment. Rocaltrol has been used successfully but is still classified as an investigational drug for this disorder.

Hypercalcemia is the chief hazard of the regimen; monthly surveillance is needed until stabilization occurs, after which 3- to 4-month intervals suffice. Rickets heals readily and satisfactory growth can be achieved, but bone radiographs show a persistent and characteristic coarse trabecular pattern. Treat-

ment must be continued even after growth ceases and epiphyses fuse, since recurrent hypophosphatemia will otherwise cause osteomalacia. Another consequence of phosphate depletion is a functional decrease in erythrocyte oxygen transport. Fatigue and malaise on this basis may precede visible bone lesions.

Rickets in Multiple Tubular Dysfunction (Renal Tubular Acidosis, Lowe Syndrome, Fanconi Syndrome)

In persistent renal tubular acidosis, urinary calcium and phosphorus are excessive; rickets may result. Alkali supplementation (sodium bicarbonate or sodium citrate, 5 to 10 meq/kg/24 hr in 3 to 4 doses) reverses renal mineral loss, and rickets heals with the usual vitamin D intake (400 IU/24 hr). It is necessary to exclude (by history) the *secondary* renal tubular acidosis of vitamin D deficiency; this responds to vitamin D alone.

In Lowe syndrome (oculocerebrorenal dystrophy), tubular dysfunction is not uniform. Correction of acidosis heals rickets in some; others require phosphate and vitamin D as in primary hypophosphatemic rickets. In Fanconi syndrome (multiple tubular dysfunction), alkali, phosphate, and vitamin D are usually required, though a few patients have shown a good response to vitamin D alone.

Tetany

WILLIAM H. BERGSTROM, M.D.

Neonatal Care. Prematurity, perinatal stress, maternal diabetes, and alkali therapy predispose to hypocalcemia within the first 72 hours of life. Carpopedal spasm, stridor, and positive Chvostek sign are uncommon; hyperirritability, seizures, and respiratory irregularities predominate. Serum phosphorus is not elevated in early tetany.

Immediate correction requires intravenous 10% calcium gluconate (1 ml = 9 mg Ca) at 2 ml/kg, given over several minutes with care to avoid bradycardia and extravasation. Plasma calcium can be sustained by intravenous infusion at 2 mg/kg/hr (0.2 ml of 10% calcium gluconate) or by oral calcium lactate (13% calcium; 0.5 gm per 4-hour feeding = 390 mg/24 hr). To ensure absorption, give 400 IU of vitamin D daily as Drisdol.

If response to these measures is inadequate, phosphorus intake should be reduced temporarily by dilution of the formula with an equal volume of 10% dextrose in water. The resulting caloric reduction (from 0.7 to 0.5 per ml) will be well tolerated for the few days necessary to deal with this transient problem.

Care in Infancy and Childhood. After the first

week of life, hypocalcemia and hyperphosphatemia are usually due to renal insufficiency, hypoparathyroidism (primary or secondary to maternal hyperparathyroidism), pseudohypoparathyroidism, or excessive phosphate intake; the latter is uncommon following the advent of proprietary formulas. Rarely, magnesium deficiency may cause tetany, either per se or by compromising parathyroid function. Rachitic tetany is seldom seen before 3 months of age. In all instances, calcium and vitamin D supplementation (together with phosphate restriction if necessary) should be used until the primary disorder is defined.

Idiopathic Hypercalcemia

WILLIAM H. BERGSTROM, M.D.

This disorder probably represents excessive endorgan response to vitamin D, with signs of toxicity at or below levels that are usually well tolerated. Severity is highly variable; hypercalcemia (12 to 18 mg/dl) resolves spontaneously but facial anomalies, vascular stenosis, nephrocalcinosis, and mental retardation, if present initially, are permanent.

In increasing order of stringency, treatments are (1) removal of dietary vitamin D and protection against sunlight; (2) restriction of dietary calcium. A milk substitute can be made from strained lamb (2 jars = 200 gm), polycose (6 tablespoons), and whipping cream (2 oz) made up to 1 quart. This provides 600 calories and 45 mg of calcium; (3) cortisol, 1 mg/kg every 6 hours; (4) furosemide (1 mg/kg every 6 hr)—urine volume must be measured and replaced with two thirds normal saline containing 20 meq of KCl per liter.

The first two measures often suffice; if hypercalcemia persists after 2 to 4 weeks, cortisol should be added. To minimize the side effects of steroid in this self-limited disorder, cortisol should be stopped for a week at 2- to 3-month intervals.

If hypercalcemia does not recur, a normal diet can be gradually resumed. Furosemide should be used only if hypercalcemia seems immediately hazardous.

Magnesium Deficiency

PHILIP SHAUL, M.D.,
and REGINALD C. TSANG, M.B.B.S.

Magnesium deficiency, which can be reflected by hypomagnesemia, results from decreased Mg intake, malnutrition, steatorrhea, specific Mg malabsorption, and decreased Mg absorption secondary to intestinal diseases including Hirschprung's disease, Crohn's disease, celiac disease, Whipple's disease, long-lasting diarrhea, and diverticulosis. Following intestinal surgery it may be associated with short bowel syndrome, jejunocolic fistula, ileostomy or colostomy. Hypomagnesemia is also seen in infants with intrauterine growth retardation, birth asphyxia, hypoparathyroidism, or hyperphosphatemia, and in infants of mothers with hypomagnesemia, hyperparathyroidism, or diabetes. Increased Mg losses take place with repeated exchange blood transfusions and with increased urinary losses from intensive diuretic therapy and hyperaldosteronism.

Hypomagnesemia often presents with hypocalcemia. Signs and symptoms include anorexia, nausea, vomiting, apathy and weakness, tremors, spasticity, generalized seizures, Trousseau's sign, and Chvostek's sign. The minimum daily requirement of Mg is estimated to be 6 mg/kg/day. Normal serum concentrations are 1.5 to 2.5 mg/dl. However serum magnesium concentrations often do not accurately reflect total body magnesium status because Mg is a predominantly intracellular cation.

Mg deficiency or hypomagnesemia is treated with magnesium salts. Calcium or vitamin D therapy may aggravate the hypomagnesemia. In most conditions with magnesium deficiency only short courses of supplementation are needed, but infants with specific magnesium malabsorption require lifelong therapy. In acute hypomagnesemia, 50% $MgSO_4$ 0.1 ml/kg or 10 mg of elemental Mg/kg can be given IM (50% $MgSO_4$ contains 100 mg Mg per ml). IV infusion should be done cautiously over a 10 minute period with electrocardiographic monitoring to detect prolongation of atrioventricular conduction time and sinoatrial or atrioventricular block. Systemic hypotension, urinary retention, hyporeflexia, CNS depression, and respiratory depression can occur with overdosage. The above dose can be repeated every 8 to 12 hours. Serum Mg concentrations should be determined every 12 hours in order to monitor the course of therapy.

Maintenance doses of Mg can be given as the sulfated salt, gluconate, lactate, citrate, or glycerophosphate. Initially, daily oral supplementation should be in the range of 20 to 40 mg of elemental Mg/kg. With 50% $MgSO_4$ solution, 0.30 ml/kg can be used daily, diluted to 10% and given in four oral doses. Normally only 55 to 75% of the Mg may be absorbed; in malabsorption, only 10% may be absorbed and the oral dosage may have to be increased. Large doses of oral Mg salts, however, may lead to diarrhea. This may be controlled by increasing the frequency of administration and decreasing individual dose size, or by reduction of the daily dose.

Zinc Deficiency

K. MICHAEL HAMBIDGE, F.R.C.P. (Ed.)

The treatment of zinc deficiency depends to some extent on the pathogenesis of the deficiency state and on the clinical circumstances. The most acute need for zinc therapy is provided by the clinical syndrome of acrodermatitis enteropathica. This term is sometimes, and more correctly, reserved for an autosomal recessively inherited disease, the clinical manifestations of which result from an inherited defect in the major pathway of zinc absorption at normal dietary zinc concentrations in the lumen of the gastrointestinal tract. Oral zinc therapy in quantities sufficient to compensate for the effects of this inherited molecular defect will result in a rapid and complete clinical and biochemical remission, which is also sustained provided the zinc therapy is continued on a life-long basis.

The quantities of zinc required usually range from 30 to 50 mg of elemental zinc per day (3 to 5 X the Recommended Dietary Allowance). This dose obviously is not related to age or size, but a smaller quantity (2 to 3 mg/kg body weight/24 hr) is recommended for infants. Human milk is the best source of bioavailable zinc for infant feeding. However, occasionally breast-fed premature infants show the typical features of acrodermatitis enteropathica from inability of the maternal mammary gland to secrete normal quantities of zinc into the milk. It is important to distinguish this syndrome, because zinc supplements are required only temporarily to correct the severe deficiency state. Moreover, the dose of zinc required is small because it is exceptionally well absorbed in the presence of human milk.

Severe acquired zinc deficiency states with acral and orificial skin lesions and diarrhea occur most commonly in patients fed intravenously.

The quantity of zinc required for treatment depends on the extent of continuing losses, which can be very high if there is persistent diarrhea or excessive losses of gastrointestinal fluids from ileostomies and so on, and can be determined accurately only by balance studies. In lieu of such studies, commence treatment with 300 to 500 μg Zn^{++}/kg body weight/24 hr intravenously and adjust on the basis of changes in plasma zinc concentrations. Recommended intravenous maintenance doses are 100 μg Zn^{++}/kg body weight/24 hr for full-term infants and 300 μg Zn^{++}/kg body weight/24 hr for premature infants. If the patient is being fed orally at the time of the severe acquired zinc deficiency state, treat temporarily as for acrodermatitis enteropathica.

Mild nutritional zinc deficiency states appear to be quite common in formula-fed infants and in young children, and probably result more from poor zinc bioavailability from some formulas and diets than from absolutely low dietary zinc intakes. These can be managed by administering 0.5 to 1.0 mg of Zn^{++}/kg body weight/24 hr for an initial period of 3 months. Secondary or conditioned zinc deficiency has been reported to occur in association with a variety of conditions and disease states. The quantity of zinc required will depend on the circumstances and especially on the extent of malabsorption of zinc or of excessive losses. In general, it is reasonable to start therapy with 1.0 mg Zn^{++}/kg body weight/24 hr, but this may need to be increased. Two mg/kg/24 hr have been recommended for infants with protein energy malnutrition.

Monitoring zinc therapy is important, particularly in the treatment of severe zinc deficiency states. Plasma zinc determinations in samples collected with scrupulous care to avoid contamination are reasonably adequate for this purpose in most cases. Plasma copper or ceruloplasmin or both also should be monitored, as copper deficiency is a complication of high-dosage zinc therapy.

Zinc absorption appears to be influenced very little by the choice of inorganic zinc salt. The sulfate and acetate, both of which are soluble, are among those most frequently used. A commercial preparation of zinc chloride is available for intravenous use. There is no evidence that expensive commercial preparations of zinc that are liganded to proteins or amino acids are absorbed any better. Foods have a major, though variable, effect on the absorption of pharmacologic quantities of zinc. Hence, for maximal absorption, zinc should be administered 1 to 2 hours before meals.

Hepatolenticular Degeneration

(Wilson's Disease)

OWEN M. RENNERT, M.D.

Wilson's disease may present in the pediatric patient without the classic clinical triad of Kayser-Fleischer corneal rings, hepatic cirrhosis, and neurologic dysfunction. Early diagnosis is paramount since effective treatment may prevent irreversible organ damage and progression of the disease. Symptoms occur as early as 4 years of age, though the second and third decades are the usual ages of onset. The mode of presentation is variable, but the hepatic form is most common in childhood. Presenting symptoms may include hand tremors, slurred speech, spasticity, decreased academic performance, and behavioral disturbances. Two neurologic variants have been identified: dystonic (predominantly seen in young patients) and pseudosclerotic; the dystonic variant appears to be less responsive to therapy.

It is important to stress the wide variability of expression of Wilson's disease. This extends to age of onset, mode of presentation, severity of organ system involvement, and response to therapy. The less common manifestations, such as renal, skeletal, hematologic, and psychiatric disturbances, may occur at any time during the disease course, and usually are preceded by hepatic or neurologic manifestations.

The liver is the *central* homeostatic organ for copper metabolism. Wilson's disease is characterized by a congenital inability to maintain normal copper homeostasis, with resultant accumulation in the liver. Impaired secretion of copper via ceruloplasmin and diminished lysosomal biliary copper excretion are associated with saturation of hepatic binding capacity and subsequent release of copper into the circulation, leading to hemolytic crisis and diffusion into the central nervous system and kidneys, giving rise to the distinctive clinical manifestations.

Therapeutic Rationale

Excessive storage of copper in viscera leads to organ system failure because the organism is unable to mobilize, utilize, and detoxify this trace metal. The principles of therapy are based upon enhancing the mobilization and excretion of copper, limiting copper intake, and monitoring the function of copper-toxic target organs. Successful therapy requires early recognition and establishment of the diagnosis.

Chemotherapy is the central approach for achieving negative copper-balance in patients. Penicillamine is the most effective and least toxic agent utilized in the treatment of these patients.

Therapy

Penicillamine. The dosage of penicillamine used in children is related to the age of the patient. Children under 10 years of age are treated with 0.5–0.75 gm/day—in adults the dose is 1.0–1.5 gm/day. Initial dosage may be calculated as 0.02 gm/kg/day, divided into 2–4 doses/day. *Treatment is lifelong.* Following initiation of therapy, cupruresis of 1000 to 5000 μg/24 hours may occur. Over a 4 to 6 month period, following initiation of therapy, the degree of cupruria gradually falls to approximately 1000 μg/24 hours. Because penicillamine inhibits pyridoxine-dependent enzymes, patients should be given daily supplements of 12.5 to 25.0 mg/day of vitamin B_6. In patients with far advanced neurologic disease L-dopa has been proposed as adjunctive therapy. Published data identify variable success of this therapeutic maneuver.

During the lifelong therapy, patients should be monitored regularly, not only for toxic side effects but also for assessment and maintenance of negative copper balance and clinical improvement. Improvement of symptomatology defines successful therapy, and demonstration on physical examination of symptom reversal usually postdates chemical laboratory evidence of betterment.

Patient evaluation includes regular assessment of serum copper and ceruloplasmin concentration, as well as 24-hour urinary copper excretion. Improvement of hepatic function is documented by measurement of prothrombin time, serum transaminases, and bilirubin determination. Renal function may be sequentially evaluated by measurement of serum BUN and creatinine; additionally, examination of the urine for the characteristic aminoaciduria and glycosuria seen as evidence of heavy metal intoxication (Fanconi syndrome) is a valuable adjunct. Recent clinical studies have documented hypercalciuria as a component of the renal dysfunction seen in Wilson's disease.

Successful therapy can be confirmed by regular slit-lamp ophthalmoscopy to document disappearance or absence of the Kayser-Fleischer corneal rings, as well as absence of the "sunflower cataracts" seen in some untreated patients. Recent reports document the potential usefulness of computed tomography to evaluate central nervous system anatomy prior to and during therapy.

Hematologic manifestations occur as a consequence of the pathologic processes of Wilson's disease itself and also as a cytotoxicity of penicillamine therapy. The hemolytic crises seen have been ascribed to a variety of pathophysiologic mechanisms, including copper inhibition of erythrocyte glycolytic enzymes, direct erythrocyte membrane damage, and oxidative denaturation of hemoglobin. During hemolytic crises, patients show marked cupriuria and elevated serum copper concentrations. Thrombocytopenia and leukopenia have been reported to occur as a consequence of hypersplenism.

Thrombocytopenia may be an early sign of penicillamine cytotoxicity. Anemia or granulocytopenia may also occur. Regular evaluation of hematologic status is required. Anemia may develop during therapy as a consequence of red cell aplasia secondary to penicillamine toxicity. The toxic hematologic sequelae of penicillamine therapy are reversed by discontinuation of the drug. Early hypersensitivity reactions have occurred in one third of treated patients; however, these usually respond to gradual desensitization under steroid therapy, usually accomplished by a two week discontinuation of penicillamine. Subsequently, the patient is started on half the calculated penicillamine dose in addition to 20 mg/day of prednisone. The steroid therapy is continued for 2 weeks, then the penicillamine dosage is gradually increased. In certain instances penicillamine dosage may have to be reduced to 50 mg/day for 7 days, rather than the simple 50% reduction, and then gradually increased.

In the past decade clinical reports have identified undesirable side effects of penicillamine therapy. These toxicities are seen infrequently; however, the nature of the reactions is diverse. Descriptions in the literature include nephrotic syndrome, immunocomplex nephritis, immune system alterations (including lupus erythematosus-like syndrome, alterations in T-cell and B-cell function), lymphadenitis, dermatologic manifestations (including elastosis perforans serpiginosa, papular eruptions, and cutis hyperelastica), myasthenia-like syndrome, defects in retinal pigmentary epithelium, and Goodpasture's syndrome. These have remitted following discontinuation of penicillamine therapy.

Alternate chemotherapy is available for the patient who develops toxic side reactions to penicillamine and who cannot be desensitized to this drug. The newly developed copper-chelator triene-2HCl (triethylene tetramine dihydrochloride)*has been shown to be a safe alternative for the treatment of Wilson's disease.

Other Considerations

To minimize copper deposition, dietary restriction of copper should be advocated. Foods high in copper that should be limited or excluded from the diet are liver, nuts, chocolate, cocoa, mushrooms, brain, shellfish, and broccoli. The average American ingests approximately 3.5 to 5.0 mg of copper per day; the patient with Wilson's disease should ingest no more than 1.5 mg per day.

Because of successful therapy of patients with Wilson's disease, it has become necessary to recognize the potential teratogenic action of penicillamine when used during the reproductive period. Penicillamine crosses the placental barrier. Considerations relating to its potential detrimental effect on the fetus are based upon three factors: (a) the drug's capacity to increase solubility of collagen and decrease intramolecular cross-linking, (b) its ability to chelate copper (and potentially other trace metals) and make it unavailable to the fetus, and (c) its structural antagonism to pyridoxine dependent enzymes. Thus, penicillamine dosage should be kept as low as possible when used in the pregnant woman.

Supportive therapy is directed at palliation and minimization of the handicaps that are a consequence of irreparable damage from copper toxicosis. These relate to treatment and rehabilitation of the neurologic sequelae and management of hepatic damage and cirrhosis. Treatment of the agi-

tation and emotional instability has involved use of benzodiazepine and phenothiazine derivatives. Treatment of movement disorders has consisted of use of trihexyphenidyl and related drugs. In the past few years two patients have been treated with liver transplantation. This is consistent with the premise that the central metabolic defect of Wilson's disease is expressed in the liver. This therapeutic maneuver is reserved for the patient with irreversible cirrhosis as a consequence of copper toxicosis.

Hyperphenylalaninemias

NEIL A. HOLTZMAN, M.D.

Long-term follow-up of infants with phenylketonuria (PKU) has established the benefit of dietary restriction of phenylalanine: mental retardation can be prevented without impairment of physical growth. The outcome is best when treatment is started early. Deficits in intellectual development are quite frequent when the diet is started after 30 days of age and grow progressively more severe and more likely the longer the delay. Nevertheless, the diagnosis of PKU *must be firmly established* before treatment is started; phenylalanine is an essential amino acid and its restriction will have dire consequences in infants with elevated levels of phenylalanine who do not have PKU.

Moderate elevations of phenylalanine accompanied by hypertyrosinemia (greater than 5 mg/dl) are observed more frequently in premature than full-term infants. These chemical alterations usually respond to reduced protein intake and oral vitamin C of 50 to 100 mg/24 hr.

Some infants in whom the low phenylalanine diet is started will prove not to have classic PKU and will not need long-term treatment. In such infants, dietary phenylalanine needed to maintain serum levels above 2 mg/dl may approach normal intakes over the first few years of life. All infants with persistent elevations of phenylalanine, *of any degree,* also should be tested for the biopterin-deficient forms of PKU.

Principles of Management

Because PKU infants differ in their requirements for phenylalanine, because requirements change as infants grow, and because of the possibility of inducing phenylalanine deficiency—which can be lethal—frequent monitoring of dietary and blood phenylalanine levels and physical growth is essential to optimal management.

Parents will greet the diagnosis of a potentially serious genetic disorder in a healthy-appearing infant with disbelief. The continued good health of the PKU infant often reinforces this denial. Consid-

---

*Investigational drug, not commercially available in the United States.

erable family education, delivered over several visits, is needed to explain the nature of the condition. When first confronted with the diagnosis in their new infant, few parents will think about recurrence risks. The implications of PKU as an autosomal recessive condition—that each of the parents is a carrier and that the recurrence risk is 25% with each pregnancy—will usually need repeated discussion.

In view of the problems of establishing the diagnosis, the need for careful monitoring, and the need for parental education and counseling, PKU infants should be managed in close and sustained consultation with experienced medical geneticists and nutritionists who have access to reliable, accurate, and prompt phenylalanine testing facilities.

Initiation of Therapy

Early onset of the low phenylalanine diet is a more important determinant of intellectual development than the actual level of phenylalanine restriction once the diet is started. Rapid reduction of phenylalanine can be accomplished by starting the PKU infant *exclusively* on a low phenylalanine product such as Lofenalac. With the exception of phenylalanine and fluoride, Lofenalac is a complete infant food. Sufficient amounts are used to meet the infant's caloric and fluid requirements. For the PKU infant this will provide about 20 mg/kg/24 hr of phenylalanine. This method should be used only when *daily* measurement of serum phenylalanine is possible; in some infants the phenylalanine concentration may fall to dangerously low levels within 1 to 2 days, while in others it may take more than a week. Hospitalization, which permits frequent monitoring, is essential for this approach. It also gives parents time to adjust to the diagnosis, partic-

ularly if they can discuss the problems repeatedly with knowledgeable staff. During the hospitalization the parents can learn to make the formula. Once the serum phenylalanine falls below 8 mg/dl, phenylalanine should be added to the formula, in the form of milk (Table 1), to provide the approximate amounts of phenylalanine indicated in Table 2. The actual intake should be adjusted to keep the serum phenylalanine between 2 and 8 mg/dl.

Alternatively, infants can be started on a mixture of Lofenalac and whole cows' milk, evaporated milk, or a proprietary formula such as Similac to provide approximately 60 mg/kg/24 hr of phenylalanine. As a rule of thumb, *about* 90% of the calories should be provided by Lofenalac in the young infant. Thus, for the 4-kg PKU infant requiring about 240 mg of phenylalanine and 480 kcal per day, 10 scoops of Lofenalac will provide 75 mg of phenylalanine and 430 kcal, and 1.5 ounces of evaporated milk will provide 158 mg of phenylalanine and 66 kcal (Table 1). Dilution of the mixture

Table 2. PHENYLALANINE, PROTEIN, AND ENERGY REQUIREMENTS IN PHENYLKETONURIA

Age (months)	Phenylalanine (mg/kg/24 hr)	Protein (gm/kg/24 hr)	Energy (kcal/kg/24 hr)
0–3	60 ± 15	3–4	120
4–6	40 ± 10	2.5–3.5	115
7–9	30 ± 10	2.5	110
10–12	30 ± 10	2.5	105
13–24	25 ± 5	2.0	100
25–36	20 ± 5	1.8	100
37–48	20 ± 5	1.6	100
49–72	20 ± 5	1.5	90

Table 1. PRODUCT INFORMATION NEEDED TO PREPARE FORMULA FOR INFANTS AND CHILDREN WITH PHENYLKETONURIA

Product	Volume	Weight (gm)	Phenylalanine (mg)	Protein Equivalent (gm)	Energy (kcal)	Water Added [ml (oz)]	Final Volume [ml (oz)]
Lofenalac (powder)	1 scoop*	9.5	9.5	1.4†	43	60 (2)	65 (2.2)
	8 oz	139	110	20.8†	640	858 (28.6)	946 (32)
Evaporated milk	1 oz	—	105	2.2	44	30 (1)	60 (2)
Whole cows' milk	1 oz	—	58	1.1	20	—	30 (1)
Similac (powder)	1 scoop*	8.7	59	1.0	44	60 (2)	66 (2.2)
Enfamil (powder)	1 scoop*	8.3	44	1.0	44	60 (2)	66 (2.2)
Phenyl-free (powder)	1 scoop*	9.85	0	2.0†	40	41 (1.3)	48 (1.6)

*Enclosed with powder; approximately 1 tablespoon.
†Deficient in phenylalanine.

to 660 ml with water will supply adequate fluid. (As long as the infant's fluid requirements are satisfied, addition of the exact amount of water is not critical.) As PKU infants vary in their response, this method requires monitoring of blood phenylalanine at least twice a week. If the phenylalanine level has not fallen to 10 mg/dl within 10 days, the amount of milk in the mixture should be reduced.

As the infant grows, phenylalanine requirements will also change (see Table 2), necessitating monitoring at approximately weekly levels and changes in formula when indicated. Fruits, cereals, and vegetables should be added at the same ages as in non-PKU infants. The phenylalanine in these foods must be included in calculating the infant's daily diet. Lists of serving sizes of foods containing 15 or 30 mg of phenylalanine are available. The very high phenylalanine content of dairy products, meats, poultry, and fish prohibits their use. As the child becomes less dependent on formula as the major calorie source, substitution of a phenylalanine-free formula, such as Phenyl-free (see Table 1), allows more liberal allotments of solid foods. Mixtures of Lofenalac and Phenyl-free can also be used.

Management of Children

The greatest problem of management will be encountered in the PKU child between 2 and 6 years of age. As a result of increasing social contacts, the PKU child will be tempted to try "forbidden" foods. Stealing of foods is not uncommon and may be detected only by monitoring of blood phenylalanine. Demands of the PKU child for a normal diet may seriously disrupt family life. In anticipation of dietary problems, the reason for the diet should be explained to the young child with PKU. Parents have a major role to play in this education.

Children in the U.S. PKU Collaborative Project who continued the low phenylalanine diet after six years of age had, on average, better performance on standardized psychological and achievement tests than children in the project who came off the diet. Because the groups were not completely randomized we cannot be confident that the differences are attributable entirely to termination of the low phenylalanine diet. Nevertheless, the prudent course is to maintain some restriction of dietary phenylalanine in older children and adolescents with PKU. Seldom is it possible, however, to maintain serum phenylalanine levels below 4 mg/dl in older children. PKU children generally prefer low phenylalanine or phenylalanine-free formulas to regular milk, and this should be encouraged.

Maternal PKU

The pregnant woman with PKU in whom serum phenylalanine levels are elevated is at increased risk of delivering an infant with mental retardation. The chance of this varies directly with the mother's serum phenylalanine concentration, but is increased even with serum phenylalanine levels in the range of 3 to 10 mg/dl. Except when phenylalanine levels are maintained at less than 10 mg/dl from *before conception,* which thus far has been reported in only three pregnancies, there is little assurance of a normal outcome.

Adolescent PKU females should be warned of the likelihood of poor pregnancy outcomes, and counseled about birth control methods and alternatives to childbearing, such as abortion and adoption. (In vitro fertilization and surrogate mothering may become options in the future.)

PKU women who want to become pregnant should be on a low phenylalanine diet. This will be easier to accomplish if a female child with PKU continues to ingest a low phenylalanine formula: people unaccustomed to these formulas often find the odor and taste unpleasant. Once pregnant, the PKU woman must be provided with adequate tyrosine and other essential nutrients, for which the requirements in pregnancy will not be satisfied by phenylalanine-free formula.

Treatment of Biopterin-Deficient Forms of PKU

The biopterin cofactor needed for the synthesis of tyrosine from phenylalanine is also needed for the synthesis of the neurotransmitters L-dopa and serotonin from tyrosine and 5-hydroxy-tryptophan, respectively. Inherited defects in the synthesis of biopterin, or in the recycling of its active form, account for between 1 and 5% of infants with persistent elevations of serum phenylalanine. The neurologic problems that appear in infancy with these variant forms, despite control of blood phenylalanine by dietary restriction, are probably a consequence of neurotransmitter deficiencies. The administration of tetrahydrobiopterin corrects both peripheral and central nervous system chemical abnormalities in these forms of PKU, but clinical improvement is not always observed. Administration of L-dopa and serotonin, as well as a dopa decarboxylase inhibitor, is also capable of correcting the chemical deficiencies in the brain: a low phenylalanine diet must also be given. Good outcomes are likely only if the diagnosis is made promptly following newborn screening, and if appropriate treatment is immediately started with careful monitoring.

Amino Acid Disorders

MARY G. AMPOLA, M.D.

Disease (and Approximate Incidence)*	Clinical Features	Abnormal Enzyme or Other Defect	Amino Acids Increased in Blood	Amino Acids Increased in Urine	Comments	Treatment
PHENYLKETONURIA						
Phenylketonuria, classic. (1:14,000)	Mental retardation; also seizures, eczema, and fair skin, eyes, and hair in some patients.	Phenylalanine hydroxylase (virtually total absence).	Phenylalanine—levels usually over 30 mg/dl.	Phenylalanine; phenylpyruvic, -lactic and -acetic acids; orthohydroxyphenylacetic acid also increased.	Increasing evidence treatment must continue well past age 5.	Low phenylalanine diet to maintain blood phenylalanine level between 3 and 8 mg/dl.
Phenylketonuria, atypical. (1:13,000)	Mental retardation; often less severe than in classic form.	Phenylalanine hydroxylase (partial defect).	Phenylalanine—levels not as high as in classic form, about 20 mg/dl.	Same as in the classic form but often in smaller amounts.	May not need treatment to maintain normal blood phenylalanine after early childhood.	Low phenylalanine diet to tolerance.
Hyperphenylalaninemia, persistent mild. (1:19,000)	Normal in all respects.	Phenylalanine hydroxylase (partial defect—more enzyme remains).	Phenylalanine—levels in range of 6–8 mg/dl.	None.	Mental and physical development normal.	None necessary.
Dihydropteridine reductase deficiency. (rare)	Progressive neurologic deterioration with hypotonia, aspiration, death usually after 2 years.	Dihydropteridine reductase.	Phenylalanine—levels from below 8 to above 20 mg/dl.	Phenylalanine (low levels of 5-hydroxyindole-acetic acid).	Low phenylalanine diet lowers plasma phenylalanine but does not alter course.	L-Dopa, L-5-hydroxytryptophan and carbidopa may be helpful if begun early.
DISORDERS OF AMMONIA METABOLISM **UREA CYCLE DISEASES**	NOTE: Glutamine elevated in blood and urine in hyperammonemia, but often difficult to detect on screening. Hemo- or peritoneal dialysis and sodium benzoate helpful for acute hyperammonemia crises.					
Carbamyl phosphate synthetase I deficiency. (rare)	Vomiting, seizures, tachypnea, coma; death in newborn period usual. Occasional patients survive, with progressive mental retardation.	Carbamyl phosphate synthetase I.	—	—	Postprandial hyperammonemia.	Low protein diet with arginine supplments; also alpha-keto acids.
Ornithine transcarbamylase deficiency. (rare)	Vomiting, seizures, tachypnea, coma; death in newborn period or later in first year in males.	Ornithine transcarbamylase.	—	—	Postprandial hyperammonemia. Inheritance as X-linked gene.	Low protein diet with argine supplements; also alpha-keto acids.
Citrullinemia. (rare)	Vomiting, seizures, failure to thrive, mental retardation; may die in neonatal period.	Argininosuccinic acid synthetase.	Citrulline, alanine.	Citrulline.	Postprandial hyperammonemia.	Low protein diet with arginine supplements.
Argininosuccinic aciduria. (1:75,000)	Ataxia, seizures, mental retardation, friable hair, hepatomegaly; may die in neonatal period.	Argininosuccinase.	Argininosuccinic acid, citrulline.	Argininosuccinic acid, citrulline.	Postprandial hyperammonemia.	Low protein diet with arginine supplements.
Argininemia. (rare)	Seizures, spasticity, mental retardation.	Arginase.	Arginine.	Arginine; lysine, ornithine, and cystine also present at times.	Postprandial hyperammonemia may be present.	Low protein diet. Also (?) lysine supplements helpful.

OTHER HYPERAMMONEMIAS

"Hyperglycinemia, ketotic form." (rare)	Periodic vomiting, lethargy, ketosis, myoclonic jerks, osteoporosis, neutropenia, and thrombocytopenia.	Not specific; deficiencies of enzymes responsible for organic acid disorders (methylmalonic and propionic acidemias; biotin-responsive multiple carboxylase deficiency).	Glycine, occasionally lysine.	Glycine, occasionally lysine.	Hyperammonemia may be present.	Low protein diet; appropriate vitamin therapy for some.
Ornithinemia (type I) (with homocitrullinuria). (rare)	Irritability, ataxia, myoclonic seizures, aversion to protein, mental retardation.	Unknown.	Ornithine.	Homocitrulline; ornithine may be normal.	Hyperammonemia.	Low protein diet.
Lysinuric protein intolerance with hyperdibasic aminoaciduria. (rare)	Vomiting and diarrhea, failure to thrive, neutropenia, aversion to protein, hepatomegaly.	Intestinal, renal tubular, and hepatocyte defect in transport of dibasic amino acids.	—	Arginine, lysine.	Usually normal intelligence. Ammonia intoxication after high protein intake.	Low protein diet with citrulline supplements to improve urea formation from ammonia.

OTHER AMINO ACID DISORDERS

Cystathioninuria. (1:60,000)	Probably benign.	Cystathionase.	Trace of cystathionine.	Cystathionine.	—	None necessary (although pyridoxine, 200 to 400 mg daily, will clear cystathionine).
Cystinosis, nephropathic. (rare)	Multiple renal tubular defects, failure to thrive, vitamin D-resistant rickets. Progressive uremia in early childhood.	Unknown.	Essentially normal, including cystine and cysteine.	Generalized aminoaciduria.	Phosphaturia, glycosuria; cystine deposits in many tissues.	General supportive treatment as problems appear. Vitamin D derivatives for rickets; renal transplantation for uremia. (?) Reducing agents helpful.
Cystinuria. (1:13,000)	Renal calculi.	Defective transport of cystine and the dibasic amino acids in kidney and intestine.	—	Cystine and dibasic amino acids.	—	High fluid intake and D-penicillamine if calculi appear. Alkalization of urine (?) effective.
Hyperglycinemia, nonketotic form. (1:150,000)	Hypotonia, seizures, spasticity, mental retardation. May need ventilatory assistance from birth.	Serine hydroxymethyl transferase.	Glycine.	Glycine; occasionally not elevated.	Spinal fluid glycine 15–30 times normal.	No effective therapy. (?) Strychinine temporarily helpful.
Hartnup disease. (1:18,000)	May be benign; light-sensitive rash, ataxia, psychosis, mental retardation in some.	Defective transport of neutral amino acids in kidney and intestine.	None; indeed, neutral amino acids about 30 per cent less than normal.	Neutral amino acids.	Indoles produced by intestinal bacteria from tryptophan are absorbed and excreted into the urine.	None necessary in some; nicotinamide for rash (up to 400 mg/24 hr); high protein diet for general nutrition.
Histidinemia. (1:18,000)	Probably benign.	Histidase.	Histidine.	Histidine.	Urocanic acid absent in skin homogenates and sweat; low serotonin in serum.	None necessary.

*Incidence figures are from the state of Massachusetts Metabolic Screening Program (courtesy of Dr. Harvey Levy) and from review of the literature. The figures presented are approximations: in many cases the disease is not detectable on routine screening and true incidence is unknown.

(Table continued on following page)

AMINO ACID DISORDERS (Continued)
MARY G. AMPOLA, M.D.

Disease (and Approximate Incidence)	Clinical Features	Abnormal Enzyme or Other Defect	Amino Acids Increased in Blood	Amino Acids Increased in Urine	Comments	Treatment
Homocystinuria. (1:300,000)	Dislocated lenses, malar flush, arterial and venous thromboses, long thin extremities, osteoporosis, mental retardation in some.	Cystathionine synthetase.	Methionine; small amount of homocystine.	Homocystine.	Two variants; pyridoxine-responsive and nonresponsive.	Up to 1 gm pyridoxine daily for responders, otherwise, low-methionine diet with cystine supplement.
Hyperlysinemia. (rare)	May be benign.	Lysine ketoglutarate reductase, saccharopine oxidoreductase, and saccharopine dehydrogenase.	Lysine.	Lysine; some also increased saccharopine.	—	Treatment probably not necessary.
Hyperpipecolatemia (cerebrohepatorenal syndrome of Zellweger). (rare)	Failure to thrive, unusual facial features, hypotonia, hepatomegaly, nystagmus. Progressive mental retardation; death by third year.	(?) Alpha-amino-adipic-delta semialdehyde oxidase.	Pipecolic acid.	Pipecolic acid.	—	None known.
Maple syrup urine disease (severe infantile form). (1:400,000)	Vomiting, progressive hypertonicity, acidosis, coma, early death.	Branched-chain keto-acid decarboxylase (absence virtually complete).	Leucine, isoleucine, valine.	Leucine, isoleucine, valine (with their three corresponding keto-acids).	Urine has odor of maple syrup.	Partially synthetic diet low in leucine, isoleucine, and valine; peritoneal dialysis during crises.
Maple syrup urine disease (intermediate and intermittent forms). (rare)	Episodic vomiting, lethargy and coma, often with infection; some normal between episodes, including IQ.	Branched-chain keto-acid decarboxylase (activity 2 to 15 per cent of normal).	Leucine, isoleucine, valine variable; worse during acute attacks.	Leucine, isoleucine, valine (with their 3 corresponding keto-acids)—may be only during acute attacks.	Odor of maple syrup when ill; disease may be fatal during crises.	Low protein diet as needed. During exacerbations 0 to 1 gm protein/kg/24 hours.
Gyrate atrophy of the choroid and retina. (rare)	Prolonged neonatal jaundice, failure to thrive, liver cirrhosis, mental retardation, retinal atrophy.	Ornithine keto-acid transaminase.	Ornithine (lysine low).	Ornithine.	Normal serum ammonia even after protein loading.	Low protein diet with lysine supplements.
Hyperprolinemia (type I). (1:300,000)	Probably benign.	Proline oxidase.	Proline.	Proline; hydroxyproline and glycine may also be elevated.	—	Necessity doubtful.
Hyperprolinemia (type II). (1:300,000)	Probably benign.	Δ^1-pyrroline-5-carboxylate dehydrogenase.	Proline.	Proline, Δ^1-pyrroline-5-carboxylate, hydroxyproline and glycine.	—	Necessity doubtful.
Sarcosinemia. (1:300,000)	Probably benign. (?) Mild mental retardation; variable clinical picture in patients reported.	Sarcosine dehydrogenase.	Sarcosine.	Sarcosine.	—	(?) Necessary; no special diet tried.
Tyrosinemia, hereditary. (rare)	Failure to thrive, vomiting, diarrhea, liver cirrhosis, renal tubular defects, vitamin D-resistant rickets.	Unknown.	Tyrosine, methionine.	Generalized renal tubular defect; including generalized aminoaciduria, especially tyrosine.	Glycosuria, phosphaturia, hypoglycemia, hypophosphatemia.	Low phenylalanine, tyrosine, and methionine diet helpful in some; vitamin D derivatives for rickets.

Inborn Errors of Carbohydrate Metabolism

NOEL K. MACLAREN, M.D.,
and MARVIN CORNBLATH, M.D.

A rich variety of enzymatic deficiencies in carbohydrate metabolism are important to the practice of pediatrics. Most patients with such disorders can be greatly helped clinically, provided the underlying disease is recognized and characterized. Galactosemia is discussed elsewhere.

THE GLYCOGENOSES

Disorders involving pathologic storage of glycogen within the body can be subdivided into two groups: those involving principally the liver and kidney—types I, III, VI, and IX—and those with skeletal muscle involvement—types II (heart) and V (limb musculature).

Hepato (Renal) Syndromes

Type I (Von Gierke Disease). The disease results from a deficiency of glucose-6-phosphatase. Since hydrolysis of glucose-6-phosphate to glucose is the common end-event for gluconeogenesis and glycogenolysis, hypoglycemia is severe. Further, new glucose-6-phosphate is diverted into glycogen deposition, to lactic acid formation, and indirectly to triglyceride synthesis following generation of diphosphopyridine nucleotide from pentose shunt activity.

HYPOGLYCEMIA. In severely affected infants, blood glucose levels regularly fall to the hypoglycemic range within a few hours of eating. Curiously, symptoms such as associated central nervous system disturbance may be blunted, presumably because of some cerebral capacity to use substrates other than glucose for its energy needs. However, symptoms of the associated sympathetic response (pallor, sweating, etc.) are more common.

Many features of the disease (such as hepatomegaly, lipemia, hyperuric acidemia, lactic acidosis, growth retardation, bruising) may improve markedly if hypoglycemia is minimized. To this end, infants must be fed every 3 hours night and day. We use Cho-Free with 10 gm/dl (10 per cent) glucose added and avoid sucrose (cane sugar) and lactose (milk sugar), since the contained fructose and galactose cannot form new glucose but rather tends to be stored as glycogen or be directed to lactic acid formation. Glucose water (10%) may be offered between feedings as needed. The diet should provide 60 to 70 percent carbohydrate (glucose, maltose starches), 12 to 15% protein, and 10 to 25% fat.

Burr, Greene, and colleagues have shown the benefits of long-term continuous intragastric feedings during nighttime periods in the older child. Such feedings consist of Vivonex* delivered via a small nasogastric tube from a continuous infusion pump (see below) over a 12-hour period to provide one third of the total daily calories. The remaining two thirds of the caloric requirement is best given as 2- to 3-hour feedings for the 12-hour period of the daytime regimen. Although there appears to be clinical improvement with increasing age, perhaps due in part to cerebral adaptive processes, hypoglycemia prevention, whether clinically apparent or not, remains the goal in therapy.

There is probably no place in therapy for drugs such as diazoxide, ephedrine, or glucagon. Portacaval shunting procedures have been reported to increase blood glucose levels, reduce hyperlipemia, diminish liver glycogen and lipid content, and improve growth. However, the procedure should be considered experimental at this time since encephalopathic changes may result, the shunts may close spontaneously with time, and simpler methods involving dietary manipulations, as outlined above, may achieve the same end.

ACIDOSIS. Lactic acidosis is not uncommon during infancy and is often associated with infections. Acidosis is worsened in the presence of dehydration. For acute acidosis (pH < 7.2), give 2 meq/kg of IV bicarbonate suitably diluted with 5% dextrose (e.g., 1 part to 5), and monitor the subsequent response. This should be sufficient to raise the serum bicarbonate level by approximately 5 meq/l. Buffering with sodium lactate is contraindicated. Parenteral glucose should also be given as indicated by the blood glucose level. For chronic acidosis, we use sodium bicarbonate, 2 to 4 meq/kg/24 hr in divided doses; that is, ½ teaspoon per feed for infants, and 0.5- to 1.0-gm tablets three to six times daily for older infants and children.

HEMORRHAGIC DIATHESIS. A tendency to increased bleeding or bruising is common, with epistaxis being the most frequent manifestation. Studies suggest that the origin of these problems is disordered platelet functioning. Application of cold compresses to the nose and face, together with rest, is all that is usually required. For severe epistaxis, nasal packing and transfusions of whole fresh blood or platelets are appropriate management. Major surgical procedures should be carefully planned and monitored.

HYPERURICEMIA. Raised blood levels of uric acid occur often and may be reduced by careful frequent feeding (as above). Transient joint pain may occur in young patients; however, gouty arthritis occurs mainly in older patients. If dietary management

---

*Vivonex—89 per cent of calories as glucose and glucose oligosaccharides, 1.8 per cent as safflower oil, and 9.2 per cent as crystalline amino acids.

cannot control uric acid levels, then allopurinol,* a methyl xanthine inhibitor, at a dose of from 5 to 10 mg/kg/24 hr (maximum 150 mg under 6 years; 300 mg/24 hr 6 to 12 years), is the drug of choice. Uric acid nephropathy should be prevented by maintaining blood uric acid levels as normal as possible and by avoiding chronic acidosis with frequent feeding regimens or alkalis.

HYPERLIPIDEMIA. In type I disease, triglyceride levels may be greatly raised with more modest elevations of blood cholesterol. Again, avoidance of hypoglycemia, with accompanying elevations of glucagon, growth hormone, and catecholamines, is associated with improved lipid levels. But, should hyperlipidemia persist, clofibrate (Atromid-S)† can be used with effect at a dose of 50 mg/kg/day in two divided daily doses, although long-term trials with the drug still need to be carried out.

Type III. This disease results from a deficiency of amylo-1,6-glucosidase (debrancher enzyme). Patients have an illness similar to but milder than that with type I disease. Fasting hypoglycemia and moderately severe hepatomegaly are the usual clinical findings. Lactic acidosis, abnormal bleeding, hyperuricemia, and hyperlipemia are not usual problems clinically. Treatment consists of avoiding prolonged fasting. A late night snack consisting of protein with carbohydrate is important. During intercurrent illnesses associated with poor food intake, carbonated drinks are useful to prevent hypoglycemia. The parents should be taught to test for ketonuria (Acetest or Ketostix), as presence of ketones provides a warning that hypoglycemia is imminent. Glucagon is of no value for treatment of hypoglycemia; however, Instant Glucose‡ or Monajel may be administered at home with effect. Diet restrictions as for type I do not apply; however, the diet should be high in protein.

Type VI and Type IX. These disorders result from deficiencies of hepatic phosphorylase and phosphorylase-activating enzymes. The latter disease is sex-linked and is associated with a defect in phosphorylase kinase. These disorders resemble type III disease clinically and are much milder clinical disorders than type I. The therapy for these types has been outlined under type III.

Type IV. This results from a deficiency of alpha-1,4 glucan:1,4 glucan 6-glycosyl transferase or brancher enzyme. Affected infants have progressive hepatomegaly with increasing signs of portal hyper-

tension and congestive failure resulting in death within 2 years of life. Therapy is supportive. Attempts at specific therapy utilizing purified alpha-glucosidase from *Aspergillus niger* have been encouraging but have not altered prognosis appreciably.

Muscle Glycogen Storage Syndromes

Type II (Pompe Disease). The disease results from a deficiency of the lysosomal hydrolase acid maltase. Lack of this enzyme allows a massive accumulation of glycogen in cardiac muscle and neuromuscular tissue. Hypoglycemia is not characteristic. Cardiac hypertrophy with attendant cardiac failure is usually unremitting, and affected infants can seldom be supported beyond 1 year of age despite the use of antibiotics, digitalis, nasogastric feedings, and the like. Specific therapy is unavailable, although alpha-glucosidase purified from a fungal source has been used with limited success.

Type V (McArdle Disease). This has been characterized as a deficiency of muscle phosphorylase. Onset is often during the second decade of life. Whereas affected patients may suffer excessive muscle fatigue on exercise, noncustomary exercise during adulthood may precipitate the characteristic muscle pains, often in the calves, associated with red myoglobinuria. Fructose ingestion (30 gm) prior to exercise may improve the capacity for exercise. Recognition of the inability of the patient to withstand much muscular exercise will permit avoidance of attacks. No specific therapy appears effective; however, apart from the rare occurrence of acute renal failure following an episode, longevity appears to be unaffected.

DISORDERS OF FRUCTOSE METABOLISM

The principal disorder involving fructose metabolism is that of hereditary fructose intolerance, and this condition needs to be distinguished from the gluconeogenic defect of fructose-1,6-diphosphatase deficiency, and benign fructosuria.

Hereditary Fructose Intolerance

Severely affected infants may suffer hypoglycemia with vomiting, apnea, and/or convulsions following sucrose-containing feedings. Continued sucrose feedings may lead to hepatomegaly with hepatic dysfunction (ascites, bleeding diathesis, jaundice, and so on), Fanconi-like syndrome following renal damage, and recurrent hypoglycemia, which may be accompanied by acidosis. Older infants and children have abdominal symptoms and hypoglycemia. The defect is one of deficiency of the enzyme fructose aldolase in liver, kidney, and intestinal mucosa. Acute hypoglycemic episodes should be treated with intravenous glucose.

Sucrose should be strictly avoided. Besides su-

---

*Manufacturer's Precaution: Allopurinol is contraindicated in children with the exception of those with hyperuricemia secondary to malignancy.

†Manufacturer's Statement: In children, insufficient studies have been done to show efficacy and safety.

‡Tubes of "Instant Glucose" in absorbable gel are available from the Diabetes Association of Greater Cleveland, 2022 Lea Road, Cleveland, Ohio 44018.

crose-containing sweets, drinks, and cookies, the following should be avoided completely: ham, bacon, lunch meats, sweet potatoes, all fruits and fruit juices, bread, sugar-containing cereals, salad dressings, most desserts, catsup, pickles, jam, preserves, and honey. Allowable foods include beef, veal, lamb, pork, fish, poultry, cheese, cabbage, cauliflower, celery, green beans, lettuce, spinach, peppers, wax beans, white potatoes, macaroni, noodles, spaghetti, rice, crackers, nonsugared cereals, dietetic gelatin and ice cream, and vegetable juices (not tomato) and soups made from allowable meats and vegetables. All processed packaged foods should be viewed with suspicion and the list of contents carefully examined.

Friends and teachers should be given a list of allowable foods and warned of the dangers of sucrose-containing food or drinks. Some potatoes, especially if fresh, certain vegetables such as broccoli, cucumber, and gourds, and some varieties of peas and rhubarb may contain small amounts of sucrose or fructose and should be viewed with caution or avoided. Invert sugar, sorbitol, or levulose must never be administered IV. Whereas some tolerance to fructose develops over time, these dieting principles will be lifelong.

Fructose-1,6-Diphosphatase Deficiency

This disease manifests with hypoglycemic attacks that may be precipitated by fasting or by ingesting fructose or glycerol. Lactic acidosis usually accompanies hypoglycemia. The disease often presents within the first months of life and hepatomegaly may be apparent. Feedings should be frequent and fasting avoided. Sucrose, fructose, and sorbitol should be eliminated from the diet. A diet consisting of 56% carbohydrate, 32% fat, and 12% protein has resulted in normal growth and development. Acute attacks must be treated promptly with IV glucose and sodium bicarbonate as required (see above), since fatalities have resulted from such episodes. Specific therapy is unavailable.

Essential Fructosuria. This is a rare and benign inborn error of carbohydrate metabolism. Fructose is a reducing sugar and reacts positively with Clinitest tablets or Benedict solution, but not to the glucose oxidase system which is specific for glucose (Testape, Clinistix, Dextrostix). No treatment is required.

OTHER MELITURIAS

Sucrosuria may occur after sucrose ingestion in association with various gastrointestinal disorders, such as gastroenteritis. Sucrose is not a reducing sugar and may be detected by testing the urine with Clinitest tablets after hydrolysis of the urine with glacial acetic acid and boiling. In itself, sucrosuria is benign.

Benign pentosuria is another rare disorder that results in urinary excretion of L-xylulose but has no associated medical problems. The urine shows a constant small quantity of reducing sugar, which can be shown to be other than glucose by specific glucose oxidase (as above). Provided the patient is not mistakenly treated for diabetes, the condition is of little consequence.

Hyperlipoproteinemia

NOEL K. MACLAREN, M.D.,
and WILLIAM J. RILEY, M.D.

Hypercholesterolemia has been shown to be one of the many risk factors for atherosclerosis. Treatments aimed at reducing hypercholesterolemia are thought to reduce the risk of an atherosclerotic outcome; however, evidence for this is incomplete. Treatment regimens are often ineffective in restoring lipid levels to normal in the genetic syndromes, and there is uncertainty as to whether the degree of improvement in circulating lipid levels that can be currently achieved will reduce atherosclerosis. The decision to treat a particular patient calls for an assessment of probable outcome as well as an appraisal of the efficacy of therapy to be initiated, since treatment is often for life.

Diet. The initial and sometimes only treatment should be dietary. For the hypertriglyceridemias, the general aim is to reduce the load of transported lipids (triglycerides and cholesteryl esters). Because of the close relationship between transport of very low-density lipoproteins (VLDL) and low-density lipoproteins (LDL), the association between elevated LDL cholesterol levels and premature atherosclerosis, and the atherogenic potential of VLDL itself, the major aim is to reduce VLDL synthesis. Thus the first principle is to avoid excesses in total daily calories, the major determinant of VLDL synthesis. Calorie-restricted diets should always be prescribed for obese patients with hyperlipidemia. Elevations in LDL can be reduced in most cases by a diet restricted in saturated fats (and cholesterol). Isocaloric amounts of carbohydrates or polyunsaturated fat (usually of vegetable origin) or both can be substituted. Diets high in polyunsaturated fats augment fecal excretion of cholesterol and bile acids and, indeed, increase the risk of lithogenicity of the bile. Fat restriction should be avoided in small infants as much as possible because of the requirement for cholesterol and essential fatty acids in early growth. Severe fat restriction may require supplementation with fat-soluble vitamins A, D, E, and K.

Bile Acid Sequestrants. These nonabsorbable cationic polymers interrupt the enterohepatic recirculation of bile acids. Cholestyramine is the most commonly used agent, while colestipol and di-ethylaminoethyl-Sephadex are rarely used for treatment of children. The major effect of these agents is to lower LDL and cholesterol levels. Cholestyramine is given in two divided daily doses, and a reduction in serum cholesterol by about one third can be achieved by total doses of 0.6 gm/kg (250 mg/kg active agent/24 hr). Questran is a palatable form of the drug and comes in packets containing 9 grams (4 gm of active agent). Side effects include bloating; constipation; malabsorption of folic acid, fat-soluble vitamins, and phosphate; and bleeding from hypoprothrombinemia. Steatorrhea may be seen if large doses are given. Supplements of folate and vitamins A and E should be provided. Since cholestyramine binds coumarin anticoagulants, digitalis glycosides, and thyroxine, these drugs should be given some hours before the sequestrant to facilitate absorption.

Clofibrate. The best-defined effect of this agent is to increase plasma triglyceride catabolism, probably by increasing lipoprotein lipase activity. It also promotes hepatic oxidation of fatty acids and has variable effects on reducing cholesterol synthesis and promoting biliary cholesterol excretion. The major effect of this agent is in lowering VLDL and triglyceride levels. It may lower LDL levels 15% or so more than diet alone in hypercholesterolemia. LDL levels are little affected by clofibrate in hypertriglyceridemia.

Clofibrate* is given in divided doses at 20 to 30 mg/kg/24 hr. Side effects include increased frequencies of cholelithiasis, nausea, diarrhea, skin rash, leukopenia, increased serum transaminases, and a syndrome of cramping myalgias with increased levels of creatine phosphokinase, especially when serum albumin levels are low. Clofibrate potentiates the anticoagulant effect from coumarin and the hypoglycemia effects of the sulfonylureas. As a possible benefit, it also reduces the hypersensitivity to adenosine diphosphate- or epinephrine-induced platelet aggregation seen in familial hypercholesterolemia, an action that may justify its adjunctive use in that disease.

Nicotinic Acid. The hypotriglyceride effect of the drug may be due to inhibition of lipolysis in adipose tissue. It has effects similar to those of clofibrate in lowering VLDL and LDL levels. Divided doses of approximately 100 mg/kg/24 hr are required for full effect. Cutaneous flushing is invariable but can be overcome by gradual increases in dose. Other side effects include nausea, hepatocellular damage, hyperuricemia, and cardiac arrhythmias.

---

*Manufacturer's Precaution: Safety and efficacy of clofibrate in children have not been established.

Other Agents. D-Thyroxine lowers lipid levels, but its use is restricted because it increases the work of the heart owing to contamination with L-thyroxine. Neomycin interferes with cholesterol absorption by the gut, an action independent of its antibiotic properties. The effect of neomycin is to lower raised plasma LDL. Para-aminosalicylic acid lowers both cholesterol and triglyceride levels, and it may have a place in treatment of familial hypercholesterolemia. β-Sitosterol reduces cholesterol absorption by the gut. Some derivatives of testosterone increase triglyceride catabolism and reduce plasma triglyceride levels. Estrogens and pregnancy worsen most hyperlipidemias.

Surgery. Excision of the terminal ileum prevents resorption of bile acids and has an effect like that of the bile acid sequestrants. It has no efficacy in the homozygous form of hypercholesterolemia; however, end-to-side portacaval shunting may have a useful effect. At present, such therapies must be considered experimental.

It is important to make as complete a diagnosis as possible of the type of hyperlipidemia present in order to determine outcome risks and thus aid in decisions of management.

PRIMARY (FAMILIAL) HYPERLIPOPROTEINEMIAS

Type I (Familial Lipoprotein Lipase Deficiency)

Accelerated atherosclerosis is not a problem, but rather there is onset of eruptive xanthomata, attacks of abdominal pains (pancreatitis), and hepatosplenomegaly during late infancy and childhood. If the diagnosis is made during "abdominal episodes," a fat-free diet (that is, < 1 gm/24 hr) should be prescribed until the serum is optically cleared. For long-term therapy, dietary fat should be reduced to a level sufficient to maintain serum triglyceride values below 1000 mg/dl, as attacks of pancreatitis are uncommon at serum triglyceride levels that fall well below this upper limit. This is achieved by diets containing 15 to 20 grams of fat per day, which will also resolve symptoms. Medium-chain triglycerides may be given as supplements to enhance palatability of the diet. Infants under 2 to 3 years of age probably should be only minimally fat restricted, perhaps by providing skimmed rather than whole cow's milk. For those maintained on fat-reduced therapeutic diets, some attention should be given to provide essential cholesterol (1 to 2 eggs/week) and fat-soluble vitamin supplements as necessary. Drug therapies are not usually necessary and are not recommended.

Type IIa (Familial Hypercholesterolemia)

The disease is composed of three subtypes, all with defects in LDL binding to membrane receptors. The gene frequency of about 1:500 persons makes this disease the most common of the hyperlipidemias. *Homozygous individuals* develop symptomatic atherosclerosis, often during the second decade, and life expectancy is not more than 30 years. Diagnosis should await laboratory confirmation at 1 year of age. The combined therapy of a low-fat diet (20 to 25% of total calories) with a polyunsaturated to saturated fat ratio of 1 : 1, cholestyramine, and nicotinic acid is recommended. To achieve significant serum cholesterol reductions, diets with a severe fat restriction (down to 1 gm/24 hr) and supplemented with polyunsaturated fats such as from safflower oil (to provide 20% of total calories) are often required. Supplements for the total regimen include cholesterol, vitamins A and E, and folate, with additional vitamin K_1 should prothrombin levels fall. Cholesterol levels are seldom maintained below 500 mg/dl, but even a partial response may improve outcome.

Heterozygous patients also have accelerated atherosclerosis, especially males. Lifelong therapies appear to be justified. Diet therapy should aim to reduce ordinary fat intake to 15 to 20 gm/daily, with substitution by polyunsaturated fat. This measure often reduces cholesterol levels by about 20%. For greater reductions to maintain plasma cholesterol levels below 250 to 300 mg/dl, additional cholestyramine is often necessary. Since compliance with long-term diets is an obvious problem, most patients are treated with the agent. Supplements should be offered as noted. Recently, a new class of experimental agents has been introduced. Drugs of this class include compactin and mevinolin and act as competitive inhibitors of HMG-COA reductase. This action results in lowering plasma LDL by decreasing hepatic LDL production and stimulating formation of LDL receptors in the liver. When either agent is given together with cholestyramine, a greater cholesterol (and LDL) lowering effect is seen. At present, such agents should be used only in a research setting. On epidemiologic data, increased levels of HDL cholesterol appear to have a protective effect, offsetting the atherosclerotic effects of elevated LDL cholesterol. Exercise and, in adults, alcohol both have the effect of raising HDL levels. It is not yet proven that such measures actually reduce atherosclerosis; however, we currently recommend both.

Type IV (Familial Endogenous Hypertriglyceridemia)

For these patients, therapy should be a weight-reducing diet. Reduction in calories or carbohydrates, or both, will usually bring lipid levels to normal. In those with continued elevations of VLDL and triglyceride, clofibrate is often also necessary usually only because of poor compliance with the diet.

Type IIb (Familial Combined Hyperlipidemia)

Dietary therapy for type IIb disease is as for type IV; however, continued elevations of cholesterol may be an indication for the addition of cholestyramine. The condition is diagnosed only unusually during childhood, and affected persons have increased rates of atherosclerosis, which effective treatment may reduce. A chronic program of daily exercise and modest daily alcohol consumption (in adults) is to be promoted as for type IIB heterozygous patients as above.

Type III (Familial Dysbetalipoproteinemia)

Therapy should include weight reduction and thyroxine as indicated. Otherwise a diet restricted in dietary fat to 40% or less of the total calories and restricted in cholesterol to less than 300 mg/24 hr is prescribed. Clofibrate is the preferred drug, and response to therapy is usually good.

SECONDARY HYPERLIPOPROTEINEMIAS

Diabetes

In insulin-dependent diabetes, the inadequately treated patient has increased VLDL and occasionally elevated cholesterol values. Adequate insulin replacement will usually correct the lipid values. Long-term diets with reduced saturated fat and cholesterol and substituted polyunsaturated fats are reasonable, but long-term compliance is often poor, and a reduced atherosclerotic outcome has not been shown. Occasional instances of severe hyperlipidemia and diabetes in the absence of ketosis (diabetic-hyperlipidemia syndrome) probably represent familial disorders, as noted.

Glycogenosis Type I
(See also article on Inborn Errors of Carbohydrate Metabolism.)

A considerable increase in VLDL and triglyceride levels is characteristic of type I disease, possibly due in part to a counter-regulatory hormone response of hypoglycemia. Thus continuous nasogastric feeding reduces these levels. In addition, dietary fat should be restricted to 15 to 30% of total calories, mainly provided as polyunsaturated fat. Clofibrate has no proved value. In type III (debrancher) and type VI (hepatic phosphorylase) glycogenoses, increases in LDL are common and can usually be managed with simple dietary measures.

Hypothyroidism

Hypercholesterolemia is common, as are IIa and III lipoprotein phenotypes. Thus hypothyroidism should always be excluded in patients with these phenotypes. Treatment with replacement thyroxine resolves serum lipid abnormalities.

Renal Disease

In nephrosis, LDL/cholesterol levels are increased due to increased hepatic synthesis of apoprotein B, while increased VLDL may also result from diminished lipoprotein lipase. Treatment is directed at the primary renal disease. Low-fat diets are not indicated, and clofibrate is contraindicated when serum albumin levels are low.

In uremic patients, hyperlipidemia and atherosclerosis are common, especially in those on renal dialysis programs. This in part may relate to high-fat diets, to uremia-induced glucose intolerance and insulin resistance, or to steroid therapies. The use of polyunsaturated fats in the diet seems justifiable in selected cases.

Obstructive Jaundice

Cholesterol levels are often extreme. Low-fat diets and cholestyramine relieve xanthomata and itching of the skin.

The Galactosemias

GEORGE N. DONNELL, M.D.

Galactosemia most often results in severe and life-threatening signs and symptoms early in infancy. If galactosemia is suspected, it is better to institute treatment than risk irreversible damage or death while awaiting confirmation of the diagnosis.

Immediate attention must be given to the frequently fulminant secondary manifestations, but specific treatment of infection, bleeding tendency, and other problems is rarely successful unless the primary disease is cared for concurrently. The basic problem presented by these infants is control of tissue accumulation of galactose metabolites, caused by the absence of activity of galactose-1-phosphate uridyl transferase, an enzyme essential in galactose metabolism. At present, no way is known to provide a functional enzyme system, thus galactose must be excluded from the diet. Dietary control of galactose intake is crucial in the management of galactosemia, but dietary restriction alone is insufficient therapy of the fulminant secondary manifestations.

DIET THERAPY

Exclusion of galactose from the diet prevents or reverses many manifestations. The most important step is elimination of milk and milk products from the diet. The substitution of a commercially prepared casein hydrolysate (Nutramigen) or soy or meat base formula has been successful.

In the past there was concern about the galactose-containing oligosaccharide content of soy formulas. Recently, soy formulas have been prepared from soy protein isolate rather than from whole soy flour. The isolate reduces the oligosaccharide content and the potential source of galactose. Experience with these formulas has not resulted in increased erthyrocyte galactose-1-phosphate levels, and these products are considered safe for galactosemic children.

The formula may be the sole source of calories until the usual baby foods are added. Many "baby dinners," soups, and puddings contain some form of milk and should not be offered. Manufacturers should be consulted if there is any doubt about the composition of their product.

Cereals, vegetables, fruits, and meat are safe to administer. There previously was some question about the advisability of feeding legumes. Peas and beans contain oligosaccharides, of which galactose is a constituent. Presumably these more complex sugars cannot be digested to free galactose, and their intake is permissible.

As the child grows older and the diet becomes more varied, caution should be used in the selection of new foods. Milk is commonly found in bread, cake, some canned puddings, and various chocolate candies. Accordingly, the labels of all food packages must be carefully examined. Other potential problems are the use of lactose as a sweetening agent in medicinal capsules and as a coating in frozen ready-to-eat foods.

Parents will need periodic advice to ensure that the diet is well balanced and contains the nutrients needed for growth and development. As these children reach school age, they will tend to reduce disproportionately their intake of the milk substitute. Water or fruit and vegetable juices may be substituted. Calcium supplement may be necessary. Meat, poultry, fish, and eggs are excellent protein sources, but certain galactose-storing organs, such as liver, pancreas, and brain, should be avoided. Labels on cold cuts and other meats commonly containing fillers should be carefully scrutinized to make sure that no milk or milk products are included.

The question arises as to how long the diet should be continued. It is essential to exclude lactose during the years of rapid growth and development. Whether or not tolerance to galactose occurs with increasing age is still unclear. Unless an objective means, such as periodic monitoring with erythrocyte galactose-1-phosphate levels, is available, one should err on the conservative side and continue to avoid galactose intake.

TREATMENT OF COMPLICATIONS

Fluid and Electrolyte Disturbances. Vomiting, dehydration, and weight loss are common in the untreated patient, especially the infant. The indications for fluid therapy are the same as those in other disorders in which similar symptoms are present.

Infection. Untreated galactosemic infants are extremely susceptible to infection. Septicemia, meningitis, and osteomyelitis are the most common. Gram-negative organisms predominate, and the choice of drugs should take this into account.

Jaundice. Onset of icterus is generally during the first week of life. Occasionally a sufficiently high level of indirect bilirubin warrants consideration for exchange transfusion. Removal of galactose from the diet and supportive treatment of infection are followed by rapid clearing of the jaundice.

Edema. Liver damage also may be reflected in hypoalbuminemia, which in turn may result in generalized edema and ascites. Whole blood, plasma or human albumin may be administered IV to correct the hypoproteinemia.

Cataracts. Cataracts of varying degrees of severity occur in most untreated patients. In the untreated patient progression to mature cataracts is variable. Patients with a late diagnosis or those improperly treated may require corrective surgery. When the diagnosis is made early, lesions usually become arrested or may even improve.

Mental Retardation. Retardation occurs in untreated patients. Although further mental impairment is arrested by treatment, the possibility of improvement with therapy depends on the age of the child. The need for early diagnosis and careful management is evident.

HYPOGONADOTROPHIC HYPOGONADISM

Recently, it has been shown that female patients with galactosemia have a high incidence of ovarian failure due to acquired ovarian atrophy. The cause is unclear. Gonadal function in males, for the most part, appears to be unaffected, but the data are insufficient to draw definitive conclusions. Treatment of gonadal failure in female patients should follow the currently accepted approaches.

GALACTOKINASE DEFICIENCY

A second rare genetic disorder of galactose metabolism has been reported in which a deficiency of galactokinase is responsible for the clinical and laboratory findings. The inability to phosphorylate galactose results in the accumulation of galactose in blood and the appearance of galactose in urine. In contrast to the well-known transferase defect type of galactosemia, the important clinical manifestations of galactokinase deficiency recognized to date are pseudotumor cerebri and cataract formation. Diet therapy is identical to that described for galactosemia.

Disorders of Porphyrin, Purine, and Pyrimidine Metabolism

PHILIP ROSENTHAL, M.D.,
and M. MICHAEL THALER, M.D.

THE PORPHYRIAS

The porphyrias are a group of disorders characterized by defects in heme synthesis resulting in excessive accumulation of heme precursors in the tissues. Most fatalities are caused by delays in diagnosis and treatment. Awareness of the clinical patterns associated with these disorders and investigation of family members of patients with porphyria will accelerate the diagnostic process and may prevent unnecessary surgery. Appropriate therapy will bring about relief from acute attacks and ensure a favorable long-term outcome.

Congenital Erythropoietic Porphyria (Günther's Disease). For this, one of the rarest inborn errors of metabolism, treatment includes avoidance of sunlight, screening window light, use of special light bulbs, protective clothing, avoidance of minor trauma to the skin, barrier skin creams, and appropriate topical and systemic antibiotics. Photosensitivity in some patients has been reduced with beta-carotene (30 to 150 mg/24 hr orally). Beta-carotene capsules may be opened and contents mixed in orange or tomato juice to aid administration in children. Recently, canthaxanthin (4,4-diketo-beta-carotene) has been utilized in doses of 25 to 100 mg/24 hr with good results. Instead of a yellow hue from beta-carotene, canthaxanthin causes a brownish discoloration of the palms and a pleasant suntanned appearance to the face.

Blood transfusions frequently are necessary to treat the hemolytic anemia. Splenectomy may reduce transfusion requirements and decrease formation of porphyrins responsible for photosensitivity. However, the increased risks of sepsis in children susceptible to repeated skin infections should be considered in the decision for splenectomy.

Erythrodontia, a pinkish-brown discoloration of teeth due to porphyrin deposition, may be improved cosmetically with dental crowns. Patients with such crowns should receive careful dental surveillance, since gingivitis may develop, forcing removal of the crowns.

Congenital Erythropoietic Protoporphyria. Congenital erythropoietic protoporphyria occurs more commonly than erythropoietic porphyria. Treatment consists of avoidance of sunlight by screening window light and by using special wavelength light bulbs (not in the 400 nm range), protective clothing, and barrier skin creams. Oral administration of beta-carotene at a dose of 30 to 150 mg/24 hr, maintaining serum carotene concentrations above 500 μg/dl over a period of months, has been found to dampen photosensitivity. Hemolytic anemia is a rare complication that may require splenectomy. Formation of porphyrin gallstones has been reported, which has been treated by cholecystectomy.

Acute Intermittent Porphyria (Swedish Type). Treatment of acute attacks includes provision of 450 to 600 gm of glucose/24 hr, infused through a central vein as 10 to 15% solution in water. Pain is treated effectively with chlorpromazine or chloral hydrate. Hyponatremia secondary to inappropriate secretion of antidiuretic hormone (ADH) often develops during an acute attack and should be managed with fluid restriction. Careful replacement of the sodium deficit with hypertonic saline may be necessary. Severe hypertension is an occasional complication and should be treated as primary malignant hypertension. Paralysis of intercostal muscles with respiratory insufficiency may develop in patients with acute intermittent porphyria in the acute phase. Paresis is often reversible with aggressive management in an intensive care unit. Treatment includes tracheal intubation or tracheostomy and mechanical respiratory support with frequent blood gas monitoring.

A recently introduced therapeutic strategy intended to reduce porphyrin production by means of IV-administered hematin* appears to be extremely effective. An IV line running normal saline is used to inject hematin as a bolus over a period of 15 minutes at a dose of 3 mg/kg body weight. The tubing is then flushed with normal saline (0.9% NaCl). Hematin administration may be repeated with 12- to 24-hour intervals depending on response, but usually is given twice daily for 3 days.

Propranolol,† administered orally or IV to adults with acute intermittent porphyria, has been reported to exert a beneficial effect on acute attacks. The IV regimen consists of 1 mg propranolol every 1 to 2 hours initially, increasing each dose to a maximum of 40 mg if necessary.

Intravenous administration of the carbohydrate levulose‡ has also been reported to reduce the severity of acute attacks in adults.

In patients whose attacks may be precipitated by menstruation, the use of ovulatory suppressants, androgens, oophorectomy, and oral contraceptives may be indicated.

Porphyria Variegata (Congenital Cutaneous Hepatic Porphyria, South African Type, Mixed Porphyria). Treatment consists of protection from sunlight (see Congenital Erythropoietic Porphyria) and careful avoidance of even trivial trauma. Cho-

lestyramine (note: dosage of cholestyramine resin for infants and children has not been established), 12 gm daily, has proved useful in the management of cutaneous manifestations. The resin binds porphyrins in the intestinal tract, thus preventing their reabsorption. Fat-soluble vitamins (such as vitamins A, D, and K) should be supplemented in patients treated with cholestyramine.

Porphyria Cutanea Tarda. For porphyrias of this type, treatment should be nonaggressive since the disease is not life-threatening. Dermatologic manifestations should be managed as previously described (see Congenital Erythropoietic Porphyria). When ingestion of toxic chemicals is discovered and discontinued, complete recovery often follows within a few months.

Other modes of therapy include attempts to increase porphyrin excretion by alkalinization of the urine and administration of cholestyramine. The antimalarial agent chloroquine forms complexes with uroporphyrin in the liver, which are readily excreted in urine. However, this form of treatment is potentially dangerous and should be avoided in most cases.

Vitamin E (alpha-tocopherol acetate), 400 IU daily, increased to 1600 IU daily, administered for several months has reduced the dermatologic complications in limited trials with adult patients.

Hereditary Coproporphyria. Treatment of hereditary coproporphyria is as described for acute intermittent porphyria.

DISORDERS OF PURINE AND PYRIMIDINE METABOLISM

Hyperuricemia. Hyperuricemia is rare in childhood. While gout is the major complication of hyperuricemia in adults, formation of urate renal stones is the most frequently observed manifestation of hyperuricemia in children.

Two categories of drugs are used in treatment: those for control of hyperuricemia and those for acute attacks of gout. Since hyperuricemia is rare in childhood, agents currently employed in treatment of hyperuricemia with or without gout have not been adequately evaluated in children. Recommended doses are the usual adult doses, unless specifically noted as designed for children.

The rapid cell turnover and breakdown of nucleic acids in neoplastic diseases such as leukemia and lymphoma induce hyperuricemia, which may lead to clinical complications, especially in the course of chemotherapy or radiation therapy. As mentioned, the major complication of hyperuricemia in childhood is formation of uric acid stones in the urinary tract. The xanthine oxidase inhibitor allopurinol (hydroxypyrazolo pyrimidine) is indicated in children with hyperuricemia due to malignancy. To ensure maximal inhibition of xanthine oxidase,

---

*Investigational drug; procedure not yet approved by FDA.
†This use is not listed in the manufacturer's official directive.
‡Investigational procedure.

treatment with allopurinol at 10 to 20 mg/kg/24 hr should be initiated several days prior to chemotherapy. When pretreatment is not possible, allopurinol in doses ranging from 120 to 500 mg/day is used concomitantly with cytotoxic agents. The actual dose of allopurinol is adjusted to body weight, monitored with determinations of serum uric acid, and reduced when renal function is impaired. Side effects of allopurinol include nausea and diarrhea, hepatotoxic manifestations, and skin rashes. Hepatic microsomal enzymes may be partially inactivated by allopurinol, resulting in prolongation of the effective half-life of other drugs metabolized by the liver. When the antileukemic agents mercaptopurine and azathioprine are used in conjunction with allopurinol, their usual doses must be reduced by two thirds to three fourths. Allopurinol and ampicillin should not be administered concomitantly because of an increased risk of serious skin rashes.

An abundant fluid intake and alkalinization of the urine to increase solubility of uric acid are important adjuncts in the treatment of hyperuricemia. This can be accomplished by the use of oral sodium bicarbonate (2 to 6 gm/24 hr) or sodium citrate (20 to 60 ml/24 hr). If renal stone formation occurs in association with diminished renal function, peritoneal dialysis or hemodialysis may be used to remove excess uric acid.

Dietary manipulation includes elimination of purine-rich foods such as organ meats (liver, sweetbreads, kidney), anchovies, sardines, wild game, meat extracts, and meat concentrates (gravies).

Acute attacks of gout are usually treated with colchicine administered orally (0.5 or 0.6 mg once hourly) until objective improvement is obtained. The drug must be discontinued when gastrointestinal complications of colchicine develop (cramping, diarrhea, nausea, vomiting). The maximum daily dose of colchicine is preferably administered IV (1 to 3 mg total dose, based on body size and weight, diluted in 20 ml normal saline) to minimize the gastrointestinal side effects. Colchicine is contraindicated in patients with leukopenia or substantial renal or hepatic disease. The drug must be injected slowly, with care taken not to infiltrate. In addition to gastrointestinal toxicity, side effects include granulocytopenia, alopecia, aplastic anemia, and respiratory depression.

The prostaglandin inhibitor indomethacin* is also effective in acute gouty arthritis at 25 to 100 mg orally every 4 hours, continued until symptomatic relief is obtained. Another regimen is to provide 75 mg initially and 50 mg every 6 hours, tapered after resolution of inflammatory signs. Side effects include anorexia, nausea, abdominal pain, bleeding peptic ulcers, headaches, dizziness, mental confusion, depression, and convulsions. Bone marrow depression has also been described.

Phenylbutazone and its analog oxyphenbutazone (contraindicated in children under 14 years of age) are potent anti-inflammatory agents useful in the treatment of gout. Usual adult dosage for acute gout is 400 mg initially, followed by 100 mg every 4 hours until inflammation subsides, usually within 4 days. The smallest dose possible should be utilized. In general, 600 mg in 4 divided doses during the first 24 hours of an acute attack is sufficient in adults. Gastrointestinal toxicity is similar to that of indomethacin (see above). Other significant side effects are aplastic anemia and salt retention.

Naproxen, ibuprofen, fenprofen, and piroxicam have been utilized with moderate success in adults to treat acute attacks of gout but have not been evaluated in children.

Lesch-Nyhan Syndrome. Severe deficiency of hypoxanthine-guanine phosphoribosyl transferase in this disorder caused marked uric acid overproduction associated with choreoathetosis, mental retardation, and self-mutilation. Hyperuricosuria and urate gravel or stone formation are treated with allopurinol* until the serum urate level and urinary urate excretion return to normal. Dosages must be individually titrated, but usually range from 100 to 300 mg daily in divided doses. Prevention of urate stones may be accomplished with increased fluid intake, which stimulates increased renal output of uric acid.

Treatment with allopurinol cannot reverse the neurologic manifestations of Lesch-Nyhan syndrome. Physical restraints (elbow splints and hand bandages) may be used to control self-mutilating behavior of patients. Lip biting may require extraction of teeth, but permanent teeth should be spared, since lip biting usually diminishes with age. Nondestructive behavior should be rewarded when possible, but attempts at self-injury should not be punished. This approach is based on reports which suggest that positive reinforcement is preferable to punishment in controlling self-destructive behavior in children with Lesch-Nyhan syndrome.

Recently, 5-hydroxytryptophan,† a precursor of serotonin, in a dose of 8 mg/kg/24 hr in four equal increments, in conjunction with the peripheral decarboxylase inhibitor carbidopa (safety in children not established), 1 to 10 mg/kg/24 hr in two to four equal portions, has been shown to reduce athetoid movement significantly and to produce a sedative effect without improvement in mood or self-multilation. Unfortunately, tolerance may develop with 1 month, with permanent loss of efficacy upon retreatment.

Xanthinuria. Xanthine accumulates owing to de-

---

*Manufacturer's Warning: Safe use in children has not been established.

†Investigational drug.

ficiency of xanthine oxidase, the enzyme that converts xanthine to uric acid. Uric acid levels are low in serum and urine, and xanthine stones form in the urinary tract. Treatment consists of reducing the intake of foods with a high purine content such as organ meats, anchovies, sardines, wild game, meat extracts, and meat concentrates (gravies). Fluid intake should be increased and the urine alkalinized to facilitate renal excretion of xanthine. These measures should be carefully monitored, since continuous alkalinization of urine may induce formation of calcium stones and may enhance susceptibility to infection with organisms that thrive in an alkaline environment. Once formed, xanthine stones may require surgical removal.

Orotic Aciduria. Hereditary orotic aciduria is due to a deficiency of two enzymes, orotidylic pyrophosphorylase and orotidylic decarboxylase. Mixtures of cytidylic and uridylic acid have been reported to produce remissions, but have not been well tolerated. Treatment with uridine, the nucleoside of uracil, in divided doses of 150 mg/kg/24 hr is readily tolerated, and has resulted in hematologic improvement and diminished urinary orotic acid excretion. A copious intake of fluids assists in dilution of orotic acid in urine and may diminish precipitation of orotic acid crystals.

Lysosomal Storage Diseases

ARTHUR L. BEAUDET, M.D.

The lysosomal storage diseases are due to the genetic deficiency or dysfunction of one or more lysosomal enzymes. This group of disorders includes the lipid storage diseases, the mucopolysaccharidoses, the mucolipidoses, glycoprotein storage diseases, and type II glycogen storage disease (Table 1). The pattern of organ involvement depends on the usual site of degradation of the accumulating macromolecules. Almost all the disorders are autosomal recessive defects, although a few are X-linked. Although these diseases are heterogeneous and often have infantile, juvenile, and adult forms associated with the same enzyme defect, the disorders regularly exhibit a progressive course. An enzyme-specific diagnosis is a prerequisite for optimal management.

Medical management of patients with these diseases is largely symptomatic and supportive, but a few specific forms of intervention are important. Hypersplenism develops frequently in adult Gaucher disease, and splenectomy is indicated for correction of significant hematologic abnormalities. The Morquio phenotype is associated with odontoid hypoplasia with instability at the atlantoaxial joint. This joint should be evaluated carefully, even in the absence of symptoms. Prophylactic cervical fusion is indicated during the first decade if instability is significant, since acute and chronic cervical cord damage is likely. Judicious use of corrective orthopedic procedures is appropriate, particularly for the mucopolysaccharidoses such as mild Hunter, Morquio, and Maroteaux-Lamy diseases in which intellectual impairment is minimal or absent. Careful cardiac and ophthalmologic follow-up also is needed for the mucopolysaccharidoses and related diseases when these organs are involved.

Myringotomy and polyethylene tubes to prevent recurrent ear infections are very important in the mucopolysaccharidoses, mucolipidoses, and similar phenotypes such as mannosidosis. Hearing can be preserved in intellectually normal patients, and recurrent episodes of fever, irritability, and family stress can be avoided in profoundly impaired children.

Fabry disease has a progressive renal impairment, and renal transplantation and dialysis should be considered according to usual criteria. Renal involvement is usually severe enough to require such intervention in hemizygous males but not in heterozygous females. Painful neuropathy occurs in males and females with Fabry disease, and symptomatic relief often can be obtained with Dilantin in usual therapeutic dosage.

Cardiac and respiratory failure occur in type II glycogen storage disease and are managed symptomatically as for any cardiac and skeletal myopathy. Many of the disorders cause intellectual impairment, and special educational and training support is indicated. At times the possibility of progressive dementia exists, but the child should be given the usual special educational support, since prognosis is never certain.

Unfortunately, many children with these diseases experience progressive and ultimately severe neurologic impairment. Proper emotional and social support for the family is very important. Some of these diseases are most tragic and burdensome

Table 1. **LYSOSOMAL STORAGE DISEASES**

G_{M1} gangliosidosis	Sialidosis
G_{M2} gangliosidosis, Tay- Sachs	Aspartylglycosaminuria
G_{M2} gangliosidosis, Sandhoff	Hurler, MPS IH*
Krabbe leukodystrophy	Scheie, MPS IS
Metachromatic leukodystrophy	Hunter, MPS II
Niemann-Pick disease	Sanfilippo A, MPS IIIA
Gaucher disease	Sanfilippo B, MPS IIIB
Fabry disease	Sanfilippo C, MPS IIIC
Wolman disease	Sanfilipo D, MPS IIID
Cholesteryl ester storage disease	Morquio, MPS IV
Farber lipogranulomatosis	Maroteaux-Lamy, MPS VI
Pompe disease, glycogenosis type II	β-Glucuronidase deficiency, MSP VII
Acid phosphatase deficiency	Multiple sulfatase deficiency
Fucosidosis	Mucolipidosis II, I-cell disease
Mannosidosis	Mucolipidosis III
	Mucolipidosis IV

*MPS, mucopolysaccharidosis.

for families. The family should be encouraged early to explore local resources for institutional care. This can be of value in the event of family illness and can allow the family vacation time. Eventual long-term institutional care should be at the discretion of the family. Assistance can be provided with some medical problems. Seizures occur in many of the disorders and can be treated routinely. Constipation is frequent and can be managed with stool softeners, laxatives, and enemas in a usual manner. Feeding is progressively difficult and may require blenderized or liquid diets. Behavioral abnormalities, which include emotional outbursts, crying out as if in pain, and failure to sleep at night, are extremely burdensome for the family. Sedative medications may assist a family in managing a child at home, but erratic responses to drugs are not unusual in the face of brain damage. Behavioral difficulties are particularly severe in the Sanfilippo mucopolysaccharidoses but occur with other juvenile disorders. Major tranquilizers such as Mellaril,*in doses up to 3 mg/kg/24 hr. may be quite helpful. Finally, there may be many difficult ethical decisions late in the course of these patients. When endless hours are required to feed the patient, tube feeding or gastrostomy may be necessary. Institution of these methods of nutritional support should be discussed with the family as they may prolong the life of a helpless child, a result that may or may not be desired by the family. The family should be involved in deciding when to hospitalize and how to manage pneumonias in terminally ill children.

Specific correction of the enzyme defects in these diseases is a subject of active research. While prenatal diagnosis and other reproductive options can prevent the disease in subsequent siblings, these diseases will continue to occur within families unless heterozygote screening, as applied to Tay-Sachs disease, can be extended to other disorders. For the present, effective therapy is a major need. Enzyme replacement is one research modality. Enzyme activity can be delivered to some organs, such as liver and spleen. There might be cause for optimism that certain non-CNS manifestations could be treatable by enzyme infusion. To be effective in treating CNS damage, enzyme replacement must overcome the additional obstacle of the blood-brain barrier. At present, enzyme replacement is not of proven effectiveness and is not standard therapy in any lysosomal storage disease. Recent reports have revived interest in bone marrow transplantation or amnion implantation as modes of therapy. Carefully planned research trials are appropriate and are in progress. Some families may wish to explore the opportunities for their children to participate in human studies, but at present there is no proof of effective treatment or prevention of central nervous system symptoms. A variety of physical and biochemical methods for targeting enzyme to affected tissues and for overcoming the blood-brain barrier are being explored. The hope of replacing the defective gene itself is still quite distant, although perhaps considerably more realistic than at the time of the last edition of this book. Rapid developments in recombinant DNA technology suggest that many of the relevant genes will be available in cloned form soon. Only β-glucoronidase has been cloned at this writing. Considerable obstacles will still remain, and the feasibility of such therapy remains in question.

The final aspect of management of the lysosomal storage diseases is concerned with the family and prevention of future cases. The first step is complete genetic counseling, including a discussion of the risk of the disease, the burden of the disease, and reproductive options. In autosomal recessive conditions, the major risk is for subsequent pregnancies of the parents of the propositus. Occasionally a sibling of the mother will marry a sibling of the father, creating a high-risk situation. Genetic counseling must be extended to maternal relatives in the case of X-linked diseases. Heterozygote detection is feasible for most of the diseases in question and can be offered to aunts, uncles, and unaffected siblings of the patients with autosomal recessive disorders. For reliable heterozygote detection, however, a laboratory should have substantial experience in assaying normal controls and obligate heterozygotes. Samples from the obligate heterozygote parents of the propositus should be assayed simultaneously to assist in family-specific interpretation of unusual laboratory data which may result from rare alleles (mutant forms of the gene) in a family. Heterozygote testing of relatives is most important in disorders in which the carrier frequency is great, such as for Gaucher or Tay-Sachs disease in the Ashkenazi Jewish population. Mass screening for heterozygotes has been applied for the prevention of Tay-Sachs disease but has not been used significantly for other lysosomal storage diseases to date.

As part of the genetic counseling process, contraception, sterilization, adoption, and artificial insemination should be discussed as alternative methods for reducing the risk of disease. Prenatal diagnosis has been accomplished or presumably could be carried out for almost all the lysosomal storage diseases. The enzyme defects routinely are demonstrable in cultured fibroblasts and amniotic fluid cells. In fact, the vast majority of biochemical prenatal diagnosis in the last decade has involved the lysosomal storage diseases, with Tay-Sachs disease, type II glycogen storage disease, Krabbe leukodystrophy, metachromatic leukodystrophy, and Hurler disease among the most frequently tested.

---

*Manufacturer's precaution: Mellaril is not recommended for children under 2 years of age.

11

Connective Tissue

Collagen Vascular Disease

J. ROGER HOLLISTER, M.D.

The treatments of collagen vascular disease in children are based on the anti-inflammatory properties of medications, the restorative qualities of physical and occupational therapy, and the support of physician and family. There are no cures for these illnesses because the causes of them have yet to be understood. The increased knowledge of pathophysiologic mechanisms has led to more rational strategies to interrupt the inflammatory sequence without specific information of a unique pathogen. In this article the medications used will be arranged in hierarchies for each disease. The underlying principle of therapy will be that treatment for a given illness should be consonant with the severity of the illness, the prognosis, and the side effects of the particular drug. For example, although steroids are necessary when the kidneys and central nervous system are affected with systemic lupus erythematosus, lesser degrees of illness can be managed with less toxic drugs. Although juvenile rheumatoid arthritis can be treated with salicylates alone, gold with its attendant side effects is indicated in patients with progressive unremitting disease, to control the inflammation and favorably alter the natural history of the disease.

JUVENILE RHEUMATOID ARTHRITIS

The prognosis for those with juvenile rheumatoid arthritis (JRA) is better than for adults with rheumatoid arthritis, and 80% of patients will lead independent, productive lives 20 years after the onset of illness. Crippling and a dependent existence occur in a small fraction of JRA patients. Therefore, treatment should be oriented to relieving pain and inflammation and to returning children to their age-appropriate lifestyle *without* toxic side effects from drugs. The goal of therapy in the treatment of JRA is to restore normal physical and emotional function in the child. The eradication of all swelling or evidence of disease may not be possible, but if the patient can run, play, and participate in age-appropriate activities, the treatment should be considered successful. In this view the presence of a limp, the nonuse of a dominant extremity, or the failure to walk is more important than the degree of swelling in any joint.

Salicylates remain the treatment of choice in the majority of JRA patients. Seventy-five per cent of all JRA patients can gain relief of symptoms and return to normal function on therapeutic doses of aspirin. Starting doses of 100 mg/kg/24 hr divided into 4 doses in children under 5 years of age and 75 mg/kg/24 hr in patients over 5 years of age will usually result in therapeutic levels without toxicity. Serum salicylate levels are not followed routinely. If compliance is a problem, or toxicity is questioned, or an inadequate effect is observed, one should achieve a serum salicylate level of 20 to 30 mg/dl measured 2 hours after a dose before considering aspirin therapy to have failed. Side effects include gastric irritation, bruising, and epistaxis. Giving the aspirin with meals or use of enteric-coated aspirin usually can help stomach distress. The side effects of bruising or epistaxis can be avoided by use of a salicylate preparation that does not contain the acetyl portion responsible for platelet dysfunction. Arthropan (choline salicylate) and Trilisate (choline magnesium trisalicylate) offer this advantage, and the prolonged serum half-life of Trilisate allows twice a day dosage. Although serum levels with both drugs are adequate, comparison studies with aspirin have not been performed to evaluate efficacy.

Children under age 7 do not experience tinnitus

as a toxic manifestation of excessive salicylate dose. Therefore, their parents should be warned of lethargy, vomiting, and hyperpnea as toxic symptoms of salicylism. If such symptoms do occur, the salicylate should be withheld for 48 hours and reinstituted at a lower dose.

The duration of salicylate therapy is determined by the activity of the arthritis. Since the salicylate is a treatment and not a cure, it need be given only as long as signs of active arthritis, such as joint swelling, pain, and morning stiffness, are present. When the arthritis is in remission, the drug can be stopped without a long tapering period.

Before describing other drugs, we will discuss physical and occupational therapy and education as cornerstones in the successful management of JRA. Physical therapy is important to maintain or regain range of motion in the affected joints and to build muscle strength. To be successful, a home program of range of motion and resistive exercises should be designed to be performed on a once or twice daily schedule. A warm bath prior to exercising helps to relieve stiffness and pain. Hot paraffin treatments may aid some children. The children should not be restricted in their activities but rather should be allowed to set their own activity level. Children rarely use their disease to avoid physical activity. Normal childhood activity does not obviate the necessity of range of motion exercises if limitations in joint mobility exist. Occupational therapy helps children develop normal responsibilities for self-care and activities of daily living as they grow up with their illness. For instance, dressing, hair combing, bed-making, and so on, should be done by children at the age-appropriate level. In addition, resting night splints made by occupational therapists may greatly relieve the contractures and pain in wrists and knees. The splints are not corrective but are supportive in a comfortable position which prevents further flexion deformity during sleep. Even in the presence of acute inflammation, range of motion exercises should be performed within the limits of pain to maintain range.

Education about JRA is important for the patient, family, and school. Because neither the cause nor the cure for JRA is known, the family will be inundated with useless advice from well-meaning relatives and friends. With knowledge about natural history, genetics, and the effects of diet and climate, the parents can more accurately interpret the advice of others. A clear understanding of the good prognosis in JRA will help the family cope during periods of disease activity. In addition, the family physician can be of great support in counseling the parents about discipline, peer relationships, and educational goals as the child matures with this chronic disease. In the optimal situation the child will reach adulthood as an independent, self-sufficient member of society, and the disease will have left no physical or emotional residua.

Treatment of JRA includes routine slit lamp examination by an ophthalmologist to direct asymptomatic iridocyclitis before the inflammation has caused secondary effects. Young females with pauciarticular JRA and a positive antinuclear antibody test run a 35% risk of developing chronic iritis within the first 2 years of their illness. Slit lamp examination should be performed every 3 months in these children. In ANA-negative pauciarticular patients, screening at 6-month intervals is sufficient. Polyarticular patients should be screened once a year. The risk of chronic iridocyclitis in systemic-onset disease is essentially nil, and slit lamp examination need not be done. If chronic iridocyclitis is found, ophthalmologic management includes topical steroids and mydriatics. The response and inflammatory activity are monitored by slit lamp examination. Although the iritis may be persistent and recurrent, the prognosis for visual acuity appears favorable. Systemic steroids are indicated if topical treatment fails.

Additional Medications

For patients who fail on aspirin, gold therapy provides an additional order of magnitude of therapy but with a consequent increase in cost and risk of side effects. Gold salts must be administered by intramuscular injection, although oral preparations may soon be available. The dose is 1 mg/kg/week. It is a slow-acting medication and may take up to 20 injections before definite benefit is observed. Side effects of eczematoid rash, proteinuria, and bone marrow depression are monitored by dipstick urinalysis and white blood cell counts. The side effects are reversible on cessation of the drug but may recur with readministration. Fully 80 per cent of JRA children who fail with aspirin therapy can be expected to respond to gold treatment. After the child responds, the frequency of injection at the same dose can be reduced to biweekly or monthly intervals. Duration of therapy should be for as long as the drug is effective, but a lengthy remission may also allow discontinuation.

Nonsteroidal anti-inflammatory drugs (NSAID) are not more efficacious than aspirin but may offer advantages in fewer side effects and more convenient dosage schedules. However, they are expensive. Tolectin (tolmetin) is the prototype of many similar drugs and is the only one currently approved for use in children. The dose is 20 to 30 mg/kg/24 hr, and stomach irritation is less than with aspirin. Other derivatives of prostaglandin synthetase inhibitors abound, but their use should be tempered by the realization that they are no more effective in JRA than aspirin.

Penicillamine and hydroxychloroquine are other anti-inflammatory agents that are effective in patients with progressive arthritis. In controlled studies with gold, penicillamine was equally effective. It requires several months to see a response. The side effects on skin and kidneys are similar, but thrombocytopenia is more frequent with penicillamine than with gold. Some unique but rare toxicities have suggested cautious use of the drug. Hydroxychloroquine, an antimalarial drug, has demonstrable anti-inflammatory effects in JRA. Retinal toxicity from doses in excess of 400 mg/24 hr has led to conservative use of the drug. The dose in children is 5 to 7 mg/kg/24 hr. Although experience is limited in children, the drug appears more potent than aspirin, but, again, several months may be necessary to gain the effect.

Steroids do not alter the natural history of JRA; therefore, the profound side effects discourage their use. As little as 3 mg/24 hr of prednisone can prevent linear growth. Recognized uses of steroids in JRA include systemic disease unresponsive to aspirin, pericarditis, chronic iridocyclitis unresponsive to topical therapy, and palliative therapy during the period necessary for a long-acting anti-inflammatory drug to take effect. It is extraordinarily difficult to discontinue steroids in this chronic, painful illness, and every-other-day therapy is seldom tolerated. Immunosuppressive agents such as azathioprine and cyclophosphamide are rarely indicated in JRA. While they are successful in adults with arthritis, the risks of sterility and oncogenesis prohibit their use in a non–life-threatening illness like JRA.

Other medicaments (e.g., DMSO), aloevera juice, and spinal manipulation have only anecdotal support and lack the controlled studies of efficacy shown for the aforementioned drugs.

Artificial joint replacement by orthopedists has provided amazing rehabilitative results in patients in whom progressive arthritis has not been controlled with medication. Young adults who would have lived a wheelchair existence are now thriving with prosthetic hips and knees. The future of such procedures for other joints looks bright.

SYSTEMIC LUPUS ERYTHEMATOSUS

The disease spectrum in systemic lupus erythematosus (SLE) is so broad that a number of therapeutic choices exist. In addition to medications, a few other treatment precepts apply. The disease is no longer uniformly lethal, although the potential exists. The most recent statistics show a ten-year survival of 85% of patients. The other popular misconception is that photosensitivity is present in all SLE patients. Only one third of patients need to protect themselves from ultraviolet rays. Topical preparations containing para-amino benzoic acid (PABA) will protect in most situations. Fatigue is a significant problem, and it is often the last symptom to respond to therapy. SLE patients need not give up schooling, employment or recreation, but they often need to adjust their schedule to allow periods of rest amid periods of activity. SLE is a mysterious disease to most patients, and the physician must spend extra time with them until their understanding permits effective coping with the illness.

When noncritical organs are involved or the symptoms are minimal, nonsteroidal medications should be used to treat SLE. Salicylates can often relieve the fever, joint symptoms, and pleuritic pain. Therapeutic doses should be used to achieve serum levels of 20 to 30 mg/dl (see JRA). Patients who do not respond to salicylates may do well on Indocin (indomethacin*), Tolectin (tolmetin‡) or Naprosyn (naproxen†), as examples of nonsteroidal anti-inflammatory drugs, but controlled studies have not shown NSAID to be generally superior to salicylates. SLE patients appear to be more susceptible to the hepatotoxic effects of salicylates, and laboratory measurements of hepatocellular damage for patients on high-dose daily therapy are indicated. Hydroxychloroquine (5 to 7 mg/kg/24 hr, not to exceed 400 mg/24 hr) appears to be particularly helpful in the treatment of rashes in SLE. It should be emphasized that SLE can be a lethal disease requiring steroids and immunosuppressives, but patients without kidney disease, central nervous system involvement, or a generalized flare of their disease may well be managed with less toxic regimens.

When steroids are indicated for treatment of SLE, the laboratory can be used to judge the response to therapy. Elevated levels of anti-DNA antibody and depressed levels of complement are associated with active renal, central nervous system, and skin disease in SLE. As SLE responds to therapy, these immunologic parameters return to normal. Subsequent worsening of the immunologic parameters may warn of a clinical flare in disease. The routine urinalysis, especially the casts and cellular elements, is the best indicator of the activity of lupus renal disease. Proteinuria may continue for several weeks after active inflammation in the kidney has subsided.

Steroids have been responsible, in part, for the improved prognosis in SLE in the past three decades. The initial dose of prednisone is 1 mg/kg/24 hr in divided doses until clinical symptoms and laboratory tests have returned to normal. Thereafter the dose may be tapered to the level that keeps the patient well. Every-other-day steroid therapy is frequently possible. It may be necessary to use aspirin on the "off" day to control minor symptoms. The duration of steroid treatment of lupus renal disease is not clearly established. If there has been no evidence of renal inflammation for 2 years and repeat renal biopsy shows no activity, it may be reasonable to discontinue steroid treatment.

---

*Safety of indomethacin in children has not been established.
‡This use is not listed by the manufacturer.
†Pediatric indications and dosage for naproxen have not been established.

Although there is no conclusive evidence that immunosuppressive drugs have prolonged life in the disease as a whole, individual patients whose disease progresses despite steroid therapy may benefit from cyclophosphamide and azathioprine.[‡] Neither medication is effective rapidly enough to be used in an acute situation. Cyclophosphamide (1 to 2.5 mg/kg/24 hr) is probably more toxic than azathioprine (2 to 2.5 mg/kg/24 hr). Leukopenia and consequent infections are major problems with either drug. Also, cyclophosphamide causes hemorrhagic cystitis, alopecia, and sterility. Azathioprine is hepatotoxic. The long-term risk of oncogenesis is unknown. Despite these toxicities, the immunosuppressant drugs may control renal or central nervous system lupus in patients unresponsive to steroid.

Two new therapeutic regimens deserve mention. Intravenous pulse steroid therapy with Solu-Medrol (methylprednisolone) (30 mg/kg/dose) given as a bolus for 3 days, has been reported to reverse rapid renal deterioration in SLE. It may be used also in other acute situations. In addition, some patients can be managed on an intermittent weekly or biweekly schedule without daily steroids and their side effects. The regimen is safe except for hypertension in renal patients. Bacterial sepsis has not been reported in children. Plasmapheresis is the other experimental therapy in recent use. The rationale is to remove circulating immune complexes, which are felt to mediate the disease. Experience is limited, but in the profoundly ill SLE patient plasmapheresis may be of benefit. Renal transplantation is feasible in patients with end stage renal disease with good control of the systemic features of their illness.

DERMATOMYOSITIS

Steroids remain the treatment of choice in childhood dermatomyositis. The dose may need to be extraordinarily high (2 mg/kg/24 hr) to gain initial control of the disease. Elevated muscle enzymes respond to treatment often before there is discernible change in muscle strength. The enzymes should return to normal within 2 to 3 weeks, followed by improved strength. As the patient regains strength, the steroid dosage can be reduced, and every-other-day dosage is frequently possible. Should the disease be exacerbated, the muscle enzymes will again become abnormal before weakness ensues, and the steroid dosage should be increased. The activity of the rash may be independent of muscle weakness and steroid dose. The total length of steroid treatment averages 1 to 2 years but usually at nontoxic doses.

Physical therapy is necessary to prevent contractures. As the patient improves, resistive exercises are added. A therapist can help in the choice of activities that regain balance and coordination. Prophylactic treatments to prevent soft tissue calcifications are discouragingly unsuccessful.

Immunosuppressant therapy is necessary in occasional patients who fail to respond to steroid therapy or who develop intolerable side effects. Although many agents appear to work, intravenous methotrexate[‡](0.5 to 1.5 mg/kg/dose every 1 to 2 weeks) has been used most often with the fewest side effects, which include leukopenia, diarrhea, stomatitis, and hepatotoxicity. It may take 8 to 12 weeks of treatment to show a definite response. With steroids and immunosuppressants, the prognosis is good; most children return to normal activity. A significant mortality and morbidity remains in some patients.

ANKYLOSING SPONDYLITIS

As an inflammatory arthropathy, ankylosing spondylitis (AS) is treated with many of the same agents previously discussed (see JRA). Salicylates in therapeutic doses can manage many of the patients, but indomethacin and phenylbutazone have been more effective in controlled studies. Both drugs have significantly more serious side effects than aspirin. Indomethacin[*]should be started at a dose of 25 mg b.i.d. or t.i.d. At doses greater than 150 mg/24 hr nearly all patients will experience gastric discomfort and severe headaches. Phenylbutazone[§] is used in doses of 100 to 400 mg/24 hr. Dose-related and idiosyncratic leukopenia are rare but troublesome. Gastric irritation and fluid retention are additional problems. Steroids and gold are felt not to be effective in AS, but experience is limited. Drugs do not appear to alter the natural history of the disease, which leads to sacroiliac fusion and ankylosis of the spinal apophyseal joints. Physical therapy is oriented toward maintenance of good posture so that spinal fusion will lead to minimal functional compromise. Back braces and neck collars are generally not effective, and supporting muscle strength may be lost with their use. For acute flares of disease, bed rest on a flat, firm surface may be most helpful. With joint ankylosis the pain ameliorates, and functional disability may be surprisingly mild. The prognosis for the peripheral joints is very good with the exception of the hips. Unfortunately, prosthetic replacement of the hips may be followed by reankylosis of the joints.

Acute iritis in AS patients should be managed by an ophthalmologist with topical steroids, and the prognosis is good. Symptomatology with acute iritis leads to early evaluation; therefore, routine slit lamp screening is not necessary.

[‡]This use is not listed by the manufacturer.

[‡]This use is not listed by the manufacturer
[*]Safety of indomethacin in children has not been established.
[§]Safety of phenylbutazone in children has not been established.

REITER SYNDROME

Of the tetrad of symptoms (iritis, urethritis, arthritis, and dermatitis), only the eye and joint involvement require specific therapy. Topical steroids and mydriatics will control eye inflammation. Salicylates and NSAIDs reduce joint inflammation. Tolmetin, an indomethacin derivative, is approved for pediatric use and has fewer side effects than the parent molecule. The dose is 20 to 30 mg/kg/24 hr. Reiter syndrome most often runs a self-limited course of a few months after which therapy can be discontinued. Recurrences are rather common, and dysenteric causes should be sought and treated. Otherwise antibiotics appear to have little influence on the inflammation.

SCLERODERMA

Until recently, scleroderma has been the least treatable of the collagen vascular diseases. Treatment failures are likely due to the fact that inflammatory and immunologic mechanisms may not be part of the pathogenesis of scleroderma. Localized scleroderma (morphea) requires little therapy and frequently runs a benign course. Systemic scleroderma may be best managed with vasoactive drugs. Recent reports have shown reversal of scleroderma renal disease, which had previously been shown to be lethal. This antihypertensive approach to the renal disease has also improved other organ system involvement. Similar to Raynaud phenomenon in this disease, other clinical manifestations may well be due to vascular compromise.

MCTD (MIXED CONNECTIVE TISSUE DISEASE)

Mixed connective tissue disease is an overlap syndrome of scleroderma, arthritis, myositis, and so on, which does not fit recognized disease categories. MCTD is defined by the presence of an antibody to extractable nuclear antigen (ENA or RNP) and a speckled antinuclear antibody (ANA) pattern. The disease is more steroid responsive than is scleroderma, but recent studies suggest significant morbidity and mortality from pulmonary and renal involvement. Prednisone (1 to 2 mg/kg/24 hr) and immunosuppressants are used.

POLYARTERITIS NODOSA

Polyarteritis (PAN) has two disease spectra in childhood. The infantile type seen in the first 2 years of life is usually an overwhelming, acute illness diagnosed at autopsy by evidence of coronary artery occlusion and vasculitis. Although steroid treatment has been used, the pathologic similarity to mucocutaneous lymph node syndrome (Kawasaki disease), which may be adversely affected by steroids, has suggested that nonsteroidal anti-inflammatory agents be used.

PAN in the older child resembles the adult disease, although neurologic involvement may be less. Recent series indicate that predisone (1 to 2 mg/kg/24 hr) is effective. The disease may have long-term remission, and the prognosis is not as grim as previously thought.

HENOCH-SCHÖNLEIN (ANAPHYLACTOID) PURPURA

The arthritis is self-limited, and responds well to salicylate therapy. Intestinal vasculitis leads to abdominal pain, melena, and occasionally intussusception. Steroid treatment is indicated for intestinal involvement, with prompt control of symptoms. Renal involvement is usually mild and runs a benign course with no long-term sequela. Early oliguric, nephrotic, or azotemic manifestations are ominous, and it is not certain that steroid or immunosuppressant treatment can change the prognosis.

12

Genitourinary Tract

Renal Hypoplasia and Dysplasia

GEORGE W. KAPLAN, M.D.,
and WILLIAM A. BROCK, M.D.

Small kidneys usually are clinically classified as either hypoplastic or atrophic, depending upon their presumed mode of development (i.e., congenital or acquired). Clinically, the hypoplastic kidney is thought to be nongenetically determined and congenitally small but otherwise normal. Whether an entity fitting this definition truly exists is unknown. Nevertheless, small kidneys are seen clinically and, when they are present, it is difficult to decide if the etiology is congenital or acquired. Acquired small kidneys are known to develop from lesions such as renal artery stenosis, renal vein thrombosis, and vesicoureteral reflux.

When present unilaterally, small kidneys usually are discovered during evaluation of urinary infection or hypertension. Although hypertension in such instances can be managed medically, nephrectomy can be curative in selected cases. When it can be shown by selective renal vein renin determination that renin is produced by the small kidney, there is a greater than 90% chance that nephrectomy will be curative. If segmental renal vein renin determinations are performed in patients with nonlateralizing main renal vein renin determinations, other potentially curable patients will be discovered. Medical management (discussed elsewhere in this volume) usually will be appropriate for patients with a small kidney and nonlateralizing main or segmental renal vein renin determinations.

Much has been written about segmental renal hypoplasia (the Ask-Upmark kidney), which also usually presents as hypertension. Patients with this lesion and hypertension have been cured by either total or segmental nephrectomy. This was ori-ginally thought to be a congenital malformation but recent thought incriminates reflux nephropathy as the usual etiologic event. The ureterovesical junction may have matured sufficiently that reflux will not be present at the time the problem is discovered, in which case surgical therapy is directed at the kidney alone. However, even if reflux is still present, ureteral reimplantation usually does not cure the hypertension.

If the presenting problem is infection, and reflux is present in association with a unilateral small kidney, therapy is determined by several factors: the patient's age, the grade of reflux, whether or not the urine can be sterilized with suppressive antibacterials (see Vesicoureteral Reflux in this section), and the degree of renal function contributed by the kidney. If surgery is indicated for treatment of reflux, nephroureterectomy may be the appropriate choice if the degree of function provided by the small kidney is minimal and the other kidney is normal.

If bilateral renal hypoplasia is present, the patient usually will present with chronic renal failure. Some hypoplastic kidneys that present in renal failure will also manifest cystic renal dysplasia. (See Chronic Renal Failure in this section.) At times percutaneous or open renal biopsy is helpful in diagnosis and in assessing genetic risk, but surgical intervention (other than renal transplantation) is of no therapeutic benefit.

The term renal dysplasia implies disordered nephrogenesis. This is a histologic diagnosis, and it is generally agreed that the presence of primitive tubules surrounded by cuboidal epithelium is required for diagnosis. In addition, most patients with histologically proven renal dysplasia are found to have cartilage in the renal tissue. Most dysplastic kidneys also contain renal cysts, but these cysts vary greatly in size and number. There is no relationship between cystic dysplasia and polycystic disease, however. Ureteral anomalies, specifically ureteral atresias or vesicoureteral reflux, are often associated with dysplastic kidneys. These kidneys may be discovered while evaluating children with urinary infection, although the dysplastic kidney (which is usually nonfunctional) rarely is the cause of the infection. Dysplastic kidneys that subtend a refluxing ureter may be of some importance in management and require surgical removal.

Another common variation of renal dysplasia is the multicystic kidney. This problem usually presents as a renal mass in infancy. Standard treatment has been nephrectomy, but in recent years there has been a trend toward observation only; whether nephrectomy is required is problematic at this time. However, we believe that elective nephrectomy is the preferred course, as the prospect of lifelong follow-up when an alternative exists is, to us, overwhelming.

Hydronephrosis and Disorders of the Ureter

SELWYN B. LEVITT, M.D.

Optimum treatment of hydronephrosis and ureteral disorders depends upon determining the nature of the primary pathology and its location. The information obtained is invaluable to the clinician when determining whether a salvage operation or a nephrectomy or nephroureterectomy is the preferred treatment.

Obstructive uropathy, particularly when complicated by infection or calculus formation, requires urgent treatment in order to preserve maximum renal function. The term *obstructive uropathy* implies an impedance to normal urinary drainage. The obstruction may be located anywhere along the course of the urinary drainage system and may be organic or functional. In neonates, infants, and children, it is usually congenital. Hydronephrosis due to obstruction at the pelviureteric junction (PUJ) is the most common upper tract obstruction encountered in children. Treatment of PUJ obstructions is surgical, regardless of the etiology, and involves plastic repair of the pelviureteric junction. Transection of the ureter below the PUJ, excision of the pelviureteric junction and redundant renal pelvis, and reanastomosis of the spatulated upper ureter to the remaining renal pelvis is the operative technique favored by most surgeons. A widely patent, dependent, and well-funneled pelviureteric junction is accomplished in most cases. An excellent clinical response, including absence of pain, infection, and complicating calculi, can usually be expected. Grossly dilated calyces, however, seldom return to

normal, although progressive dilatation and further renal functional impairment are prevented.

Some surgeons prefer splinting of the anastomosis and temporary nephrostomy tube drainage, particularly in severely hydronephrotic kidneys. These tubes, when employed, should be connected to closed catheter drainage in order to minimize the incidence of bacteriuria. Should bacteriuria supervene, specific antibiotic treatment, beginning 24 to 48 hours before mobilization and removal of the tubes, is mandatory if acute pyelonephritis and bacteremia are to be avoided. Prophylactic chemotherapy with nitrofurantoin or sulfisoxazole is generally prescribed for the first 6 weeks following surgery pending normal healing of the repair. Nephrectomy is occasionally necessary in severe cases, but most kidneys can be salvaged by reparative surgery, thereby preserving useful renal function. Even severely impaired obstructed kidneys, particularly in young children, are capable of significant functional recovery after successful reconstructive surgery.

Ureteral dilatation secondary to demonstrable organic obstruction is termed *hydroureter*. The ureterovesical junction is the most common site of obstruction. A ureterocele (submucosal dilatation of the distal end of the ureter) is the most frequently encountered cause of hydroureter at this location. Ureteroceles usually occur in the ectopic ureter draining the upper pole moiety of a completely duplicated collecting system. In most instances the segment of renal parenchyma at the upper end of the ureterocele is severely dysplastic and poorly functioning. Heminephroureterectomy of the dysplastic parenchyma and its dilated ureter down to the level of the bladder is generally the treatment of choice. The ureterocele is thereby decompressed. Relief of the ipsilateral and contralateral ureteral obstruction as well as bladder outlet obstruction, if present, is thereby accomplished.

Some surgeons advise excision of the ureterocele only if, after decompression, it is associated with obstruction of the bladder outlet, persistent vesicoureteral reflux into the ipsilateral or contralateral ureters, recurrent urinary tract infections, or incontinence. Others believe that these complications occur often enough to warrant routine simultaneous or planned sequential excision of the ureterocele with repair of the associated posterior bladder wall defect, which invariably accompanies a large ureterocele. Reimplantation of the ipsilateral ureter is also necessary following excision of a large ureterocele in order to repair the bladder defect and protect the ureter from vesicoureteral reflux. In those cases with contralateral vesicoureteral reflux, the opposite ureter or ureters are also reimplanted in an antireflux manner.

Heminephroureterectomy may be too risky in the sick neonate or septic baby. Temporary percutaneous or formal open nephrostomy tube drainage of the pyonephrotic upper pole may be required in these babies several days prior to definitive hemi-nephroureterectomy. This is preferable to un-roofing the ureterocele by an endoscopic proce-dure or an open suprapubic operation. Such a procedure will result in massive vesicoureteral reflux into the ectopic ureter. Occasionally both segments of the duplicated system are so severely dysplastic or complicated by obstruction that ne-phroureterectomy of the duplication is necessary. In the unusual case with good renal function in the upper pole parenchymal cap, excision of the ureterocele, repair of the bladder defect, and an-tireflux reimplantation of both ipsilateral ureters is preferable to ablation of the upper pole. Pyelopye-lostomy (anastomosis of the upper pelvis to the lower pelvis) with excision of the dilated upper pole ureter with or without ureterocelectomy and reim-plantation of the ipsilateral lower pole ureter is a satisfactory alternative method of treatment in these cases.

Simple ureteroceles obstructing single collecting systems are less frequently encountered in children than are ectopic ureteroceles. The renal paren-chyma in these cases is generally well preserved, and in most instances there is a significant amount of renal function present. Ureterocelectomy and antireflux ureteral reimplantation is the preferred treatment in these cases.

Ureteral strictures at various levels or valves ob-structing the ureter are best treated by simple exci-sion, spatulation of both cut ends of the ureter, and reanastomosis, thereby restoring continuity of the ureter. Extensive strictures of the ureter or ac-quired lesions involving long segments of ureter require more complex procedures in order to sal-vage the affected kidney. The ureteral gap can be bridged by a variety of ingenious techniques, de-pending upon the segment of ureter involved. Hitching the bladder to the psoas muscle with or without tubularizing a flap of bladder will bridge most lower ureteral defects. Transureteroureteros-tomy (transferring a healthy upper ureter across the abdomen and allowing it to drain into the contralat-eral normal ureter) is a satisfactory alternative. A good kidney with even more extensive ureteral pa-thology can still be salvaged either by total replace-ment of the ureter with an isolated tapered segment of bowel reimplanted into the bladder by non-refluxing technique, or by autotransplanting it into a pelvic location.

Ureteric dilatation, without an obvious anatomic obstruction, is commonly referred to as *megaureter.* It is seen clinically in two forms: (1) with free vesicoureteric reflux, and (2) without reflux. In refluxing megaureter, severe ureteral dilatation is seen on excretory urography as well as on retro-grade cystourethrography. Severe hydronephrosis

and marked parenchymal atrophy are the rule. The urinary bladder is frequently enlarged, the combi-nation being referred to as "megaureter-megacystis syndrome." The bladder is smooth walled and lacks trabeculation. Despite its large size, it is capable of complete emptying, although it refills rapidly from the return of urine that flows back from the large ureters following voiding. No obstructive abnor-mality at the bladder neck has been identified.

Surgical correction involves tapering the distal portion of the dilated ureters and reimplanting them into the bladder so as to reconstitute the nor-mal antireflux ureterovesical junction. The direct hydrostatic effect on the kidneys that results from changing bladder pressures is thereby eliminated. Antegrade urine flow from the bladder eliminates the large residual urine volumes that previously effluxed into the bladder after micturition; less sta-sis within the urinary tract reduces the predisposi-tion to infection. A successful antireflux operation prevents lower urinary tract infections, should they occur, from ascending to the kidneys. The long-term beneficial effects from surgery in these cases, particularly when renal impairment is already evi-dent, are uncertain. Some children seem to progress inexorably toward renal failure regardless of therapy.

Primary obstructive megaureter is a dilated ureter that has neither reflux nor mechanical ob-struction at the ureterovesical junction. Conserva-tive management may be indicated in mild cases in which there is bulbous dilatation of the lower ureter associated with a well-preserved calyceal system or when the pressure gradients across the ureterovesi-cal junction, determined by flowmetry, are equivo-cal. However, excision of the obstructive segment with ureteral remodeling and reimplantation is rec-ommended in patients with calyceal blunting, re-current urinary tract infections, and loin pain, or when pressure gradients across the ureterovesical junction are unequivocally obstructive. Good re-sults can be expected in most patients, with im-provement in the pyelographic appearance, freedom from infections, and alleviation of symp-toms. Nephroureterectomy is occasionally neces-sary when the kidney has been destroyed by hydronephrotic atrophy.

Ureteral ectopia is usually seen in association with complete duplication of the kidney and ureter, al-though ectopic ureters occurring in single collect-ing systems are well documented. The ectopic ureter is subject to ureterocele formation, which should be treated in the manner already outlined. In the absence of a ureterocele, the dilated ectopic ureter may either reflux or be "functionally" ob-structed. Severe hydroureteronephrosis or dys-plasia or both of the renal segment served by the ureter are common. Heminephroureterectomy is usually required, although, on occasion, preservation of a functioning renal segment is possible by ureteral reimplantation or by ipsilateral ureteroureterostomy or pyelopyelostomy.

Ureteral duplications not associated with ectopia, impaired drainage, ureterocele formation, or reflux require no treatment.

Malignant Tumors of the Kidney

WILLIAM A. CAMPBELL, III, M.D.

The treatment of Wilms' tumor has been greatly refined in the past decade, thanks to the National Wilms' Tumor Study (NWTS) series. NWTS III was initiated in 1981 to further clarify treatment via protocols, generally in regional referral centers, and numbered clinical stages. Central referral seems a proven reward through combined experience in a relatively uncommon (400 per year) tumor.

Wilms' tumor is described basically by extent, and the treatment is correlated. The clinical stage is decided by the operating room surgeon and is confirmed by the pathologist, who also evaluates the histology; this differs somewhat from the previously used grouping method:

In Stage I, the tumor is limited to the kidney and is completely excised.

In Stage II, the tumor extends beyond the kidney and is also completely excised.

In Stage III, there is residual non-hematogenous tumor confined to the abdomen.

Stage IV includes hematogenous metastases.

In Stage V, there is bilateral renal involvement at diagnosis.

Unfavorable histology (UH), a further important grading, occurs in 12% of patients and includes focal anaplasia, diffuse anaplasia, "rhabdoid" sarcoma, and clear cell sarcoma, not seen in the favorable histology (FH) group. The FH group on the whole enjoys an 89% survival rate, while the UH group shows only 39%.

Therapy is usually initiated with surgical exploration, but preoperative radiation therapy is a consideration. This decreases the incidence of tumor spillage and with it the need for wider field postoperative radiation therapy and its complications; however, preoperative diagnosis of Wilms' tumor is in error in 5% of patients. At surgery the opposite kidney is explored for bilaterality, lymph nodes are biopsied or removed, the surrounding organs are inspected, and the kidney is removed if necessary.

Only with microscopic examination of the kidney can mesoblastic nephroma, the primary differential diagnostic possibility, become evident. This congenital fetal renal hamartoma is essentially benign but it has produced recurrence and death. In the older literature it was not delineated from Wilms'

tumor; thus the prognosis for kidney tumor removal in the infant was confused.

The treatment protocols for NWTS III, which are based on the positive findings of Studies I and II, test whether chemotherapy and radiation therapy can be reduced for early stage disease with FH. High-risk children will be treated with increasing intensity of therapy:

Stage I-FH: Children are given actinomycin and vincristine and are randomized between courses of 10 weeks and 6 months; no radiation therapy is administered.

Stage II-FH: Randomization to receive actinomycin and more intensive vincristine or triple agent therapy of vincristine, actinomycin,*and Adriamycin. Therapy in both cases lasts 15 months. Postoperative radiation is 2000 rads or more.

Stage III-FH: The chemotherapy scheme is identical to that of the preceding, while postoperative radiotherapy tests 1000 vs 2000 rads.

Stage IV (all histologies) or UH (any stage): All children receive postoperative radiation therapy, with escalating doses for increasing age. Children are randomized to triple agent vs quadruple agent (adding cyclophosphamide) chemotherapy for 15 months.

These refinements assume great importance not only in potential cure rate but also in producing minimum cost to survivors. The pediatrician will see in these stages a real incidence of scoliosis, renal failure, bowel obstruction, and hepatic, splenic, and gonadal dysfunction. Second cancers may occur. The treatment protocols have reached an encouraging level that furthers the goal of enhanced cure rate and preservation of normal functions.

Glomerulonephritis

WALLACE W. McCRORY, M.D.

Glomerulonephritis (GN) occurs in a variety of unrelated conditions. With the advent of renal biopsy we can now establish the specific histopathologic findings in each type of GN. We also know something about the natural history of those forms in which the etiology has been established (poststreptococcal GN, "shunt" nephritis, lupus nephritis, etc.). As a result, current diagnostic terminology combines the etiology and histopathology when known (e.g., acute proliferative poststreptococcal GN). This gives information of value to predict short-term outcome and long-term prognosis and thus aids in management. Glomerular disease may exist without other systemic organ

---

*Manufacturer's warning: Actinomycin should not be given to children under 6 months of age because of greater frequency of toxic effects.

involvement (primary GN) or in association with systemic disease (secondary GN) such as found in systemic lupus erythematosus (SLE) or Henoch-Schönlein purpura (HSP). The distinction between these two forms of GN is important, since clinical problems in GN all relate to the renal damage, while the problems associated with extrarenal involvement (hematologic, gastrointestinal, CNS in SLE or HSP) may overshadow the renal problems. The clinical problems occurring in children with GN depend on the extent and severity of the alterations in renal function consequent to glomerular damage. Therapy is thus primarily symptomatic.

GENERAL TREATMENT MEASURES

Hospitalization is indicated when circulatory or fluid and electrolyte imbalances are present or suspected and when the diagnosis is uncertain. Management of patients in the acute stage is accomplished easiest in the hospital. When the condition is stable and gross hematuria, hypertension, edema, and azotemia have cleared, ambulation and discharge are indicated. In mild forms the patients could be observed at home but careful monitoring by parents would be essential.

Hypertension. This is a fairly common complication during the acute course of glomerular disease, particularly if the glomerular filtration rate (GFR) is reduced. The cause of hypertension in acute forms of glomerulonephritis remains uncertain. Hyperreninemia is not a common finding. The major alteration documented has been hypervolemia secondary to fluid retention, which may be accompanied by signs of circulatory congestion (increased pulmonary circulation and cardiac enlargement on chest x-ray). Children who seem entirely well prior to onset of acute glomerular disease should not have signs of long-standing hypertension, such as cardiac hypertrophy or hypertensive retinopathy. Finding either of these suggests that the patient has long-standing hypertension and possible pre-existing renal disease. Antihypertensive therapy should include three components: 1) measures to decrease body fluid volumes by diuresis, 2) prevention of fluid retention by restriction of water and salt intake, and 3) antihypertensive agents when necessary. In cases in which the only abnormal finding is a mild elevation of BP, bed rest, restriction of sodium intake, and administration of a diuretic (furosemide, 1–4 mg/kg/day) will usually suffice. In patients in which there is progressive elevation in BP in spite of antihypertensive therapy or in which hypertension is associated with symptoms of encephalopathy or impending cardiac failure, acute blood pressure lowering therapy is indicated. The drug of choice is diazoxide.* This is injected in-

travenously as a bolus dose of 5 mg/kg up to a maxiumum of 300 mg with very rapid injection, since it is rapidly protein-bound. Onset of fall in BP should be within 5 to 10 minutes and duration is usually 4 to 6 hours if an effective response occurs. If this fails to lower BP within 1 hour, the dose can be repeated. An effective alternative is nitroprusside drip intravenously 0.1–8.0 μg/kg/min, run at whatever rate is necessary to lower diastolic BP to below 90 mm Hg. This solution must be protected from light. Once BP control has been obtained, one should institute a program of continued BP medication employing other agents.

When hypertension is not life-threatening (associated with encephalopathy and/or pulmonary or circulatory congestion) a stepwise program of control can be used. The aim is to lower diastolic BP below 90 mm Hg. The administration of the diuretic furosemide 1 to 4 mg/kg IV can be quite helpful if urinary output is adequate. The combination of hydralazine, 0.15 to 0.4 mg/kg, and reserpine, initial dose 0.07–0.1 mg/kg IM is usually successful. The reserpine provides tranquilization that facilitates lowering of BP. Hydralazine can be continued at 4 to 6 hour intervals orally (0.7–3.0 mg/kg/day) as required to maintain diastolic BP below 90 mm Hg. If this is not effective in a few hours, methyldopa (Aldomet), 5 to 10 mg/kg, can be given and the dosage increased to 50 mg/kg/day if required. Some combination of these agents given at appropriate intervals will usually control BP (diastolic below 90–100 mm Hg).

Hypertension will usually abate as renal function improves, edema clears, and weight decreases.

Edema. Edema occurs because of hypoalbuminemia or reduced GFR. Distinction between these factors requires measuring plasma total protein and A/G ratio and cholesterol; quantitating daily urine protein excretion; and measuring blood urea nitrogen and serum creatinine to evaluate the GF level. In all patients with edema, dietary sodium chloride intake should be limited (1–2 gm/day) and diuretics should be used. It is important to monitor serum and urine electrolytes daily with vigorous diuretic therapy. Significant urinary losses of sodium and/or potassium may result in hyponatremia, hypokalemia, or metabolic alkalosis. Diuretics should be continued until weight has been stable for 1 to 2 days, indicating that the patient has achieved dry weight. The hypoalbuminemia is usually of short duration (2–3 weeks) and no treatment is required. If the nephrotic syndrome does evolve (plasma albumin less than 2.5 gm/dl, significant proteinuria, and hypercholesterolemia) and lasts more than 4 weeks, specific treatment would be indicated (see Nephrotic Syndrome).

Fluid and Electrolyte Disturbances. Glomerular damage may be sufficient to markedly reduce urine output (oliguria), and measures must be instituted to avoid sustained expansion of extracellular fluids

---

*Manufacturer's precaution: Safety in children has not been established.

and blood volume as will occur if intake is not adjusted to the level of output. Routine fluid restriction is not necessary unless there is marked edema, oliguria, or cardiovascular congestion; thirst can be a reliable guide to intake.

The most life-threatening problems in fluid and electrolyte imbalance are related to acute renal failure (ARF), evidenced by oliguria. These include hyponatremia, hypervolemia, hyperkalemia, metabolic acidosis, and hypocalcemia. Successful therapy of ARF requires a medical care team well versed in intensive care of acutely ill children and experienced in dialysis techniques.

Oliguria. Oliguria is the hallmark of ARF. It is present when daily urinary output is less than 350 ml/m^2 S.A./day in the presence of a normal fluid intake without abnormal fluid losses (vomiting, diarrhea). Azotemia (BUN greater than 50%, creatinine greater than 2.5 mg/dl) is always associated but may be present without a decreased urinary output (nonoliguric ARF). Since oliguria may have a prerenal component (shock, dehydration, and/or salt depletion), it is important to ensure an adequate plasma volume before limiting fluid intake to replacement of urine output plus estimated insensible water losses (IWL). If the patient is not clearly overhydrated and does not have documented normal fluid intake in the preceding 24 hours, a normal fluid intake should be provided initially and discontinued if there is evidence of overhydration and weight gain without return to normal urinary output within 12 to 24 hours. If urine output fails to increase IV furosemide (1–2 mg/kg) or 20% mannitol (0.2–0.5 gm/kg) can be administered. No response to these measures (greater than 50% increase in urine volume within 2 hours) is clear evidence of intrinsic renal failure, and restriction of fluid intake to cover insensible water loss and urine output becomes mandatory.

Fluid Balance. Restriction of fluid intake to match urinary output must be continued as long as anuria or oliguria persists. The intake should be matched to replace the previous 8 to 12 hour output plus IWL, with calculations monitored to avoid weight gain and to lose 1.5 to 1.0% of body weight/day. Fluids can be given as a 10% dextrose solution without potassium unless plasma levels are low and sodium in maintenance amounts (30 meq/L) unless hypo- or hypernatremia is present, which requires careful correction. Providing an appropriate water and electrolyte intake requires daily measurement of blood and urinary electrolytes.

Hyponatremia. Hyponatremia usually reflects overhydration from continued intake or administration of hypotonic fluids (water, fruit juices, soda, 5% dextrose, etc.) in the face of severe oliguria or anuria. Marked hyponatremia (serum Na less than 120–125 meq/L) can be associated with mental obtundation, headache, and seizures, and may require partial correction to relieve symptoms. This can be accomplished by intravenous administration of 3% NaCl in amounts calculated to raise the serum Na to 130 meq/L. The remainder of the correction should be accomplished by fluid restriction or, in the case of anuria, by peritoneal dialysis.

Hyperkalemia. Hyperkalemia is a medical emergency that can cause fatal disturbances in cardiac activity. Metabolic acidosis and acidemia accentuate the effects of hyperkalemia. An electrocardiogram (ECG) should be obtained to see if signs of cardiac depression are present. If serum potassium is below 6.5 meq/L and the ECG does not show signs of serious hyperkalemia, an attempt to lower serum potassium by removal from the gut can be made using sodium polystyrene sulfonate (Kayexalate) in a dose of 1 gm/kg to decrease serum potassium 1 meq/L over a period of 1 to 3 hours. It can be given rectally or orally as a 20 to 30% solution. Sorbitol may be added to prevent constipation. For serum potassium concentrations above 6.5 meq/L, more rapid treatment is necessary. Temporary relief may be obtained by administration of sodium bicarbonate, 2 to 3 meq/kg IV; 1 unit of insulin/3 to 4 gm of glucose IV; sodium lactate, 2 to 3 meq/kg IV; or calcium gluconate, 100 to 300 mg/kg IV. These maneuvers merely transfer potassium from one body compartment to another, or counteract its cardiotoxic effects, and do not effect a net removal from the body. Hence, they must be supplemented by use of an exchange resin or peritoneal dialysis to correct potassium excess.

Hypocalcemia. Occasionally, hypocalcemia manifests as tetany or convulsions, particularly as acidosis is rapidly corrected. Symptomatic hypocalcemia can be treated with intravenous calcium gluconate, 50 to 100 mg/kg/dose given over 4 to 6 hours and repeated as required until the desired serum calcium level is obtained and then start oral calcium gluconate 2 to 6 gm/day in divided doses.

Metabolic Acidosis. This is a common problem in ARF and is usually tolerated to bicarbonate levels of about 10 to 12 meq/L. Sodium bicarbonate or sodium lactate given intravenously in amounts sufficient to maintain serum bicarbonate between 15 and 20 meq/L will allow reasonable correction without overloading the patient with sodium. One must remember that therapy for the relief of metabolic acidosis or hyponatremia with sodium-containing solutions may contribute to hypervolemia. The persistence of hyperkalemia, hyponatremia, severe metabolic acidosis, or marked hypervolemia is an indication for peritoneal dialysis, and the patient should be in a medical facility where this can be done.

Diet. Catabolism of tissues contributes significantly to endogenous water production, acidosis, hyperkalemia, and hyperphosphatemia. Patients usually eat very poorly, but provision of minimal adequate calories is essential. This can be accomplished if 20 to 30 calories/kg/day are given as carbohydrate or lipid and this will minimize tissue breakdown.

Restriction of protein intake to 1 gm/kg/day is indicated only with azotemia and oliguria. In the presence of anuria, protein intake should be eliminated with a progressively rising BUN but can be allowed if intermittent peritoneal dialysis is employed. When hyperphosphatemia is present, milk should be avoided and aluminum hydroxide (Amphogel, Basalgel) given orally (50–100 mg/kg/24 hours) in divided doses. Potassium-containing foods should be avoided with marked oliguria or anuria.

TREATMENT REGIMENS FOR SPECIFIC TYPES OF GLOMERULONEPHRITIS

Acute Poststreptococcal GN. There is no specific therapy for glomerulonephritis. If the patient has a positive throat culture for group A beta hemolytic streptococci, a 10 day course of penicillin (900,000–1,200,000 units/day or single dose of 600,000–1,200,000 units of benzathine penicillin IM) should be given, or erythromycin if the patient is sensitive to penicillin. There is no indication for continuous antibiotic prophylaxis during convalescence.

Hemolytic Uremic Syndrome (HUS). This form of nephritis is discussed separately.

Nephritis in Henoch-Schönlein Purpura (HSP). Evidence of a glomerular disease (proteinuria and hematuria) is very common (greater than 40%) in HSP. While the renal disease may be quite severe, it is mild in most cases and spontaneously resolves. There is no evidence from controlled studies that treatment with steroids or immunosuppressive agents with or without anticoagulants favorably alters the course of the nephritis, though they have been recommended. Drugs used have included corticosteroids, azathioprine, cyclophosphamide, heparin, and dipyridamole. In view of the good outlook from studies of the natural history of HSP nephritis, the use of potentially dangerous drugs is not justified unless there is evidence of severe glomerular damage by renal biopsy. Treatment with steroids, immunosuppressants, and/or anticoagulants is experimental and should be supervised by a pediatric nephrologist experienced in use of these agents in such patients.

Rapidly Progressive Glomerulonephritis. The clinical term rapidly progressive glomerulonephritis (RPGN) applies to a particularly fulminant form of glomerular disease. The disease presents with an acute onset and pursues a progressive course to renal failure in weeks or months. The characteristic feature of the renal lesion is abundant formation of glomerular crescents. While there is no absolute percentage of crescentic glomeruli that indicates a poor prognosis, it appears that when more than two thirds of glomeruli have crescents the prognosis for

recovery is poor and end-stage renal failure is likely. Patients with preceding streptococcal infection have much better prognosis than those with no apparent etiology. There is no unequivocal evidence that corticosteroids, cytotoxic and/or immunosuppressive agents, anticoagulants, and antifibrinolytic agents alone or in combination have a favorable effect on the course of RPGN but the subject is controversial. Recently, plasmapheresis has been used in combination with some or all of these agents with some reports of benefit, but this also is uncertain and can be hazardous. In view of the lack of established response of RPGN to available therapies, supportive regimens to permit survival of the patient to stable chronic renal failure are the key to therapy. Consultation with a pediatric nephrologist should be obtained if new modes of therapy are to be considered.

Nephritis in Systemic Lupus Erythematosus (SLE). Glomerular disease is an important, frequent, and potentially serious complication of SLE. A renal biopsy should be done early in all patients with signs of renal involvement to establish its type and severity. A variety of forms may be seen, and it is important to distinguish between them because aggressive therapy is needed in some while no specific therapy may be required in others.

Therapy for *mesangial* and/or *focal proliferative* lupus nephritis should be aimed at control of nonrenal manifestations and at normalizing serologic and immunologic abnormalities. If worsening of urinary findings (proteinuria, hematuria, or slow elevation of BUN and/or serum creatinine) occurs, follow-up renal biopsy should be done and aggressive treatment considered, depending on whether transformation or progression to a more serious type of nephritis has occurred.

In *diffuse proliferative* lupus nephritis, specific therapy is indicated. Daily prednisone 1 to 2 mg/kg/day in divided doses for 1 to 2 months followed by gradual introduction of single dose alternate day programs should be used. Azathioprine (Imuran) or cyclophosphamide (Cytoxan) may be added to this regimen, though the benefits of this combined therapy are still controversial. In patients with rapidly progressing renal failure (RPGN), pulse therapy with methylprednisolone (Solu-Medrol), 5 mg/kg bid IV for 3 days, and plasmapheresis are also being used with some promising results. These forms of therapy are still in the experimental stage and should be supervised by physicians experienced in such treatments. This acute therapy is followed by daily prednisone and gradual introduction of alternate day therapy with careful monitoring of renal function, quantitative proteinuria and hematuria, and serologic signs of lupus activity. Long term therapy is necessary to obtain maximal benefits. Abrupt withdrawal of steroid therapy is to be avoided since acute relapse and

RPGN not responsive to therapy can occur. The effect of therapy on the signs of glomerular disease (serum creatinine/BUN levels, proteinuria) is the best indication of short-term benefits and the potential for long term improvement.

Membranoproliferative Glomerulonephritis (MPGN). Patients presenting with acute onset are managed symptomatically as outlined above. Those who present a nephrotic picture (hypoalbuminemia and proteinuria) would be treated as discussed in Nephrotic Syndrome. Persistent hypertension is not uncommon and should be treated in an attempt to delay the development of secondary renal vascular changes. The value of long term treatment with corticosteroids is controversial but one should consider a trial of such therapy in patients with histologically proven Type I MPGN before they show evidence of decreased renal function, since favorable effects have been observed. Such treatment has not been beneficial in Type II or III or in patients with reduced renal function (GFR less than 70% of normal).

Glomerulonephritis Associated with Infected Shunts for Hydrocephalus, Heroin Abuse, Osteomyelitis, Sepsis, Syphilis, or Hepatitis. In these patients, the most important part of treatment is the recognition that the GN is due to the underlying infection. Appropriate treatment to eliminate the infecting organism will usually lead to resolution of the glomerular disease.

Drug- or Toxin-Induced Glomerulonephritis. The physician must be alert to the possibility of the drug- or toxin-induced GN (associated with hematuria, proteinuria, and azotemia) since resolution or improvement requires cessation of exposure to the offending agent.

Convalescence. Hospitalized patients can be discharged when they have normal body weight, normal blood pressure without restriction of salt intake, and require no antihypertensive agents. They can ambulate normally since there is no evidence that this will adversely affect convalescence. They should be followed until urinary abnormalities have cleared.

The long-term prognosis for complete recovery of poststreptococcal and postviral GN is excellent; that of HSP nephritis is also good but more variable in respect to likelihood of complete recovery. The acute clinical episode is usually self-limited, and evidences of immunologic activity (C_3 levels) usually return to normal within 6 weeks. Gross hematuria will usually disappear by 6 weeks and microscopic hematuria by 1 year in 90% of cases. Proteinuria may take somewhat longer to clear. Factors influencing outcome are age at onset (poorer outcome in adults), degrees of reduction in renal function, and severity of the histologic picture on renal biopsy (crescentic GN being associated with poorest outcome). It is generally believed that severity of the disease initially correlates with the development of chronicity.

When plasma creatinine and BUN levels are normal, creatinine clearance is within normal range, renal concentrating ability is normal (sp. gr. of 1.025 or higher with fluid restriction), and there is no hematuria or proteinuria, complete recovery has occurred and there is no risk of subsequent development of chronic nephritis. If the patient has persistence of elevation of BUN or serum creatinine levels or edema associated with significant proteinuria beyond 4 weeks, renal biopsy should be done. Renal biopsy should also be done if the presentation is atypical or the plasma C_3 concentration remains abnormally low beyond 6 months or if hematuria and proteinuria persist beyond 1 year.

Chronic Glomerulonephritis. At present there is no treatment that favorably affects the underlying glomerular disease. Until signs of renal insufficiency develop, no treatment is indicated, but early recognition of specific problems (metabolic acidosis, hypocalcemia and hyperphosphatemia, renal osteodystrophy, etc.) is of great importance since treatment of these complications prolongs the child's ability to engage in normal physical activities and maximizes the potential for continued skeletal growth into the pubertal period. These measures are discussed elsewhere (Chronic Renal Failure). Hypertension is quite frequent and its management can be achieved by appropriate combinations of diuretics (furosemide), vasodilators (hydralazine), and adrenergic blockers (propranolol, methyldopa, clonidine). Restriction in physical activity or changes in diet before the appearance of signs of renal insufficiency or cardiovascular disease secondary to hypertension seems to have no discernible long term benefits and will only heighten concern about the long term outlook.

Nephrotic Syndrome

THOMAS E. NEVINS, M.D.,
and ALFRED F. MICHAEL, M.D.

The nephrotic syndrome is a clinical diagnosis made in patients with significant albuminuria, hypoalbuminemia, and edema. The syndrome may occur during the course of virtually any renal disease associated with glomerular capillary injury and increased permeability to protein. In children, the etiology is usually unknown and in this discussion is included under the designation idiopathic nephrotic syndrome (INS).

In a child presenting with edema, two questions commonly arise: 1) Should the patient receive prednisone? 2) Is a renal biopsy indicated?

In typical patients with INS, prednisone therapy may be initiated in a daily divided dose of 60 mg/m². Renal biopsy is reserved for atypical patients (> 10 years of age; features of glomerulonephritis —gross hematuria, hypertension, renal insufficiency) and those not responding to daily divided-dose steroids.

Prednisone therapy will induce a complete remission with diuresis and loss of proteinuria in about 95% of INS patients within approximately 4 weeks. However, INS is a polyrelapsing disease, and up to 80% of patients will undergo one or more relapses in the course of their disease. The relapses are usually steroid-responsive and may be associated with mild intercurrent infections. Since infection may lead to steroid unresponsiveness, a patient with INS who has been previously steroid-responsive but becomes unresponsive should be carefully searched for occult infections (osteomyelitis, urinary tract infection, and so on).

The general therapy of INS is directed at restoring a more normal sodium and water balance. Although dietary salt and water restriction is necessary to some degree in all patients, it is rarely effective as the only means of controlling edema. Chlorothiazide in a dose of 10 to 40 mg/kg/24 hr usually will produce a prompt diuresis. In more resistant cases, furosemide orally (1 to 10 mg/kg) or intravenously (2 to 6 mg/kg) may be required.* If continued diuretic therapy is necessary, the addition of spironolactone (3 mg/kg/24 hr) will moderate the hypokalemia induced by diuretics and secondary hyperaldosteronism. Certain patients with massive edema may require intravenous therapy with 25% human albumin (1 gm/kg). This treatment has transient benefit and carries the risk of volume overload with hypertension and congestive heart failure. However, in patients with serious bacterial infections, marked decrease in GFR, or severe edema with skin breakdown, infusions of albumin may be quite useful to rapidly restore a normal circulating volume.

Although the overall prognosis for children with INS is excellent, the specific prognosis depends on the patient's response to steroid therapy and the histologic definition of the renal lesion. Precisely because patients with typical steroid-responsive INS have excellent prognoses, they deserve careful follow-up, aggressive evaluation, and therapy of complications.

Complications

Complications include growth retardation, altered coagulation, renal failure, and hypertension. The therapy for hypertension is presented elsewhere in this text.

---

*Manufacturer's Note: Oral doses of furosemide greater than 6 mg/kg in children are not recommended.

Infections. With the loss of immunoglobulins and certain serum complement components (e.g., Factor B), nephrotic patients have an increased incidence of serious bacterial infections. The most frequently occurring organisms have been pneumococcus, *Hemophilus influenzae*, and *Escherichia coli*. These infections often occur in sites compromised by edema, causing peritonitis, cellulitis, and pneumonia. Owing to their immunosuppressed state, patients with INS should be observed carefully for evidence of infection. Appropriate cultures should be taken early and therapy begun pending the culture results. Prophylactic antibiotics may prevent certain specific infections (e.g., penicillin for pneumococcus) but usually are not necessary. Pneumococcal vaccine may benefit these patients.

Frequent Relapses. Some patients will frequently relapse and consequently develop serious signs of steroid intoxication. Others become steroid-dependent and require continuous steroid therapy in order to maintain protein-free urine. In these patients short-term (2 months) cytotoxic therapy with cyclophosphamide† (2.5 mg/kg/24 hr) or possibly chlorambucil† may reduce the steroid dose required and prolong the duration of the remission. The short-term risks of this therapy include alopecia, leukopenia, infection, hemorrhagic cystitis, and seizures. While gonadal injury with sterility has been documented, especially in males, the long-term risks of cytotoxic agents are not completely known but may include cancer and genetic abnormalities in future generations. Since steroid-responsive INS has a good prognosis for complete recovery, the use of cytotoxic drugs in these patients should be individualized and restricted to those in whom the benefits exceed both the known and potential risks.

Other Causes of Nephrotic Syndrome

As noted above, various immune-mediated glomerular lesions may produce significant proteinuria and should be considered in the differential diagnosis of atypical nephrotic syndrome in children. The general therapy for all of these diseases includes dietary salt and fluid restriction and diuretic therapy to control edema and hypertension. Albumin therapy is not appropriate because the intravascular volume is usually expanded.

With the exception of lupus nephritis, the use of steroids and cytotoxic drugs in other types of glomerulonephritis associated with the nephrotic syndrome is controversial.

---

†This use is not listed by the manufacturer.

Renal Venous Thrombosis

THOMAS L. KENNEDY, M.D.,
and ROBERT H. McLEAN, M.D.

The term renal venous thrombosis is anatomically more accurate than renal vein thrombosis, since the thrombus rarely originates in or is restricted to the renal vein. The distinction may appear trivial but is useful in understanding the etiology of this condition and in deciding on therapy. The thrombus generally forms in one or more of the small intrarenal vessels and may then extend to involve the renal vein.

Treatment initially should be preventive. That is, the infant or child at risk for renal venous thrombosis must be recognized and have the predisposing condition (e.g., hyperosmolality) corrected. Once the diagnosis is suspected or established, treatment is supportive and directed at continuing to correct the underlying disorder and disturbances resulting from impaired renal function. The efficacy of anticoagulants, specifically heparin, in the therapy of renal venous thrombosis is unproven. We have restricted the use of heparin to patients in whom a hypercoagulable state has led to diffuse systemic thromboses, patients whose disease is associated with pulmonary embolism, and patients with evidence of uncontrolled consumption coagulopathy. Although the duration of oligoanuria is frequently short, the degree of metabolic derangement at the time of diagnosis may occasionally be severe and require dialysis.

The role of surgery in the treatment of renal thrombosis remains controversial. We believe thrombectomy is rarely if ever indicated and should be avoided in unilateral cases. Nonetheless, some physicians believe that thrombectomy may be helpful when bilateral renal venous thrombosis resulting in acute failure has been promptly detected. Unfortunately, no controlled surveys with results to support either opinion exist. There is general agreement that acute nephrectomy is never warranted.

Follow-up data on infants with renal venous thrombosis are limited. A variety of renal functional and structural abnormalities may result, and these may mimic other conditions. Functional changes may be both glomerular and tubular. Glomerular injury results in a diminished filtration rate, which varies from mild to severe but is usually not progressive. Tubular injury may result in impaired concentrating capacity, glucosuria, aminoaciduria, hyperkalemia, and bicarbonate wasting. Hypertension may also occur as a late complication of renal venous thrombosis. The elevation of blood pressure is usually not severe and may not be permanent.

Structural changes include focal or generalized atrophy of one or both kidneys, with or without intrarenal calcification. Focal atrophy is usually accompanied by caliectasis and may be mistaken for the focal scar of pyelonephritis or segmental hypoplasia. Generalized atrophy may be indistinguishable radiographically from congenital renal hypoplasia or dysplasia.

Chronic Renal Failure

RICHARD N. FINE, M.D.

The technical advances in the area of dialysis and renal transplantation during the past 25 years have stimulated considerable interest in the symptoms associated with declining renal function. The potential for prolonging life once end-stage renal disease (ESRD) ensues has mandated the need to dissect each potential adverse consequence of uremia and to attempt to avoid the progression of symptoms.

Almost every organ system is affected by uremia. Unfortunately, there is no direct relationship between the degree of reduction in renal function and the development of uremic toxicity. Because of the wide range of signs and symptoms associated with uremia, a specific "uremic toxin" has been sought, delineation of which would facilitate development of a direct therapeutic approach, thereby avoiding the many clinical problems consequent to uremia. Unfortunately, one or more factors that directly correlate with uremic symptomatology have not been identified. Therefore, the current therapeutic approach to the child with chronic renal insufficiency is toward alleviating the clinical manifestations of uremia.

CLINICAL MANIFESTATIONS

Sodium

Sodium excretion is impaired in children with renal insufficiency leading to salt and water retention, edema, and hypertension. Dietary sodium restriction and the judicious use of diuretics are advantageous.

The degree of restriction varies with the kidney's ability to excrete sodium. In general, sodium intake is limited to 2.0 gm daily in older children and adolescents and to 1.0 to 1.5 gm daily in infants and younger children. A potent diuretic, such as furosemide (Lasix), 1.0 mg/kg once or twice daily, will enhance sodium excretion in the face of significant chronic renal insufficiency.

Urinary sodium loss occasionally accompanies the pathologic process, causing progressive renal insufficiency. Dietary sodium restriction can produce a sharp drop in renal function. Occasionally, supplementation with sodium chloride tablets is required. The amount of supplementation can be determined by calculating the 24 hour urinary excretion of sodium.

Potassium

Hyperkalemia occurs in patients with renal insufficiency as a result of an increase in extracellular potassium due to catabolism and acidosis in addition to decreased renal excretion. Provision of adequate caloric intake to minimize catabolism, correction of acidosis, and limitation of foods high in potassium are recommended to avoid the potentially disastrous consequences of hyperkalemia. Routine administration of a cation exchange resin (Kayexalate) is sometimes desirable. It should be noted, however, that this resin exchanges sodium for potassium and will result in increased sodium absorption.

Dietary potassium intake is usually limited to 1.5 gm in older children and adolescents and 1.0 gm in infants and younger children. The cation exchange resin can be administered orally in a dose of 1.0 gm/kg once or twice daily, sprinkled on food or dissolved in liquid.

Acidosis

Variable degrees of reduced net acid excretion accompany the decline in renal function. The resulting systemic acidosis may lead to clinical signs of tachypnea as well as accentuate the development of hyperkalemia. Correction of acidosis with supplemental alkali therapy is often required. Sodium intake is increased by such therapy.

The amount of alkali therapy required will vary with the degree of acidosis. In a stable child with chronic renal insufficiency approximately 2 meq/kg/day of alkali is required to buffer the acid production. Alkali therapy is available as sodium bicarbonate tablets (10 or 20 grains) or as Bicitra liquid (1 meq sodium citrate per ml). The amount of alkali prescribed should be adjusted continuously to maintain the CO_2 content of serum at 22 to 24 meq/l.

Glucose

Glucose intolerance accompanies renal insufficiency, producing an abnormal glucose tolerance test and occasional hyperglycemia. Presumably, this results from inhibition of cellular glucose uptake because plasma insulin levels are elevated. The hyperglucagonemia that occurs may contribute to the hyperglycemia. This intolerance should be considered when prescribing dietary carbohydrate supplementation. Hyperglycemic coma can occasionally occur when a moderate glucose load is administered to a child with severe chronic renal insufficiency.

Lipids

Decreased hepatic lipase activity is thought to account for the hypertriglyceridemia of renal insufficiency, which may be associated with the accelerated atherosclerosis seen in adult patients with ESRD. Similar abnormalities have been reported in children undergoing hemodialysis. Although the relationship between the lipid abnormalities and the eventual development of vascular disease in children is unknown, it has been demonstrated that children with ESRD who die while undergoing hemodialysis or following renal transplantation exhibit coronary artery lesions that are preatherosclerotic. Carbohydrate supplementation to increase caloric intake in children with renal insufficiency, which may enhance the hypertriglyceridemia, should be undertaken with caution.

Water

Fluid balance is difficult to maintain in the child with renal insufficiency because the renal diluting and concentrating mechanism is often absent. The resultant isosthenuria dictates that fluid intake equal urinary output in order to avoid dehydration. Similarly, excessive fluid intake will easily lead to volume overload because of the limited ability of the damaged kidney to excrete an adequate urine volume. Daily fluid intake should be limited to 400 mL/m² plus the child's daily urinary output.

Anemia

Exogenous testosterone has been effective in increasing the red blood cell mass in postpubertal adolescents and adult patients with ESRD; however, its use in prepubertal children is limited because it may accelerate bone maturation without a comparable increase in height.

Splenic sequestration of red blood cells in patients may exacerbate the anemia. Splenectomy has been effective in decreasing transfusion requirements in these patients.

Symptomatic anemia requires blood transfusions. However, excessive blood transfusions should be avoided in the child with renal insufficiency because of the potential for iron deposition and hemosiderosis.

The serum ferritin level is a good indicator of body iron stores. Serum ferritin should be monitored periodically in the child with chronic renal insufficiency who does not require transfusions in order to detect iron deficiency, which may result from excessive blood drawing for analysis. If the serum ferritin level is low, oral iron therapy should be prescribed.

Hypertension

Hypervolemia due to salt and water retention is the primary factor in increased blood pressure in children with renal insufficiency. Diuretic therapy and dietary restrictions of sodium and fluid intake are beneficial.

Overproduction of renin by the diseased kidney may contribute to the hypertension. Salt and water restriction may exacerbate the degree of hypertension by increasing renal renin production consequent to reduced renal perfusion.

Mild to moderate hypertension can usually be controlled by the use of a diuretic (furosemide, 1–2 mg/kg, 2–4 times a day) and hydralazine (0.5 to 2 mg/kg, 2–4 times a day) and/or propranolol* (1–2 mg/kg, 2–4 times a day). The combination of hydralazine and propranolol is particularly effective because the latter blunts the tachycardic response to the former.

With severe hypertension, especially in a child with elevated plasma renin activity, captopril† (0.1–0.4 mg/kg/dose in the neonate and 6.25–50 mg 2–4 times a day in children and adolescents) or minoxidil (0.1–1.4 mg/kg/day) is effective. Diuretics should be given with either of these antihypertensive drugs because of the potential for fluid retention. Captopril may be associated with reduced renal function, which usually remits spontaneously despite continuation of the drug. The major drawback to the use of minoxidil is the development of hirsutism, which is extremely annoying to the older child or adolescent. Because of this minoxidil is usually reserved for patients whose hypertension is resistant to captopril therapy.

Cardiac Dysfunction

Congestive heart failure in children with renal insufficiency is attributable to both hypervolemia and hypertension. Adherence to sodium and fluid restrictions and control of hypertension can limit this complication.

Cardiomegaly and episodes of congestive heart failure unrelated to hypervolemia and hypertension are rare in children with renal insufficiency.

Pericardial effusion may occur in severe uremia. The effusion is typically serosanguineous. Dialysis usually leads to resolution within a short period of time. Persistence of the effusion or development of tamponade may necessitate pericardiocentesis. Instillation of a nonabsorbable corticosteroid (triamcinolone) into the pericardial space is effective in patients with persistent effusion despite repeated pericardiocentesis.

---

*Manufacturer's note: Data on the use of propranolol in children are too limited to permit adequate directions for use.

†Manufacturer's note: Safety and effectiveness in children have not been established. Captopril should be used in children only if other measures for controlling blood pressure have not been effective.

Renal Osteodystrophy

Decreased production by the kidney of the active metabolite of vitamin D, 1,25 dihydroxycholecalciferol (1,25 dihydroxy D_3), results in decreased calcium absorption from the intestine. The unavailability of adequate amounts of calcium leads to osteomalacia, which in the growing bone is manifested radiologically as rickets. Relative hypocalcemia stimulates parathormone production and the radiologic lesions of osteitis fibrosa.

The severe clinical manifestations of renal osteodystrophy are valgus deformities of the lower extremities, slipped capital femoral epiphyses and metastatic calcification.

The use of phosphate binders to lower the serum phosphate level and the administration of an analog of vitamin D should prevent development of the osseous lesions and resolve the lesions once they have developed.

Magnesium-containing phosphate binders should *not* be used because of the prevalence of hypermagnesemia in patients with chronic renal insufficiency. Aluminum hydroxide (Amphojel) and aluminum carbonate (Baseljel) are available in tablet and liquid preparations. The amount of binder prescribed is varied to maintain the serum phosphate level within normal limits; however, the dose is usually 4 to 6 gm daily. It is advisable to prescribe the binders after meals when the maximal reduction in phosphate absorption is effective. In general, children resist taking phosphate binders because of their chalky taste; therefore, constant reinforcement of the need to take the binders is necesssary and frequent monitoring of the serum phosphate level is required to ensure compliance. A watermelon-flavored aluminum hydroxide liquid preparation (Nephrox) is, at times, better tolerated by small children.

The vitamin D deficiency of chronic renal insufficiency is treated with either dihydrotachysterol, 0.125 to 0.75 mg/day (Hytakerol), or 1,25 dihydroxy D_3, 15 to 60 ng/kg/day (calcitriol). Hytakerol is available in both liquid and tablet form, whereas calcitriol is available only in capsules; therefore, for infants and small children Hytakerol is usually prescribed. For children who can take tablets, either 0.2 mg of Hytakerol daily or 0.25 μg of calcitriol daily is prescribed initially. The serum calcium level is monitored and the dosage increased every 2 weeks until the serum calcium level approaches 11.0 mg/dl or the serum alkaline phosphatase level is within the normal range for the patient's age, indicating resolution of the renal osteodystrophy. Additional phosphate binders are usually required with 1,25 dihydroxy D_3 therapy because this drug enhances gastrointestinal phosphate absorption.

Profound hypocalcemia or hypocalcemia that persists despite vitamin D therapy requires supplemental oral calcium administration. The daily dosage of elemental calcium varies between 0.5 and 2.0 gm daily.

Peripheral Neuropathy

Paresthesias of the palms of the hands and/or soles of the feet are the initial clinical manifestations of uremic peripheral neuropathy. Abnormalities of the nerve conduction time may occur in the absence of clinical manifestations. This complication is rare in children with renal insufficiency. The lesion is indicative of severe uremia and of the need to initiate dialysis. Resolution may require several months of dialysis.

Mental Retardation

The onset of uremia during the first year of life, when significant brain development is proceeding, may result in mental impairment. Recently, brain dysfunction has been described in 20 of 23 children who had onset of renal insufficiency during the first year of life. If these data are corroborated, it may be important to identify the child with impaired renal function as early as possible during the first year of life and to initiate dialysis at an earlier age in order to maximize brain development.

Growth Retardation

The etiology of the growth retarding effects of renal insufficiency is unknown. Although multiple factors have been implicated, a precise relationship has not been shown. The factors proposed are age at onset of renal insufficiency, etiology of primary disease, acidosis, energy malnutrition, renal osteodystrophy, and uremic inhibitors.

Approximately one third of the child's growth occurs during the first 2 years of life. Any interruption of the growth pattern during infancy will have a profound effect on the child's ultimate stature unless significant "catch-up" growth occurs once the cause of the interruption is alleviated.

Children with congenital abnormalities have more severe growth retardation than those with acquired renal lesions. Since the onset of renal insufficiency in those children with congenital lesions is usually at an earlier age, it is difficult to determine whether the age at onset or the primary renal disease is the significant factor.

Children with renal insufficiency who were acidotic manifest growth retardation. Because correction of acidosis in children without renal insufficiency leads to improved growth velocity, attempts should be made to correct the acidosis in children with renal insufficiency.

It has been suggested that low calorie intake contributes to the growth retardation of renal insufficiency. Optimal caloric intake should be attempted in children with renal insufficiency, although a beneficial effect on growth velocity remains to be verified.

It seems obvious that renal osteodystrophy has an adverse effect on growth. Recent studies have demonstrated that treatment with 1,25 dihydroxy D_3 improves growth. However, not all investigators have validated this concept. In any case, prevention of renal osteodystrophy is desirable and it is possible that treatment with one of the new vitamin D analogs may be advantageous.

Somatomedin mediates the growth-promoting effects of growth hormone on bone. A uremic inhibitor of somatomedin activity coincident with reduction in the glomerular filtration rate has been proposed as a possible mechanism of growth failure with progressive renal insufficiency. The presence of such an inhibitor could obviously adversely affect growth. Until the inhibitor is definitively characterized, it is difficult to devise methods to minimize the potential adverse effects.

INDICATIONS FOR INITIATING DIALYSIS

Prior to the widespread availability of hemodialysis for children and the development of newer techniques of peritoneal dialysis, definitive treatment of the child with ESRD did not begin until life-threatening complications of uremia were apparent. This led to severe symptomatology involving multiple organ systems, which was at times either irreversible or only partly reversible following initiation of dialysis. Consequently, the objective of early identification and serial evaluation is prevention of the consequences of uremia and determination of the expectant need for dialysis before severe symptomatology occurs.

The child with progressive renal insufficiency may manifest an accelerated decline in renal function for various reasons, such as dietary indiscretions or a superimposed infectious process. Indications for initiating dialysis in this child are similar to those in the child with acute renal failure. In many instances, symptoms emanating from involvement of a single organ system may predominate and dictate the need for dialysis. These are absolute indications to commence dialysis because they either are potentially life-threatening or can lead to irreversible organ damage.

The absolute indications for dialysis in a child with chronic renal insufficiency are 1) uncontrollable hypertension with hypertensive encephalopathy or congestive heart failure; 2) congestive heart failure, especially in the presence of a myocardiopathy; 3) pericarditis with or without tamponade; 4) peripheral neuropathy manifested by paresthesias or motor dysfunction; 5) renal osteodystrophy; and 6) bone marrow depression with either severe anemia, leukopenia, or thrombocytopenia.

In the child with progressive renal insufficiency who does not manifest absolute indications, it may be difficult to determine the proper time to initiate dialysis. The general functioning of the child must be utilized in this situation. A child who is apathetic, anorexic, and not engaged in age-appropriate activities can probably benefit from dialysis, despite the absence of clear-cut indications. Once renal function deteriorates to a glomerular filtration rate of < 5 ml/min/$1.73 m^2$, the need for dialysis should be considered imminent and discussion should be initiated regarding placement of a dialysis access. It is advantageous that such peritoneal or vascular access be created prior to the immediate need for dialysis so that the surgical procedure can be performed in the optimal clinical setting.

Peritoneal Dialysis

DONALD E. POTTER, M.D.

Acute peritoneal dialysis is commonly used to treat acute renal failure and is sometimes used to treat poisonings. It is much simpler to perform than hemodialysis on an acute basis. Chronic peritoneal dialysis is becoming an increasingly popular alternative to hemodialysis for the treatment of children with end-stage renal disease.

ACUTE PERITONEAL DIALYSIS

Indications. The commonest indications for starting dialysis in a child with acute renal failure are 1) A BUN level greater than 100 to 120 mg/dl or a rapidly rising BUN level accompanied by neurologic symptoms; 2) fluid retention resulting in severe hypertension and/or pulmonary edema; and 3) a serum potassium level greater than 6.0 meq/liter. Less common indications are severe acidosis (serum CO_2 less than 15 meq/liter) and severe hypocalcemia (serum calcium less than 7.0 mg/dl).

Although peritoneal dialysis is effective in removing many poisons from the body (e.g., salicylates, barbiturates), in children with normal renal function dialysis is rarely indicated, and the primary emphasis of treatment is supportive care.

Technique. This is usually performed in an intensive care unit. A peritoneal dialysis tray (Trocath) contains the peritoneal catheter and other supplies used in inserting the catheter. An acute pediatric catheter is used in children who weigh less than 15 kg. In larger children an adult catheter is used and the intra-abdominal segment is cut to the proper length (the distance from the umbilicus to the pubis). In newborns a 10 or 12 French chest tube in which additional side holes have been cut may be tailored more specifically to the size of the infant. After the bladder is emptied, a 5-mm skin incision is made in the midline, one third of the distance from the umbilicus to the pubis. A 16 Angiocath or Intracath needle is inserted through the peritoneum, and approximately 30 ml per kg of dialysate solution is instilled to distend the abdomen. The Angiocath is removed and the peritoneal catheter is inserted over a stylet. After the peritoneum is punctured, the stylet is removed and the catheter advanced caudally into one of the colic gutters.

Dialysis is performed with dialysate solutions in two-liter bottles (Dianeal, Inpersol, Peridial) which are warmed to body temperature. The solutions vary in their electrolyte concentrations. A typical example is sodium 132 meq, chloride 102 meq, lactate 35 meq, calcium 3.5 meq, and magnesium 1.5 meq per liter. Two concentrations of glucose, 1.5% and 4.25%, are available. Potassium chloride can be added as needed. The use of prophylactic antibiotics in the dialysate is not recommended.

The optimum volume of dialysate is approximately 1200 ml/m^2, but this volume may cause respiratory embarrassment in some patients, and it is best to start dialysis with slightly smaller volumes. A dialysis cycle consists of an inflow phase of 2 to 5 minutes, a "dwell" phase of 20 minutes, and an outflow phase of 5 to 10 minutes. Inflow and outflow, which are accomplished by gravity, should be as rapid as possible. Cycles with longer dwell times can be used for the sake of convenience but are less efficient. Since the initial outflows after catheter placement are usually bloody, and clotting of the catheter may occur, heparin, 500 U/liter, is added to the first one or two bottles.

Results of Treatment. Peritoneal dialysis is less efficient than hemodialysis in removing urea and other toxic substances from the body. It takes approximately 24 hours to lower a child's BUN level by 50%. Peritoneal dialysis is usually performed for 48 hours in acute renal failure and BUN levels typically decrease from 120 to 150 mg/dl to 25 to 35 mg/dl.

Serum potassium levels are easily controlled and acidosis is rapidly corrected with dialysis. Although total serum calcium levels increase with dialysis, the more rapid correction of acidosis can result in a decrease in ionized calcium and, rarely, tetany or convulsions have been observed.

Ultrafiltration of excessive extracellular fluid is accomplished by adjusting the dialysate glucose concentration. With 1.5% glucose, ultrafiltration per cycle is usually less than 10% (outflow volume exceeds inflow volume by $< 10\%$). With 4.25% glucose, ultrafiltration is 15 to 25%. Several liters of fluid can easily be removed from a small child during 12 to 24 hours, and peritoneal dialysis is superior to hemodialysis in this regard. The complications of ultrafiltration are hypernatremia and hyperglycemia. Hypernatremia is treated by increasing the dwell time to 45 to 60 minutes. Severe hyperglycemia (blood sugar > 400 mg/dl) is rare and is managed by discontinuing 4.25% glucose cycles or, if ultrafiltration is imperative, cautiously alternating 4.25% and 1.5% glucose cycles. Insulin can be used if necessary.

Complications. The commonest complications are outflow obstruction, leaking around the catheter, and peritonitis. Perforation of the bowel, bladder, or major blood vessel during catheter insertion is rare. Outflow, or one-way obstruction usually results from entanglement of the catheter with bowel and can be relieved by repositioning the patient, by stimulating bowel activity with an enema or suppository, or by irrigating the catheter. Leaking occurs when a portion of the perforated segment of the catheter lies outside the peritoneum. This is treated by advancing the catheter. More commonly, however, leaking indicates an excessively large hole in the peritoneum and, if persistent, is an indication for insertion of a new catheter at a different site.

Peritonitis is treated with antibiotics, either intravenously or intraperitoneally. Cephalothin, 50 mg per liter, in each bottle of dialysate is started until the results of culture and sensitivities are known. Peritonitis is not an indication for removing the catheter unless it proves resistant to treatment or unless the infection is caused by Candida.

The risk of peritonitis developing increases when the catheter is left in place longer than 48 to 72 hours. In most centers the catheter is removed after this interval, and if subsequent dialysis becomes necessary, a new catheter is inserted. In situations where several weeks of dialysis are anticipated, an alternative plan is to initiate dialysis with a chronic (Tenckhoff) catheter, which requires surgical implantation, and removal, under general anesthesia. These catheters are associated with a much lower risk of peritonitis and can be used indefinitely.

CHRONIC PERITONEAL DIALYSIS

Chronic peritoneal dialysis is almost always performed in the home. Intermittent peritoneal dialysis is similar to acute peritoneal dialysis but is performed with a machine that cycles dialysate into and out of the abdomen every 30 to 40 minutes. Children are usually treated for 12 hours, overnight, three times a week. A more popular technique is continuous ambulatory peritoneal dialysis (CAPD). Four times a day dialysate is introduced into the abdomen by gravity from a plastic bag attached to the catheter by IV-type tubing. The empty bag is folded up and worn around the waist under the clothing. The fluid remains in the abdomen and dialysis takes place while the child pursues normal activities. At the end of each cycle the dialysate is returned to the plastic bag, which is discarded, and a new cycle is started. Thus dialysis takes place continuously except during the four bag changes, which can be performed in a variety of settings, in and out of the home, and which take approximately 30 minutes to perform. In contrast to hemodialysis, which is performed in a medical center for 4 hours three times a week, this technique is performed without a machine and allows children more freedom and more responsibility for their own care.

Dialysate bags for CAPD come in volumes of 250, 500, 750, 1000, 1500, and 2000 ml. Glucose concentrations of 1.5, 2.5, and 4.25% are available. Children tolerate dialysate volumes similar to those used in acute peritoneal dialysis (e.g., 1000 ml in a 25-kg child) with minimal change in their appearance, and are able to take part in vigorous activities, including swimming.

CAPD is equally effective as chronic hemodialysis in controlling the biochemical and clinical manifestations of uremia. The average BUN level of children undergoing CAPD is approximately 70 mg/dl. Ultrafiltration sufficient to control extracellular fluid volume is achieved in most children by using three bags of 1.5% and one bag of 4.25% glucose per day. Most children on CAPD are allowed unrestricted diets and their calorie intakes are supplemented by glucose absorbed from the dialysate, approximately 2.5 gm per kg per day. Protein is lost in the dialysate, however, 0.2 gm per kg per day. There is some evidence that children on CAPD have better growth than those on hemodialysis.

Complications. The most important complication of CAPD is peritonitis. Its incidence varies from one episode every four patient months to one episode every 13 patient months in different centers. It is diagnosed by the presence of cloudy dialysate, with or without abdominal pain, which contains greater than 100 white blood cells per mm^3 and a preponderance of neutrophils. Peritonitis is treated by adding cephalothin to the dialysate, 500 mg per liter in the first bag, followed by 250 mg per liter in each bag for 10 days. Tobramycin, 1.7 mg per kg in the first bag, followed by 8 mg per liter in each bag for 8 days, is commonly used for peritonitis resistant to cephalothin. Heparin, 500 U per liter, is added to each bag as long as the dialysate remains cloudy. With adequate treatment the dialysate should clear and symptoms disappear within 2 to 3 days. For peritonitis resistant to treatment the catheter is removed, antibiotics are administered intravenously for 10 to 14 days, and a new catheter is inserted. Most episodes of peritonitis can be treated in the home.

Complications of CAPD related to the catheter include obstruction, leaking of dialysate around the catheter, infection at the site where the catheter enters the skin, and erosion through the skin of the subcutaneous Dacron cuff attached to the catheter. Treatment frequently necessitates catheter replacement. Hernias, both ventral and inguinal, and hydroceles are other complications of CAPD.

CAPD is rapidly becoming the preferred method of dialysis for children who require long-term treatment. Improvements in technology will hopefully reduce the present high rate of complications with this therapy.

Hemodialysis

RICHARD N. FINE, M.D.

INDICATIONS

Acute Hemodialysis. Two primary situations in which acute hemodialysis has been used are accidental poisoning and acute renal insufficiency. The number of children requiring hemodialysis after accidental poisoning is minimal. Peritoneal dialysis (PD) is preferable for water-soluble substances because of its easy accessibility; however, for profound toxicity requiring rapid intoxicant removal, charcoal hemoperfusion is indicated. Hemodialysis can be used to treat acute renal failure in children; however, with the exception of severe intraperitoneal bleeding consequent to a coagulopathy, such as may exist with the hemolytic-uremic syndrome, PD can be easier and safer.

Chronic Hemodialysis. The number of patients in the pediatric age group with end-stage renal disease (ESRD) has been reported to vary from 1 to 3.5 per million population per year. Indications for initiating extended hemodialysis are variable and depend somewhat upon available facilities. The indications are similar to those described in the article on peritoneal dialysis. Although age is not a contraindication to hemodialysis, peritoneal dialysis is preferable for young children.

TECHNICAL ASPECTS

Vascular Access

Initially, the silicone rubber–polytef arteriovenous cannula was used. Although special pediatric cannulas have been designed and utilized, the adult type of cannula is acceptable. The largest cannula that fits comfortably without compromising the intima of the vessel is inserted. The radial artery and forearm vein are cannulated in older children (over 30 kg), the brachial artery and cephalic vein in younger children (under 30 kg), and the superficial femoral artery and saphenous vein in very small children (under 10 kg). The posterior tibial artery and saphenous vein can be cannulated to facilitate home dialysis.

The disadvantages of the external cannula are shunt infections and clotting episodes, requiring frequent revisions. In addition, the presence of an external cannula may inhibit activity and, in some children, is a source of anxiety. The internal arteriovenous fistula, anastomosing a forearm vein to the radial artery, has been used successfully in a number of children, the youngest of whom was 7 years of age.

The internal arteriovenous fistula may result in insufficient blood flow because of the small caliber of the forearm veins. An alternate internal arteriovenous fistula can be created using either a bovine graft or synthetic material (polytetrafluoroethylene). The primary site for creating an internal arteriovenous fistula in older children is the forearm, utilizing the radial artery at the wrist and the cephalic vein in the antecubital fossa. For younger children, the brachial artery and axillary vein in the arm are used.

Dialyzer

The ideal dialyzer for children requires a fluid volume to fill both dialyzer and blood tubing that does not exceed 10% of a child's blood volume, since blood loss of such an amount when commencing dialysis is well tolerated without producing serious hypotension. Many commercially available parallel-flow or hollow-fiber dialyzers can be used to hemodialyze children. The surface area of the dialyzer is used to determine its appropriateness for use, depending upon the patient's weight: 0.25 m^2 dialyzer for children weighing less than 10 kg; 0.5 to 0.6 m^2 dialyzer for children weighing 10 to 20 kg; 0.9 to 1.0 m^2 dialyzer for children weighing 25 to 35 kg; and 1.3 to 1.6 m^2 for adolescents weighing more than 40 kg.

Delivery Systems

No special modifications of existing delivery systems are required for use with pediatric patients. The delivery system mixes tap water with commercially prepared concentrate so that the final dialysate solution has the following composition: calcium, 3.5 meq/1; potassium, 1.0 or 2.0 meq/1; sodium, 135 meq/1; chloride, 100 meq/1; magnesium, 1.5 meq/1, and acetate, 38 meq/1. If the child exhibits evidence of acetate intolerance, specially prepared equipment is available to substitute bicarbonate. Ultrafiltration is facilitated by a positive displacement effluent pump, which allows a negative pressure adjustment from 0 to 450 mm Hg.

Technique of Dialysis

The dialyzer and arterial and venous tubing are primed with a normal saline solution containing heparin. Blood is not used. The quantity of priming solution administered is inversely proportional to predialysis blood pressure and weight. Total body heparinization is used exclusively. Aqueous heparin sodium, 500 to 2000 units, is given intravenously when beginning dialysis. Venous blood specimens are obtained hourly and a one-tube Lee-White clotting time test is performed. Additional heparin is administered continuously for maintenance of a clotting time between 30 and 60 minutes. When dialysis is carried out within 96 hours of a surgical procedure, heparin dosage is adjusted to maintain the clotting time between 15 and 20 minutes. A patient is weighed prior to, halfway through, and at termination of each dialysis or continuously using a bed scale. Hypotensive episodes are treated with normal saline via venous drip chamber. Blood pressure and pulse are monitored frequently during the initial 15 minutes of dialysis and at 30- to 60-minute intervals after stabilization. At termination of dialysis, the arterial tubing is rinsed with a small volume of normal saline following disconnection from the cannula, and a column of air is used to return blood in the dialyzer and tubing to the patient.

Various treatment schedules have been advocated. We treat all children thrice weekly for periods of 4 to 6 hours, depending upon the child's weight, the fluid accumulation between dialyses, and the predialysis level of blood urea nitrogen.

Diet. The need for dietary restrictions during extended dialysis in children is onerous for patient, parent, and staff. Certain limitations are necessary in most patients to prevent catastrophic situations and facilitate adequate dialysis. These restrictions, however, must not prevent intake of adequate calories. An effort should be made to maximize the number of calories ingested while limiting sodium, potassium, phosphorus, protein, and fluid to an extent needed for weight gain and linear growth without compromising the clinical status or precipitating catastrophic complications.

Daily dietary recommendations are calories, $2000/m^2$; protein, 1.5 to 2.5 gm/kg, which can be increased to 3 to 4 gm/kg in small children weighing less than 10 to 15 kg; sodium, 40 meq/m^2; potassium, 30 meq/m^2; and fluids, 500 ml/m^2 plus an amount equal to urine volume. In addition, supplemental B complex vitamins and folic acid, 1 mg daily, and phosphate-binding gels (Amphojel or Basaljel, 1 to 3 capsules three times a day with meals) are given to reduce the serum phosphorus level.

Ultrafiltration. The degree of ultrafiltration is varied according to the desired weight loss during dialysis. This depends upon the predialysis blood pressure and the weight gain between dialyses. Excessive ultrafiltration (greater than 3 kg for adolescents or 2 kg for younger children) is frequently necessary because of dietary indiscretion and may cause nausea, vomiting, severe headache, and leg cramps. Leg cramps usually improve after intravenous administration of normal saline or 5% sodium chloride, and other symptoms may respond to small doses of sedatives and reduction of ultrafiltration.

In the edematous child with a reduced serum albumin level (less than 3.0 gm/dl), ultrafiltration will not effect fluid removal until the serum albumin is raised to more than 3.0 gm/dl with intravenous administration of albumin.

Profound hypotension may occur with ultrafiltration, preventing the ability to remove fluid. Diafiltration—dialysis without dialysate flow—for 1 hour at the initiation of dialysis will effectively remove fluid without lowering the blood pressure.

Hypertension. This usually responds to dietary fluid and salt restriction and fluid removal by ultrafiltration during dialysis. Occasionally, antihypertensive drugs are adjunctive in controlling hypertension. Infrequently, hypertension does not respond to these measures or worsens with ultrafiltration. This has been labeled renin-dependent hypertension and is associated with elevated plasma renin activity. Bilateral nephrectomy may be required to control this hypertension. However, the use of potent antihypertensive agents, such as minoxidil or captopril, may control the blood pressure, thereby obviating the need for bilateral nephrectomy.

Anemia. A spontaneous rise in hematocrit and maintenance at a level greater than 20% can be obtained in chronically dialyzed children. However, most children undergoing chronic dialysis require periodic blood transfusions to maintain the hematocrit at more than 20%.

Because of blood loss in the dialyzer and blood sampling for laboratory determinations, iron deficiency may develop. However, because of the frequency of transfusions, iron overload also may occur. Therefore, supplemental oral or intravenous iron dextran should be administered with caution. Serial determinations of the serum ferritin level are the best indicators of the need for iron supplementation. A serum ferritin level of less than 50 mg/dl indicates iron deficiency.

In adolescents with fused epiphyses, supplemental parenteral androgen (nandrolone decanoate* [Deca-Durabolin], 100 mg IM every week or nandrolone phenpropionate* [Durabolin], 50 to 100 mg IM every week for boys and every 2 weeks for girls) is administered to patients who fail to respond to iron therapy.

Because of the adverse effect of bilateral nephrectomy on maintenance of the hematocrit level, such a procedure should be deferred unless indicated for treatment of uncontrollable hypertension or the need to remove infected kidneys or correct lower urinary tract abnormalities.

Osteodystrophy. Two types of roentgenographic lesions have been noted: rickets-like lesions (osteomalacia) and subperiosteal bone resorption (secondary hyperparathyroidism or osteitis fibrosa). Generalized demineralization has also been observed.

Significant bone disease is probably present in all children with chronic renal disease, even in the absence of roentgenographic abnormalities. Serial determinations of serum calcium, phosphorus, and parathormone levels are helpful in developing an appropriate therapeutic approach to the prevention and treatment of renal osteodystrophy.

---

*These dosages exceed manufacturer's recommended dosages.

The serum calcium level is maintained with dihydrotachysterol, 0.2 to 0.4 mg daily, and supplemental oral calcium (Os-Cal, 500 to 2000 mg daily). Persistent hypocalcemia at the initiation of dialysis can be corrected by increasing the dialysate calcium concentration to 7.5 to 8.0 mg/dl. The serum phosphorus level can be lowered with phosphate-binding gels (Amphogel, Basaljel, Dialume).

With maintenance of the serum calcium and phosphorus levels at normal values, the degree of hyperparathyroidism as indicated by an elevated serum parathormone level may be minimized. The use of 1,25-dihydrocholecalciferol (Rocaltrol[†]), 0.25 to 0.50 μg daily, is indicated with persistent hypocalcemia or persistent hyperparathyroidism.

If the roentgenographic lesions of hyperparathyroidism fail to heal or the extraosseous lesions (pruritus, metastatic calcification) persist despite this therapeutic approach, parathyroid extirpation may be necessary. Osseous deformities resulting from renal osteodystrophy that prevent optimal ambulation are particulary troublesome in pediatric patients. Correction of deformities is often mandatory in order to effect rehabilitation. It is important to demonstrate healing of roentgenographic lesions of osteodystrophy prior to correcting deformities. Deformities will recur if osteodystrophy is not healed. Parathyroid extirpation may also be necessary in these circumstances.

Pericarditis. Pericarditis occurs with varying frequency in the uremic child. Three to four weeks of dialysis are usually curative. Heparin dosage should be monitored carefully to avoid increasing effusion and precipitating tamponade.

COMPLICATIONS

Seizures. Convulsions occurring either during or after hemodialysis are particularly vexing because of anxiety produced in both patient and family. Fear that subsequent dialyses will lead to recurrence is especially prevalent in children who had not experienced a seizure prior to dialysis.

In most instances, a specific etiology cannot be identified and seizures are attributable to dialysis disequilibrium syndrome. This syndrome appears to be due to cerebral edema consequent to generation of idiogenic osmoles in the brain, an event that occurs when the BUN is lowered rapidly.

Mannitol infusion (1 gm/kg per dialysis) during dialysis is recommended to prevent the disequilibrium syndrome in children with elevated predialysis BUN levels (greater than 125 mg/dl).

Prophylactic anticonvulsant therapy (phenobarbital) is advisable prior to and occasionally during hemodialysis for a child who has a history of previous seizures or who has had a convulsion consequent to hemodialysis. This is of special benefit during the initial period of hemodialysis, when large variations in serum osmolality can be expected.

Hepatitis. The incidence of hepatitis in children treated with chronic hemodialysis is similar to that in adults (10%). Monthly serum glutamic oxalic transaminase, serum glutamic pyruvic transaminase, serum bilirubin, and hepatitis B antigen levels should be obtained as a precaution.

The following measures are used to curtail development and spread of hepatitis: 1) isolate equipment used for any patient who becomes HB$_s$Ag-positive; 2) instruct nursing personnel to use gloves and gowns when handling blood during a dialysis procedure; and 3) maintain routine serial testing of both patient and staff to identify asymptomatic carriers of HB$_s$Ag. Patients who become HB$_s$Ag-positive should be dialyzed separately to avoid spread to other children in the unit.

The significant incidence of "e" antigenemia in children with persistent hepatitis B antigenemia who are undergoing dialysis indicates the potential for infectivity in these patients.

Elevations in the serum glutamic oxalic/pyruvic transaminase levels in the absence of hepatitis B antigen may indicate hepatitis A or non-A–non-B hepatitis infection. Recommendations to curtail the spread of the latter are not available at the present time.

Dietary Indiscretions. Episodes of pulmonary edema, hyperkalemia, and volume-dependent hypertension are usually related to dietary indiscretions. They can be prevented by adherence to dietary restrictions previously delineated and are treated by emergency dialysis.

Renal Transplantation

RICHARD N. FINE, M.D.

CRITERIA OF ACCEPTABILITY

Age

Although age should not be a factor in the deliberations concerning the treatment of a child with end-stage renal disease (ESRD), pediatric nephrologists believe that children less than 5 years of age, and especially those less than 1 year of age, require special consideration. In our experience, the results of transplantation of young children with cadaver donor allografts are somewhat poorer than our overall results; however, others have shown results similar to those obtained with older children. The reason for the decreased allograft survival is not apparent; however, the incidence of technical problems is not increased.

Age as a criterion of acceptability for transplantation, therefore, is a philosophic consideration. Is

---

[†]Safety and efficacy of Rocaltrol in children have not been established.

the potential prolongation of life justified by extraordinary means? Parents of young children are confronted with this question and can make a decision only with dispassionate counseling.

Mental Status

Children with severe mental retardation to the degree that they are not educable and always will require custodial care pose a significant problem. Children with milder degrees of mental retardation respond less well to the rigors of dialysis and transplantation. Extensive parental counseling is necessary prior to the formulation of a therapeutic approach for mentally retarded children. If conservative, nonlife-saving management is elected, the family will require a great deal of psychoemotional support. There is no unequivocal contraindication to embarking upon ESRD treatment in a mentally retarded child; however, extensive parental counseling should be undertaken prior to deciding upon the treatment plan.

Psychoemotional Status

Children with behavioral or psychiatric problems and ESRD require significantly more involvement of the health care team in creating and implementing a treatment program. If appropriate psychoemotional support is not available, it is futile to undertake the care of children with psychoemotional disorders. The major difficulty following transplantation in psychoemotionally disturbed patients is the inability to assure compliance with the therapeutic regimen.

The significant incidence of noncompliant patients and the uniformly poor allograft outcome in them indicate the need to evaluate the psychoemotional status of all patients prior to embarking upon transplantation. Unfortunately, prospective analysis to identify the potential noncompliant patient and possibly to intervene psychotherapeutically may not be totally effective. However, it seems advisable to attempt to identify potential noncompliant patients to avoid the wanton loss of allografts. Transplantation should be deferred until the patient's psychoemotional status is such that it is reasonable to assume that the post-transplant therapeutic regimen will be followed.

Generalized Infection

The presence of a generalized infectious process prevents transplantation because of the potential for dissemination once immunosuppressive drug therapy is started. If the potential for eradication of the process exists, a trial of dialysis should be considered.

Multisystem Disease

A multisystem disease may involve vital organs other than the kidney, and the systemic process that damaged the native kidneys could potentially involve the allograft. Patients with systemic immunologic diseases, such as lupus erythematosus, or those with a generalized metabolic disease, such as cystinosis, require consideration.

Persistent clinical disease activity in patients with lupus erythematosus is justification for deferral of transplantation. The presence of clinical symptomatology, not merely abnormal immunologic parameters, indicates that the patient is a poor risk to withstand the potential complications of transplantation. Transplantation should be deferred until clinical symptoms have abated and the patient no longer requires immunosuppressive medication to control symptomatology.

Malignancy

The previous existence of a primary malignancy involving either the kidneys or other organs is a potential risk factor because of the possibility of recurrence following transplantation. Bilateral Wilms tumor is the primary renal malignancy necessitating ESRD treatment in pediatric patients. Of the 13 recipients with this entity reported to the ACS/NIH Transplant Registry, only 1 died from recurrent tumor following transplantation. However, only 5 recipients survived more than 6 months, and death was frequently attributable to generalized infection. Previous chemotherapy and irradiation were causally related to the latter.

Transplantation in children with prior nonrenal malignancies is possible; however, it is advisable to wait at least 1 year following removal of the primary malignancy before transplantation, to ensure that recurrence or metastasis does not occur.

Lower Urinary Tract Abnormalities

Although an uncommon cause of renal failure in adult patients, obstructive uropathy is diagnosed in almost one fourth of children with ESRD. Typically, these patients have a prolonged course of renal insufficiency prior to the development of ESRD and have undergone multiple operative procedures to correct urinary tract abnormalities. Temporary or permanent urinary diversion has been frequent. Consequently, when ESRD ensues, the bladder is often scarred and contracted. The efficacy of renal transplantation in such patients has been questioned because of the potential for anatomic and infectious complications following transplantation.

The results of our experience indicate that the outcome of renal transplantation in patients with obstructive uropathy is similar to that of other pediatric recipients even if an ileal loop is required in patients with a nonfunctional or neurogenic bladder. Post-transplant urologic complications occur with increased frequency; however, with appropriate management, allograft function is not adversely affected. Therefore, the presence of an abnormal bladder is not a contraindication to acceptability for transplantation.

Recurrence

In renal allografts, recurrence of the disease affecting the recipient's native kidneys is a consideration for determining acceptability for transplantation. In pediatric recipients, the principal diseases to consider are membranoproliferative glomerulonephritis (MPGN), focal glomerulosclerosis (FGS), cystinosis, and congenital nephrotic syndrome. The latter entity has been shown not to recur.

Membranoproliferative Glomerulonephritis. Type 2 MPGN or dense deposit disease recurs frequently in the transplanted kidney. However, we have not observed any relationship between recurrence of the histologic lesion and allograft function. Therefore, the presence of MPGN is not a contraindication to transplantation.

Focal Glomerulosclerosis. If the following criteria for recurrence of FGS are adhered to, the incidence of true recurrence is quite low (5.6%): 1) idiopathic nephrotic syndrome in the recipient, with evidence of the lesion of FGS in the native kidneys; 2) immediate (less than 1 month) recurrence of the nephrotic syndrome following transplantation; 3) demonstration of the lesion of FGS in the allograft without concomitant chronic rejection. Since the incidence of recurrence is low, it seems reasonable to consider all potential recipients with FGS as acceptable candidates for transplantation. Immediate recurrence in an initial allograft indicates a substantial risk for recurrence in subsequent allografts.

Cystinosis. This is a metabolic disorder with an autosomal mode of inheritance, characterized by intracellular deposition of cystine crystals in various organs. Childhood cystinosis results in uniform progression to ESRD by the end of the first decade of life. The Fanconi syndrome does not recur following transplantation. Cystine crystals are observed in the interstitial tissue of all allografts, and the free cystine content of white blood cells, cultured skin fibroblasts, and allograft tissue is elevated. Despite successful transplantation, the extrarenal manifestations of cystinosis persist. Growth following successful transplantation in cystinotic children is similar to that in other allograft recipients.

Donor Source

Kidneys from adult donors can be transplanted into children as young as 2 years of age and who weigh 10 kg. Usually, the allograft can be placed extraperitoneally in the iliac fossa; however, if the donor is excessively large, it is occasionally necessary to place the kidney intraperitoneally, with anastomoses of the allograft vessels to the recipient aorta and vena cava. The decision to utilize a parental or sibling donor allograft for a young child is a parental one and should be made only after dispassionate counseling of the parents using current factual data. Sibling donors must have reached adulthood prior to being considered as potential donors.

Kidneys from a pediatric cadaver donor are an excellent allograft source for both pediatric and adult recipients. One kidney from a young donor provides sufficient function; anatomic hypertrophy occurs within a few weeks of transplantation.

Histocompatibility Testing

HLA A, B, C, and DR Matching. Transplants between HLA identical siblings (similar HLA A, B, C, and DR antigens) are associated with a more than 90% long-term survival (± 5 years) of renal allografts. Consequently, these antigens, which can be determined serologically with results available within 4 hours, have been considered transplantation antigens. Allografts from parents to offspring or from one-haplotype identical siblings have a long-term survival of approximately 75% and those from cadaver donors a long-term survival of 40 to 50%. Attempts to improve cadaver donor allograft survival by improved HLA A, B, and C matching between donor and recipient have not proved uniformly efficacious. However, recent data have indicated an improvement in allograft survival rates of cadaver donor allografts when there are no mismatched DR antigens between donor and recipient.

Mixed Lymphocyte Culture (MLC). The MLC presumably detects antigenic differences between donor and recipient that are similar to the DR antigens. HLA A, B, C, and DR identical siblings are usually nonstimulatory (unresponsive) in the MLC test. Since the standard MLC test requires 5 days to perform, it is impractical for cadaver donor transplants. However, decreased responsiveness between one-haplotype identical parents or siblings and potential recipients is associated with improved allograft survival.

Cross Match. Preformed lymphocytotoxic antibodies in the recipient against donor HLA A and B antigens, which are acquired from a blood transfusion, previous transplant, or prior pregnancy, are associated with immediate (hyperacute) rejection of the allograft. Thus, a negative cross-match test utilizing donor T lymphocytes and recipient serum is a prerequisite to transplantation. Preformed antibodies against DR antigens detected on B lymphocytes are not deleterious to allograft outcome. Therefore, a positive B cell cross match is not a contraindication to transplantation.

Blood Transfusion and Allograft Survival

Recipients who receive a renal allograft without a prior blood transfusion have a significantly decreased allograft survival rate. The mechanism by which blood transfusions have a salutary effect on allograft survival is unknown; however, it is desirable to have the potential recipient receive at least 3 to 5 units of blood prior to transplantation.

Immunosuppressive Therapy

Corticosteroids and azathioprine are the primary immunosuppressive drugs used for renal transplantation. The dosage of prednisone is initially 3 mg/kg/24 hr, tapered to 2 mg/kg/24 hr by the third post-transplant week, 1 mg/kg/24 hr by the sixth post-transplant week, and 0.5 mg/kg/24 hr by the ninth post-transplant week. Subsequently, the dosage is tapered, depending upon adequate allograft function, to 7.5 to 15 mg by the sixth post-transplant month. At 1 year post-transplant, alternate-day corticosteroid therapy is introduced at twice the daily dose.

The dosage of azathioprine (Imuran) is initially 2 to 3 mg/kg/24 hr and is maintained at that level unless allograft function is diminished (oliguria) or toxicity (leukopenia < 4000 mm^3 or hepatic dysfunction) ensues, at which time the dosage is decreased to 0.5 to 1.0 mg/kg/24 hr.

Adjunctive immunosuppressive therapy with antithymocyte globulin, cyclophosphamide, splenectomy, thymectomy, and local X-irradiation has been utilized with equivocal results.

A new immunosuppressive agent, cyclosporin A, has been used experimentally, and the initial results are promising. However, the drug is not available for routine use at present.

Rejection Treatment

Acute rejection episodes are treated with intravenous methyl-prednisolone, 10 mg/kg/24 hr in a single bolus for 3 days. No treatment is available for hyperacute or chronic rejection. If acute rejection episodes are not controlled with 3 to 4 treatments during the initial 3 post-transplant months, it is advisable to discontinue treatment to avoid toxicity. Steroid-resistant rejection episodes are treated with antithymocyte globulin, 15 mg/kg, for 5 to 10 days (Upjohn Co., Kalamazoo, Mich.).

Growth

Growth retardation in children with renal insufficiency has been appreciated since the last century. Despite the institution of dialysis and presumed reversal of uremic milieu, growth retardation persists. Following successful renal transplantation, normal linear growth occurs infrequently. Normal growth occurs in only 12.5% of recipients receiving daily corticosteroid therapy. The factors implicated are poor growth potential at transplantation, allograft function, and corticosteroid therapy. Children with a bone age greater than 12 years at transplantation grow minimally following transplantation. The ad-

verse effect of impaired allograft function on growth is indicated by the fact that recipients with a glomerular filtration rate of less than 60 ml/min/1.73 m^2 grow poorly.

The precise mechanism by which corticosteroids suppress growth is unknown; however, the introduction of alternate-day corticosteroid therapy has been associated with improved growth. At present, linear growth can be maximized following transplantation by maintenance of optimal allograft function and utilization of alternate-day corticosteroid therapy if possible.

Retransplantation

If the optimal therapeutic modality for children with ESRD of successful transplantation is to be achieved, retransplantation will be required with increasing frequency. At 5 years post-transplant, the actuarial survival rate for the second and third allografts is similar to the first (± 45%). The primary factor influencing retransplant allograft survival is patient responsiveness as reflected by sensitization with preformed lymphocytotoxic antibodies. Actuarial allograft survival rates for nonpresensitized (< 5%) and moderately presensitized (5 to 50%) recipients are significantly better than those of highly presensitized (> 50%) recipients. Although HLA A, B, and C antigen histocompatibility does not have a statistically significant effect on retransplant outcome, it appears to influence allograft survival in the highly presensitized recipients.

Long-Term Outcome

There are few reports describing the long-term follow-up of pediatric allograft recipients. Our experience of 69 children who received 81 renal allografts between 1967 and 1972 and were at risk for a minimum of 5 and a maximum of 10 years indicated that 78% of the patients were alive and 68% were surviving with a functioning allograft. The 5-year actual survival rate for 26 live donor first allografts, 42 first cadaver donor allografts, and 13 second cadaver donor allografts was 73%, 39%, and 62%, respectively. These data indicate the potential for long-term allograft survival in pediatric recipients.

Hemolytic-Uremic Syndrome

WARREN E. GRUPE, M.D.

The hemolytic uremic syndrome (HUS) comprises the familiar triad of hemolytic anemia, thrombocytopenia, and acute renal failure. In many areas, it is the most common cause of acute renal failure, while in others, it is the most common cause of bloody diarrhea. In most cases a precise etiology is elusive, but in some HUS appears in conjunction with viral infections, bacterial infections, drugs and chemicals, pregnancy, hypertension, immune deficiency syndromes, and carcinomatosis.

The usual case involves kidneys and blood; however, the colon, liver, heart, brain, and pancreas may also be involved to variable degrees. The common underlying injury appears to be small vessel endothelial damage that involves at least the glomerular capillary but can extend to larger renal vessels or to vessels in other organs. The mediator of the endothelial injury is not clear.

There is no specific treatment. Many therapeutic measures have been attempted, including heparin and other anticoagulants, steroids, exchange transfusion, fresh frozen plasma, plasmapheresis, splenectomy, antithrombin III, prostacyclin, streptokinase, urokinase, aspirin, and dipyridamole. Each measure has had proponents and reports of putative success, but none has clearly withstood the challenge of controlled study and none has been broadly accepted. The most successful results have been obtained when early vigorous supportive care has been provided.

Gastrointestinal Involvement

For most children, vomiting and diarrhea, with or without blood or mucus in the stool, precedes the onset of the full triad by a few days to a few weeks. Many of the infectious agents associated with HUS are also common causes of gastroenteritis, including shigella, salmonella, *Escherichia coli,* campylobacter, yersinia, coxsackie virus, and echovirus. Enteric pathogens should be sought by appropriate blood and stool cultures and treated suitably when found. Therapy for the diarrhea, other than bowel rest, is not required. Antispasmodics, antacids, or cimetidine do not alter the course of the disease. In fact, with altered renal function, magnesium-containing antacids are frankly contraindicated. Inevitably, the disease manifestations are limited to the colon. Management of dehydration follows the general principles of fluid and electrolyte therapy, both oral and parenteral.

Marked abdominal symptoms occur in 20% of the children. Occasionally, severe colonic disease can mimic ulcerative colitis, including classic radiographic alterations; gastrointestinal bleeding can require transfusion. At times, signs of acute peritoneal irritation are paramount, accompanied by dilatation and altered bowel sounds, suggesting bowel perforation. Severe complications have always been colonic, with the small bowel spared. Bowel changes have included ischemia and infarction, pseudomembranous colitis, toxic megacolon, and colonic perforation. On occasion, surgical exploration cannot be avoided, even though actual colonic perforation is quite rare. In these instances, a com-

promised and discolored colon, either diffusely or segmentally, is found, which suggests excision to the surgeon. This urge should be restrained, however, since most colons will recover completely when decompressed by a temporizing colostomy. Rarely, colonic stricture can develop at a later date. Severe colonic disease is not generally considered a part of HUS. The triad, in fact, may not have developed at the time of severe gastrointestinal disease and, unfortunately, may appear only after surgical intervention. That such can occur emphasizes that repeated, careful observation and a high index of suspicion is demanded.

Hepatocellular involvement is evidenced by an elevation in the serum levels of liver enzymes during the acute phases of the disease, often accompanied by hepatosplenomegaly. Jaundice is uncommon. No therapy is required. Diabetes mellitus, requiring insulin, has also been described; it usually disappears with resolution of the acute disease but may persist.

Hematologic Involvement

Coombs negative hemolytic anemia is almost always present, accompanied by thrombocytopenia and a peripheral smear that shows characteristic erythrocyte fragmentation. Anemia requires correction when the patient becomes symptomatic. Slow transfusion of packed red blood cells is used to keep the hematocrit above 16 to 18%. Thrombocytopenia appears to be the product of increased platelet consumption and decreased platelet production. Since transfused platelets are usually rapidly destroyed, platelet administration is restricted to periods when invasive procedures are required.

The presumption of a localized intravascular coagulopathy has greatly influenced the types of therapy tried. Although coagulation abnormalities have been demonstrated, the usual case has no evidence of disseminated intravascular coagulation at the time seen by a physician. Thus, there is little factual basis for anticoagulation, the results of which have been disappointing. Until recently, heparin has been the most commonly used agent. However, no significant differences have been found in the recovery of patients treated with or without heparin and the best results with heparin are no better than the results obtained with good supportive care alone. Many studies have noted a high incidence of hemorrhagic complications from anticoagulation and some reports have even claimed an increased mortality associated with the use of heparin.

Streptokinase and urokinase have been offered as activators of plasminogen to induce lysis of intravascular clots. No study has clearly shown an alteration in the acute disease and only one study has suggested that there is a late beneficial effect on the subsequent development of proteinuria and hypertension.

Although one uncontrolled report suggested that aspirin and dipyridamole were effective in 2 patients, a subsequent controlled study in 16 severely affected children failed to attenuate the clinical course by any parameter measured, including dialysis requirement, platelet count, evidence for hemolysis, normalization of blood pressure, or mortality. It is not clear that inhibition of platelet aggregation should be effective or that the thrombocytopenia has any relation to the mediators of endothelial injury. It has not been shown, for example, that maintenance of a normal platelet count favorably affects the outcome of the disease.

It has been postulated that the intravascular injury results from either the deficiency of a plasma component or the presence in the plasma of a toxic factor. The missing plasma factor has been postulated to be related to prostacyclin metabolism. Plasma exchange has been proposed as a means of either removing the toxic factor or replacing the essential plasma component. Plasma exchange and plasma infusion have been thought by some to improve platelet count and normalize antiplatelet aggregating activity, but to have no effect on renal function. Other studies, however, have failed to find the value of plasmapheresis in children. There is no evidence that steroids are useful.

Renal Involvement

Acute renal failure is the major challenge in HUS. Prompt and appropriate management of acute renal failure and its complications has produced the best effect on morbidity and mortality. The extent of renal insufficiency and the degree of derangement in renal metabolic regulation vary considerably between patients with HUS. The severity of the renal involvement can range from minor urinalysis abnormalities to frank bilateral cortical necrosis. The most threatening problems include hypertension, hypervolemia, hyperkalemia, metabolic acidosis, and hypocalcemia. The approach to therapy involves the integration of several interrelated facets. Successful therapy requires a team of physicians and nurses well versed in the intensive care of children and experienced in dialysis techniques.

Initial Supportive Measures. The severely oliguric patient may still have a prerenal component although hypervolemia is a more common condition in HUS. If renal resuscitation with fluid and electrolytes has already been adequate, attempts to ensure an adequate plasma volume need not be pursued. When present, hypovolemia should be corrected with IV replacement of 10 to 20 ml/kg over a 2- to 4-hour period of 5% dextrose containing 75 meq Na^+, 50 meq Cl^-, and 25 meq HCO^- (as $NaHCO_3$, Na-lactate, or Na-acetate) per liter, allowing for a definite rise in central venous pressure or an increase in weight. If urine output fails to increase with this effort, mannitol, 0.2 to 0.5 gm/kg IV as a 20% solution, may be infused, or furosemide, 1 mg/kg, may be given parenterally. No response to these two measures is clear evidence of an intrinsic renal problem, and any further attempts to increase urine flow by further overhydration invite calamity from cardiac failure or acute water intoxication.

Fluid Balance. Restriction of intake to match output capabilities now becomes mandatory. Fluid for a 6- to 8-hour time block should match the urine output and insensible loss of the previous 6- to 8-hour period. The calculation should be monitored through accurate weights, aiming to allow the child to lose 0.5 to 1% of body weight per day. During this period, fluid is generally administered as 10% dextrose in water. Solute may not be required in the first 24 hours and should be added thereafter according to demonstrated need through changes in serum levels and urinary losses. Other fluids given, such as plasma or blood, should be carefully counted in the total volume of intake.

Sodium Requirements. Sodium balance is usually maintained with 1 meq/kg/day or less. Provided fluid balance is accurately determined and maintained, sodium requirements can be determined by changes in the serum level and urinary output. Hyponatremia usually is a reflection of overhydration, although it can result from gastrointestinal losses or inadequate intake.

Hyperkalemia. Limitation of potassium intake in both diet and IV fluids to no more than urinary losses is mandatory; in practice, it is unusual in renal insufficiency that any exogenous potassium is required. Removal of potassium can be effected with sodium polystyrene sulfonate; 1 gm/kg of this ion exchange resin will decrease serum potassium 1 meq/l over a period of 1 to 3 hours when administered rectally as a 20 to 30% solution. Sorbitol may be added to prevent constipation.

For serum potassium concentrations above 6.5 to 7 meq/l, a more rapid effect is necessary. Other forms of treatment include sodium bicarbonate, 2 to 3 meq/kg IV; 1 unit of insulin per 3 to 4 gm of glucose IV; sodium lactate, 2 to 3 meq/kg IV; or calcium gluconate, 100 to 300 mg/kg IV. These maneuvers merely transfer potassium from one body compartment to another or counteract its cardiotoxic effect and do not effect a net removal from the body. Hence they are temporary and must be supplemented by exchange resin or dialysis.

Metabolic Acidosis. Acidosis usually can be managed by administration of 1 to 3 meq/kg/day of sodium bicarbonate or sodium lactate IV, or the same amount of sodium bicarbonate or citric acid/sodium citrate orally. The goal is to maintain serum bicarbonate levels between 15 and 20 meq/l; attempts to correct the serum bicarbonate totally or to correct it too rapidly can produce unwanted complications. Acidosis is generally well tolerated to serum bicarbonate levels below 10 meq/l.

Therapy for both hyperkalemia and acidosis involves sodium-containing agents. Unless the sodium is included in the patient's total intake, hypervolemia, hypernatremia, pulmonary congestion, or cardiac failure may result. Often dialysis for hyperkalemia or acidosis is dictated by the patient's inability to tolerate the sodium load of such therapy rather than specific problems with either potassium or hydrogen ion.

Diet. Catabolism contributes significantly to endogenous water production, acidosis, hyperkalemia, and hyperphosphatemia. As important as limiting intake and pharmacologic measures is the provision of adequate calories. A minimum of 20 to 30 cal/kg/day as carbohydrate and/or lipid is needed to minimize tissue breakdown. As much as 60% of the usual daily requirement may be necessary to reduce endogenous urea nitrogen generation.

Hypocalcemia. Occasionally hypocalcemia manifests as tetany or convulsions, particularly as acidosis is vigorously corrected. Symptomatic hypocalcemia can be treated intravenously with 10% calcium gluconate, 0.5 ml/kg over 4 hours, followed by oral calcium, as tolerated, in doses of 10 to 20 mg elemental calcium/kg/day.

Hyperphosphatemia. Serum phosphate is controlled by reduced protein intake and aluminum hydroxide, 50 to 150 mg/kg/day orally with meals.

Dialysis is indicated for 1) intractable hypervolemia with impending pulmonary edema, cardiac failure or uncontrolled hypertension; 2) hyperkalemia unresponsive to therapy; 3) metabolic acidosis unresponsive to therapy; 4) uremic symptoms of stupor, disorientation, or seizures; 5) serum sodium concentration < 120 meq/l or > 160 meq/l when more conservative management is unsuccessful. The choice of peritoneal dialysis or hemodialysis depends on the size of the patient and the experience of the medical team. In general, peritoneal dialysis is the method of choice, particularly in infants and younger children.

Neurologic Involvement

Central nervous system dysfunction is usually manifested as seizures, irritability, drowsiness, coma, or paresis. Frank hemorrhage is more common in patients treated with anticoagulants. Seizures are usually managed with anticonvulsants: diazepam, 0.2 mg/kg IV, for acute control and phenytoin, 5 to 10 mg/kg/day, for longer term management. Hypertensive encephalopathy, however, is best managed by a more stringent control of fluid balance and antihypertensives: diazoxide,* 3 to 5 mg/kg as a rapid IV bolus for acute control and either hydralazine, 0.5 to 5.0 mg/kg/day, and/

or propranolol,[†]1 to 10 mg/kg/day, for extended management.

Uremic metabolic encephalopathy is improved by intensive dialysis. Hyponatremia, the most common electrolyte abnormality, is usually the result of overhydration. A rapid fall in the serum sodium level accompanied by lethargy, stupor, or convulsions requires IV correction with 3% sodium chloride; a dose of 12 ml/kg should raise the serum sodium level by 10 meq/l.

Prognosis

With adequate management, acute mortality is less than 10%, and most children recover completely. Gastrointestinal and central nervous system sequelae are rare and progression to chronic renal failure occurs in less than 6%. A few patients have an unrelenting course with persistent hematologic abnormalities and a progressive loss of renal function; some in this group require bilateral nephrectomy to return the platelet count to normal. For a few others, a severe acute phase produces bilateral renal cortical necrosis wherein chronic renal insufficiency is retained even though the other aspects of the syndrome resolve completely. Recurrence has been reported following renal transplantation.

The early identification of those likely to have an unfavorable result is not assured. Nevertheless, some initial clinical findings are associated with a poor outcome. Anuria, malignant hypertension, and severe central nervous system involvement, alone or collectively, denote a more severe disorder. Isolated anuria or oliguria lasting more than 3 weeks often indicates a poor renal recovery.

Familial occurrence of HUS is associated with a poor prognosis when siblings develop the syndrome more than a year apart, while the appearance in siblings within a few days of each other does not increase mortality. The absence of a prodrome, an age over 5 years, and recurrent disease also imply a poor outcome. Sequelae of persistent proteinuria, hypertension, or a reduced creatinine clearance occur in 6 to 20% of cases. The long-term prognosis in these children is not clear.

Perinephritis and Perirenal Abscess

C. W. DAESCHNER, M.D.

Bacterial infection of the perirenal tissue is characterized by the acute onset of high septic fever, chills, malaise and *intense* local pain. The pain is unilateral, but localization to the flank, hip, psoas,

---

*Manufacturer's precautions: Safety in children has not been established.

†Manufacture's note: Data on the use of propranolol in the pediatric age group are too limited to permit adequate directions for use

or abdominal area depends upon the site and distribution of the primary process. The infection may originate from rupture of a septic renal cortical abscess, primary cellulitis of the perirenal tissue, or penetrating trauma. Although etiologic bacteria may vary widely, the staphylococcus is the most common offender. Broad antibiotic coverage is indicated unless the specific etiologic agent is known. Frequently surgical drainage will be necessary to release loculated pus before signs and symptoms are relieved. In recent years perinephritic infections have been uncommon.

Urinary Tract Infections

ALLAN J. WEINSTEIN, M.D.

GENERAL CONSIDERATIONS

Decisions regarding the treatment of urinary tract infections in children must be based on the age of the patient, the severity of symptoms, and the presence or absence of underlying structural defects of the genitourinary system. Neonates with urinary tract infections should be hospitalized and treated for sepsis, because of the high incidence of bacteremia associated with such infections. Neonatal urinary tract infection is more common in boys, and vesicoureteric reflux is present in approximately one half of the patients. Ampicillin (100–200 mg/kg/24 hours) and an aminoglycoside (gentamicin or tobramycin) should be administered. Ampicillin is administered in two divided doses in children less than 1 week of age and in three divided doses in older children. Gentamicin and tobramycin are given in doses of 5 mg/kg/24 hours in two divided doses in children less than 1 week of age and 7.5 mg/kg/24 hours in three divided doses in older children. Amikacin is not currently recommended for routine use in children.

Children with pyelonephritis should be hospitalized. After cultures have been obtained, antibiotic therapy should be administered to the infant or child with fever and other findings indicative of acute pyelonephritis. In such instances, the parenteral administration of full therapeutic doses of ampicillin (100–200 mg/kg/24 hours in four divided doses) is appropriate initial therapy. Gentamicin or tobramycin (5–7.5 mg/kg/24 hours in two to three divided doses) should also be given. Alterations in such therapy must be based on the results of culture and sensitivity studies and on the clinical response. Symptomatic treatment of fever and vomiting may be necessary. Adequate fluid intake is important. The therapy of pyelonephritis should be 10 to 14 days.

Children with less severe systemic symptoms and those with complaints limited to the lower urinary tract should receive supportive and symptomatic care. Antibacterial treatment may be initiated im-

mediately or may be withheld until the results of the urine culture are available. The initial selection of an antimicrobial agent may be guided by the results of a Gram-stain smear of the urinary sediment. Gram-positive cocci identified in the sediment usually are staphylococci or enterococci. These bacteria usually are susceptible to penicillin, ampicillin, amoxicillin, or nitrofurantoin. The gram-negative bacilli that produce urinary tract infections usually originate in the intestinal tract. If the patient has not recently received an antibacterial agent, infections due to such organisms are likely to be eradicated by sulfisoxazole, trimethoprim-sulfamethoxazole, nitrofurantoin, or ampicillin.

Relief of symptoms occurs within 48 hours when the organism is sensitive; if it is not, the sensitivities should be available to guide a change of the antibiotic. A follow-up urine culture should be obtained 2 to 4 days after the initiation of therapy. Bacteriuria is almost always eradicated within 24 to 48 hours following institution of effective treatment. Persistence of the bacteriuria usually indicates that the antimicrobial agent is ineffective in vivo and that a different agent should be selected. Urine cultures should be sterile before the medication is discontinued. Additional cultures should be taken 1 week and 6 weeks later. Subsequent urinalyses and cultures should be obtained for at least 2 to 3 years, since most recurrences develop during this period. The initial course of therapy should last 10 to 14 days. Failure to eradicate the infection or early emergence of a resistant organism suggests the presence of obstruction, calculus, or severe vesicoureteric reflux.

Supportive measures include a high fluid intake, which reduces renal medullary ammonium and osmolar concentrations, thereby enhancing phagocytosis and discouraging protoplast formation. The high urinary flow rate, aided by frequent bladder emptying and double micturition, may help to speed the elimination of bacteria from the urinary tract. Chronic constipation predisposes to recurrent infection and should also be treated. Vulvovaginitis, which may have precipitated the infection, usually responds to local management with neomycin cream, daily saline baths, and a change from nylon to cotton underwear.

ANTIBIOTIC SELECTION

The drugs regularly included in sensitivity testing for children with urinary tract infections are ampicillin, tetracycline, one of the cephalosporins, nalidixic acid, nitrofurantoin, trimethoprim-sulfamethoxazole, and the aminoglycosides. Specific features of some of the antibiotics deserve mention: Ampicillin is the recommended penicillin derivative for treating uncomplicated infections. This compound may be associated with the production of skin rash in non-penicillin allergic patients and may produce diarrhea. Amoxicillin is less irritating to the gastrointestinal tract. The tetracyclines should be avoided in children less than 8 years of age because they may cause a permanent yellow discoloration of the teeth. The cephalosporins are active against *Escherichia coli, Proteus mirabilis,* and many strains of *Klebsiella pneumoniae.* Cephalexin and cefadroxil are usually reserved for the treatment of infection produced by resistant organisms or for patients who cannot tolerate other drugs. Nalidixic acid* may be useful. However, repeated courses of therapy may be associated with the development of bacterial resistance, and nalidixic acid may produce increased intracranial pressure in children less than 3 months of age. Enteric bacteria usually remain susceptible to nitrofurantoin despite many courses of therapy; this is apparently related to the fact that very little of the drug appears in the stool. However, the nitrofurantoins may produce hemolytic anemia in children less than 1 month of age. Drugs containing sulfonamides are contraindicated in children less than 2 months of age, since enzymes that acetylate sulfonamides are poorly developed in newborns. Sulfonamides also may be associated with the development of bone marrow suppression and Stevens-Johnson syndrome. Antimicrobial suppression with methenamine mandelate is ineffective, and it is generally not administered to children with urinary tract infections.

Short-Course Therapy

Since most antibiotics used to treat urinary tract infections are excreted by the kidneys, high and relatively prolonged concentrations of these agents are achieved in the urine. Following a single large dose, or a conventional dose, drug concentrations in the urine may reach 1000 times that of the peak serum concentration and may exceed the minimal bactericidal concentration for many pathogens for 24 hours or longer. Such pharmacologic factors have been exploited in adults with lower urinary tract infections, and short course (3 days) or single dose therapy has become accepted practice in such individuals.

The advantages of short course therapy are improved compliance, lower drug costs, and fewer untoward effects of treatment. Furthermore, since a short course of therapy may place less selective pressure on bacteria colonizing the intestine and perineum, susceptible organisms are less likely to be replaced by more resistant strains, thus diminishing the likelihood of the subsequent development of an urinary tract infection due to resistant bacteria.

There is not yet adequate information to permit the utilization of short course therapy for urinary

tract infections in children. Short course therapy is effective for certain patients, those with infection limited to the lower urinary tract. However, at present there is no practical and reliable clinical or laboratory technique for precise identification of this group of children.

Recurrent and Persistent Infections

Ten to 14 days of therapy usually are as effective as longer courses in preventing recurrent infections. In the group of children with recurrent infections, which may range from 36 to 80% of patients, 20% will be cured of subsequent urinary tract infections with each succeeding treatment. The development of three or more urinary tract infections per year may be an indication for the institution of long-term antimicrobial prophylaxis.

Twenty to 35% of girls with asymptomatic bacteriuria have vesicoureteral reflux. Persistent asymptomatic bacteriuria in a girl with a radiologically normal urinary tract probably is the most common urinary tract disorder of childhood. Many of these patients have had symptomatic urinary tract infections before asymptomatic bacteriuria has been detected and they may have developed episodes of clinical cystitis on subsequent occasions. Treatment appears to have no effect on the emergence of symptoms, the clearance of vesicoureteral reflux, the growth of kidneys, or the progression of renal scars. It is unusual for girls with persistent asymptomatic bacteriuria and radiologically normal urinary tracts to develop acute clinical pyelonephritis or renal scars. Some have suggested that asymptomatic bacteriuria in a school-age girl with a radiologically normal urinary tract should not be treated since elimination of the bacteria may predispose these children to reinfection with more pathogenic microorganisms and subsequent symptomatic recurrences. Although long-term data are not available, no therapy may be a reasonable alternative to continuous therapy or repeated courses of treatment for asymptomatic bacteriuria in the school-age girl with a radiologically normal urinary tract.

Low-dose antibiotic treatment for months or years has been advocated to encourage normal growth of the remaining healthy tissue in children with scarred kidneys, to prevent scarring in those with vesicoureteric reflux, as previously noted, and to relieve symptoms in those with incapacitating recurrent infections. Such programs reduce the number of recurrences but have not been shown to prevent renal scarring. Intermittent therapy appears to have little effect upon the development of new renal scars or upon the renal growth rate in the presence of reflux. Although reflux may cause infection to persist in the untreated child, there is little evidence to suggest that reflux or scarring significantly increases the susceptibility to recurrent

*Manufacturer's precaution: Until further experience is gained, nalidixic acid should not be administered to children younger than 3 months.

infections. Long-term antibiotic prophylaxis should be administered to children with significant vesicoureteric reflux, those with frequent recurrent symptomatic urinary tract infections, and those with recurrent infections superimposed on impaired renal function. Surgical therapy may be indicated if infection cannot be controlled or when there is significant renal scarring.

Eighty per cent of acute or chronic urinary tract infections are produced by organisms that originate from the bowel or this periurethral flora, and the antibiotic selected for prophylaxis should not induce antibiotic resistance in them. Trimethoprim-sulfamethoxazole reduces the number of coliform bacteria while leaving the sensitivity of the remaining microorganisms unaltered, and resistant bowel flora rarely appear during treatment with nitrofurantoin or methenamine mandelate. However, the emergence of resistant organisms is frequently associated with sulfonamide or nalidixic acid therapy. The failure of trimethoprim-sulfamethoxazole and nitrofurantoin to provoke resistance correlates well with their ability to prevent urinary infections in girls. However, reinfections in boys originate from the preputial sac, and changes in bowel microflora may be less important.

Long-term therapy should be used with caution in patients with chronic renal failure, and some drugs, such as nitrofurantoin, should not be given. Nalidixic acid also is unsuitable because of the risk in children of intracranial hypertension. Ampicillin is inadvisable because of its association with the rapid development of bacterial resistance. In the event of a "break-through" infection, prophylactic therapy should be interrupted by a 2-week course of the appropriate antimicrobial agent administered at full dose.

Urolithiasis

GEORGE W. KAPLAN, M.D.,
and WILLIAM A. BROCK, M.D.

The treatment of stone disease in children, as in adults, can be divided into phases. The management of the acute aspects of stones is dictated largely by the presence or absence of urinary infection or urinary obstruction as well as the control of pain. When a child presents acutely with a stone, the pain is often severe. Consequently, potent narcotics are usually necessary for adequate pain relief. In our opinion, morphine in full therapeutic doses affords the best pain relief and is thus the drug of choice. Although morphine theoretically causes smooth muscle spasm and might be thought to delay stone passage, in practice this does not seem to be a factor. The pain of the acute passage of a stone may cause severe vomiting and, for this reason, in-

travenous fluids may be desirable during this phase. Also, good hydration tends to produce a diuresis which may aid in stone passage.

Urinalysis and urine culture should be obtained early, to look for specific evidence of urinary infection as well as crystalluria. Urine pH may also provide a clue to the type of stone present. If the patient is febrile, infection should be considered present until proved absent, and antibiotics should be given promptly. An intravenous urogram or renal ultrasound study should be obtained early in the course to determine the presence or absence of urinary tract obstruction. Additionally, knowledge of the radiodensity of an obstructing stone is a clue to its composition.

Although urinary obstruction may lead to renal damage over a period of time (weeks to months), in the short term it does not seem to be harmful. Inasmuch as many small stones (less than 5 mm in longest diameter) will pass spontaneously even in small children, one may often use expectant therapy, provided adequate pain relief can be afforded during this period. Despite the fact that obstruction is well tolerated for short periods of time, the combination of obstruction and infection is not, and it can rapidly lead to renal deterioration or sepsis. In these situations urgent intervention may be necessary.

Large stones in the renal pelvis and intravesical calculi rarely present as an acute problem. Acute problems usually are produced by impacted ureteral or urethral stones. Ureteral stones usually impact at either the ureteropelvic junction or the ureterovesical junction. If intervention is deemed necessary, one may either temporize by providing urinary drainage (by percutaneous or open nephrostomy, ureteral catheterization, or cystostomy, depending on the location of the stone) or definitively remove the stone. If removal of the stone is chosen, direct operative removal is usually necessary in children. The endoscopic techniques that are so applicable to the adult are rarely employed in children, as the complication rates in children, in our opinion, far outweigh the benefits.

In patients with larger stones presenting as chronic problems of either obstruction or infection, operative removal is usually necessary. Large staghorn calculi are best removed surgically rather than left in situ, as their long-term presence leads to renal deterioration in most cases. It is axiomatic that the presence of urinary infection in the face of stone disease is unlikely to be resolved until the stone is removed.

A discussion of the types of operative procedures employed in the removal of stones is beyond the scope of this presentation, but the procedures include nephrolithotomy, pyelolithotomy, ureterolithotomy, cystolithotomy, and urethrotomy. Stone fragments that remain following removal of large struvite stones often can be dissolved with solutions such as hemiacidrin or Suby's G solution through indwelling nephrostomy or cystostomy tubes. Great care must be taken to ensure that the urine is sterile and that there is no obstruction to outflow if these adjunctive techniques are employed. (Hemiacidrin [Renacidin] is not approved by the FDA for supravesical use. Nonetheless, it has been demonstrated to be both safe and efficacious when properly used [JAMA 215:1470, 1971].)

Although stone disease often presents as an acute event, some patients with stones will experience recurrence of their problem; for this reason one must search for clues to the etiology of the stone's genesis. Analysis of the recovered stone to determine its composition is essential to further management, as this is an excellent clue to etiology. If it is anticipated that a stone will be passed spontaneously, all urine should be strained so that the stone may be recovered after it is passed and then submitted for analysis. Stones removed operatively should be analyzed and cultured.

Urinary stasis may predispose the patient to stone disease; consequently, any congenitally obstructing lesions present in association with stone formation (for example, ureteropelvic junction obstruction) should be corrected surgically to prevent further stone formation. Similarly, a urinary infection with *Proteus* species may predispose the patient to stone formation; once such a stone has been removed the patient should receive vigorous antibiotic therapy to eradicate infection, if possible. Patients receiving corticosteroids and those immobilized for fractures experience bone demineralization; these patients may form stones because of the increased urinary calcium levels produced. Renal tubular acidosis type I similarly is associated with nephrolithiasis and occasionally with stone formation. A secondary form of renal tubular acidosis occurs in children receiving Diamox (carbonic anhydrase inhibitor) for seizure disorders or glaucoma, and stones have been reported in such patients.

Two other metabolic disorders that produce stones are important to identify because the stones produced are both preventable and treatable by medical means. Patients with cystinuria often form stones; these stones may be prevented by high fluid intake and urinary alkalinization. Similarly, cystine stones have been noted to dissolve on such a regimen in patients with known cystine stone disease. In recalcitrant cases of cystinuria, D-penicillamine may be effective.

Uric acid stones are produced in patients with hyperuricemia (e.g., patients with large amounts of tissue breakdown due to malignancy or those with Lesch-Nyhan syndrome). Uric acid stones, again, can be prevented by forced fluids and urinary alkalinization. Allopurinol, by preventing uric acid formation, is also helpful in the management of uric

acid urolithiasis. A rare metabolic form of calculous disease is xanthinuria, which is also occasionally seen in patients receiving allopurinol to prevent uric acid stones. Xanthine stones may be prevented by forced fluids and urinary alkalinization, but, unfortunately, these stones are very poorly soluble and consequently cannot usually be dissolved, once formed.

Hyperoxaluria may occur on either a dietary or a familial basis. Additionally, hyperoxaluria is seen in patients with inflammatory bowel disease. Oxalate stones occasionally can be prevented by the use of cholestyramine, vitamin B_6, or inorganic phosphates, but once they have formed they are treatable only surgically, as they are not dissolvable. The various hypercalciuric states so commonly seen in adults are uncommon in children in our experience. Hence only in patients with calcium oxalate or calcium phosphate stones and no other predisposing causes for stones (e.g., stasis, immobilization) is a metabolic evaluation for these types of problems warranted.

Vesicoureteral Reflux

TERRY W. HENSLE, M.D.,
and KEVIN A. BURBIGE, M.D.

The understanding and management of vesicoureteral reflux (VUR) continues to stir controversy, as evidenced by the ever expanding literature. The prevalence of silent VUR in the general population is probably on the order of 0.5%. However, it may be detected in up to 75% of children undergoing urologic evaluation for recurrent urinary tract infection and in up to 25% of their siblings. Infection, then, would seem to be the marker for identifying a population at risk.

Abnormalities of the normal passive valve mechanism of the ureterovesical junction that predispose to VUR include a deficiency of the longitudinal muscle layer of the submucosal ureter (short tunnel), an ectopic insertion of the ureter into the bladder, and deficient muscular support of the submucosal ureter (paraureteral diverticulum). The ratio of submucosal tunnel length to ureteral diameter would seem to be the major determinant in preventing VUR. VUR is generally accepted as a primary lesion of the ureterovesical junction and is not due to obstruction at the bladder neck, as was once thought.

The diagnostic tools best suited for detecting VUR and determining its severity are the excretory urogram, the voiding cystourethrogram, and, to a much lesser extent, cystoscopy. The radionuclide cystogram is a very adequate means of following VUR once it has been identified on a standard voiding cystourethrogram. The radionuclide study can

Table 1. VESICOURETERAL REFLUX GRADING SYSTEM

Grade I—VUR into the lower ureter only

Grade II—ureteral and pelvic filling without caliceal dilatation

Grade III—ureteral and pelvic filling with mild caliceal blunting

Grade IV—marked distention of pelvis, calices, and ureter

Grade V—massive VUR associated with severe hydronephrosis

be done with much less radiation exposure but cannot be used to quantify VUR initially. Radiologic evaluation of the child with a history of urinary tract infection is best done when the urine is sterile after antibiotic treatment. The degree of VUR is characterized by a grading system (Table 1).

The aim of treatment is preservation of renal parenchyma, maintenance of renal function, and elimination of urinary infection. Factors to be considered when planning treatment are the grade of VUR, chronicity of the symptoms, number and severity of infections, presence of anatomic urinary tract abnormalities, and the patient's ability to adhere to a treatment program.

MEDICAL MANAGEMENT

It has yet to be shown that sterile VUR in the absence of increased voiding pressures causes renal damage. Therefore, if medical management is chosen it is extremely important that a sterile urine be achieved and continuous antibiotic prophylaxis be maintained until the VUR has subsided. Children with less than Grade III VUR are usually managed medically, since there is about an 80% probability of spontaneous resolution. As somatic growth progresses, the submucosal ureter will lengthen and VUR will often cease.

During this period of waiting, a sulfamethoxazole/trimethoprim*combination (Bactrim, Septra) or nitrofurantoin (Furadantin)† is most commonly used for prophylaxis, at about half the usual therapeutic dose. In the elixir form these are well tolerated by most children, have a high concentration in the urine and vaginal epithelium, and do not significantly alter bowel flora. In following patients, a urine culture should be obtained every 4 to 8 weeks and can be done at home by a dip slide method. A CBC should be done routinely every 3 months in children suppressed with sulfamethoxazole/trimethoprim in order to detect early signs of bone marrow depression, which is infrequent but must be recognized.

An excretory urogram and voiding cystourethrogram (conventional or radionuclide) should be done once a year to monitor renal growth and persistence or absence of VUR. Adjunctive measures such as good perineal hygiene and a frequent voiding schedule may also help to prevent lower tract infection in the female child who is an infrequent voider. Repetitive cystoscopy, meatotomy, urethral dilatation, and internal urethrotomy should be avoided unless significant pathology can be demonstrated radiologically and on urodynamic evaluation.

SURGICAL TREATMENT

The major indications for antireflux surgery are the presence of a significant anatomic abnormality at the ureterovesical junction, recurrent urinary tract infection despite continuous antibiotic therapy, high grades of VUR, noncompliance with medical therapy, intolerance to antibiotics, and VUR after puberty in the female. Children with high grades of VUR and dilated ureters due to VUR (grades IV and V) have only a 40% probability of spontaneous cessation of their VUR. Surgical intervention is generally required earlier in this group than in children with a lesser degree of VUR.

The Cohen cross trigone and Politano-Leadbetter methods of ureteral reimplantation are the most reliable and most often performed antireflux procedures. Creation of an adequate submucosal tunnel can be accomplished by either procedure; the success rate is over 97% when done by surgeons with appropriate pediatric urologic experience.

Cystitis may occur in approximately 20% of children following antireflux surgery but pyelonephritis is rare. Postoperatively antibiotics are continued until a voiding cystourethrogram demonstrates a successful result with no further VUR. Excretory urograms are done prior to discharge from the hospital, and at 3 months, 1 year, and 3 years after surgery to assess renal growth. Interestingly, accelerated renal growth may be observed in some children after successful surgery.

The medical and surgical managements of VUR are not competitive, and there are clear indications for each. The goal is the same, to protect renal parenchyma and maintain renal function.

Neurogenic Bladder

KEVIN A. BURBIGE, M.D.,
and TERRY W. HENSLE, M.D.

Neuropathic voiding dysfunction in childhood can be secondary to many different primary etiologies (Table 1); in general, however, myelomeningocele is the most common cause in children. Our treatment approach is based on the myelodysplastic child; however, the general principles are applicable to most forms of neurogenic bladder. Ex-

---

*Manufacturer's warning: Not recommended for children less than 2 months of age.

†Manufacturer's warning: Not recommended for children less than 1 month of age.

Table 1. VOIDING DYSFUNCTION IN CHILDREN

Neurological
  Myelomeningocele
  Sacral agenesis
  Spinal cord trauma
  Spinal cord tumors
  CNS tumors
  Spinal dysraphism
  CNS inflammation

Functional
  Enuresis
  Non-neurogenic neurogenic bladder
  Urinary tract infection

Anatomic
  Exstrophy
  Severe epispadias
  Posterior urethral valves
  Lower urinary tract trauma
  Urethral stricture

perience has proved that a coordinated multidisciplinary effort by the pediatrician, neurosurgeon, orthopedist, and urologist will provide the best overall care for the myelodysplastic child. Just as critical is the presence of nursing and support personnel specifically skilled in the care of these patients. The goals of urologic treatment of the myelodysplastic child are basically three: preservation of renal function, control of urinary tract infection, and socially acceptable urinary continence.

The bony abnormality of myelomeningocele occurs most commonly in the lumbosacral region (80%) but the level of neurologic impairment may vary. A differential growth rate of the bony somites and developing vertebral arches in relation to the neural tube accounts for the apparent foreshortening of the spinal cord in the developing fetus with myelomeningocele. Nerves at or below the level of the bony defect are generally most affected, but owing to this differential growth rate, proximal nerve root damage may also occur. Most children with myelomeningocele will have a lower motor neuron lesion of the bladder (detrusor hyporeflexia), although an upper motor neuron lesion (detrusor hyperreflexia) is seen in almost 30%.

The urologic evaluation of the myelodysplastic child should begin in the neonatal period, and should include a urinalysis, urine culture, and renal function studies as well as an excretory urogram or renal ultrasonography. The vast majority of these babies will have normal renal function and normal appearing urinary tracts by either imaging technique. Careful follow-up at regular intervals will facilitate early detection of renal deterioration; therefore, repeat excretory urography or ultrasonography should be done at 6 months of age and then yearly until age 10 years, when follow-up should be individualized. A voiding cystourethrogram should be part of the evaluation if there is a history of urinary infection, and probably should be performed in all myelodysplastic children along with the annual upper tract studies in order to assess bladder configuration and emptying.

Urodynamic testing may provide important information relative to bladder management in the child with a neurogenic bladder. This testing should include measurement of intravesical pressure during filling and voiding (cystometrogram phase) as well as simultaneous measurement of urinary flow rate (uroflow) and electromyography of the external urinary sphincter. These studies combined with measurement of a urethral pressure profile constitute a full urodynamic evaluation. The goal of urodynamic testing is to identify neuromuscular abnormalities not readily definable by routine neurologic examination or standard radiographic evaluation.

Simply stated, the bladder has two primary functions, urine storage and urine emptying, and both can be adversely affected in myelodysplastic children. In order to facilitate urine emptying, several options are available. In some few infants and young children the Credé maneuver, manual expression of bladder urine by suprapubic pressure, may be effective. Credé, however, has inherent drawbacks, and if post-Credé residuals become elevated or if there are signs of upper tract deterioration, another method should be selected. Credé is definitely contraindicated in the presence of vesicoureteral reflux or if significant outlet resistance is present. Just as outmoded are medications such as bethanechol chloride (Urecholine), which have been used to facilitate bladder emptying and have proved to be of little benefit in the hyporeflexic bladder.

Clean intermittent catheterization is the single most important advance in bladder emptying and has largely altered the treatment of children with neuropathic voiding dysfunction secondary to myelomeningocele. The bladder is emptied at regular intervals by means of a small caliber catheter, using clean but not sterile technique. Clean intermittent catheterization is a simple and straightforward procedure easily performed by the parent or child, and urine sterility can be monitored on a routine basis by an inexpensive home culture method.

In terms of urine storage, adjunctive pharmacologic therapy is usually required to facilitate continence, and the use of these drugs should be based on both clinical and urodynamic findings. If uninhibited bladder contractures (hyper-reflexia) are producing incontinence, an anticholinergic medicine (Pro-Banthine, Ditropan) may be helpful. When outlet resistance is low, an alpha adrenergic agent (Ornade, Ephedrine) may increase outlet resistance. If continued incontinence is due to poor bladder emptying (overflow) or there is any upper tract dilatation, then clean intermittent catheterization is indicated in association with the use of these drugs. These medications, used alone or in combination with clean intermittent catheterization, will in most cases produce a reasonable degree of continence. Low dose prophylactic antibiotics are often added to the regimen; however, their use is not universally advocated. Procedures designed to lower bladder outlet resistance, such as transurethral resection of the bladder neck, sphincterotomy, and overdilatation of the urethra, should be avoided since they may damage whatever continence mechanism is present.

In general, urinary incontinence is no longer an absolute indication for permanent urinary diversion. In selected instances diversion by means of a nonrefluxing colon or ileocecal conduit may be required if clean intermittent catheterization is not technically feasible or upper tract deterioration continues despite appropriate conservative therapy. Temporary urinary diversion may be a reasonable alternative in a very young infant until the age of expected continence, when clean intermittent catheterization can be instituted, and cutaneous vesicostomy is probably the best method for this temporary diversion.

In summary, the urologic care of the child with neuropathic bladder dysfunction requires a thorough evaluation including clinical, radiologic, and urodynamic modalities. Follow-up evaluation is lifelong and therapy is directed at the preservation of renal function, the control of urinary infection, and establishing socially acceptable urinary continence.

Exstrophy of the Bladder

PANAYOTIS P. KELALIS, M.D.,
and CHARLES N. GLASSMAN, M.D.

Exstrophy is nearly always associated with complete epispadias. Only rarely is the penis formed, and then the open bladder needs to be dealt with. If the infant who has been born with exstrophy can be cared for within the first 48 hours of life, the bladder should be closed primarily. The quality of the mucosa is satisfactory and the presence of maternal circulating hormones makes closure of both the bladder and the abdominal wall with a few sutures much easier; osteotomy is therefore obviated. Otherwise, treatment should be deferred, provided the excretory urogram shows that the kidneys are normal.

Some time during the first year of life, re-evaluation is done. If the bladder is of good size and is easily inverted and the mucosa is of satisfactory quality, primary closure again should be attempted; this will convert the problem to one of complete epispadias. We use this approach without osteotomy, and we use abdominal wall flaps to breach the suprapubic defect. Almost always, elongation of the penis will be necessary, after which repair of the epispadias is carried out several months later. Reflux is universal, and some form of antireflux surgery will also become necessary; this should be carried out in combination with vesical neck plasty in an attempt to produce continence. All attempts at reconstruction should be completed before school age, and the goal should be to provide a boy with a good-sized penis, urinary control, and normal kidneys.

In female patients, the urethra is closed at the time of the anti-incontinence procedure, and the bifid clitoris is corrected by rotation of skin flaps in order to improve cosmetic appearance and distribution of hair in the suprapubic area. A vaginoplasty may be necessary some time after puberty; the possibility of hematocolpos always exists.

It is imperative that one follow the integrity of the upper urinary tract closely, and any deterioration indicates the need to abandon efforts at achieving continuity of the urinary conduit in favor of a sigmoid conduit diversion with antireflux ureterocolonic anastomosis.

Of course, if the bladder is not satisfactory for primary closure because it is too small or fibrotic, a permanent urinary diversion should be considered from the start. Ureterosigmoidostomy some time after age 2 years, together with simultaneous cystectomy and closure of the urethra, is one of the choices, provided that anal prolapse or other difficulties with fecal control have been excluded with certainty. Some evidence suggests that in children with this type of urinary diversion somatic growth is generally well below normal. For this reason we prefer a diverting procedure via the sigmoid conduit with an antireflux anastomosis of the ureters to this unit. This appears to prevent the difficulty with growth, provided that the kidneys are normal and the presence of ureteral reflux has been excluded by a sigmoidogram. An undiversion is carried out where the sigmoid loop is anastomosed to the sigmoid colon by an end-to-side anastomosis. This is done some time before puberty to prevent the untoward psychologic effects of the urinary stoma and external appliance.

Patent Urachus and Urachal Cysts

PANAYOTIS P. KELALIS, M.D.,
and CHARLES N. GLASSMAN, M.D.

If the urachus, the fibrous remnant of the allantois, has not been obliterated at birth, it will often become sealed within the neonatal period. Only rarely will there be failure of complete urachal closure. Depending on where failure occurs, one of four types of urachal anomalies will result.

The most common type, *patent urachus,* results when complete communication exists between the bladder and the umbilicus. Urine is seen leaking from the umbilical area, and the disorder can be confirmed by demonstrating intravenously administered dye appearing on the abdominal wall. However, cystourethrography is recommended, not only to outline the fistula but also to evaluate the urethra, for up to 25% of these patients have some degree of outlet obstruction. Early treatment is recommended in order to avoid the complications of urinary tract infections, sepsis, and calculus formation. Elimination of the infravesical obstruction, if present, and complete extraperitoneal excision of the tract, including umbilicus and bladder cuff, have yielded the most success.

When the urachus fails to become obliterated at its most caudal attachment to the bladder, a *vesicourachal diverticulum* will result. Again, cystourethrography will outline this beaking of the bladder dome. As in patent urachus, this disorder may appear in conjunction with bladder outlet obstruction, but it is unique in its frequent association with prune-belly syndrome. These diverticula are rarely symptomatic, and they should be locally excised only when associated with infection resulting from poor diverticular emptying.

An *external urachal sinus* occurs when only the vesical communication of the urachus closes. The patent umbilical end often has a chronic or intermittent discharge and is prone to omphalitis with granuloma formation. Rarely, with temporary plugging of the umbilical side, an infected sinus will dissect retrograde and empty into the bladder. A fistulogram is useful in determining the extent of the sinus, and cystoscopy occasionally will demonstrate a reddened area of the bladder dome. Because of the frequency of recurrent infection, complete excision is recommended. It is often difficult to distinguish this entity from remnants of the vitelline duct, and one should therefore be prepared to identify and remove such structures if they are encountered.

Finally, when the urachal lumen is incompletely obliterated along its tract, this potential epithelium-lined space makes possible the development of a *urachal cyst.* These cysts generally remain small and asymptomatic, but they become apparent when their size or a secondary infection leads to symptomatic complaints. Such cysts are usually found in adults, often with the resected cyst dissecting to create a urachal sinus. Urachal cysts are best treated initially by incision and drainage followed by complete excision, as previously described.

Tumors of the Bladder and Prostate; Disorders of the Lower Urinary Tract

MOHAMMAD H. MALEKZADEH, M.D.

BENIGN TUMORS

Benign tumors of the bladder in children, although rare, include hemangioma, lymphohemangioma, neurofibroma, fibroma, fibromyoma, and papilloma.

The presenting symptoms are those of urinary tract obstruction if the tumor invades the vesical neck or ureters, plus hematuria.

Treatment consists of cystoscopic examination with transurethral resection or surgical excision, depending upon the age of the child and the site of the tumor. Surgical intervention is mandatory for hemangiomas because life-threatening bleeding is possible. Papillomas are considered Grade I carcinomas and should be resected or excised. There should be a follow-up by periodic roentgenologic and cystoscopic examinations. Recurrence is uncommon and has only been reported in a few children.

RHABDOMYOSARCOMA OF THE BLADDER AND PROSTATE

The bladder is the most common urologic site of this tumor, with a male to female ratio of 2:1. Most reported cases are in children less than 5 years of age, with the majority less than 3 years of age.

Rhabdomyosarcomas of the prostate are similar to those arising from the bladder, but are more solid, rather than the botryoid type. The age of onset is usually between 3 and 5 years of age. Characteristically, the symptoms are those of obstruction, often complicated by infection and only rarely by hematuria.

Treatment involves radical surgical extirpation of the tumor and adjacent structures along with radiotherapy and a triple chemotherapeutic regimen of actinomycin D, cyclophosphamide, and vincristine. The survival rate is very poor. Radical surgical approach offers survival of from 8 to 10 months. The multitherapeutic approach has increased the survival rate fourfold.

DISORDERS OF LOWER URINARY TRACT

Presenting symptoms and signs of lower urinary tract disorders in children include repeated urinary tract infection, dysuria, hematuria, frequency, incontinence, abdominal mass, and poor urinary stream, often requiring thorough urologic investigation. Evaluation includes urinalysis, urine culture, renal function tests, renal ultrasound, renal scan with Lasix washout, urinary cystourethrogram, intravenous pyelography, and urodynamic studies. Cystoscopic examination may be indicated in selected patients.

Urinary tract dysfunction with vesicoureteral reflux can be due to an anatomic abnormality or to incoordination between the bladder and the urinary sphincter.

Anatomic abnormalities of the bladder and sphincter are as follows: a) short or absent intravesical ureter, seen in girls with larger than expected bladders and infrequent voiding; b) ureteral ectopia; c) paraureteral diverticula with or without bladder neck obstruction; and d) iatrogenic abnormalities following incision of ureterocele or after ureteral reimplantation. Surgical correction is determined by the following factors: reflux persisting beyond the first decade of life; failed conservative management of urinary infections; dilation of collecting system with blunting of calyceal tip; golf-hole ureteral orifices with minimal or totally absent submucosal tunnel; and lack of family willingness to cooperate and noncompliance with a long-term medical regimen. All these conditions are indications for surgical intervention.

In neurologically normal children, the disorders of vesicourethral function that are significant enough to cause urinary tract infection and reflux represent abnormalities of toilet training and disturbances in the development of normal urinary control.

These problems can be subdivided according to whether the dysfunction occurs during bladder filling or bladder emptying. The infantile, or so called uninhibited, bladder is common in childhood. Because uninhibited contractions are involuntary and unsuppressible, the child in attempting to maintain continence during such contractions must voluntarily and tightly constrict the urinary sphincter. One sign frequently observed in little girls that is almost pathognomonic of detrusor-sphincter dysergia is the Vincent curtsy, so named because while the child is playing, she suddenly squats and, with the heel of one foot, compresses the perineum and urethra to prevent urinary leakage.

Urinary tract infection due to high intravesical pressure is a frequent complicating event. In addition, trabeculation, diverticula, and abnormalities of ureteral orifices with reflux in the absence of anatomic obstruction have been observed regularly.

Anticholinergic drugs are used to reduce detrusor hyperactivity, to enlarge the functional capacity of the bladder and to increase intravesical threshold, which delays the initial desire to void. Oxybutynin, a long acting anticholinergic and antispasmodic medication, is now being used. The initial dosage is 5 mg two or three times a day. The dosage should be titrated against anticholinergic side effects. In addition, frequent micturition and fluid restriction help to minimize bladder volume and residue.

Detrusor-sphincter dysfunction during bladder emptying occurs in meningomyelocele with neurogenic bladder and in children without neurologic problems.

Children with neurogenic bladders often have involuntary sphincter constriction during bladder contractions. Children with non-neurogenic, neurogenic bladder have incontinence, fecal retention, soiling, and emotional disturbances. Bladder trabeculation, diverticula, reflux, and hydronephrosis are often present. Treatment consists of intermittent bladder catheterization, frequent voiding with double or triple micturition, pharmacotherapy, biofeedback techniques, hypnosis, and bladder retraining.

Neurogenic bladder is always present in meningomyelocele, spina bifida, sacral agenesis, spinal cord tumors, traumatic paraplegia, transverse myelitis, and spinal dysraphism. Because of inadequate emptying, urinary stasis and urinary infection are common. Hydronephrosis may be present at birth. Reflux is uncommon in newborns but increases with age. An intravenous pyelogram should be performed as soon as possible and should be repeated every 2 years.

Monthly urinalysis and urine culture should be done. Urinary tract infection should be treated with appropriate antibiotics. Once the meningomyelocele closure has healed, bladder emptying with the Credé maneuver at regular intervals should be done. Males with incontinence by age 5 can be fitted with a suitable penile appliance. In females with urinary incontinence by age 5, urinary diversion is indicated. A thick walled, trabeculated bladder may produce an obstruction at the ureterovesical junction such that resection of the bladder neck and external sphincter will not produce improvement. In this situation, urinary diversion is indicated, even in males. The major criterion in the decision concerning urinary diversion is preservation of renal function; therefore, supravesical diversion is indicated in any child with neurogenic bladder who shows progressive biochemical, radiographic, and clinical changes in the upper tracts.

Abdominal muscle deficiency, severe urinary tract abnormalities, and cryptorchidism together form a condition known as prune-belly syndrome in which there is abrupt transition from an extremely wide prostatic urethra to a narrowed distal portion of urethra, caused by agenesis or hypoplasia of the prostate. In fact, intravesical pressure is abnormally low in prune-belly syndrome. Management should be conservative to prevent urinary tract infection. Urinary diversion is seldom necessary and should be done only after careful urodynamic studies that document anatomic obstruction.

Infants with posterior urethral valves usually need prompt attention. There is increased intravesical pressure with varying degrees of hydronephrosis. In severe obstruction, the newborn may develop urinary ascites. Uremia, electrolyte abnormalities, failure to thrive, and infection may be present. Management is directed toward fluid and electrolyte correction, treatment of documented infection, and urinary decompression. Once the infant's condition has been stabilized with proper fluid and electrolyte balance, control of infection, and improvement of renal function, surgical resection of valves should be attempted. If successful, urinary undiversion should be done, if previous diversion had been necessary. Prognosis depends on the degree of obstruction, degree of associated renal dysplasia, and adequacy of renal function. If renal dysplasia is severe, renal function will not improve and a chronic renal failure regimen should be instituted.

Nephrogenic diabetes insipidus is due to end organ unresponsiveness to antidiuretic hormone, leading to marked polyuria. The mode of inheritance is X-linked dominant with varying expressivity in the heterozygous female. Marked and prolonged polyuria results in bladder enlargement with an overloaded reservoir. Repeated voluntary retention and increasing tolerance of an overfull bladder are aggravating factors. Relative indistensibility of the ureter in the presence of a marked increased urine flow will lead to a functional obstruction, causing greatly distended ureters and upper tracts. This condition is managed with a low salt diet, diuretics to reduce free water clearance and increase osmolar clearance, and frequent double or triple micturition.

The surgical approach to management of exstrophy of the bladder depends on the size of the bladder. If the bladder is large, primary closure is attempted. Bilateral iliac osteotomies at the time of vesicoplasty aid in this procedure. The vesical neck should be reconstructed with ureteroneocystostomies. If infection and hydronephrosis occur, urinary diversion is necessary. When a child is not a candidate for vesicoplasty because of a small fibrotic bladder, urinary diversion with ureterocolonic anastomosis is performed at the age of 18 to 24 months.

The bladder can be injured by blunt trauma, by fractures of the bony pelvis, penetrating wounds, or iatrogenic injuries. If the extraperitoneal tear is small, bladder injury can be treated with catheter drainage. Almost all other ruptures require surgical intervention.

Urethral stenosis in boys is treated with meatotomy; urethral ring in girls is treated by calibration or internal urethrotomy. The treatment of hypospadias is surgical and depends upon the location of the urethral orifice and the degree of chordee. Surgery is staged and is performed when the child is 2 years of age. Epispadias with incontinence in girls and boys needs surgical correction.

Posterior urethral injury is usually secondary to trauma involving the pelvis, with fractured pubic rami. The anterior urethra can be injured by blunt trauma to the external genitalia, crushing the urethra against the pubic arch. Injuries of the posterior and anterior urethra can be iatrogenic. Treatment involves urinary diversion and urethral realignment.

Undescended Testes

ABDOLLAH SADEGHI-NEJAD, M.D.

Treatment of undescended testes has three theoretical goals: to decrease the high rate of infertility, to diminish the increased, albeit small, risk of testicular malignancy, and to alleviate the potential psychological problems. The optimal form of treatment and its timing, however, remain controversial. Unfortunately, the efficacy of any form of therapy in terms of testicular function (virilization and fertility) is not known. Furthermore, it is clear that treatment might not alter the risk of malignant transformation. There is still no unanimity as to whether spontaneous descent occurs and if so how often; whether an undescended testis is primarily defective or whether the morphologic and functional abnormalities are a consequence of its abnormal position; and whether treatment improves gonadal function and if so at what age the damage, if present, is irreversible.

Testicular maldescent is present in 1 to 4% of full-term newborns and in a larger number of prematures. In the majority, spontaneous descent occurs in the first year of life. There is general agreement, therefore, that no treatment is indicated before age 1 year. After this age, spontaneous descent is less likely. The trend has been toward treatment at an earlier age and the optimal time, at present, is thought to be at about age 2 years. Although it is not known whether this earlier treatment improves testicular function, it is probably of psychological benefit to the patient.

Retractile Testes. This is caused by an overactive cremasteric reflex, which develops at about age 2 years and is active through childhood. These testes remain in the scrotum post-pubertally. Accordingly, no treatment is indicated.

Bilateral Undescended Testes. It must be emphasized that it may be difficult to distinguish a retractile testicle from a maldescended one. Therefore, repeated and careful examinations are required before treatment is undertaken.

In a pubertal child, or in a prepubertal child with testicular maldescent and an inguinal hernia, surgical correction is the treatment of choice. A dysplastic testicle requires surgical removal and insertion of a prosthesis. In all others, an attempt should be made to preserve the blood supply and to stabilize the testicle in the scrotum. It cannot be overstated that here the skill and the experience of the surgeon are of great importance.

In a prepubertal boy, before surgical correction is considered, a 6-week course of human chorionic gonadotropin (hCG 250–1000 units intramuscularly two to three times per week) should be administered. Measurement of serum testosterone after hCG serves to distinguish cryptorchidism from bilateral anorchia, and in up to a third of patients the testes descend with treatment. If descent occurs, no further treatment is required; if not, surgical correction is indicated. It has been argued that the testicle that descends with hCG is a retractile testicle and not a truly maldescended one. Even if this were true, medical treatment would be worthwhile since it might prevent unnecessary surgery in a large number of patients. Although the potential long-term complications of hCG are not known, it is unlikely that this form of therapy is significantly hazardous.

Recently good results have been reported with the use of gonadotropin-releasing hormone and its analogs. This form of treatment at the present time is still investigational and more data are needed to assess its efficacy.

Unilateral Testicular Maldescent. As in bilateral undescended testes, before surgical correction is undertaken, treatment with hCG should be tried. In a patient who requires orchidectomy and insertion of a prosthesis, the contralateral testis, if normal, is adequate for virilization and fertility. It should be kept in mind that the maldescended testis is at higher risk for malignant transformation, even after surgical correction, as is its descended scrotal partner.

Circumcision and Disorders of the Penis and Testis

GEORGE T. KLAUBER, M.D.

PENIS

Circumcision and Penile Hygiene. An uncircumcised penis is a normal penis. Presence of a foreskin and the need for penile hygiene are not considered indications for circumcision and the procedure itself should not be considered "routine." If circumcision is requested for nonreligious reasons, adequate counseling should be a prerequisite; however, when parents strongly favor circumcision, their request should not be denied. Circumcision, if elected, should be performed during the neonatal period in order to obviate the need for general anesthesia.

Normal penile hygiene for the uncircumcised infant penis consists of gentle washing with soap and water. Retraction of the foreskin is not necessary and should only be carried out if it can be performed easily.

Preputial Adhesions. The foreskin is normally adherent to the glans penis in the infant. At birth, such adherence is close to the urethral meatus; gradual separation occurs with time and is usually complete by age 6 to 8 years. The foreskin should not be forcibly retracted in the infant or young child because separation invariably occurs naturally. Forcible retraction may result in splitting the foreskin, with subsequent phimotic scarring. Penile skin bridging is somewhat different; it occurs between the shaft and the glans penis. It is a complication of circumcision consisting of epithelialized adhesions that may or may not cover trapped smegma. Sharp dissection under local or general anesthesia is usually required.

Phimosis and Paraphimosis. Phimosis is a narrowing of the foreskin preventing retraction over the glans penis. It is normal in infants and little boys and usually disappears as the child grows and the distal prepuce dilates. Occasionally the preputial opening is narrow enough to obstruct the urinary stream and cause ballooning of the foreskin with voiding. Severe phimosis can be relieved by the Heineke-Mikulicz procedure, dividing the constricting outer preputial skin vertically and suturing transversely. This is an acceptable alternative to a circumcision, which remains the more popular treatment for phimosis.

Paraphimosis occurs when the foreskin is somewhat narrow and after retraction cannot be brought back over the glans penis. Edema occurs secondary to lymphatic obstruction. Reduction of paraphimosis can usually be achieved manually be squeezing the edematous foreskin and rolling it upon itself. If this cannot be carried out, immediate circumcision is the optimum therapy.

Balanitis. Balanitis is an inflammation of the glans penis and the inner aspect of the prepuce in the uncircumcised male, often associated with phimosis. Topical antibiotic ointments will usually cure the acute episode, but occasionally parenteral broad-spectrum antibiotics may be required if severe cellulitis occurs. Circumcision or a dorsal relaxing incision in the foreskin to permit retraction should be considered if balanitis recurs.

Meatal Stenosis. The most common complication of circumcision, meatal stenosis usually presents as a delicate web of epithelium producing a partial obstruction across the inferior portion of the meatus. This causes dorsal deviation of the urinary stream. The web variety of meatal stenosis can be dilated in the office using a forceps and lidocaine (Xylocaine) jelly. Stenosis that does not reduce the caliber of the urinary stream does not require therapy. Surgical meatotomy is indicated only for a very small or scarred meatus associated with a poor urinary stream.

Hypospadias. This refers to ventral ectopia of the urethral meatus anywhere from the ventral glans penis to the perineum. Hypospadias, especially the coronal or glandular variety, can now usually be corrected in infancy. A minihypospadias repair is little more than a modified circumcision combined with an advancement urethral meatoplasty.

Most cases can be corrected by a one-stage operation that must include chordee excision, complete straightening of the penis, and construction of a neourethra, with the meatus as close as possible to the tip of the penis. Staged repairs are still preferred by some surgeons, especially by the occasional operator.

Boys recognize the importance of their genitalia at a very early age, and standing erect to void is an important skill in western society. Severe psychologic disturbances are common in boys if definitive reconstruction is delayed beyond school age.

Epispadias. This very rare defect affects the dorsum of the penis. Surgical reconstruction is always indicated and should include penile and urethral lengthening plus bladder neck reconstruction when necessary.

Micropenis. By definition a micropenis should be more than two standard deviations smaller than the norm. Two distinct types can be recognized. Corpus cavernosus tissue is present in the more common variety, which is often associated with intracranial pathology. Endocrine evaluation should be performed and therapy with topical or parenteral testosterone considered. A normal penis will never develop in boys with a micropenis that consists of skin and urethra alone and lacks corporeal tissue. In this event, a serious case can be made for amputation of the penis and female gender assignment.

Concealed Penis. This is a penis of normal size hidden within the suprapubic fat pad. It can occur naturally in some obese boys and requires no treatment. Retraction of the penis and circumferential cicatrix formation of the shaft skin over the glans occurs as a complication of neonatal circumcision. Surgical release of the glans is required; this can be performed as an office procedure in the neonate. A partially concealed penis, pseudomicropenis, also a complication of circumcision, is caused by excessive removal of penile shaft skin. If the condition is recognized immediately, the skin edges should be separated and the denuded penile shaft allowed to epithelialize. If recognized later in childhood, surgical correction may be necessary.

SPERMATIC CORD AND TESTES

Torsion. Acute painful swelling of the scrotum should always be considered a torsion of the spermatic cord or testis until proven otherwise, as should the painful groin swelling associated with ipsilateral undescended testis. Surgical treatment, which is always required for torsion, consists of bilateral trans-scrotal exploration and orchidopexy, except in infants or in the presence of primarily groin symptomatology, when an inguinal approach is preferred. Viability of the testicle depends upon prompt treatment. Surgery can be temporarily delayed if manual detorsion is successful; the contralateral testicle should always be anchored.

Torsion of the Appendix Testis. Scrotal exploration is mandatory if there is any doubt in the diagnosis. Symptoms usually subside spontaneously in approximately 1 week; however, boys are often less incapacitated by prompt surgical excision, which allows them to resume normal activities within 24 to 48 hours.

Epididymitis and Orchitis. Both conditions are rare in childhood; they must be differentiated from testicular torsion, and thus diagnosed with caution. Treatment for both consists of bed rest, scrotal elevation, and ice packs. A broad-spectrum antibiotic such as ampicillin for 10 to 14 days should be added in the treatment of epididymitis. Subsequently, investigative urographic studies should be performed. Steroid prophylaxis may be useful in mumps orchitis to preserve future spermatogenesis.

Trauma. If the trauma is severe and testicular rupture is suspected, scrotal exploration should be performed. A hematoma or hematocele can be evacuated and a ruptured tunica albuginea repaired.

Testis Tumors. In children, these tumors usually present as firm, painless scrotal masses that do not transilluminate. Surgery is always indicated unless the child has leukemia. Preoperative studies should include serum alpha fetoprotein, beta-subunit of human chorionic gonadotropin, carcinoembryonic antigen, testosterone, luteinizing hormone, and follicle-stimulating hormone estimations, as well as excretory urography, chest x-ray, and a metastatic series. Speckled calcification in the neonatal scrotum strongly suggests prenatal meconium peritonitis.

Seventy per cent of pediatric testicular tumors are of germinal origin, and 80% of these are malignant embryonal cell carcinomas. However, leukemia relapses presenting as testicular tumors are common.

Testis tumors should be explored through the groin. The spermatic cord is cross-clamped with vascular instruments before the testicular mass is examined. If there is any question about the diagnosis of malignancy, a frozen section is performed; otherwise, a radical orchiectomy is indicated. CT scanning should be performed to evaluate the retroperitoneal lymph nodes (RPLN). The role of RPLN remains controversial; if preoperative tumor markers are elevated and fail to return to normal levels, RPLN dissection is indicated; otherwise, evidence that this procedure improves survival is inconclusive. Cancer chemotherapy is indicated for most germ cell tumors except for the rare cases of seminomas, for which radiation therapy remains the treatment of choice. Intermittent courses of a combination of vincristine, actinomycin D, and cyclophosphamide (Cytoxan) have increased the long-term survival rate to more than 80%. Leukemia of the testicle does not require biopsy and should be treated aggressively with radiation and chemotherapy.

Hernias and Hydroceles

ARNOLD H. COLODNY, M.D.

Surgical repair of a hernia or hydrocele is the most common indication for major surgery in infants or children. Incarceration is the most serious preoperative problem, and while most incarcerations can be reduced nonoperatively, sequelae such as atrophy of the ipsilateral testicle secondary to thrombosis of the spermatic vessels may occur.

Inguinal Hernia. Inguinal hernias in children are invariably indirect (99%) and represent a persistent patent processus vaginalis, an outpocketing of the peritoneum that develops during the third month of gestation as the testicle descends from high in the abdomen to its final resting place in the scrotum. Ordinarily, it is obliterated during the last trimester of pregnancy or the first year of life; if not, the baby is born with a hernia sac, a potential space that can be compared to a "finger on a glove," which communicates with the abdominal cavity. When eventually some abdominal content gets into it, a swelling is seen. This is the hernia. Hernias are more common in small prematures and are much more common in males, with a ratio of approximately 6 to 1. Sixty percent are right-sided, approximately 20% are bilateral when first seen, and overall approximately 15% are incarcerated. Most incarcerated hernias can be reduced by use of the head-down position, sedation with sodium pentobarbital (Nembutal) and/or meperidine (Demerol), application of an ice pack, and gentle pressure. Picking the infant up by his feet and suspending him with his head down will maximize the effect of gravity and facilitate reduction in some patients who cannot be reduced by the usual methods. If the incarceration cannot be reduced, immediate surgery should be done to prevent strangulation and gangrene of the intestine. Even in those whose incarceration has been successfully reduced, a significant incidence of testicular atrophy secondary to thrombosis of the spermatic veins by pressure from the incarcerated hernia will occur. If the incarceration can be reduced completely, surgery is postponed for 24 to 48 hours to allow edema and inflammation to subside. Once a diagnosis of inguinal hernia is made, surgical repair is indicated unless there are strong contraindications. In the infant group this should be done within a few days of diagnosis to minimize the possibility of incarceration. In the asymptomatic older child, repair may be scheduled at a time of convenience. In infants and children, the most common viscus found in a hernia is the small intestine. Occasionally, omentum will herniate into the sac and may actually adhere to it or even be infarcted, necessitating removal with the hernia sac. The tip of the appendix may be seen at the time of hernia repair, but appendectomy during a standard repair is not recommended. However, if the mesoappendix and appendix are actually part of the wall of the hernia sac (sliding hernia) they may have to be removed to complete the repair. In the female infant the most common viscus in the hernia is the ovary or the fallopian tube. Often the ovary cannot be reduced. Unless there is unusual swelling or tenderness, this does not oblige one to do an emergency operation; however, the procedure should be undertaken promptly to prevent any damage to the ovary.

Diagnosis is sometimes difficult. Two techniques may be helpful. One is to ask the child to blow up a thick-walled balloon, promising him he can take the balloon home with him if he can blow it up. Many children will cooperate and may pop out the hernia. Another technique is to pump the abdomen with the palm of the hand while the child is in the upright position. If neither technique is successful, one may feel a thickened cord in the inguinal region at the level of the pubic tubercle, by rolling the spermatic cord structures under the fingertips. The examiner can compare it with the normal cord on the opposite side. However, sometimes one has only the word of a reliable observer of a swelling in the groin that comes and goes. The only thing that can mislead the examiner is a retractile testicle.

Inguinal hernias may disappear transiently and then reappear but do not disappear permanently. Surgical repair is the only successful treatment. The surgical repair should be straightforward. However, in the young infant, the operation may be trying for a surgeon who is not expert in this area. Most of these patients can be operated on in ambulatory surgery and can be discharged approximately 2 hours after completion of the operation. Ambulatory surgery repair of hernias has many benefits, including the fact that the parents can be with the child the entire time except during the actual operation. They frequently are allowed into the operating room for induction of anesthesia and are in the recovery room when the child wakes up. The psychologic advantages of this are as obvious as the economic benefits.

The surgical procedure consists of high ligation

of the sac; no formal repair is necessary. In the female infant a portion of the wall of the sac may in actuality be the fallopian tube (sliding hernia). High ligation of the sac would result in resection of a portion of the tube. Thus, a different type of repair is necessary. The inguinal incision is closed in anatomic relationships. Subcuticular sutures are used so that no stitches go through the skin. The resultant scar is much more pleasing and the child does not have to undergo the unpleasant experience of having sutures removed. The appendix testis should be removed if the testicle is visualized during a hernia repair. We have seen five patients who presented after hernia repairs with acute swelling of the scrotum. Each was found to have torsion of the appendix testis. Therefore, if a pedunculated appendix testis is seen, it should be removed at the time of the repair. If a boy presenting with an inguinal hernia also has an undescended testicle, an orchidopexy should be carried out at the time of hernia repair.

The main controversy in the surgery of inguinal hernias is whether the contralateral side should be explored if there is no history or physical evidence of a hernia on that side. The available statistics pro and con are invalid. It is certainly distressing to all concerned when a child who has had a unilateral repair presents within a few years with a clinical hernia on the other side, necessitating another anesthesia and operation. The main arguments against contralateral operations are that there may occur additional morbidity and complications such as injury to the vas deferens or spermatic vessels. I believe that if one is worried about injuring the vas or spermatic vessels on the contralateral side, one should not undertake to repair the hernia on the involved side. There should be no complication except possible wound infection on the contralateral side. This, of course, would not happen if one had not explored the contralateral side. However, wound infections after inguinal hernia repair are quite rare, much less than 0.5 per cent. If repair of the initial side has been expeditious and there are no anesthesia problems, it seems reasonable to explore the other side in an infant when finding a hernia sac is a reasonable expectation. The younger the patient at the time of unilateral hernia repair, the greater is the chance of finding a hernia sac on the opposite side. Bilateral hernias are more common in premature infants, in females, and when a unilateral hernia is on the left side. We recommend exploration of the opposite side in males under 2 and in females under 6 years of age.

Postoperative complications are unusual. There is a certain minimal irreducible incidence of wound infection after any clean operation. Hematomas are unusual and most do not require therapy except initial application of an ice pack followed by warm compresses. A hydrocele may appear postopera-

tively but usually absorbs in a few weeks. Recurrences are extremely rare and most are direct hernias. Since direct hernias are uncommon in this age group, one must consider the possibility that they are iatrogenic and related to improper surgical technique. Atrophy of the testicle due to injury to the vessels occasionally occurs. Iatrogenic undescended testicle is more common than reported and is due to the testicle being pulled up into the incision during hernia repair and then not properly replaced in the scrotum. If the patient has an active cremasteric reflex (retractile testicle), this may lead to retraction and fixation of the testicle postoperatively. Division of the cremasteric fibers will prevent this. At the conclusion of the operation, the surgeon should verify that the testicle(s) is well down in the scrotum. If it is in an improper position, this is the best time to replace it in the scrotum since it will never again be as easy to do. If it is left in the groin, it will become fixed in the scar tissue and will require a secondary procedure to bring it down into the scrotum.

Injury to the urinary bladder may occur during hernia repair because the infant's bladder is very close to the internal inguinal ring ("bladder ears"). This complication is accounted for by the fact that if one dissects the sac too high, one may include the lateral aspect of the urinary bladder when ligating the sac.

Inguinal hernias occasionally are seen in association with diseases such as hydrocephalus with ventriculoperitoneal shunts, congenital cytomegalic inclusion disease, exstrophy of the bladder, Ehlers-Danlos syndrome, and Hurler-Hunter syndrome. They require a formal anatomic hernia repair. In the female, a sliding hernia frequently involves various parts of the genital tract, including ovary, fallopian tube, and/or uterus.

Rarely, in an apparent female infant with inguinal hernia, the testicular feminization syndrome (TFS) will be present. Although the patient will have a completely normal phenotypic female appearance the gonads and chromosomes will be male. The müllerian derivatives (tubes, uterus, cervix, and upper vagina) will not develop because of the elaboration of müllerian inhibiting substance by the testes. The external genitalia will be female in appearance. It is important to recognize this syndrome because the retained testicles, which may achieve feminization during puberty, have a high incidence of malignant degeneration and should eventually be removed. I believe that TFS, although its incidence is low, must be definitely ruled out. This can be done by performing a buccal smear or by inserting a pediatric cystoscope into the vagina at the conclusion of the operation. If a normal cervix is seen at the top of the vagina, TFS is not present. Visualization of a completely normal fallopian tube in the hernia sac will also rule out TFS. The presence of a normal testicle and vas deferens in the hernia sac would confirm the diagnosis of TFS. Palpation of a cervix by rectal exam would tend to rule out TFS. Doubtful observations can be confirmed by a karyotype. It would be 46XY in TFS.

If the vas deferens is absent at the time of hernia repair in a male, cystic fibrosis should be suspected and a sweat test carried out. Patients with cystic fibrosis have either a poorly developed or absent vas deferens.

HYDROCELE

Accumulation of fluid within a patent processus vaginalis results in a hydrocele. These are frequently seen in neonates, and the majority absorb and cause no problems. Persistence beyond 4 to 12 months or a definite variation in size indicates a communication with the peritoneal cavity through a patent processus vaginalis and requires surgical repair. If fluid from the peritoneal cavity gets into and acutely enlarges a patent processus vaginalis, it may be necessary to differentiate this from an incarcerated inguinal hernia. If the swelling is clearly around the testicle, one can be relatively certain that this is a hydrocele. If there is any doubt about the diagnosis, the differentiation should be made in the operating room. Operative repair should be undertaken through the groin. If a hydrocele is found, ligation of the processus at the level of the internal ring will prevent reaccumulation of fluid. A partial excision of the hydrocele sac and evacuation of its contents is also carried out.

Disorders of the Vulva and Vagina

MARTIN FARBER, M.D.,
and AMOS MADANES, M.D.

The white vaginal discharge that collects in the vulvar folds of the neonate in the first few days of life should not be regarded as pathologic. It is nonodorous and composed of desquamated vaginal cells mixed with endocervical mucus resulting from maternal estrogen stimulation. This physiologic discharge subsides after several days of life.

Nonspecific Vulvovaginitis. The most common gynecologic disorder of the prepubertal girl is chronic, nonspecific vulvovaginitis. The syndrome is usually primarily a vulvitis and is due to poor vulvar, perineal, and perianal hygiene. A culture and a sensitivity test are not necessary (the organisms most commonly are mixed coliforms), and the symptoms are ameliorated by warm water sitz baths and cleansing of the involved areas with bland soap. The skin is blotted dry, exposed to warm, dry air, and covered with powdered starch. Both the patient and her parents are taught the necessity for mechanical removal of smegma from areas of entrapment and the proper technique for perianal wiping poststool (from front to back). The patient is advised to wear white, cotton, loose-fitting panties. Estrogen vaginal cream is applied to the vulva only if symptoms persist for more than a month despite meticulous attention to cleanliness of the affected area.

Acute edematous nonspecific vulvitis is symptomatically relieved by frequent sitz baths in cool water or physiologic saline or an aqueous solution of bicarbonate of soda or starch. In several days the involved areas are intermittently painted with a bland solution such as calamine lotion. When the acute phase is resolved, an antipruritic cream (hydrocortisone cream 1%) is applied daily, followed by iodochlorhydroxyquin ointment or cream (Vioform) at night.

Bacterial infections of the vulva transmitted from extragenital primary sites (nasopharynx, intestine, skin) are treated in accordance with the sensitivity of the offending organism.

***Trichomonas Vaginalis* Vulvovaginitis.** The prepubertal child with *Trichomonas vaginalis* vaginitis is given metronidazole (Flagyl),*125 mg tid for 5 days. In the adolescent female, the dose of metronidazole is 250 mg tid for 7 days; if she is coitally active, her male partner should be similarly treated.

***Monilia* Vulvovaginitis.** This may be precipitated by the prior ingestion of broad-spectrum antibiotics or may be one of the presenting symptoms of diabetes mellitus and is commonly present in women who ingest oral contraceptives. Therapy for the prepubertal girl consists of the application of nystatin cream or ointment to the vulva tid for 2 weeks. When the infection is recurrent, nystatin cream may be applied intravaginally or, alternatively, 1 ml of nystatin suspension (100,000 units/ml) may be administered tid intravaginally, using an eyedropper. In the adolescent, nystatin (Mycostatin) vaginal suppositories should be inserted bid for 2 weeks and Mycolog cream (nystatin–neomycin sulfate–gramicidin–triamcinolone acetonide) applied to the vulva bid as long as the vulvitis persists.

***Hemophilus Vaginalis* Vulvovaginitis.** The treatment in the adolescent girl is controversial; no single therapeutic regimen is rewarded by success in all cases. Ampicillin, 500 mg qid for 10 days, is advocated by some, while metronidazole† (Flagyl), 250 mg tid for 7 days, is prescribed by others. There is uniform agreement that Sultrin Triple Sulfa Cream is not effective, and that the male part-

---

*Manufacturer's precaution: The safety and effectiveness of metronidazole in children have not been established.
†This use of metronidazole is not listed by the manufacturer.

ner should be treated when the patient is sexually active.

Pinworm Vulvovaginitis. Vulvovaginitis due to pinworms *(Enterobius vermicularis)* may be treated with piperazine citrate (Antepar) tablets or syrup as a single daily dose of 65 mg (hexahydrate equivalent)/kg of body weight/24 hr for 7 consecutive days (maximum daily dose, 2.5 grams). Other agents such as pyrantel pamoate[†] (Antiminth) oral suspension in a single dose of 11 mg/kg (maximum dose, 1 gram), pyrvinium pamoate (Povan) tablets or suspension in a single dose of 5 mg/kg, or mebendazole (Vermox) as a single dose of one chewable tablet are also effective. All of these regimens may be repeated if the child is not cured in 3 weeks, after checking all other family members for infection.

Gonococcal Vulvovaginitis. Uncomplicated gonococcal vulvovaginitis in children who weigh less than 100 pounds should be treated with amoxicillin, 50 mg/kg orally, or with probenecid, 25 mg/kg (maximum 1 gram). Alternatively, aqueous procaine penicillin G, 100,000 units/kg IM, plus probenecid may be used. If the child is allergic to penicillin, spectinomycin,[‡] 40 mg/kg IM, may be given, or, if the child is older than 8 years, tetracycline, 40 mg/kg/24 hr, may be administered orally in four divided doses for 5 days. Children with complicated infections such as peritonitis or arthritis should be hospitalized for the intravenous administration of aqueous crystalline penicillin G, 100,000 units/kg/24 hr for 7 days; when meningitis is present, the dose of penicillin is increased to 250,000 units/kg/24 hr for 10 days.

Herpes Vulvitis. This condition is treated symptomatically with sitz baths and antibiotics when necessary for systemic manifestations of secondary bacterial infection.

Condyloma Acuminata. For condyloma acuminata in the prepubertal child, biopsy should be performed for a histologic diagnosis and then the lesion removed by electrodesiccation. In the adolescent girl, a careful speculum examination of the vagina and anoscopy should be performed to search for a potential nidus that will cause recurrence. Vulvar warts may be painted with podophyllin resin (25%) in tincture of benzoin, but the vaginal and anal lesions are best electrodesiccated.

Lichen Sclerosus et Atrophicus. In the vulva, this disease is unusual in prepubertal girls. Cases that spontaneously went into remission at puberty have been reported. Estrogen creams usually do not help, while corticosteroid creams occasionally provide some relief. Testosterone creams have been used successfully in some cases but these are not routinely available and must be specially prepared by the pharmacist.

Foreign Body. A persistent, profuse, bloody, purulent, foul-smelling vaginal discharge frequently is caused by a foreign body. A pelvic radiograph may be negative since toilet tissue is most commonly the cause. When there is a high index of suspicion, the Robertson cystoscope utilizing a fiberoptic light source and sterile water to distend the vagina permits excellent visualization of the entire vagina and cervix for removal of the foreign body and assessment of the degree of tissue trauma. As adolescence is approached it is necessary to remember that vaginal synechiae from a chronic infection may totally obstruct the vagina and lead to cryptomenorrhea.

Agglutination of the Labia Minora. This condition prevents visualization of the hymen and may be so extensive as to cause urinary retention by obstructing the external urethral meatus. The cause of the lesion, found between ages 2 and 6 years, is unknown. Manually tearing the labia apart is sometimes necessary when there is urinary retention, but in most cases the labia will separate subsequent to the daily application of estrogen vaginal cream for 2 weeks.

Imperforate Hymen. This may lead to mucocolpos, which presents prepubertally as a painless abdominopelvic mass that points between the labia minora. Cruciate incisions in the hymen are necessary for drainage. Postmenarchially, hematocolpos due to an imperforate hymen causes cyclically recurrent intractable pelvic pain, a palpable pelvic mass, and amenorrhea. The hymen should be excised and a Heineke-Mikulicz perineorrhaphy should be performed to widen the vaginal introitus. Microperforation of the hymen is a slight variation associated with a small opening in the hymen (usually situated just inferior to the external urethral meatus and 2 to 3 mm in diameter) and accompanied by extreme hypomenorrhea and dysmenorrhea. The surgical treatment is the same as that for imperforate hymen.

Transverse Vaginal Septum. This condition has the same symptoms as imperforate hymen. They are alleviated by resecting the septum and suturing the vaginal mucosal edges together.

Vaginal Agenesis. In 1 of 5000 women, the vagina is congenitally absent. The normally formed fallopian tubes end in rudimentary muscle nubbins laterally situated in folds of the broad ligaments that extend across the pelvis to form a hammock that contains the bladder. Their normal secondary sexual characteristics due to normal hypothalamic-pituitary-ovarian function reflect their normal 46,XX karyotype. This symptom complex, the Rokitansky-Kuster-Hauser syndrome, presents primary amenorrhea without cyclically recurrent pel-

---

[†]Safety and efficacy of pyrantel pamoate in children under 2 years of age have not been established.

[‡]Manufacturer's Warning: Safety for use in infants and children has not been established.

vic pain. Primary amenorrhea is *not* arbitrarily diagnosed when menarche fails to occur by age 18 but is diagnosed and intensively investigated when menarche fails to be established within 3 years of thelarche. Intravenous pyelography should be performed in all these patients (45% of them will be found to have a significant renal anomaly), and they should be karyotyped to differentiate this from the androgen insensitivity syndrome (testicular feminization syndrome).

When the patient desires, a vagina can be created by the daily insertion of dilators in graduated sizes (Frank's nonoperative technique) or by surgical construction. McIndoe's procedure, which employs split-thickness skin placed over a mold and inserted into a space dissected between the bladder and rectum, is widely accepted. A vagina should be created only when the patient desires one and has completed her somatic growth. The best postoperative anatomic and functional results accrue to young women who are adequately prepared psychologically preoperatively. Postoperatively, it is necessary to insert a vaginal mold daily to keep the newly created vagina open until coital frequency is such as to maintain patency of the neovagina.

In less than 10% of women with ostensible vaginal agenesis, the vagina is only partially absent and there is a functioning uterus. These potentially fertile women have primary amenorrhea and cyclically recurrent pelvic pain. Dissection between the bladder and rectum will lead to an apical vaginal segment, which must be mobilized and sutured to the mucosa of the vestibule. Normal menstrual function, fertility, and vaginal delivery have resulted in women promptly diagnosed and surgically corrected.

Benign Tumors of the Vulva and Vagina. Hemangiomas are the most common tumors of the vulva. Grossly, they assume a port wine, strawberry, or cavernous appearance. They are benign and should be resected only if the diagnosis is in doubt or if they are expanding and causing increasing deformity of the external genitalia. A lymphangioma presents as a colorless swelling of the vulva and should be excised only when symptomatic. Similarly, lipomas, papillomas, and leiomyomas are benign and may be kept under observation. A hidradenoma presents as an umbilicated lesion on the vulva overlying a small, cystic, subcutaneous tumor and should be removed only if the diagnosis is uncertain. A cyst of the canal of Nuck presents as a painless cystic swelling of the labia majora and should be excised only when large or symptomatic. It is caused by cystic dilatation of the leading end of a hernial sac, with fibrous obliteration of the proximal portion of the sac.

Epithelial inclusion cysts, polyps, or hemangiomas of the hymen are resected only if they are large and causing symptoms.

Cystic remnants of the mesonephric ducts (Gartner duct cysts) are lesions of variable size on the anterolateral vaginal walls. They are usually asymptomatic and require no surgical therapy. When extremely large, they may partially obstruct egress of the menstruum or interfere with coital function, and they may be aspirated, marsupialized, or excised. Benign vaginal lipomas, fibromas, lymphangiomas, and papillomas have all been described and should be biopsied only when the diagnosis is in doubt.

Diethylstilbestrol (DES). The ingestion of DES by pregnant women before the 18th week of gestation is associated with an increased incidence of benign changes of the vagina and cervix of their daughters. These changes include vaginal transverse fibrous ridges and cervical ridges (cockscomb cervix, cervical hood, cervical pseudopolyp) in 20% of DES daughters, vaginal adenosis in 35%, and a cervical erosion or ectropion in 90%. Unusually, clear cell adenocarcinoma of the vagina or cervix is found (range of incidence is 0.14 to 1.4/1000 DES daughters). Progression from benign adenosis to clear cell adenocarcinoma has not been demonstrated. The peak incidence of vaginal and cervical malignancies in this population at increased risk occurs at age 19 years (greater than 90% of the tumors have occurred in females 14 to 23 years of age). Twenty per cent of the patients with tumors have had false-negative Pap smears. Therefore, all DES exposed daughters should be screened initially at age 14 or just following menarche and then yearly, with a pelvic examination, Papanicolaou smear, colposcopy, and iodine staining of the vagina and cervix, with biopsy of all suspicious lesions. Symptoms such as abnormal bleeding or discharge warrant an interim assessment or an initial examination at an earlier age. These young girls are best managed at medical centers equipped to offer emotional support to them and their mothers, as well as with colposcopists sophisticated enough to properly evaluate the anatomic lesions. If the lesion is malignant, depending on the stage of the disease the patients are treated with radical pelvic surgery, radiation therapy, or a combination of both.

Carcinoma of the vulva is very unusual in children and has a poor prognosis. Radical vulvectomy, superficial inguinal lymphadenectomy, and deep pelvic node dissection (when indicated) is the indicated surgical treatment.

Sarcoma botryoides of the vagina has been reported in patients from a few days old to 5 years of age. Bleeding or discharge leads to discovery of a polypoid mass at times large enough to fill the vagina and protrude from the introitus. Radical surgery (pelvic exenteration, vaginectomy, simple vulvectomy, and complete pelvic lymphadenectomy with ovarian preservation) may be used to treat the tumor, and radiation therapy or chemotherapy or both may be used exclusively or adjunctively.

Disorders of the Uterus, Tubes, and Ovaries

MARTIN FARBER, M.D.,
and AMOS MADANES, M.D.

PRIMARY AMENORRHEA

Primary amenorrhea is diagnosed when menarche has not arrived within 3 years of thelarche. Subsequent to a diagnosis of hypergonadotropism, these patients should be started on estrogen therapy to effect full maturation of their secondary sexual characteristics. Diethylstilbestrol, 0.5 mg; ethinyl estradiol, 0.05 mg; Premarin, 1.25 mg; or Estrace, 2 mg, may be given by mouth once daily for 3 weeks with the addition of medroxyprogesterone acetate (Provera), 10 mg, concomitantly for the last week. After a hiatus of 1 week during which vaginal bleeding occurs, the same steroid regimen is repeated. After full maturation of secondary sexual characteristics (usually 3 years) the estrogen dose may be reduced by one half.

Hypogonadotropism and failure of puberty to occur by age 13 years is most commonly idiopathic (constitutional delayed puberty) and occurs in 1 of 160 girls. Hypogonadotropism with anosmia (Kallmann syndrome) is due to congenital absence of the hypothalamic centers responsible for secretion of luteinizing hormone-releasing hormone, together with congenital absence of the olfactory lobes. Congenital defects in the ability of the adenohypophysis to synthesize each of the gonadotropic hormones have also been reported. Hypogonadotropism may coexist with hyperprolactinemia and may be secondary to neoplasms of the adenohypophysis or pituitary stalk (prolactinoma, craniopharyngioma).

Girls with constitutional delayed puberty may be given a 3-month course of ethinyl estradiol (0.01 mg daily) to initiate early maturation of secondary sexual characteristics. The steroid regimen may be repeated if puberty does not spontaneously ensue after a 6-month hiatus. Other hypogonadotropic states may be treated with a steroid regimen as described for hypergonadotropism. Remember, however, that the ovulation may be induced in hypogonadotropic hypogonadal states by the sequential administration of intramuscular follicle-stimulating hormone (Pergonal) and human chorionic gonadotropin (biologically analogous to luteinizing hormone) when the patient wants to become pregnant. Hyperprolactinemic hypogonadism without a radiologically demonstrable pituitary tumor should be treated by the administration of the dopamine agonist bromocriptine (Parlodel), 7.5 mg daily for 6 months. Neoplasms may be resected or treated with radiotherapy or with a similar dose of Parlodel.

Primary amenorrhea in the presence of eugonadotropism commonly is due to a congenital anomaly of the müllerian ducts, as described in the article on anomalies of the vulva and vagina. At times luteinizing hormone is found to be elevated and follicle-stimulating hormone to be in the normal or low-normal range. This gonadotropin profile, together with other stigmata, such as obesity, acne, hirsutism, and seborrhea, suggests primary hypothalamic pituitary dysfunction (polycystic ovarian syndrome). Medroxyprogesterone acetate (Provera), 10-mg tablets, should be administered to these patients every third month to induce menses and reverse the constant estrogenic stimulus of the endometrium.

SECONDARY AMENORRHEA

Secondary amenorrhea is quite common in the first 2 postmenarcheal years and reflects immaturity of the hypothalamic-pituitary-gonadal axis. If a thorough history and physical examination followed by a pregnancy test fail to uncover an obvious cause, no further investigation is warranted, and the treatment is expectant for 6 months. At that time, in the presence of euprolactinemia, medroxyprogesterone acetate (Provera), 10 mg a day, should be given for 5 days every third month until menses spontaneously resume. Failure to menstruate subsequent to Provera administration suggests hypoestrogenism, most commonly due to psychogenically induced hypogonadotropism. After the patient is biochemically categorized by the assay of gonadotropins, she is placed on the sequential steroid regimen described for hypergonadotropic primary amenorrhea. In the unlikely event a specific endocrinopathy is identified (thyroid, adrenal, pituitary), the symptom may be etiologically treated.

HYPERMENORRHEA

Hypermenorrhea at irregular intervals is usually due to anovulation and may be associated with anemia. In all cases, pregnancy and a coagulopathy should be ruled out. At times these patients will develop mild degrees of adenomatous hyperplasia of the endometrium. The administration of medroxyprogesterone acetate (Provera), 10 mg for 5 days each month, is usually sufficient to reverse the histologic pattern. If bleeding is persistent and heavy and anemia is present, the patient should be hospitalized, provided with whole blood transfusions if necessary, and given a combined estrogen-progestin pill in sufficient quantity to stop the bleeding. Initially Enovid (norethynodrel, 10 mg + mestranol, 0.150 mg), 10 mg, is given orally and the dose increased by daily increments of 5 mg until bleeding is markedly reduced or stopped. Curettage of the uterus is rarely necessary but should be performed in the presence of pharmacologically uncontrollable brisk hemorrhage. After cessation of uterine bleeding, the patient is maintained for 3 weeks on that steroid dose initially necessary to control the hemorrhage. Iron supplements are given to promote hematopoiesis. In subsequent cycles the steroid dose is reduced and then discontinued (usually after 3 months) in the hope that ovulatory menses will ensue.

Cyclically repetitive hypermenorrhea is unusual in adolescent girls, is associated with ovulation, and, in the absence of a coagulopathy, is due to an anatomic lesion of the endometrium or uterus (fibroid, polyp). Hysterosalpingography followed by hysteroscopy and curettage is often needed to make the diagnosis and treat the lesion.

DYSMENORRHEA

Cyclically repetitive dysmenorrhea should not be assumed to be primary (without an anatomic basis) until a thorough pelvic examination has been performed. Anomalies caused by incomplete fusion of the müllerian ducts and unilateral obstruction to the egress of the menstruum cause a palpable and sometimes visible pelvic mass. Resection of the nonpatent but functioning müllerian ductal segment or connecting it to the contralateral segment to permit free egress of the menstruum cures the patient.

If the pelvic examination is normal, the patient may be provided with acetaminophen when necessary (not a narcotic), advised to apply warm heat to the lower back or anterior abdominal wall, and counseled as to the necessity of continuing the daily performance of her usual activities (attendance at school, and so on). When contraception is a concern (the history is best elicited without the parents present), primary dysmenorrhea will most often be eradicated by the administration of an oral contraceptive. Tablets containing 1 mg of norethindrone with 0.035 mg of ethinyl estradiol (Norinyl 1 + 35, 28-day tablets) may be tried and the dose increased to Norinyl 1 + 50, 28-day tablets (containing 1 mg of norethindrone and 0.050 mg of mestranol), if breakthrough bleeding occurs. When contraception is not a concern, a prostaglandin synthetase-inhibiting agent should be prescribed, such as naproxen sodium (Anaprox), 275-mg tablets. On the first day of menses, two tablets are taken initially and then three more tablets during the remainder of the day. Three tablets a day are continued for an additional 1 to 2 days as required.

A patient who fails to respond to these modalities of therapy requires diagnostic laparoscopy. Although it has been reported that endometriosis is commonly found (though not histologically proved) in these patients, this has not been our experience. However, the importance of endoscopy should not be minimized in light of the frequent amelioration of symptoms after the patient and her parents are told that no anatomic lesion has been identified.

CONTRACEPTION

By age 19 years, 55% of young women have had sexual intercourse, but only half of them will utilize contraception. The "pill" is most commonly used, with barrier methods (condom and diaphragm), coitus interruptus, and the intrauterine device (IUD) used in order of decreasing frequency. Each method's failure rate for the first year of use is inversely related to age. There is also an inverse relation between age and termination rates for each method. The sexually active teenager must therefore be carefully evaluated and then motivated to properly utilize the contraceptive method prescribed by her gynecologist.

Oral contraceptives are ideal for most teenagers and should initially be prescribed as preparations that contain less than 50 micrograms of the estrogenic steroid. Brevicon (0.035 mg ethinyl estradiol + 0.5 mg norethindrone) or Norinyl 1 + 35 (0.035 mg ethinyl estradiol + 1 mg norethindrone) is satisfactory for most patients. Persistent breakthrough bleeding may be managed by prescribing Norinyl 1 + 50, which increases the dose to 0.050 mg of mestranol + 1 mg of norethindrone. Packages containing 28 pills should be prescribed (the last 7 tablets are placebos) to induce habituation and thus decrease the failure rate.

Dysmenorrhea, hypermenorrhea, and spontaneous expulsion occur less often with copper-containing IUDs than others. The copper-containing IUD thus may be tried in the teenage patient, but the seven-fold increase in the rate of acute pelvic inflammatory disease associated with this mode of contraception, together with the increased incidence of pelvic abscess formation and ectopic pregnancy, makes this contraceptive method the least frequently employed by this age group.

Barrier methods (diaphragm and condom) have gained increasing acceptance by the teenage population. The condom used with spermicidal jelly is not as efficacious as the diaphragm but offers some protection against the acquisition of gonorrhea.

GONORRHEAL CERVICITIS

Adolescent women who reportedly have contacted gonorrhea (with or without cervicitis) should have a cervical and urethral specimen taken for culture of the organism. They should be treated with aqueous procaine penicillin G, 4.8 million units intramuscularly, with 1 gram of probenecid orally. Alternatively, tetracycline hydrochloride, 0.5 gram qid for 5 days; ampicillin, 3.5 grams; or amoxicillin, 3.0 grams, with 1 gram of probenecid, may be given orally. Cervical cultures should be repeated 3 to 7 days after treatment is completed.

SALPINGITIS

Adolescent women with acute salpingitis should be hospitalized for intravenous antibiotic therapy. Ampicillin (2 gm/24 hr intravenously in 4 divided doses) is a satisfactory drug to be used initially, but, in the absence of clinical improvement in 48 hours, gentamicin (3 mg/kg/24 hr in 3 divided doses) and Cleocin Phosphate (600 to 1200 mg/24 hr in three divided doses) should be added for broader aerobic and anaerobic antibacterial therapy. Keen clinical judgment is required to manage pelvic abscess formation, and extirpative surgery is employed only when the infection is unresponsive to antibiotics and is life threatening.

ECTOPIC PREGNANCY

The triad of menstrual irregularity (not always amenorrhea), unilateral pelvic pain, and a positive assay for the beta subunit of human chorionic gonadotropin are diagnostic of oviductal pregnancy. The lesion may be laparoscopically identified and, in the presence of a normal contralateral fallopian tube, should be treated by salpingectomy. Every effort should be made to preserve the ipsilateral ovary. If the contralateral fallopian tube is surgically absent and it is technically feasible, the involved segment of tube may be resected and an anastomosis of the remaining tubal segments be performed by a tubal microsurgeon at another time. When the extent of damage warrants complete resection of the remaining tube, the uterus may be left intact, depending on the preoperative choice of the patient in light of recent advances in in vitro fertilization and embryo transfer.

Tumors of the Uterus, Tubes, and Ovaries

MARTIN FARBER, M.D.,
and AMOS MADANES, M.D.

Endometrial adenocarcinoma and sarcoma are extremely rare in the pediatric age group and are usually treated by radical surgery or radiotherapy. Biopsy should be performed on all lesions of the cervix, such as leukoplakia, polyps, papillomas, hemangiomas, leiomyomas, condylomas, and endometriomas, to establish their histologic diagnosis. Yearly Papanicolaou smears should be performed when teenage women become sexually active. Dysplasias should be investigated colposcopically and biopsy performed on suspicious areas. Cryotherapy or radial hot cautery is utilized to treat various severities of cervical dysplasia.

Squamous cell carcinoma of the cervix is very rare in this age group and is treated by radical surgery or radiotherapy or both. A primary malignancy of the fallopian tube has not been reported in a child.

Ovarian tumors are the most common genital neoplasms in young women. However, they account for only 1% of neoplasms in girls less than 16 years old. Although 20% of ovarian "tumors" histologically are follicular cysts, 30% are benign cystic teratomas and about 30% are malignancies. The latter fact, together with the observation that the incidence of ovarian torsion due to neoplasia is very high (30%), suggests the need for quick surgical intervention when an ovarian enlargement is felt.

The most common symptom produced by an enlarged ovary is abdominal or pelvic pain, with vomiting, constipation, discomfort on voiding, and isosexual or heterosexual precocious puberty being occasional accompaniments. The most common sign is a pelvic or abdominal mass. The normal ovaries of children and adolescents are not usually felt on rectoabdominal examination when they are awake and frequently are not palpated when they are anesthetized. Therefore, it should be assumed that any adnexal mass found on rectoabdominal examination is neoplastic. It is to be noted that in an infant or small child an ovarian tumor less than 4 cm is not likely to be felt abdominally and requires a rectoabdominal examination for its palpation.

All ovarian enlargements in neonates as well as in premenarchial girls should be resected. An ovarian cyst 6 cm or less in a postmenarchial girl may be followed clinically for 3 months, during which time Norinyl* 1 + 50 (norethindrone, 1 mg, with 0.050 mg mestranol) is cyclically administered to suppress the "functional" cyst. Persistence of the cyst for 3 months or enlargement of it during the period of observation necessitates surgical excision. All solid ovarian neoplasms in postmenarchial girls should be surgically excised.

Small follicular cysts observed incidentally at laparotomy in premenarchial girls should be left alone and not punctured. Unilateral ovarian cysts should be resected by oophorocystectomy (whenever technically feasible) and solid tumors by oophorectomy, and the tissue submitted for histologic examination of frozen sections. If the specimen is histologically benign, the contralateral ovary is bivalved when indicated (when the incidence of bilaterality is significant). If the lesion is well encapsulated, grossly confined to one ovary, and "borderline" or frankly malignant by histologic examination of frozen sections, a salpingo-oophorectomy is performed; the contralateral ovary is bivalved and a biopsy is taken, peritoneal washings

---

*This use of Norinyl is not listed by the manufacturer.

are sent for cytologic examination, and a decision regarding additional surgical therapy is deferred until the examination of permanent histologic sections. Further management of the patient should be pursuant to consultation with a gynecologic oncologist. In general, if the lesion is a well-differentiated Stage IA serous or mucinous cystadenocarcinoma or dysgerminoma, no further surgery is necessary. If the lesion is poorly differentiated, consideration should be given to resection of the uterus and remaining tube and ovary.

13

Bones and Joints

Craniofacial Malformations

HENRY K. KAWAMOTO, Jr., M.D., D.D.S.

The treatment of craniofacial malformations has undergone a remarkable revolution during the past decade. A child with a disfiguring, "untreatable" facial anomaly now has a brighter prospect. The stigmata of the deformity can be erased sufficiently to allow the child a relatively normal life.

Craniofacial anomalies are rare. They present problems that are extremely complex and demand the skills of multiple specialists. To receive optimal care, *children with craniofacial anomalies should be referred to centers that deal with these problems daily.*

The cardinal principle in treating craniofacial anomalies is to establish the underlying framework on which one can build. Abnormally located craniofacial skeletal parts must be returned to their normal position. Absent parts must be constructed, using autologous materials whenever possible.

Once the osseous structure is in proper order, attention can be directed toward redraping and modifying the overlying soft tissues.

Mental retardation should not be used as the sole criterion to withhold treatment. If a child can perceive his or her deformity as a source of taunts by peers, correction of the disfigurement should be considered.

The vast number and individual variations of craniofacial anomalies make it impractical to describe the treatment of every deformity. However, sufficient overlap exists to permit a discussion of concepts as they relate to the major groups.

CRANIOSYNOSTOSIS

Early release of a prematurely closed cranial suture is the treatment of choice. This recommenda-

tion is dictated by the rapid growth of the brain, which triples its weight and obtains 80 per cent of its adult size during the first year of life.

Premature fusion of an isolated suture may not create problems associated with increased intracranial pressure. However, the calvaria will be distorted. Furthermore, premature arrest of coronal and metopic sutures has a pronounced effect on the growth and development of the face. Early intervention minimizes the disfigurement.

When multiple sutures are involved, the danger of increased intracranial pressure increases. Papilledema, optic atrophy, and mental retardation can be added to the craniofacial deformity if treatment is delayed.

Scaphocephaly. Premature closure of the sagittal suture produces a cranium with an elongated anteroposterior dimension and an inverted-boat–like appearance.

An early sagittal or bilateral parasagittal strip craniectomy is recommended. Depending upon the neurosurgeon's preference, the edges of the craniectomy can be left open or covered with a sheet of silicone to discourage refusion.

Trigonocephaly. A triangular cranium as viewed from the vertex is the result of premature obliteration of the metopic suture. A prominent ridge occupies the midline of the forehead, and both superolateral orbital rims are symmetrically recessed.

The deformity can be totally corrected in one stage with an intracranial approach performed in early infancy. A frontal craniotomy is made. The superior orbital rims are repositioned to their normal location. The frontal bone flap is trimmed and rotated 90 degrees to reproduce a normal curvature of the forehead.

Plagiocephaly. Unilateral premature fusion of

the coronal suture can produce the severest asymmetry of the cranium and face. The facial midline takes on a "C"-shaped curvature, with the convexity pointing toward the involved side.

On the ipsilateral side, the vertical dimension of the face is increased and the frontal area and the supraorbital rims are flattened and recessed. The fused half of the coronal suture is palpable as a ridge.

Contralaterally, the forehead is bossed, the facial height is lessened, and the orbit is displaced caudad.

Through a coronal incision, a frontal craniectomy is made. The involved suture is removed and the strip craniectomy is prolonged caudad along the sphenozygomatic suture into the inferior orbital fissure. A transverse osteotomy across the orbital roof is required to advance the recessed superior orbital rim to its normal position and to negate any restrictive influence of possible frontoethmoidal and frontosphenoidal sutural involvement.

The frontal bone flap is rotated to restore the most favorable contour. The rapid expansion of the developing brain favors restoration of the normal craniofacial relationships.

Complexity, risks, and length of operation are greatly increased if treatment is deferred beyond the early months of life.

Craniofacial Dysostosis (Crouzon Syndrome) and Acrocephalosyndactyly (Apert Syndrome). The coronal suture is the principal site of premature closure. The sagittal and lambdoidal sutures can also be involved. The malformations are inherited in an autosomal dominant manner.

Although distinct as entities, sufficient clinical similarities exist between the two syndromes to permit a joint discussion. The forehead is flattened and recessed. The entire midface is hypoplastic and retruded, giving the mandible a pseudoprognathic appearance. The shallow orbits house normal-sized globes, thus producing exorbitism. Telorbitism is of a mild degree. Nasal airway exchange is limited by the constricted nasal cavity and a posteriorly displaced soft palate that fills the cramped nasopharynx. Cor pulmonale and sleep apnea can occur in severe cases.

The ideal time for treatment, again, is during the first months of life. An intracranial approach is used to advance the forehead and the superior orbital rims. The coronal craniectomy is extended along the sphenozygomatic suture into the inferior orbital fissure. This release allows the anterior cranium and midface to move downward and forward in response to the expanding brain.

If the golden period of treatment is allowed to slip by, the beneficial effect produced by the enlarging brain is lost. Strip craniectomy may still be re-

quired to prevent the detrimental consequences of increasing intracranial pressure. When the pressure is normal, correction can be deferred until the age of 5 or 6 years. A combined intracranial and extracranial approach is used to advance the forehead, orbits, and midfacial mass. In Apert deformity, a facial bipartition with a midline trapezoidal resection may be added to correct the orbital extorsion and the constricted maxilla. Earlier intervention is indicated if the risk of corneal exposure or severe upper respiratory obstruction occurs.

The trend clearly favors early correction. Nevertheless, there remains a large group of older patients who have had only limited craniectomies that prevented problems associated with increased intracranial pressure but left a disfiguring retruded midface. Treatment of these individuals is often postponed until the eruption of the permanent teeth. An extracranial approach is used to separate the face from the calvarium (Le Fort III type of osteotomy). The midfacial mass is advanced to its normal position and is supported by autologous costal and iliac bone grafts. A facial bipartition modification is often required to correct the Apert syndrome.

TELORBITISM

Abnormal interorbital distance should be regarded as a clinical sign and not as a syndrome. When the distance is excessive, the term *hyper*telorbitism is used; when it is less than normal, *hypo*telorbitism exists.

Indications for operation are cosmetic improvement and restoration of binocular vision. Abnormal displacement of the orbits is frequently accompanied by strabismus and disuse amblyopia. The question is yet unanswered whether early operation can restore binocular vision. When the deformity is grotesque, correction can be recommended as early as 2 years of age. In others, treatment can be postponed until the age of 5 or 6 years.

Mild-to-moderate forms of hypertelorbitism can be treated, using extracranial procedures that bring in the medial canthi and medial orbital walls and augment the dorsum of the nose.

Severe expressions of hypertelorbitism require an intracranial approach to correct the deformity. Osteotomies are made to remove the excess interorbital structures and to free the orbital cavities anterior to the orbital cone and the superior orbital fissure. The "useful" orbits can then be easily repositioned to correct the deformity.

BRANCHIAL ARCH DEFORMITIES

Structures derived from the first and second branchial arches include the mandible, the maxilla, and the external and middle ear. Hemifacial microsomia and mandibulofacial dysostosis are two representative craniofacial anomalies that feature a constellation of deformities of these embryologic arches.

Hemifacial Microsomia (First and Second Branchial Arch Syndrome). Removal of the ear tags and correction of the macrostomia can be performed in early infancy. The timing of the reconstructive procedures of the remaining defects will depend a great deal on the severity of the mandibular deformity.

When the condyle is absent, the first major procedure can be undertaken around the age of 5 or 6 years. A costochondral graft is used to construct a condyle and ascending ramus. A glenoid fossa must also be provided.

With milder forms, early orthodontic treatment can be recommended. An intraoral appliance is inserted to stimulate growth of the hypoplastic ascending ramus and the associated musculature. The extent of surgical intervention can be minimized and deferred until adolescence and the eruption of the permanent dentition. If needed, the mandible and maxilla can then be surgically repositioned.

Construction of an external ear is usually begun between the ages of 6 and 8 years. An autologous costal cartilage graft or a silicone prosthesis is used as a framework, depending upon the surgeon's preference. When the zygomatic arch is involved, it should be properly relocated prior to the ear construction. An attempt to restore conductive hearing with middle ear operations is presently not recommended since binaural hearing is usually not achieved.

Mandibulofacial Dysostosis (Treacher Collins Syndrome). Unlike hemifacial microsomia, which is usually unilateral, this malformation is bilateral in nature. It is inherited in an autosomal dominant manner with variable penetrance.

When a cleft of the palate is present, closure of the defect is usually performed between 12 and 18 months of age. Treatment of the remaining deformities is generally started around the age of 5 to 6 years or deferred until adolescence.

If early intervention is chosen, attention is directed toward constructing a zygoma and establishing the orbital skeletal base. The use of cranial bone grafts is well suited for this purpose.

When correction is deferred to the adolescent period, autologous costal and iliac bone grafts are used to construct the underlying skeleton. The mandible and chin are also advanced at this time. In patients with an anterior open bite, maxillary repositioning should be considered.

The ear deformity is treated in a manner like that of hemifacial microsomia.

Disorders of the Spine and Shoulder Girdle

JACK K. MAYFIELD, M.D.

DISORDERS OF THE SPINE

Treatment of spinal disorders falls into three areas: (1) observation, (2) bracing, (3) surgery. At various times in the natural history of these disorders, one or more treatment modalities may have to be utilized.

Scoliosis. In *idiopathic scoliosis,* early detection by school screening is useful. Approximately 3% of children have demonstrable scoliosis. Once detected, curves of less than 25 degrees should be observed for progression at 4- to 6-month intervals with standing posteroanterior roentgenograms. If curves progress, bracing is necessary. The usual time for curve progression to occur is during the adolescent growth spurt. The orthotic devices available are the Milwaukee brace and a plastic underarm brace, both of which are worn 23 hours each day, with 1 hour brace-free for skin care and exercises. Bracing must be maintained until skeletal growth ceases (usually age 15 in girls and age 17 in boys). The brace is discontinued gradually, with a weaning process over about a year to nights only, then the brace is discontinued after 1 additional year of wearing the brace for nights only if curve correction is maintained. Some patients demonstrate continued curve progression with or without bracing. With progressive scoliosis and scoliosis over 40 degrees in a skeletally immature patient, a posterior spinal fusion with Harrington rod instrumentation is recommended.

In *congenital scoliosis,* early recognition of vertebral malformation (unilateral unsegmented bar, hemivertebrae, and mixed anomalies) is essential. The unilateral unsegmented bar is associated with relentless progression leading to severe deformity and sometimes early death. Early surgery is frequently necessary in order to stop curve progression. Spinal bracing with carefully timed surgery is the usual mode of treatment. The Milwaukee brace or underarm brace may be indicated.

Scoliosis due to *neuromuscular* etiologies (myelomeningocele, cerebral palsy, spinal muscular atrophy, muscular dystrophy, and so on) is much more difficult to treat. Paraplegia or quadriplegia in children under age 10 is associated with progressive spinal deformity in almost all cases. A bivalved plastic interlocking and lined body jacket can be used to control curve progression until skeletal age 10 or 12, at which time spinal fusion is usually necessary. Both anterior and posterior fusion are necessary, with anterior instrumentation (Dwyer cable or Zielke rod) and posterior instrumentation (Harrington rods). Since approximately 85% of the total length of the spine has been achieved by growth by age 10, spinal fusion is usually delayed until then to avoid excessive torso shortening.

Kyphosis. Kyphosis (roundback) frequently occurs as a separate entity from scoliosis. *Scheuermann kyphosis* is usually diagnosed during early adolescence, and Milwaukee bracing has resulted in excellent permanent correction of the deformity. The best results are in children in whom bracing is started at an early age. The brace must be worn 23 hours a day with 1 hour brace-free for skin care and exercises. Maximal correction usually occurs after 12 months, and weaning can be started earlier than in idiopathic scoliosis. The need for surgery is uncommon if Milwaukee bracing is started early. If kyphosis due to Scheuermann disease is detected late, when little growth remains, when the cosmetic deformity is unacceptable, or when there is unacceptable pain, surgical correction with instrumentation and spinal fusion may be necessary.

Congenital kyphosis can be associated with severe deformity or paraplegia due to spinal cord compression. Spinal bracing is rarely helpful. Surgical correction and fusion are usually necessary. Early recognition and fusion are imperative to avoid the development of paraplegia or deformity or both.

In 16% of children who have received radiation therapy to the axial skeleton for neuroblastoma or Wilms tumor, *postradiation kyphosis* will develop, most frequently in the thoracolumbar spine. Most prone to develop kyphosis are children who received radiation before age 2, received over 3000 rads, and had radiation directed through combined anterior and posterior fields. It is recommended that these children be followed at 6-month to yearly intervals with spine roentgenograms. Curve progression will require spinal bracing. Spinal fusion and instrumentation, both anteriorly and posteriorly, are often necessary.

In kyphosis due to myelomeningocele and after laminectomy for spinal tumors, spinal fusion and instrumentation are frequently necessary. Spinal bracing postoperatively is customary.

Spinal Trauma. Spinal trauma in children can be associated with bony or epiphyseal injury with or without spinal cord damage. Without spinal cord damage, cast immobilization frequently will lead to healing in stable injuries. With paraplegia or quadriplegia, spinal deformity can be expected to develop. In the preadolescent child with spinal cord injury, paralytic scoliosis or kyphosis or both can be expected to develop in 90% of cases. Spinal bracing with a plastic body jacket can control curve progression, but spinal fusion and instrumentation probably will be necessary by skeletal age 12.

Severe spinal trauma in adolescent patients is commonly associated with spine fractures or fracture-dislocations, much as in the adult. Spinal cord damage with paraplegia or quadriplegia in the adolescent patient, however, is not usually associated with paralytic spinal deformity. Surgery is usually necessary for unstable injuries and incomplete neurologic deficits. In these circumstances a standard posterior fusion with Harrington rod instrumentation is usually sufficient.

Spondylolysis and Spondylolisthesis. Spondylolysis (pars interarticularis defect without vertebral slippage) should be observed for vertebral slippage in children with bilateral defects. In children with back or radicular pain or hamstring tightness, underarm bracing may be necessary. Lumbosacral fusion in children with painful spondylolysis unrelieved by bracing is occasionally necessary. Children with spondylolisthesis (bilateral pars interarticular defects with vertebral slippage) should be followed at 6-month to yearly intervals with standing lateral roentgenograms of the spine for possible progression of deformity. The most frequent time for progression to occur is during the adolescent growth spurt. All Grade III slippage should be fused posteriorly because of the high incidence of further slippage. Grades IV and V slippage will frequently require correction of the deformity with anterior and posterior spinal fusions.

Herniated Intervertebral Disc. Rupture of the intervertebral disc in children is not common and thus may be missed when present. The symptoms and signs are usually the same as in adults and are usually seen in adolescents. Treatment should be conservative, including bed rest, traction, analgesics, and local heat. Surgery occasionally is necessary in patients who do not respond to conservative treatment, especially if rupture is associated with persistent or progressive neurologic deficits. Surgery consists of laminectomy and disc excision. A posterior spinal fusion may be necessary concomitantly if spinal instability exists.

Intervertebral Disc Space Infection and Vertebral Osteomyelitis. In children, these are associated with marked back and occasionally radicular pain. Every attempt should be made to isolate the type of organism, either by needle biopsy, open biopsy, or blood cultures. Treatment should utilize intravenous antibiotics, bed rest, analgesics, and heat. Plaster-cast immobilization may be useful. Treatment should continue until constitutional signs and symptoms of infection have subsided and there is radiographic evidence of healing. Disc space narrowing is a usual sequela in follow-up.

Intraspinal and Axial Skeletal Tumors. Any child with persistent back pain should be evaluated for an intraspinal or axial skeletal neoplasm. The most common tumors that involve the spine in children are 1) astrocytoma, 2) ependymoma, 3) medulloblastoma, and 4) neuroblastoma. Orthopedic management is directed toward 1) spinal instability associated with tumor resection or decompression, 2) paralytic spinal deformity, and 3) radiation-induced scoliosis and kyphosis. In some children one or more spinal problems may exist. Early spinal bracing and judicious and appropriately timed spinal fusion are imperative.

Sacral Agenesis. Children with partial or complete sacral agenesis frequently have associated congenital vertebral defects in the lumbar spine. Complete sacral agenesis is usually associated with absence of the fourth or fifth lumbar vertebrae, or both. The major orthopedic problems often associated with sacral agenesis are spinopelvic instability, scoliosis, myelomeningocele, hip dislocation, hip and knee contractures, and foot deformity. Orthopedic treatment of resultant spinal instability is spinal fusion and instrumentation with postoperative bracing at age 3 or 4.

Klippel-Feil Syndrome. Failure of segmentation of the cervical spine, or Klippel-Feil syndrome, is clinically associated with a short and webbed neck and reduced neck motion. Associated deformities, such as elevation of the scapula (Sprengel deformity) and cervical ribs and scoliosis may require surgical management. Treatment of the spinal abnormality per se is not indicated unless there is associated instability of the cervical spine above or below the fused spinal segment. Spinal fusion may be indicated for this particular problem since instability in this area may result in severe, accidental neurologic deficits.

DISORDERS OF THE SHOULDER GIRDLE

Sprengel Deformity. Congenital high scapula or Sprengel deformity is an embryologic failure of descent and imperfect formation of the shoulder girdle, usually unilateral. The scapula is deformed and elevated and may be attached to the vertebral column by a fibrous, cartilaginous, or bony bridge (omovertebral bone). Associated abnormalities of the shoulder girdle musculature, hemivertebrae, fused ribs, and Klippel-Feil syndrome may be present. The clavicle is also frequently deformed. The entire shoulder girdle is frequently smaller than the normal side. Surgery is commonly necessary between the ages of 4 and 7. Treatment at ages older than 10 can be associated with brachial plexus palsy and insufficient correction. Treatment consists of surgical morselling of the clavicle; resection of the bony, cartilaginous, or fibrous bridge to the spine; removal of the upper portion of the scapula; and transfer of the scapula with its muscular attachments distally. The transfer is maintained with a cable passed through the bony scapula and attached to a Milwaukee brace or cast. A Milwaukee brace with appropriate pads is used after primary correction to mold the neck line and maintain correction.

Congenital Pseudarthrosis of the Clavicle. This condition is uncommon, is usually right-sided, and is associated with some disfigurement due to a local mass. The deformity usually increases with growth. There is little or no functional impairment. Surgical treatment with internal fixation and bone grafting may occasionally be indicated.

Chest Wall Deformities

MARC I. ROWE, M.D.,
and DAVID A. LLOYD, M.D.

Pectus Excavatum (Funnel Chest)

This deformity is marked by sharp, posterior recession of the body of the sternum, and is the most common congenital chest wall deformity. The effect of this lesion on pulmonary and cardiac function is hotly debated. However, there is little question that in many children the lesion represents a grave cosmetic defect which interferes with their quality of life. Controversy also exists regarding the optimal age for operation. In infancy, the procedure is simpler and more rapid, but at this age the child is unable to take part in the decision as to whether or not operation is indicated, or to cooperate in postoperative exercises. Most surgeons in the United States prefer to operate between the ages 2 and 7 years.

Operation consists of excision of the abnormally shaped costal cartilages on either side of the sternum, and straightening the sternum by osteotomy. Fixation of the sternum is usually accomplished by means of bone blocks, sutures, or metal pins. External fixation devices are no longer used. Recurrence is rare and the cosmetic result is usually satisfactory.

Protrusion Deformities

Protrusion deformities of the sternum are less common than pectus excavatum in a ratio of 1 : 6 to 1 : 10. There are two types. The pouter pigeon breast is a prominent forward-tilting of the manubrium, distal to which there is a depression so that the sternum is "Z" shaped. More common is the pigeon breast, where there is prominence of the body of the sternum with lateral depression of the ribs and costal margins on each side.

The pouter pigeon deformity can be corrected by subperichondral excision of the costal cartilages and sternal osteotomy to correct the angle of the sternum. Many procedures have been suggested for correction of the pigeon breast deformity; the authors favor that described by Ravitch. This operation consists of subperichondral resection of the deformed cartilages on both sides of the sternum; reefing sutures take up the slack in the perichondrium, obliterating the lateral depression. Usually, nothing further is required.

Sternal Clefts

Upper and total sternal clefts are the most common. The cleft involves the upper sternum only or the entire sternum down to the xiphoid. The defect is covered by skin and in the low lesion the pulsation of the heart can be seen. These defects have been repaired in infancy. Repair may be by direct suture or by sliding osteotomy or chondrotomy; occasionally, mesh prostheses have been used to bridge the defect.

Ectopia cordis is restricted to those instances where there is a sternal cleft and the naked heart is completely exposed outside the chest. In almost all cases, the heart is so seriously malformed that survival is impossible.

Distal clefts are usually part of the *pentalogy of Cantrell*. Other associated anomalies include omphalocele, absence of the central tendon of the diaphragm, absence of the lower pericardium, and cardiac septal defects. Treatment consists of closing the omphalocele and repairing the diaphragmatic and pericardial defects. Survival depends on the adequacy of pulmonary function and the severity of the congenital heart lesion.

Miscellaneous

Poland's syndrome is unilateral absence of the second to fourth costal cartilages as well as variable portions of the adjacent ribs. This is associated with absence of the pectoralis minor and part of the pectoralis major muscles. The breast tissue is absent, although the nipple and areola are present. In the complete syndrome there are associated deformities of the hand with short or absent middle fingers, prominent webbing, and brachysyndactyly. With localized absence of the rigid chest wall there is paradoxical respiration and frequently the appearance of a "lung hernia."

Correction is accomplished by placing rib grafts across the defect, which is covered with Malex mesh or dural grafts. In girls, augmentative mammoplasty is done at an appropriate age.

Asphyxiating Thoracic Dystrophy of the Neonate (Jeune's Syndrome). In this syndrome there are shortened horizontal ribs and a narrow rigid thorax. The chest is immobile, narrow, and cylindrical or bell shaped. In the severe form, death rapidly occurs due to respiratory insufficiency. Operation is seldom successful.

Orthopedic Disorders of the Extremities

ALVIN H. CRAWFORD, M.D.

UPPER EXTREMITIES

Sprengel's Deformity (Congenital Elevation of the Scapula). The patient presents because of an elevation of the shoulder with a small, high-riding scapula. Abduction of the affected arm is usually limited. There may be a bony or fibrous connection of the scapula to the neck that restricts motion of the arm. One must be aware of associated conditions such as thoracic scoliosis, Klippel-Feil syndrome, and renal and cardiac anomalies. Nonoperative management has not resulted in correction of this deformity. Surgical management may be directed toward correcting the basic deformity by releasing and reattaching the scapula inferiorly to its normal position, or limited surgery may be carried out to remove the anterior overhang of the scapula and improve shoulder motion.

Congenital Dislocation of the Shoulder. This is a rare condition, most commonly associated with Larsen's syndrome or multiple joint dislocations. Treatment is supportive. Rarely is operative intervention required.

Recurrent Dislocation of the Shoulder. This is rare prior to skeletal maturity. The arm is usually in forced abduction and external rotation when dislocation occurs. Treatment, following reduction of the initial dislocation, is strapping of the arm in adduction and internal rotation. Physical therapy and rehabilitation are then carried out. If dislocation recurs surgery is usually required to limit the amount of abduction and external rotation of the shoulder.

Unicameral Bone Cyst. The child may complain of occasional or intermittent pain in the shoulder or arm after trivial or sustained athletic activity. The presence of a cystic lesion in the proximal humerus on x-ray is diagnostic. The current recommended treatment is multiple aspirations and injection of methylprednisolone acetate. The early results following treatment are encouraging, especially when one considers the high recurrence rate following surgical excision, curettage, and bone grafting.

Congenital Pseudarthrosis of the Clavicle. This condition is infrequent and is most often of cosmetic significance only. It occurs primarily on the right side, except when it is associated with dextrocardia. The proximal fragment usually presents as a bump in the midclavicular region. Function is quite good and surgery is rarely necessary. When operative management is recommended, it is carried out by placing a bone graft between the proximal and distal fragments. Parents should be warned that they are replacing a bump with a scar. Function, however, is usually not improved. Bilateral pseudarthrosis of the clavicle or absence of the midportion of the clavicle is usually diagnostic of cleidocranial dysostosis.

Osteochondritis Dissecans of the Elbow. This may represent an overuse syndrome in the child. It is usually noted in throwing athletes such as pitchers, catchers, or first basemen. There may be a cystic appearance of the lateral humeral condyle on x-rays. Diagnosis is usually made following a history of elbow locking. Occasionally a small osteochondral bone fragment is seen on x-ray. Treatment is surgical excision of the loose fragment, followed by drilling of the cystic lateral humeral condyle.

Congenital Radioulnar Synostosis. This unusual condition rarely causes problems. It may not be diagnosed prior to age 6 or 7, when the child begins to engage in group sports activities and is noted to throw a ball with unusual motions. One 3-year-old presented because his father noted difficulty when trying to teach him to give a high five. The child could not rotate his forearm to slap his palm. Rarely is treatment indicated, and the only surgery performed should be the occasional corrective osteotomy to improve the fixed position.

Radiohumeral Synostosis. This extremely rare condition has been called "boomerang arm" because of its x-ray appearance. There is usually a severe angulation of the radiohumeral joint. Surgery may be indicated to improve the angular position, but arthroplasty is usually unsuccessful. Thoracic scoliosis has been associated with this condition and should be ruled out.

Congenital Dislocation of the Radial Head. It is important to definitively confirm that the dislocation is congenital rather than acquired. A line drawn down the radial shaft usually points to the capitellum on x-ray. The congenital condition will have a globe-shaped radial head, whereas in the acquired condition the head maintains its normal concave shape. There may be associated limitation of pronation and supination; however, flexion and extension of the elbow are rarely limited and surgery is not usually indicated.

Congenital Absence of the Thumb. The thumb may be totally absent or a rudimentary thumb may be present. Most surgical procedures to improve function of the rudimentary digit have not been successful. When the thumb is completely absent, surgery may be indicated to pollicize one of the remaining digits to perform the function of opposition and improve pinch for the patient. These patients sometimes do surprisingly well with no surgery.

Syndactyly. This is one of the most common deformities of the hand. Most often, a web occurs between the ring finger and the small finger. Surgery to release the webbing is indicated; however, the timing is dependent upon whether there is tethering of one finger on the other with a progressive angular deformity. If tethering and angulation occur, surgical release should be carried out directly. If there are multiple syndactylies, three adjacent fingers should not be corrected simultaneously because of the possibility of compromise to the blood supply.

Gigantism of the Fingers (Macrodactyly). Historically this condition has been felt to be associated with neurofibromatosis, but conclusive association has not been verified. The condition may be managed surgically by reduction of soft tissue and phalangeal growth arrest.

Camptodactyly. This is an interphalangeal joint contracture that is felt to be related to an abnormal shortening of the flexor digitorum sublimus. Serial casting has been beneficial and tends to cause compensatory hyperextension of the MP and DIP joint, rather than to correct the flexion contracture of the interphalangeal joint. Tendon lengthening does not always resolve the deformity. It is best to treat the child with repetitive stretching exercises in the newborn period.

Clinodactyly. This deformity is usually found on the small finger, which is curved toward the thumb. Passive stretching and splinting do not completely correct the deformity. Interference with hand function is the only indication for surgical correction, which, fortunately, is rarely necessary.

Constriction Bands (Streeter's Dysplasia). This is felt to result from the limb of a digit being trapped between the chorionic and amniotic membranes. The deformity is seen in the neonatal period as a circumferential soft tissue constriction. The urgency of treatment is directly related to whether or not edema is present and there is compromise of venous return. Treatment is primarily surgical and is usually carried out in two stages. Only one side or 180 degrees of the ring should be released at one time. The function of the digit or extremity is usually quite good if there has been no vascular compromise.

Trigger Thumb. This is a most rewarding diagnosis to make because the treatment is usually quite successful. The history is usually that of the thumb cocking or trapping in acute flexion of the distal interphalangeal joint. The thumb can be passively extended; however, the infant has difficulty flexing and extending the joint. Absence of the thumb extensor (congenital clasped thumb) as the cause of lack of extension must be ruled out. A small nodule is usually palpable in the flexor tendon over the metacarpal phalangeal joint. I find surgical correction of this deformity so overwhelmingly effective that I no longer recommend stretching exercises, injection, or serial casting.

Madelung's Deformity. Congenital Madelung's deformity, a relatively rare condition characterized by excessive prominence of the distal ulna at the wrist, is found most commonly in females. Radiographically one sees a triangulation or upside-down pyramidal shape of the carpal bones. The deformity is primarily cosmetic and may require no treatment other than advice or assurance to the patient and parent.

Acquired Madelung's deformity is usually secondary to a growth arrest following a distal radial epiphyseal fracture. In the growing child, treatment consists of a segmental shortening ostectomy and an epiphyseal arrest of the distal ulna. An angulation osteotomy of the distal radius is occasionally necessary to restore wrist alignment.

Lobster Claw Hand. This condition is usually unilateral. There is absence of the inner (second through fourth) digits of the hand or variations thereof. The peripheral digits may be syndactylized. The child may have very little difficulty with the deformity; but if he or she has trouble in handling large objects, it may be necessary to deepen the web-space to improve grasp and pinch. The excellent sensation and functional length of the hand will usually cause the child to resist any attempt at prosthetic fitting.

Congenital Absence of the Radius. This usually causes progressive deviation of the hand to the radial side. The hand may or may not have its full complement of five digits. Concern must be addressed very early to the possibility of a hematologic disorder such as thrombocytopenic purpura if the thumb is not present. All of our very diligent efforts to splint the hand when the child is very young have not resulted in significant correction. If the deformity is bilateral it may be best to leave it alone surgically and persist with splinting. If the deformity is unilateral and the elbow is stable, I recommend performing a centralization procedure (putting the hand on the end of the ulna) to better align the hand on the forearm. The parents should be forewarned that the procedure might require more revision after the initial surgery. Continuous splinting at night until skeletal maturity is reached is essential for a good result.

Below Elbow Amputation. This is the most common congenital amputation of the upper extremity. The left forearm is most often affected. These children should be considered very early for prosthetic fitting; when the child is able to sit independently, a passive forearm and hand device is applied. An articulated prosthesis such as a Northwestern ring over-the-shoulder prosthesis with a CAPP (Childhood Amputee and Prosthetic Project) hand is applied when the child can control the shoulder device. The child may or may not accept the prosthesis; however, one should always attempt prosthetic fitting early and allow the child the option.

Phocomelia (Seal Flipper). In this extremely rare condition, which is noted in the newborn nursery, a small remnant of the upper extremity, usually the hand, is attached to the shoulder. These patients accommodate quite well and will tend to use their feet for feeding, typing, writing, and even driving. Prosthetic fitting should be attempted in unilateral cases; however, in bilateral phocomelia, prosthetic fitting is rarely successful. The advent of soccer as a public school sport in this country has presented a tremendous athletic outlet to these patients and they tend to excel in this sport.

Congenital Absence of the Ulna. This is much less common than absence of the radius. There will occasionally be absence of fingers. Children with bilateral deformity tend to get along better with surgery or prosthetic fitting. Passive splinting at night is significantly beneficial. Surgery to centralize the hand over the radius will improve cosmesis.

LOWER EXTREMITIES

Rotational Deformities. Metatarsus adductus, internal tibial torsion, and femoral anteversion compose a triad of rotational problems that present clinically as in-toeing or "ding toes," one of the most common lower extremity complaints seen by the pediatric orthopedist. The emphasis on corrective measures of different types has possibly been overdone. Spontaneous resolution of these problems following a natural course of time has been quite impressive to me. All of these conditions cause the child to toe-in when walking, and treatment is directed toward derotating or causing the child to externally rotate the affected foot to the normal 20 to 30 degree externally rotated foot progression angle.

In *femoral anteversion,* characterized by in-toeing, the child usually sits in the so-called TV squat positions, which can be described as Type I and Type II. Type I is the classic TV squat position ("W") or reverse tailor position, as opposed to the Type II position, in which the child sits on his feet, which are tucked under his buttocks. This causes the feet to be in more adduction and presents as the worst of the two deformities.

To determine if the child should be treated, the child is placed in the supine position and the log-roll test is given, that is, the femoral shaft is externally rotated with the hips in extension. The femur can usually be internally rotated to approximately 90 degrees; however, external rotation is limited. If external rotation is greater than 20 degrees, the child will be able to compensate and should not require treatment. I have discontinued treatment with the Denis Browne bar in favor of trying to alter the sleeping pattern (most of these children sleep in the prone position with their feet tucked under them, which aggravates the deformity). The Denis Browne bar will alter the position but is not tolerated well by child or parent and can give rise to valgus deformities of the knees. As a result, we recommend sleeping shoes with the heels tied together by a shoelace with approximately one inch play between them. This will allow the child to sleep with the feet together or toes out, but will not allow him to toe-in.

For the late adolescent child who has no compensatory external rotation, and who may be made fun of because of his deformity, we recommend the supracondylar derotation osteotomy. Rarely is this procedure performed.

The diagnosis of *internal tibial torsion* is confirmed by flexing the knee to 90 degrees and observing the bimalleolar relationships. The medial malleolus is normally 20 degrees anterior in the transverse plane to the lateral malleolus. If the malleoli are level or the internal malleolus anterior, the diagnosis is confirmed. The treatment of internal tibial torsion is primarily observation of the natural course. Corrective shoeing has not produced a dramatic response with resolution of the problem but continues to be advocated by many groups. Surgical correlation by derotation of this deformity is to be frowned upon.

I recommend dividing *metatarsus adductus* into three types and basing the treatment on the type. The adducted foot presents as a "C" on its *outside border,* unlike the "V" of the normal foot.

Type 1 is a "C" foot that corrects to a "V" when its outer margins or the distal lateral leg is stroked. No treatment is necessary for this very supple deformity.

In Type 2 the deformity will not correct when stroked on its lateral surface but can be passively manipulated to the "V" position. This foot can be treated by repetitive passive manipulations of approximately 20 times with each diaper change during the waking hours.

Type 3 deformity cannot be corrected to neutral with passive manipulation and requires serial casting. Usually two or three casts over 6 to 8 weeks will resolve the problem.

Physiologic Bowleg. This presents at approximately 15 to 20 months and is usually associated with early walking. Physical examination reveals a significant amount of internal tibial torsion. Standing x-rays should be taken of all children whose femoral intercondylar distance is greater than 10 centimeters with the ankle malleoli held together. Those patients with intercondylar (between the knee) distances less than 10 centimeters are observed at approximately 4- to 6-month intervals and usually self-correct, whereas those with distances greater than 10 centimeters should be placed in a Blount's bowleg brace at night. It is important to discuss with the parents the natural history of bowleg deformity, which is normal up to 3 years of age, as is knock knee tendency between 3 and 6 years of age.

Tibia Vara (Blount's Disease). This deformity may be unilateral or bilateral. When it is bilateral, an x-ray is necessary to differentiate it from physiologic bowing. With Blount's disease there is fragmentation of the proximal medial tibial metaphysis. The initial management of Blount's disease is by bracing; however, parents should be informed that surgery is usually necessary and that recurrences are frequent and require further surgery.

Knock Knee Deformity. IDIOPATHIC. Children usually undergo a progressive valgus alignment between ages 3 and 6. Treatment is determined by the amount of between the ankle distance present with the knees together. If more than 10 centimeters, a treatment program is begun. This usually consists initially of night splinting in an A-frame brace. If the deformity is progressive under this treatment, one must consider medial femoral epiphyseal stapling to allow the child to self-correct with growth. If there is not enough growth remaining, tibial fibular osteotomy may be necessary to correct alignment.

ACQUIRED KNOCK KNEE DEFORMITY. Unilateral progressive valgus deformity and overgrowth may follow proximal tibial fractures in young children. Observation is initial treatment. If the valgus angulation exceeds that of the opposite side by 20 degrees, a proximal tibial osteotomy and fibular ostectomy may be required. Epiphyseal stapling should be considered if there is enough growth remaining to allow the child to correct the deformity himself.

Congenital Angulation of the Tibia. There are two basic angular deformities: 1) Posterior medial bowing, "kyphoscoliosis tibia," is a fairly benign condition that usually resolves without treatment. The child may present initially with a calcaneovalgus deformity of the foot. X-rays show the posteromedial angulation with an increase in bone density. The primary complication is residual shortening that may amount to as much as 1 to 2 inches at skeletal maturity. Recently, some authors have recommended early surgical correction for the deformity in the interest of preserving length. I recommend careful longitudinal follow-up with bracing if angulation progresses. A skeletal growth chart should be plotted to monitor limb lengths.

2) Anterior lateral bowing is potentially malignant and occasionally results in spontaneous fracture and pseudarthrosis tibia. Every effort should be made to prevent fracture in these cases because of their poor healing potential. Early bracing and electric stimulation have been helpful for us in the management of this disorder. Bone grafting and plating have not been rewarding for the cases that have undergone fractures. We have had limited success with microvascular fibular transplantation in cases of frank pseudarthrosis tibia. Von Recklinghausen neurofibromatosis has been found to be associated in approximately 45 to 55% of patients with pseudarthrosis tibia, even though no café-au-lait spots need be present when the diagnosis is made.

Congenital Absence of the Tibia. Complete absence of the tibia is usually associated with absence of several toes on the medial aspect of the foot. The limb is quite short, and usually amputation and conversion to prosthetic fitting is the treatment of choice. Some authors have attempted to articulate the proximal fibula with the femur. This is a reasonable alternative if there is a functioning quadriceps mechanism and the patella is present. Most of these children are converted to prosthetic wear when they start to stand and walk so their progress is not delayed.

In partial absence, if the proximal tibia is present it can be fused to the fibula to provide a longer limb. Amputation and prosthetic fitting are required because of the shortening. Most surgeons try to preserve the calcaneus and its weight-bearing skin when amputation is performed.

Congenital Absence of the Fibula. This condition may be associated with partial loss of the foot and a foreshortened femur. There also may be a ball-and-socket joint of the ankle. Treatment is directed toward equalizing the length of the limbs. Lengthening of the involved extremity may be considered for severe limb length discrepancies, and contralateral epiphyseal arrest for moderate discrepancies.

Chondromalacia Patella. The patient usually presents with vague aching symptoms around the inferior pole of the patella. The pain usually follows activity, although it may accompany activity without limiting participation. Pain is made worse by walking up or down stairs. There is considerable stiffness and discomfort after prolonged sitting. Activity modification and simple aspirin compose the initial treatment. A knee immobilizer may be required. A vigorous quadricep strengthening program is strongly recommended.

Recurrent Dislocation/Subluxation of the Patella. The dislocation usually occurs to the lateral side of the knee joint and may be traumatic or congenital and spontaneous. The traumatic type is usually followed by an effusion. X-rays should be examined very carefully to rule out the presence of a small osteochondral fracture, which usually occurs off the medial patellar facet or lateral femoral condyle. This fragment may subsequently become a loose body or joint mouse. The knee is aspirated for comfort and if a fracture is suspected, arthroscopy is performed and small fragments removed. The knee is rigidly immobilized for 3 weeks, followed by rehabilitation. If there are repeat dislocations following rehabilitation, then surgery consisting of a lateral release or medial reinforcement and alignment may be necessary.

Subluxation of the Knee. This is very difficult to diagnose or manage. It is most frequently found in teenage females. The symptoms are accentuated by physical education requirements. There is a positive patellar apprehension sign (performed by attempting to displace the patella laterally with the knee in extension). The surgical management of this problem has not been rewarding. I recommend that these patients be excused from physical education.

Congenital Dislocation of the Patella. In this condition there is either a small, high-riding patella or a deficiency of the lateral supracondylar femoral articular surface. The patient may have a history of spontaneous dislocation but no serious physical disabilities. Surgery has not been overwhelmingly successful and we now recommend soft-ware bracing during symptomatic periods or when the child engages in vigorous athletic activities. Surgical realignment of the patella by soft tissue combined with a lateral release is the treatment of choice if splinting, bracing, and physical therapy are unsuccessful.

Congenital (Recurvatum) Dislocation of the Knee. This condition usually presents in the newborn nursery. There is a history of breech delivery and the foot positions are either submandibular or axillary. The knee may be hyperextended, subluxated, or completely dislocated. Recommended treatment is serial casting of the knee into progressive flexion, which can usually be achieved over a 6-week period, followed by night splinting in 30 or 40 degrees of flexion for perhaps 6 months. When treatment is started early, surgery is rarely necessary.

Bipartite Patella. This variation of patellar ossification has until recently been an x-ray diagnosis only. The symptomatic patient presents with superior lateral patellar pain, and direct pressure over this area reproduces the pain. If arthroscopy shows a step-off, then removal of the accessory ossicle may resolve the symptoms.

Discoid Meniscus. This usually presents by age 2 to 3, with a history of a popping/snapping mass over the lateral aspect of the knee. If there is no history of locking, such as would occur with a torn meniscus, I recommend observation and assurance to the parents. If there is a history of locking, direct surgical removal is recommended. Arthroscopic surgery has recently been advocated for this lesion; however, it is too early to evaluate the results.

Osteochondritis Dissecans. This condition is one of retropatellar pain with activity that is relieved by rest. X-rays are completely diagnostic and show the characteristic lesion to be on the lateral aspect of the medial femoral condyle in the region of the intercondylar notch. Initial treatment should consist of cylinder cast immobilization with the knee in flexion, followed by rehabilitation. If symptoms persist, arthroscopic drilling has been successful in resolving the problem. If the osteochondritic fragment becomes loose and falls into the joint, the patient may experience locking. Direct operative excision to remove the loose fragment is then recommended.

Osgood-Schlatter's Disease (Tibial Tubercle Apophysitis). There is pain to palpation directly over the patellar tendon insertion. There may be significant swelling—"knobby knees." This probably represents one of the "overuse syndrome" or "growing pains" disorders. Discontinuing all athletic activity for a period of time is the initial treatment of choice. If the symptoms do not improve, a knee immobilizer or cylinder cast is recommended. Injection of steroids is definitely contraindicated. Surgery is reserved for the older adolescent or young adult noted to have a small painful ossicle remaining as the residual of active childhood disease.

Popliteal Cyst (Baker's Cyst). The cyst is usually found on the medial aspect of the posterior knee joint by the parent while bathing the young child. The mass is totally asymptomatic. Most authors recommend aspiration or no treatment of the small lesion. Surgery may be performed for the larger lesions, usually greater than 2 or 3 centimeters. The parents should be forewarned of the high recurrence rate following excision. If there is pain associated with the mass, one must be aware of the possibility of a dissecting popliteal cyst (associated with rheumatoid arthritis), which requires diagnostic studies.

Equinovarus (Clubfoot) Deformity. When the newborn child presents with a severely inverted and rotated foot deformity, efforts should be made to manipulate the foot into the neutral position, no matter how rigid the deformity. If the foot can be passively brought into the neutral position and the heel brought down, the treatment is the same as that outlined for metatarsus adductus. If the heel cannot be brought down, the diagnosis of clubfoot should be established and serial casting started. The parents should be forewarned that surgery may be necessary and that following surgery extensive aftercare such as shoeing and/or repeat casting may be necessary to ensure a good foot at skeletal maturity.

Flatfoot. Most flatfeet are familial. It is most important to distinguish the supple versus the rigid flatfoot deformity. The young infant usually has the flexible flatfoot, which looks even worse because of the medial fat pad. If the foot is flat when the child is standing but an arch appears when suspended, the patient can be assured that the condition will resolve. If the arch does not appear with suspension, the flatfoot is considered rigid. For the non-painful, rigid flatfoot, a heel seat cup provides adequate medial support and can be worn in any shoe, as opposed to the more expensive orthopedic corrective shoe. The painful or rigid flatfoot should be thoroughly investigated by radiography for inflammatory arthritis or tarsal bone abnormalities. Computed tomography has been especially beneficial in identifying occult lesions causing a painful flatfoot. No treatment is recommended for the flexible flatfoot.

Pes Cavus "High Arches." Idiopathic or congenital pes cavus is extremely rare and is most often associated with a neurologic condition. There might be associated clawing of the toes. It is the responsibility of the treating physician to make the correct diagnosis. Primary treatment is usually directed toward the neurologic condition. When the neurologic condition has been verified as either static or progressive, then attention can be directed to the foot. The first stage of treatment should include release of the tight plantar fascia and serial casting. In the older child, metatarsal osteotomy and calcaneal osteotomies may be necessary. The associated cock-up and claw-toe deformities may also require surgery.

Osteochondrosis of the Foot. Several pain problems about the foot are manifestations of osteochondrosis.

KOEHLER'S DISEASE. This condition presents in the 5- to 7-year-old as pain on the medial side of the foot with weight-bearing. There may be subtle swelling over the tarsal navicular region. An x-ray will usually show a characteristic increase in density of the tarsal navicular bone, representing avascular necrosis. If the foot is extremely tender, a short leg walking cast may be required. If the child is only moderately symptomatic, a firm shoe will suffice.

FREIBERG'S INFARCTION. In this condition, pain can be isolated directly under the head of the second metatarsal and x-rays show avascular necrosis of the head. Treatment is a firm supportive shoe. Occasionally a short leg walking cast may be necessary. The metatarsal head may undergo flattening with arthritic changes. No surgical treatment is usually required in the pediatric age group.

SEVER'S DISEASE (CALCANEAL APOPHYSITIS). Sever's disease is usually found in a very athletic youngster and probably represents an overuse syndrome. At one time x-rays were considered diagnostic; however, x-rays of all children in this age group are similar, and the disease has no unique radiographic characteristic. Treatment may consist of resting the pull of the tendo-achilles on the calcaneus with a shoe lift or of insertion of a powder sponge in the heel of the shoe. If the pain is severe, the child may be placed temporarily in a short leg walking cast with the foot in equinus.

Calcaneovalgus Foot. This occurs in the newborn, with the foot maximally dorsiflexed against the tibia. One must differentiate this condition from congenital vertical talus. The primary distinction is the mobility of the heel. In congenital vertical talus, the heel is firmly fixed in equinus, but it is quite mobile in calcaneovalgus foot. Treatment of this condition consists of passive stretching exercises. Serial casting is very rarely necessary if the parents are not afraid to perform the plantar flexion stretching exercises.

Congenital Vertical Talus (Rocker Bottom Foot, Persian Slipper Foot, Congenital Convex Pes Valgus). This condition presents in the newborn nursery as a severe flatfoot with the heel in equinus and the forefoot in marked dorsiflexion. The head of the talus can usually be found presenting as a bulge on the medial aspect of the foot. Casting may be attempted early, but surgery is almost always required to obtain a complete correction.

Tarsal Coalition (Peroneal Spastic Flatfoot). The child with this condition has a history of repeated ankle sprains and strains. Physical examination shows limited subtalar motion. The foot may be fixed in pronation with peroneal muscle spasm, hence the oft-used term peroneal spastic flatfoot. The x-rays may be diagnostic by showing a failure of separation of some of the tarsal bones. At our center the most common coalition is the calcaneal navicular bar. The initial treatment should be a 3- to 6-week period of cast immobilization followed by rehabilitation. If this fails, surgical excision of the bony bridge should be attempted if there is no evidence of arthritis of the other foot joints. Infrequently, a triple arthrodesis may be necessary for relief of pain.

Congenital Shortening of the Achilles Tendon. This condition is most frequently bilateral and the child is noted to walk on his toes most of the time, hence the term "habitual" or "idiopathic" toe-walker. Cerebrospasticity and other neurologic conditions must be ruled out. Initial treatment may consist of a negative heel-walking cast, the heel of which is placed under the toes in an attempt to have the child stretch out the heel cord with walking, similar to the position of the heel with Earth shoes. If this treatment is unsuccessful, a limited heel cord lengthening is performed.

Pump Bumps. The patient presents with heel pain from the pressure of the shoe-heel counter. These patients have an unusual bony prominence of the posterior superior aspect of the calcaneus at the insertion of the achilles tendon. The term pump bump originates from a type of woman's shoe (pumps) causing the irritation. Surgical excision of the bump ensures correction of the deformity.

Accessory Navicular (Symptomatic). It is not uncommon to see on x-ray an accessory ossification center of the tarsal navicular with a symptomatic accessory navicular. There is pain on the inside of the arch, and a prominence of the medial border of the foot at the insertion of the posterior tibialis tendon into the navicular bone. The child is usually quite athletic. I feel this represents an overuse syndrome. Initial treatment is rest of the foot in a short leg cast. If the child continues to be symptomatic, it may be necessary to remove the accessory ossicle.

Bunions. This condition usually is a cosmetic deformity and a problem with shoe wear rather than with pain. A family history is quite frequent. Nonoperative management by changing the type of shoe is occasionally successful. For progressive bunion deformity, surgical correction is recommended.

Subungual Exostosis. This is a resistant or recurrent fungating ingrown toenail. X-rays are diagnostic and show a bony spur just under the nail bed on the lateral view. Direct excision usually results in complete relief.

The Hip

LYNN T. STAHELI, M.D.

Hip problems in childhood are unusually serious for several reasons. First, the hip is normally only marginally competent; degenerative arthritis frequently occurs without known cause. Second, hip problems are often more difficult to diagnose than other joint disorders because of the hip's deep location under layers of muscle. Third, the blood supply to the proximal femoral epiphysis is tenuous. Trauma, inflammation, or compression can obstruct flow, cause necrosis, and permanently damage the hip in as short a time as 6–8 hours. Thus, early diagnosis of hip problems is critical. With early diagnosis and skillful management, deformity and disability can usually be prevented.

CONGENITAL DYSPLASIA OF THE HIP (CDH)

CDH includes a variety of deformities, from shallow acetabulum to frank dislocation. Effective management requires early diagnosis, which is not easy. The hip is primarily cartilaginous in the newborn, making radiography unreliable. Physical findings are subtle, and CDH can be missed by even the most skillful examiner. Thus, it is essential that the search for the problem continue throughout infancy.

Newborn Screening. The infant should be quiet and relaxed for the screening examination. The examiner employs Ortaloni's or Barlow's maneuvers to detect instability. "Clicks" are insignificant. "Clunks" or "jerks" are signs of instability felt by the examiner as the femoral head slides in and out of the socket. If screening is negative, the hip should be re-examined when the infant is next seen. If a "click" is heard, the infant should be examined at the next two or three visits to be certain that it is insignificant. If a "clunk" is felt, treatment is indicated. If the hip is stable in abduction, a simple, soft abduction splint is applied. If the hip is unstable, a "Pavlik harness" should be used. This harness is the most effective splint available.

If one is uncertain whether it is a "click" or a "clunk," the infant is either treated or referred. It is prudent to overtreat when in doubt. Triple diapers are not helpful and are often harmful. They become compressed between the thighs and provide little or no abduction. More importantly, they create the illusion that treatment is in progress when in fact valuable time is being wasted.

Early Infancy (1–3 Months). The physical findings change during the first weeks after birth. Hip instability signs, which are most reliable in the neonatal period, tend to disappear and are replaced by signs of limited abduction and limb shortening, which become more pronounced with increasing age.

HIGH RISK INFANTS. The incidence of classic CDH is about 0.1%. The chances increase 30 times when a positive family history is present. It is about 10 times more likely to occur in infants with metatarsus adductus. CDH is found in about 20% of infants with torticollis. Infants at risk should have a single AP radiograph of the pelvis taken at 3 months of age. Some infants with a negative examination will have definite radiographic findings of CDH. Without treatment these children face early degenerative arthritis, perhaps as early as their teen years.

Radiography. Radiography in the newborn period is reliable in only about half of the cases. Reliability rapidly improves over the next 3 months, when it becomes the most definitive diagnostic method. A single AP radiograph of the pelvis is adequate for routine screening and follow-up evaluations. The slope of the acetabulum (acetabular index) is measured as an indicator of acetabular dysplasia. The relationship of the upper femur and acetabulum is assessed for evidence of dislocation. Ossification of the proximal femoral epiphysis, which normally occurs during the first 6 months, is often delayed in CDH. In its absence, the position of the upper femoral metaphysis is compared with the acetabulum. If the hip is reduced, the metaphysis will fall medial to a line (Perkin's) drawn vertically from the lateral margin of the acetabulum and at right angles to a line that passes through both triradiate cartilage clear spaces (Hilgenreiner's). If the epiphyseal ossification center is seen, it should fall in the inner lower quadrant created by the intersection of Perkin's and Hilgenreiner's lines.

The end point of treatment is a normal radiograph. After the hip is reduced, the physical examination becomes normal. Acetabular dysplasia may persist and must be corrected to ensure a lasting satisfactory result. This can only be assessed radiographically.

Older Infants and Children. Limited abduction, shortening of the limb, and limp are classic findings. Whenever the diagnosis is seriously considered, a radiograph should be taken.

Referral

The role of the primary care physican is diagnostic. Treatment should be provided by an orthopedics specialist. Objectives include achieving a concentric reduction, correcting acetabular dysplasia, and avoiding avascular necrosis. At present, Pavlik harness treatment is appropriate in infants under 6 months of age. Traditional traction, closed reduction under anesthesia, and cast immobilization are indicated if dislocation persists after a trial with the Pavlik harness, and for children first seen after 6 months of age. Open reduction is indicated if closed reduction fails or if the child is seen after about 2 years of age.

SEPTIC ARTHRITIS

Bacterial infection of the hip joint is one of the most urgent problems in orthopedics. It not only can damage the articular cartilage but also can obstruct the circulation to the epiphysis, causing avascular necrosis. The sequelae of necrosis include a severely shortened leg and a fused hip.

Early Infancy. Most sequelae of septic arthritis result from hip infections that occur during the neonatal period or early infancy. At that age diagnosis is difficult; systemic and localizing signs are few. The only reliable sign is "pseudoparalysis" of the involved limb. Spontaneous hip movement is absent. The cause should be determined. Trauma and true paralysis must also be considered.

Joint fluid examination is the only reliable method of establishing the diagnosis. Other studies are unreliable. When in doubt, the joint is aspirated under image intensifier guidance. A negative study should be confirmed by arthrography. After aspiration, dye is instilled into the joint and a permanent radiograph is made. This confirms that the joint was entered.

In later infancy and childhood, diagnosing septic arthritis is less difficult. The patient is often ill, has guarding of the hip, resists rotational movement, and shows an elevated sedimentation rate. Again, these findings mandate the need for a diagnostic arthrocentesis. Studies such as bone scanning delay diagnosis and usually are of little help.

Radiography is of limited value. Fat pad signs are not reliable. It is a common mistake to rely on negative radiographs. Only a negative arthrocentesis documented with an arthrogram can rule out the presence of septic arthritis.

If purulent fluid is obtained from the arthrocentesis, the joint should be surgically drained. An open procedure makes certain the joint is completely evacuated and will remain free of fluid. Incomplete drainage by needle aspiration is too risky to be justified. The potential for disability is too great. About 20% of purulent drainage will be culture and Gram stain negative. This is to be expected. Open drainage and antibiotic treatment should be provided. The antibiotic is selected empirically, using the age of the patient as a guide.

TOXIC SYNOVITIS

Toxic synovitis or "observation hip syndrome" is a benign inflammatory problem of the hip of unknown etiology. It commonly occurs in late infancy and childhood, and in 1 to 3% of cases leads to Perthes' disease.

The major diagnostic problem is clearly separating this benign condition from septic arthritis. Differentiation is made by considering several factors: 1) The patient with synovitis is usually not as ill as the child with arthritis. The child's fever, malaise, and activity level are helpful guides. 2) In septic arthritis joint guarding is more pronounced and the patient will usually refuse to walk. 3) The ESR is usually slightly elevated in synovitis and moderately or severely elevated in septic arthritis. Leukocytosis is variable in both. 4) If the diagnosis remains uncertain, an arthrocentesis is indicated. It should be re-emphasized that radiographs and bone scans are seldom helpful in making this differentiation.

Synovitis is managed by rest. Traction on the limb is unnecessary and theoretically harmful. The hip joint capsule is most relaxed and, thus, the joint capacity greatest, when the hip is flexed, slightly abducted, and laterally rotated. The patient will assume this position while resting. Traction is likely to alter this position, increasing the intra-articular pressure and possibly impairing circulation to the epiphysis.

Bed rest is continued until hip rotation is free and unguarded. A follow-up check should be made in a month or so to ensure that motion has completely returned. Persisting stiffness is an indication for a radiograph to rule out Perthes' disease.

PERTHES' DISEASE

Perthes' disease is commonly referred to as LCP disease, a name derived from the initials of those first describing the disease (Legg-Calvé-Perthes). LCP is an idiopathic avascular necrosis of the femoral capital epiphysis that occurs spontaneously during midchildhood. Healing occurs consistently but slowly over 2 to 3 years. Residual deformity may lead to degenerative arthritis in adult life. LCP tends to occur in some families, in children of delayed skeletal age, and occasionally following toxic synovitis. It affects males most frequently, and in most cases the cause is unknown. During midchildhood, circulation to the femoral epiphysis is even more tenuous than at other ages, being almost totally provided by the lateral retinacular vessels. These may be obstructed by trauma, inflammation, coagulation defects, or other causes.

LCP disease results from one or more ischemic episodes occurring at different sites in the vascular network. In mild cases only the anterior portion of the head is involved; in severe cases the whole head is involved. The disease is also more serious in the older child.

Clinical Features. Onset is usually insidious. It commonly occurs in one hip of a boy between 4 and 8 years of age but may occur in either sex between ages 3 and 14 years. The child presents with a limp and mild discomfort. Often the symptoms are present for months before the family seeks medical attention. The physical findings include limitation of abduction and medial rotation of the affected hip. Radiographic features vary according to the stage of the disease. *Synovitic stage:* This stage has usually passed by the time the child is first seen. If the child is seen very early in the disease process, the radiographs may show slight joint space widening. *Necrotic or collapse stage:* The earliest definitive sign is a crescentic radiolucency just under the subchondral bone of the epiphysis on the lateral projection. More commonly there is a flattening, irregularity, and increased density of the epiphysis. *Fragmentation stage:* Replacement of necrotic bone with preossified fibrous tissue produces a "motheaten" appearance characteristic of this stage. *Consolidation stage:* Reossification progresses with increasing homogenicity of the epiphysis. Widening of the neck and head (coxa magna), and flattening of the epiphysis (coxa plana) are frequently seen.

These stages take several years to run their course. Treatment is usually started during the necrotic stage and continues through the fragmentation stage. This requires about 12 to 18 months.

Management. Treatment is controversial, but current management trends are conservative. Individualized management, fewer operative procedures, and shorter treatment periods with less cumbersome braces are currently favored. The first step is restoration of motion by rest. Activity causes microfractures of the soft, ischemic epiphysis. These fractures induce synovitis, which causes stiffness and adductor contracture. Rest reduces this inflammation and allows return of motion. Active motion is encouraged. Traction to immobilize the child and gently stretch the tight adductor muscles is appropriate in some cases. This can be done at home or in the hospital. The objective is to maintain the sphericity of the femoral head during the healing process by providing "containment." The uninvolved firm acetabulum is utilized as a mold to maintain the shape of the head. This requires that the hip be maintained in abduction, usually with an abduction brace. Currently the smaller, lighter braces are most favored because they allow the child to maintain a nearly normal activity level.

No treatment is required for mild LCP disease. For severe cases, treatment is much less effective. In some cases, maintaining containment by operation is appropriate. The procedures alter the shape of the upper femur or acetabulum so that containment is provided with the child standing in the normal weight-bearing attitude.

SLIPPED CAPITAL FEMORAL EPIPHYSIS (SCFE)

SCFE is a fracture of the capital femoral epiphysis that usually occurs in the pubescent male and gradually produces progressive displacement (chronic slip). Occasionally, acute injury produces varying degrees of slip. Often these are superimposed on the chronic form.

SCFE is a serious condition. The slipping not only produces deformity but also stretches the vessels to the epiphysis. Prognosis depends upon the severity of displacement, which in turn is dependent upon the duration of the problem. Early diagnosis is critical.

SCFE is suspected when the pubertal patient complains of hip or knee pain. As the obturator nerve innervates both the hip and knee, referred pain to the knee is common. The physical examination demonstrates limited medial rotation of the hip. This is best evaluated with the patient prone and the knees flexed to a right angle. Both thighs are then rotated in (feet going out), while the pelvis is held in a level position. Asymmetry of rotation is consistent with the diagnosis. Diagnosis is established by a lateral radiograph. A so-called "frog lateral" of the pelvis is ordered. This view will demonstrate the characteristic posterior displacement of the femoral epiphysis relative to the neck. In addition, diffuse rarefaction of the metaphysis and widening of the physis are seen.

After the diagnosis is established, the patient should be hospitalized without delay, since further slipping can occur at any time and fixation of the epiphysis by operation is essential. Fixation is achieved by passing two or three threaded pins across the physis. This promotes fusion, preventing further displacement.

Idiopathic Cortical Hyperostoses

(Infantile Cortical Hyperostosis [Caffey's Disease], Familial Cortical Hyperostosis, and Related Conditions)

RICHARD B. GOLDBLOOM, M.D.

Accumulating evidence suggests that idiopathic cortical (subperiosteal) hyperostosis may occur in infants and children under several different circumstances, possibly reflecting a common response to different disease processes. The best known of these conditions is infantile cortical hyperostosis, or Caffey's disease. A striking decline in prevalence of this condition had been observed during the period since the 1960's, but sporadic reappearance of the disease has been reported from several centers over the past 2 years.

Typically, symptoms first appear before 6 months of age, though prenatal radiographic diagnosis has been reported. Since the cause is unknown and the course is most often one of progressive spontaneous resolution without sequelae, treatment is symptomatic, and often no therapy is required. Signs and symptoms that may require treatment include fever, refusal of food, irritability, and swelling and tenderness over affected bones. The mandible is involved in virtually all cases, thus increased salivation may be associated with feeding difficulty.

During the acute phase, the child should be handled gently, since the affected bones may be very tender to pressure. If bottle feeding is utilized, because of mandibular involvement a cross-cut nipple may be used to reduce the effort and discomfort of sucking.

Local and systemic manifestations usually improve spontaneously, sometimes even during the first week of illness. If fever and irritability are pronounced, acetaminophen (30–60 mg/kg/24 hours) every 4 to 6 hours by mouth may be given for a few days only. Acetylsalicylic acid should be used with caution in young infants. If necessary, it can be given for 1 or 2 days in a dose of 30 to 60 mg/kg/24 hours, in divided doses, but preferably not to infants under 6 months of age. Sedation is rarely required.

Corticosteroids may alleviate the systemic manifestations of the disease but do not appear to affect the course of the hyperostosis. Thus, their use should certainly be restricted to cases in which the signs and symptoms are unusually severe and fail to respond to the measures described earlier. In such instances, cortisone may be given in a dose of 5 to 10 mg/kg/24 hours in divided doses, or prednisone, 1 to 2 mg/kg/24 hours. The duration of steroid therapy should be as short as possible, e.g., until the child has been afebrile for a few days, whereupon the dosage should be reduced gradually and discontinued.

Parents should be advised of the generally favorable outlook, despite possible involvement of additional bones. Although there are occasionally recurrences, most infants recover progressively without sequelae. Recovery may take weeks or months.

Familial occurrence has been reported on several occasions, sometimes with strong evidence of autosomal dominant inheritance, with variable (sometimes subclinical) expression and/or non-penetrance. Individuals with the familial disorder appear to be less subject to mandibular involvement and more to tibial lesions than those with typical sporadic Caffey's disease. Whether these represent two distinct etiological entities with a similar phenotype is not known. From a practical viewpoint, the possibility of familial occurrence should be recognized; if suspected, relatives who have tibial bowing should be x-rayed for evidence of the disease, and parents should be made aware of both the recurrence risk in siblings and the generally good prognosis. A few individuals with tibial involvement in the familial form have shown persistent tibial bowing as a sequela of the acute disorder. Late recurrences are also possible.

Idiopathic cortical hyperostosis with raised immunoglobulins has been described in older children and also as a familial disorder. This condition also undergoes gradual spontaneous remission. Most recently, cortical hyperostosis (without mandibular involvement) has been described in infants with cyanotic congenital heart disease following long-term administration of prostaglandin-E_1 (PG E_1). Though the mechanism of this phenomenon is not understood, the cortical thickening subsides following cessation of PG E_1 therapy.

Osteomyelitis and Suppurative Arthritis

JOHN D. NELSON, M.D.

When possible, medical and surgical management of bone and joint infections should be a joint effort of the pediatrician and orthopedic surgeon. Because the day-to-day aspects of management are primarily medical, it is generally preferable that the pediatrician be the primary physician and the orthopedic surgeon the consultant.

ACUTE BACTERIAL INFECTIONS

Surgical Management of Arthritis. Surgical evacuation of pus is necessary in all cases of suppurative arthritis. This can often be effected by needle aspiration with or without saline irrigation. (It is inadvisable to irrigate with antibiotic solutions since they are usually irritating to synovium.) In most cases, two or three daily aspirations suffice. If substantial amounts of pus persist after a few days, open surgical drainage is performed.

There are at least three situations in which needle aspiration of joint fluid is not satisfactory. 1) With rare exceptions, open surgical drainage of hip joint pus should be performed immediately. The joint is especially vulnerable to permanent damage from pus itself and from vascular compromise due to pressure. 2) If the history suggests the possibility of foreign body in the joint, open surgical drainage and exploration are advisable. 3) In my experience, the elbow joint seldom is thoroughly evacuated of pus by needle aspiration. The use of drains and the types of drains employed are a matter of personal preference of the surgeon and have not been subjected to the scrutiny of controlled trials.

Joints should be immobilized in a functional position of extension by sand bags, splints or casts until pain is alleviated and range of motion exercises can be carried out.

Surgical Management of Osteomyelitis. The optimal surgical management of acute osteomyelitis is controversial. The information that follows has been our practice for many years; it is possible that a less aggressive surgical approach would be as beneficial.

If frank pus is encountered in a diagnostic aspiration, the patient undergoes surgical decompression through an oval cortical window. There are exceptions to this. In very young infants, metaphyseal pus often decompresses spontaneously into the contiguous joint, whence it can usually be removed by repeated needle aspirations. If the infected area abuts the growth plate, surgical intervention could conceivably cause damage.

If the diagnostic aspiration yields only bloody material rather than pus, generally antibiotic therapy alone suffices.

The need for casts and immobilization must be determined in individual cases. If there is extensive involvement of a bone in the legs, weight bearing is prohibited to avoid the possibility of pathologic fracture.

Medical Management. Fluid and electrolyte therapy and medication for relief of pain are given as necessary.

Initial antibiotic therapy in about half the cases can be guided by the results of Gram stained specimens of joint fluid or pus interpreted by an experienced microbiologist. Otherwise, initial therapy is empirical and based on likely pathogens at various ages (Table 1).

Table 1. ETIOLOGIC BACTERIA IN ACUTE SUPPURATIVE BONE AND JOINT DISEASES

Ages	Arthritis	Osteomyelitis
Neonates	**Group B streptococci*** *Staphylococcus aureus* Coliform bacilli Gonococcus	*Staphylococcus aureus* **Group B streptococci** Coliform bacilli Pseudomonas
Infants	*Haemophilus influenzae b* **Pneumococcus** Other streptococci Salmonella Staphylococcus aureus	*Staphylococcus aureus* Streptococci *Haemophilus influenzae b*
Children	*Staphylococcus aureus* Pneumococcus Gonococcus	*Staphylococcus aureus* Streptococci

*The most common causes are shown in bold face type.

In the newborn infant, group B streptococci and staphylococci are the major pathogens, but coliform bacilli must be considered. Initial therapy with methicillin and an aminoglycoside antibiotic is advisable. If cultures confirm group B streptococcal or gonococcal infection, treatment is changed to penicillin G or ampicillin. Pseudomonas infection is rare and part of a picture of sepsis and cutaneous lesions. It is treated with ticarcillin or mezlocillin along with an aminoglycoside.

Arthritis in infancy is most often due to *Haemophilus influenzae* b, but a variety of organisms are encountered. Initial therapy with nafcillin and chloramphenicol or with cefuroxime alone would be appropriate. Osteomyelitis in infancy is usually due to *Staphylococcus aureus* or streptococci. Unless gram-negative bacilli are seen in the Gram stained specimen, an antistaphylococcal penicillin is given initially.

Beyond infancy most cases of arthritis and osteomyelitis are due to gram-positive cocci, but gonococcal arthritis must suspected in sexually active youngsters.

Antibiotic therapy is tailored to the culture and susceptibility test results. Suggested dosages are given in Table 2. Customarily, antibiotics are given parenterally, for the entire course of treatment. However, several studies have shown that large-dosage oral antibiotic regimens can be successfully employed under rigidly monitored conditions. Af-

Table 2. SUGGESTED DOSAGES OF ANTIBIOTICS TO TREAT BONE AND JOINT INFECTIONS

Antibiotic	Parenteral Dosage	Oral Dosage*
Beta-lactam Antibiotics		
Amoxicillin	—	150 mg/kg/day q6h
Ampicillin	150 mg/kg/day q6h	—
Bacampicillin or cyclacillin	—	100 mg/kg/day q6h
Cefaclor	—	150 mg/kg/day q6h
Cefazolin or cefuroxime	75 mg/kg/day q8h	—
Cefotaxime or moxalactam	100 mg/kg/day q6h	—
Cephalexin or cephradine	—	100 mg/kg/day q6h
Cloxacillin	—	100 mg/kg/day q6h
Dicloxacillin	—	75 mg/kg/day q6h
Methicillin	200 mg/kg/day q6h	—
Oxacillin or nafcillin	150 mg/kg/day q6h	—
Penicillin	150,000 u/kg/day q4–6h	100 mg/kg/day q6h
Ticarcillin or mezlocillin	200–300 mg/kg/day q4–6h	—
Aminoglycosides		
Amikacin or kanamycin	15–22.5 mg/kg/day q8h	—
Gentamicin	6 (children)–7.5 (infants) mg/kg/day q8h	—
Miscellaneous		
Chloramphenicol	75 mg/kg/day q6h	50–75 mg/kg/day q6h
Clindamycin	30 mg/kg/day q8h	30 mg/kg/day q6h
Vancomycin	40 mg/kg/day q6h	—

*These dosages are greater than those recommended by the manufacturers for less serious infections.

ter several days, when the clinical condition has stabilized, an appropriate oral antibiotic is selected and given in dosages two to three times greater than those recommended for less serious infections (Table 2). Approximately 1 hour after a dose, the serum bactericidal titer against the pathogen isolated from the patient is tested. It should be at least 1:8 against *S. aureus* and *H. influenzae* and 1:32 or greater against streptococci. Approximately 10% of patients have poor gastrointestinal absorption of antibiotics and cannot be treated successfully by the oral route. The large dosages of drugs are well tolerated and do not cause gastrointestinal side effects.

Response to therapy is judged by resolution of fever and local signs and by normalization of the erythrocyte sedimentation rate (ESR). Persistent elevation of the ESR, even though clinical signs have improved, should prompt investigation for undrained pus or sequestrum.

Duration of antibiotic therapy varies with the type of bacteria. For *S. aureus* and coliform bacilli, a minimum of 21 days is suggested, while 10 to 14 days generally suffice for disease due to streptococci or *Haemophilus*. A 3 day regimen has been reported successful for gonococcal arthritis, but most authorities recommend at least 7 days of therapy. Ten to 14 days is adequate for *Pseudomonas* osteomyelitis, provided that thorough surgical debridement has been performed.

SPECIAL SITUATIONS

In children with *sickle cell disease,* aseptic bone infarction can mimic osteomyelitis, and vice-versa. Bone infarctions tend to be multiple, there is little fever, no bandemia, and the ESR is normal. Osteomyelitis usually affects one bone, fever is higher, bandemia may be present, and the ESR becomes elevated. When in doubt, a diagnostic aspiration can be done. Infection is usually due to streptococci, *Salmonella,* or other coliform bacilli.

Sacroiliitis is indolent on presentation and occurs in older children. It is almost always staphylococcal.

Discitis, a syndrome of unknown etiology, affects infants and young children and resolves spontaneously within a few weeks. It must be differentiated from vertebral osteomyelitis, which occurs in older children and is associated with more severe symptomatology. It is most often due to staphylococci, but *Pseudomonas* infection occurs in intravenous drug abusers.

Brodie abscess, a subacute or chronic staphylococcal infection, can occur in the metaphysis or diaphysis. It can be difficult to differentiate from bone tumor without surgical curettage. If surgical removal is not done, I treat Brodie abscess with antistaphylococcal antibiotics for several weeks or months until there is roentgenographic resolution of the lesion.

Granulomatous diseases due to mycobacteria, fungi, or *Brucella* tend to be indolent processes that cross the epiphyseal plate and cause disabling sequelae. Cases are treated with long-term antimicrobial drugs.

Chronic staphylococcal osteomyelitis is treated by surgical removal of sequestrum, when necessary, and with prolonged courses of oral antistaphylococcal drugs in dosages adjusted to produce serum bactericidal titers of 1:8 to 1:16. If a thorough sequestrectomy has been done, I treat with antibiotics for at least 3 months; otherwise, I treat for 6 to 12 months, depending on the clinical and roentgenographic responses.

Malignant Bone Tumors

MARK E. NESBITT, JR., M.D.

The most common primary malignant tumors of bone seen in children and adults are osteogenic sarcoma and Ewing's sarcoma. Chondrosarcoma, a tumor of cartilaginous origin, will not be dealt with in this section even though it can be as frequent as osteogenic sarcoma. Treatment regimens for both Ewing's and osteogenic sarcoma are still evolving. Newer therapeutic modalities that appear promising in small series of patients must be studied in large clinical trials before being recommended for widespread use. Because of the relatively low incidence of these tumors and the necessity for long intervals of observation, an extended period of time can elapse before a therapy is proven to be efficacious.

EWING'S SARCOMA—NON-METASTATIC

An integrated approach using surgery, radiotherapy, and chemotherapy has significantly improved disease control and survival in Ewing's sarcoma of bone. Most of the primary tumors can be controlled by radiotherapy. The effectiveness of radiation therapy has recently been improved by a) increasing the amount of bone and surrounding tissue included in the irradiated volume, b) using supervoltage machines, and c) using a dose of radiation to the primary tumor of greater than 4000 rads.

Therapy should be started as soon as possible after surgery and in consultation with the surgeon. Patients who have had complete resection without microscopic residual should not receive radiation therapy. However, if adequate margins are not present or if the tumor is entered at the time of surgery, radiation therapy should be administered. The primary lesion should receive 4500 rads to the whole bone, including both epiphyseal growth centers to ensure inclusion of the metastases in the 90% isodose region. All soft tissue should include a 5 cm margin. The portals should be reduced to include all evidence of tumor extent (radiographs of bone and soft tissue and isotope bone scans), with a 5 cm margin in all directions to a dose of 5000 rads. Thereafter, the area of tumor extension should be boosted to an additional 500 rads, using a 1 cm margin in all directions. In the pelvis, the entire bony hemipelvis and/or sacrum should be included, with all soft tissue extensions present at the time of initial diagnosis with a 2 cm margin. Thereafter, the portals should be reduced to include all evidence of tumor extent, as determined by routine radiographic studies and CT scan examination to a dose of 5000 rads with a 5 cm margin. Subsequently, the area of tumor extent should be boosted by an additional 500 rads using a 1 cm margin in all directions. CT scans prior to surgery are mandatory for evaluation of soft tissue extension.

Though the local failure rate with radiotherapy is usually around 15%, the increasing incidence of late effects with the use of higher doses of radiotherapy supports the recent evaluation of surgery for treatment of the primary tumor. Surgical resection should be considered for lesions in expendable bones. Complete surgical resection is preferred. The resulting disability would be acceptable for example in lesions of the foot, fibula, rib, forearm bones, clavicle, and scapula. The role of amputation is controversial. It is recommended for the following lower extremity lesions: a) a huge destructive lesion, b) a pathologic fracture, and c) a primary lesion located in the region of the distal femoral epiphysis or distally in a child less than 6 years of age. Lesions that arise in the pelvis are usually too large or diffuse for one to consider surgical resection at time of diagnosis. However, surgery in this location can be considered after initial therapy with chemotherapy alone. Lesions in the wing of the ilium, the sacrum, or the pelvic bones can often be surgically resected without resulting in major functional deficit.

More often failure in achieving a cure is due to distant metastases that are undetected at time of diagnosis. The addition of effective chemotherapy programs to surgery and radiation therapy has resulted in improving disease-free and overall survival. Various chemotherapeutic agents have shown effectiveness in metastatic disease: cyclophosphamide, vincristine sulfate, Adriamycin, actinomycin-D and 5-fluorouracil. There are presently large clinical trials being conducted by cancer centers and cooperative study groups (Children's Cancer Study Group and Pediatric Oncology Group) to determine the best multiagent chemotherapy and the length of chemotherapy to be used to treat

Ewing's sarcoma. A patient with Ewing's sarcoma should be treated at a center by a team of orthopedic surgeons, radiotherapists, and pediatric or medical oncologists.

The survival rate for Ewing's sarcoma is still disappointing when compared to cure rates for Wilms' tumor, Hodgkin's disease, or retinoblastoma. Furthermore, patients who are surviving have a high risk of having either a significant orthopedic problems or developing a secondary tumor. For these reasons, alternatives to the above plan are now being explored, which include the following: 1) Induction chemotherapy prior to treatment of the primary tumor with radiotherapy or surgery. 2) More liberal use of surgical resection of the primary lesion. 3) Decreasing the dose and size of the irradiation field for control of the primary. 4) Decreasing the length of maintenance chemotherapy. 5) Exploring the use of total body irradiation and half body irradiation with or without autologous marrow transplantation.

METASTATIC EWING'S SARCOMA

The presence of metastatic disease at the time of diagnosis complicates a treatment plan. After establishing the diagnosis, multiagent chemotherapy (vincristine, actinomycin-D, cyclophosphamide, and adriamycin) should be started. Radiation therapy should be given to the primary lesion and, if possible, to all metastatic sites. If undue myelosuppression occurs, radiation therapy can be delayed so as not to unduly interfere with optimum chemotherapy. Additionally, if the areas of metastases involve more than 30% of the myeloproliferative tissue, radiation therapy should be given sequentially to various metastasis sites. No more than 60% of myeloproliferative tissue (bone marrow) should be irradiated. The use of an aggressive surgical approach to the primary in patients with distant metastases is not indicated. However, in patients with rib lesions and pleural effusion and/or localized pleural metastases, surgery should be considered. Studies are under way to determine whether delaying radiation therapy to later in the course of therapy as well as the addition of newer chemotherapeutic agents such as 5-fluorouracil or melphalan may improve survival in patients with metastatic disease at time of diagnosis.

OSTEOSARCOMA

As in Ewing's sarcoma, the treatment of osteogenic sarcoma needs the consultation of the orthopedic surgeon, medical or pediatric oncologist, and radiotherapist. Most of the treatment is surgical and chemotherapeutic, while the role of radiotherapy is usually allocated to patients with metastases.

Treatment of Localized Disease. Amputation has generally been considered the treatment of choice, as most primary tumors are in the extremities. For lesions that cannot be easily resected, radiotherapy can be used to treat the primary. The dose necessary for control is over 6000 rads. Removal of the whole bone at or above the contiguous joint is recommended for treatment of the primary lesion. In lesions of the femur, where removal of the whole bone causes significant orthopedic problems, cross bone resections are considered safe if there is a 7 cm tumor-free margin.

Recently, in certain selected cases there appears to be as good local control for patients treated by a limb salvage procedure as for those undergoing conventional amputation surgery. The criteria for selection of a patient for a limb salvage are still being established, but the three most important variables are as follows: 1) The surgeon must make a judgment that, initially or after effective systemic chemotherapy, the tumor can be excised with a wide margin (5–7 cm or more of normal marrow above the level of the tumor) with a plane of soft tissue around the tumor; 2) the age of the child; and 3) the size and site of the lesion. It is generally felt that limb salvage procedures should be considered only in skeletally mature children. Children with significant further growth potential are not good candidates because the procedure would result in a marked leg length discrepancy. As far as the site of the tumor, in certain expandable bones, complete surgical removal can be accomplished without significant disability and would be preferable to a limb salvage procedure.

The fibula, ulna, and radius can be sacrificed without extensive functional loss. In the distal femur, proximal femur, and proximal humerus, a limb salvage procedure seems the treatment of choice if the other criteria are met. When the primary tumor occurs in the distal tibia and foot, a below the knee amputation would generally be the surgical procedure of choice. The size of the tumor is probably also important. Tumors that are well localized within the bone and have not broken through the cortex are most suitable for limb salvage; those that are extremely large and involve a lot of soft tissue are not.

With the increasing use of preoperative chemotherapy, the selection criteria for a limb sparing technique might liberalize with a reduction in the tumor size. There is, however, a certain risk in those nonresponders who are allowed to have tumor growth prior to definitive surgery for the primary lesion.

Chemotherapy. As in other tumors, the initial use of certain chemotherapeutic agents has produced significant regression of tumor masses. The most effective chemotherapeutic agents for osteogenic sarcoma have been high dose methotrexate with leucovorum rescue, cyclophosphamide, Adriamycin, and cis-platinum, as well as multiple drug combinations of bleomycin, cyclophosphamide, and actinomycin-D (BCD), and cyclophosphamide, vincristine, melphalan, and Adriamycin (COMPADRI).

Recently, several large series of patients have reported improved survival in patients with osteogenic sarcoma who have been treated with surgical removal of the primary in combination with chemotherapy for a total of 12 to 18 months. With this experience, and the suggestion that there might be some variability in response with certain drug combinations from patient to patient, the use of preoperative chemotherapy has been piloted. After approximately a month of chemotherapy, the assessment of response of the tumor to the chemotherapy can be evaluated. For nonresponders, the chemotherapeutic agents can be changed and the ineffective agent or agents dropped. The use of preoperative chemotherapy has also improved the probability of limb salvage by allowing time for construction of an endoprosthesis as well as increasing the number of patients who can fit the general criteria for such a procedure.

The use of adjuvant chemotherapy has brought about an improvement in survival in patients with osteogenic sarcoma. For this reason most centers provide adjuvant chemotherapy. There is some question, however, on how much adjuvant chemotherapy has really added to this improvement in survival. Several authors have reported similar results, approximately 50% survival, in series of patients treated without adjuvant therapy.

Certainly an alternative approach to the treatment of localized osteosarcoma would be initial surgical resection and close follow-up. At the first evidence of pulmonary disease, which is the most common metastatic site, thoracotomy would be performed and the patient treated with chemotherapy. Most programs now popular for adjuvant chemotherapy are using maximally tolerated sched-ules and doses of our most toxic chemotherapeutic agents. If 50% of the patients do not need chemotherapy and another 20 to 30% can be cured with surgery and delayed chemotherapy, then initial surgery only might be preferable to having all patients treated with intensive chemotherapeutic regimens. The obvious answer is a prospectively controlled trial of adjuvant therapy. A large multi-institutional group is presently undertaking such a trial. For the physician who is responsible for a single patient, it is recommended that the patient be referred to a center that is either participating in such a trial or at least is evaluating in an organized manner a therapeutic question on the treatment of this tumor.

METASTATIC DISEASE

An important question in treating patients with osteogenic sarcoma is how to handle patients with clinically detectable metastases. Several cancer centers have in the past reported the use of resection of pulmonary metastases to salvage patients with metastatic disease. The practice of aggressive metastasectomy is now widely accepted. For patients with recurrent lung metastases, sequential thoracotomies, as many as 9 or 10, should be considered, until this procedure is shown to be a failure. Though adjuvant chemotherapy is often given following surgery there are no studies to support that this procedure is warranted. Usually the longer the delay from the original diagnosis to the appearance of metastases, the better will be the result with thoracotomy. Most of the benefit is probably derived from the fewer metastases that occur with later relapse. At the present, it would be reasonable for patients with recurrence later than 9 months to have metastasectomy without postoperative chemotherapy. For patients with earlier metastases, preoperative chemotherapy followed by metastasectomy should be done. For responders, postoperative chemotherapy can be given.

14

Muscles

Congenital Muscular Defects

THOMAS S. RENSHAW, M.D.

Congenital absence of a voluntary muscle may be partial or total and is usually unilateral. Virtually any muscle may be absent. The most common defects are noted in the shoulder girdle, the neck, the thigh, the upper arm, and the hand. The most commonly absent muscles are the pectoralis major and trapezius, although absence of these is usually of no functional significance, exercises are of no therapeutic value, and reassurance is all that is needed. With absence of the pectoralis major, particularly its sternal part, one should look for the Poland syndrome, which includes syndactyly, upper extremity defects, cardiac abnormalities, and often rib anomalies. Absence of one sternocleidomastoid muscle frequently leads to torticollis and, if so, should be treated by surgical release of the remaining sternocleidomastoid, a procedure that may require repeating during the growth period.

Absence or severe hypoplasia of abdominal muscles can be associated with "prune belly syndrome." This condition has a high incidence of gastrointestinal and genitourinary anomalies, congenital dislocation of the hip, and possible spinal deformities. Respiratory problems, sometimes severe, can also occur. Treatment consists of an external abdominal support and attention to the other anomalies.

Absence of the quadriceps femoris causes profound interference with gait but may be improved by transferring medial and lateral hamstring muscles to the patella and augmenting, if necessary, with a brace. Absence of muscles that stabilize the foot or ankle usually causes progressive imbalance and deformity and should be evaluated by gait analysis, including dynamic EMG studies, followed by appropriate orthotic or surgical treatment to reestablish muscle balance. Absence of the plantaris and/or palmaris longus musculature is significant only in that these muscles have tendons highly suitable as donor graft material.

Finally, absence of extraocular muscles requires ophthalmologic procedures for visual improvement.

Torticollis

THOMAS S. RENSHAW, M.D.

Although torticollis, or "wry neck," is usually a benign cosmetic problem secondary to muscle tightness and responds successfully to stretching exercises during infancy, one must realize that there are causes of torticollis for which an exercise program could bring about catastrophic results. These include traumatic or congenital spinal lesions producing instability between the occiput and C-1, or C-1 and C-2, such as congenital hypoplasia or aplasia of the odontoid, nonunion of an odontoid fracture, rupture of the transverse alar ligament of C-1, and subluxation of C-1 on C-2. Torticollis can also result from a tumor in the bony vertebral column or spinal cord. Infections in the neck, involving the retropharyngeal space, a disc space, or upper respiratory tract have also caused torticollis. It is, therefore, essential in the evaluation to have good radiographs of the entire cervical spine in both frontal and sagittal planes, as well as dynamic flexion and extension views to assess the stability from the occiput to C-2.

Idiopathic muscular torticollis is a condition that usually presents in early infancy but can develop at any time during childhood. In children under age 1 year, who have little or no facial asymmetry, an exercise program is almost always successful. The specific exercise is designed to place maximum distance between the ipsilateral sternoclavicular joint and mastoid process and is done by bending the neck laterally *away* from the torticollis and then slowly providing maximal rotation of the head *to* the side of the torticollis. This position should be held for about five seconds and then released and repeated 10 times, at least 4 times a day, or better yet, with each diaper change. Another conservative therapeutic method involves positioning the infant prone in the crib with the normal side toward the wall, which may cause some rotation toward the affected side and help with the stretching exercise program. The exercises are worth trying in children beyond age 1 year, but often by that time surgical treatment will be necessary. There is a high failure rate with the exercise program at any age when the torticollis is accompanied by significant facial asymmetry and/or the restriction of neck rotation exceeds 30° when compared with the normal side.

When surgical treatment is indicated, the treatment of choice is a distal release of both the sternal and clavicular attachments of the sternocleidomastoid muscle. As long as the incision is placed 1.5 to 2 cm above the clavicle, the cosmetic result is quite acceptable. It is rarely necessary to do bipolar tenotomy or a single release at the mastoid area. Surgical results are not age-dependent and a good result may be expected up to and beyond age 10 years. Postoperative management consists of a cast or a brace for a period of approximately 4 weeks.

There is a 10 to 20% incidence of congenital hip dysplasia associated with infantile idiopathic torticollis. In addition, approximately 15% of all torticollis is on an ophthalmologic basis, the most common cause being amblyopia.

Congenital Hypotonia

ANDREA MORRISON, M.D.

Congenital hypotonia may be produced by a variety of disorders that affect the nervous system. Abnormalities of muscle, nerve, spinal cord, brain, or myoneural junction may all produce hypotonia, as may chromosomal abnormalities, metabolic disorders, endocrine disturbances, systemic infections, trauma, and anoxia. These patients are noted at some point between birth and the end of infancy to be "floppy," with decreased muscle tone, real or apparent muscle weakness, unusual posture, decreased resistance to passive joint manipulation, increased joint range of motion, and, if symptoms last long enough, delayed motor development. Frequently, by the time patients are initially recognized as hypotonic, it is impossible to discover if the disorder was congenital. Serial observations may then be required to decide if the problem is progressive, static, or improving. Investigation begins with historical information and clinical examination, followed by evaluation of the clinical course. It may never proceed further, or may be broadened to include computed tomography (CT), electromyography (EMG), nerve conduction velocity (NCV), chromosomes, metabolic studies, muscle, nerve, or brain biopsy, cultures, or lumbar puncture. The aim is obviously to establish a diagnosis beyond "hypotonia," which is only a descriptive term. Careful assessment cannot always lead to diagnosis, but exclusion or establishment of hereditary, basically treatable, or progressive disorders is possible in most patients (Table 1).

A complete history is mandatory, but some questions are particularly important: Is there a family history of children with similar findings? If so, what happened to them? What neurologic, endocrine, hereditary, or congenital problems have been noted in other family members? Is there parental consanguinity? What was the pregnancy like? Did the infant move less in utero than previous children, or move less actively at some point during the pregnancy? Were there any difficulties at delivery or in the neonatal period? Were any abnormalities noted at birth, or since? Is there anything unusual about this child (odor, appearance, twitchy tongue, strabismus, large head)? Has there been retrogression? Has the child's development "plateaued" or improved rapidly at any time? Was there an acute insult when symptoms were first noted? Has the child seemed uncomfortable? Alert? Does he appropriately attempt to manipulate his environment and respond to stimuli? Is there anything that the physician should be aware of which has not been asked? What tests have already been done?

Once this information has been reviewed, a full general physical examination and as complete a neurologic examination as possible are necessary. Simply observing the infant in bed or in his mother's arms is often quite useful, since severe hypotonia is readily apparent. The extremely hypotonic child lies with limbs relaxed in a "frog-leg" position when supine, but with hips extended when prone, so that his buttocks are not raised off the bed by hip flexion. Spontaneous movements are decreased in number and amplitude. When he is pulled from a supine to a sitting position, his arms remain extended, with little or no traction response, and his head lags, with poor control. When lifted with the examiner's hands under his arms, he "slips through," because he does not clamp his upper arms down on the examiner's hands or fix his scapulae. When held in the air, prone, with the examiner's hands under his chest, he achieves less than the normal newborn's usual posture. His head and limbs dangle loosely, with the head seldom brought up to horizontal, and the limbs flexed little,

Table 1. CAUSES OF CONGENITAL HYPOTONIA

METABOLIC AND DEGENERATIVE DISORDERS*

Isovaleric acidemia
Lactic acidosis
Methionine malabsorption (Oast House syndrome)
Homocystinuria with defective methylation
Hyperpipecolatemia
GM2 gangliosidosis, type I (Tay-Sachs and congenital Tay-Sachs)
GM2 gangliosidosis, type II (Sandhoff)
GM1 gangliosidosis, generalized, type I (neurovisceral lipidosis)

Hyperlysinemia
Hyper-B-alaninemia
Infantile Gaucher's disease
Fahr's disease
Galactosemia
Canavan's disease
Pelizaeus-Merzbacher disease
Leigh's subacute necrotizing encephalomyelopathy
Triose phosphate isomerase deficiency
Ataxia telangiectasia

CHROMOSOMAL ABNORMALITIES*

Trisomy 13
Trisomy 10 p
Down syndrome
Deletion of short arm of chromosome 4
Deletion of short arm of chromosome 18

XXXY
XXXXY
XXXXX
Partial deletion of short arm of chromosome 5 (cri du chat)

SYNDROMES WITH ABNORMAL PHYSICAL APPEARANCE*

Achondroplasia
Blepharophimosis
Coffin-Sirus syndrome
Cohen syndrome
Congenital laxity of ligaments
Ehlers-Danlos syndrome
Langer-Giedion syndrome
Lowe syndrome
Marfan syndrome
Marinesco-Sjogren syndrome
Miller-Dieker syndrome

Neurofibromatosis
Osteogenesis imperfecta
Pena-Shokien II syndrome
Prader-Willi syndrome
Pseudo-vitamin D dificiency
Rickets
Shprintzer syndrome
Stickler syndrome
Thanatophoric dysplasia
Tuberous sclerosis
Zellweger syndrome

FETAL EXPOSURE TO ABNORMAL ENVIRONMENT

Aminopterin
Alcohol
Hyperthermia, severe
Maternal myotonic dystrophy

Maternal myasthenia gravis
Maternal drug overdosage
Intrauterine infections
Maternal hypothyroidism

SYSTEMIC DISORDERS

Sepsis
Dehydration
Severe renal gastrointestinal, or cardiac disease
Malnutrition (rickets, kwashiorkor)
Hypercalcemia
Hypothermia, severe
Recurrent seizures

Drug overdosage
Brain deterioration in advanced chronic lung disease of prematurity
Asphyxia
Hypothyroidism
Hypoadrenalism

DISORDERS OF MUSCLE*

Carnitine deficiency
Glycogenosis, Type II, Pompe's disease
Glycogenosis, Type III, Cori's disease
Glycogenosis, Type IV, Andersen's disease
Congenital muscular dystrophy
Congenital myopathies:
   Central core disease
   Minicore disease

Congenital myopathies (continued):
   Nemaline myopathy
   Myotubular myopathy
   Congenital fiber type disproportion
   Myopathies with abnormal subcellular organelles
   Myopathies with minimal pathologic change
   Reducing body myopathies
Polymyositis (rare in this age group)

DISORDERS OF MYONEURAL JUNCTION

Infantile botulism

Myasthenia gravis

DISORDERS OF NERVE

Guillain-Barré (rare in this age group)

Hypertrophic neuropathy of infancy

DISORDERS OF SPINAL CORD

Infantile spinal muscular atrophy (Werdnig-Hoffman and intermediate types)*
Poliomyelitis
Coxsackie infection resembling poliomyelitis clinically

Trauma, including secondary subdural and epidural hematomas
Malformation: *arteriovenous malformation*, congenital abnormality, syringomyelia, *meningomyelocele*
Tumor (especially neuroblastoma)

DISORDERS OF BRAIN

Congenital malformations*
Trauma
Infection (meningitis, encephalitis, abscess)
Arteriovenous malformation
Hydrocephalus

Mental retardation and hypotonia, nonspecific
Precursor of choreoathetosis, cerebellar signs, or spasticity
Hemorrhage (intraventricular, intracerebellar, intracerebral)
Seizures, recurrent*

*Genetic Counseling Suggested.
 Disorders in italic type are potentially treatable.

if at all. Held in a standing position, his legs do not support his weight or do so only briefly. Manipulation of the limbs reveals decreased muscle tone and increased range of motion of joints, except in infants who were so severely hypotonic in utero that they have joint contractures at birth. The muscles feel normal, flabby, or woody to palpation and may be normal, enlarged, or small in bulk, although this is often hard to establish in plump infants. Deep tendon reflexes, clonus, and plantar responses must be carefully noted and the tongue and other muscles watched for fasciculation. Sensory testing is often omitted but pinprick and even tickling light touch with a cotton wisp can be easily checked. Most infants respond to these stimuli if they are awake and alert. Sensory level or obvious paraplegia is important to establish. Level of responsiveness and manipulative skills for age level must be judged and weighed against the parents' observations. The head circumference should be plotted, and the child should be carefully examined for anomalies, systemic disease, and skin lesions of phakomatoses. The examination should be well described in the chart for future comparison.

Following these maneuvers, the diagnosis is often obvious. A history of perinatal asphyxia, kernicterus, intraventricular hemorrhage, hydrocephalus, trauma, meningitis, or encephalitis may establish the etiology. Confirmatory evidence is found in records of the perinatal course and by following the child's clinical progress. Hypotonia resulting from such early brain injury is nonprogressive and is not treatable in the usual sense. However, nonprogressive illness may show itself in different ways as the child grows older. The originally hypotonic child may remain hypotonic, or may develop superimposed spasticity, rigidity, choreoathetosis, or cerebellar signs as his "cerebral palsy" changes with brain maturation. He may or may not be mentally retarded. Treatable complications may develop. Seizures may occur if cerebral abnormality is present. Shunts for hydrocephalus may malfunction, come apart, or become infected. A child acutely hypotonic after head injury may have unrecognized subdural hematomas and develop progressive subdural hygromas, with increasing head size and cerebral dysfunction. A mildly hypotonic child with tuberous sclerosis or neurofibromatosis may develop a brain tumor. Cardiac disease may become increasingly limiting with age. Therapy must be addressed to these and other specific complications; they are discussed under appropriate headings elsewhere in this volume.

Other diagnoses are also made relatively easily. In particular, onset of hypotonia during systemic illness lends itself to rapid diagnosis, as in congenital heart disease, severe infection (especially overwhelming sepsis, meningitis, and encephalitis), severe head trauma, and dehydration. Slightly less obvious clinical syndromes are associated with hypothyroidism, the hypoadrenal state, or renal disease. All are potentially treatable to some degree. Physical examination may reveal Down's syndrome, various other syndromes of multiple anomalies, neurofibromatosis, or tuberous sclerosis. These are basically untreatable but their complications may be treated.

Some children present more of a diagnostic puzzle, particularly those with primary disease of the nervous system. After determining whether the disorder is progressive, static, or improving, the most useful step is to localize the disorder within the nervous system. A few simple aids are quickly listed. Patients with absent or markedly diminished reflexes usually have muscle or nerve disease. Exceptions are children with anterior horn cell disease, acute spinal shock, and acute brain injury. Excessively brisk deep tendon reflexes result from brain disease or from irritation of, or pressure on, the spinal cord; they are rarely seen with significant nerve or muscle disease. Hypotonic patients with delayed motor development, but who are obviously alert and intelligent, usually have nerve, muscle, or spinal cord disease. Patients who appear dull, with delayed social and intellectual skills, usually have brain disease. Seizures, abnormal primitive reflexes, or abnormal postures such as "cortical thumbs" or "I surrender" upper limb posturing strongly suggest that the brain is involved.

When muscle disease is suspected, laboratory investigations must be planned carefully. Blood tests (CPK, aldolase, SGOT, sedimentation rate, thyroid function tests) should be done prior to EMG, since "muscle" enzyme values may be elevated markedly and for a prolonged period by EMG. Enzymes are also raised by recent intramuscular injections or grand mal seizures. After blood studies have been done, EMG and NCV are done. Often these are done routinely on the right side of patients with generalized involvement, so that muscle biopsy, if required, can be done routinely on the left side. This prevents the possible biopsy of an EMG site, which will show inflammation and may lead to an incorrect diagnosis of polymyositis, the only really treatable primary muscle disorder. Muscle biopsy must be performed by a surgeon who can prepare the tissue for the pathologist; the pathologist should have access to histochemical techniques and electron microscopy and be capable of interpreting the biopsy. It is the clinician's responsibility to suggest the site of muscle biopsy, preferably an involved muscle that is not totally paralyzed.

When nerve disease is suspected, EMG, NCV, and muscle and nerve biopsy are often required. Patients should also have spinal taps (for spinal fluid protein), and CPK and aldolase should be checked before the EMG is done, in case the diagnostic impression is incorrect.

Unless children with proven polymyositis or polyneuropathy are already improving, they should receive a trial of steroid therapy. One acceptable regimen is oral prednisone as follows: on day one, the child is given 5 mg/kg in 3 divided doses. The dosage is then decreased daily by 1 mg/kg, still in divided doses, for 2 days, until a maintenance dose of 3 mg/kg/day is reached. This is continued for a total of 10 days. If no benefit is apparent, the drug is tapered and discontinued over another week. If the patient has improved, but has not recovered completely, or worsens as the drug is decreased, prednisone may be continued, using alternate day dosage (6 mg/kg/day, every other day, in 3 divided doses), making periodic efforts to decrease and discontinue the medication. The parents must be made aware of the possible side effects of this regimen. Again, this treatment is best supervised by a specialist who has experience with it.

When disease of the myoneural junction is considered, only three disorders are likely: transient neonatal myasthenia gravis, congenital myasthenia gravis, and infantile botulism. If myasthenia is suspected, an edrophonium (Tensilon) test should be done by a physician experienced in its performance and ready to handle complications. The total dosage used is 0.5 mg (0.05 ml) in neonates and small infants. One tenth of the dose is given intravenously, and the patient is observed for 2 to 3 minutes. If the child does not develop diarrhea, vomiting, bradycardia, shock, or hypotension, the rest of the dose is given slowly intravenously. Within 2 or 3 more minutes, the myasthenic child will improve markedly in hypotonia, weakness, and (if present) ptosis. Treatment of myasthenia gravis is discussed elsewhere. The child with infantile botulism will not respond to the Tensilon test. When that diagnosis is made clinically, it is confirmed by the finding of the organism and/or its toxin in the stool. The baby with infantile botulism does not require specific antitoxin and will recover completely with supportive therapy. Death is unlikely as long as respirations are supported and aspiration is prevented.

Spinal cord disease may cause hypotonia in a variety of ways. Trauma, tumor, syringomyelia, pressure on the cord from blood clot, abscess, or anomaly may occur; usually these disorders are associated with brisk reflexes, sphincter abnormalities, and sensory deficits. When such disorders are suspected, the neurologist, neurosurgeon, and neuroradiologist should help in the decision-making process. The choice of standard myelography versus metrizamide myelography with CT is best left up to such specialists. Frequently, EMG and NCV's are performed in such patients early in the course; they demonstrate denervation without evidence of nerve conduction deficit.

In anterior horn cell disease, progressive hypotonia is associated with decreased and decreasing deep tendon reflexes and sometimes with visible fasciculations. Progressive spinal muscular atrophy (Werdnig-Hoffman disease) is basically untreatable.

If a brain disorder is being considered, the use of ultrasound (if the fontanel is open widely enough) or CT may establish the presence of congenital anomalies or other abnormalities. The use of contrast material with CT scanning is not usually necessary, unless tumor, AVM, abscess, or other diagnosis requiring contrast is being considered.

The brain may be affected by many metabolic disorders; when appropriate, urine and blood should be examined for amino and other organic acids. Some congenital infections may be evaluated with TORCHS titers and cord IgM. When progressive degenerative disorders are suspected, specific enzymes may be measured, or biopsy of skin, muscle, nerve, rectum, or brain may be required. Immunologic studies may identify early ataxia telangiectasia, although this diagnosis is usually made much later, when characteristic vascular lesions, ataxia, chorea, and unusual eye movements are added to hypotonia.

Once diagnosis has been made, specific treatment is, of course, vital; when it is not available vigorous and well-informed physical therapy can help prevent contractures and increase muscle strength and functional ability regardless of diagnosis. Even a child with a progressive, ultimately fatal illness will benefit. Speech and occupational therapy may greatly help in teaching the patient to function despite his handicap. Genetic counseling is important when indicated. Orthopedic evaluation and follow-up are necessary in most children, not only to help prevent contractures and to help oversee physical therapy but also to avoid or treat scoliosis. Emotional support is vital and psychologists, social workers, and psychiatrists may be most helpful. Appropriate education referral is important for children whose hypotonia is the result of cerebral lesions that also affect intellect, learning ability, or attention span. A handicap may prevent attendance at a normal school. Most children who can be "mainstreamed," however, should be, so that they can function in the nonhandicapped world as early in life as possible. Involvement in research projects can be most helpful to some parents, who need to feel that they are providing all possible therapy for their children. Other parents prefer only supportive care until definitive treatment has been fully evaluated. When seizures complicate the clinical picture, therapy is very important.

It is vital to help families avoid reliance on quackery. Many parents whose children have neurologic symptoms or deficits are easily convinced that megavitamins, patterning exercises, treatment for nonexistent hypoglycemia, acupuncture, or herbal remedies are useful. Some "alternative therapies" are harmless, but they take time and effort, and divert financial resources from truly potentially helpful treatments. Other programs are too rigorous for anyone to follow perfectly, but parents are told that success will always result if they do as they are instructed, thus setting up predictable failure and subsequent guilt reactions. Megavitamin therapy may be particularly hazardous. Children who develop severe, progressive hypotonia with secondary respiratory embarrassment or chronic pulmonary disease must be treated with appropriate suctioning, respiratory therapy, antibiotics when necessary, and at times, respirator support. When to terminate heroic support for these unfortunate children must be decided by physicians and parents together.

Benign congenital hypotonia deserves a word. Affected children are of normal intelligence, have hypotonia with normal reflexes in most cases, and gradually improve, usually becoming completely normal by age 5 at the latest. Often there is a family history of parents or close relatives who were similarly affected and are now normal. When there is no indication of any other disorder, and the child can be carefully watched, such patients are best treated by "tincture of time."

Muscular Dystrophy and Related Myopathies

IRWIN M. SIEGEL, M.D.

Muscular dystrophy is the general term for a group of chronic diseases that have in common abiotrophy with progressive degeneration of skeletal musculature, leading to atrophy and weakness, often contracture and deformity, and motor disability.

GENERAL THERAPY

Management of the patient with a muscle disease should be aggressive and multidisciplined. Treatment is best administered by a team including pediatric, neurologic, genetic, physiatric, and orthopedic consultants. Additionally, occupational therapists, physical therapists, and medical social workers or psychologists can assist the patient and the family. Speech and dietary therapy, as well as subspecialty consultation (for instance, gastrointestinal and cardiopulmonary care), provide a thorough approach to the problems of comprehensive management.

Medications. Except in those myopathies due to the absence of a specific metabolite, for which replacement therapy will sometimes help (e.g., muscle carnitine deficiency), or in muscle disease

secondary to endocrinopathy (e.g., hypothyroidism) in which appropriate therapy of the primary condition can alleviate the secondary myopathy, there is no effective drug treatment for muscular dystrophy. Although the myotonia of dystrophia myotonica can be relieved by a variety of agents, the dystrophia (weakness) remains. Agents used are phenytoin (Dilantin), 100 mg two to three times a day, or quinine,* 200 mg three times daily. Both procainamide and prednisolone, though mentioned in the literature, have undesirable side effects and are not suggested.

Cardiac. Cardiomyopathy is said to be present in over 80% of patients with Duchenne muscular dystrophy (DMD), but the child may not show clinical evidence of heart disease because his restricted activity maintains a precarious status quo. Treatment is along conventional lines, with the administration of cardiac glycosides and diuretics when indicated.

Respiratory. Pneumonitis, secondary to decreased pulmonary function and poor respiratory toilet with aspiration, is frequently encountered in those with advanced stages of the muscular dystrophies, and periodic evaluation to monitor restrictive pulmonary disease is an integral part of any treatment regimen. Reduction in chest compliance, secondary to progressive weakness of respiratory musculature, requires an ongoing program of pulmonary rehabilitation. This may include diaphragmatic breathing exercises, postural drainage, chest percussion, proper humidification, and training in the use of various respiratory aids. Vigorous treatment of upper respiratory infections requires pharyngeal suction and intermittent positive pressure breathing as well as appropriate antibiotic therapy. Mechanical ventilation of patients in the terminal stages of DMD often can be managed at home without a tracheostomy, utilizing apparatus such as the rocking bed, plastic wrap ventilator, chest-abdomen cuirass respirator, and pneumobelt.

Dietary. Because obesity accelerates functional disability, nutrition should be carefully monitored throughout the course of muscular dystrophy but particularly after wheelchair confinement. A well-balanced vitamin-supplemented diet of no less than 1200 calories is suggested. Patients are encouraged to choose fruits and vegetables as alternatives to high-caloric snacks, and high fiber foods and fruit juices to aid in maintaining normal elimination. Only small amounts of dairy products are included because of their mucus-producing tendency.

When deglutition is difficult because of posterior pharyngeal and upper esophageal weakness, swallowing can be assisted by instruction in proper positioning, eating slowly, sitting upright for a time after meals, and introducing soft foods into the

---

*This use of quinine is not listed by the manufacturer.

diet. Myotonic patients should avoid cold foods or fluids, which may cause pharyngeal myotonia.

Psychosocial. In addition to coping with the psychologic problems imposed by a progressively disabling disease, children with muscular dystrophy face the same problems of peer interaction, body image, family adjustment, and sexuality that all normal youngsters must resolve in the process of maturing. Supportive psychiatric intervention made available at times of psychosocial crises can avert critical emotional damage, and empathic counseling of both the patient and family throughout the course of the illness is an important part of total management.

A higher incidence of mental retardation and decreased intellectual function has been noted in patients with DMD than in normal or other control groups. However, whenever possible, it is desirable to keep the child in the mainstream in the regular neighborhood school. Finally, in the treatment of muscular dystrophy the family is the patient. Group therapy has proved valuable in assisting parents and normal siblings by helping them develop insight and increasing communication through experience-sharing.

MOTOR DISABILITY

Physical Therapy/Occupational Therapy. Because muscular activity enhances protein synthesis (the danger of rapid loss of strength because of inactivity in DMD is well documented), it is imperative that the patient with muscular dystrophy be kept as mobile as possible for as long as feasible. The physical therapist systematically assesses weakness, imbalance, and contracture, and provides submaximal exercise, gait training, and contracture stretching. As the child grows, surface area increases by the square of each linear increment and volume by its cube. This "scale effect" explains why a child with a condition limiting the ultimate muscle mass may eventually lose the ability to ambulate, even though the disease is arrested or only slowly progressive. Gradient measurement of strength and functional ability by the physical therapist aids in indicating appropriate times for contracture release and bracing.

The occupational therapist determines the patient's ability to attend to the tasks of daily living, assisting him or her through a variety of techniques and devices, such as life and transfer equipment, clothing adaptations, special mattresses, and so on.

Wheelchair Care. Wheelchair confinement is a critical incident, both physiologically and psychologically, in the life of a patient with muscular dystrophy. Special wheelchair adaptations—for example, balanced forearm orthoses facilitating the use of the hands for feeding, writing, as well as other utilitarian tasks—can be prescribed to increase both comfort and function. Electric wheelchairs are available for those patients with insufficient strength to manage the standard model.

ORTHOPEDIC MANAGEMENT

Orthopedic complications are found in most of the muscular dystrophies. Central core disease (one of the congenital myopathies) can present at birth with congenital dislocation of the hips. Neonatal dystrophia myotonica is frequently complicated by severe clubfeet. In addition to weakness and contracture, particularly of the heel cords, children with dermatomyositis often develop subcutaneous or intramuscular calcification or both. In DMD, lower extremity contracture progresses until equinovarus and weakened pelvic balance, produced by hip flexion contracture, prohibit ambulation. Patients develop a stance and gait typified by hip flexion and abduction, increasing lumbar lordosis, and equinocavovarus. Eventually, they no longer can maintain a line projected from their center of gravity behind the center of rotation of their hips, in front of that of their knees and within their base of support. Ambulation stops at this point.

Properly timed surgery and bracing have helped selected patients to continue standing and walking anywhere from 2 to 5 years, thus significantly delaying confinement to a wheelchair with its inevitable downhill course.

Surgical management should permit early postoperative mobilization, as even brief restraint can lead to rapid loss of strength. Anesthesia must be closely monitored with particular attention to preventing gastric dilatation or potassium overload, to assuring adequate ventilation, and to the singular danger of malignant hyperthermia in this class of disease.

For the patient experiencing increased difficulty with walking because of lower extremity contracture, percutaneous hip flexor, bipolar tensor fascia lata, and heel cord tenotomies, followed by extremity bracing, have proved effective in maintaining ambulation. Percutaneous tarsal medullostomy or osteoclasis with soft tissue release has been successful in treating late equinocavovarus with rigid bony deformity. Isolated forefoot adduction is corrected by percutaneous metatarsal osteotomy. Postsurgical orthotic management employs molded plastic appliances that are considerably lighter than steel or aluminum braces, yet equally sturdy. In those cases of facioscapulohumeral dystrophy in which shoulder weakness significantly interferes with upper extremity function, scapular stabilization has been performed.

Scoliosis. Because paraspinal weakness is symmetric, spinal curvature is unusual in the walking Duchenne dystrophic or the child with limb girdle dystrophy. Asymmetric muscle weakness, leading to scoliosis in the ambulatory patient, can occur in the Becker form of muscular dystrophy, sometimes in childhood dystrophia myotonica, and often with childhood facioscapulohumeral dystrophy. These spinal curves, when severe and progressive, can be surgically stabilized.

Most patients with DMD develop paralytic scoliosis as a complication of wheelchair confinement. A variety of external spinal containment systems, such as thoracic jackets or special wheelchair seating, designed to keep the pelvis level and to shape and hold the spine in the upright extended position, can retard such deformity.

Spinal fusion has been successfully used to correct and stabilize scoliosis in heritable neurologic conditions such as spinal muscular atrophy, familial dysautonomia, Charcot-Marie-Tooth disease, and Friedreich's ataxia. Such surgery is being increasingly performed in properly selected wheelchair-confined Duchenne dystrophics with rapidly decompensating scoliosis.

Fractures. Fractures in muscular dystrophy are most frequently seen in the long bones and are more common in patients falling from wheelchairs than in braced patients still ambulating. Such fractures are usually only slightly displaced, and there is not much pain as there is little muscle spasm. They heal without complication in the expected time and should be treated with minimal splintage (mold and sling for humeral fractures, light walking casts for fractures of the femur), encouraging continued independent function as long as possible.

Myasthenia Gravis

SUSAN T. IANNACCONE, M.D.,
and FREDERICK J. SAMAHA, M.D.

Myasthenia gravis is an autoimmune disorder in which a circulating antibody attacks a portion of the specialized postsynaptic membrane of muscle, the acetylcholine receptor. Fatiguability, a hallmark of neuromuscular junction dysfunction, is the most common presenting complaint. Typically, the levator palpebrae and extraocular muscles are affected first. When no other muscles are involved, the patient is classified as having *ocular myasthenia*. The prognosis is better and remission rate higher for this group so that treatment should be conservative in these cases.

More often, the neuromuscular junction defect, which can be documented by electrophysiologic studies, spreads to nasopharyngeal, axial, and appendicular muscles. Virtually all skeletal musculature may be involved in *generalized myasthenia*. Symptoms may evolve over days, weeks, or months and may cause respiratory failure if not treated appropriately.

Transient Myasthenia. Myasthenia gravis can occur at any age although the spontaneous remission rate is higher during childhood (about one fifth). Neonatal or transient myasthenia is present at birth and is caused by the transplacental circulation of acetylcholine receptor antibody. These infants are born to mothers with myasthenia gravis. Although the mother may be asymptomatic, either in remission or not yet diagnosed, the infant develops paralysis of bulbar musculature with feeding difficulties and respiratory failure as a result of elevated serum antibody levels. These levels generally fall by 6 weeks of age but management before then is crucial.

Affected infants should be monitored carefully to prevent aspiration pneumonia or respiratory insufficiency. While symptomatic, they should be treated with anticholinesterases: neostigmine (Prostigmin) at 2 mg/kg/day in 3 to 6 divided oral or intramuscular doses. Pyridostigmine bromide (Mestinon) can be given orally as an elixir (12 mg/ml), 1 mg/kg/dose every 3 to 6 hours. These doses must be titrated against the infants' requirement, which will decrease almost daily. The cholinergic side effects—increased oral secretion, increased stools, abdominal cramps—can be reversed with atropine but are best managed by decreasing the dosage of anticholinesterase. In babies with elevated acetylcholine receptor antibody levels who require exchange transfusion for hyperbilirubinemia, the antibody level comes down rapidly after only one exchange. Such infants may require anticholinesterase therapy for less than 2 weeks.

Infants who are born to myasthenic mothers taking anticholinesterases during pregnancy and who do not have neonatal myasthenia may show clinical evidence of the cholinergic effects of the mother's medication. These effects are short lived, 24 to 48 hours. The most troublesome are copious oral secretions, which can be managed by frequent suctioning or atropine, 0.01 mg/kg/dose orally or subcutaneously every four hours as needed.

Congenital Myasthenia. Children who acquire myasthenia gravis before age 2 years are generally classified as having congenital myasthenia, while patients over 2 years are juvenile myasthenics. Congenital myasthenia is still a controversial classification since it represents a very small group of patients who may differ considerably from other myasthenics. Infants with acquired myasthenia tend to lack acetylcholine receptor antibodies. They tend to have affected siblings and may in fact show electrophysiologic and morphologic abnormalities of the presynaptic nerve endings at the neuromuscular junction. These rare patients may respond to steroid therapy, which will be discussed in a later section.

Juvenila Myasthenia. At present, data concerning various therapies for juvenile myasthenia are sparse. Most studies include one or two children in a large group of adult patients so that it is not yet clear whether juvenile myasthenics should be handled differently from adult patients. One fact is clear—the spontaneous remission rate for myasthenia acquired in childhood is high. For that reason, conservative medical therapy is indicated for at least 1 year following diagnosis. (Most remissions occur 6–12 months after onset of symptoms.)

The young child with complete ptosis will be at risk for amblyopia. Therefore, ophthalmologic consultation can be helpful. Eyeglasses with lid crutches are sometimes useful. Orbicularis oculi weakness may produce ophthalmologic complication by exposing conjunctiva and cornea to irritation. This can be managed by artificial tears or eye patching during sleep.

Anticholinesterases. The anticholinesterase drugs are the primary treatment for juvenile myasthenia gravis. Edrophonium chloride (Tensilon) is the most short acting (30–60 second duration) and is usually given as a test dose, 0.2 mg/kg intravenously, the "Tensilon test." Response to Tensilon may be difficult to interpret. Therefore, this test should be performed under controlled conditions in the presence of an experienced physician, usually a neurologist. Pyridostigmine (Mestinon) is given orally, 10–60 mg/dose, its peak effect at one hour, duration 3–4 hours. Neostigmine (Prostigmine), with a slightly longer duration of action, can be given orally 2 mg/kg/day or intramuscularly 0.04 mg/kg/dose. All of the drugs must be given to asthmatics with caution. All must be titrated carefully so that the patient receives the maximum benefit with a minimum of side effects. Many patients do better on smaller, more frequent doses than on larger doses given 6 to 8 hours apart. Most patients do not require medication while at rest, i.e., overnight. Patients should be examined for muscle strength before their dose and 1 hour afterward in order to determine the appropriate size and frequency of anticholinesterase medication for them.

Steroid Therapy. As myasthenia progresses, the patient may require larger and larger doses of anticholinesterase. This is an indication for more aggressive therapy, namely steroids. Prednisone is the drug of choice, 2 mg/kg/day orally, but methylprednisolone may be given intravenously in a similar dosage. Steroids should be instituted while the patient is hospitalized under close observation by someone (usually a neurologist) expert in handling myasthenia, since the patient may experience an exacerbation of the myasthenia or a marked increase in weakness during the first 7 to 10 days of steroid therapy. Weakness may be severe enough to require mechanical ventilation. Steroids should be given in conjunction with anticholinesterases but the latter must be titrated carefully as the steroids exert their effect. The patient's requirement for anticholinesterase will decrease as the steroid improves his myasthenia, presumably by decreasing production of acetylcholine receptor antibody.

High-dose steroids should be maintained until the patient's strength improves or until undesirable side effects appear. Improvement may occur in days but very often takes several weeks. The patient can then be tapered to an every other day regimen, ideally 2 mg/kg of prednisone every other day. Such dosage can be maintained for years in some patients without complications. The dosage should be tapered to that required to maintain strength without causing hypertension, osteoporosis, diabetes, or gastrointestinal bleeding.

Occasionally patients who do not respond to steroids have been treated with immunosuppressants: azathioprine, cyclophosphamide, and methotrexate. Some data indicate that adult myasthenic patients who have been refractory to other therapies may respond to one or more of these medications. The use of immunosuppressants in juvenile myasthenia must be considered experimental at this time.

Thymectomy. The third acceptable line of treatment for the young myasthenic is thymectomy. As many as 80% of adult patients experience improvement or complete remission following thymectomy. It is not yet completely understood why thymectomy works. The thymus gland may be the source of abnormal lymphocytes, which either are directly responsible for producing the acetylcholine receptor antibody or which fail to suppress its production by other lymphocytes. Cultures of thymic tissue from myasthenic patients have produced cells that seem to attack the neuromuscular junction in vitro. There is evidence that thymic tissue shares an antigen with the acetylcholine receptor. This antigen may stimulate production of abnormal lymphocytes. Each mechanism is consistent with the sometimes delayed and frequently prolonged effect of thymectomy.

Computed tomography of the anterior mediastinum prior to thymectomy has helped to identify enlarged thymus, ectopic thymic tissue, and thymoma. Since all thymus tissue must be removed in order to obtain remission of myasthenia, a sternal splitting procedure should be done. The thoracic surgeon should be experienced at clearing the anterior mediastinum of thymic tissue. Postoperatively, the patient may require much less anticholinesterase medication and therefore requires careful monitoring at this time to prevent cholinergic crisis. Most patients now recover easily from thymectomy. Steroid and anticholinesterase therapy can be titrated to the patients' needs following thymectomy. We do not yet know the possible immunologic risks of thymectomy in children under 4 years of age.

Plasmapheresis. The severely ill myasthenic requiring ventilatory assistance may benefit from plasma exchange or plasmapheresis. This procedure removes acetylcholine antibody from the circulation with the patient's plasma. Antibody levels drop rapidly following exchange, and clinical improvement may be apparent within 24 hours. However, effects are short lived, most adult patients requiring two-volume exchanges 2 to 3 times each week for up to 6 weeks. The risks are much greater in a child, whose blood volume may be less than one fourth that of the adult. They include hypotension, volume overload, sepsis, and cardiac arrest. This procedure is used in some medical centers on a limited number of patients to improve clinical status prior to thymectomy or as a last resort in patients who have been refractory to other forms of treatment. It must be considered experimental therapy in juvenile myasthenia at this time.

Drugs that May Worsen Myasthenia. Most medications that act at the neuromuscular junction to block acetylcholine transmission are contraindicated for use in myasthenia gravis except under special circumstances. They include the aminoglycoside antibiotics, lactate, quinidine, quinine, procainamide, phenytoin, propranolol, lidocaine, and curare. Moreover, sedatives and narcotics that might interfere with normal respiratory function should be used with caution.

The prognosis for most children with myasthenia gravis is very good. For those who do not respond to anticholinesterase therapy, steroids and immunosuppressants may offer improvement or remission. Surgical management through thymectomy should be considered for children whose disease persists for more than 1 year.

Periodic Paralysis

ROBERT C. GRIGGS, M.D.

Recognition and accurate diagnosis are often the major challenges in the treatment of periodic paralysis. Most patients present in childhood—usually in the first weeks of life for paramyotonia and hyperkalemic periodic paralysis and by adolescence in hypokalemic periodic paralysis. When diagnosis is first considered, careful exclusion of other disorders associated with weakness and abnormality of potassium (K) is necessary. Initial attacks require careful documentation before treatment is initiated. Provocative testing is necessary in most patients to establish diagnosis.

HYPOKALEMIC PERIODIC PARALYSIS

Acute Attacks. During paralytic episodes, potassium is invariably low, and, unless the patient is unable to swallow or is vomiting, potassium should be administered orally. A preparation of KCl that is free of sucrose and other carbohydrate should be chosen. A dosage of 0.5 meq/kg as 25 per cent KCl is usually indicated and may have to be repeated. During severe attacks, serum electrolytes and electrocardiogram (ECG) should be monitored at half-hourly intervals until the attack resolves. The exact dosage of potassium depends on the severity and duration of the attack and on the response to the initial dosage of potassium.

If patients are unable to take oral potassium, intravenous KCl may be necessary. The diluent for such treatment is of concern since both 5% glucose and physiologic saline will cause a transient lowering of serum potassium. A concentration of at least 60 meq/l of KCl must be used if either of these diluents is employed. Intravenous treatment is reserved for severely affected patients and requires careful monitoring of electrolytes, ECG, respiratory function, strength, and urinary output. Intravenous KCl-containing solutions should be administered slowly.

Prevention of Attacks. The prophylactic administration of potassium salts is seldom successful in preventing attacks, even when given in large doses on a daily basis. Patients subject to frequent attacks merit a trial of agents to prevent attacks. I have found that most patients respond to the carbonic anhydrase inhibitor acetazolamide with complete cessation of attacks. Treatment is usually effective within 24 to 48 hours, and attacks recur promptly after treatment is discontinued. The dosage is quite variable but is usually that required to produce metabolic acidosis, as indicated by serum chloride elevation and bicarbonate depression. In severe cases, an every-6-hour schedule is necessary.

In occasional patients acetazolamide may produce sufficient hypokalemia to worsen the disorder. In these patients, potassium-sparing agents such as triamterene may be effective. Dietary management, including the avoidance of carbohydrate and sodium loads, may be effective—occasionally as the sole, and often as adjunctive, treatment.

Chronic acetazolamide treatment presents certain hazards, most notably the occurrence of renal calculi. Patients on acetazolamide should have periodic abdominal radiographs and should maintain a high urine output. Sulfonamides should not be prescribed concurrently since a sulfonamide nephropathy may be produced. Frequent but less troublesome side effects include dysgeusia for carbonated beverages, paresthesias, mild anorexia, and osteomalacia.

Treatment and Prevention of Progressive Weakness. Patients with frequent attacks of all types of periodic paralysis may develop persistent interattack weakness after repeated attacks. Acetazolamide prevents and improves such weakness in many patients. Patients unresponsive to acetazolamide may respond to the chloruretic carbonic anhydrase inhibitor dichlorphenamide.

Thyrotoxic hypokalemic periodic paralysis rarely occurs in childhood, and its treatment is markedly different from that of other hypokalemic periodic paralysis. Potassium administration is indicated for acute attacks, but acetazolamide markedly worsens patients. Treatment consists of management of underlying thyrotoxicosis. Propranolol is strikingly effective in preventing attacks, even while patients remain thyrotoxic.

HYPERKALEMIC PERIODIC PARALYSIS

Acute Attacks. Hyperkalemic periodic paralysis is often a misnomer since the serum potassium may remain within the normal range during attacks. The disorder is, therefore, defined by the development of weakness with potassium-loading. Acute attacks are often so mild that treatment is unnecessary. Oral carbohydrate administration in the form of sugar solutions is preferable to potassium-containing fruit juices and soft drinks. Attacks are seldom severe enough to require intravenous therapy. If a severe attack does occur, it will respond to standard measures used to treat hyperkalemia—intravenous glucose, insulin, or sodium bicarbonate.

Prevention of Attacks. Many patients do not require chronic treatment, particularly those with slight, infrequent attacks. Acetazolamide in dosage sufficient to produce a mild kaliopenia (usually 3 mg/kg, 2 or 3 times a day) will prevent attacks and has the added benefit of ameliorating myotonia. Side effects (particularly paresthesias) often limit patient acceptability, and for this reason I have found thiazide diuretics the agent of choice. Chlorothiazide in a dosage of 10 mg/kg in two divided doses prevents attacks; *hypo*kalemia and weakness can develop in these patients as in normal people. Dosage should be kept low enough to prevent this occurrence.

Normokalemic Periodic Paralysis. There are few, if any, well-documented cases of patients with so-called normokalemic periodic paralysis who have not been found to have features identical to those of hyperkalemic periodic paralysis, and treatment is similar.

PARAMYOTONIA CONGENITA

Myotonia is the more disabling feature of paramyotonia, and episodic weakness is usually mild and infrequent. If the disorder requires treatment, it is important to distinguish the two types: (1) true paramyotonia, and (2) paralysis periodica paramyotonica. Patients with the latter disorder are worsened by potassium administration and respond to agents such as acetazolamide and thiazides, which are kaliopenic. True paramyotonia is worsened by such treatment, and patients may develop quadriplegia with acetazolamide. Tocainide,

an investigational drug recently used for treatment of cardiac arrhythmias, is useful for the myotonia and weakness of paramyotonia congenita. Simple maneuvers to avoid cold exposure are usually adequate treatment for mild cases of paramyotonia.

Myositis Ossificans

FREDERICK J. SAMAHA, M.D.

Two types of myositis ossificans are recognized, one follows trauma to muscle and the other is a rare genetically determined progressive disease.

In the former condition, an injury usually involves crushing or shredding of muscle fibers in association with hemorrhage; connective tissue proliferates with metaplasia and subsequent osteoid formation. Calcification of this osteoid concludes the formation of heterotopic bone. The patient will usually relate the occurrence of a crushing injury, as might occur from a high fall, or of repeated minor trauma such as pitching a baseball. Following the injury a tender, firm mass gradually appears over several weeks. As bone formation occurs the mass hardens. The x-ray study of the mass will show the typical feathery calcification. Avoidance of further trauma and physical therapy are all that is needed in mild cases. The persistence of pain or discomfort and the breaking down of overlying skin may require surgical removal of the mass.

The clinical features of progressive myositis ossificans are characteristic. Most of the cases begin in the first decade, and more than 90% have their onset in the first 20 years of life. There appears to be no sex predilection, and in less than 5% of cases a family history of myositis ossificans may be obtained. The latter observation, along with a 90% incidence of digital abnormalities in these patients and the occurrence of digital abnormalities alone in the family history, provide the basis that progressive myositis ossificans may be genetically determined. The most common anomaly is microdactyly or adactyly.

The initial complaints are those of a painful, swollen, tender area, probably following minor trauma, which may be associated with erythematous skin. The pain subsides over several weeks and a firm lump gradually becomes ossified. The heterotopic bone formation occurs in the connective tissue of skeletal muscles, tendons, ligaments and capsules of joints. As in the case of traumatic myositis ossificans, the basic lesion is one of proliferating connective tissue followed by metaplasia, osteoid formation and calcification. The lack of classic inflammatory changes and the lack of direct involvement of muscle cells have moved some clinicians to note that "myositis ossificans" is a misnomer. It is more characteristically a fibrodysplasia. In this regard a case of myositis ossificans has been reported in association with polyostotic fibrous dysplasia.

The prominent areas of involvement are the muscles in the neck, paravertebral area, shoulders and arms, head, face, jaw, hips and legs, in decreasing order of frequency. The episodes of painful swelling and heterotopic bone formation recur over three to four decades until the patient becomes totally immobilized as a "stone man." When intercostal and masseter muscle involvement occurs, death may occur because of respiratory failure and inanition.

Over the last 10 years treatment attempts with ethylenediaminetetraacetic acid (EDTA), parathyroid extract, triiodothyronine, propylthiouracil, corticosteroids, vitamins and low dietary calcium have failed. On the other hand, physical therapy that attempts to maintain full range of joint motion has been of significant value.

A few patients with progressive myositis ossificans have been treated with sodium etridonate (EDHP),* 10 mg/kg/day by mouth. In these patients either the disease has stabilized or the patient has progressively improved. The few therapeutic studies allow some preliminary observations: (1) No serious side effects were encountered. (2) The rates of normal and pathologic bone accretion and resorption decreased. These preliminary conclusions are consistent with in vitro studies on the effects of EDHP on hydroxyapatite formation and dissolution and in studies on in vivo deposition of pathologic calcification in rats. It is also of interest to note that one case of calcinosis universalis occurring in association with dermatomyositis was dramatically helped with EDHP. Since this experimental drug represents the only possible therapeutic approach and since its toxicity is apparently low, patients with documented progressive myositis ossificans might benefit by being referred to centers using EDHP.

---

*EDHP is an experimental drug and is available only on this basis.

_15_
Skin

Topical Therapy: A Dermatologic Formulary for Pediatric Practice

JO DAVID FINE, M.D.,
and KENNETH A. ARNDT, M.D.

Most common childhood dermatoses can be effectively managed by the pediatrician. Unusual diagnostic or therapeutic problems can be referred to a consultant dermatologist for future evaluation as deemed necessary.

GENERAL PRINCIPLES

Acute Versus Chronic Inflammation. The ability to distinguish between acute and chronic inflammatory states will simplify diagnosis and initial skin care. Acute processes are often exudative, vesicular, and crusted and respond best to wet dressings, powders, lotions, and creams. Chronic eruptions often are dry, scaling, and lichenified and require more occlusive preparations, such as ointments, to lubricate the skin and to enhance the percutaneous absorption of the active ingredients.

Role of Infection. The possibility of primary or secondary infection should be considered when initially evaluating a skin eruption. Information obtained from gross examination of the lesions may be sufficient to make a clinical diagnosis of an infectious process. For example, the presence of honey-colored or yellow crusting or exudate, frequently accompanied by a history of recent exacerbation of an underlying or concomitant dermatosis, suggests secondary bacterial impetiginization. The use of appropriate systemic antibiotics to treat streptococcal and staphylococcal infections will result in marked improvement of the patient. At other times cultures of the lesion (exudate; contents of pustules, vesicles, bullae) or mass (skin biopsy with half the specimen for cultures and half for histology) may be required. Bacterial, fungal, viral, and occasionally mycobacterial cultures may be indicated.

Surface Area to Volume Ratio. Children have an increased surface area to volume ratio compared with adults. Percutaneous absorption following application of topical agents over large body areas may result in systemic drug levels and subsequent acute toxicity or unwanted systemic effects. The former is seen with boric acid soaks (gastrointestinal symptoms, renal or hepatic failure, cardiovascular collapse, central nervous system stimulation or depression), while the latter is illustrated by adrenal suppression secondary to topical corticosteroid applications. In addition, marked temperature lability may occur when large surface areas are treated with wet compresses. To avoid significant chilling and hypothermia due to surface evaporation of water, only small areas should be treated simultaneously (i.e., a limb or part of the trunk).

Barrier Function and Penetration. In normal skin, intact stratum corneum serves as a barrier to absorption of external agents as well as loss of internal fluids. Barrier function is altered, however, when inflammation is present or when fissures or denuded areas develop. Skin hydration also affects barrier function—substances are absorbed more readily through hydrated than through dry epidermis.

Ointments are more effective vehicles than creams for promoting percutaneous absorption, presumably by increasing surface hydration via occlusion. Similarly, the use of plastic gloves, vinyl exercise suits, or plastic wraps as occlusive dressings with topical corticosteroids will be advantageous in selected nonexudative dermatoses such as psoriasis, chronic eczema, and lichen planus. However, occlusion may also increase skin maceration, particularly in acute vesiculobullous and sec-

425

ondarily impetiginized disorders, and therefore are contraindicated in these situations.

When excessive scale is present (i.e., psoriasis), efficacy of corticosteroids may be enhanced by prior or concomitant use of keratolytic agents under occlusion (see Corticosteroids later in this article).

Frequency of Application. Little is known about the optimal number of applications needed per day of most types of topical medications for effective treatment of a given skin disease. Some studies suggest that single daily applications of topical corticosteroids, with or without occlusion, may be as effective as multiple daily applications. Despite this, most authorities still recommend the latter approach.

Tachyphylaxis. The continued and uninterrupted use of topical corticosteroids may result in temporary diminution in their effectiveness. This may occur as early as 2 weeks into the course of treatment, but responsiveness returns after corticosteroids have been discontinued for 1 or more weeks. Intermittent use is best both to insure optimal results and to decrease the risk of any adverse effects.

Adverse Systemic Effects. The prolonged use of even low-concentration topical corticosteroids over large surface areas may result in pituitary-adrenal axis suppression. Growth retardation in children has also been reported. Application of potent fluorinated corticosteroids can result in atrophy, telangiectasia, and striae formation within 1 month of use. Areas such as the face and genital and intertriginous areas are particularly at risk; therefore, corticosteroids must be used judiciously in these sites.

Boric acid compresses may result in significant systemic toxicity and should no longer be used.

Elevated phenol levels in blood and urine may result from application of carbol-fuchsin solution (Castellani paint) in children. Although an excellent astringent agent for macerated or fissured intertriginous skin folds or web spaces or intertriginous candidiasis, it should be used only in very select situations.

Absorption of silver sulfadiazine (Silvadene) from extensively burned skin may result in hyperosmolality from the propylene glycol in its vehicle and may thereby add to the metabolic instability of such patients.

Appropriate Selection of Quantities by Prescription. Careful thought must be given to the amount of topical medication needed by each patient to ensure that enough is dispensed to last for days or weeks and also to decrease the cost of the prescription. In an adult, 30 to 60 gm of an ointment or cream are required to cover the entire body in a single application. Most preparations are less expensive when purchased in larger prepackaged containers than in multiple small tubes or jars. If appropriate amounts are dispensed, the overall cost of care is reduced and patient compliance will be improved.

Fixed Combination Preparations. One can usually provide more versatile and at least as effective therapy by using single-component preparations in concert rather than fixed-combination medications. Furthermore, use of many of the latter may result in unwanted side effects. As an example, an impetiginized inflammatory lesion may be better treated with oral antibiotics and topical corticosteroids than with a fixed combination of neomycin with steroid. Use of neomycin may actually exacerbate some skin disorders as a result of development of allergic contact dermatitis. Positive patch test reactions have been reported in up to 20% of patients subsequent to use of neomycin on inflamed skin.

TYPES OF TOPICAL PREPARATIONS

"Wetness" provides benefit by cooling and drying through surface evaporation of water. *Wet dressings* also clean the skin of surface exudates and crusts and help drain infected sites. They are the principal form of therapy for acute exudative inflammation. *Powders* increase skin surface area, thereby enhancing drying and reducing maceration and friction. They are especially useful in body fold areas. *Lotions* are suspensions of powder in water. After the aqueous phase evaporates, a layer of protective or therapeutic powder is left on the skin.

Creams are emulsions of oil in water; they are less occlusive and more drying than corresponding ointments. *Ointments* either are suspensions of water droplets in oil or are inert bases such as petrolatum. They may not be miscible with water. *Gels* are transparent colorless emulsions that liquefy when applied to skin.

Pastes are combinations of powder and ointment and are of stiffer consistency than ointments. Cornstarch is frequently the powder used, as in zinc oxide paste. Since application of cornstarch to intertriginous sites may enhance the overgrowth of yeast, pediatricians should be careful to use zinc oxide ointment rather than paste as a perianal barrier; otherwise secondary *Candida albicans* infection might result.

FORMULARY

This formulary contains a representative list of commonly available topical agents that are beneficial in dermatologic therapy. Although more inclusive lists are available, we believe that this formulary is adequate for general pediatric use.

Acne Preparations

Benzoyl Peroxides. These preparations contain 2.5 to 10% benzoyl peroxide. They are bacteriostatic for *Propionibacterium acnes* as well as mildly comedolytic. They are usually applied thinly once or twice daily to all acne areas, but should be used less frequently or discontinued if excessive redness or dryness develops. The lower concentrations should be used initially to avoid unnecessary irritation. Higher concentrations of benzoyl peroxide should be used with caution in darker-complexioned individuals, because excessive irritation may lead to postinflammatory hyperpigmentation.

An oil base lotion is Benoxyl (Stiefel), which is available in 5 and 10% concentration. Benzagel (Dermik, 5 and 10%) and PanOxyl (Stiefel, 5 and 10%) have an alcohol gel base. A lotion with acetone gel base is Persa-Gel (Ortho, 5 and 10%), while an aqueous gel base can be found in Desquam-X(Westwood, 5 and 10% gel, 10% wash) and PanOxyl AQ (Stiefel, 2.5%).

Retinoic Acid (Vitamin A Acid; Tretinoin). This agent is useful in comedonal acne because of its loosening effect on cellular debris impacted within sebaceous gland and follicular ostia. Used nightly or every other night on acne sites (except eye and lip areas), retinoic acid induces comedones to be expelled. A transient flare in activity may be seen approximately 3 to 6 weeks into treatment. Because of the risk of exaggerated sunburn and possible photocarcinogenicity, retinoic acid preparations should be used with caution, if at all, during summer months. Lower concentrations and creams are initially used; in oilier skin, the gel may be more efficacious. Commonly used forms are Retin-A (Ortho Pharmaceutical) cream (0.05 and 0.1%) and gel (0.01 and 0.025%).

Topical Antibiotics. These agents may be quite effective in mild-to-moderate acne and are used often in conjunction with benzoyl peroxides or retinoic acid. Clindamycin, erythromycin, and tetracycline are all effective against *P. acnes* and may be obtained either commercially prepared and prepackaged or extemporaneously compounded by the physician and pharmacist. Their effectiveness is generally in the order just cited. Topical tetracycline may cause a temporary yellow hue to the skin and also fluoresces when viewed under ultraviolet light; this may make it less desirable for adolescent patients. Although pseudomembranous colitis has been seen in only a very few patients treated with topical clindamycin, its use is contraindicated in patients with ulcerative colitis, Crohn disease, or pseudomembranous colitis, and its use should be discontinued in otherwise healthy patients who develop persistent diarrhea.

Preparations commercially available include clindamycin (Cleocin-T, Upjohn, 30-ml package); erythromycin (Staticin, Westwood, 60 ml) and others; and tetracycline (Topicycline, Proctor and Gamble, 70-ml package). Alternatively, one can extemporaneously formulate an approximately 1% clinda-mycin solution in the following ways: one 600 mg Cleocin hydrochloride capsule in 50 ml of Neutrogena Vehicle/N, or one 600 mg capsule of Cleocin hydrochloride in 54 ml of 70% isopropyl alcohol and 6 ml of propylene glycol.

Acne Cleaners. Many products contain combinations of sulfur, salicylic acid, resorcinol, alcohol, and insoluble or slowly dissolving particles. These have at best only a minor role in acne therapy, providing mild drying and peeling of the skin. It must be emphasized that dryness and superficial peeling are not the desired end point of topical acne therapy. They are side effects of most of the effective topical agents and are not necessary for successful treatment. We do not suggest these agents routinely, but they may be used at the patient's discretion, with care to avoid excessive dryness and irritation.

Anesthetics (Topical)

Although usually ineffective in alleviating pain or itching of inflamed skin, topical anesthetics may be beneficial in some inflammatory mucocutaneous conditions (aphthous stomatitis, herpes simplex infection of the oral cavity or anogenital area, oral erosive lichen planus). However, benzocaine-containing preparations should be avoided because of their tendency for allergic contact sensitization.

Topical anesthetics include dyclonine hydrochloride (Dyclone) (Dow Pharmaceuticals), 0.5 or 1.0% solution, 30 ml; diphenhydramine hydrochloride (Benadryl elixir) (Parke-Davis), 4 oz; and lidocaine (Xylocaine) (Astra), as a 2% viscous solution (100 ml), and 2.5 and 5.0% ointment (35 gm). These agents may be applied locally to the lesion(s), or in the case of elixirs, may be used as mouth rinses, four to six times daily as needed for symptomatic relief.

Antibacterial and Antiseptic Agents

Several preparations are available in both liquid and ointment form that contain bacteriostatic or bactericidal agents. Although most pyodermas are better treated with systemic antibiotics (i.e., penicillin for ecthyma and streptococcal impetigo, erythromycin or dicloxacillin for staphylococcal impetigo), localized superficial wounds often may be adequately treated with topical preparations. Such conditions include surgical sites, burns, areas of localized folliculitis, and abrasions.

Combination formulations often broaden the effective antibacterial spectrum. Although a very effective antistaphylococcal agent, neomycin often causes an allergic contact sensitization, with subsequent worsening of the dermatosis. Systemic absorption and toxicity are very improbable for these agents, owing to their poor percutaneous permeability.

Liquids/Surgical Cleansers. Chlorhexidine is antibacterial for both gram-positive and gram-negative organisms; it has immediate as well as continuing antibacterial effects and is not inhibited by the presence of blood. It is available as Hibiclens (Stuart), in a 4-oz package. Povidone-iodine has antibacterial coverage similar to Hibiclens. However bacterial killing with povidone-iodine requires several minutes of direct contact with the skin and may be inhibited by blood. Furthermore, it may leave a slight yellow tint to the skin if it is not thoroughly removed by rinsing. It is available as Betadine (Purdue Frederick) as well as other brands, in the following liquid forms: solution, surgical scrub, shampoo, and douche.

Ointments. Bacitracin is bactericidal, especially for gram-positive organisms like streptococci and staphylococci. It may be dispensed simply in 15-gm tubes or in combination, as in Neosporin ointment (Burroughs Wellcome) (containing 5000 units of polymyxin B sulfate, 400 units of zinc bacitracin, and 3.5 mg of neomycin sulfate per gm), 15 gm; Neo-Polycin ointment (Dow Pharmaceuticals) (containing 8000 units of polymyxin B sulfate, 400 units of zinc bacitracin, and 3 mg of neomycin sulfate per gm), 15 gm; and Polysporin ointment (Burroughs Wellcome) (containing 500 units of zinc bacitracin and 10,000 units of polymyxin B per gm), 30 gm.

Neomycin sulfate is effective against most gram-negative and some gram-positive organisms, but it has a significant potential as a contact allergen. It is available either alone in generic forms (15 gm) or in combination, as previously noted.

Polymyxin B is effective against most gram-negative organisms, but not *Proteus* and *Serratia*. It is available in combinations, as noted.

Povidone-iodine is also available in ointment form (30 gm) as Betadine or a generic brand.

Gramicidin is bactericidal against gram-positive organisms. It is available in combination with neomycin (Spectrocin ointment, Squibb) and polymyxin B (Neosporin-G cream, Burroughs Wellcome).

Any of these agents can be applied (or used as cleansers if liquid) four to six times daily to the affected sites, as needed.

Antifungal Medications

Dermatophyte Infections. Any agent listed below may be used twice daily for localized dermatophyte infections. Treatment is continued until approximately 2 weeks after all clinical signs of infection are gone—the average duration is about 1 month. However, systemic griseofulvin is necessary for adequate treatment of dermatophyte involvement of hair and nails, when large surface areas of skin are involved, or for recalcitrant, persistently recurrent infection.

Clotrimazole is available as either Lotrimin (Schering) or Mycelex (Miles Pharmaceuticals); cream (30 gm) is usually used, but solution (30 ml) may be preferred for moist, macerated sites, such as interdigital web spaces of toes. Miconazole is similar in structure and mode of action. It is available as Monistat-Derm (Ortho Pharmaceutical), 30 gm of cream or 30 ml of solution. Haloprogin is available as Halotex (Westwood), 30 gm of cream or 30 ml of solution. Tolnaftate (Tinactin, Schering) is available as 1% cream in a 15-gm package; as solution, 10 ml; as powder, 45 gm; and as aerosol, 100 gm. Generic brands are also available.

Candida Infections. Clotrimazole, miconazole, or haloprogin can be used, as just described.

Nystatin is found in many brands of medications, including Mycostatin (Squibb). The most commonly used forms are ointment, cream, and powder. All are available in 15-gm sizes. The use of topical nystatin in our experience seems to result in a slower clinical resolution of active lesions, and we therefore prefer initially the use of the broader-spectrum antifungal agents previously described.

For *Candida* paronychial infections, any of the above preparations may be tired; occlusion under a fingercot may increase their effectiveness. If this treatment is unsuccessful, 2 to 4% thymol in absolute alcohol (prescribed 30 ml) may be compounded; this is applied 2 to 3 times daily to the nail fold areas until healing is complete. The area must be kept dry at all times during the latter nonaqueous therapy.

For oral *Candida* infection (thrush), nystatin oral suspension (100,000 units/ml; 2 ml for infants, 4 to 6 ml for older children and adults) may be swished in the mouth four times daily and swallowed. An alternate therapy is 1 to 2% gentian violet solution painted in the oral cavity 1 to 2 times a day.

Iodochlorhydroxyquin (Vioform, CIBA), 3% cream or ointment (30 gm), may be used alone or combined with 1% hydrocortisone (Vioform-Hydrocortisone, CIBA, 20 gm); generic preparations are also available. This agent has mild antifungal and antibacterial properties and is frequently used in diaper dermatitis, especially when the skin is mildly eczematous, impetiginized, or secondarily infected with yeast. Clothing and skin may be stained yellow by its use.

Topical amphotericin B (available as Fungizone cream, ointment, and lotion, Squibb) is effective against *Candida* but not dermatophytes. Its use has no advantage over other anti-*Candida* therapies, and its yellow-orange color may stain.

Tinea Versicolor. This superficial infection, caused by *Malassezia furfur*, may be treated in many ways. Some effective approaches are (1) 2.5% selenium sulfide suspension (available as Selsun, Abbott, and as Exsel, Herbert Laboratories). This lotion is applied daily to all skin areas from the neck to the knees and showered off after 15 to 30 minutes. This routine is repeated daily for 10 to 14 days. The scalp also should be shampooed with this solution on the first night of treatment; (2) shampoos containing zinc pyrithione (e.g., Head and Shoulders) applied 5 to 10 minutes nightly for 10 to 14 days; (3) 25% sodium hyposulfite (available as Tinver lotion, Barnes-Hind). This is applied twice daily for about 2 weeks to the affected areas; and (4) clotrimazole, miconazole, haloprogin, or tolnaftate preparations.

Antipruritic Agents

If significant itching is present, the use of oral antihistamines as well as topical agents is helpful. For localized pruritic processes, however, drying and cooling preparations can be beneficial when applied 4 to 6 times a day. Examples of the latter include (1) Schamberg lotion (somewhat oily), which contains menthol, 0.5 gm; phenol, 1 gm; zinc oxide, 20 gm; calcium hydroxide solution, 40 ml; and peanut oil to make 100 ml. (2) Menthol, 0.25 gm, and phenol, 1 gm. in Eucerin cream (Beiersdorf) to make 100 gm (lubricating). (3) Calamine, or phenolated calamine lotion (drying). Caladryl (Parke-Davis) cream or lotion, frequently self-prescribed, should be avoided since diphenhydramine when applied topically is both ineffective and a contact allergen. Sarna lotion (Stiefel), 0.5% each of camphor, phenol, and menthol in an emollient lotion vehicle.

Antiviral Agents

Acyclovir (ACV). ACV is a recently released antiviral compound shown to be effective against herpes simplex. The drug is an acyclic nucleoside of guanine. Following phosphorylation by thymidine kinase it becomes antiviral, exerting inhibition of herpes simplex DNA polymerase. ACV is also somewhat effective against varicella-zoster virus.

This drug may be beneficial topically in the first episode of genital herpes but is ineffective in recurrent disease. It is also effective intravenously in primary genital herpes and may be useful in bone marrow recipients to prevent or attenuate the course of cutaneous herpes infections.

ACV is available as 5% ointment (Zovirax, Burroughs Wellcome, 15 gm).

Burn Preparation

One of the most frequently used agents for first, second, and third degree burns is silver sulfadiazine (available as Silvadene, Marion, in 50- and 400-gm packages). It is bactericidal against a wide spectrum of organisms, allowing wound healing to occur under rather sterile conditions. However, it should be avoided in sulfa-allergic patients because of its potential for systemic absorption and subsequent allergic response.

Corticosteroids

Topical corticosteroids are often the most effective single therapy for a variety of inflammatory and hyperplastic cutaneous disorders. The pediatrician will have most frequent need of them in eczematous dermatitis (including allergic contact dermatitis and atopic dermatitis) and psoriasis. Sensible and effective use of these agents necessitates not only a correct diagnosis but also an understanding of tachyphylaxis, the use of occlusion, and the potential for systemic and cutaneous side effects, all of which have been discussed earlier. Although many preparations exist, it is necessary to become familiar with only a few of these in order to effectively treat steroid-responsive dermatoses.

Table 1 lists the corticosteroids. All of these creams and ointments may be applied thinly two to four times daily to affected skin areas. They are most effective if applied to well-hydrated skin. Corticosteroid solutions are applied one to two times daily after shampooing and drying of the scalp; they are used for 7 to 14 days as needed and for psoriasis should be occluded overnight by use of a plastic showercap. After a few days of treatment with potent topical corticosteroids, facial, genital, and intertriginous areas are more safely treated with 1% hydrocortisone in order to avoid steroid side effects.

Moist or vesicular lesions (acute inflammatory lesions) are better treated with creams, while cortico-

Table 1. REPRESENTATIVE TOPICAL CORTICOSTEROIDS FOR DERMATOLOGIC DISORDERS

High Potency	Fluocinonide 0.05%. Lidex cream and ointment. Lidex E cream (Syntex) and Topsyn gel (Syntex) available in 15, 30, and 60 gram sizes.
	Halcinonide 0.1%. Halog cream and ointment (Squibb), Halciderm cream (Squibb) available in 15, 30, and 60 gram sizes. Halog also comes as 0.1% solution (2 oz) as well as 240 grams in both cream and ointment.
Middle Potency	Betamethasone valerate 0.1%. Valisone (Schering), 15 and 45 grams cream and ointment; 60 ml solution.
	Fluocinolone acetonide 0.025%. Synalar (Syntex), available in 30, 60, and 425 grams in both 0.025% cream and ointment; 2 oz as 0.01% solution.
	Hydrocortisone valerate 0.2%. Westcort cream and ointment (Westwood), in 15, 45, and 60 gram cream and ointment.
Low Potency	Hydrocortisone 1%. Nutracort (Owen), 120 gram cream and ointment; Hytone (Dermik), Synacort) (Syntex), 30 and 120 gram cream and ointment; others.

steroid ointments are better suited for dry lichenified areas (chronic inflammatory or hyperplastic lesions). If excessive scale is present (i.e., psoriasis, hypertrophic lichen planus), pre- or concomitant treatment with Keralyt gel (Westwood, 30 gm) under occlusion (i.e., plastic gloves, bags, or wraps) for 2 to 4 hours will enhance the effect of subsequent corticosteroid applications.

Emollients

Many emollients are readily available and inexpensive. If hydrophobic (greasy) substances are applied to skin surfaces after adequate hydration (immersion in water for at least 10 minutes), they will add to the surface barrier and impair water loss. In pediatric practice they are most frequently used for children with atopic dermatitis. By decreasing dryness, they help prevent further fissuring, itching, and subsequent inflammation and possibly impetiginization. Some emollients are greasier in texture than others; choice of emollient will depend on expense and cosmetic acceptance. Commonly used emollients include lotions—for example: Alpha Keri (Westwood), U-Lactin (T/I Pharmaceutical), Lubriderm (Ortho), Cetaphil (Parke-Davis), Lubrex (T/I Pharmaceutical), and Wibi (Owen); creams, such as Nivea (Beiersdorf), Eucerin (Beiersdorf), Carmol (Syntex), and Keri (Westwood); and ointments—Aquaphor (Beiersdorf) and hydrated petrolatum USP.

Keratolytics

Propylene glycol solutions with or without added salicylic acid are excellent agents for loosening and removing scales; they are especially effective when applied to affected skin for 2 to 4 hours under plastic wrap occlusion after adequate prior hydration by soaks or bathing. Patients with conditions such as ichthyosis (vulgaris and X-linked), psoriasis, hypertrophic lichen planus, and tinea manuum and pedis will benefit from this treatment. Available preparations include Keralyt gel (Westwood, 30 gm) or 40% propylene glycol solution, the latter prepared by a pharmacist. Whitfield ointment (as half-strength concentration, 3% salicyclic acid and 6% benzoic acid, in 30-gm tube) is mainly used either alone or in conjunction with other antifungal creams for the treatment of hyperkeratotic dermatophyte infection of the palms and soles. In isolated cases of dense scalp psoriasis, nightly treatment under a plastic shower-cap with either Keralyt gel or P&S liquid (Baker) helps in scalp debridement.

Scabicides and Pediculocides

Gamma benzene hexachloride (Kwell lotion or shampoo, Reed and Carnrick, 60 ml, and other generic brands) is effective for both mites (scabies) and lice (pediculosis). When treating scabies, all skin below the angle of the jaw is covered; medication should be applied to dry skin (i.e., the patient should not shower first) and washed off 8 hours later. The treatment may be repeated in 7 days to protect against possible reinfection by hatched larvae. Because of its potential for percutaneous absorption, lindane is contraindicated in pregnant women, in neonates and very young children, and in those with widespread cutaneous disease and an abnormally permeable skin barrier; isolated case reports of central nervous system side effects in children have been reported.

Pediculosis pubis is treated by application of lindane to the groin and other affected areas, with rinsing after 8 hours. Pediculosis capitis may be treated with single lindane shampooing, although some advocate repeat treatment in 4 to 7 days.

Crotamiton (Eurax cream and lotion, Westwood, 60 gm and 2 oz packages) is an alternative to lindane for the treatment of scabies. This is applied twice daily for 2 days.

Six to 10% precipitated sulfur in petrolatum (30 or 60 gm), the initial antiscabetic therapy in pregnancy and infancy, is applied daily for 3 days. It is messy and malodorous, but has no risk of systemic side effects.

Effective over-the-counter alternate treatments for pediculosis are pyrethrin-containing agents such as A-200 Pyrinate liquid (Norcliff Thayer) and RID (Pfipharmecs).

Involved eyelashes may be treated by careful application of petrolatum twice daily for 8 days, 0.025% phosphostigmine ophthalmic ointment (5 gm) or yellow oxide of mercury.

Shampoos

Although nonmedicated shampoos are certainly useful in local scalp hygiene, shampoos containing selenium sulfide, zinc pyrithione, tar or salicylic acid-sulfur are more beneficial for seborrheic dermatitis and psoriasis. These are initially used daily with a second application after the first rinsing; after the scalp improves in appearance, shampooing may be performed every other or every third night as necessary. Useful agents include selenium sulfide, available as Selsun (Abbott) and Exsel (Herbert Laboratories); zinc pyrithione—Zincon (Lederle) and Head and Shoulders (Procter and Gamble); tar (particularly useful in psoriasis)—Sebutone (Westwood), Pentrax (Coopercare), T-Gel (Neutrogena), and others; and salicylic acid-sulfur—Sebulex (Westwood), Vanseb (Herbert Laboratories), TiSeb (T/I Pharmaceutical), and others.

Soaps

Children with eczema or atopic dermatitis may develop skin irritation from harsh soaps. The least irritating soap has been found to be Dove, followed by a group including Aveenobar, Purpose, Dial, Alpha Keri, Neutrogena, Ivory, and Oilatum.

Sunscreens

Sunscreens are agents containing chemicals that absorb ultraviolet light from the sunburn spectrum. Use of sunscreens permits increased exposure time to sunlight without development of sunburn. Their use is especially important in sunlight-aggravated diseases such as lupus erythematosus and polymorphous light eruption. The individual usefulness of a sunscreen to prevent sunburn depends on its relative efficacy in blocking or absorbing UVB radiation (280 to 320 nm), as well as its SPF (sunlight protection factor) rating. Two of the more effective sunscreens are PreSun 15 (Westwood) and Total Eclipse (Herbert Laboratories). A very effective sunscreen that does not contain para-aminobenzoic acid is TiScreen (T/I Pharmaceutical). Most sunscreens should be reapplied after sweating or swimming. For total sunlight exclusion, sunshades containing opaque substances can be used; these include zinc oxide paste, A-Fil (Texas Pharmacals), and Reflecta. Lipstick sunscreens are also available.

Tar Compounds

Coal tar preparations have been long known to be effective in psoriasis and eczematous dermatitis, although their exact modes of action are still unknown. Tars are anti-inflammatory, inhibit DNA synthesis, and photosensitize to longwave (UV-A) ultraviolet light. Among commonly used preparations are the following:

Liquids. For chronic hand or foot eczema, soaks or compresses for 30 minutes twice daily with Balnetar (Westwood, 8 oz) or Zetar emulsion (Dermik, 6 oz) are useful, especially if areas are fissured. When more widespread areas are involved, as in generalized atopic dermatitis or psoriasis, tar baths twice daily, followed by application of other medication or emollients, are beneficial.

Gels. Beneficial in psoriasis in conjunction with topical corticosteroids and/or ultraviolet light therapy or both. T/Derm (Neutrogena) or Estar gel (Westwood, 90 gm) is applied daily to the individual lesions. Similarly, tar-containing gels can be applied simultaneously with corticosteroids and/or Vioform to refractory hand eczema, one to two times a day; the hands are then loosely covered with porous white cotton gloves to decrease the messiness of this combination. These gels contain alcohol and can sting on application.

Ointments and Pastes. In some patients, better response occurs when tar ointments or pastes are used. Two frequently prescribed forms are 5% crude coal tar or Zetar ointment (Dermik). These preparations are quite messy and malodorous and will stain clothing and sheets if not adequately re-moved; mineral oil may be useful in cleansing them from the skin.

Tar Shampoos. These have been previously discussed. Descriptions of other multicompound formulations containing tar can be found in any of the current dermatology textbooks or monographs.

Wart Remedies

Many modes of therapy are available for warts, depending on types, location, number of lesions, and previous responses to treatment. These include chemicals, liquid nitrogen application, and electrodesiccation and curettage.

Condylomata acuminata usually respond to application of podophyllin, but there is high potential for cutaneous burns and possible systemic toxicity secondary to overaggressive treatment.

Isolated common warts can be self-treated with daily applications of combined salicylic and lactic acids in collodion (Duofilm, Stiefel, 15 ml; Viranol, American Dermal Corp., 10 ml; Ti-Flex, T/I Pharmaceuticals). Two to four drops daily are applied to the wart after prior hydration (5 to 10 minutes of soaking in warm water). The lesion is then covered with adhesive or plastic tape for 12 to 24 hours. If the area becomes red and tender, treatment is withheld for a few days. The resultant whitened surface of the wart is gently filed down daily with a callus file or pumice stone and the medication reapplied. Using this approach, the majority of warts can be cured, but at least 6 to 12 weeks of daily applications may be required. Plantar warts can be treated similarly, or by the daily application of 40% salicylic acid plaster carefully cut to just cover the area of the wart. This is then covered with tape, and the wart should be frequently debrided.

Wet Dressings, Compresses

Weeping, exudative, crusted, and vesicular eruptions require the use of wet dressings to aid in drying and surface debridement. As mentioned previously, boric acid solutions are no longer used because of the risk of absorption and toxicity. We do not use potassium permanganate solutions because of the difficulty in mixing, the potential for chemical burn from undissolved crystals, and the rather dramatic and persistent staining of skin and nails.

Wet dressings of comfortable temperature are applied using several layers of sterile gauze, Kerlix, or clean old linens. The dressings are removed, remoistened, and reapplied every 5 to 10 minutes for a total of 15 to 30 minutes three to four times a day as needed. As mentioned, in children only small surface areas are treated simultaneously to avoid chilling due to evaporative heat loss. Solutions include (1) Aluminum acetate (Burrow solution)—available as Domeboro powder or tablets (Dome Laboratories, box of 12). Use one tablet or packet to a pint of water (makes a 1:40 solution). A fresh solution should be remade daily, but it can be refrigerated for storage; however, it should be allowed to warm to room temperature prior to application. (2) Acetic acid solution—0.25 to 1%. The higher concentration has been suggested to have the added benefit of killing *Pseudomonas aeruginosa*. (3) Normal saline. (4) Betadine—this is less advantageous than the others because of its color, which may make subsequent wound observation somewhat more difficult unless the wound is first irrigated.

Cosmetic Masking Agents

Some vascular or pigmentary congenital lesions are cosmetically unsightly and deforming. An excellent approach to therapy is the use of Covermark makeup (Lydia O'Leary, 22.5 and 85.5 gm cream). Many of these lesions can b completely masked in this manner.

Skin Diseases of the Neonate

NANCY B. ESTERLY, M.D.

The skin of the normal newborn infant requires no special care other than gentle cleansing. As in any age group, the skin serves as an effective protective barrier to ingress of organisms and harmful or toxic substances. It is the outermost layer in particular, the stratum corneum, that constitutes the critical layer for barrier function, and its efficacy as a limiting structure depends on preservation of its integrity. Mechanical removal or maceration and injury to this layer will reduce barrier function and provide a portal of entry for pathogenic organisms and potentially damaging chamicals. In general, principles of skin care applicable to the term infant are also acceptable for the preterm infant, although earlier in gestation the integument is thinner, more fragile, and probably more permeable to certain substances. These infants are, therefore, more vulnerable to the effects of trauma, occlusion, maceration, and moisture.

The purpose of cleansing the newborn skin can be regarded as three-fold: 1) for aesthetic reasons; 2) to remove excess vernix, blood, meconium, urine, and stool; and 3) to discourage colonization and proliferation of pathogenic organisms. Cleansing should be postponed until the body temperature has become stable. Warm sterile water will adequately remove soiled vernix, blood, and meconium on the head and perineum. Vernix may be left elsewhere on the skin and will gradually disappear during subsequent days. Incomplete removal of the vernix caseosa probably is not detrimental, for this lipid covering more than likely provides an additional physiologic protective barrier. During the remainder of the nursery stay, urine and stool can be removed from the diaper skin in a similar fashion; the use of a mild, nonmedicated toilet soap is also acceptable provided all traces are rinsed away thoroughly. However, it should be remembered that contaminated liquid or bar soaps have the potential for acting as a source for dissemination of bacteria. Cord care is important in order to limit colonization by pathogenic organisms. Several effective regimens include local applications of triple dye, alcohol, or antimicrobial agents such as bacitracin ointment and silver sulfadiazine cream.

Although daily baths with detergents containing hexachlorophene were once standard nursery procedure, the use of this agent has been abandoned except during outbreaks of staphylococcal infection because of the potential neurotoxicity of the compound, if absorbed. However, in the event of such an outbreak, hexachlorophene bathing may be reinstituted for control provided it is carried out in an appropriate manner. The infant should be thoroughly washed with a warmed 3% hexachlorophene-detergent cleanser (pHisoHex) and the skin thoroughly rinsed with warm, sterile water. Particular attention should be paid to the skin-cord pocket, which can serve as a moist repository for proliferating organisms. Neither soap nor alcohol should be used concomitantly since both will wash off or dissolve the hexachlorophene, thereby limiting its effectiveness. Hexachlorophene bathing should be used only on term infants. Additional appropriate surveillance measures and epidemiologic investigations should be instituted in the involved nursery. Meticulous handwashing by nursery personnel, using antibacterial preparations such as iodophors, is always critical but particularly important during outbreaks of infection.

Desquamation of the skin may be prominent in some neonates during the latter part of the first week in life. The temptation to lubricate these infants should be resisted since application of oils, lotions, creams, or ointments serves no useful purpose and may, in fact, diminish barrier function. Likewise, exposure to an excessively humid environment or the use of occlusive dressings and tape may macerate the skin, compromising barrier function and predisposing the infant to infection.

Birth Trauma

A difficult labor and delivery may be reflected by the presence of areas of intense erythema, bleeding into the skin (petechiae, ecchymoses, and hematomas), contusions, and erosions. In some infants these lesions may contribute to the development of anemia and hyperbilirubinemia. Absorption of blood occurs spontaneously during the first few weeks of life and usually requires no intervention. When the complications of anemia and jaundice supervene, phototherapy or exchange transfusion may be indicated.

Pressure necrosis may occur if there is cephalopelvic disproportion or in the unusually large term infant, such as infants of diabetic mothers. Common areas of involvement are the skin overlying the bony prominences of the head and face, particularly the parietal bosses and the zygomata. At times these erosions are mistaken for cutis aplasia (congenital absence of skin). Generally they heal spontaneously in an uncomplicated fashion and with a small, unobtrusive scar. Treatment is aimed at preventing infection and minimizing scar formation. Exudate should be examined for cells and organisms and cultured for pathogens. The presence of normal flora is not an indication for either local or systemic antibiotic therapy. Routine care should include saline compresses for moist or exudative lesions to remove purulent matter and debris. Once clear, the area should be kept dry and permitted to heal by granulation and re-epithelialization. In the event of secondary infection, choice of antibiotic should be determined by the identification of pathogens on culture.

Caput succedaneum is a diffuse, edematous swelling of the presenting part, most often the scalp, but, in the infant delivered by breech extraction, sometimes the vulval or scrotal skin. The overlying skin may be studded with petechiae or display extensive ecchymoses. Both the edema and hemorrhage, even when alarmingly extensive, will subside spontaneously during the first few days of life. Complications are rare; associated erosions should be treated conservatively. Compresses and ointments may only further macerate the skin and facilitate penetration of pathogenic organisms.

Cephalhematomas may occur independently or in association with a caput succedaneum. These lesions result from rupture of the blood vessels that traverse the cranial periosteum and produce a swelling sharply limited to the surface of one cranial bone because of adherence of the periosteum at the suture line. Bilateral lesions may also occur and are detectable by a central depression corresponding to the periosteal attachment at the bony margin. Resolution is slow, usually requiring 3 to 6 weeks, and is usually uncomplicated. Aspiration is contraindicated as infection may be introduced by the needle. Massive hemorrhage resulting in severe anemia is an indication for transfusion. Hyperbilirubinemia due to absorption of bilirubin may also complicate the course. Linear fractures, which occur in approximately 25% of infants with cephalhematomas, rarely cause a problem but should be followed with appropriate radiologic studies. Depressed fractures are an indication for neurosurgical consultation. In the rare event of secondary infection, systemic antibiotics should be administered, based on the identification of the organism cultured from aspirated material.

Nevi

A variety of nevoid lesions may be apparent at birth and are often of considerable concern to parents. *Sebaceous nevi* are yellow-pink, hairless plaques that occur most commonly on the scalp but may also involve the skin of the face and pinnae. Although of no consequence in the newborn period or early childhood, ultimately they require removal owing to their propensity for verrucous change and for the development of secondary tumors, including benign adnexal neoplasms and basal cell carcinomas, during adolescence and adulthood. These lesions may be identifiable clinically or histologic identification may be obtained from a biopsy.

Congenital pigmented nevi of all sizes are now believed to pose an increased risk for the development of malignancy, although the incidence of melanomas arising in small lesions is still unknown. It is extremely important for the neonatologist to document the presence of these lesions at birth, including site, size, color, and morphology, so that appropriate counseling can be given to parents regarding management later in life. All too often, because of incomplete records, it is impossible to verify whether these lesions were present at birth, which is information critical to proper management.

Vascular nevi (hemangiomas) of various types usually cause no problems in the newborn period. Two exceptions are nevus flammeus in the trigeminal area, which dictates a careful ophthalmologic examination to detect possible associated glaucoma, and the presence of an extensive cavernous hemangioma, which may herald onset of Kasabach-Merritt syndrome (thrombocytopenia and disseminated intravascular coagulation).

TRANSIENT LESIONS OF NEWBORN SKIN

Milia. Milia are superficial epidermal inclusion cysts, 1 to 2 mm in diameter and pearly white in color, that are found most commonly on the upper two thirds of the face of term infants. These lesions require no therapy since they exfoliate spontaneously during the first few weeks of life. Occasionally they develop elsewhere on the body or are larger, as are those that occur occasionally on the foreskin. They may also form as a secondary phenomenon in scarring conditions, such as epidermolysis bullosa, or in surgical scars.

Sebaceous Gland Hyperplasia. These lesions are pinpoint-sized, closely grouped yellow or white spots that may appear in profusion on the nose, nasolabial folds, forehead, and malar areas of the term infant. They are frequently confused with milia but simply represent the large sebaceous glands of the infant that have been stimulated by the maternal androgens. Parents can be reassured that they will disappear during the first several days of life.

Miliaria Crystallina. These are the most superficial lesions signifying sweat retention and result from blockage of the sweat pore due to hygroscopic swelling of the stratum corneum. The lesions are tiny, round or irregularly shaped, noninflammatory vesicles filled with clear fluid, which rupture easily with gentle pressure. Miliaria occurs with increased frequency in infants subjected to high ambient temperature or phototherapy. The condition is harmless and requires no therapy save alteration of the environmental temperature and humidity. Ointments, creams, and oils are contraindicated—they will simply cause maceration of the skin and further plugging.

Sucking Blisters. Occasionally solitary blisters are noted at birth or shortly thereafter on the radial surface of the forearm or the dorsum of the hand and fingers. These are in response to vigorous sucking activity and are readily explained by observation of the infant. They are harmless and may be ignored provided infections and congenital blistering disorders can be excluded as possibilities.

Erythema Toxicum. This is a benign, self-limited, extremely common skin eruption that appears in some measure in approximately 50% of newborns. Although it has been observed at birth, most commonly it affects infants during the first to fourth days of life. Lesions range from blotchy erythematous macules to a frank pustular eruption easily confused with staphylococcal or candidal infections as well as pustular melanosis. The most typical lesion, however, is a small, ivory-colored papulopustule set on a wide erythematous base. Since the histologic lesion is that of a perifollicular subcorneal or intraepidermal pustule filled with eosinophils, a smear of the intralesional contents will contain these cells in profusion and readily distinguish this eruption from others of the newborn period. Cultures are always sterile. The lesions may be sparse or profuse, or widely scattered or grouped, but are always evanescent and asymptomatic. The infant is healthy, and no treatment is indicated.

Transient Neonatal Pustular Melanosis. This is another benign, self-limited disorder of the neonate, seemingly occurring predominantly in black infants. Lesions are almost always present at birth and often are noted on examination in the delivery room. Any or all of the three characteristic types of lesions may be present: 1) vesicopustules of 1 mm to 1 cm on a nonerythematous base or with a narrow rim of erythema, 2) ruptured vesicopustules identifiable by their characteristic collarette of scale, and 3) hyperpigmented macules. Sites of predilection are forehead, anterior neck, submental

area, lower back, and soles. Smears of the subcorneal pustules show few to no eosinophils, variable numbers of polymorphonuclear leukocytes, and cellular debris. Cultures are sterile. Affected infants are usually healthy term neonates, and parental reassurance is all that is necessary. The macules may persist for up to 3 months but always fade completely.

Cutis Aplasia (Congenital Absence of Skin). These lesions may be superficial, representing absence of only epidermis and dermis, or may reflect loss of subcutaneous tissue and periosteum as well. When the defects are small, the course is usually benign with epithelialization resulting in an atrophic or hypertrophic scar devoid of appendageal structures. Complications, usually of deeper or extensive lesions, include secondary infections, meningitis, and septicemia, which should be diagnosed promptly and treated appropriately. A skull film is advised since an underlying bony defect is rather frequent. Most important is the recognition that these defects may be falsely attributed to obstetric trauma, with obvious medicolegal ramifications. In those instances, a biopsy of the lesion or margin of the defect demonstrating absence of normal skin architecture and appendages may be extremely helpful. Although a course of expectant observation is always preferable, in instances of nonhealing after several weeks it may be prudent to intervene. Open lesions should be kept clean and dry. If purulent drainage is noted, compressing with Burow solution may suffice; cultures should always be obtained, and true infection treated with the appropriate antibiotic. Excision with primary closure or grafting may be required. Plastic repair may be desirable at an older age if an unsightly scar has formed.

Acne Neonatorum. This term is often used to describe the facial papular eruption common in young infants that represents plugged follicular pores. True acne neonatorum is distinguished by the presence of inflammatory papules, open and closed comedones, and, rarely, nodulocystic lesions. It occurs almost exclusively in male infants and, although attributed to maternal androgens, may well reflect an abnormal response to his own androgens in an infant with a hereditary hyperresponsive end-organ (sebaceous follicle and gland). Treatment in the small infant should be conservative since the process is self-limited and rarely scars. It is particularly important to anticipate and forewarn parents about the hazards of applying over-the-counter preparations that may aggravate the condition. A mild benzoyl peroxide preparation (2½ or 5%) in a lotion vehicle or water-based gel applied once or twice daily may suffice. If the comedonal element is marked, the addition of a low potency topical vitamin A acid (Retin-A) may be effective. Topical antibiotics in a vehicle appropriate for the patient with acne, newly available, are also acceptable for once or twice daily application (erythromycin 1 to 2%).

Scleroma Neonatorum. Occurring primarily in preterm or debilitated infants, this skin change is characterized by a diffuse, nonpitting, woody consistency. It may reflect the presence of a life-threatening condition such as sepsis, gastroenteritis, or pneumonia but has also been attributed to hypothermia. Supportive care and treatment of the associated disorder are all that is required. The skin changes will resolve spontaneously and without sequelae as the infant improves. Corticosteroids are of no value in this condition, which should be regarded as a cutaneous marker of serious systemic disease.

Subcutaneous Fat Necrosis. The lesions usually occur in healthy term newborn infants and are tender, sharply circumscribed nodules or plaques which may be skin-colored or have a violaceous hue. Common sites are the cheeks, back, upper arms, buttocks, and thighs. Although they have been attributed to hypothermia, asphyxia, or obstetric trauma, in fact the etiology is unclear. Occasionally infants appear ill and are hyperthermic. In most instances, the lesions resolve spontaneously and without residual changes during the first few weeks of life. If deposition of calcium in the nodules is extensive, liquefaction of tissue leading to rupture and drainage may result in scarring. Uncomplicated lesions require no therapy. Careful needle aspiration is advisable only for fluctuant lesions to reduce scarring; however, the physician must recognize the possibility of introducing infection. Rarely, associated hypercalcemia and visceral calcification may require vitamin D and administration of systemic corticosteroid therapy.

Eruptions in the Diaper Region

GARY M. GORLICK, M.D.

General Measures

These measures are aimed at the prevention of the most common diaper rashes as well as their early treatment by simple, effective, and safe measures.

Most importantly, parents must be educated in correct cleaning, bathing, and diaper-care of the infant; they in turn, must transmit this to the infant's baby-sitters and/or day-care and nursery school personnel, especially when a rash is present. After birth, the umbilicus should be cleaned with isopropyl alcohol tid–qid and continued for approximately 1 week after it has detached and become dry at the stump, to prevent a focus from which bacterial dermatitis might develop. Signs of

infection at the umbilicus or circumcision must be brought to the physician's attention and treated. Tub-bathing is not begun until the umbilicus is dry and fully healed. Either type of diaper, permanent (cloth) or disposable, is currently acceptable inasmuch as there is inadequate evidence at this time that one type predisposes to increased incidence of rash. If a disposable type is used, the plasticized outer covering should be folded away from the baby's skin at the back, front, and thigh regions if not pleated. Cloth diapers are best washed in Ivory Snow and rinsed thoroughly. Fabric softeners should not be used if a rash develops. The diaper is to be removed and changed as soon as stooling is noted; with the onset of a rash, quickly changing the diaper after urination also becomes important, as does a change late in the evening hours. The infant's room should not be overheated and should be kept at normal humidity. Skin cleansing is best done with cool or tepid water on a soft and nontraumatic (not heavy and rough-surfaced) washcloth or cotton pledgets. Particular care is necessary to clean and dry all creases well. If soap is used, a mild one is recommended, such as Dove or Neutrogena Baby Soap. Oils should not be used, particularly in the diaper region. Avoid overdressing the infant; consequent heat and sweat retention may lead to miliaria and/or intertrigo. When early chafing or eruption is noted, allow open air exposure as often as feasible, decrease the use of outer plastic pants, and apply a protective ointment such as Desitin, A and D, or zinc oxide to the involved areas.

There appears to be a role for diet management in some diaper eruptions. The infant should have adequate fluid intake. Some rashes respond to water supplements alone. At times, empiric stopping of juices will clear the eruption. The prevention and treatment of diarrheal stools by diet manipulation (e.g., adding banana or rice foods for a binding effect, decreasing or stopping juices or other known diarrhea-producing agents) will often help. Although there is strong evidence against "ammoniacal dermatitis," at least as a primary entity, oral cranberry juice bid–tid may be tried. Any new food introduced and soon followed by a rash should be discontinued and reintroduced carefully when the rash has abated. Cow's milk should not be introduced until an infant is at least 6 to 12 months of age (the American Academy of Pediatrics recommends 12 months) and dermatitis should be carefully watched for at any area of the body including the diaper region. Obesity should be prevented; the friction of opposing skin creates a greater than normal propensity for intertrigo to develop.

Many contactants must be avoided. Oils applied directly to the skin or placed in the bath water should be avoided, as should "bubble-bath" in the young child. The infant's skin should be kept free of cosmetics and other skin and hair preparations. Creams, ointments, oils, talcs, and emollients being used at the time of an eruption may be etiologic and should be empirically stopped. Careful review of all aspects of bathing, cleansing, and diaper care may be necessary to identify contactants that are causing a dermatitis.

SPECIFIC MEASURES

These measures are aimed at the treatment of the listed conditions below. Reference to *Topical Therapy: A Dermatologic Formulary for Pediatric Practice* is herein made for dosage schedules not repeated in this section.

Chafing, Irritant Dermatitis, Intertrigo, and Perianal Dermatitis. Ointments such as Desitin, A and D, Diaparene, and zinc oxide may be applied as often as each diaper change. Talcum power is useful, especially in the creases, but must not be used if the skin is denuded, and care must be taken that it is not inhaled by the infant, as it is easily airborne. Corn starch is less likely to be inhaled but may enhance the growth of *Candida albicans* (monilial dermatitis).

Monilial Dermatitis. Therapy consists of applying mycostatin cream or ointment bid–qid to the rash. Another technique is to alternate the application of hydrocortisone cream 1% with either mycostatin cream or mycostatin dusting powder at each diaper change. The dusting powder can also be applied bid to tid when the skin is clear in the infant who is prone to repetitions of this condition. Oral mycostatin is added to the local treatment in the following situations: when thrush is present; when the baby is breast-fed and the mother has monilial mastitis; when the diaper eruption is extensive; when there is nonresponse to local therapy alone; or when the eruption recurs soon after local treatment. One to 2 ml of oral mycostatin is given tid to qid until finished (60 ml bottle), with particular attention to its contact with all areas of thrush before being swallowed. A mother with active monilial vaginitis may be a source of reinfection and should be treated. The treatment of oral lesions with topical gentian violet is messy and is rarely used today. Oral ketoconazole is *not* to be used for simple monilial dermatitis. In addition to mycostatin, there are many topical antifungals that are applied bid and are active against *C. albicans:* e.g., clotrimazole (Lotrimin, Mycelex), miconazole (Monistat-Derm), haloprogin (Halotex, Tinactin). As of this writing a topical form of ketoconazole is not available.

Seborrheic, Atopic, and "Psoriasiform" Dermatitis. Apply hydrocortisone cream 1% on a "least-often" as necessary basis, that is, once to qid prn. Stronger topical corticosteroids are rarely necessary, but if they are, use one from the next higher potency group and stop it as soon as response is noted and return to the very safe hydrocortisone

1% cream. Never use fluorinated corticosteroids or oral/parenteral steroids, nor occlusive technique, in the diaper region. The therapeutic role of Biotin for generalized seborrhea (not Leiner's) is uncertain at the present time.

Bacterial Dermatitis. Controversy exists over the therapeutic effectiveness of topical antibiotics for skin infections. In addition, the potential for allergic contact sensitization is of concern. However, if the diaper dermatitis area is small, topical Neosporin-G *cream* (not ointment) qid alone may suffice. Since *Staphyloccocus aureus* is by far the most common cause of diaper area bacterial infection, cloxicillin sodium (Tegopen) is given orally at 25 to 50 mg/kg/day in four divided doses for 7 to 10 days when more than local treatment is necessary.

"Ammoniac Dermatitis." As mentioned before, controversy exists as to whether ammonia causes dermatitis, or if it exacerbates an existing dermatitis. Some clinicians, however, believe the following measures may be efficacious: oral cranberry juice or oral methionine (Pedameth), and/or Caldesene Medicated Powder or Ointment. Pedameth liquid contains 75 mg of racemethionine per 5 ml, and the recommended dosage for infants 2 to 6 months old is 5 ml tid (in formula, milk, or juice) for 3 to 5 days. For infants 6 to 14 months of age the same dosage is given but at a qid frequency and also for 3 to 5 days.

Psoriasis. The ideal therapy for the infant and very young child with psoriasis in the diaper region has not yet been established. Corticosteroids probably should be avoided as much as possible. Treatment with tars such as 2% crude coal tar in a zinc oxide ointment (removed with warm mineral oil) once or twice a day has been effective. Estar, a 5% coal tar, may also be used once or twice a day. Should corticosteroids be used because of nonresponse to the above, it is best to attempt control with mild 1% hydrocortisone ointment. Since this dermatitis is often chronic, it might be best to treat only flare-ups with these specific agents. Preventing Koebner reaction by the most atraumatic hygienic methods is important.

Granuloma Gluteale Infantum. In this uncommon condition symmetrical nodular lesions occur in the diaper region following diaper dermatitis with or without candidiasis and previously were often treated with fluorinated steroids. It resolves without therapy, and therefore all agents should be stopped. In some cases it is best to taper corticosteroid agents gradually from those of strongest to those of mildest potency to avoid a "flare-up" when they are abruptly stopped.

Recalcitrant Diaper Eruptions. Rule out pinworms and/or urinary tract infection when appropriate. Rule out *Tinea corporis* infection on rare occasion. Consider dermatitis medicamentosa—especially when Mycolog *cream* has been used, for this contains a potent corticosteroid as well as potential allergic sensitizers. Look for signs of telangiectasis or bleeding within the rash, and for anemia, fever, hepatosplenomegaly, and intractable diarrhea, in the child who shows signs of failure to thrive, for these may herald serious systemic conditions such as congenital syphilis, acrodermatitis enteropathica, Wiskott-Aldrich syndrome, or Letterer-Siwi disease.

Agents Not to Be Used. Boric acid, baking soda, mercurials, hexachlorophene, fluorinated corticosteroids, and oral ketoconazole should not be used to treat diaper eruptions. The *cream* form of Mycolog should be avoided; if the physician wishes to use Mycolog, the *ointment* form is strongly advised, as is the precaution to stop as soon as the rash improves and to continue therapy with hydrocortisone cream 1% with or without anticandidal therapy as necessary.

Contact Dermatitis

STEPHANIE H. PINCUS, M.D.

The term contact dermatitis refers to an acute or chronic inflammatory process of the skin that is due to interaction between the skin and an exogenous substance. It is further divided into two types of contact dermatitis: irritant and allergic. The irritant type, sometimes known as primary irritant dermatitis, is the result of damage to the skin by toxic chemicals such as alkalis and detergents. Allergic contact dermatitis refers to the specific lymphoctyemediated reaction that occurs in sensitized individuals. Whenever possible, irritant dermatitis should be distinguished from allergic dermatitis since prevention of these conditions may depend on differing environmental factors.

IRRITANT CONTACT DERMATITIS

Severe irritant dermatitis can develop in all persons exposed to strong acids, potent alkalis, or other toxic chemicals. The treatment of all irritant dermatitis is similar, regardless of the cause. The most important treatment is avoidance of the irritating substance itself. Diaper dermatitis was discussed in the preceding article. The irritant dermatitis seen in older children, again, should be treated by avoidance of the irritating substance and use of emollients such as Nivea cream, Keri cream, and so on. If severe erythema, cracking, or fissuring is present, it may be necessary to add a topical steroid. In such a case, one of the moderate-strength steroid creams, such as triamcinolone cream (0.025 or 0.1%) or betamethasone cream, should be selected. This medication should be applied only as long as necessary. Usually therapy is initiated four times a day and decreased to twice a day as toler-

ated. In a typical case, treatment for 10 to 14 days is adequate. When the eruption has persisted for a considerable time and resulted in a thickened, lichenified skin, an ointment is preferred. An intermediate-potency ointment such as Valisone is usually adequate. The high-potency fluorinated medications should be reserved for refractory cases since cutaneous atrophy and telangiectasias may result from excess usage.

ALLERGIC CONTACT DERMATITIS

Allergic contact dermatitis is a specific lymphocyte-mediated eruption. It requires that the child be exposed to a sensitizing dose; upon reexposure, the dermatitis typically develops 48 to 72 hours later. The area of dermatitis is confined to the area of contact, and this explains the peculiar distribution sometimes seen.

Treatment of acute allergic contact dermatitis depends upon the severity of the eruption. For most cases, topical treatment is adequate. During the acute phase, which is manifested by erythema, weeping, oozing, or vesicle formation, drying may be promoted by the use of cool, wet dressings. Burow solution diluted 1:20 for young children and 1:10 for teenagers should be used. Wet dressings should be applied for 15- to 20-minute periods three of four times a day. Wet dressings will promote evaporative cooling and remove serous exudate and crust. During the acute phase, steroid creams may be applied. In children under the age of 2 years, 1% hydrocortisone is frequently adequate. In older children, it is usually necessary to use a stronger fluorinated steroid, such as 0.1% triamcinolone cream (Kenalog or Aristocort) or betamethasone (Valisone or Benisone). Newer non-fluorinated steroid compounds have been developed to lessen possible atrophy and stria formation. When the weeping and oozing have subsided, steroid cream should be applied three or four times a day. The frequency of application of steroid cream may be gradually tapered after 7 to 10 days. For control of itching, it may be useful to use antihistamines such as Benadryl, Atarax, or Vistaril.

Severe contact dermatitis involving large areas of the body, the face, or the male genitalia requires treatment with systemic steroids. These agents are most effective when given at the onset. Hospitalization may be necessary when there is extensive acute contact dermatitis. The usual initial dose is 1 or 2 mg/kg of prednisone. After 1 day the dose should be reduced to 1–0.5 mg/24 hr. This dose should be maintained for 3 to 5 days and the medication gradually tapered over a 2-week period. Thus, 3 weeks of therapy are usually necessary. A common problem is the exacerbation of contact dermatitis after inadequate courses of systemic steroids (5 to 7 days). When systemic steroids are employed, topical steroids are an adjunctive measure.

A common complication of acute contact dermatitis is development of secondary bacterial infection with *Staphylococcus aureus* or streptococcus. The development of purulent lesions or an exacerbation after initial clearing should suggest secondary infection, as does fever or erythema. In such instances, a culture should be obtained and appropriate systemic antimicrobial therapy given. Topical antibiotics are not adequate to treat such infections. In the treatment of contact dermatitis, it is important to avoid sensitizing agents such as topical antihistamines, topical benzocaine, or topical neomycin, which may lead to the development of a second contact dermatitis. Frequent offenders are topical antipruritic sprays, ointments, and lotions.

Atopic Dermatitis

ALVIN H. JACOBS, M.D.

Atopic dermatitis is a genetically determined abnormality of the skin that often occurs in association with allergic diseases, probably as linked inheritance. It is manifest as dry, itchy skin, which is subjected to many internal and external factors that tend to increase the pruritus, thereby stimulating the "itch-scratch" cycle. These factors include environmental temperature changes, stimulation of sweating, external irritants such as rough clothing, bacterial infection, emotional stress, antigen-antibody reactions, bathing with soap and water, and many others.

In managing patients with atopic dermatitis the physician must recognize that the only primary skin manifestations are pruritus, dryness, and a generalized "goose-pimple" appearance. All other skin findings, such as oozing, weeping, crusting, or cracking, are secondary to scratching and rubbing.

GENERAL MANAGEMENT

Psychological. Successful management is time consuming for both parents and physician. At the outset the parents must understand that this is a chronic disorder for which there is no complete and quick cure; rather, the therapy is aimed at controlling factors that contribute to the eruption and its attendant discomforts.

During the introductory discussions, the physician must be alert to the mother's emotional reactions to her child's disorder, since in many mothers guilt feelings arise from the fear that they are in some way responsible for the skin problem, as well from their frequent feelings of rejection of the child and his ugly skin. The mother's emotional involvement if further complicated by the consumption of time in taking care of this crying, fussing, irritable, scratching infant or child. The physician must try to relieve the mother of her guilt feelings and express understanding of the rejection phenomenon. The treatment program must take into account the time the mother will have to devote to the care of her child's skin problem and must allow her periods of relief when she may be away from the child and without anxiety. I feel quite strongly that maternal anxiety transmitted to the infant or child may make the itching worse and aggravate the disease.

Infection. When first seen, most patients with atopic dermatitis have secondary infection, usually due to *Staphyloccus aureus*. This presents as oozing, crusting, and fissuring of the skin. This infection must be adequately treated before other steps will be effective. Locally applied antibiotics are of little use in this situation. Systemic antibiotic therapy should be given for a period of 10 days to 2 weeks to adequately eliminate the secondary infection. Recurrent infection is a common occurrence, requiring prolonged antibiotic therapy with eventual reduction to a maintenance dose. The most useful antibiotic is erythromycin in a dose of 50 mg/kg/day. Occasionally it is necessary to use cloxacillin in the same dosage.

Clothing. The individual with eczema has a tremendous tendency to itch and anything that irritates the skin will cause him to scratch. He should, therefore, avoid irritating materials, especially woolens. Cotton and some of the softer synthetics are preferable for the atopic patient. Wool upholstered chairs and wool carpets are also a source of irritation.

Sweating. Another important factor in the stimulation of pruritus is perspiration. Atopic dermatitis is always associated with a degree of sweat retention that will produce itching. Therefore, excessive clothing, high environmental temperatures, and over activity will increase perspiration and promote itchiness.

Antipruritic Sedation. Since the worst scratching is done at night, it is wise to give these patients night-time sedation until their skin condition is under control. Diphenhydramine given in doses of 25 to 50 mg about 1 hour before bedtime is an effective antipruritic sedative. In severe cases it is also advisable to give a daytime medication such as hydroxyzine (Atarax), 10 to 25 mg three times daily. *Systemic corticosteroids should rarely be given.*

Diet. Dietary management is helpful only in the first year or two of life. Since cow's milk is the most common allergen in infancy, eliminating it from the baby's diet will often make the dermatitis more easily controllable. In the older patient, food elimination is less often of help, although a complete dietary history and use of a food diary will occasionally bring out revealing information.

Hyposensitization. Skin test and hyposensitization therapy are of very little use in the management of the patient with atopic dermatitis, since there seems to be little relationship between the positive tests and causation of flares of the dermatitis.

Topical Therapy

When eczema is first seen in the acute phase, with inflammation, oozing, and crusting, it is important to recognize that secondary infection is present and systemic antibiotic therapy must be promptly instituted (vide supra). Reduction of inflammation and removal of crusts and exudate is best done with intermittent cool wet dressings applied by the open method. Two or three layers of gauze, Kerlix, or linen are thoroughly moistened with Burow's solution and loosely applied to the involved areas without occlusion. One half to one hour of application four times daily is usually sufficient, with remoistening by complete removal of the dressing every 10 minutes to prevent drying and sticking. Burow's solution, 1:40, is prepared by dissolving one tablet or packet (Domeboro tablets and powder packets) in one quart of cool tap water. *Wet compresses should not be used for longer than 3 days.*

At this point, or if the patient is first seen in the dry itchy phase, one may proceed with the modified Scholtz regimen, the prime feature of which is the *complete avoidance of bathing with water.* The dry skin of atopic dermatitis is due to a lack of sufficient water in the stratum corneum. The drier the skin, the greater is the pruritus. Washing with water removes the water-soluble substances that retain the water in the horny layer, thus resulting in increased dryness and itchiness after bathing.

The modified Scholtz regimen is instituted as follows:

1. No bathing with either soap or water is allowed. The only exception to this rule is the use of a moist wash cloth to cleanse the groin and axillary areas if necessary.

2. The entire skin surface is cleansed at least twice daily with a nonlipid cleansing lotion consisting primarily of cetyl alcohol, sodium lauryl sulfate, propylene glycol, and water (Cetaphil lotion, Owens Laboratories). The lotion is applied liberally and rubbed in until it foams. It is then gently wiped off, leaving a film of the lotion on the skin. This film aids the retention of water in the horny layer of the skin.

3. No oily or greasy lubricants are allowed, since these will further occlude sweat pore openings and contribute to sweat retention.

4. Inflamed or pruritic areas of the dermatitis are treated by topical corticosteroids in a solution or cream formulation, not an ointment base. In relatively mild or moderate cases, 1% hydrocortisone cream is effective. However, some generic preparations of hydrocortisone do not have a satisfactory base and may even be irritating. Several hydrocortisone preparations have been found to have smooth, nonirritating vehicles (1% Nutracort, 1% Hytone, and 1% Synacort). In more severe cases a medium strength steroid, such as 0.1% Triamcinalone cream, may be used. However, as soon as improvement is evident, one should shift down to hydrocortisone. In any case, only 1% hydrocortisone should be used on the face, groin, and genitalia.

All acutely inflamed areas can be cleared with the topical steroid preparation. If the entire program is followed, clearing usually occurs in 2 to 3 weeks. After the acutely inflamed areas have responded, it is possible to maintain the improvement by adhering to the no-bath and Cetaphil cleansing. The topical steroid is then needed only occasionally when there is a brief flare of the dermatitis.

5. When the skin has remained clear of eruption for several months, a brief cool bath is allowed once or twice monthly, always followed immediately by liberal application of Cetaphil lotion. Most patients are eventually able to tolerate a brief, not hot, bath as often as once weekly after they have remained clear for several months. It is essential that they learn never to bathe more often than once weekly, and that they continue indefinitely to use the Cetaphil lotion for daily cleansing and lubrication.

Urticaria

VICTOR D. NEWCOMER, M.D.

Urticaria or hives is a vascular reaction pattern of the skin characterized by evanescent wheals, which represent localized leakage of plasma from small blood vessels into the connective tissue of the dermis.

The *single most important step* in the management of acute urticaria is the identification and removal of the causative agent. With a complete history and review of systems, the causative agent can be identified in about 20 to 30% of all patients with urticaria.

Aggravating factors should be avoided whenever possible. The patient should remain quiescent and avoid strenuous activities as much as possible. Excessive heat, sunbathing, and cold showers should be avoided. Vasostimulatory foods and beverages such as tea, coffee, and alcohol should be avoided. Emotional stress should be minimized. Aspirin, which is present in many proprietary preparations, should be avoided, particularly in chronic urticaria, as over 50% of this latter group can be made worse by its administration.

Antihistamines are the mainstay in the management of urticaria of all types and provide symptomatic relief in about 80% of patients. They are particularly indicated if the sympathomimetics are contraindicated because of cardiovascular problems. They may be divided into six pharmacologic groups. In general, their properties are similar, and there are few comparative studies to give guidance as to which is the most effective. The choice is largely empirical. Antihistamines block the action of histamine at the receptor site and thereby interfere with the action of histamine on the capillaries. The blocking effect is clinically gradual, and, once obtained, the continued suppression of skin reactivity is of great importance if exacerbations are to be prevented. It is often necessary to maintain the dosage to the point of drowsiness to achieve the greatest benefit. When an antihistamine is ineffective or its side effects are troublesome, one should choose the next agent from another subgroup. Hydroxyzine hydrochloride (Atarax) (0.5 mg/kg q 4–6h for children) has been used increasingly for urticaria.

Cyproheptadine hydrochloride (Periactin) (0.1 mg/kg/q 4–6 h for children) has been especially effective in cold urticaria. β-Adrenergic drugs are the agents of choice in severe and acute attacks on urticaria or where angioedema is developing.

Aqueous epinephrine (Adrenalin) 1:1000, 0.01 ml/kg q 3 to 4 hours subcutaneously, offers prompt relief. Epinephrine suspension (Sus-Phrine) 1:200, 0.005 ml/kg, may be used where prolonged suppression is desired. Ephedrine sulfate, 25 mg qid, may be used but is slower in action. Anxiety and tachycardia are common side effects with the use of all these agents.

Systemic corticosteroids are the drugs of choice in the treatment of severe forms of serum sickness and severe acute attacks of urticaria. Since they require hours for a therapeutic effect, anaphylactic urticaria and angioedema affecting the upper respiratory tract are most effectively treated with the β-adrenergic drugs. Systemic corticosteroids are not advised for chronic recalcitrant urticaria; any possible benefits are more than outweighed by the potential hazards of prolonged treatment. They are of value, however, when used for a short period, in the control of acute, incapacitating exacerbation of chronic urticaria. Topical treatment with steroids is of no value.

The value of *tranquilizers and sedatives* is still debatable, but they may be helpful in patients with an emotional or stress component. Usually, the sedative effect of the antihistamine is all that may be required or tolerated. Hyposensitization has no role in the treatment of urticaria except for insect stings and urticaria due to inhalants such as pollens, dust, and molds. In general, topical agents are of little value in the management of urticaria. Cala-mine lotion, containing the antipruritic phenol 0.5% and menthol 0.25%, is still used.

Patients who develop hoarseness and do not respond promptly to measures to provide relief from severe pruritus should be admitted to the hospital for close observation and possible endotracheal intubation. *Hereditary angioedema* caused by a low or functional deficiency of an inhibitor of the first component of complement should be ruled out. Diagnosis is made by history and laboratory evidence of a deficiency of C esterase inhibitor and/or low serum complement. Antihistamines, corticosteroids, and epinephrine have no effect. Sublingual methyltestosterone increases the activity of the inhibitor with subsequent decrease in severity or frequency of attacks. Recently, testosterone ethanate (Danazol) has proved more effective in preventing attacks of angioedema and has the advantage of producing few if any masculinizing effects. Epsilon aminocaproic acid (Amicar) and tranexamic acid* (Cyclokapron), an epsilonaminocaproic acid analog, are also effective treatments. The long-term effects of testosterone ethanate and tranexamic acid in humans are unknown and as a rule children and pregnant women have not been treated.

If the larynx is affected repeatedly, a permanent tracheostomy may be required to sustain breathing.

Erythema Nodosum

LAWRENCE SCHACHNER, M.D.

Erythema nodosum is not a simple clinical diagnosis, nor is it an entity whose pathogenesis is well understood. It is believed to be a Type 3 hypersensitivity reaction to a myriad of agents, including infectious diseases, inflammatory diseases, drug reactions, and disorders that may frequently be of undiagnosed or unknown origin. The clinical appearance of erythema nodosum may be mimicked by various focal infections and inflammations of the subcutaneous fat and soft tissues with a predilection for the lower extremities.

On clinical examination in the acute stage, one will note multiple tender red nodular lesions. Although the lesions are most frequent and obtain their greatest size on the lower extremities, more generalized lesions, including facial erythema nodosum, have been seen. A characteristic color change from red to blue to yellow-green before resolution is probably commensurate with the degree of focal subcutaneous hemorrhage. Fever and malaise may precede the cutaneous lesions and/or accompany the acute stage of these lesions. Patients often complain of arthralgias, usually in the lower

---

*Investigational drug in the United States; it is used in Europe.

extremities, during the acute course of this disorder. While all ages and races, and both sexes, may be involved, there is an increased incidence in females versus males and in young people versus old people.

The etiology of erythema nodosum cases seen by a pediatrician may be determined by the ages and even the socioeconomic class of the patients he or she sees. For example, a practitioner who sees many school-age children may see many cases of streptococcus-evoked erythema nodosum. A practitioner who services indigent populations or an area with a recent influx of immigrants from South America or Asia may see a fair amount of tuberculosis-associated erythema nodosum. Similarly, a pediatrician with a large adolescent practice may find many cases of oral contraceptive associated erythema nodosum.

THERAPY

The intial therapeutic approach should be conservative but strict. At least 2 to 3 weeks of bed rest is usually optimal when patients are seen at the onset of disease. Every 3 hours throughout the day, cool water soaks should be placed wet over the lesions and allowed to dry for 20 minutes. If fever, malaise, or joint pain are significant, salicylates in dosages appropriate for age should be administered. It should be stated here that the most effective therapy for the specific case of erythema nodosum requires discovery of the etiology of the underlying infection.

Of the many etiologies of erythema nodosum, perhaps those most appropriately diagnosed are the infectious diseases. The most common causes, such as group A beta hemolytic streptococcal infection, may be diagnosed by throat culture or streptozyme titer. A purified protein derivative (PPD) test is worth applying to any previously PPD-negative erythema nodosum patient. *Yersinia* species have been associated with gastrointestinal complaints and erythema nodosum.

Lymphogranuloma venereum, cat scratch fever, and deeper fungal infection including coccidioidomycosis, blastomycosis, histoplasmosis, and deep trichophyton infections may also be associated with erythema nodosum. Frequently associated inflammatory disorders include sarcoidosis, regional enteritis, ulcerative colitis, and Behçet's syndrome. Various medications have been associated with eruptions of erythema nodosum, and many contemporary cases have accompanied the use of oral contraceptives, phenytoin, and halogens.

A minimal diagnostic work-up would include a streptozyme test, a PPD, a chest x-ray, and skin tests for fungi, and a skin biopsy to rule out the various infections and inflammatory conditions that mimic erythema nodosum clinically but can be distinguished histologically.

Bed rest, wet soaks, and salicylates will usually alleviate pain and tenderness. Rarely, one finds persistent erythema nodosum in a patient whose clinical diagnosis has been confirmed by biopsy and in whom both infectious and noninfectious etiologies have been ruled out. In these rare instances, the use of intralesional corticosteroids may hasten involution of the lesions and relieve discomfort. Although the use of oral corticosteroids has been advocated in the literature, I have not found them to be necessary.

Drug Reactions and the Skin
LAWRENCE SCHACHNER, M.D.

Cutaneous drug reactions include both immunologic reactions of all classes of hypersensitivity and nonimmunologic reactions. The class of hypersensitivity reaction in the immunologic type often determines the appropriate therapy. In Type 1 hypersensitivity reactions, IgE antibodies are produced and reactions ranging from urticaria to angioedema and anaphylaxis may occur. In Type 2 reactions, drugs may form an antigenic complex with the surface of red blood cells or platelets. Thrombocytopenic purpura may be observed. Type 3 hypersensitivity reactions with drugs inducing an antigen-antibody and complement immune complex may result in cutaneous signs such as urticarial vasculitis. Indeed, a Type 3 reaction may be manifested by the persistence of urticarial-wheal type lesions that may progress to purpura. Severe cutaneous reactions of erythema multiforme, Stevens-Johnson syndrome, and toxic epidermal necrolysis might also be examples of Type 3 reactions. Further immune-complex mediated cutaneous reactions to medications include specific reactions, such as fixed drug reaction and erythema nodosum. Type 4 cell-mediated hypersensitivity may occur as an eczematous dermatitis with eruptive distribution in areas where topically applied medications have been used. Photoallergic reactions may be induced by either internal or external use of various medications.

In the pediatric population, the drugs most often associated with immediate or Type 1 hypersensitivity drug reaction are the penicillins, which may also be associated with Type 3 hypersensitivity drug reaction. In addition, numerous other drugs can produce a serum sickness syndrome with urticarial vasculitis and/or angioedematous components. These drugs include the commonly used childhood medications phenytoin and the sulfonamides. In Type 2 hypersensitivity reactions, again penicillin and the more rarely used quinidine class drugs may be associated with characteristic reactions. Topical medications may induce a Type 4 or cell-mediated drug reaction, including antibiotics such as neomycin as well as numerous ointments with parabens and ethylenediamine as components.

Nonimmunologic drug reactions may take several forms. Long term use of gold or mercury based drugs may lead to cutaneous or mucous membrane changes. Drugs may also be capable of a nonimmunologic activation of mast cell and complement mediated pathways inducing cutaneous reactions such as acute and chronic urticaria and angio-edematous changes.

One may see among the common drug eruptions not only urticarial and vasculitic lesions but also acne type lesions, erythema multiforme, erythema nodosum, exanthem type lesions, eczematous dermatitis, fixed-drug eruptions, lichen planus–like eruptions, lupus-like eruptions, photosensitive eruptions, pigmentary changes, and blistering reactions.

THERAPY

Whenever the diagnosis of a drug eruption is made, if possible, the offending agent should be replaced by a non–cross-reacting medication. Many drug reactions are mild and require little more than discontinuation of the offending medication, followed by simple supportive measures. When pruritus is intense, oral antihistamines as well as mentholated topical preparations can offer considerable relief. The combination of hydroxyzine (Atarax) and pseudoephedrine (Sudafed) has been particularly successful in our more pruritic patients with drug reactions. Mentholated petrolatum or calamine with 0.25% menthol is also quite soothing.

In drug reactions of more emergent nature such as the various severe hypersensitivity reactions, therapy must be individualized. A patient with a Type 1 hypersensitivity reaction of the anaphylaxis class, will require emergency preservation of airway supplemental oxygen, and intravenous use of epinephrine, benadryl, and systemic steroids as the clinical manifestations mandate. Patients in whom the drug reaction may provoke considerable loss of cutaneous surfaces, such as drug induced toxic epidermal necrolysis or Stevens-Johnson type erythema multiforme, may require fluid and electrolyte monitoring identical to patients with extensive burns. Indeed the epidermal barrier function may be equally as disturbed as in a severe burn. In such patients we have used wet to dry soaks and Silvadene as topical therapy. In severe drug reactions, antibiotic treatment for secondary infection is often necessary. Although controversial, toxic epidermal necrolysis associated with several medications, including Dilantin reactions and Stevens-

Johnson syndrome invoked by a number of medications, may necessitate the use of systemic steroids as a life-saving step.

Lastly, cutaneous reactions to topical medication may be approached as any eczematous dermatitis. In the acute stage, it is important to apply wet to dry soaks to induce drying of the lesions. This may be followed with topical steroid cream preparations to induce added drying and decrease inflammation. Concomitant utilization of oral antihistamines may hasten the patient's relief.

Erythema Multiforme

JAMES E. RASMUSSEN, M.D.

Erythema multiforme is a poorly understood process with a broad spectrum of presentations: minor forms show only erythematous papules and targetoid lesions on the extremities, while the major varieties consist of widespread blisters, severe erosions of the mucous membranes (the Stevens-Johnson syndrome), and a more generalized loss of the epidermis (toxic epidermal necrolysis). A wide variety of causes have been incriminated, such as drug allergies, recurrent herpetic infections, tumors, and mycoplasma. Children with erythema multiforme do not usually have a readily identifiable cause for their disease, however.

The therapy for erythema multiforme can be conveniently directed toward the major or minor forms.

Minor. This is a common manifestation of erythema multiforme, often occurring after recurrent herpetic infections (which is not a common problem in childhood). My approach to these patients is to employ a diligent history and physical examination searching for drug allergies and infections. Usually no specific therapy is indicated. Antihistamines such as Atarax and Vistaril can be used for their antipruritic and sedative effect.

Major. These severe forms of erythema multiforme are usually quite symptomatic and can occasionally be life-threatening. Consequently, there is more of a sense of urgency involved in their therapy, which can be divided into specific and general categories.

SPECIFIC. Systemic corticosteroids in high dosages are usually suggested as the therapy of choice for patients with severe erythema multiforme. The rationale for their use is straightforward and plausible—erythema multiforme probably represents an antigen-antibody complex disease with the resulting severe inflammation causing epidermal death and separation. Corticosteroids are anti-inflammatory and consequently have been accepted for many years as the treatment of choice for this condition. Many reports testify to the "life-saving" qualities of these drugs, but there is no proof in the literature that these remarkable responses would not have occurred in untreated patients. I have seen erythema multiforme of major and minor variety develop in patients who had been on corticosteroids for other preceding diseases; conversely, the great majority of patients with severe erythema multiforme whom I have treated with corticosteroids have not shown remarkable recoveries. Consequently, I reviewed the records of children admitted to the Buffalo Children's Hospital with the diagnosis of severe erythema multiforme, Stevens-Johnson type, to determine whether treatment with corticosteroids had significantly shortened hospitalization times. Exactly the opposite was true. Those patients treated with systemic corticosteroids had a far greater incidence of side effects (infection and bleeding) than did those patients offered only supportive care. From that point on, I have not used corticosteroids in the treatment of erythema multiforme and have never regretted this decision.

Regardless of the reader's position on the use of corticosteroids in erythema multiforme, it should be realized that the inflammatory phase of the disease is extremely short—certainly not more than a week. If corticosteroids are employed, their use should be limited only to the inflammatory phase of the disease and they should not be continued during active wound healing. Corticosteroids decrease wound healing and make the patient a prime target for bacterial infection. The reader should also understand that the majority opinion strongly favors the use of corticosteroids with severe erythema multiforme. Prednisone or equivalents may be used in a dosage ranging from 0.5 to 1.0 mg/kg. Topical steroids have little or no place in the treatment of erythema multiforme.

An ophthalmologist should be consulted to manage every patient with erythema multiforme involving the ocular conjunctiva. These patients are prone to develop keratitis sicca, decreased visual acuity, corneal scarring, and, when the affection is severe, blindness. These sequelae may be seen regardless of the choice of systemic or topical care for the eye, however.

GENERAL. The general management of patients with severe erythema multiforme differs little from the care of those patients with other types of widespread damage to the skin and mucous membranes:

(1) The responsible physician must maintain adequate fluid, electrolyte, and caloric intake. Water lost from the skin is not great unless patients have shed a significant portion of their epidermis (which is commonly seen in patients with toxic epidermal necrolysis). The situation of these patients is similar to that of burn patients. In addition, inflammation of the mucous membranes makes oral intake all but impossible. Fortunately, severe erythema multiforme is not a common problem in children, and toxic epidermal necrolysis is rarer still. It is imperative to monitor fluid and electrolyte intake with the standard modalities, such as serum electrolytes, hematocrit, blood pressure, pulse, central venous pressure, and urinary output. Acute renal failure is not rare and may result from hypovolemia with resulting acute tubular necrosis, as well as glomerulonephritis.

(2) Wound care—patients with extensive bullous erythema multiforme or toxic epidermal necrolysis should be treated as though they have been burned. Localized blistering can be treated on the nursing floor or in an intensive care unit with compresses and local antiseptics such as Silvadene. More extensive widespread loss of the epidermis usually requires admission to a burn unit where the choice of topical antiseptics versus biologic dressings will rest with local experience and expertise, but grafting is rarely necessary. Severe cutaneous pain is frequently minimized with such aggressive treatment.

(3) Monitor for infection—patients with severe erythema multiforme may be septic on admission, and such an infection may actually be the causative factor in the development of their cutaneous disease. In addition, patients may develop sepsis from localized contamination of denuded skin and mucous membranes. Blood and lesional cultures should be done, based on the patient's history, physical examination, and course in the hospital. Broad-spectrum prophylactic antibiotics are advocated by some experienced physicians, but I prefer to treat only when physical and laboratory evidence suggests the development of an infection. If antibiotics are given in a prophylactic fashion, then one that will cover staphylococcus, streptococcus, and pneumococcus should be used. These are the most common causes of sepsis in patients with Stevens-Johnson syndrome. Broad-spectrum topical antibiotics, especially those containing neomycin, should not be used in patients with substantial damage to their epidermal barrier. The resulting increase in percutaneous absorption of these drugs has been associated with substantial toxicity.

(4) Analgesia—major varieties of erythema multiforme are usually quite symptomatic: the common prodromal pharyngitis, tender skin, and painful erosions. Unless otherwise contraindicated, analgesia should be offered to every patient in the form of salicylates, acetaminophen, and narcotics. Pain may persist in the cutaneous and oral lesions until healing takes place in 7 to 14 days. Denuded areas of the skin are particularly uncomfortable and frequently respond remarkably to biologic dressings. Oral erosions are less easily treated, and, while effective local analgesics are available, patients are usually unable or unwilling to use them. Hemorrhagic crusting on the lips can be treated

with cool compresses or with ice chips held in a cloth diaper. If the patient is old enough to cooperate, sucking on the ice chips will produce analgesia as well as a moderate source of fluid. Older and less severely affected patients may be able to use a milk of magnesia or an elixir of Benadryl mouthwash, which will provide some local anesthesia before meals.

Papulosquamous Disorders

RONALD C. HANSEN, M.D.

PSORIASIS

Psoriasis tends to be chronic, recurrent, and sometimes quite refractory to therapy. Accordingly, a full understanding by patient and family of the disease, the goals of therapy including therapeutic limitations, and the central importance of compliance are necessary prerequisites for successful therapy.

Localized Psoriasis. Localized psoriasis is often best managed by twice daily applications of a high potency topical corticosteroid. Examples include halcinonide (Halog 0.1%), betamethasone dipropionate (Diprosone 0.05%), and fluocinonide (Lidex or Topsyn 0.05%). Where necessary in refractory cases, night-time occlusion with Saran wrap or similar synthetic material will increase the efficacy of the steroid preparation. A convenient alternative for occlusive therapy is Cordran tape, which is a plastic tape impregnated with a potent topical steroid.

Alternatively, or as adjunctive therapy, tar preparations such as Estar gel, or T/Derm may be applied. Sun exposure is also helpful, especially after the application of one of the above mentioned tar-gel preparations.

Generalized Psoriasis. Where numerous lesions cover the body, topical therapy is obviously a much larger project, with consequently greater problems in compliance and follow through. Potent topical steroids remain a major therapy, as described under localized psoriasis. However, where a high percentage of the body surface is to be treated, or where extensive occlusion is employed, significant amounts of the potent fluorinated steroid may be absorbed. Therefore, one should caution the family to apply the corticosteroid only to lesional skin, and only in small amounts which disappear into the psoriatic plaque as the agent is thoroughly rubbed into the lesion. For lubrication purposes, one should rely on Eucerin or Nivea cream, and this can be applied to all lesional and nonlesional skin after the corticosteroid cream is applied to the lesions. The corticosteroid should never be used as an emollient or lubricant, as this will encourage abuse of the agent. Corticosteroid creams never need be used

more often than twice daily, even in refractory psoriasis.

Daily tub baths with warm water and ordinary soaps, or a tar bath made by the addition of Zetar emulsion or Balnetar to the bath water, may assist in removing scales and facilitating therapy. Tar preparations may be effective when applied to the individual psoriatic plaques, and are especially helpful when followed by ultraviolet B exposure, either through artificial lights, or sunlight, approximately 2 hours after the tars are applied. For home use, Estar gel and T/Derm are easy to use, relatively inoffensive as far as odor, and need not be washed off prior to sun exposure. Sun exposure should be cautiously undertaken, in view of the photosensitizing properties of the tars, so as to avoid sunburn. A sunburn injury can, in fact, flare one's psoriasis through the so-called Koebner or isomorphic response to skin injury seen in this disease.

For refractory, generalized psoriasis, one should consider hospitalization if progress is not being made as an outpatient. Hospitalization can facilitate the carrying out of the traditional Goeckerman regimen, wherein 2 to 5% crude coal tar is applied to the whole body, left in place 2 to 4 hours, removed with mineral oil, and followed by suberythemic doses of ultraviolet-B phototherapy. Although it may take 2 to 3 weeks to completely clear the psoriasis, a remission achieved by this method may last as long as 6 to 12 months. Hospitalizations may be shortened by concurrent use of topical steroids under sweat suit or Saran wrap occlusion, or by the use of anthralin paste. In general, hospitalization for psoriasis should be supervised by a dermatologist, given the complexities of management.

Psoriasis of the Scalp. Thickened scalp scales are anchored by hair, and are much more difficult to loosen than body plaques. They are most readily softened by applying either mineral oil or Baker's P and S solution to the individual plaques overnight, occluding with a shower cap. Vigorous shampooing, using brisk, mechanical action with the fingertips and fingernails, with a tar-based shampoo such as Neutrogena T/gel or Sebutone, is then much more effective. After repeated softening and shampooing over a period of days, enough scales will have been removed to allow topical steroid lotions such as triamcinolone or betamethasone to penetrate the lesions and induce their anti-inflammatory and antiproliferative effect. Gel preparations such as Topsyn gel are also effective and reasonable to use in the hairy areas.

Nail Psoriasis. Psoriasis of the nails is notoriously difficult to treat. The effect of potent topical steroids applied to the nail folds, while sometimes beneficial, is not predictable. Intralesional injections of the nail matrices with corticosteroid suspensions is unthinkable because of the pain involved, and systemic therapy is seldom warranted, even for generalized psoriasis in childhood. These latter two approaches are really the only ones reliably effective in nail psoriasis.

Psoriasis Therapies That Are Hazardous or Controversial in Childhood

Systemic Steroids. Oral prednisone or triamcinolone injected intramuscularly will cause improvement in psoriasis but this approach is seldom justified. The psoriasis will predictably rebound, sometimes with ferocity, when the steroids are tapered. Of course, one is additionally concerned about all of the problems associated with the chronic usage of steroids in a growing child.

Potent Topical Steroids Under Sweat Suit Occlusion. Although this method may control generalized psoriasis, even in an outpatient, it must be very cautiously approached. Systemic absorption of topical steroids is significant when generalized occlusion is used; hence, one may incur any of the problems associated with chronic use of systemic steroids in childhood. I usually reserve sweat suit occlusion of topical steroids for inpatient purposes only.

Psoralens Plus Ultraviolet A Therapy (PUVA). This type of photochemotherapy has been effective over the past 10 years in adults, and has recently been approved by the FDA for those purposes. However, there remain significant concerns relative to its use in childhood, and it should probably be discouraged until more is learned about the potential side effects during the years of maturation. At least three levels of concern exist. First, there is little doubt that this type of therapy encourages the development of skin cancers. Secondly, experimental data in animals raises serious concerns about development of cataracts of the lens with long term usage. Thirdly, because of the way in which psoralens bind to DNA, causing so-called photo-adducts, with possible crossed-linkage problems, other theoretical objections to this therapy in childhood have been raised. Nonetheless, where life-ruining or life-threatening psoriasis exists and has been unresponsive to conventional therapy, PUVA may be preferable to other approaches, including methotrexate and systemic steroids. Additional data on long term follow-up are needed.

Methotrexate. In adults, only liver fibrosis and cirrhosis are frequent problems in the long term usage of methotrexate for generalized and recalcitrant psoriasis. However, in childhood, chronic use is much less desirable. Its use in children can rarely be justified.

Synthetic Retinoids. Formerly, toxic and near-toxic doses of vitamin A were occasionally thought to be of benefit in severe psoriasis. Obviously, neurotoxicity and hepatotoxicity limited this approach, which never found favor in childhood. Newer generations of synthetic retinoids may hold some promise in keratinizing disorders including psoriasis. Of these, the currently available 13-cis retinoic acid (Accutane), approved for use in cystic acne, is relatively less effective against psoriasis and the other papulosquamous disorders than is its cousin, etretinate, the aromatic retinoid which has been mainly studied in Europe. Whether either of these compounds will find meaningful application to childhood psoriasis is conjectural.

SEBORRHEIC DERMATITIS

Seborrheic dermatitis in infancy is usually self-limited, a fact to be remembered as treatment is outlined. The limited scalp form, or cradle cap, may be treated by merely increasing the vigorousness of mechanical removal of scale. Often this can be done with simple baby shampoos, provided the mother uses her fingertips vigorously. Alternatively, one can use special shampoos, such as Sebulex, which will be slightly more beneficial in scale removal. If necessary, soaking the scalp for a few minutes with mineral oil, or Baker's P and S solution will help to loosen the scale prior to vigorous shampooing. Corticosteroid lotions may occasionally be necessary for scalp seborrheic dermatitis, and, where the infantile hair is thin enough, creams may even be feasible.

Facial seborrheic dermatitis may also be helped somewhat by gentle removal of scale with baby shampoo. Here 1% hydrocortisone cream is virtually always potent enough to manage the dermatitis; likewise, nonfluorinated steroids such as 1% hydrocortisone cream can usually manage seborrheic dermatitis in the diaper area. It is prudent to remember that seborrheic dermatitis is frequently superinfected with *Candida albicans* in the diaper area, necessitating a combination of 1% hydrocortisone cream and a topical antiyeast agent such as miconazole or clotrimazole.

PARAPSORIASIS

The term parapsoriasis describes a disparate group of disorders that have nothing to do with psoriasis and really are not that readily confused with it. Three of these may be seen in childhood. The first, pityriasis lichenoides et varioliformis acuta, often presents in childhood, and is generally a temporary phenomenon, lasting several months or less. It resembles chronic insect bites or "recurrent chickenpox." When treatment is necessary, oral tetracycline or erythromycin in the child over age 8 years, or erythromycin in the younger child, may be helpful. Graduated exposure to increasing amounts of sunlight may also be useful. Methotrexate has been effective in adults who are very symptomatic with pruritus in this disease, but its use in children cannot be justified.

Guttate parapsoriasis is a more superficial process, and does not seem to respond to the above mentioned antibiotics. It is probably best treated by emollient or lubricating creams, and is seldom helped much by topical steroids. Fortunately, it also disappears with time.

Parapsoriasis en plaques, frequently a precursor to the cutaneous T-cell lymphoma mycosis fungoides, rarely presents in childhood or in the teen-age years. Treatment is simply symptomatic, and the really important feature is to recognize this as potentially premalignant.

Pityriasis Rosea. Most patients with pityriasis rosea need no treatment. Of special importance here is to do no harm, as by applying drying agents such as calamine lotion or Selsun shampoo, mistaking the process for fungal or yeast infections, thereby aggravating the inflammatory response. The patient should be bathed carefully to prevent xerosis, and lubricated freely. Sunshine may cause the lesions to resolve and reduce itching. Topical steroids are minimally helpful for patients who experience itching. Night-time sedation with Benadryl or Atarax may be necessary for the pruritic patient.

Pityriasis Rubra Pilaris. This entity is notoriously difficult to treat, and is fortunately rare. Inherited forms may be seen in early childhood or infancy. Topical steroids are of little benefit. Topical vitamin A acid (retinoic acid or Retin-A) may help some patients. Lubrication and keratolytic agents such as salicylic acid may be of some assistance. The aromatic retinoid etretinate may be quite useful, provided that it is ultimately released for use in this country.

Lichen Striatus. This condition is seldom symptomatic and usually needs no treatment. Patients who are dramatically itchy may be treated with potent topical steroids.

Lichen Nitidus. Although this disease is classically nonsymptomatic, itching does occur in some patients. They are relieved by the use of topical steroids, and need only intermittent therapy. It is possible that in these patients, there is a combination of atopic dermatitis and lichen nitidus.

Lichen Planus. Fortunately rare in childhood, this disorder can be treated with moderate success with topical steroids. The disease waxes and wanes and, hence, treatment must be tailored to individual symptoms.

Vesiculobullous Disorders of Childhood

SIDNEY HURWITZ, M.D.

EPIDERMOLYSIS BULLOSA

The term epidermolysis bullosa refers to a group of five distinct genetic disorders, characterized by bullous lesions that develop spontaneously or as a result of friction or trauma. The conditions can be divided into two major groups: those that produce scars and those that result in complete healing without scarring.

The scarring forms are the most distressing. They are divided into dominant and recessive forms. In *dominant dystrophic epidermolysis bullosa*, lesions usually appear in infancy but in mild cases may be delayed. Bullae generally appear on the dorsal aspect of the extremities, milia are frequently present, red atrophic scars appear, and hypertrophic nail changes are common.

Recessive dystrophic epidermolysis bullosa is a severe distressing disease with widespread dystrophic scarring and deformity and severe involvement of mucous membranes. Erosions and blisters usually appear at or shortly after birth. Bullae are often followed by atrophic scars, which may fuse the fingers and toes, causing pseudosyndactyly or mitten-like deformities. Blisters and erosions in the oral mucosa may limit eating and immobilize the tongue; esophageal stricture may result and laryngeal bullae may produce respiratory stridor. The teeth are malformed and carious, anemia due to chronic blood loss and malnutrition occurs, and failure to thrive is common, as is secondary bacterial or candidal infection of the skin.

The nonscarring variants include epidermolysis bullosa simplex (autosomal dominant), epidermolysis bullosa letalis (autosomal recessive), and recurrent bullous eruptions of the hands and feet (autosomal dominant). In *epidermolysis bullosa simplex* the bullae heal without scarring, the mucous membranes and nails are rarely affected, and the disease often improves at puberty. In *epidermolysis bullosa letalis* (junctional epidermolysis bullosa or Herlitz disease) there are large areas of erosion and spontaneous bullae, which usually occur on the legs at birth or shortly thereafter. About 50% of cases result in death within the first year or two of life; if the infant survives, the disease tends to improve and resembles epidermolysis bullosa simplex. *Recurrent bullous eruptions of the hands and feet* (Weber-Cockayne disease) is an autosomal dominant disorder that requires a higher threshold of frictional trauma to induce blister formation. Bullae frequently do not appear until adolescence or early childhood, are often associated with hyperhidrosis and are generally confined to the hands and feet. In young children, blisters occasionally develop on the knees from the trauma of crawling.

It is the responsibility of the physician to inform parents of the risks associated with transmitting genetic abnormalities. Treatment is palliative, with avoidance of trauma and control of secondary infection. Since blisters result from mechanical injury, measures should be taken to relieve pressure and avoid trauma. A cool environment, avoidance of overheating, and lubrication of the skin to decrease the coefficient of friction help to reduce blister formation. Extension of blisters may be prevented by aseptic aspiration of blister fluid. The roofs of blisters should be trimmed with a sterile scissors whenever feasible, and no ragged edges should be left under which organisms can flourish and lead to secondary infection.

A water mattress and soft fleece covering will help limit friction and trauma. Daily baths, topical protective antibiotic dressings, or sterile petrolatum-impregnated gauze applied with sterile precautions may help reduce bacterial infection and assist spontaneous healing. Large denuded areas should be treated, when possible, by the open method (as in treatment of burns) with intravenous fluids and appropriate systemic antibiotics when indicated. In severe dystrophic forms, prophylactic antibiotics lessen the tendency to local infection, sepsis, and severe scarring, and help reduce the risk of glomerulonephritis secondary to cutaneous streptococcal infection.

Dysphagia is a major symptom of esophageal involvement in recessive dystrophic epidermolysis bullosa. Softening the diet may improve symptoms, but if conservative management fails, bougienage or surgery, or both, should be considered.

A recent development in the management of severe recessive dystrophic epidermolysis bullosa has been the use of oral phenytoin (Dilantin).*The rationale for its use is that it inhibits the action of collagenase and, in dosages of 2.5 to 5.0 mg/kg of body weight per day, to a maximum of 300 mg per day (a dosage high enough to obtain serum levels of 5 to 12 mcg per milliliter), it seems to help reduce the number of bullae and subsequent cicatricial damage.

Nursing care in severe epidermolysis bullosa is time-consuming and difficult. Restoration of function in severe fusion and flexion deformities of the hands and feet may be helped by physiotherapy and plastic surgery. Mild cases of the dystrophic and nondystrophic types may be compatible with a nearly normal existence. Severe forms, however, are often frustrating and require cooperation by patient, parents, and physician.

DERMATITIS HERPETIFORMIS

Dermatitis herpetiformis is a chronic recurrent disease characterized by intensely pruritic papulovesicular and, at times, bullous eruptions that respond dramatically to oral doses of sulfones or sulfapyridine. Usually occurring during the second to fifth decades of life, it is relatively uncommon in infancy and childhood and affects males more frequently than females. In children the disorder usually occurs in those over 8 years of age, persists into adulthood, and is fundamentally the disease seen in adults.

Characteristic are an extremely pruritic symmetrically grouped papulovesicular eruption, excoriations, and at times, erythematous plaques that affect the extensor surfaces, particularly the elbows, knees, sacrum, buttocks, and shoulders. The pathogenesis is still not clearly understood but it includes morphologic and immunologic skin and small bowel changes.

The histology of cutaneous lesions consists of subepidermal blisters; the most important diagnostic criterion is the demonstration of IgA immunofluorescence in a granular or linear band along the basement membrane of normal appearing skin.

Sulfapyridine is generally considered to be the drug of choice for treatment. The initial dose for children is usually 100 to 200 mg/kg/day in four divided doses (with a maximum of 2 to 4 gm a day).* Once existing lesions have been suppressed, the dosage may be tapered at weekly intervals, with a maintenance level of 0.5 gm or less as the daily required dose. A screening test for glucose-6-phosphate dehydrogenase (G6PD) deficiency should be performed prior to initiation of therapy, with close observation of the patient and pretreatment and follow-up blood counts at monthly intervals.

Various sulfone derivatives of 4,4-diaminodiphenyl sulfone (dapsone, DDS) are better tolerated and more economical than sulfapyradine. Their side effects, however, are more severe and because of an increased tendency to hemolytic anemia in patients with G6PD deficiency, a screening test should be done prior to initiating therapy. Dapsone (available in 25 and 100 mg tablets as Avlosulfon) may be initiated with 2 mg/kg/day, with an increase or decrease in dosage depending upon the clinical response and associated side effects.†If side effects do not occur, a maximum of 400 mg a day may be reached (the required dosage, however, is usually in the range of 50 mg three times daily). Once a favorable response is achieved (usually within a week) the dose is decreased gradually to a minimum level (generally 25 to 50 mg daily). In patients who do not respond to therapy, a gluten-free diet for 8 to 12 months may help bring the disease under control when used in combination with sulfapyridine or dapsone. In this way many patients can lower their required dosage of sulfapyridine or dapsone and some patients may be able to control their condition by diet alone.

JUVENILE BULLOUS PEMPHIGOID

Juvenile bullous pemphigoid is an acquired chronic bullous eruption that on rare occasions affects young children below 8 to 10 years of age. The clinical features of this disorder are characterized by mild pruritus and by large tense, sometimes hemorrhagic bullae that measure 0.5 to 2.0 cm in

---

*This use of Dilantin is not listed by the manufacturer.

---

*This dose may exceed that recommended by the manufacturer.

†This dosage of Dapsone is not listed in the manufacturer's directive.

diameter and generally involve the lower abdomen, anogenital region, posterior aspect of the thighs, and sometimes the face. Lesions may appear on normal skin or on an erythematous base, and they frequently occur at the periphery of annular or polycyclic erythematous plaques.

Response to treatment is variable. Systemic corticosteroids may suppress the eruption. In severe and resistant cases, a combination of sulfones or sulfapyridine in conjunction with corticosteroids may be helpful.

BULLOUS DISEASE OF CHILDHOOD

Chronic bullous dermatosis of childhood usually occurs in the first decade of life, with onset most frequently during the preschool years and spontaneous remission after several months to 3 years.

Characteristic are large, tense, annular or sausage-shaped, clear or hemorrhagic bullae that measure 1.0 to 2.0 cm in diameter and overlie a normal or erythematous base. The eruption is widespread and areas of predilection are the face, scalp, lower part of the trunk (including the genitalia and pubis), buttocks, inner thighs, legs, and dorsal aspects of the feet. Pruritus is variable.

Sulfapyradine is the drug of choice. In cases where the response to sulfapyradine is inadequate, dapsone may be utilized.

PEMPHIGUS

Pemphigus, extremely uncommon in childhood, is a severe, chronic, sometimes fatal autoimmune blistering disease characterized by flaccid bullae on normal-appearing skin and mucous membranes. Cutaneous lesions of pemphigus vulgaris favor the seborrheic areas (face, scalp, neck, sternum, axillae, groin, and periumbilical regions) and pressure areas of the feet and back. In more than half of the patients this disorder begins with erosions of the oral mucosa, and mucous membranes are affected in 95% of patients. Pemphigus vulgaris tends to be chronic and, although spontaneous remissions and even permanent healing may occur, it usually ends fatally if not treated with systemic corticosteroids.

Adverse reactions associated with prolonged high-dose corticosteroid therapy are a major hazard in long-term management. Once a maintenance dosage is attained, therefore, treatment should be reduced about 20% every 2 weeks, and alternate day therapy is preferred once the disease has been controlled. Immunosuppressive drugs (methotrexate, azathioprine, or cyclophosphamide)*may be used as ancillary agents for patients with severe disease who cannot be controlled by steroids alone or when prolonged high-dose steroids are undesirable. Because of potential adverse effects, cytotoxic agents should be used with caution in children.

---

*This use of these drugs is not listed by the manufacturer.

FAMILIAL BENIGN PEMPHIGUS

Familial benign pemphigus (Hailey-Hailey disease) is an autosomal dominant genodermatosis characterized by recurrent vesicles and bullae, which most commonly appear on the sides and back of the neck, in the axillae, the groin, and the perianal regions. The primary lesions are small vesicles that occur in groups on normal or erythematous skin. These may enlarge to form bullae, which rupture easily leaving an eroded base, exude serum, and develop crusts resembling impetigo or pyoderma.

As yet there is no effective treatment. An effort should be made to avoid precipitating factors of heat, humidity, and the friction associated with tight or ill-fitting clothing. Topical antibiotics and topical corticosteroids may be helpful, and systemic antibiotics chosen on the basis of bacterial culture and sensitivity appear to be the most effective form of therapy.

HERPES GESTATIONIS

Herpes gestationis, an uncommon dermatological complication of pregnancy and the postpartum period, is associated with an increased risk of fetal morbidity and mortality. Its cause is unknown and the pruritic eruption consists of grouped erythematous edematous papules and plaques, grouped vesicles on erythematous bases, and tense bullae. Onset of eruption most commonly occurs during the fourth or fifth month of gestation but has occurred as early as 2 weeks after conception and as late as the day before delivery, and even during the first few weeks of the postpartum period. The course is cyclic but generally abates spontaneously during the last few weeks of gestation. Although the etiology remains unknown, a hypersensitivity or toxic reaction to fetal or placental products or to hormones or their metabolites must be considered.

Fetuses of women with this disorder may be premature or stillborn, or suffer herpes gestationis themselves. Therapeutic goals include controlling maternal pruritus and blister formation and lessening the risk of fetal complication. Although systemic corticosteroids and pyridoxine have been reported effective for some pregnant women with this disorder, their effect on the morbidity and mortality of the fetus requires further study.

Discoid Lupus Erythematosus

RONALD C. HANSEN, M.D.

The skin lesions of discoid lupus erythematosus characteristically appear in the chronic cutaneous form of the disease but may also be found in systemic and neonatal lupus erythematosus. The lesions should be approached as a separate problem when associated with the systemic disease.

Although the degree of induction or aggravation of the cutaneous lesions by sunlight varies from patient to patient, it is prudent to assume that photosensitivity is a feature in each case. Hence, a sunscreen lotion with a sun protection factor (SPF) of 15 should be applied to all lesional and exposed skin on a daily basis. Caution in sun exposure must be advised as well.

Topical corticosteroid creams are the mainstay of therapy. Here one is forced to use potent fluorinated steroid creams, even on the face, since the disease is difficult to control. It is advisable to review the possibly poor outcome of the lesions, noting that atrophy and telangiectasia are usually the results of the disease rather than of the therapy. Cordran tape is a convenient method by which to occlude a topical steroid.

In refractory cases, intralesional corticosteroid injections can be very beneficial. Intralesional steroids produce temporary atrophy, and this must be discussed in the context of an atrophy and scarring-prone disease such as discoid lupus erythematosus. Antimalarial agents such as hydroxychloroquine (Plaquenil)*can be very helpful when the above measures have failed. However, there are finite risks, chiefly retinal toxicity requiring close ophthalmologic follow-up. Hence, antimalarials should be prescribed only by physicians who are knowledgeable about these agents and experienced in the management of childhood lupus erythematosus.

A brief course of systemic steroids is of occasional value in bringing an acute flare of discoid lesions under control, but systemic steroids have no place in chronic therapy of discoid lupus erythematosus in childhood. When systemic steroids are used for other organ system involvement, there is likely to be concurrent improvement in the discoid lesions.

Kawasaki Syndrome

(Mucocutaneous Lymph Node Syndrome)

MARIAN E. MELISH, M.D.

Truly effective therapy for Kawasaki syndrome awaits discovery of its etiology and pathogenesis. For the present, a carefully conducted management program designed to detect complications is indicated. Supportive therapy can be offered based upon a consideration of pathology. Although serious, for most patients the disease is self-limited and can be divided into three stages. Stage I, the acute febrile period, lasts for approximately 12 days. Stage II encompasses the period characterized by resolution of fever, desquamation, and thrombocytosis. Arthritis and carditis, when present, usually appear in this period. This period has the highest risk for sudden death due to coronary thrombosis and lasts until approximately day 30 of illness. Stage III, or the convalescent period, lasts from clinical recovery to the time when the sedimentation rate returns to normal, usually 8 to 10 weeks from onset. Patients must be carefully monitored through their illness with visits to the physician at least two times per week during Stages I and II and weekly through Stage III. An electrocardiogram and a chest radiograph should be obtained at the onset and repeated if there are any clinical signs of cardiac decompensation. Repeated physical examinations are superior to repeat electrocardiograms in detecting cardiac abnormalities, the most important complication of Kawasaki syndrome.

During the acute febrile phase, aspirin in standard anti-inflammatory doses of 80 to 100 mg/kg/24 hr may reduce the duration of fever. We monitor the salicylate level at 48 hours after starting aspirin, aiming for a level between 18 and 28 mg/dl, and we adjust the dose upward or downward as indicated. Once fever, rash, and acute symptoms have been controlled, we *decrease* the aspirin to a dose of 10 mg/kg/24 hr or less. Low-dose aspirin is more effective in preventing thrombosis during Stages II and III as it decreases platelet aggregation without stimulating vascular thrombogenic factors. It is important to reduce the aspirin during the period when platelet count is elevated as most fatalities are due to thrombosis during a period when vasculitis is declining.

If two-dimensional echocardiography is available, patients should be studied during Stage II; approximately 20% of patients will have coronary artery dilatation detected by this technique. This will identify a high-risk group who should be followed longer and more carefully. In selected children, especially those with pericarditis, myocarditis, congestive heart failure, or myocardial infarction, cardiac catheterization with selective coronary artery angiography may be indicated. This invasive technique should not be employed routinely as echocardiography will reveal 80 to 90% of the abnormalities detected by angiography and carries essentially no risk.

We have been adding dipyridamole (Persantine*), another inhibitor of platelet aggregation, to low-dose aspirin for patients known to have coronary aneurysms. As no dosage recommendations for this drug are available, we calculate the dose using the formula: patient surface area (m²)/1.7 X 150 mg (adult daily dose) = patient's daily dose. The drug is given in three divided doses. In patients

---

*This use is not listed by the manufacturer.

*This is an investigational use of Persantine.

with coronary aneurysms, we continue aspirin and dipyridamole for 1 year or until aneurysms resolve on repeat study. For patients with no evidence of heart disease and normal echocardiogram, we continue low-dose aspirin alone for 8 to 10 weeks until the sedimentation rate is normal.

Cardiac arrhythmias, congestive heart failure due to myocarditis, transient mitral insufficiency, or myocardial infarction must be treated in hospital with monitoring, digitalis, and anti-arrhythmia drugs. Arthritis is self-limited, usually lasting less than 2 weeks, but may require continuing high-dose aspirin. Gallbladder hydrops, presenting clinically as a right upper quadrant mass, can be confirmed by diagnostic ultrasound and monitored until natural resolution occurs. Surgical removal is not necessary as this complication is also self-limited.

Although Kawasaki syndrome is a disease characterized by vasculitis, corticosteroids are specifically *contraindicated* because of a carefully conducted controlled study indicating that corticosteroids increase the frequency of aneurysms compared with aspirin or no anti-inflammatory therapy. Less carefully conducted studies in Japan have shown a higher mortality rate in steroid-treated children compared with those treated with aspirin.

As the cause of death is nearly always coronary thrombosis, the patients' primary need is for careful monitoring and antiplatelet aggregation therapy throughout the period of greatest risk.

Fungal Infections

LAWRENCE SCHACHNER, M.D.

The use of creams and lotions with combined antifungal and anti-yeast action, such as miconazole (MicaTin) clotrimazole (Lotrimin) and haloprogin (Halotex) have made the treatment of superficial mycosis somewhat simpler. However, their appropriate use, as well as that of griseofulvin in tinea capitis and tinea unguium, can maximize their effectiveness and enhance the rate at which the patient is helped. Adjuncts that enhance the therapeutic action of these medications in specific mycosis, and the substitution of often less expensive preparations such as selenium sulfide (Selsun) or sodium thiosulfate (Tinver) in tinea versicolor have also been very effective.

Specific diagnostic tests for cutaneous fungal infections should not be allowed to become a lost art. Correct performance of potassium hydroxide (KOH) preparations and Wood's lamp examination can lead to immediate and inexpensive confirmation of the diagnosis of cutaneous fungal infections. Fungal cultures, particularly in tinea capitis, can lead to confirmation that a clinical finding such as alopecia is appropriately attributed to a dermatophyte and is not a clinical sign of severe underlying disease.

It is worth reiterating briefly the technique of KOH preparation. Hair specimens, scale from the border of the cutaneous eruption, nail scrapings, or blister roofs are placed on a microscope slide and cover slip. Ten to 20% KOH may be added to the side of the cover slip and will disperse itself equally over the covered material by flowing under the edge of the cover slip. KOH solutions free of dimethylsulfoxide (DMSO) should be heated until they begin to boil. If the KOH solution contains DMSO, the preparation should not be heated. Scanning the field under low power, with the condenser lowered to a position that allows for reduced amounts of illumination, will often aid in finding characteristic hyphae in dermatophytes, or pseudohyphae and budding spores in candidiasis.

The Wood's lamp is a valuable diagnostic tool in a number of cutaneous and systemic diseases, not the least of which are tinea capitis and tinea versicolor. In a totally darkened room, the patient's scalp or skin is illuminated with the Woods lamp. The microsporum species causing tinea capitis reveals a characteristic green fluorescence that is most notable in the areas of inflammation and loss of the acral hair shafts. The Wood's lamp produces an orange or yellow fluorescence over areas of involvement of the skin with tinea versicolor.

There are several media to choose among when preparing fungal cultures. Dermatophyte test medium (DTM) is a reliable diagnostic adjunct. The presence of a dermatophyte is confirmed not only by colony growth but also by the change in color of the media from gold to red in the presence of a dermatophyte. Mycosel agar is another good diagnostic culture medium for identifying dermatophytes and *Candida albicans*.

THERAPY

Two dermatophytoses that always require griseofulvin therapy are tinea capitis and tinea unguium. Tinea capitis, caused by species of *Trichophyton* and *Microsporum*, presents as an inflammatory or noninflammatory scalp disorder featuring scaling and alopecia. Inflammation, when present, can vary from mild to a suppurative boggy mass, replete with pustules and swelling, called a kerion. Griseofulvin should be started in doses of 10 to 20 mg/kg in the microcrystalline forms and half that dose in the ultra-microcrystalline griseofulvins, such as Gris-PEG. Since griseofulvin absorption seems to be enhanced by fatty food, I recommend that it be given after meals including milk or ice cream products. Griseofulvin should be given for a minimum of 4 weeks and preferably for at least 2 weeks after all clinical signs of disease have abated. Additional benefit may be gained by the use of keratolytic shampoos, such as Sebulex, which have been reported to decrease dissemination of spores and infected particles to the patient, and to others who may physically contact the patient. Topical antifungal solutions including clotrimazole, haloprogins, and miconazole preparations may enhance the rate of clinical improvement.

When tinea capitis has evolved to the point of kerion formation, the choice of therapies to clear the infection and minimize permanent hair loss and scalp scarring takes on added importance. In addition to griseofulvin, a course of prednisone at 1 mg/kg/day for 1 to 2 weeks will greatly decrease the inflammation and help attenuate the course of the kerion. Although the subject is certainly controversial, I among others feel that a 10 day course of oral antibiotics such as cloxacillin or erythromycin also may be helpful when kerions are present.

Tinea unguium is a chronic fingernail infection that is fortunately rare in childhood. Culture and KOH can help distinguish onychomycosis caused by *Trichophyton* or *Epidermophyton* from that caused by *Candida albicans.* The latter often is limited to the nails of the upper extremities, and concurrent paronychial inflammation is characteristic. Topical medications are effective in candidal nail infections, and any of the medications mentioned above, such as clotrimazole or nystatin preparations, would be useful. The onychomycoses due to *Trichophyton* and *Epidermophyton* species require long-term griseofulvin therapy. Similar dosages as for tinea capitis are appropriate; however, therapies must extend for at least 4 to 6 months for potential cure.

Tinea corporis, tinea cruris, tinea faciei, and tinea pedis, when acute, merit wet to dry soaks to decrease the inflammation and the oozing associated with the eczematous state. Tap water soaks are both effective and most inexpensive; if soaks are applied for 20 minutes every 4 hours for 2 days, most patients with these forms of tinea are ready for topical therapy. Most will respond nicely and completely to 2 to 3 weeks of twice daily therapy with clotrimazole, haloprogin, miconazole, or tolnaftate (Tinactin) though the latter is effective only against dermatophytes and is not active against *Candida albicans.* Recurrences of tinea may be decreased by the prophylactic administration of topical antifungal creams or powders. Only the most chronic severe and unresponsive forms of the above-mentioned tineas will require the addition of griseofulvin.

Tinea versicolor is a common chronic cutaneous infection that may be entirely asymptomatic. Although any of the above-mentioned topical antifungal preparations can be effective, the widespread distribution of the lesions makes selenium sulfide (Selsun) or sodium thiosulfate (Tinver) an effective and less expensive therapeutic approach. Overnight applications of either of these preparations to the entire affected area for a period of 2 weeks often leads to resolution. Pigment changes will take longer to resolve. Prophylactic therapy with these two preparations or with the above-mentioned antifungals can prevent recurrence, especially in more temperate months and climates.

Candidiasis, whether of the oral mucous membrane, the perineum, the flexural surfaces of the body, or the nails or interdigital spaces of the upper extremities, is responsive to nystatin preparations. Oral administration of nystatin suspension is useful not only in thrush but also in decreasing the bowel contamination that can seed candidal diaper dermatitis. The candidal dermatitis of the newborn infant is also nystatin responsive as is candidal vulvovaginitis, which can be treated with vaginal preparations. Much previous enthusiasm for Mycolog cream and similar polyformulary preparations has waned because of the presence of topical corticosteroids and sensitizing compounds in their formulation.

Warts and Molluscum Contagiosum

STEPHEN E. GELLIS, M.D.

WARTS

Warts are viral skin tumors commonly seen in children. Their appearance may vary with their location on the body. On the face, they may be flat or filiform. Around the hands and nails, they often become keratotic. Over the plantar aspect of the feet, they appear as localized thickened keratotic areas that may be confused with corns and calluses. Treatment in children should be governed by the understanding that most warts eventually resolve spontaneously. Treatment should be attempted only for painful or cosmetically objectionable lesions, or lesions in immunosuppressed patients which, left untreated, may disseminate. The choice of treatment depends on the age of the child and the location of the warts.

Lesions on the hands and around the fingers respond best to repeated freezing with liquid nitrogen applied with a disposable cotton-tipped applicator (Q-tip). The interval between treatments should not exceed 3 weeks. One should pare the bulk of the lesion with a sterile blade prior to treatment. In younger children, application of a salicylic acid–lactic acid combination (Duofilm, TiFlex, Viranol) nightly can be helpful. This method may require many weeks. Each night the involved area should be pared, soaked for 5 minutes, dried, and then covered with several drops of the medication, which is left to dry. Following this, the wart should be covered with a waterproof bandage.

Flat warts, particularly of the face, can be treated best by brief, 5- to 15-second freezes with liquid nitrogen applied with a Q-tip. Overly vigorous treatment may produce pigmentary changes. In small children who may not tolerate this method, a daily application of topical retinoic acid cream (Retin A* cream 0.05%) may be tried. Applications should be discontinued if too much irritation is produced.

Plantar warts are often the most difficult form to eradicate. The least painful approach is by topical salicyclic acid–lactic acid applied nightly as outlined above. Another approach is the use of a 40% salicylic acid plaster applied daily. In both forms of treatment, it is important to remove the softened wart with a pumice stone or an emory board prior to applying the medication. Care should be taken to avoid application to normal skin of either the liquid medication or the plasters. Treatment may be required for many weeks.

Condylomata acuminata are verrucous lesions appearing on the mucous membranes of the genitalia. They are rarely seen in small children and, when encountered, should raise the possibility of sexual abuse. Treatment consists of applications of a topical preparation of 25% podophyllin in tincture of benzoin at weekly intervals. Care must be taken to avoid applying the preparation to uninvolved skin. At the beginning of the treatment, the podophyllin should be removed after 1 to 2 hours to prevent a severe reaction. As the treatment progresses, the podophyllin can be left on for up to 6 hours. Other forms of treatment include liquid nitrogen freezing, electrosurgery, and curettage.

MOLLUSCUM CONTAGIOSUM

Molluscum contagiosum, a viral skin disorder commonly seen in young children, is characterized by firm umbilicated papules, often on the trunk and face. The lesions are spread by scratching with autoinoculation. Although the lesions will eventually resolve spontaneously, this may not occur for months. Treatment should be attempted only if it can be done without trauma. Any preparation causing irritation can promote a resolution. Gentle freezing by application of liquid nitrogen with a Q-tip for 2 to 3 seconds may be effective when repeated weekly. Expressing the keratotic core of a lesion with a comedo extractor after incising it with a sterile needle is effective in older children. In small children, daily careful application of an unoccluded salicylic acid–lactic acid preparation may produce good results. Treatment should continue until the lesions either become irritated and red or begin to dry.

---

*This use is not listed by the manufacturer.

Scabies and Pediculosis

LAWRENCE SCHACHNER, M.D.

SCABIES

Scabies is still a common infestation of infants, children, and adults. When a pediatrician sees a patient with a pruritic new eruption, a most useful question is: "Are there other people with this itchiness at home?" Often a history of concurrent itchy family members or frequent visitors will help to make the diagnosis.

On clinical examination, a child will often exhibit vesicles or bullae on the palms and soles. Children often have scabies lesions above the neck; this area must be treated in infants and children. Children have a propensity for longstanding lesions, usually in flexural distribution, including the axillae and groin, with formation of large nodular lesions that appear to be infiltrative and worrisome.

Since the advent of over-the-counter steroid preparations, many patients present with "scabies incognito," in which much of the inflammation is reduced but no cure has been effected.

A rapid confirmation of diagnosis can be accomplished by using a mineral oil preparation. The pediatrician may use a scalpel with a # 15 blade or a small curet, to scrape at least six lesions. He or she should choose the newest, unexcoriated lesions. The scalpel is dipped in mineral oil and then gently used to abrade the roofs and the very superficial base of the lesion. The scabies mites, eggs, and stools are all found in the very superficial epidermis; there is no need to create major excavations. When the lesions have been abraded, a cover slip can be put over the material collected in mineral oil on a routine laboratory slide. The mites are often found alive and mobile within the oil.

The therapy of scabies infestations has evoked considerable controversy vis à vis the question of neurotoxicity of gamma-benzene-hexachloride preparations such as lindane (Kwell). In fact, with the very widespread use of Kwell preparations for scabies, there have been a very small number of neurotoxic events documented, which in most cases represented misuse of the medication. For children over 3 years of age a 1% Kwell preparation would appear to be the therapy of first choice. However, several factors militate against use in younger children and infants: the increased surface area to body weight in this age group; the increase in severe, self-inflicted excoriations in this age group; and the propensity for sucking and licking of fingers, toes, hands, and feet in this age group, which lead to an increased potential for absorption and for untoward effects. Five per cent sulfur in petrolatum is a safe and effective therapeutic agent for those in this age group. Crotamiton (Eurax) has also been used and has the additional benefit of being a topical antipruritic. Our most successful experience in children under 3 has been with the use of sulfur in petrolatum.

Lindane creams and lotions are recommended by the manufacturer as curative with one application. Our experience has shown an increased efficacy by substituting for the recommended 12-hour or overnight treatment two 6-hour applications of the medication from the head to the toes of children over 3 years of age. At the end of 6 hours, the medication is removed by a thorough bathing. A second 6 hour application on day 2 may enhance the curative effect. Treatment of children under 3 also involves application of medication from the head to the toes. We have found three successive overnight applications of 5% sulfur in petrolatum to be effective.

Severe excoriations and secondary infection are sequelae of the intense pruritus provoked by scabies. We use an antihistamine such as Benadryl elixir and, when indicated, an oral antibiotic. Scabies therapy should include treatment of all household members and visitors who have frequent contact with the child. The family must realize that, although the infestation may be eradicated, the pruritus may persist for several weeks after beginning treatment. After completion of the treatment period, one may continue to utilize the oral antihistamine. Occasionally a topical steroid is useful if inflammation and pruritus persist. Although the garments and bed clothing are only rarely vectors of disease, most families feel better after thoroughly laundering them.

HEAD LICE

Pediculosis humanus capitis has become a very frequent disease of childhood. Clinically after a child has acquired the infestation initial complaint will be that of pruritus. On physical examination the children often show a predominance of lesions in the retroauricular and occipital areas of the scalp. Usually the scalp is marked by areas of excoriation that may be impetiginized. There may be matted scalp hair in this area accompanied by lymphadenopathy. A few live adult organisms may be present, but one is most likely to notice many nits. Magnification with a hand lens will reveal that the eggs are plump and have an operculum; they are easily distinguishable from dandruff or seborrheic scales.

Lindane shampoo (Kwell) is a safe and effective therapy. One tablespoon or approximately 15 ml of 1% Kwell shampoo is massaged into the scalp until the scalp is moistened. When the hair is thoroughly wet, a small amount of water may be added and worked into a lather. Shampooing is continued for 4 minutes and is followed by a thorough rinsing. A second application of Kwell 1 week later may increase the cure rate. With the emergence of Kwell-resistant head lice in Europe and reports of potential Kwell toxicity, alternative therapies have been explored. Pyrethrins combined with piperonyl butoxide (A-200, RID) have also been found to be safe but may be less effective.

An alternative treatment is malathion (Prioderm) in a 0.5% lotion. This has a 10 year history of safety and efficacy as therapy for head lice in Europe. The scalp is well moistened with Prioderm, preferably before going to bed at night. The hair is then allowed to dry naturally overnight. The next morning, the hair is thoroughly shampooed and rinsed. A fine-tooth comb may be used to remove the dead lice and nits. Reapplication 1 week after the first treatment will improve the cure rate.

Itching, the main complaint, can be treated with antihistamines. Secondary bacterial infection, a major complication, may merit a course of oral antibiotics. Unlike scabies infestation, head lice infestation does not necessitate treatment of all household members. However, all should be examined for head lice or nits and those afflicted should be treated. Washable clothing, towels, and bedding should be laundered in hot water cycles for at least 20 minutes; machine drying at maximal heat will kill nits within 20 minutes. Nonwashable clothing should be dry cleaned, and nonwashable items such as combs and brushes should be disinfected for one hour by soaking in the pediculicidal shampoo.

Disorders of Pigmentation

DAVID B. MOSHER, M.D.

HYPERMELANOSES

Café-au-lait macules are discrete, flat, pale brown, 2- to 20-cm, oval macules found in 10% of normal people and in those with neurofibromatosis, Albright syndrome, and Watsons syndrome Isolated macules occur in many normal people, but six or more lesions 1.5 cm or larger in diameter are considered diagnostic for neurofibromatosis. No therapy is available.

Ephelides or freckles are 0.1- to 0.5-cm, oval, medium-to-dark brown macules occurring on sun-exposed areas of light-eyed, fair-skinned, light-haired individuals who generally tan poorly. Use of highly efficient broad-spectrum sunscreens, such as Total Eclipse (creamy) 15 or PreSun 15, may retard some pigmentary darkening of freckles. Hydroquinone-containing bleaching creams are generally ineffective.

Lentigines are uniformly or variegated-colored, 0.5 cm, brown macules found on any cutaneous surface, including palms, soles, and mucous membranes, and associated with electrocardiographic abnormalities, ocular hypertelorism, pulmonary stenosis, abnormal genitalia, growth reduction, and deafness (leopard syndrome). There is no treatment for established lesions.

Melasma is a facial hypermelanosis found primarily in women on oral anovulatory agents or pregnant women. It is more apparent in summer than in winter because of sun-induced delayed pigmentary darkening, particularly of involved skin. Wood light examination will distinguish epidermal hypermelanosis of melasma from dermal melanoses that do not respond to therapy. Effective treatment requires use of sunscreens, hydroquinone, and Retin-A. The sunscreen should be an opaque formulation (Reflecta, Clinique). Twice daily application of 4% hydroquinone cream and Retin-A 0.05% cream together should lead to pigmentary lightening in 6 to 8 weeks. Regular sunscreen usage and periodic hydroquinone may have to be maintained until the problem resolves. Discontinuation of oral contraceptives often results in clearing.

Photodermatoses, including berloque dermatitis, result from uv irradiation after topically applied photosensitizer, including psoralen-containing cosmetics, vegetables, or plants. Application of 2 or 4% hydroquinone twice daily and avoidance of offending agents is the treatment of choice.

Postinflammatory hypermelanosis is a pigmentary darkening that may follow resolution of many dermatoses. Those postinflammatory hypermelanoses that are epidermal (they contrast with normal surrounding skin heightened with Wood light exam) may resolve spontaneously and no therapy is usually required. Particularly in dark-skinned individuals, postinflammatory hypermelanoses may be dermal and thereby lighten slowly if at all. There is no effective treatment for dermal postinflammatory hyperpigmentation.

Mongolian spots or dermal melanocytosis (nevus of Ito and nevus of Ota) refers to blue-gray pigmentation found particularly on the face (unilaterally) or the lumbosacral skin, particularly in mongolians, polynesians and blacks. These lesions are congenital or arise shortly after birth. Opaque cosmetics may provide acceptable coverup. These lesions do not spontaneously resolve.

HYPOMELANOSES

Oculocutaneous albinism is an autosomal recessive, diffuse hypomelanosis characterized by pallid skin that does not tan, white-to-yellow hair, and ocular abnormalities. Because albinos are unable to synthesize significant amounts of melanin to protect them from solar irradiation, they are exquisitely sensitive to acute sunburn reaction and highly prone to develop chronic actinic changes, including tumors, by their second or third decade. Avoidance

of midday sun exposure and daily use of highly efficient broad-spectrum sunscreens such as Pre-Sun 15 or Total Eclipse 15 are mandatory.

Phenylketonuric children, if not diagnosed early by neonatal testing and placed on low phenylalanine diets, may develop irreversible mental retardation. Such individuals are often fair-skinned and fair-haired compared with other unaffected family members. Sunscreens are the only topical agents required because of the pigmentary dilution.

Vitiligo is a common, acquired, progressive depigmentation of the skin, often with a positive family history and associated in some cases with thyroid disease, diabetes mellitus, pernicious anemia, and Addison disease, as well as cutaneous disorders including alopecia areata, halo nevi, and premature graying of hair.

There are several options for therapy. Simple reassurance may be all that is required. But as one cannot predict exact prognosis, the patient and parents must understand that vitiligo is most likely to progress, with new macules developing and older ones enlarging, and very unlikely spontaneously to repigment to an acceptable degree. Parents and physicians must be encouraged to address themselves to the psychologic and developmental needs of the child first and treat the vitiligo only if it begins to present psychosocial problems for the child. In any event, use of sunscreens such as Eclipse 10 will prevent acute sunburn reaction and should be applied daily and more often after swimming or sweating. Cosmetics (Covermark) or dyes (Dy-O-Derm, Vitadye) may be applied to vitiliginous macules if temporary camouflage is required.

In younger patients, particularly those with constitutively dark skin color, attempts at repigmentation may be desirable for social reasons. Hydrocortisone 2.5% cream applied topically bid may occasionally be effective; occlusion overnight may increase the response rate. In patients over 12 years of age and in rare younger patients, trimethylpsoralen (Trisoralen), 0.6 mg/kg, plus sunlight or high-intensity UVA (PUVA) given twice weekly with careful physician supervision, may lead to successful repigmentation. With such therapy, up to 70% of patients should repigment the vitiliginous macules of the head and neck; the trunk, arms, and legs do nearly as well but the dorsal digits and feet do so poorly as rarely alone to justify attempts at repigmentation. Completely repigmented macules have a 90% chance of remaining filled in. PUVA does not necessarily keep new macules of vitiligo from developing and should never be construed as a cure.

For the very rare child who develops aggressive vitiligo that spontaneously depigments over 90 per cent of the skin, removal of the remaining normally melanized color may be accomplished by application of 20% monobenzylether of hydroquinone

(Benoquin) twice daily for 9 to 12 months to accomplish irreversible depigmentation. Such individuals must be able to forgo any hope of future tanning.

Piebaldism and Waardenburg syndrome are characterized by irreversible congenital amelanotic macules. Protection with sunscreens is obligatory. Cosmetic coverup as with vitiligo may be attempted. A uniform appearance may be achieved by application of Benoquin to depigment normally melanized skin. This may require 12 or more months of twice daily application.

Nevus depigmentosus, unlike segmental vitiligo, is congenital, hypomelanotic (not amelanotic), and stable. No effective therapy is available.

Tuberous sclerosis in up to 95% of cases is characterized by the presence of congenital thumbprint or lance-ovate hypomelanotic macules. Confetti or segmental macules also may be observed. The presence of three or more such discrete macules at birth is virtually diagnostic of tuberous sclerosis and antedates by several years the appearance of seizures, mental retardation, or cutaneous findings including shagreen patches and adenoma sebaceum. No treatment for the hypomelanotic macules of tuberous sclerosis has been described, but their presence in a child necessitates examination of parents and other siblings for evidence of genetic transmission (25%) as opposed to spontaneous mutation (75%).

Incontinentia pigmenti achromians or hypomelanosis of Ito is a bizarre, bilateral, faint-to-moderate hypomelanosis of the trunk and extremities. IPA presents as swirls of hypomelanosis appearing after the age of 2. Musculoskeletal and central nervous system abnormalities, including seizures and mental retardation, have been reported in many patients. There is no known treatment for the hypomelanosis, which is often a mild cosmetic defect.

Pityriasis alba is a common hypomelanosis associated with a powdery scaling of macules of the face, arms, and sometimes legs. Probably an eczematous process, pityriasis abla is more noticeable among darkly pigmented races and is a self-limited disorder. Therapy with 1% hydrocortisone cream twice daily or emollients is usually moderately effective.

Postinflammatory hypomelanosis develops at the site of resolved lesions of psoriasis, eczema, or other dermatoses. Spontaneous repigmentation is usual, and no specific therapy is necessary to reverse the pigmentary dilution.

Tinea versicolor is a chronic, recurrent, asymptomatic dermatosis attributed to a lipophilic yeast, *Pityrosporum orbiculare*. The upper chest and back are the sites most commonly affected by these scaling, hypopigmented, sometimes raised macules, which may fluoresce yellow-green under the Wood light. Application of selenium disulfide (Selsun) daily for 3 weeks (rinsed off in 15 minutes to prevent development of irritant eczematous dermatitis), or miconazole (MicaTin) or clotrimazole (Lotrimin) twice daily is often curative. After effective treatment, the hypomelanosis may resolve completely only after ultraviolet irradiation adequate to stimulate delayed melanogenesis. Tinea versicolor tends to recur.

Halo nevus refers to the development of a macule of leukoderma around a pre-existing pigmented nevus. The appearance of a concentric white ring around a normal-appearing nevus should be viewed as a benign evolutionary process that is usually followed by spontaneous disappearance of the central nevus and then, but not always, repigmentation of the remaining macule of leukoderma. No therapy is required. However, the appearance of an eccentric halo of leukoderma or a halo around an atypical-appearing lesion should be viewed with suspicion; biopsy of such lesions may be indicated to exclude the halo phenomenon surrounding a melanoma.

Nevus anemicus is a congenital vascular anomaly that mimics a hypopigmented lesion. Pressure with a clear glass slide causes it to become inapparent; these lesions, in contradistinction to all circumscribed hypomelanoses, disappear under the Wood light. Nevus anemicus is usually subtle in appearance, fortunately, for there is no treatment.

Photodermatoses

BARBARA A. GILCHREST, M.D.

Photodermatoses are diseases caused by or exacerbated by exposure to particular wavelengths of ultraviolet (UV) or visible light. They are distinguished clinically by a distribution usually restricted to exposed areas of the body and an often obvious temporal relationship to sun exposure.

Because protection against causative wavelengths of light is central to the treatment of most photodermatoses, it is important to define these spectral bands for the diseases under consideration and to classify sunscreens according to their ability to block light of these wavelengths. (See Table 1.)

Sunburn. Sunburn is without doubt the most commonly encountered adverse reaction to sunlight. Reactions requiring medical intervention are usually the result of accidental overexposure to UVB, such as falling asleep under a sunlamp or at the beach. Erythema first appears 3 to 6 hours after exposure and peaks at approximately 24 hours, but may persist for several days. Treatment consists of cool compresses or baths. Aspirin is a useful analgesic and, as a cyclo-oxygenase inhibitor, may actually reduce the severity of the reaction, especially if administered early in the course. Neither topical nor oral corticosteroids have any docu-

Table 1. COMMON SUNSCREENS

Commercial Name*	Major Ingredients	Protective Spectrum†	Appropriate Usage
PreSun Pabanol	5% para-amino-benzoic acid (PABA)	UVC, UVB, some UVA	sunburn, freckling
Block Out Eclipse Sungard Sundown Pabafilm	2.5–5% PABA esters and derivatives	UVC, UVB, some UVA	sunburn, freckling
PreSun 15 Supershade Total Eclipse	5% PABA and benzophenones	UVC, UVB, UVA	LE, PMLE, solar urticaria, photosensitivity
Uval Solbar Piz Buin #6	benzophenones, cinnamates	UVA, some UVB	photosensitivity, PABA allergy
A-fil RVPaque Reflecta	titanium dioxide, zinc oxide	UVC, UVB, UVA, visible light	melasma, EPP, PCT

* Selected products are representative and widely available; undoubtedly many equally effective sunscreens are omitted.
† UVC 200–290 nm "germicidal" light
  UVB 290–320 nm sunburn spectrum, shortest wavelengths penetrating the earth's ozone layer
  UVA 320–400 nm "black light," shortest wavelengths transmitted through window glass
  Visible 400–700 nm shortest wavelengths transmitted through the ocular lens

mented value in the treatment of severe sunburn, despite positive anecdotal reports.

Painful conjunctivitis also may result from sufficient exposure to UVB or more commonly UVC (germicidal light) and has a time course similar to the sunburn itself. Severe reactions benefit from patching both eyes closed for 12 to 14 hours and, if this gives insufficient relief, from local instillation of proparacaine, 0.5%, or other topical anesthetic.

Ephelides (Freckles). These 1- to 2-mm brown macules appear on the face and other exposed body sites of most fair-skinned individuals, especially those of celtic ancestry, during the first years of life. They darken during periods of frequent sun exposure and fade but never disappear after weeks to months without exposure. Because the hyperpigmentation is epidermal in location, hydroquinone 2 to 4% cream (Artra, Eldoquin, Eldoquin Forte) is effective in lightening freckles. A broad-spectrum UV blocker or opaque makeup is essential to prevent immediate reappearance in sunny climates.

Melasma (Mask of Pregnancy). This macular, reticulated brown hyperpigmentation may occur at any time after puberty. The lateral cheeks and forehead are most commonly involved. Women are affected much more often than men, and lesions usually first appear during pregnancy or while using an oral contraceptive, but may persist indefinitely. Melasma is more common and more prominent in dark-skinned individuals. As with freckles, pigmentation is epidermal and does not occur in the absence of sun exposure. Treatment is identical. In difficult cases, a 6-week course of twice daily applications of hydroquinone 4%, retinoic acid 0.05%, and hydrocortisone 2.5% creams plus an opaque sunscreen is usually successful.

Polymorphous Light Eruption (PMLE). PMLE is an intensely pruritic eruption that predictably appears 2 to 48 hours after sun exposure, affects some but not all exposed skin surfaces, and resolves without scarring in 1 to 2 weeks. The disorder must be distinguished from lupus erythematosus, photoexacerbated eczema, and allergic contact or photocontact dermatitis (e.g., to sunscreens). Treatment consists of appropriate sunscreens, usually a combination of both UVB and UVA blockers such as PABA and benzophenones (PreSun 15, Total Eclipse, Supershade). In patients with severe photosensitivity, oral use of antimalarial agents may be justified.

Hydroxychloroquine (Plaquenil*), 3 to 5 mg/kg/24 hr given as 200 mg tablets, frequently produces a marked increase in the exposure time necessary to induce lesions within 6 weeks of initiating therapy. Because retinal toxicity is total dose-dependent, the drug should be used only during the spring and early summer or other high-risk periods. Patients should undergo a complete ophthalmologic exam including field testing in the paracentral area with red test objects every 6 months while on therapy. Chloroquine (Aralen*), 3 to 6 mg/kg/24 hr given as 250 mg tablets, is equally effective and has virtually no associated retinal toxicity but produces a distinctly lemon-yellow color in white skin at therapeutic doses, restricting its usefulness to blacks and other dark-skinned patients.

Photochemotherapy with the psoralen compound methoxsalen, 0.6 mg/kg, followed 2 hours later by filtered UVA in gradually increasing doses (approximately 3 to 15 J/cm^2), has benefited many patients, but requires special facilities and a dermatologist's supervision. PUVA appears to protect patients by stimulating a dark tan or "natural sunscreen" with UV wavelengths not capable of inducing PMLE. Therapy should be given 2 or 3 times weekly for at least 2 weeks before a trial of intentional sun exposures. PUVA is not helpful for patients whose abnormal sensitivity includes the UVA as well as the more common UVB wavelengths, since the therapeutic exposures themselves then precipitate lesions.

Hydroa Aestivale and Hydroa Vacciniforme. Hydroa aestivale and hydroa vacciniforme resemble PMLE clinically and histologically but are much

---

*This use is not listed by the manufacturer.

less common and display more scarring and a greater tendency to "harden" with repeated sun exposure. Treatment principles are the same as for PMLE.

Solar Urticaria. In this rare disorder, skin exposed to sunlight develops hives, clinically indistinguishable from "standard" hives, usually within minutes of receiving a sufficient ultraviolet dose. EPP should be excluded by quantitation of plasma and erythrocyte porphyrin levels.

Broad-spectrum sunscreens may be helpful, but often patients are so exquisitely sensitive that lesions still develop during routine outdoor activities. Antihistamines are similarly disappointing. The best approach currently is "desensitization"—brief, carefully monitored, daily UV exposures to natural sunlight or phototherapy bulbs. It is presumed that these exposures progressively degranulate cutaneous mast cells at a rate too slow to induce symptoms. Since mast cells can completely regranulate within a few days, the brief daily exposures are necessary indefinitely if the skin is to remain unreactive to intermittent larger UV doses.

Photosensitivity to Drugs. Certain oral and topical drugs may cause abnormal cutaneous responses in sun-exposed skin. Treatment consists of eliminating the causative drug or, if this cannot be done, minimizing sun exposure. A special case and one occasionally encountered in teenagers being treated for acne is that of photo-onycholysis due to tetracycline. The nail plate appears to act as a lens, focusing light on the underlying nail bed and producing painful separation of the nail plate due to local edema. Clinically detectable phototoxicity involving the skin surface is much less common. Photo-onycholysis can be prevented by use of nontranslucent (colored) nail polish.

Lupus Erythematosus (LE). Discoid LE, other cutaneous manifestations of LE, and indeed systemic manifestations of LE are frequently precipitated or exacerbated by sun exposure; in many patients skin lesions are distributed almost entirely in sun-exposed areas. For such patients, broad-spectrum, highly efficacious sunscreens are central to therapy. Nonscarred discoid lesions usually resolve completely after less than 1 week of two to three times daily application of a potent corticosteroid cream or ointment. Fluocinonide, halcinonide, and betamethasone dipropionate are all appropriate to use in this manner even on facial lesions, since inadequately treated DLE may progress to scarring within a few weeks. Patients with widely disseminated or very frequent lesions or both are candidates for treatment with oral chloroquine* or hydroxychloroquine (see PMLE discussion). Prednisone, 0.5 to 1.0 mg/kg/24 hr, also rapidly suppresses lesions in most patients but is difficult to justify in the absence of major systemic disease manifestations.

Erythropoietic Protoporphyria (EPP). This autosomal dominant disorder is the second most common of the porphyrias and by far the most common in children. Lesions occur when porphyrins in the cutaneous microvasculature are activated by wavelengths in the Soret band, 400 to 410 nm (blue light), and hence may follow exposure through window glass and despite use of PABA sunscreens (see Table 1). Symptom-free sun exposure times are frequently increased 10-fold by use of the singlet oxygen quencher, oral β-carotene (Solatene), approximately 1 to 3 mg/kg daily, to achieve a serum carotene level of 600 to 800 μg/dl, although intentional sun exposure still should be limited to minimize late cutaneous sequelae.

β-Carotene has proved completely safe in extensive clinical trials, although rusty orange diarrhea may occur and therapeutic doses usually produce an obvious yellow-orange discoloration of the skin, especially the palms. Patients should be followed annually for the possible development of cholelithiasis (up to 12% of cases) or hepatic cirrhosis (rare). Many patients have also been noted to have a mild hemolytic anemia, although this rarely requires therapy. Genetic counseling is appropriate.

Other Porphyrias. Erythropoietic porphyria (EP), or Günther disease, is an extremely rare autosomal recessive disorder due to uroporphyrinogen cosynthetase deficiency. Treatment of the cutaneous disorder is complicated by the extreme photosensitivity, but opaque sunscreens and oral β-carotene may be helpful. Splenectomy per se has been reported to reduce the photosensitivity in some patients.

Porphyria cutanea tarda (PCT) is the most common porphyria among adults and occurs rarely even in prepubertal children. The disorder, a deficiency of uroporphyrinogen decarboxylase, is probably inherited in an autosomal dominant manner but not expressed in most patients in the absence of hepatic injury, iron overload, or elevated estrogen levels. Photosensitivity is subtle and many patients fail to relate their lesions to sun exposure. Skin fragility and bullae on the dorsa of the hands are the most common finding; patients may also develop fine excess facial hair or rarely sclerodermatous changes in exposed skin. Treatment consists of phlebotomy every 2 weeks of 500 ml of whole blood in an adult or a proportional volume in a child until symptoms resolve and urinary porphyrin excretion approaches normal levels. In adults, oral chloroquine,* 125 to 250 mg (approximately 2 to 4 mg/kg) twice weekly, has also proved safe and effective, but hepatotoxicity may result and

---

*This use is not listed by the manufacturer.

liver enzymes should be monitored at monthly intervals during therapy. Chloroquine, 500 mg daily for 7 to 8 days only, is also effective in adults with PCT but frequently produces abdominal pain, jaundice, and marked hepatocellular dysfunction due to massive porphyrin release. Both phlebotomy and chloroquine therapy require several months to over a year to eliminate clinical and laboratory evidence of disease. Remissions usually last several years and may be permanent if the precipitating factor can be removed.

Nevi and Nevoid Tumors

ARTHUR J. SOBER, M.D.

A nevus is a proliferation of one or more cutaneous elements within the skin. These lesions may be either congenital or acquired. For therapeutic considerations, nevi are subdivided into those of melanocytic (nevocytic) origin, those of vascular origin, and those originating from other cutaneous elements. A 10 X hand lens and bright room illumination are most helpful in facilitating diagnosis. Consultation with a dermatologist may be useful if the diagnosis is unclear.

MELANOCYTIC NEVI

Junctional, compound, and *dermal nevi* usually require no therapy as long as they can be reliably distinguished from cutaneous melanoma (relatively rare in prepubertal children). When treatment of these nevi is indicated for cosmetic considerations alone, or for chronic irritation, then total excision or shave excision can be performed at the discretion of the physician. Histopathologic examination of all melanocytic nevi removed for whatever reason is essential since an unsuspected melanoma may occasionally be removed as a "benign" nevus.

Halo nevi occur frequently in pediatric populations and are usually of no pathologic significance.

Congenital melanocytic nevi fall into two categories: (1) giant—about which there is general agreement that a malignant potential exists that may express early in life, and (2) congenital nevi of the smaller variety—about which there is debate about the malignant potential. The presence of hair is of no help in the management of pigmented nevi. For giant congenital nevi, early full-thickness removal of the entire lesion is recommended. This usually can be accomplished by a combination of staged excisions and grafting. Dermabrasion is not recommended since this procedure will not remove the nevus cells located in the lower reticular dermis or subcutaneous fat. Melanomas have been observed arising in the dermis of giant congenital nevi.

For the smaller congenital nevi, I have been recommending prophylactic removal at an age convenient for surgery, since I have seen melanomas arising in association with them. The overall frequency of such occurrences is not clear and the risk of not removing an individual lesion is at present unknown but is probably relatively low. Other experts on melanomas feel strongly that the prophylactic removal of congenital nevi of the smaller type is unwarranted. I have been recommending full-thickness excision with close margins for congenital raised pigment nevi greater than 1.5 cm in size. Therapeutic recommendations for congenital nevi of the smaller type are evolving, so the reader should check the current literature for subsequent opinions.

Spitz nevi (benign juvenile melanoma, compound spindle cell nevus, epithelioid cell nevus, and so on) need no therapy if recognizable as such. Since this lesion may be difficult for the pathologist to distinguish from malignant melanoma, the slides of any lesion diagnosed as malignant melanoma in a prepubertal child should be sent to an expert melanoma pathologist for confirmation. The physician and patient may be rewarded with the good news that the previously diagnosed "melanoma" was actually a benign lesion (Spitz nevus). No treatment is needed for Spitz nevi, but simple excision with close margins is adequate should removal be desired. Any confusion on clinical grounds with malignant melanoma (since some Spitz nevi may be darkly pigmented) warrants a biopsy.

Therapy is unnecessary for a *blue nevus,* a benign lesion, unless the physician suspects malignant melanoma in which case excisional biopsy with narrow margins is the procedure of choice.

No treatment is needed for a *mongolian spot,* since these lesions usually disappear spontaneously. Of those that fail to disappear, most occur in covered locations and require no therapy. For the rare patient with a mongolian spot of cosmetic concern, the lesion can be effectively covered with an opaque cosmetic (Covermark) matched in color to the patient's skin and applied daily.

VASCULAR NEVI

A plethora of diagnostic terms for these lesions in part contributes to the management confusion.

Capillary nevi (salmon patches, plane nevus, nevus flammeus, telangiectatic nevus, port-wine nevus) usually require no treatment. With the exception of port-wine lesions, capillary nevi on the eyelids fade rapidly and almost all will disappear by the end of the first year of life. Patches on the forehead fade more slowly. Over 50% of lesions on the nape of the neck are still visible at age 1 year, but these present little cosmetic problem. Port-wine lesions increase in size with the growth of the child and have little tendency to fade. Involvement of the trigeminal area may be associated with Sturge-Weber syndrome. Opaque cosmetics matched to the skin tone (Covermark) have been remarkably helpful in hiding the disfigurement. Experimental therapy with the argon laser (especially on the deeper-colored lesions) appears promising.

Cavernous nevi (hemangioma, angiomatous nevi) in the majority of patients require no active therapy. Most important in the management of these lesions is to establish a trusting rapport with the parents. The management of each lesion should be individualized and therapy based on the likelihood of resolution with good cosmetic results without treatment. Regular followup is advised at frequent intervals during periods of rapid growth and at progressively longer intervals when resolution is occurring. Serial photographs of the lesion are helpful in following the course and in the instruction of other parents in what they should expect from their own child's lesion.

The nevi composed of superficial vessels alone can be expected to resolve with good cosmetic results in at least 90% of patients. Those nevi with deeper vessel involvement will involute less frequently, but still the majority (50 to 70%) will undergo complete resolution. Folds of atrophic skin may remain after the deeper lesions have involuted. Resolution is less likely to be complete when mucosal surfaces are involved or when the lesion is large. Serial monitoring with an ultrasonic flowmeter to determine whether arteriovenous fistulae are persisting or decreasing has been reported predictive of spontaneous regression. Fewer than 10% of cavernous nevi ultimately result in any cosmetic handicap, according to Rook. Surgical excision in selected cases may be of use in the late management of noninvoluting lesions.

Therapeutic intervention is triggered by the presence of complications, which include hemorrhage, ulceration, malignant change, encroachment on a vital structure, or thrombocytopenia. Hemorrhage following trauma is rare. Ulceration is of no immediate significance but may result in a more conspicuous scar. Local care includes wet to dry dressings with saline or Domeboro solution three to four times daily followed by local application of bacitracin ointment. Malignant change is extremely rare. Thrombocytopenia and encroachment on vital structures have led to the use of systemic prednisone (2 mg/kg/24 hr per one source or $\geq$ 20 mg/24 hr per another source), with improvement usually noted in 2 to 3 weeks. After 3 to 4 weeks of the high doses, the steroid levels can be tapered over an additional 4 weeks. Relapse may require reinstitution of systemic steroids. Therapy also may be necessary for complications resulting from internal organ involvement (rare) by a vascular nevus associated with a cutaneous nevus. X-ray therapy is no longer recommended for management of hemangiomas.

Treatment of *lymphangiomas* by surgery is deceptive, with recurrences frequently resulting even with full-thickness excision and grafting. Lymphangiomas are often best left without treatment.

NEVI OF OTHER CUTANEOUS ELEMENTS

Nevus sebaceus—prophylactic excision with close margins is recommended to prevent the subsequent development of basal cell carcinoma.

Connective tissue nevi (shagreen patch, and so on) —other stigmata of tuberous sclerosis should be sought. Examination of the entire skin with longwave ultraviolet light (Wood light) is recommended. Management is that of the underlying disease. The connective tissue nevus per se needs no treatment.

Epidermal nevi—excision where possible is recommended since these lesions may give rise to basal cell carcinomas. Dermabrasion frequently results in recurrence of the lesion.

Other Skin Tumors

GUINTER KAHN, M.D.

Skin tumors, other than nevi and vascular anomalies, are uncommon in childhood. Even though most are benign, they are important for three reasons: 1) they may create cosmetic defects; 2) they occasionally are associated with systemic disease; and 3) they must be separated into subgroups needing immediate attention (malignancies), eventual removal (cosmetic defects), or observation only (evanescent, self-healing masses).

BASAL AND SQUAMOUS CELL CARCINOMA

Basal and squamous cell carcinomas in children differ from those in adults only in their rarity. They occur primarily on the head and neck (sun-exposed areas) and are distinguished by their histology rather than their clinical appearance.

Never treat skin tumors of children with irradiation. The object of therapy is to destroy the lesions with the least inconvenience and the best cosmetic result for the youngster. Size and number of lesions often determine the optimal method. Large lesions are best removed surgically, grafting when necessary. Multiple lesions are best removed by curettage and electrodesiccation or cryosurgery, depending upon the experience and facilities of the physician. No single method of therapy is applicable to all patients. The goal is for a cure rate of more than 95%.

The key to the treatment of these lesions is prevention. Prevention begins with the avoidance of the ravages of sunlight by limiting exposure and by appropriate shielding. Sunlight between the hours of 9 A.M and 4 P.M. causes most of the degeneration that leads to skin cancer. The harmful effects of sunlight begin in the pediatric age group and accumulate to cause skin cancer in later years. Doctors need to emphasize more strongly to the sun-susceptible population that *avoidance of sunlight must begin in the early years of childhood.*

BENIGN EPIDERMAL TUMORS

Epidermal nevus is also called nevus unius lateris and verrucous nevus. These papillary elevations occur as linear or patchy, narrow or widespread, pigmented lesions that may wax and wane as the seasons come and go. They seldom resolve spontaneously. They may involve most of the body, even the oral and vaginal mucosae. Widespread lesions may be associated with skeletal, vascular, and central nervous system anomalies.

Treatment is for cosmetic reasons. It is often unsatisfactory because removal is often followed by scars or recurrences. Therapy should be withheld until adolescence to allow for full development of the condition. Dermabrasion, electrodesiccation, and grafting all may leave cosmetically unacceptable scars. Chemical peeling as done for wrinkles may be effective in selected patients. It is best to attempt the procedure on a small test area to forecast the patient's response.

Seborrheic keratoses occur primarily in blacks as *dermatosis papulosa nigra,* presenting as small black papules on the cheeks. Treatment for pedunculated lesions is to snip the base with curved iris scissors. Sessile lesions can be lightly electrodesiccated or frozen with liquid nitrogen. Painting with bichloracetic acid also gives satisfactory results. Malignant-appearing seborrheic keratoses must be biopsied prior to removal. Problems result in dark-complexioned children with the formation of keloids and also hyper- and hypopigmentation, so that multiple lesions are removed only upon request in patients with black skin.

Epidermal cysts are removed rapidly via punch biopsy, after which strong pressure is applied to the edges of the cyst to insure the appearance of the sac, which is then pulled out with a hemostat. The size of the punch is tiny (2 mm whenever possible), especially for removal of lesions on the face. For larger cysts, larger punches are used, and the wound may be closed with a suture. In patients with multiple epidermal cysts, the possibility of malignant intestinal polyps associated with the Gardner syndrome must be ruled out.

Tiny epidermal cysts, like *milia,* are removed with a comedo extractor. In the neonate these lesions are ignored since they resolve without therapy.

EPIDERMAL APPENDAGE TUMORS

Nevus sebaceus of Jadassohn is a flat yellow growth on the scalp and upper face of the neonate. It becomes thickened and papillated by adolescence. After puberty, about 20% of the lesions develop sweat gland tumors, and 10% develop basal cell epitheliomas. Early complete excision gives gratifying cosmetic results; it "cures" the bald, yellow patches and precludes the formation of tumors in them. Central nervous system abnormalities have been noted in patients with extensive sebaceous nevi associated with the epidermal nevus syndrome.

Trichoepitheliomas may be solitary and look like basal cell carcinoma. When the lesions are multiple, a confirmatory biopsy of one lesion can serve as a guide to management of subsequent ones.

In general, multiple appendageal tumors are dominantly inherited, while single lesions occur on a sporadic, nongenetic basis. Single lesions are removed easily and successfully by complete excision, while multiple lesions are extremely difficult to eradicate because the lesions continue to recur and results sometimes are cosmetically worse than the original lesions. Electrocautery, electrodesiccation, and dermabrasion all may result in minimal-to-moderate improvement. Advise the patient that recurrences in or near scars might replace the removed tumor.

These rules also apply to *syringomas,* which are small, benign, flesh-colored papules that occur in the periorbital area, primarily during adolescence, and to *steatocystoma multiplex.*

Supernumerary nipples enlarge around the time of puberty and can be excised at the patient's request.

DERMAL TUMORS

Keloids occur primarily on the chest, shoulders, and ears in children, especially in blacks. Pedunculated keloids can be excised deeply at the base and injected immediately after the excision and at 6-week intervals if lesions continue to grow.

Most sessile keloids are treated with steroid injections in an attempt to flatten them. Large keloids are best treated by surgeons experienced in plastic repair and steroid physiology. Irradiation may be advocated as a last resort to prevent grotesque deformities from occurring. The larger the lesion, the more difficult is the treatment.

Dermatofibromas occur most often on the limbs, mainly the legs. The lesions dimple when compressed laterally, and the surrounding skin rides up over the edges. Because they tend to become darker and firmer with age, it is best to remove them upon request. Most conform to the circular pattern of a punch biopsy, so that usually a single suture will hold the edges of the lesion together in healing position.

Skin tags (*fibroepitheliomas*) are found in the intertriginous areas of obese children and adults. Pseudoacanthosis nigricans may be a concomitant finding. Tags are gently pulled perpendicularly from the skin and the base is snipped and lightly electrodesiccated.

Adenoma sebaceum is a dominantly inherited condition in which flesh-colored papules (angiofibromas) begin in the nasolabial area at puberty. The lesions spread on the cheeks and are often confused with unrelenting acne. Dermabrasion or light electrodesiccation is of variable and sometimes of only temporary value. More important is genetic counseling and avoidance of hydantoin derivatives, estrogens, and pregnancy. The hydantoin drugs produce fibrosis and cause the tumors associated with this condition to grow.

Neurofibromatosis is another dominantly inherited condition in which patients need genetic counseling. Here, too, they should avoid hydantoins, estrogens, and pregnancy. Large lesions require surgical intervention. Enlarged plexiform lesions should be removed to reduce even the small incidence of subsequent fibrosarcoma.

Juvenile xanthogranulomas are yellow-tan nodules, which appear between 2 and 20 months of age and resolve spontaneously, often before the child starts school. Because ocular and internal lesions can occur (which also resolve spontaneously), slit lamp examination, chest radiographs, and examination of the testicles are also recommended as part of the management. After the diagnosis is established, no therapy is required other than ophthalmologic followup.

Urticaria pigmentosa, in the nodular stage, can appear identical to juvenile xanthogranuloma. Urtication after stroking is diagnostic, but histologic confirmation by biopsy is better. The majority of cases occur in the first year of life, mostly as single lesions. Bullous lesions occur in the early months; the lesions at that time may be more symptomatic than after 1 to 2 years. Parents should be advised that the symptoms abate after about 2 years of age, but that lesions may remain until puberty. Children with numerous lesions should avoid morphine and related narcotics, aspirin, alcohol, and polymyxin, as these may cause mast cell degranulation and the symptoms of vasodilation. Infants and children with numerous lesions should be screened by bone scan and, if symptomatic, should undergo gastrointestinal survey and hematologic evaluation.

SUBCUTANEOUS TUMORS

Lipoma is a raised, soft, mobile, flesh-colored mass that usually does not dimple when it is moved. Stable, small, asymptomatic lesions require no therapy unless the patient desires removal. Cosmetic excision of large lesions may result in a slightly depressed area.

Infantile digital fibromatoses are benign, invasive, skin-colored nodules on the dorsal or lateral surfaces of the distal fingers and toes. Most occur in infants less than 1 year of age. The lesions may be solitary or multiple and are often asymptomatic. They can be destructive and cause flexion deformities of the distal digits. Diagnosis is confirmed by histology. After local excision, 60% of lesions re-

cur; occasionally the lesions regress spontaneously. Therefore, in cases of nongrowing, asymptomatic lesions it is best to observe the lesion for many months before advising surgery.

Collagenoma and *juvenile elastoma* are connective tissue nevi, that is, localized malformations of either collagen or elastic fibers. Some are inherited. They appear as clusters of slightly raised, skin-colored, ovoid lesions scattered symmetrically over the abdomen, back, buttocks, arms, and thighs. After histologic confirmation, no therapy is required or effective.

Mucosal neuroma syndrome (Sipple syndrome) is a dominantly inherited condition in which patients with a marfanoid habitus have multiple tiny nodules of the outer third of the tongue, extending onto the buccal mucosa and to the commissures of the lips. Ocular and gastrointestinal abnormalities are also commonly found. Of extreme importance is the high incidence of medullary thyroid carcinoma associated with high calcitonin levels, pheochromocytoma, and hyperparathyroidism—the latter probably representing a compensatory response to the high levels of circulating calcitonin. Management is by periodic screening for the associated malignant tumors.

The Genodermatoses

JOSEPH C. ALPER, M.D.

Although many of the heritable cutaneous diseases are not amenable to specific therapy, recent advances in basic pharmacologic research combined with clinical trials have enabled us to treat diseases which, only a few years ago, could be no more than palliated. For those disorders that do not respond to specific drug therapy, the approach is still that of classic clinical genetics.

Before addressing the therapy of individual genodermatoses, it is important to discuss briefly a relatively new class of drugs that is going to be used in the near future to treat both genetic and nongenetic skin disease. These agents will have particular use in heritable cutaneous disorders associated with excess production of stratum corneum. Within this group of diseases are found the most common and most severely disfiguring of the genodermatoses.

These new drugs are referred to as the substituted aromatic retinoids. They are formed by a variety of chemical alterations either on the side chain or on the aromatic ring of retinoic acid. Although these drugs are available for experimental use only, preliminary data indicate that the different structural variants have slightly different side effects and that their effectiveness varies depending on the type of disease being treated.

The exact mechanism of action of these compounds in diseases of excess or abnormal keratinization is unknown. Numerous effects of the various derivatives have been elucidated, one of which is to allow normal cellular differentiation. This might explain the benefits seen in the disorders under consideration here.

The dosage varies from 0.5 mg/kg to about 4 mg/kg for most of the congeners. Unlike naturally occurring vitamin A compounds, the new synthetic analogs are not stored in the liver but are rapidly metabolized and excreted. Thus, toxicity is less than with the natural vitamin.

Side effects are quite common but are usually mild and do not require cessation of the drug. The two most prevalent toxic manifestations are cheilitis and conjunctivitis, which are seen in almost every patient. Next in order are skin fragility, facial dermatitis, xerosis, rhinitis sicca with nose-bleed, and fingertip peeling. Unusual side effects include itching, headache, appetite change, hair loss, urethritis, dry mouth, and punctate corneal keratitis. However, the actual incidence of these manifestations does vary from one study to another and also varies with the type of analog used.

Very few children have been treated with this new class of drugs and, therefore, long-term toxicity has not been assessed. For the time being, these agents are not being recommended for use in children or in women of childbearing age unless they are following contraceptive measures. As more experience with the drugs is gathered, these recommendations may change.

THE ICHTHYOSES

Although a large number of congenital disorders are associated with generalized ichthyosis, the pediatrician is likely to encounter four main types: ichthyosis vulgaris (autosomal dominant), sex-linked ichthyosis, epidermolytic hyperkeratosis (bullous congenital ichthyosiform erythroderma—autosomal dominant), and lamellar ichthyosis (non-bullous congenital ichthyosiform erythroderma—autosomal recessive).

The rationale behind most therapy directed at the ichthyoses is similar; hydration of the stratum corneum and removal of the scale. In addition, attempts at slowing epidermal turnover are made in the two hyperproliferative disorders. General principles of therapy will be discussed first and, whenever appropriate, therapy of a specific ichthyosis will be discussed next.

Since hydration of stratum corneum is of paramount importance, the therapy of all the ichthyoses should begin with soaking. This can be accomplished in a tub or shower, with optimal hydration occurring in about 15 minutes (as evidenced by wrinkling of the skin of the palmar surfaces of the fingertips). After this hydration has occurred, the skin is softer and will remain pliable as long as it is hydrated. In addition, any medication applied to the skin surface will penetrate moist stratum corneum more readily than dry.

The easiest and least expensive method of treating the normoproliferative ichthyoses is to apply plain petrolatum to the skin surface after soaking. This can be done once or twice a day and will keep the skin surface moist and supple. Additional benefit can be obtained by adding 3 to 6 per cent salicylic acid to the petrolatum. The only drawback to this form of therapy is that it is very greasy and messy. Therefore, it is poorly tolerated by most children.

Because of the messiness of petrolatum, a number of other vehicles with a variety of medicaments have been formulated. These include vanishing cream bases and gels (clear cellulose jellies). Urea can be incorporated into a variety of vanishing creams in concentrations of 10 to 20%. When applied to hydrated skin, urea imparts a feeling of smoothness, ostensibly by increasing the water content of the stratum corneum. It can be used once or twice a day with excellent success in the mild-to-moderately severe normoproliferative ichthyoses.

The α-hydroxy acids have also been used with good results in ichthyosis vulgaris, X-linked ichthyosis, and mild lamellar ichthyosis. Lactic acid in concentrations of 2.5 to 5% is most commonly used; one proprietary lotion, called U-Lactin, is combined with 10% urea. Application to hydrated skin is important to avoid irritation. The mechanism of action is probably keratolysis (removal of stratum corneum), similar to that of salicylic acid.

Propylene glycol in concentrations of 40 to 60%, either alone or in combination with 3 to 6% salicylic acid, is an excellent keratolytic agent, particularly for ichthyosis vulgaris, X-linked ichthyosis, and lamellar ichthyosis. It must be applied to hydrated skin while the skin is dripping wet. As it is rubbed in, large sheets of stratum corneum will come peeling off. Keralyt is available as 60% propylene glycol and 6% salicylic acid in a gel base and is particularly effective in X-linked ichthyosis. After 4 or 5 nights of Saran Wrap occlusion over Keralyt, the ichthyosis essentially disappears and will remain clear for about 1 to 2 weeks without further therapy. At this point, it is important to indicate that any salicylic acid preparation should be applied to the skin of young children with extreme caution, particularly when used under Saran Wrap occlusion. It is possible to cause salicylate toxicity in this setting. It is recommended that no more than one tube of Keralyt be used per day and that only limited areas of the body be occluded at any one time.

Vitamin A acid (retinoic acid) in a vanishing cream base in concentrations of 0.05 to 0.1% can be very effective in lamellar ichthyosis, particularly on the face. It is started at the lower concentrations and used once or twice a day to tolerance. The most frequent side effect is skin irritation.

In epidermolytic hyperkeratosis, the most frequent cause of morbidity associated with the ichthyosis is infection within the crypts of the keratotic furrows. When this produces objectionable odor or blistering, either topical or systemic antibiotics can be used.

The drugs which, it is hoped, will revolutionize the therapy of the hyperproliferative ichthyoses are the synthetic retinoids. Lamellar ichthyosis has been treated very successfully to almost complete clearing in some patients. Unfortunately, epidermolytic hyperkeratosis has not responded as well. Perhaps other substituted retinoids will be more effective. It should be re-emphasized that long-term toxicity in children has not yet been determined.

PALMOPLANTAR KERATODERMAS

These are a large, heterogeneous group of disorders with either punctate or diffuse thickening of the stratum corneum of the palms, soles, or both. Therapy is similar to that of the ichthyoses but the keratodermas are much more difficult to treat effectively. Since the palms and soles are frequently exposed to friction and trauma, there is a continual stimulus to produce more thickening. Therefore, mechanical removal of thickened stratum corneum is often necessary to create an optimal response. This can best be accomplished by first soaking the hands or feet, then applying a good keratolytic agent such as Keralyt gel and rubbing lightly with a pumice stone, all done while the skin is wet. An alternative to the pumice stone is actual paring with a blade, but this is obviously fraught with more hazard.

Topical application of retinoic acid cream, 0.05 to 0.1%, alternating on opposite nights with Keralyt under Saran Wrap occlusion may be quite helpful in softening and removing excess stratum corneum.

DARIER DISEASE (KERATOSIS FOLLICULARIS)

Darier disease is an autosomal dominant disorder with usual onset at the end of the first decade of life. Topical therapy with retinoic acid cream is remarkably effective, particularly when used under Saran Wrap occlusion. This form of therapy, however, is limited by irritation. Salicylic acid (3 to 6%) in cream or gel base can also be effective when used on hydrated skin under occlusion as described in the section on the ichthyoses. Ointments are to be avoided since they become trapped in the crypts of verrucous plaques with subsequent maceration and rancidity. Occasionally, the verrucous plaques of the scalp, ears, or trunk may become infected.

Treatment is then initiated with either topical or systemic antibacterial agents.

Systemic therapy with large doses of vitamin A (200,000 units or more) either alone or in combination with vitamin E has been used with variable results. Because of the significant hepatotoxicity associated with high doses of vitamin A, this form of therapy cannot be recommended for use in Darier disease. Several series have been reported with the use of the synthetic retinoids, however. Thus far, the results have been excellent, with marked improvement in the majority of patients who were treated. Very few side effects were noted, particularly with one specific congener. It is hoped that a structural form of the drug that can be used safely in children will become available.

PACHYONYCHIA CONGENITA

Pachyonychia congenita is an autosomal dominant disorder of which the major manifestation is marked thickening of the nail beds, usually beginning shortly after birth. Ordinarily, all 20 nails are involved. During childhood, management of the nail disorder is difficult. Nails should be kept well-trimmed, and subungual debris should be removed as completely and as carefully as possible. In spite of careful attention to the nails, subungual and paronychial infections do occur. Both pyogenic bacteria, such as *Staphylococcus aureus,* and the fungus *Monilia* can be found. Cultures should be obtained and appropriate therapy instituted. Systemic antibiotics are required for staphylococcal infections and topical antiyeast solutions, such as Lotrimin lotion, for *Monilia.*

If recurrent infections of the nails become troublesome or if the degree of thickening interferes with fine function of the fingers, surgical ablation of the nail beds can be performed. Often, this leads to dramatic relief of symptoms.

Blistering of the skin is best controlled by attempting to minimize trauma. The skin should be kept well-lubricated to prevent drying with increased fragility. As the child begins to walk, it is imperative to have well-fitted shoes. On occasion, consultation with a podiatrist or rehabilitation medicine physician with a special interest in sports medicine should be sought. Speical shoes can be made that will redistribute stress on the foot so that small areas are not subjected to all the friction of weight bearing.

The hyperkeratotic lesions that develop in the older child and adolescent are treated as described in the discussion of palmoplantar keratodermas. In addition, special shoes should be made for these patients. On occasion, it is necessary for a person who develops marked keratoderma of the soles (sometimes associated with blistering underneath the thickened stratum corneum) to severely curtail all activity such as walking or even standing. As these people get older, they often require a sedentary job in order to reduce friction on the soles.

EPIDERMOLYSIS BULLOSA (MECHANOBULLOUS DISORDERS)

The term epidermolysis bullosa is actually a generic one and encompasses at least five distinct genetic disorders. These include three nonscarring variants and two scarring types. The former include epidermolysis bullosa simplex (autosomal dominant), epidermolysis bullosa letalis (autosomal recessive), and recurrent bullous eruption of the hands and feet (autosomal dominant). The latter two include autosomal dominant and autosomal recessive dystrophic forms. Certain modalities of therapy are used commonly in all the variants and will be discussed first. Where appropriate, specific therapy for individual disorders will be discussed next.

Most of the morbidity in these diseases is caused by blistering and erosion of the skin. This occurs most prominently over areas exposed to friction and trauma and is particularly severe during infancy and early childhood. Therefore, therapy should initially be directed at preventing the formation of blisters. A great deal of effort must be expended by the parents to arrange the infant's and young child's environment to reduce frictional trauma of the skin. As the children grow, they usually learn what types of activity they must avoid in order to reduce the amount of blistering.

For the infant, the entire crib must be padded with soft material and a soft covering put over the mattress. Only soft, well-washed cloth diapers should be used and closed with tape rather than pins. If possible, rubber pants should be avoided, particularly ones that fit tightly around the waist and thighs. Clothing should be of a soft cloth material and should be loose-fitting. Strollers and carriages should also be padded. Only soft or pliable toys should be used. A soft, nonabrasive surface should be provided when the infant begins to crawl. As the child begins to walk, it is important to have well-fitting, cushioned shoes. Consultation with a sports medicine podiatrist or rehabilitation medicine physician may be necessary.

When blisters do form, they should be aspirated aseptically with needle and syringe. The blister roof is left intact to provide a covering over the denuded base. A new water vapor-permeable membrane called Op-Site has recently become available in the United States. Studies that may prove very useful in epidermolysis bullosa are under way at present with this wound dressing.

If superficial erosions become infected, the crusts should be gently soaked off with sterile saline. The area should be patted dry and an antibiotic or povidone-iodine ointment applied. Neomycin-containing ointments should be avoided for long-term use because of their sensitizing potential.

In general, blistering appears to be worse during warm weather. Therefore, the environment should be kept as cool as possible and the child not overdressed.

Oral erosions are troublesome during infancy in all forms of epidermolysis bullosa. However, oral disease is much more severe, persists in adult life, and is associated with esophageal erosion in the recessive, dystrophic variety. During infancy, extreme caution must be observed during feeding. Only soft rubber syringes should be used rather than the standard rubber nipple bottle. The bulb syringe used for feeding infants with cleft palate before repair is often helpful.

As the infant with the recessive dystrophic disease grows, cereal thinned with milk must be used. Later, puréed foods have to be utilized to decrease mechanical trauma to the mouth and esophagus. In spite of all these measures, however, oral and esophageal stricture does occur and may require esophageal bougienage.

Because of the difficulty in eating and also because of loss of nutrients from eroded skin, children with recessive, scarring epidermolysis bullosa often have difficulty maintaining adequate nutrition. Therefore, they require dietary supplementation with high-protein liquid substances and also liquid vitamin preparations that contain therapeutic amounts of iron.

Large doses of systemic vitamin E have been used in the past in the two dystrophic varieties of the disease. The results are extremely variable, and most investigators are unable to confirm beneficial results in large numbers of these patients.

Systemic steroids have been used with some benefit in essentially all the groups of epidermolysis bullosa. In general, the long-term side effects far outweigh the benefits. In epidermolysis bullosa letalis, however, they can be used for short periods to control the intermittent flares of the disease. In this particular setting, systemic steroids can often be life-saving.

Plastic surgical repair of the disfiguring "glove of skin" manifestation that occurs in the recessive scarring variety must be done early and repeatedly. Otherwise, the disease that occurs is associated with resorption of the phalanges and permanent loss of function of the hand.

Lastly, on a more positive note, some cases of recessive dystrophic epidermolysis bullosa have responded successfully to systemic drug therapy. It has been determined in this variant that there is an increased production of an abnormal type of collagenase. This has occurred both in vivo and in fibroblast cell cultures derived from skin biopsies of these patients. It is also known that phenytoin can inhibit collagenase. This drug was used to treat 17 unselected patients with the disease from two separate institutions. The published results were quite dramatic, with at least a 45% reduction in blistering in 12 of the 17 patients. Five patients did not respond. It is hoped that further elucidation of the biochemical defect in this and the other variants of the disease will allow rational therapy of more people with this group of disorders.

HAILEY AND HAILEY DISEASE (BENIGN FAMILIAL PEMPHIGUS)

Hailey and Hailey disease is an autosomal dominant blistering disorder with usual onset in the second and third decade. However, on occasion, with appropriate stimuli, the disease may appear in children. Exacerbations commonly occur during the hot summer months and appear as small vesicles or, more usually, as superficial crusted erosions in intertriginous areas.

Therapy should be directed at the environmental factors that tend to cause the disease to flare. Bacterial superinfection often causes worsening of symptoms. Either topical or systemic antibiotics can be useful. If topical antibiotics are used, they should be in a solution vehicle since ointments only tend to cause moisture trapping, maceration, and deterioration of the disease. Although systemic tetracycline tends to be the drug of first choice, bacterial resistance occurs rapidly. Therefore, cultures with sensitivities should be obtained before initiating therapy. *Monilia* infections can complicate the disease and should be treated with appropriate antiyeast creams.

The intertriginous areas should be kept as cool and dry as possible. Excessive exercise should be avoided, and loose-fitting cotton clothing should be worn. If possible, the house or, at least, the bedroom should be air conditioned during the summer. The predisposed areas should also be kept clean by light washing with an antibacterial soap. When disease begins to flare, an excellent drying agent is a 10% aqueous solution of aluminum chloride. This may sting slightly during the first few applications. Once it is well tolerated, the concentration can be increased to 15, 20, or even 25%.

Corticosteroids have been used with variable success. Systemic administration is to be avoided because of severe rebound flare of the disease upon tapering. Topical steroids seem to have only transient benefit and should be used for only short periods of time.

ACRODERMATITIS ENTEROPATHICA

Acrodermatitis enteropathica is an autosomal recessive disorder of abnormal zinc absorption. All of the symptoms of severe diarrhea, acral and orifical erosions, alopecia, and emotional disturbances can be explained by zinc deficiency. It appears that a specific zinc-binding ligand is absent from the affected child's intestine but is supplied by breast milk.

Although the disease is essentially "cured" by systemic zinc administration, it is of interest to briefly review the historical therapy of the disease. The drug diiodohydroxyquinoline was first used in the early 1950s with good success and continued to be the main modality of therapy for about 20 years. Its use became sharply curtailed with the advent of several reports of optic atrophy and corneal opacities secondary to its use. It has recently been hypothesized that the ocular lesions may, indeed, be secondary to zinc deficiency and not the drug. Human breast milk has also been used as therapy in the past, either by prolonging breast feeding or by obtaining breast milk and bottling it.

In the early 1970s, it was found that the patients all had low serum zinc levels and that the disease responded dramatically to zinc supplementation. Therapy can be started with 100 mg to 150 mg daily of zinc sulfate. (Lower doses may be adequate in some patients.*) After complete improvement, the drug can be tapered to the lowest effective dose. Improvement in temperament and irritability usually occurs within 1 to 2 days of initiating therapy. Appetite increases in a few days, and the skin begins to improve in 2 to 3 days. Diarrhea decreases in a few days, and hair growth begins in 2 to 3 weeks. An increase in growth occurs in about 2 months. Thus far, there has been no toxicity associated with zinc administration.

MISCELLANEOUS DISORDERS

In several other genodermatoses, therapeutic intervention offers little or no benefit. They are mentioned here for the sake of completeness and in the hope that future editions of this volume will have more to offer.

Anhidrotic Ectodermal Dysplasia. This is an X-linked disorder with partial expression in the carrier females. Absence of sweating, hypotrichosis, abnormal teeth, and deficient lacrimation are the most striking features of the disorder. The patients also have frontal bossing and hypoplasia of the midface, giving them a characteristic facies. The lacrimation defect can easily be treated by the use of artificial tears. The anhidrosis leads to more serious problems, particularly hyperpyrexia during warm weather. During this time of the year the children should be kept cool, often having to spend many hours soaking in a cool tub. Air conditioning may be a necessity. Excessive exercise should be avoided, and febrile illnesses should be treated aggressively with antipyretics. With attention to these details, a normal life is possible.

Hidrotic Ectodermal Dysplasia. In this autosomal dominant disorder, sweating is normal or only slightly decreased. Other characteristic features are hypoplasia of the nails, sparse hair, and hyperkeratosis of the palms and soles. Therapy of the

---

*The manufacturer's recommended dosage for adults is 15 to 20 mg daily.

latter is the same as described for the palmoplantar keratodermas.

Goltz Syndrome. This disorder is either X-linked dominant with lethality in the male or autosomal dominant with sex limitation. The hallmark of the disease is linear areas of thinning of the dermis, with herniation of the underlying fat through the thin skin. Other findings are red papillomas around the mouth, anus, vulva, gingiva, and tongue; a variety of eye anomalies; mental retardation; and a host of limb reduction anomalies, particularly of the upper extremities. Only the papillomatous lesions are amenable to therapy. Various destructive modalities can be tried, including liquid nitrogen, bichloracetic acid, electrodesiccation, or 25 per cent podophyllin resin. However, recurrences are frequent.

Incontinentia Pigmenti. Incontinentia pigmenti is also either X-linked dominant or sex-limited autosomal dominant. A bullous and a verrucous stage are present in infancy and give way to the typical swirly truncal pigmentation at about 6 months of age. Other anomalies include ocular defects, skeletal abnormalities, faulty dentition, and central nervous system problems. At present, there is no effective therapy for any part of the syndrome except for genetic counseling of the carrier females.

Disorders of the Hair and Scalp

ANNE W. LUCKY, M.D.

INFECTIOUS DISEASES

Bacterial Folliculitis and Impetigo of the Scalp. Scalp folliculitis is most commonly caused by *Staphylococcus aureus* and less commonly by Group A *beta hemolytic streptococci.* Clinically the primary lesions are pustules surrounding hair follicles, but secondary erythema, oozing, crusting, edema, tenderness, and ultimately, abscess formation with cervical lymphadenopathy are common. Predisposing factors include occlusion by greasy hair preparations, impetigo, and trauma. Bacterial folliculitis must be distinguished from a kerion, a hypersensitivity reaction to fungal infection. A diagnosis of folliculitis is confirmed by culturing the pustules. Fungal and bacterial disease may coexist. Treatment should be tailored to the particular bacterial organism found on culture using systemic antibiotics such as erythromycin in doses of 30 to 50 mg/kg/day or dicloxacillin in doses of 25 to 100 mg/kg/day orally for *S. aureus* and penicillin V in doses of 250 to 500 mg/kg/day for streptococcal infections. A 10 to 14 day course is usually sufficient but may be prolonged if infection lingers. Adjunctive local care should consist of a keratolytic shampoo (see seborrheic dermatitis) when scale is present and warm soaks with an antiseptic such as

Burow's solution to remove accumulated crusts. The family should be instructed in careful hygiene, separating the infected patient's personal items (i.e., towels, combs, and hats) from those of other family members until infection has cleared. Resistant or recurrent cases may result if pathogenic organisms are harbored in the nasopharynx or on the skin of the patient or close contacts. Nasopharyngeal colonization requires topical therapy with an antibiotic ointment such as bacitracin or polymyxin (Polysporin).

Seborrheic Dermatitis, Eczema, and Psoriasis. Seborrheic dermatitis (cradle cap) and atopic dermatitis (eczema) involving the scalp are similar clinically and pathogenetically and will be considered together. "Cradle cap" of infancy is responsive to therapy. If scaling and pruritus persist or appear in later childhood we often consider that the entire picture had been a manifestation of atopic dermatitis. The typical lesions are adherent, greasy, white to yellow scales, which appear first in patches on the scalp and eventually may cover the entire scalp surface. The scalp is pruritic, and secondary excoriations with infection are frequent. There is erythema, scale, fissuring and weeping behind the ears. Greasy yellow scales and erythema can be found in the eyebrows, along the nasolabial folds, in the neck folds, axillae, and groin. Tinea capitis due to *Trichophyton tonsurans* must always be considered in the differential diagnosis of seborrheic dermatitis. Treatment consists of antiseborrheic shampoos that may contain any of a number of products to reduce itching, scaling, and erythema. Such products include sulfur and salicylic acid, pyrithione zinc, coal tar, and selenium sulfide. The shampoo should be applied daily to the scalp and left on for at least 5 minutes before washing off. This should be continued until all scale is removed. Shampooing can be reduced in frequency as clinical improvement occurs. In persistent cases, overnight applications of a phenol and saline solution (Baker's P&S) is helpful in removing excessive scale. If antiseborrheic shampoos irritate the scalp, a mild, bland shampoo plus topical steroid lotions such as 1% hydrocortisone lotion or, in severe cases, 0.1% triamcinolone lotion will hasten resolution and rapidly bring relief of pruritus.

Psoriasis may appear in childhood as single or multiple stubborn plaques of scale in the scalp or as generalized scaling. Erythematous plaques with silvery scale may be present on elbows, knees, genitalia, and intergluteal clefts and diaper area in infants. Nails are often studded with 1 mm pits. Psoriasis is usually not as pruritic as atopic dermatitis. Scalp lesions may be the only sign of psoriasis in childhood. Treatment of scalp psoriasis is similar to that outlined for seborrheic dermatitis with tar shampoos and topical steroids being especially useful.

Tinea Capitis (Scalp Ringworm). Tinea capitis is fungal infection of the scalp and hair shaft. *Trichophyton tonsurans* is now the infective agent in over 90% of cases in many areas of the U.S.A., whereas *Microsporum audouinii* once was the primary dermatophyte. A few cases acquired from kittens and puppies are caused by *Microsporum canis*. The most common presentation is diffuse scaling mimicking seborrheic dermatitis with patchy and diffuse hair loss. Since *T. tonsurans* invades the hair shafts (endothrix infection), hairs becomes fragile and break at the level of the scalp, leaving characteristic "black dots." *T. tonsurans* differs from *Microsporum* infection in that it does *not* fluoresce with Wood's light examination and is *not* limited to prepubertal children. *T. tonsurans* is a chronic disorder, carried asymptomatically by many children. It can produce lesions on the skin (tinea corporis) which serve as reservoirs of infection. In some cases, an inflammatory reaction, a kerion, may occur. A kerion is a boggy, erythematous, tender mass studded with perifollicular pustules. These pustules may be sterile or contain *S. aureus*. A kerion is the host's cellular immune response to the fungal infection. Systemic symptoms such as fever, diffuse maculopapular rash (or "id"), leukocytosis, and lymphadenopathy may accompany a kerion.

The only effective treatment is systemic griseofulvin. Topical antifungal agents are ineffective. Griseofulvin (microsize) is given in doses 10 to 20 mg/kg/day. It is available as a suspension (Grifulvin V, 125 mg/tsp) or appropriately sized capsules may be opened and fed to young children who cannot swallow tablets. Absorption is enchanced by a fatty meal (i.e., milk, ice cream, yogurt). Adjunctive therapy includes 2.5% selenium sulfide lotion (Selsun Brown, Excel) used as a shampoo twice weekly. This acts as a sporicidal agent and reduces shedding of spores significantly. The role of topical antifungal agents, such as clotrimazole (Lotrimin, Mycelex), haloprogen (Halotex), and miconidazole (MicaTin) is unclear. With systemic griseofulvin treatment it usually requires 6 to 8 weeks for fungal cultures to become negative. In refractory cases, the dose of griseofulvin should be raised and the length of treatment increased. Complete blood counts and liver function tests may or may not be measured when treatment is initiated, but should certainly be followed with prolonged therapy or therapy at increased dosage. Treatment of a kerion requires griseofulvin and systemic antibiotics if secondary infection with *S. aureus* is documented. Systemic or intralesional glucocorticoids have been advocated by some physicians to hasten resolution of kerions, but there are no data to support the contention that kerions resolve faster or that scarring is reduced. Ketoconazole is a relatively new systemic agent that may be useful for tinea capitis but is not yet approved for this purpose.

SCARRING ALOPECIAS

Cutis Aplasia Congenita. Congenital absence of the skin in single or multiple patches on the scalp leaves a thin, shiny, parchment-like hairless scar that is prone to breakdown and secondary infection and crust formation. Such lesions are often mistaken for trauma secondary to a fetal monitor. Underlying bony defects may be present and skull x-rays should be taken. In later life, excision of small lesions that do not have underlying skeletal defects may be warranted for cosmetic purposes. Nonhealing lesions may require excision and primary closure or grafting in infancy.

Nevus Sebaceus of Jadassohn. Nevus sebaceus is a benign skin hamartoma. There is overgrowth of sebaceous and apocrine elements and underdevelopment of hair follicles. Such lesions are present at birth and are usually found on the scalp and face. Nevus sebaceus is one of the main causes of localized congenital alopecia. The lesions are yellow to orange pebbly plaques that become more prominent at puberty. In the fourth and fifth decades of life tumors such as basal cell epitheliomas or squamous cell carcinomas may develop. Because of the cosmetic appearance and the malignant potential, excision in the prepubertal years is recommended. Excision prior to that time may not fully remove the lesion since the borders may be difficult to define.

Other Scarring Alopecias. Scarring alopecias may occur as a result of a number of infections and inflammatory disorders affecting the scalp such as bacterial folliculitis and tinea capitis. Systemic disorders such as lupus erythematosus, morphea, and lichen planus can result in permanent hair loss. Scarring alopecia of unknown etiology leaving a "footprint in the snow" pattern has been termed pseudopelade of Brocq. Traction from tight braids or pony tails may at first cause transient hair loss, but eventually will permanently destroy hair follicles. No therapy short of localized hair transplantation is effective.

NON-SCARRING ALOPECIAS

Alopecia Areata. Alopecia areata is one of the most common causes of alopecia in childhood. It is probably autoimmune in origin. There is a spectrum from single to multiple coin-sized areas of spontaneous complete hair loss (alopecia areata), to total loss of all scalp hair (alopecia totalis), to universal loss of scalp and body hair (alopecia universalis). Occasionally diffuse hair loss precedes the patchy lesions. Histopathologically, alopecia areata is characterized by swarms of lymphocytes surrounding the hair bulb. Other autoimmune disorders such as vitiligo, Hashimoto's thyroiditis, diabetes, and hypoparathyroidism may be associated with alopecia areata. Many patients will have characteristic linear pitting of the nails. Alopecia areata has spontaneous remissions and exacerbations. Theories that alopecia areata is a psychosomatic disorder have not been well substantiated. As a rule, the younger the child and the more extensive the hair loss, the less likely it is that regrowth will occur. Loss in the ophiasis pattern, around the margins of the scalp, also indicates a poor prognosis.

Treatment must be individualized and is often not successful. Therapy with intralesional steroids (triamcinolone acetonide, 1 ml of 5 to 10 mg/ml suspension) can be successful in limited cases, but may require multiple and repeated courses of therapy. No more than 10 mg of triamcinolone should be given every 4 to 6 weeks to avoid systemic effects from the intralesional steroids. High-potency topical steroids may be useful in a child too young or too afraid to cooperate with intralesional injections. Systemic steroids are *not* recommended in growing children. There are serious side effects, not the least of which is growth retardation. Even if systemic steroid therapy is successful in allowing regrowth of hair, when the steroids are tapered hair loss usually recurs. Newer forms of therapy promoted in the recent literature include sensitization to dinitrochlorobenzene (DNCB) with subsequent application of DNCB to the affected areas of the scalp to produce a contact dermatitis and hypersensitivity reaction. (This form of therapy has raised questions about potentially stimulating the immune system and causing malignancy.) Simple irritation of the scalp with such substances as topical retinoic acid (Retin-A) have met with moderate success. Although some groups have advocated the use of systemic psoralens and ultraviolet A light (PUVA), the efficacy and safety of this procedure in childhood has not yet been established. Psychological adjustment of the child to alopecia areata is best reflected by the attitude of the parents and the physician. Support and encouragement without specific therapy is often the best treatment.

Traumatic Hair Loss. Traumatic hair loss is usually either self-induced by compulsive hair pulling (trichotillomania) or inappropriate use of hair cosmetics or hair styling. Hair loss secondary to trauma is usually nonscarring and is a combination of traction from the bulb and breakage of the shaft. Repeated trauma to the hair bulb may eventually cause permanent scarring alopecia. Trichotillomania appears as isolated or multiple areas of alopecia. It is identified by the presence of fractured, unevenly broken off, short hairs. It is a sign of underlying emotional or psychologic conflict and if persistent and severe, the family should be referred for appropriate counseling. It is often impossible to obtain a positive history of compulsive hair pulling from parent or child. Traction alopecia occurs primarily in small children whose hair is kept in tight braids or pony tails. Rubber bands can sever the hair shafts, but the traction itself will cause disrup-

tion of the hair bulb and a permanent hair loss pattern, especially around the scalp margins. The only treatment is advice on hair styling. Overzealous cosmetic treatments can produce broken hairs, secondary to increased fragility. Home permanent waves, chemical hair straighteners, blow dryers, and hot combs are major causes of traumatic hair loss. In this condition the number and density of hairs in the scalp are normal but the hairs are broken. Discontinuation of all treatment to the hair except a mild shampoo and conditioner is warranted. Conditioners render the hair easier to comb with fewer tangles. Hair is more fragile when wet and thus combing should be done after drying.

Diffuse Hair Loss. Diffuse hair loss may result from a wide variety of causes. Normal hair loss occurs at the rate of 100 hairs per day. Thinning of the scalp hair may not be noticeable until a large percentage of scalp hair is gone, and thus increased shedding of hair may be the initial complaint. Telogen effluvium is the term used for the phenomenon of a large number of hairs going into the resting (telogen) stage of growth at the same time and then falling out. Telogen effluvium may follow 2 to 3 months after a severe illness with high fever (e.g., typhoid fever, scarlet fever, or Kawasaki disease). It is physiologic in infants and their mothers approximately 3 months postpartum. Occasionally alopecia areata may begin with diffuse hair loss. Endocrine causes such as hypo- or hyperthyroidism and excessive masculinizing levels of androgens from ovarian or adrenal origin may present with diffuse hair loss. Female pattern baldness or so-called "androgenetic" alopecia consists of thinning of the hair predominantly over the crown of the scalp. It may be a familial trait or result from elevated circulating plasma androgens in teenage girls. Deficiencies of trace elements such as zinc or iron, essential fatty acids, proteins, or multiple nutritional losses such as seen in marasmus or anorexia nervosa can produce diffuse hair loss. Finally, a careful history of drug exposure including thallium, mercury, propranolol, and chemotherapy or radiation therapy must be considered in differential diagnosis. Treatment depends on discovering the underlying cause.

Disorders of Sebaceous Glands and Sweat Glands

ANNE W. LUCKY, M.D.

DISORDERS OF SEBACEOUS GLANDS

Acne. Acne vulgaris affects nearly all adolescents at some time during puberty, starting as early as 8 years of age. The basic lesion is a *comedo*, which is a plugged sebaceous follicle. Comedones may be closed (whiteheads) or open (blackheads) to the surface of the skin. Comedones form under the stimulatory influence of androgens on the sebaceous glands at puberty. Increased growth of bacterial flora of the face *(Propionibacterium acnes)* and an acceleration of the immune response on the part of the host to this infection results in inflammation and pustule formation producing *papules* and *pustules.* When papules or pustules from single follicles coalesce into groups with multiple follicular openings and invade deep into the dermis, *nodules* and *cysts* are formed. The acne-prone areas of the body are the face, anterior chest, and back. The earliest acne lesions are comedones in the external ears and on the nose. Girls will often note flares of their acne 1 or 2 weeks prior to onset of menstrual periods. Acne usually improves dramatically in summer. Stress precipitates acne flares. Although acne is characteristically transient, there is a broad spectrum of severity.

There is no best treatment just as there is no single cause for acne. The causes are multiple and include endocrine, infectious, and immunologic factors. Occlusion with oily makeup or hair grease may exacerbate acne. There is little evidence that diet or dirt are factors. Therapy for the individual patient depends on the severity of the disease and the predominant type of lesion. The number of acne preparations available, both over the counter and by prescription, is overwhelming. It is advisable to become familiar with one or two products of each type. Therapy will be discussed on the basis of mild, moderate, and severe acne.

Mild acne is primarily comedonal with occasional papules and pustules. Benzoyl peroxide gels (2.5, 5, and 10%) are the first choice for treatment. Gels are more effective than lotions or washes but may cause more irritation. Benzoyl peroxide acts as a topical antibiotic to reduce local skin flora and seems to have anticomedonal action. Most often patients are started on a preparation of 5% benzoyl peroxide gel twice daily with increase or decrease in strength and/or frequency of applications depending on tolerance. Major side effects are redness and dryness of the skin. A small percentage of patients develop true contact allergy to benzoyl peroxide. Fair skinned individuals are more sensitive to benzoyl peroxide.

For more persistent or more numerous comedonal lesions, the use of topical retinoic acid (tretinoin; Retin-A) has made a marked difference in acne therapy in the last decade. Topical retinoic acid acts to prevent comedo formation by altering the faulty keratinization process that plugs the follicular orifice. Without comedones, there is no chance for secondary papules, pustules or cysts to develop. Topical retinoic acid comes in a cream (0.05% and 0.10%), a gel (0.01% and 0.025%), and a liquid (0.05%) form, which is the strongest. The cream is tolerated with the least amount of irritation. Therapy is begun with 0.05% Retin-A cream or 0.01% Retin-A gel once every second or third night. Application is advanced in strength and frequency to a nightly application as tolerated. Patients must be forewarned that they will look worse for the first few weeks of treatment because of erythema, peeling, and appearance of more acne lesions. The skin develops tolerance to the drug in the first month and the strength of the preparation can be increased. The back and chest are less sensitive than the face. It takes 3 months to judge whether the therapy is successful in preventing formation of new comedones. The combination of topical benzoyl peroxide and retinoic acid, each used once daily, appears to be very effective. Because of increased sensitivity to sun and a theoretical tumorigenic potential in animals when retinoic acid is used with ultraviolet light, many dermatologists discontinue topical retinoic acid during the summer months or at other times of intense exposure to sunlight.

Many topical antibiotics have become available in the past few years. Tetracycline, erythromycin, and clindamycin are all commercially available in alcoholic solutions. Their primary action appears to be to reduce bacterial colonization of the skin. Topical antibiotics can be applied once or twice daily alone or in combination with benzoyl peroxide or retinoic acid, or they may be reserved for cases in which the former combination is not tolerated. Topical tetracycline may fluoresce with "Disco" black lights.

For *moderate acne,* which includes more persistent and numerous papules and pustules in addition to comedones, systemic antibiotics are essential. They should be used in conjunction with the topical medications described above. The mainstay of systemic treatment for acne is tetracycline. It is used starting at 1 gram daily divided into four doses. Tetracycline is poorly absorbed with food and must be taken 30 minutes before or 2 hours after a meal. Dairy products are especially inhibitory to absorption. Minocycline,* close cogener of tetracycline, does not need to be taken on an empty stomach but is many times more expensive. It can be used in a dosage of 50 mg once or twice daily. Limitations of the use of the tetracyclines are gastrointestinal intolerance and vaginal candidiasis in some women. The latter may be treated with local antifungal preparations (nystatin, clotrimazole, or miconidazole) and the tetracycline continued. Tetracycline induces hepatic enzymes that also metabolize estrogens, and warnings that oral contraceptives may become less effective and that breakthrough bleeding may occur must be given to patients. Although tetracycline has been used safely in an enormous number of patients continuously for many years

---

*The use of tetracyclines during tooth development (last half of pregnancy to the age of 8 years) may cause permanent tooth discoloration.

without ill effect, there are occasional severe reactions such as photosensitivity and liver and renal abnormalities. In patients who do not tolerate tetracycline, erythromycin in a dose of 250 mg four times daily may be equally effective. As acne improves, the dose of medication is slowly reduced to a maintenance of 250 mg once daily of tetracycline or erythromycin, or 50 mg once daily of minocycline (Minocin). A course of oral antibiotics usually requires 9 to 12 months and premature withdrawal may result in exacerbation or recurrence of acne. In a rare few patients treated with long-term antibiotics, the facial flora may change to gram-negative organisms such as *E. coli, Pseudomonas,* or *Klebsiella.* Antibiotics such as trimethoprim and sulfamethoxazole (Bactrim) may be useful.

Severe acne, which is most often cystic in nature, is the most devastating and most difficult form to treat. It can be psychologically and socially crippling. It is most severe in males and is often familial. Cystic acne may take a chronic severe form called *acne conglobata* or an acute explosive form termed *acne fulminans.* In addition to high doses of systemic antibiotics, such as tetracycline or erythromycin, and topical treatment with benzoyl peroxide, retinoic acid, and topical antibiotics, systemic treatment with glucocorticosteroids or dapsone may be necessary to reduce acute inflammation in extreme cases. Individual cystic lesions respond well to cautious intralesional injections of steroids (triamcinolone acetonide 5–10 mg/ml), reducing the inflammatory response and hopefully preventing severe scarring. In September of 1982, an oral preparation of 13-cis-retinoic acid (Accutane) became available. A limited course of this potent drug lasting 10 to 16 weeks has produced prolonged remissions of severe cystic acne in clinical trials. However, there are troublesome side effects such as cheilitis, dry skin, and hypertriglyceridemia. It is extremely expensive. The use of Accutane should be limited to severe cystic acne treated by practitioners who use the drug enough to become familiar with the dosages and side effects.

There are many adjunctive treatments for acne that may help but are not essential to successful treatment. These include comedo extraction for cosmetic purposes, abrasive scrubs (which may be useful in some patients but often irritate and worsen lesions), sulphur preparations either in liquid form or as a mask, and various alcohol-containing astringents. Oil-containing makeup and/or hair grease should be eliminated from use. Although there are many so-called "acne" soaps on the market, patients should be advised simply to wash their faces two or three times daily with any mild soap. For scarring that remains after acne has become quiescent, new techniques such as dermabrasion, plastic repair, collagen implants, and autotransplants of plugs of skin may be useful. In some

females excessive production of androgenic hormones from the ovary (polycystic ovarian disease) or adrenal gland may contribute to acne flares or persistence of acne. Careful specific hormonal treatment such as estrogens (oral contraceptives) or low-dose glucocorticoids may be of use in well-documented selected cases of this type.

Sebaceous Hyperplasia of Infancy/Neonatal Acne. Infants in the first 6 months of life may have prominent sebaceous follicles and/or frank acneiform lesions, both of which spontaneously resolve. Maternal and endogenous androgen stimulation of sebaceous glands in the young infant are the presumed cause of these disorders. When hormone levels became normal in the first year of life, the skin lesions disappear. No treatment is necessary but 2.5 or 5% benzoyl peroxide may be appreciated in severe cases.

DISORDERS OF SWEAT GLANDS

Miliaria. Miliaria is caused by obstruction of the sweat ducts. *Miliaria crystallina* is seen often in the newborn as tiny (1 mm) crystal-clear vesicles that can be ruptured by gentle pressure on the skin surface, leaving a fine collarette of scale. It is caused by sweat duct obstruction high in the stratum corneum of the skin. Obstruction of the sweat ducts at a slightly lower level produces *miliaria rubra,* known as "prickly heat" or "heat rash." Miliaria rubra presents as 1 to 2 mm punctate red papules in occluded sweaty areas such as underarms, neck, chest or back. It may be quite pruritic. Treatment of both types of miliaria includes keeping the skin dry and cool. *Miliaria profunda* is deep obstruction in the eccrine ducts producing white papules on the skin and inhibition of normal sweating. It is seen in adolescents and young adults after extensive exercise and may lead to profound heat retention and collapse. Fortunately it is rare. Susceptible persons should avoid heat and strenuous exercise.

Hypohydrotic Ectodermal Dysplasia. The most common form of hypohydrotic ectodermal dysplasia is an X-linked recessive trait affecting only males. Patients are unable to sweat and have associated defects in hair, nails, and teeth. Such children may present in infancy with hyperpyrexia. It is important to recognize this disorder in order to prevent central nervous system damage. Patients should be counseled to avoid heat and strenuous exercise and to have immediate cooling in febrile illnesses by physical methods such as cold water and alcohol baths, as well as antipyretics.

Hyperhydrosis. Hyperhydrosis is exaggerated sweating of the palms, soles, and underarms. It is triggered by emotional as well as thermal stress. Aluminum chloride 20% (Dry Sol) applied once daily at bedtime may be very useful.

Pyodermas

JAMES J. LEYDEN, M.D.

Until relatively recently, there has been a great deal of confusion in the literature regarding which forms of pyoderma are caused by *Staphylococcus aureus* and *Streptococcus pyogenes*. The major sources of confusion and argument resulted from the frequent secondary colonization of streptococcal infections by *S. aureus*. Clinical-microbiologic correlations have been sufficiently studied that accurate clincal diagnosis and appropriate therapy should present little difficulty.

STAPHYLOCOCCUS AUREUS PYODERMAS

Folliculitis. Superficial follicular pustules with an areola of intense erythema are seen. This form of pyoderma can range from low grade (scattered pustules) to widespread (tender pustules with intense erythema). Localized forms will usually respond to tap water compresses (5 to 10 minutes tid), followed by topical antibiotics such as Neosporin cream or bacitracin or Polysporin ointment. More severe, widespread forms usually require compresses and systemic antibiotic therapy, such as erythromycin, 250 mg qid for 7 to 10 days, sodium oxacillin, 250 mg qid for a similar period.

Furuncles. Boils may range from isolated or scattered, relatively indolent lesions to angry, deep-seated, expanding lesions that may have associated fever and systemic toxicity. Localized nonaggressive lesions often respond to simple drainage or to warm compresses in conjunction with erythromycin or oxacillin, 250 mg qid for 10 days. More virulent, rapidly progressive lesions require penicillinase-resistant penicillin, such as oxacillin, 250 to 500 mg qid, or erythromycin 250 to 500 mg qid. The strain of *S. aureus* responsible for the latter is highly contagious, and one should inquire into the occurrence of boils in family members and sexual contacts. These strains also frequently colonize the anterior nares, and, when present, long-term (often 1 month or more) systemic antibiotic therapy along with topical antibiotics such as Neosporin or bacitracin applied twice daily to the anterior nares is required. Chronic furunculosis, in the absence of a reasonable explanation such as contact with someone with boils, is an indication to evaluate the patient for diabetes mellitus.

Bullous Impetigo. The hallmark of this condition is a superficial blister that rapidly ruptures and leaves behind a half-dollar-sized area with a second degree burn or scalded-skin look. This lesion results from the action of a particular toxin produced by a Group II phage type 71 *S. aureus*. If sufficient toxin is liberated, a generalized "scalded-skin syndrome" can result. Such patients are acutely ill and present the same problems that a widespread, second degree burn victim faces. Bullous impetigo should be treated with erythromycin or oxacillin, 250 to 500 mg qid for 7 to 10 days. Cool tap water compresses twice daily, followed by a topical antibiotic, help speed the recovery of superficial erosions. The scalded-skin syndrome may require hospitalization, systemic oxacillin (IV if the patient is so toxic that oral medication cannot be tolerated), attention to fluid and electrolyte balance, and careful observance for signs of infections. Fortunately this condition is usually short-lived (in contrast to the form induced by drug reactions), and recovery is expected.

STREPTOCOCCAL INFECTIONS

Ecthyma. This form of pyoderma is often improperly called "impetigo," a term which should be reserved for *S. aureus* bullous impetigo. This lesion characteristically occurs on the lower legs as a punched-out ulceration that develops a thick serous crust. Lymphadenopathy and fever are early signs and frequently present even when minimal lesions occur. There is a definite seasonal predilection (hot, muggy months), and local abrasions and insect bites are common associated findings. Lesions with fever and lymphadenopathy require erythromycin, 250 mg qid for 7 to 10 days, local tap water compresses to soak off the crust (*never scrub* away crusts: abrading skin retards wound healing), followed with topical bacitracin or Polysporin ointment. Localized superficial streptococcal lesions can be treated with compresses and topical antibiotics. There is no evidence to support the generally taught principle that systemic therapy will prevent postinfection glomerulonephritis if the strain is a so-called "nephritogenic" streptococcus.

Cellulitis. Deep-seated, infiltrative areas of tender erythema with fever and lymphadenopathy occur. Penicillin and erythromycin are extremely effective (e.g., phenoxymethyl penicillin or erythromycin, 250 to 500 mg orally qid for 7 to 10 days).

SECONDARILY INFECTED DERMATOSES

Chronic inflammatory processes, such as atopic dermatitis, or severe acute dermatitis, such as allergic contact dermatitis, rather commonly become secondarily infected. *S. aureus* is the usual culprit. The strains colonizing and then infecting the dermatitic strain appear to be less virulent than those causing furunculosis, bullous impetigo, and severe folliculitis. As such, fever and toxicity are rare. Treatment of these secondary infections ranges from local, cool tap water compresses, plus a topical steroid-antibiotic preparation such as Neo-Synalar cream three times daily, to systemic erythromycin, 250 mg qid, for more extensive or severe infections.

Miscellaneous Dermatoses

STEPHEN E. GELLIS, M.D.

Juvenile plantar dermatosis is a condition seen in children ages 3 to 10 that appears symmetrically in the weight-bearing areas of the feet as shiny and fissured skin. It is thought to result from the chronic exposure of the feet to a humid environment produced by occlusive footwear. The condition may also have an association with atopic dermatitis. Treatment consists of the avoidance of occlusive footwear such as running shoes and rubber boots. The purchase of well-aired shoes and the placement of insoles may be helpful. In acute flare-ups, topical steroids and soaks in an oil and tar preparation (Polytar, Balnetar) are somewhat useful.

Peroral dermatitis is an eruption of unknown etiology that appears as small asymptomatic papules and scaling surrounding the skin of the nose and mouth. It is usually seen in young females and younger children and may be a variant of acne. A brief course of tetracycline 250 mg twice a day for 3 weeks will clear most cases. For children under age 12, tetracycline should not be prescribed because of its potential for producing dental staining. In this age group, topical keratolytics such as benzoyl peroxide and topical antibiotics may be tried. Topical steroids may aggravate the condition and should be avoided.

Keratosis pilaris is a common condition in children who have either a personal or family history of atopy. It consists of keratotic papules 1 to 2 mm in size over the extensor aspect of the arms, the thighs, and occasionally the cheeks. At times, entrapped hairs may be seen within the papules. The eruption is more prominent in dry environments. Treatment consists of the use of emollients, particularly those containing urea or lactic acid (U-Lactin, Nutraplus, Lacticare, Aquacare). Increasing the humidity in the bedroom at night with a vaporizer or humidifier is also effective. In extensive cases, a keratolytic gel (Keralyte), applied with plastic occlusion overnight, will remove the keratotic papules temporarily. Manual removal by rubbing with a pumice stone while the skin is wet may also be tried.

16
The Eye

The Eye

ARTHUR L. ROSENBAUM, M.D.,
and PETER C. GRUENBERG, M.D.

OCULAR EXAMINATION

Premature Infant

The success of the neonatal intensive care unit has resulted in a dramatic improvement in the survival rate of premature infants. Consequently, the frequency of retrolental fibroplasia also has increased. The possible occurrence of this disease mandates careful and methodical ocular examination of premature infants. It is not possible to accurately assess visual acuity subjectively in a premature infant. One must rely on pupillary responses and the observation of a clear red reflex to ensure that the ocular media are normal. Because vitreous haze may be present immediately following birth, it is difficult to observe the retina initially in the premature infant. Thus, it is advisable to routinely examine all children whose birth weight is less than 2000 grams at approximately 1 month of age with indirect ophthalmoscopy and scleral depression.

In premature infants, the normal pattern of vascularization of the retina usually is not developed to the periphery of the retina. The nasal retina usually is completely vascularized before the temporal retina because the vessels have less distance to grow nasally in order to reach the retinal periphery. The acute changes of retinopathy of prematurity (ROP) occur at the junction of the vascularized and nonvascularized retina. This is usually in the retinal periphery and is impossible to see without an indirect ophthalmoscope. Approximately 80% of cases of ROP resolve without serious sequelae. However, careful serial evaluation is necessary for cases that do not resolve, in order to intervene before severe retinal detachment or secondary glaucoma can develop.

The effect of vitamin E on oxygen-induced retinopathy has been studied extensively in a kitten model. Vitamin E is a naturally occurring antioxidant. Animal data demonstrate a clearly inhibitory effect of vitamin E on oxygen-induced retinopathy. The effectiveness of vitamin E in human premature infants is still unclear. The first randomized clinical trial of vitamin E for the prevention of retrolental fibroplasia (RLF) was published by Hittner et al.* However, the sample size of several affected infants was too small to make definitive conclusions. Large, double-masked carefully controlled trials are now in progress. Since the disease usually resolves spontaneously, the efficacy of vitamin E treatment must be proved conclusively before the drug is administered to thousands of premature infants who ordinarily would not require therapy.

There are several differences between premature and full-term newborns that will aid in the ocular assessment. It is not uncommon for the pupillary membrane, the vascular net originating from the iris and lying anterior to the lens, to be visible in the premature infant. A circular, lacelike pattern is seen in the red reflex. The iris vessels are usually somewhat more prominent and may give the impression of neovascularization of the iris or rubeosis when these are not actually present. Frequently, the dilator muscle of the iris is incompletely developed in the premature infant. Consequently pupillary dilatation may be difficult.

Full-Term Infant

Careful evaluation of the newborn is essential in order to obtain early diagnosis of several ocular

---

*Hittner, H.M., et al.: N. Engl. J. Med. *305*:1365–1371, 1981.

conditions that must be treated immediately. The recent Nobel prize-winning research by Hubel and Wiesel has clarified our understanding of form deprivation amblyopia, which probably develops during the first 2 months of life because a contrasting image is not presented to the retina. It is irreversible if not detected and treated during the first few months of life.

The most important disease that may cause this amblyopia is congenital cataract. New surgical techniques have greatly improved the ophthalmologist's ability to remove these cataracts. However, the visual result depends completely on the age at which the cataract is diagnosed and surgery is performed. Frequently these cataracts are unilateral, so the child's vision appears normal and the only way to detect this type of cataract is by examination.

The most important aspect of ocular examination in the newborn is observation of the red reflex. This can best be done by using the direct ophthalmoscope with a power of approximately +6.00 diopters at a distance of about 1 foot from the infant. The red reflex then can be observed from the retina. If there is asymmetry in the quality of the red reflex between the two eyes, a congenital cataract or some abnormality of the vitreous or retina should be suspected and the child should be immediately referred to an ophthalmologist. Most pediatricians diligently attempt to use the direct ophthalmoscope to view the fundus. This is often difficult and frustrating, and will not provide as much information as a careful assessment of the red reflex—a technique that can be mastered easily.

It is also extremely important to suspect congenital glaucoma during the neonatal period. This disease is very uncommon, occurring in 0.05% of all newborns. Most cases are bilateral, and there is a slightly higher incidence in males. One third of cases are present at birth, and 80% occur prior to 1 year of age. Therefore, it is imperative to recognize the early signs of glaucoma rather than the classic later signs. The early signs include excessive lacrimation, photophobia that may be noted at first only in bright sunlight, and blepharospasm. The presence of any of these symptoms warrants immediate referral to an ophthalmologist. Since most tearing will be caused by congenital nasolacrimal duct obstruction, one should observe the nostril on the side of the eye with an epiphora. In congenital nasolacrimal duct obstruction, the nostril should be dry and the eye wet, since the passage between the eye and the nose is obstructed. If both eye and nostril are wet, one should suspect congenital glaucoma.

Congenital glaucoma is caused by a developmental abnormality in the iridocorneal angle of the eye that impairs outflow of aqueous humor from the eye. This occurs in the third to sixth month of gestation when the canal of Schlemm, the scleral spur, and the trabecular meshwork are becoming differentiated. It may be inherited as an autosomal recessive with variable penetrants, or there may be no hereditary pattern. Later signs include corneal edema, corneal enlargement, and cupping and atrophy of the optic nerve.

Therapy is usually goniotomy, a delicate operation that depends on good visualization of the chamber angle and a clear cornea. Therefore, early diagnosis is essential.

Well-Child Examination

Subjective assessment of visual function is the most important part of the ocular examination of infants and toddlers. The presence of photophobia, constant rubbing or manipulation of the eyes, and nystagmus or roving eye movements are signs of visual impairment at any age, and when noted should suggest in-depth evaluation of the visual system.

When these signs are not present, it is necessary to know certain subjective visual milestones in the child's development in order to recognize a potential visual problem.

By age 1 month, the child usually dislikes bright light and will prefer to turn his head toward a subdued light. At 4 to 6 weeks of age, the child should be attentive and will watch his mother's face and objects held directly in front of him. Eye movements become increasingly more conjugate, and by age 3 months the child should be able to maintain fixation. He will look at the movements of his hands and should be able to fixate and follow equally well with each eye.

Testing the child's tolerance to monocular vision is a mainstay in evaluating visual acuity. Alternately patching one eye and then the other will allow observation of the fixation pattern of each eye. The child usually will not object to occlusion of one eye if vision in the other is good. However, if there is dense amblyopia or organic visual impairment, the examiner will observe an asymmetric emotional response when patching one eye as opposed to the other. Poor vision in one eye can also be suspected if the ability to maintain fixation or to follow a small object is asymmetric. Symmetry of performance is often more important than the actual level observed. It is usually better to test the suspected worse eye first in case the child's cooperation is poor.

In addition to observation of the visual milestones, pupillary response and corneal light reflex testing are helpful.

Visual Acuity Testing. Subjective visual responses, mentioned above, are the mainstay of assessment for visual acuity between birth and age 2. At about age 2 years, it is possible to actually test the visual acuity of children. A new test has been developed, called the Dot Visual Acuity Test, that quantitatively records visual acuity in children as young as 2 years of age. This test requires the child to touch identify illuminated dots that vary in size from 20/800 to 20/20. At about age 4, the illiterate E game may be used.

During the past several years, a number of new tests have been developed to assist in evaluating visual acuity in infants and young children. They are the visually evoked cortical response (VER) and the forced-choice preferential looking tests. The VER is a subset test of the electroencephalogram that involves recording the signal generated from the occipital cortex in response to a visual stimulus. Since the macular area is "over-represented" in the occipital cortex, this signal may be used to assess macular function or visual acuity. By using a flash stimulus, the examiner can record the integrity and latency of the response. An alternating checkerboard stimulus of decreasing size permits testing of the discriminating capacity of the visual system. The VER is most useful in testing acuity differences between the two eyes, as in amblyopia and cataracts.

The forced-choice preferential looking test is used to assess subjective visual responses in infants and young children. The infant is held in front of two targets, one with stripes of various widths and the other with no pattern. Usually the child will prefer the striped pattern, and as the stripe width is decreased, assessment of visual acuity may be recorded. Initially a laboratory research tool, this test is gaining increasingly wide clinical acceptance.

SPECIFIC OCULAR DISEASES

Congenital Nasolacrimal System Obstruction. The most common abnormality of the infant lacrimal system is congenital impatency of the nasolacrimal duct. This occurs in 1 to 5% of newborns and usually is caused by blocking of the juncture of the nasolacrimal duct and nasal cavity by a thin membrane. Pressure over the nasolacrimal sac usually elicits mucopurulent material from the lower punctum. Epiphora is usually present and is greater when the child is emotionally upset or crying. A chronic conjunctivitis with varying degrees of mucopurulent material is almost always present, occasionally complicated by acute fulminant dacryocystitis.

Conservative initial management is always indicated. Between 70 and 90% of these obstructions will clear spontaneously with conservative management in the first 6 months of life. Initial therapy is massage over the lacrimal sac area three to four times a day. A technique to increase the hydrostatic pressure on the lacrimal sac area and encourage transmission of this pressure into the nasolacrimal duct recently has been repopularized. The index finger is placed over the superior aspect of the nasolacrimal sac and pressure is exerted downward. This downward pressure ruptures the membranous obstruction at the bottom of the nasolacrimal sac. This technique seems more effective than simple massage.

If there is evidence of secondary conjunctivitis, topical antibiotic therapy consisting of sodium sulfacetamide 10% or Neosporin drops four times a day is indicated. The antibiotic should be discontinued when the mucopurulent discharge subsides, in order to avoid the development of either resistance or sensitivity to the medication.

If obstruction remains after age 6 months despite conservative therapy, nasolacrimal duct probing is indicated. This procedure has a very high degree of success, approaching 90% to 95% after one probing.

Acute Dacryocystitis. Acute infection of the lacrimal sac occurs when there is distal obstruction to outflow of tears, as mentioned above, accompanied by rampant infection and secondary obstruction of the punctum. This results in swelling, redness, and tenderness of the lacrimal sac, and should be treated promptly. The infection almost always is bacterial, and the child is in definite distress. Acute dacryocystitis may be confused with early orbital cellulitis but is initially localized to the lacrimal sac area only. Cultures should be obtained, and appropriate systemic and topical antibiotics are necessary. Once the inflammation has subsided, nasolacrimal probing can be performed. If acute dacryocystitis has occurred, the duct should be probed rather than waiting for it to open spontaneously.

The Red Eye. The pediatrician is frequently called upon to diagnose and treat a child with a red or irritated eye. This involves skillful differentiation between causes that may range from mild to very serious. The initial evaluation should determine whether the red eye is secondary to lid, conjunctival, or intraocular disease. Each of these possibilities will be considered separately.

BLEPHARITIS. Chronic inflammation of the eyelid margin is called blepharitis. It is probably the most frequent external disease problem in children and runs a chronic course of exacerbation and remission. It is extremely difficult to treat and may recur many months after it is thought to have disappeared. Symptoms include chronic redness of the lash margin, an itching sensation, and mild narrowing of the palpebral fissure. Examination reveals small white scales at the juncture of the lash follicle.

Seborrheic blepharitis is the most common type. It is usually associated with seborrheic dermatitis of the scalp. Superimposed staphylococcal infection may occur concomitantly. Treatment consists of vigorous scrubbing of the lid margin with moistened cotton-tip applicators and instillation of topical antibiotics such as sodium sulfacetamide 3 times a day for 7 days. The scalp condition also must be treated with appropriate shampoos.

STY. A sty, or hordeolum, is a localized infection of the eyelash, usually caused by *Staphylococcus aureus*. An external hordeolum involves one of the superficial glands of the skin, and an internal hordeolum involves the meibomian gland of the tarsal plate. Children frequently exhibit recurrent sties, which may indicate chronic staphylococcal infection, frequently associated with blepharitis. Rarely, it also may indicate general physical debility, such as anemia or diabetes mellitus.

Moist, warm compresses should be applied for 5 to 10 minutes several times a day, and topical antibiotic drops are used for 7 to 10 days.

CHALAZION. A chalazion is caused by obstruction of one of the meibomian glands, which normally secrete an oily substance necessary for the tear layer of the eye. A chronic inflammation develops behind the obstruction, causing a painless, localized mass in the lid. Warm, moist compresses are used with topical antibiotics, although usually no infection is present. If the chalazion does not reabsorb spontaneously, surgical removal may be indicated for cosmetic reasons.

ORBITAL CELLULITIS. This serious, possibly life-threatening, bacterial infection usually is caused by *Staphylococcus* or *Hemophilus influenzae*. The latter organism is found frequently in children between 3 and 8 years of age, and often is secondary to infection of the ethmoid sinus. Symptoms include fever and lid edema with orbital pain, tenderness, and proptosis developing soon after the initial signs. Frequently there is limitation of extraocular rotation, and pain on movement. X-rays may be confirmed by computed tomography (CT). Severe complications may result, involving the optic nerve and cavernous sinus, if the infection is not treated aggressively. Blood cultures should be obtained, and appropriate intravenous antibiotics against both above-mentioned organisms should be begun. With prompt hospitalization and aggressive treatment, the success rate in recent large series has been excellent.

Occasionally the bacterial infection is confined to the eyelids anterior to the orbital septum. This is called preseptal or periorbital cellulitis. The globe is not involved, and there is no proptosis or limitation of movement. A specific type of preseptal cellulitis may be caused by *H. influenzae* in infants and young children. Some believe that a specific purple discoloration of the lid is characteristic of this organism. Appropriate intravenous antibiotic therapy is indicated.

CONJUNCTIVITIS. Conjunctivitis is the most frequent cause of a red eye. The pediatrician must distinguish among the viral, bacterial, and allergic etiologies as well as differentiate this cause of red eye from intraocular inflammation and glaucoma. The possibility of a foreign body or corneal abrasion must also be considered.

Viral Conjunctivitis. It is important for the pediatrician to be able to distinguish between viral and bacterial conjunctivitis, since viral conjunctivitis without corneal involvement usually can be successfully managed by the pediatrician. Viral conjunctivitis may resemble bacterial conjunctivitis symptomatically. Usually the discharge is more watery and less mucopurulent in viral conjunctivitis. The palpebral conjunctiva is inflamed in a follicular pattern as opposed to the papillary appearance of bacterial conjunctivitis. The presence of a palpable preauricular lymph node usually suggests viral etiology. The most common types of viral infection are epidemic keratoconjunctivitis and pharyngeal conjunctival fever. Both last 2 to 3 weeks, and the patient may remain infectious for as long as 7 to 14 days. There is no effective treatment, but care must be taken to isolate the child as much as possible from other members of the family to avoid dissemination of the disease.

Bacterial Conjunctivitis. Bacterial conjunctivitis may be indistinguishable symptomatically from the viral type. The discharge is usually more mucopurulent and the conjunctival reaction is in a papillary pattern. Usually no palpable preauricular node is present. The most common organisms are *S. aureus*, *Hemophilus*, and *Streptococcus pneumoniae*. Appropriate cultures and smears are obtained, and specific topical antibiotic therapy such as Neosporin is instituted. The antibiotics should be continued for 7 days.

Allergic Conjunctivitis. The child with allergic conjunctivitis is usually in marked distress. The most prominent symptom is relentless itching, with the child constantly rubbing his eyes. There may be moderate to marked photophobia and a scanty mucoid discharge.

Vernal conjunctivitis is a chronic bilateral conjunctival inflammation that goes through long periods of exacerbation and remission. It is worse in the spring and summer, and frequently there is a history of atopic allergy. Clinically it presents with giant papillae on the upper tarsal conjunctiva, which can be observed with lid eversion. Occasionally, mild corneal changes occur. If the diagnosis is unclear, conjunctival scraping may be easily performed to reveal eosinophils. Treatment consists of supportive measures to reduce itching, including antihistamines and cold compresses. The mainstay of treatment has been topical steroid drops, which usually control the disease quite well. The weaker steroid preparations should be used initially, since this is a long-term treatment program.

Cromolyn sodium 4% ophthalmic drops have been shown to be a significant benefit in the treatment of most symptoms. The effect on cobblestone papillae is less marked. Atopic patients with elevated serum IgE levels demonstrated more consistent improvement with cromolyn therapy. Acute exacerbations of the disorder often require additional topical steroid therapy, although the dose required for long-term management of this disease can be substantially reduced or eliminated. Cromalyn is, therefore, a useful addition to or substitute for steroids, reducing the inherent risk of topical steroid therapy. If initial enthusiasm is sustained, this drug will become the treatment of choice, since it does not have the serious side effects of glaucoma and cataract that may be precipitated by long-term topical steroids.

Neonatal Conjunctivitis. Since 1973, according to a statement prepared by the National Society to Prevent Blindness (NSPB) Committee on Ophthalmia Neonatorum, silver nitrate solution has been the primary recommendation for the prophylaxis of ophthalmia in neonates. These guidelines recently have been revised to reflect concern for gonococcal ophthalmia neonatorum and *Chlamydia* ophthalmia neonatorum. In some centers, erythromycin 0.5% ointment has replaced silver nitrate as the treatment of choice for a newborn eye prophylaxis.

Current recommendations of the NSPB include the following: 1) A prophylactic agent should be instilled in the eyes of all newborn infants. 2) Acceptable agents that prevent gonococcus neonatorum are silver nitrate solution 1% in single-dose ampules, erythromycin 0.5% ophthalmic ointment or drops in single-use tubes or ampules, and tetracycline 1% ophthalmic ointment or drops in single-use tubes or ampules. 3) Acceptable agents that prevent *Chlamydia* ophthalmia neonatorum are erythromycin 0.5% ophthalmic ointment or drops and tetracycline 1% ophthalmic ointment or drops. Silver nitrate does not prevent chlamydial infections. 4) Prophylaxis agents should be given shortly after birth. Delay of up to 1 hour is usually acceptable and may facilitate maternal-infant bonding. 5) The importance of performing the instillation so the agent reaches all parts of the conjunctival surface is stressed, and can be accomplished by careful manipulation of the lids with fingers to ensure spreading. If medication reaches only the eyelid and lid margins but fails to reach the cornea, the instillation should be repeated.

Prophylaxis should be applied as follows:

1. Silver nitrate: Carefully clean the eyelids and surrounding skin with sterile cotton, which may be moistened with sterile water. Gently open the baby's eyelids and instill 2 drops of silver nitrate on the conjunctival sac. Allow the silver nitrate to run across the whole conjunctival sac. Carefully manipulate the lids to ensure spread of the drops. Repeat in the other eye. Use 2 ampules, 1 for each eye. After 1 minute, gently wipe the excess silver nitrate from the eyelids and surrounding skin with sterile water. Do not irrigate the eyes.

2. Ophthalmic ointment (erythromycin or tetracycline): Carefully clean the eyelids and surrounding skin with sterile cotton, which may be moistened with sterile water. Gently open the baby's eyelids and place a thin line of ointment, at least ½ inch (1–2 cm), along the junction of the bulbar and palpebral conjunctiva of the lower lid. Try to cover the whole lower conjunctival area. Carefully manipulate the lids to ensure spread of the ointment. Be careful not to touch the eyelid or eyeball with the tip of the tube. Repeat in the other eye. Use one tube per baby. After 1 minute, gently wipe excess ointment from the eyelids and surrounding skin with sterile water. Do not irrigate the eyes.

The eye should not be irrigated after instillation of the agent. Irrigation may reduce the efficacy of prophylaxis and probably does not decrease the incidence of chemical conjunctivitis. Infants born to mothers infected with agents that cause ophthalmia neonatorum may require special attention and systemic therapy as well as prophylaxis. A single dose of aqueous crystalline penicillin G, 50,000 units per kilogram of body weight for term and 20,000 units for low-birthweight infants, should be administered intravenously to infants born to mothers with gonorrhea. The detection and appropriate treatment of infections in pregnant women that may result in ophthalmia neonatorum is encouraged.

The most common etiology of ophthalmia neonatorum is inclusion conjunctivitis caused by *Chlamydia oculogenitalis.* Symptoms of conjunctival injection and a mucopurulent discharge develop 5 to 10 days after birth, and this etiology must be distinguished from gonococcus. Diagnostic conjunctival scrapings reveal cytoplasmic inclusion bodies. Treatment is effective with topical tetracycline ointment for 2 to 3 weeks.

Gonococcal conjunctivitis usually presents 2 to 4 days following birth as a purulent conjunctivitis. It is not common but must be recognized because of the serious corneal and intraocular complications that may develop, since this organism is virulent enough to penetrate corneal epithelium. The diagnosis may be confirmed by conjunctival scrapings, which reveal gram-negative diplococci. Treatment is aggressive and consists of intravenous aqueous penicillin and topical penicillin or erythromycin therapy. Cultures are taken, but treatment must be started before obtaining the culture reports to minimize the risk of corneal ulceration and blindness.

Chemical conjunctivitis secondary to Credé prophylaxis usually occurs in the first 48 hours of life, and resolves promptly without treatment. Occasionally, other organisms such as *Staphylococcus* and

Pseudomonas may cause conjunctivitis during the newborn period.

Herpes Simplex. Primary ocular herpes infection may occur in infants and young children. The primary infection can occur on the eyelids and surrounding facial skin, and may even result in a systemic viremia. Conjunctivitis and blepharitis may occur with typical vesicular formation. Dendritic keratitis, which is best seen with fluorescein staining of the cornea, may occur during the primary infection.

Treatment consists of topical antiviral medication specific for herpes simplex, such as idoxuridine (IDU), or other similar antiviral drugs, such as ara-A (vidarabine) and acyclovir* (Zovirax). The medication must be continued for 1 to 2 weeks. Recurrent herpetic corneal infection may occur at any time, but subsequent infections usually do not involve the lids and adjacent skin. Recurrent herpetic keratitis is treated with the same medications.

Trifluoridine (Viroptic) is a new antiviral agent indicated for the topical treatment of dendritic keratitis due to herpes simplex virus types I and II. In clinical trials, 95% of patients treated healed with complete corneal re-epithelialization by 14 days. This is a slightly higher rate of recovery than with idoxuridine. It also is valuable in resistant or hypersensitive cases. Recommended is a dosage of 1 drop every 2 hours while awake until re-epithelialization occurs. If no improvement occurs after 7 days, another form of therapy is recommended.

Uveitis. It is important to differentiate iritis or uveitis, which is a noninfectious intraocular inflammation, from conjunctivitis. Iritis can cause decreased visual acuity because of the light scattering and glare associated with intraocular inflammation. Usually there is conjunctival injection but it has a characteristic perilimbal flush which is distinguished from the generalized conjunctival redness seen in conjunctivitis. Exact diagnosis requires slit-lamp examination to visualize the cellular and exudative reaction in the anterior chamber or vitreous. The presence of iritis in a child necessitates careful medical history and workup to document any etiologic agent or system illness. The differential diagnostic list is long and beyond the scope of this report. Children suspected of having iritis should be referred promptly to an ophthalmologist. Treatment includes pupillary dilation to prevent synechiae formation and usually topical steroid administration to control the inflammation.

Strabismus. In the condition known as strabismus the visual axis of each eye is not directed simultaneously to the same object in space. Tropia is defined as a manifest deviation of the visual axes

and phoria as a latent tendency of the visual axis of one eye to deviate. If strabismus is suspected, the initial evaluation consists of observation of the light reflex on the cornea from a penlight held approximately 1 meter in front of the patient. With the child looking at the light, the corneal reflex of the light should be just nasal to the center of the pupil in both eyes. If it is centered in one eye and off to the side in the other, strabismus is probably present. This can be confirmed by the cover-uncover test. The examiner should watch for movements of the uncovered eye. If the eye moves outward, he should suspect esotropia. If the eye moves inward, he should suspect exotropia. Occasionally, an eye with poor or no vision will not respond to the cover test, and the examiner will observe no movement of the eye even when the child has strabismus.

If these two simple and quick tests are performed, strabismus can be differentiated from pseudostrabismus. Pseudostrabismus in infants is most commonly due to prominent epicanthal folds, which give the appearance of esotropia. However, the light reflex test will reveal the light to be centered equally in each eye. Other causes of pseudostrabismus are hypertelorism, facial asymmetry, and retrolental fibroplasia.

Strabismus may be idiopathic or due to unknown causes. It also may be secondary to refractive errors, cranial nerve palsy, or organic lesions of the eye resulting from poor vision, such as retinoblastoma, retrolental fibroplasia, optic nerve abnormalities, congenital cataracts, and congenital glaucoma.

Because strabismus may be caused by such potentially dangerous diseases a child suspected of having strabismus should be referred to an ophthalmologist if the pediatrician is convinced that there is a constant or persistent deviation of ocular alignment, particularly after age 3 months. A head turn or tilt or any other abnormal head posture may indicate strabismus. These findings may be present in lateral rectus paralysis or superior oblique paralysis, or may be a compensatory mechanism for obtaining good vision in congenital nystagmus. If a child does have an abnormal head posture, one eye should be patched and the head position observed. If the head tilt remains, it is probably not caused by an extraocular muscle problem but is most likely a true torticollis. If the head straightens when one eye is patched, strabismus should be strongly suspected.

The consequences of strabismus include amblyopia and the disruption of binocular vision. Amblyopia is reduced visual acuity without ophthalmoscopically detectable anomalies of the fundus. It may be due to strabismus, unequal refractive errors between the two eyes, or stimulus deprivation. Stimulus deprivation amblyopia is caused by lack of a formed or contrasting visual

---

*Manufacturer's warning: Acyclovir is for cutaneous use only. Do not use in the eye.

image reaching the retina in infancy, and is usually the result of congenital cataracts or severe ptosis. Stimulus deprivation amblyopia is usually irreversible unless treated in the first 2 months of life and results in very severe visual impairment. Amblyopia secondary to strabismus or refractive error is reversible. The treatment of choice is usually patching of the good eye for various lengths of time, depending on the severity of the amblyopia. Prognosis for successful treatment depends primarily on time of onset in relation to time of treatment. The shorter the time that elapses between onset and start of therapy, the better is the prognosis.

The treatment is varied, and depends on the underlying cause. If refractive errors are present, glasses usually are prescribed, and frequently this treatment alone will eliminate the strabismus. This is especially true in farsighted children whose strabismus occurs as a consequence of this refractive error. Occasionally, miotic eye drops or orthoptic exercises are helpful.

When these conservative measures are not appropriate, surgery may be necessary. Very recently, botulinum toxin injections have been introduced as an alternative to conventional muscle surgery. The toxin acts by irreversibly blocking the binding sites for acetylcholine at the neuromuscular junction. This weakens the rectus muscle as is done by conventional rectus muscle recession surgery. This alters the balance of forces between opposing rectus muscles and may result in realignment of the strabismic deviation. For example, in esotropia, the medial rectus muscle is injected and becomes weakened. The opposing lateral rectus muscle therefore secondarily contracts and the eye is shifted outward.

The injection can be administered to a fully awake patient on an outpatient basis with only topical anesthesia. A small needle is inserted subconjunctivally in the area of the muscle to be injected. A special electromyographic lead is installed in the tip of the hypodermic needle. As the needle is passed subconjunctivally, the recording of an electromyogram signal is observed in order to monitor when the needle has entered the muscle. When the needle reaches the desired location, the botulinum toxin is injected. In children, light anesthesia is necessary. The dose of toxin injected ranges from 10^{-4} to 10^{-3} micrograms, well below the lethal dose, estimated to be approximately 1 microgram.

This new botulinum therapy may offer a major new development in the treatment of selected cases. The recorded side effects of the drug are minimal, but problems have developed, such as spread of the drug to adjacent rectus muscles and occasionally to the levator palpebral muscle of the upper lid, causing ptosis. The treatment seems much more conducive to horizontal rectus muscle disorders than to rectus or oblique muscle problems. This therapy is very new, and further extensive clinical trials will be necessary before adequate conclusions can be drawn.

OCULAR TRAUMA

Chemical Burns. Strong acid and alkali burns may be devastating to ocular tissue. This is a true emergency and must be treated immediately to avoid serious corneal damage. Immediate, copious irrigation must be performed. Parents should begin irrigation even before bringing the child to an emergency room, even if the exact source of the chemical insult is unknown. Tap water should be used, and care should be taken to open the lids to ensure that the water contacts the conjunctiva and cornea. Irrigation should be continued for 10 minutes at home.

Upon arrival in the doctor's office or emergency room, the irrigation should be repeated for 20 minutes. Topical anesthetic should be applied, and at least 2000 ml of water or saline should be used for irrigation. Any particulate matter retained in the recesses of the conjunctiva or under the upper lid should be removed with moist cotton swabs. It is convenient to utilize an intravenous set with saline or sterile water. No needle is required, but the infusion tubing allows controlled and copious flow of fluid without the need for special equipment. It is important to use a Desmarres or other lid retractor to doubly evert the upper lid when irrigation is being performed in order to reach the conjunctival tissue in the superior fornix and to be able to remove any particulate matter in this area. Litmus paper or the pH test on a urine test stick may be used to touch the conjunctiva and measure the acidity or alkalinity level. This is a good way to determine whether irrigation should be continued. Ideally, the pH should be neutral before irrigation is stopped. After the irrigation has been completed, the child should be referred immediately to an ophthalmologist in order to assess the degree of ocular damage. Iritis, glaucoma, secondary infection, and cataracts are unfortunate consequences of severe chemical burns. The corneal epithelium may be very slow to heal following chemical insult and must be monitored closely with slit lamp and fluorescein staining. Prompt, effective treatment of chemical burns may preserve vision and avoid severe corneal scarring, which can result in severe or even total loss of vision.

Corneal Abrasion. Corneal abrasion is probably the most frequent type of ocular trauma encountered by the pediatrician. The abrasion may be caused a variety of agents, including contact lenses, fingernails, and foreign bodies. This injury is exquisitely painful, since the corneal epithelium contains many nerve endings to detect pain. A drop of topical anesthetic should be applied to relieve pain and permit careful ocular examination. Large abrasions can be seen with oblique penlight illumination and fluorescein staining. A cobalt blue disposable penlight is inexpensive and extremely helpful for visualizing corneal abrasions stained with fluorescein. The fluorescein dye adheres in areas where the epithelium is interrupted or removed. A careful search for a foreign body must include eversion of the upper lid, as mentioned in the section on chemical burns. If a foreign body is encountered superficially, it should be removed with a moist cotton-tip applicator. If the foreign body is seen to be embedded in the cornea, the pediatrician should refer the patient to an ophthalmologist rather than attempt to remove the foreign body himself. Frequently, a small foreign body may have been washed from the eye by tears and only the corneal abrasion will be visible. Treatment consists of applying topical antibiotics such as erythromycin or neosporin. Commercial products containing antibiotics and steroids should be avoided. A firm eye patch should be applied for 24 hours. The purpose of the eye patch is to prevent opening the upper lid, which will rub over the epithelium and retard healing. If the abrasion is not completely healed in 24 hours, or if symptoms of pain or redness continue, further examination by an ophthalmologist is necessary.

Blunt Ocular Injury. A contusion injury of the eye and surrounding structures frequently is encountered in children. The pediatrician is faced with the dilemma of whether this extremely frequent injury should be referred to an ophthalmologist. This question is understandably legitimate, since the injury may be relatively minor and not result in significant ocular insult. On the other hand, the potential sequelae of contusion injury include hyphema, dislocated lens, traumatic iritis, blowout fracture of the orbital floor, and even retinal tear and detachment. In severe contusion injury, actual globe rupture also may occur. Some experts believe that any contusion injury should be referred to an ophthalmologist. If there is any sign of direct insult to the eye itself, consultation should be requested. Specifically, reduced visual acuity, marked conjunctival injection, inability to fully rotate the globe in all positions, and diplopia are serious findings that must be investigated by a complete ophthalmologic examination including dilated funduscopy.

Penetrating Ocular Injury. Treatment of a penetrating or perforating ocular injury is beyond the scope of this presentation. However, it is important that the pediatrician recognize the possibility of this serious insult and refer the child immediately if there is any suspicion that penetration of the globe has occurred. A high index of suspicion must always be present, even when the history may seem vague or even contradictory, since children frequently will not reveal the complete history surrounding serious eye injury, owing to fear of punishment. Detection of this type of injury is also a problem for the ophthalmologist, since there are no guidelines or signs that definitively exclude the possibility of injury, including the presence of 20/20 visual acuity. Occasionally, a sharp foreign body may pass through clear cornea or sclera in a self-sealing manner.

If a penetrating injury is suspected, it is best to avoid direct pressure or excessive manipulation of the globe, since intraocular contents may be extruded. Even antibiotic ointments should be avoided if penetration is suspected. A protective plastic or metal shield should be applied to avoid additional trauma, and the child should be referred immediately to an ophthalmologist.

OTHER OCULAR DISORDERS

Capillary Hemangiomas of Orbit and Eyelid. Capillary hemangiomas may be present at birth or may appear in the first few months of life. They vary from tiny insignificant lesions to large tumors that involve the lid and orbit and that may produce serious visual sequelae, primarily from ptosis, proptosis, and mechanical displacement of the globe. Any large lesion, especially if it involves the upper lid and causes a secondary ptosis, should be referred immediately. The ptosis actually may obstruct the visual axis or cause astigmatism, which may result in severe amblyopia. Recently, myopia has been associated with ptosis with the upper lid, which may be an additional cause of amblyopia. These lesions tend to progress during the first year of life; many then regress spontaneously over the next several years. Because of the high incidence of spontaneous regression, treatment should be reserved for hemangiomas that are visually threatening. A 4- to 6-week course of oral prednisone at a dose level of 2 mg/kg may induce partial remission. Recently, local injection of steroids into the hemangioma has become more popular, and it may be more effective and may avoid the systemic complications of steroids. These injections must be performed under general anesthesia, and can be repeated if necessary. Low dosages of radiation have been used with varying degrees of success.

Juvenile Rheumatoid Arthritis. Anterior uveitis or iritis is a common complication of juvenile rheumatoid arthritis (JRA). Frequently JRA children are asymptomatic; therefore, routine slit-lamp examination should be performed at 3-month intervals. Uveitis is more common in children with oligoarticular types of JRA. The uveitis is frequently associated with posterior synechiae, cataract, and band keratopathy. Topical steroid treatment is frequently effective in controlling the anterior uveitis, and pharmacologic pupillary dilation may prevent the development of posterior synechiae.

Retinopathy Associated with Sickle-Cell Disease. Recent studies have stressed the important finding that children with sickle-cell (S-C) disease may develop severe and even blinding forms of neovascular and hemorrhagic retinopathy. This is particularly true in children with S-C disease. These children should be followed routinely by ophthalmologists for careful fundus evaluation. Most of the changes are neovascular fronds, present primarily in the retinal periphery, and are therefore difficult to see with a direct ophthalmoscope. Dilated funduscopy and careful indirect ophthalmoscopy are necessary to detect these potentially treatable lesions.

17
The Ear

Foreign Bodies in the Ear

MELVIN D. SCHLOSS, M.D.

Foreign bodies in the external auditory canals of young children are not uncommon. It must be noted that they are more commonly seen in the ear canals of retarded children. The foreign bodies are of all shapes, sizes, and varieties. There are three major groups found in the external auditory canal.* The first is of vegetable and related matter. These include beans, peas, absorbent cotton, and rubber erasers. The second group is mineral. These are either smooth or irregular in shape and include beads, pebbles, sand, plaster of paris, hooks, and jacks. The third group is of animal matter. These insects such as moths, mosquitoes, and beetles.

It is not uncommon for a child to present to a physician's office without symptoms related to the foreign body in the ear canal. If the foreign body is smooth or if there is no reaction in the external canal secondary to trauma the foreign body will probably go unnoticed. A piece of cotton may be present in the ear canal for months before the parents become aware of its presence. With moisture and secondary infection, there is a resultant hearing loss and odor with or without discharge which usually brings the child to the physician's office.

Removal of the foreign body should be done quickly with the least amount of psychic and physical trauma. The child should be mummified in a sheet with the parent restraining the lower part of the body and a nurse holding the head firmly above. The child requires reassurance and the foreign body should be removed quickly with proper lighting, with or without an otological microscope.

The basic instruments required for removal in the office are an Oto-Microscope, proper lighting source, curets, micro-picks, alligator forceps, fine suction catheters, and an irrigating device. The technique of removal depends on the type of foreign body. Irrigation should not be used for vegetable and related matter. These objects will swell in the canal with the absorption of the water and will make removal much more difficult. Animal foreign bodies may be flushed out using solutions of chloroform or ether. It must be emphasized that there is usually only one chance to remove the foreign body in the child, thus it is of utmost importance to restrain the child adequately. If the patient is totally uncooperative, general anesthesia may be considered, as trauma to the external ear canal, tympanic membrane, and middle ear may ensue if the child is moving.

If infection secondary to the foreign body is present the child should be treated with a topical otologic solution and/or systemic antibiotics after removal of the foreign body.* If there is a laceration of the external auditory canal secondary to the foreign body or removal, the child probably should be treated with a topical otologic solution. If there are no obvious signs of inflammation or infection of the ear canal or middle ear space, there is usually no need for antibiotics. It is important to advise the parents to keep the ear canal dry for a period of 1 week to allow for healing. A small piece of cotton dipped in vaseline is a suitable plug for the meatus of the external auditory canal. This should be removed after bathing and shampooing. If the for-

---

*Senturia, B. H., Marcus, M.D., Lucente, F. E.: Diseases of the External Ear. An Otologic-Dermatologic Manual. New York, Grune and Stratton, 1980.

---

*Shambaugh, G. E. Jr.: Surgery of the Ear. Edition 2. W. B. Saunders Co., Philadelphia, 1967.

eign body cannot be adequately visualized and if the proper instruments and restraining techniques are unavailable, attempts to remove foreign bodies should not be made. The child should be referred to an otolaryngologist.

Otologic Infections

RICHARD H. SCHWARTZ, M.D.

Otitis Externa

Otitis externa (OE) is a dermatitis of the external auditory canal that may include the squamous portion of the tympanic membrane. It is usually caused by a loss of local protective mechanisms as a result of water in the external canal. Frequently, secondary infection with *Pseudomonas* or, less commonly, *Staphylococcus, Streptococcus,* or fungi occurs although contact dermatitis without a secondary infection may also present as OE. In advanced cases the meatus and lumen of the ear canal become narrowed by inflammatory edema, and even the skin of the pinna may be markedly swollen, tender, and red. Treatment must begin with gentle aural lavage if there is desquamated skin or cerumen in the canal. Unless such debris is removed, topical otic antibiotic drops may be ineffectual, as the drug cannot penetrate the debris to reach the infection site. In milder forms of OE, the patient should avoid getting water in the ear canals for a few days. A mild antiseptic containing Burow's solution, alcohol, or topical antibiotic drops containing polymyxin with hydrocortisone instilled in the canal several times a day may be helpful. Without proper treatment, inflammatory edema can become worse, and it may be necessary to insert a cotton wick or an expandable otic wick deeply into the ear canal to allow the antiseptic solution to reach the medial part. In such severe cases, a moderate analgesic such as codeine may be necessary for pain control. After the edema has subsided, the patient may get the ears wet again but after each episode, Burow's solution or a vinegar-alcohol mixture should be instilled in the canals as prophylaxis. Some patients do not improve with such therapy and I find this is most often the result of inadequate aural cleaning or failure to control inflammatory edema by use of a mildly acidic ear drop. Occasionally the patient may develop contact dermatitis from neomycin-containing ear drops. There are several topical antibiotic drops that do not contain neomycin, for example, Pyocidin-Otic. Propylene glycol–containing otic solutions may irritate inflamed skin and cause a burning sensation. Oral antibiotic therapy is necessary for Streptococcal OE.

Less common causes of OE are infections by *Monilia,* which looks like cottage cheese in the ear canal, or *Aspergillus niger,* which looks like black specks on the wet, blotting-paper–appearing desquamated skin of the canal. Otitis externa caused by these organisms is unresponsive to the above measures. After obtaining a Gram stain and culture of the material of patients unresponsive to the usual topical otic antibacterial solutions, nystatin (for monilial infections) or amphotericin B (Fungizone) topical solution (for *A. niger* infections) should be prescribed.

Because the squamous layer of the eardrum is reddened and opacified by the OE, it may be difficult to ascertain if a concomitant otitis media is present. Unless the eardrum is bulging, I suggest that the status of the middle ear be re-evaluated after a few days of treatment for the OE. After the inflammatory edema has subsided, the physician can use the pneumatic otoscope to see if there is impaired mobility of the reddened eardrum. Dermatosis such as furunculosis or herpetic or varicella-zoster infections are, in general, treated no differently than such infections that occur elsewhere on the skin.

Otitis Media

The treatment of otitis media has four major objectives: 1) recognition of those physical signs of middle ear inflammation that correlate best with a bacterial infection; 2) knowledge of primary and alternative choices of antibacterial agents with proven effectiveness against the common middle ear pathogens; 3) identification and appropriate treatment of the child with suppurative complications of acute otitis media (AOM); and 4) identification, on re-evaluation visit, of persistent otitis media with effusion (secretory otitis media) and differentiation of this entity from persistent AOM.

Most children will experience at least one middle ear infection before they reach their third birthday and one child out of five may experience three or more recurrent attacks of AOM during infancy.

Acute otitis media is best defined by the presence of a bulging, opacified, grossly discolored, red, yellow, or gray eardrum through which neither the handle of the malleus nor the malleolar short process (the ossicular landmarks) can be delineated otoscopically. Of paramount importance in diagnosis of AOM is the decreased or absent mobility of the eardrum to pneumatoscopy. Erythema, loss of light reflex, or decreased mobility of the tympanic membrane (TM) alone is not definitive of AOM. It is essential that color, contour, and medial-lateral mobility of the TM *all* be impaired for AOM to be present. Proper examination of the eardrum requires optimal illumination, preferably by a halogen light; meticulous removal of any cerumen or flakes of skin that obscure the full view of the TM; firm but compassionate restraint of infants and young, frightened, wiggly children; and consistent and proper use of a good quality otoscope.

Medical Management of AOM. The drug of choice in treating AOM is still ampicillin, 50 to 75 mg/kg/day in four divided doses, or its congener amoxicillin, 30–40 mg/kg/day in three divided doses, for 10 days. Amoxicillin has a more convenient dosage schedule, has demonstrably better absorption, and is less likely to produce diarrhea than is ampicillin. Both drugs are cost-effective choices where ampicillin-resistant strains of *Hemophilus influenzae* or *Branhamella catarrhalis* are not a significant problem. Because *H. influenzae* is the causative agent of at least 20% of cases of AOM in adolescent patients, amoxicillin or a suitable alternative drug should be prescribed for all patients with AOM.

Bacampicillin (80 mg/kg/day in two doses)*or cyclacillin (50 mg/kg/day in four doses), two newer ampicillin-like drugs, while better absorbed than ampicillin, are too expensive to be considered as drugs of choice and neither has shown any clear advantage over amoxicillin.

While most children and adolescents may be treated with an oral preparation of amoxicillin, a child who appears ill or who has persistent vomiting or complicating conditions should be given the first dose of the antibiotic intramuscularly if there is no suspicion of meningitis. Bullous myringitis, AOM with a blister of the eardrum, should be treated with amoxicillin. Neonates treated in the intensive care nursery (ICN) for AOM may require tympanocentesis to diagnose those with gram-negative enteric or group B *Streptococcus* infection. Acute otitis media in a baby in the ICN should be treated, at least initially, with ampicillin and an aminoglycoside antibiotic administered intravenously.

Acute otitis media secondary to ampicillin-resistant strains of *H. influenzae* is usually diagnosed when the patient responds poorly to amoxicillin. In such cases, antimicrobial agents such as trimethoprim-sulfamethoxazole (TMP-SMZ),†erythromycin ethylsuccinate (Pediazole), or cefaclor (Ceclor) are equally effective.

Ceclor (40 mg/kg/day in 3 divided doses) has shown promise in the treatment of AOM and is the best-tasting of the antibiotics, but the cost is greater than that of TMP-SMZ or Pediazole and about two to three times greater than that of amoxicillin. Cefaclor has enhanced anti-*Hemophilus* activity and is not inactivated by the penicillinase produced by ampicillin-resistant *H. influenzae*. It is well absorbed even when given with meals, reaches high middle ear concentrations, and appears effective against all of the common middle ear pathogens (including ampicillin-resistant *H. influenzae*). In addition, the incidence of persistent otitis media with effusion occurring after cefaclor treatment of AOM may be lower than that occurring after treatment with ampicillin. A disadvantage of this drug besides its greater cost is that a substantial number of children have developed an erythema multiforme rash during cefaclor therapy. *Branhamella catarrhalis,* a middle ear pathogen of importance in some areas of the country, may not be sensitive to cefaclor.

Cephalexin in the usual prescribed doses does not reach adequate concentrations in the middle ear to be effective in the treatment of AOM.

Erythromycin alone is not effective against middle ear infections secondary to *H. influenzae,* but a fixed combination of erythromycin and sulfisoxazole (Pediazole) has been approved for the treatment of AOM. Pediazole (50 mg/kg/day of the erythromycin component)* given four times a day, is as effective as amoxicillin in initial treatment of AOM, and is particularly effective against ampicillin-resistant strains of *H. influenzae*. It is well absorbed from the stomach, even in the presence of food, but the erythromycin component has caused abdominal pain and nausea in 10 to 15% of children who received the drug.

While there is consensus that antimicrobial treatment of AOM is prudent, the most desirable drug, the optimal duration of treatment, and whether to use ancillary measures (e.g., myringotomy, or a course of decongestants) are still much debated.

Symptomatic Relief. In addition to antibiotic treatment, the primary care physician should ameliorate any pain (often nocturnal) associated with ear infection. Glycerin or vegetable oil heated to body temperature is an effective, heat-retaining ear drop (however, oily ear drops are contraindicated if the tympanic membrane has ruptured). A warm electric heating pad held against the ear may also reduce pain. Paregoric tincture, 2 drops per kg for infants under 2 years of age, or a codeine syrup (1 mg/kg/dose) at 4 hour intervals for one or two doses only, can alleviate all but the most severe pain. However, it may take as long as 30 to 40 minutes for these analgesics to become effective.

For the treatment of intractable pain of otitis media, a myringotomy may be necessary. Additional indications for myringotomy in AOM include presence of fever and toxicity, especially in an infant; an immunocompromised host; or failure to ameliorate significant symptoms of fever and toxicity after 48 hours of antibiotic therapy.

Most studies fail to demonstrate any benefit of decongestants in hastening the resolution of AOM or preventing residual middle ear effusion. I do not

---

*This dose of bacampicillin may exceed that recommended for children by the manufacturer.

†Not recommended for children less than 3 months of age.

*Pediazole should not be administered to infants under 2 months of age.

recommend such agents unless a significant amount of rhinorrhea is present.

Suppurative Complications. If signs of toxicity persist after 48 hours of therapy, the child should be re-evaluated promptly. The key factor in the avoidance of the common, grave, suppurative complications of AOM (such as meningitis) or such rare complications as coalescent mastoiditis, lateral sinus thrombosis, cranial nerve palsy, labyrinthitis, and brain abscess is the timely recognition of clinical signs and symptoms of deterioration in the patient's condition. Such sinister symptoms and signs as prolongation of high fever beyond 48 hours after institution of therapy, persistent irritability or lethargy, and a general appearance of toxicity merit a prompt and thorough re-evaluation of the child's overall condition. Performance of a lumbar puncture must be considered. More commonly, signs of persistent AOM (completely bulging, immobile eardrum with loss of ossicular landmarks) during antimicrobial therapy are due to noncompliance, impaired absorption of the prescribed antibiotic, or prescription of an antibiotic ineffective against the strain of organisms causing the AOM. If extraotitic complications have *not* occurred, educating the parent to communicate at once any worsening of the disease and changing the antibiotic to one of the many alternatives seems reasonable.

After the child has finished the prescribed 10 days of antimicrobial therapy, it is advisable to re-examine him within the next 30 days, even though symptoms of pain or fever may be absent. Persistence of middle ear effusion medial to a nonbulging but immobile eardrum that causes a mild hearing loss can be detected in 40 to 60% of children younger than 5 years and in 35% of older children at the time of such re-evaluation. However, unless a properly sealed pneumatic otoscope head or the more sophisticated Tympanometer is used in physical diagnosis of persistent OME, fluid in the middle ear cleft may be overlooked because the eardrum appears to be normal upon visual examination alone. A common error is to equate the physical signs of persistent OME with those of an inadequately treated persistent AOM in which the eardrum is markedly bulging and immobile, and appears yellow because of the purulent exudate medial to it. Although there is some overlap, the clinician usually should be able to differentiate persistent AOM from the more frequent persistent OME (middle ear effusion) in which there is also loss of mobility but there is no bulging or loss of ossicular landmarks.

The child who still has a bulging immobile, opacified eardrum at the completion of the initial antibiotic course should receive an alternative antimicrobial agent in full doses for an additional 10 day course of therapy. The child who has a nonbulging (in neutral or retracted position) but poorly mobile eardrum may do well with no additional antibiotic therapy if he or she has not been otitis-prone. The otitis-prone child (two or three episodes of AOM in the previous 3 months) who has persistent middle ear effusion after antibiotic therapy for AOM may benefit from a single bedtime dose of sulfisoxazole (30 mg/kg) or trimethoprim-sulfamethoxazole (40 mg/kg of the sulfa component). I am in favor of a therapeutic trial of low dose antimicrobial prophylaxis for these children. The next follow-up visit for children with persistent middle ear effusion may be scheduled for 4 to 6 weeks later.

Serous effusions have low viscosity and are therefore more likely than mucoid effusions to drain into the nasopharynx via the eustachian tube. Such drainage of serous fluid may be assisted by the use of the Politzer technique; after the patient's nose has been cleared of any retained secretions, he takes a sip of water and holds it in his mouth; then, a clean 1 ounce Davol infant nasal syringe is firmly seated in one nostril, the other nostril is occluded by an index finger, and while the patient swallows the water, the nasal bulb is squeezed. When properly performed, this maneuver causes a bolus of air to traverse the nasal passages, open the eustachian tube, and enter the middle ear. The air pressure this bolus of air causes in the middle ear causes fluid of low viscosity to drain down the eustachian tube into the nasopharynx. Politzerization can be performed by the patient two to three times daily at home.

A mucoid middle ear effusion is more difficult to treat. Because pathogens can be isolated from only 15 to 25% of mucoid middle ear effusions compared with 70% of persistent acute middle ear effusions, patients with persistent OME may not benefit from a second complete course of antibiotic therapy, while patients with persistent AOM may. However, during the otitis season, 15% of young children with OME will soon develop symptoms of pain and signs of a bulging eardrum, which are diagnostic of recrudescent AOM. As a means of preventing this, I suggest that sulfisoxazole*be administered prophylactically (30 mg/kg in a single bedtime dose) for 3 to 4 weeks to a child with OME. Amoxicillin (10 mg/kg as a single dose at bedtime) also may be used. After this 3 to 4 week period another visit is scheduled in order to evaluate the status of the affected middle ear. Only 10% of children with OME have been found to have middle ear effusions persisting for longer than 3 months, so unless there are symptoms of recrudescent AOM during this 3-month observation period, visits to the physician should be at infrequent intervals,

---

*Manufacturer's precaution: Not recommended for infants less than 2 months of age.

such as every 4 to 6 weeks. Sulfisoxazole prophylaxis may be given for the whole period or observation alone may be recommended. Because tympanometry provides significant objective evidence of the presence of otitis media with effusion, patients who have OME persisting for more than 2 months should have a tympanogram and, if the patient is old enough to cooperate, an audiogram as well. A flat (type B) tympanogram pattern obtained from a patient with diminished eardrum mobility is strongly supportive evidence of OME. I believe that such a diagnostic instrument is a worthwhile investment.

Persistent OME

When middle ear effusion persists beyond the 3 to 4 month observation period, the practitioner should obtain otolaryngologic consultation. The decision to recommend ventilation tube placement must be individualized. Patients with a pre-existing hearing loss or additional serious handicapping condition should be referred earlier. Persistent bilateral OME and particularly OME associated with a moderate or severe bilateral hearing loss as determined by audiologic testing should also be referred earlier. Ventilation tubes are also indicated if there have been several episodes of recurrent AOM undiminished in frequency by sulfonamide prophylaxis. There is no compelling evidence that ventilation tube placement earlier than 3 months after diagnosis of OME is helpful unless other risk factors are present.

Prednisone, given in a short course (7 to 10 days) to selected patients with chronic OME (2 to 3 months' duration) may effectively promote drainage of mucoid fluid in 50 to 60% of patients thus treated. Barring contraindications or parental objection, prednisone (1 mg/kg/day)* as tablets, or prepared as a 5 mg/5 ml suspension in four divided doses, is given for 4 days, then a single morning dose is given for the next 6 days, for a total dosage of 10 mg/kg over 10 days. Sulfisoxazole (30/mg/kg/dose) is given twice daily in addition to the prednisone as a means of preventing recrudescent AOM. The parents must be instructed to promptly report symptoms of severe persistent headache, otalgia, or high fever in a child treated with prednisone for persistent OME. All children so treated must be re-evaluated several weeks later, as rebound OME can occur, although infrequently (in 20% of those whose OME clears with a course of prednisone). Because a nasopharyngeal neoplasm may masquerade as an innocent middle ear effusion, a thorough otolaryngologic examination including visualization of the nasopharynx should be done when the physician encounters unilateral persistent OME in older patients.

Ventilation Tubes. Ventilation tubes have become a widely accepted therapy for chronic OME, for prevention of recurrent AOM in otitis-prone children, and for severe persistent underaeration (atelectasis) of the middle ear. The tubes are unquestionably efficacious if patent and in situ, and their placement is rapidly becoming the most frequently performed pediatric surgical procedure in the United States. General anesthesia is usually advised, but several otologists have been able to use in-office lidocaine (Xylocaine) iontophoresis anesthesia of the tympanic membrane, particularly if the patient is able to cooperate. Although it is widely believed imperative to protect the ear canal from entry of water, several prominent otologists believe that earmolds or earplugs are unnecessary if the patient does not swim deeply under water or dive off the high board. Middle ear infection, even in the unprotected ear with a functioning tympanostomy tube, occurs infrequently and it is easily controlled by the instillation into the ear canal of topical otic antibiotic drops.

Because many tympanostomy tubes are designed to extrude in about 6 to 9 months, 20% of otitis-prone children will need to undergo a second procedure at a future date. Otorrhea through a functioning tube is the most frequent complication of ventilation tube use and can be expected to occur in 10 to 20% of children. Otorrhea associated with an upper respiratory infection is usually self-limited and treatment should include a course of amoxicillin or an alternative antibiotic, with or without topical otic drops instilled into the ear canal.

Chronic otorrhea, refractory to simple measures, will occur in 4% of children with ventilation tubes. It is the most frequent significant complication of ventilation tube use and can be very difficult to control. The instillation of topical antibiotic drops (such as corticosporin suspension) into the affected ear, followed by gentle intermittent pressure on the tragus in an attempt to force the drops through the lumen of the tube, may be effective. In recalcitrant cases of otorrhea, particularly if culture shows it to contain *Pseudomonas,* a course of gentamicin or another antipseudomonas drug administered intramuscularly or intravenously in hospital or practitioner's office may be efficacious but well designed studies upon which to judge this suggestion are unavailable. As a last resort, persistent otorrhea may be treated by excision of granulation tissue in the middle ear cleft or mastoidectomy.

Adenoidectomy as treatment for OME or recurrent AOM is of unproven efficacy although the removal of adenoids may be of value when there is roentgenographic or endoscopic evidence of encroachment on the airway by persistently hypertro-

---

*Manufacturer's precaution: Not recommended for infants less than 2 months of age.

phied adenoids. In the absence of such upper airway obstruction, an adenoidectomy is unlikely to prevent the need for additional middle ear surgery.

The role of allergy is unclear. If there is a strong family or personal history of allergic disease and if some screening tests such as IgE determination, a nasal eosinophil count (cytogram), selected skin tests, or RAST tests are significantly elevated above normal values for the patient's age, referral may be made to an allergist.

Prophylaxis of Recurrent Otitis Media. Infants who are otitis prone should be fed in an upright position. A 2 to 3 week trial of a hypoallergenic (milk-, peanut-, and egg-free) diet may be of benefit in identifying the course of the otitis. Several controlled studies have demonstrated that chemoprophylaxis using low-dose sulfisoxazole (30 mg/kg/dose)* or sulfamethoxazole (20 mg/kg/dose) given twice daily or in a single bedtime dose during the otitis media season (December through April), may significantly reduce the frequency of recurrent AOM in otitis-prone children.

Chronic Otitis Media

Persistent otitis media with effusion medial to an intact eardrum that has been present for at least 3 months has been termed chronic OME. When the effusion of chronic OME appears to be gun-metal blue, suggestive of cholesterolosis, or when there is a deep retraction pocket in the eardrum or adhesive otitis media, surgical intervention is almost always imperative. A cholesteatoma in the middle ear cleft associated with chronic OME with effusion must always be treated by surgical intervention.

Chronic otitis media may be also associated with chronic otorrhea. Persistent middle ear drainage through a perforation in the eardrum may be caused by *Pseudomonas* or other gram-negative pathogens, *S. aureus,* pharyngeal anaerobes, *Mycobacterium tuberculosis,* or fungal species. Chronic otorrhea may also be caused by a middle ear or nasopharyngeal mass such as a cholesteatoma, rhabdomysarcoma, or histiocytosis X. A thorough radiologic and surgical evaluation may be necessary if the draining ear is unresponsive to a trial of medical management.

Mastoiditis

Acute mastoiditis is the extension of a suppurative otitis media into the mucous membrane lining of the mastoid air cell system. Far-advanced mastoiditis leads to coalescence of the honeycomb–like mastoid septa. Mastoiditis in its early stages is characterized by otalgia, inflammation of the skin above the mastoid prominence, and swelling, tenderness, and redness of the posterior auricular area, which has the consistency of dough. The eardrum in cases of acute mastoiditis will always be opacified, poorly mobile, and completely bulging outward. Myringotomy and suction aspiration of middle ear pus should be performed at once, and an appropriate antibiotic effective against the pneumococcus and group A streptococcus must be given intravenously. A sample of middle ear pus should be obtained for Gram stain and bacteriology. If there is no improvement in the patient's condition after 24 to 48 hours of antimicrobial therapy or if signs of a subperiosteal mastoid abscess or facial paralysis have developed, the mastoid must be completely drained surgically.

Labyrinthitis

ROBERT J. RUBEN, M.D.

Labyrinthitis is an uncommon but treatable form of inner ear disease. Before the advent of antibiotics, labyrinthitis was primarily due to an infectious process entering the inner ear either from the middle ear or secondary to meningitis with spread to the inner ear from the statoacoustic nerve, the cochlear aqueduct, and/or the vessels entering the inner ear. This form of labyrinthitis was and still is essentially untreatable.

The pediatrician today will see patients with labyrinthitis the symptoms of which will not necessarily be only those of sudden deafness. Therefore, the differential diagnosis is important. Recognition of the various forms of labyrinthitis can result in successful treatment.

The symptoms and signs can involve any portion of the inner ear; the most common primarily involve the vestibular labyrinth. The child may have episodes of vomiting, tilting of the head, loss of motor skills and balance, dizziness, a feeling of rotation and/or movement (i.e., true vertigo), and nystagmus. Additionally there may be sudden, progressive, or fluctuating hearing loss.

Approximately 9% of all children who have bacterial meningitis will have an associated hearing and vestibular impairment of some degree. The amount of labyrinthine involvement may be more severe in children in whom therapy was started later in the course of meningitis. Months or years later the hearing may improve but in some cases will get worse. There is no known treatment for this progressive loss. It is necessary to monitor the loss in these children for a number of years so that proper habilitation measures can be taken.

The hearing loss found in children with congenital rubella also is from a form of labyrinthitis. There are still occasional cases of congenital rubella deaf-

---

*Manufacturer's precaution: Not recommended for infants under 2 months of age.

ness, and a large number of adolescents who have had congenital rubella hearing loss. This hearing loss also can be progressive. The need for audiologic follow-up of these children is the same as in those with hearing loss from bacterial meningitis.

Many of these children will have a vestibular impairment, which must be documented, as it can result in a severe problem, especially during the adolescent years. Those with severely impaired vestibular functions are unable to orient themselves when swimming underwater and some have drowned. Thus, any child with a vestibular impairment must be watched carefully when swimming and should be encouraged not to participate in aquatic sports.

The most frequently diagnosed acquired viral labyrinthitis is from mumps. Usually this is unilateral, but it can be bilateral. There is no effective intervention for this. Two aspects of "mumps" labyrinthitis are important for the well-being of the child. The first is accuracy of diagnosis. Often a unilateral hearing loss is discovered during a hearing screening test and is incorrectly attributed to a history of mumps. Further exploration will often show that the child has an autosomal dominant hearing loss that may have variable penetrance. A hearing loss can be progressive and thus needs continual audiologic assessment. Genetic counseling also should be considered.

The second important aspect of unilateral hearing loss is the need for amplification and identification of sound. Many children with unilateral hearing loss have significant school problems, in that they do poorly in linguistic cognitive skills. This may be ameliorated or avoided by use of a Cross hearing device, which can transmit sound from the deaf ear to the hearing ear. The child can then effectively hear from both sides and does not miss the information going to the deaf side. Children with unilateral hearing loss are now routinely fitted with Cross hearing aids. The younger the child is when fitted, the more acceptable are the results. In addition, the school should be informed of the problem so that the child has proper seating, with the better ear closest to the teacher. Although there are no firm data to show that these interventions will ameliorate the cognitive defects, they are believed to be effective. The Cross hearing aid is used for other forms of unilateral deafness following labyrinthitis, such as that from skull fracture that involves the temporal bone, and other forms of trauma to the inner ear.

Chronic middle ear infection such as cholesteatoma that has eroded the bony capsule of the inner ear or the persistent infection found in chronic tympanomastoiditis can cause labyrinthitis. The treatment for both of these conditions is surgery to remove the cholesteatoma or chronically infected bone and granulation tissue of the mastoid and middle ear cleft.

Awareness of a treatable form of childhood labyrinthitis has come about during the last decade. This labyrinthitis is associated with a loss of perilymph from the inner ear to the middle ear. The perilymph leak, or fistula, can come from either the round window or the oval window, or both. The most common cause of perilymph fistula is a congenital defect in the round or oval window that allows the inner ear fluid to escape into the middle ear. The second most common associated condition is severe malformation of the bony capsule of the inner ear, as demonstrated by imaging. The third appears to be pressure changes from increased strains such as lifting heavy weights. A child who is straining may have a sudden loss of hearing with or without associated vertigo. The fistula can also be found in cases of temporal bone fracture and erosion of the bony capsule of the temporal bone by cholesteatoma.

Symptoms can be either dramatic or subtle. A sudden hearing loss shortly after exercise is suggestive of a rupture of either the round or oval window. Recurrent meningitis following otitis media is very suggestive of congenital dehiscence of either the round or oval window. Recurrent meningitis from a fistula is life-threatening and must be corrected. Children with fluctuating or progressive sensorineural hearing loss may also have fistulas. The probability of a fistula is greatly increased in children with fluctuating or progressive hearing loss, or both, if the child also has a malformation of the bony inner ear with or without craniofacial abnormalities, or vestibular symptoms.

Episodic vestibular symptoms and signs are common manifestations. Vestibular symptoms may or may not be associated with a recurrent middle ear effusion. These children will present differently at different ages. Infants and toddlers may show motor ability retrogression associated with vomiting and at times with head tilt to the affected side. The older child can articulate his dizziness or true vertigo. Some children will be unable to get out of bed because of dizziness. Vomiting can be so severe that intravenous replacement of fluids and electrolytes will be required. These children may or may not have associated sensorineural hearing loss.

Diagnosis of perilymph fistula has also been made following a myringotomy for middle ear effusion. The fluid found was clear and continued to drain. The fluid was a perilymph and not the effusion from the middle ear. The perilymph can be easily differentiated from the exudate and transudate that occur in middle ear effusion. Perilymph is very similar to cerebral spinal fluid and does not contain many of the mucous elements found in middle ear effusions.

All of these fistulas must be surgically closed to prevent meningitis and to stop the debilitating vestibular symptoms. There is also evidence to indicate that closure of the fistula may prevent further hearing loss. Surgical repair is done through a tympanotomy incision—reflecting the tympanic membrane, exploring the round and oval windows for a leak, and then sealing the round or oval window, or both, with an autogenous graft of fat or perichondrium. The procedure is relatively safe and standard with very little morbidity. The results of sealing the fistula have been excellent in children who have had recurrent meningitis and/or severe vestibular symptoms. The procedure is life saving in children with recurrent meningitis. The hearing results have been marginal and the best that can be expected is to halt further progression of the hearing loss. There have been cases in which the hearing losses became worse after the procedure. Whether this is due to the procedure or to other factors is not known.

Exploratory tympanotomy for fistula is recommended for all children in whom there is evidence of labyrinthitis secondary to perilymph leak, and especially for those with severe vestibular symptoms or recurrent meningitis. The benefits far outweigh the minor surgical risks.

Injuries of the Middle Ear

COLLIN S. KARMODY, M.D.

Perforations of the Tympanic Membrane. Traumatic perforations of the tympanic membrane are caused either by sharp penetrating injuries or by a blow on the pinna with a flat surface—for example, the palm of the hand. Generally, traumatic perforations of the tympanic membrane heal spontaneously. Small or moderate sized clean dry perforations should be left alone. Ear drops should not be used unless infection supervenes. Larger perforations are examined with high magnification, using an operating microscope. If the edges are inverted, that is, rolled under, they may be everted back into normal position and held there with a patch of gel foam. If, after 2 months, there is no evidence of spontaneous closure of the perforation, a myringoplasty is necessary. A medially placed free graft of temporalis fascia is usually successful.

Ossicular Discontinuity. Discontinuity of the ossicular chain of the middle ear might be caused by penetrating transcanal injuries or might be associated with fractures of the temporal bone. The discontinuity might be the result of a dislocation or fracture and cause a conductive hearing loss of about 50 decibels. The incus and stapes are usually involved, the malleus rarely so. Dislocations are corrected by repositioning the ossicles into their anatomic positions and splinting them in place with gel foam. The end results are variable.

Dislocation of the stapes is likely to cause a sensorineural hearing loss and might cause vertigo. If the residual hearing is useful, a stapedectomy is performed using a prosthesis of stainless steel wire and soft tissue. Alternatively, the footplate of the stapes might be only partially displaced with fistulization of the oval window. These patients complain of dizziness. If the rest of the ossicular chain is intact, then the fistula should be sealed with tissue, e.g., fat, after the edges are freshened.

If the incus is severely dislocated, ossicular discontinuity might be achieved only by turning the incus so that the body of the incus makes contact with the head of the stapes and the long process with the handle of the malleus.

Fractures. The malleus is rarely fractured. Fractures usually involve the long process of the incus and the component parts of the stapes, usually the crura, occasionally the footplate. Fractures of the incus require repositioning of the remaining body of the incus to achieve ossicular continuity. Alternatively, the incus can be bypassed by a prosthesis between the handle of the malleus and the head of the stapes. Fractures of the footplate of the stapes require a stapedectomy because of the tendency for persistence of the fracture and leakage of perilymph and complaints of vertigo.

Fractures of the promontory of the middle ear may remain open, with leakage of perilymph and risk of meningitis. If there is suspicion that such a fracture exists, the middle ear must be explored and the open fracture plugged with fat taken from the lobule of the pinna.

Hearing Loss

ARNOLD E. KATZ, M.D.,
and HUBERT L. GERSTMAN, D. Ed.

MEDICAL AND SURGICAL MANAGEMENT OF CONDUCTIVE HEARING LOSS

The external and middle ears compose a system that gathers and transmits sound to the inner ear. This system is connected and suspended in an optimal manner so that its mass and tension characteristics efficiently transmit sound. Addition of mass (e.g., wax, fluid, tumors) or alterations in tension (e.g., otosclerosis, adhesions) impair the efficiency of the system and result in hearing loss. Conductive hearing impairments are usually treatable, medically, surgically, or both. They are also frequently effectively treated with amplification (hearing aids).

Congenital Conductive Hearing Loss

Congenital conductive hearing losses may be unilateral or bilateral. Although the maximum conductive loss can be no greater than 60 decibels or so, bilateral losses in this range can impair greatly the child's ability to develop speech. The severity of congenital impairment must be considered in outlining therapy. Surgical correction of total aplasia of the external auditory canal or middle ear is fraught with the real possibility of facial nerve injury. Surgical correction of anomalies of the ossicles is accompanied by a much smaller risk of facial paralysis. These risks must be fully discussed with the patient's family. In unilateral conductive losses, surgery should probably be delayed until the child is able to participate in the selection of therapy. Amplification is frequently a good choice.

Inflammatory Conductive Hearing Loss

External Otitis. This infection may cause a conductive hearing loss, depending on how much inflammation and debris are in the canal. When the canal is filled with debris, pain is usually a major symptom and must be controlled with salicylates or codeine. Removal of debris is accomplished with a gentle suction and small wisps of cotton wound on metal cotton carriers. A wick must also be inserted so that the otic drops used will reach the site of infection. The otic drops usually employed and quite effective contain hydrocortisone, polymyxin B, and neomycin; 4 drops four times a day. After the swelling of the canal has decreased, the wick may be eliminated; however, the drops should be continued at least 3 days after the relief of pain. Recurrences may be prevented by routine use of acid-alcohol drops (mix white vinegar and rubbing alcohol 50/50) after swimming or bathing. Any signs of systemic involvement necessitate the culturing of the exudate and the immediate institution of systemic antibiotics. *Staphylococcus aureus* group A, beta-hemolytic streptococcus, micrococci, diphtheroids, and *Pseudomonas aeruginosa* are the organisms most usually encountered.

Secretory Otitis Media. The therapy of this most common cause of hearing loss must be based on the knowledge of the natural history of this disease. By far most of these patients will experience spontaneous remission without any treatment. Medical or surgical therapy should not be instituted until the patient has been followed for at least 1 month without improvement in symptoms.

If the fluid persists for over a month, one must then ask how this fluid is affecting the patient. If speech has developed normally and the child is doing very well in school, one can feel comfortable about following the child. It would be wise to advise the school that the child may suffer from an intermittent increase in the severity of the hearing problem. He or she should be seated in the front row with the better ear toward the teacher, and any deterioration of the child's work should be brought to the attention of parents and physician.

If speech or school work is suffering (even if the hearing loss is 25 decibels or less) aggressive therapy should be instituted in the following order:

1. The child should be instructed to perform the Valsalva maneuver several times a day.
2. The chewing of sugarless gum should be recommended.
3. If the child is atopic, antihistamines or decongestants or both may be of value. If there is no response to these for 1 month, they should be discontinued. If the fluid clears while the child is taking this type of medication, parents should be instructed to reinstitute this therapy at the first sign of a running nose or other clinical symptoms of increased antigenic exposure. No group of drugs has enjoyed such widespread advocacy without demonstration of efficiency as have antihistamines and decongestants. It is highly likely that if these drugs are effective, they are only of value in a minority of patients with this disease. It has been estimated that less than 30% of patients with chronic secretory otitis media have an underlying allergic etiology.
4. Although advocated by some, the efficiency of prophylactic antibiotics in this disease has not been established. If the fluid is associated with recurrent attacks of acute suppurative otitis media, trimethoprim/sulfamethoxazole or sulfisoxazole,* 100 mg/kg/24 hr, may be of value.
5. Myringotomy with aspiration of fluid and placement of a ventilating tube is remarkably effective in immediately relieving the hearing loss caused by this disease. Unfortunately, the ventilating tubes remain effective for only about 6 months to a year. Occasionally, after the tubes are obstructed or expelled, the fluid re-collects. In these patients, replacement of the tubes is sometimes necessary. It must be remembered, however, that amplification (hearing aids) remains a viable option in the treatment of these very difficult management problems. Adenoidectomy, with or without tonsillectomy, probably does not affect the natural history of this disease.

Acute Suppurative Otitis Media. Treatment of this entity is discussed on page 485.

Chronic Suppurative Otitis Media. Intermittent foul-smelling drainage from one or both ears usually heralds a perforation of the tympanic membrane or a cholesteatoma. Both of these conditions are usually accompanied by a conductive hearing loss and the patient should be referred to an otolaryngologist. Surgery is indicated to remove the infected bone of the middle ear and mastoid, which frequently accompanies this disease.

Traumatic Causes of Conductive Hearing Loss

Foreign Bodies. These may cause a conductive hearing loss in various ways. Their presence may

---

*Sulfisoxazole is contraindicated in infants less than 2 months of age.

prevent sound from reaching the tympanic membrane. They may also cause a conductive hearing loss by perforating the tympanic membrane or fracturing or dislocating the ossicles. If there is no damage to the tympanic membrane or ossicles, removal of the foreign body will restore hearing. If there is middle ear damage, further surgery may be necessary to restore hearing. Foreign bodies in the ear of a struggling child should be removed by an otolaryngologist, frequently with general anesthesia.

Trauma to the Tympanic Membrane or Ossicles. Blast injuries or penetrating wounds to the external ear can result in conductive hearing loss. Immediate treatment should include examination under a microscope, if possible, and assessment of the amount of hearing loss. Most traumatic perforations heal spontaneously. Parents should be advised to keep water out of the ear during bathing or washing the child's hair. This is best accomplished by placing a cotton ball to which has been applied a small amount of petroleum jelly in the external canal to seal it. Do not fill the canal with petroleum jelly. Dry cotton will act as a wick and allow water to contaminate the middle ear. Antibiotic drops are also helpful in preventing or treating an ear infection while the tympanic membrane is healing.

If a conductive hearing loss persists after the eardrum is healed, one must suspect ossicle damage. Exploratory tympanotomy with an ossiculoplasty may be necessary to restore the hearing.

Fractures of the External Auditory Canal. Fractures of the external auditory canal may accompany other types of facial and temporal bone trauma. Trauma to the mandible may result in a posterior displacement of the anterior wall of the canal with obstruction. Sound is prevented from vibrating the tympanic membrane, and a conductive hearing loss will result.

If this fracture is diagnosed early (within 7 to 10 days) it can be reduced easily with a nasal speculum. The speculum is inserted into the canal and opened. If weeks elapse between the time of the fracture and the time of the diagnosis, much more extensive surgery is necessary to enlarge the canal.

Neoplastic Causes of Conductive Hearing Loss

Benign and malignant tumors of the external and middle ears may reach sufficient size to cause a conductive hearing loss. If the tumor is benign (e.g., osteoma), local surgical excision is indicated. If it is malignant, treatment of the malignancy must assume prime importance. Treatment of the malignancy will probably necessitate sacrifice of hearing in the affected ear. Malignancy must be suspected in a chronic external otitis with pain and blood-tinged purulence, and a biopsy must be performed on the canal. Even in the absence of the hallmarks of malignancy, a firm, granular-appearing external canal should have a biopsy to rule out an early squamous cell carcinoma or a rhabdomyosarcoma.

Conductive Hearing Loss—General Considerations

In general, pure conductive hearing loss is defined by the fact that the patient has normal "cochlear reserve." When the sound is loud enough, the hearing loss is compensated for by amplification. Thus, when medical or surgical treatment fails to fully restore hearing, a mild amount of gain in a hearing aid may be safely used. In chronic otitis, as in other conditions characterized by intermittent reductions in hearing acuity, a hearing aid is sometimes utilized on an "as needed" basis.

Except in rare cases, "pure" conductive pathologies seldom require significant other supportive treatment. However, if the illness is a concomitant, subsequent or consequent condition to etiologies affecting motor speech, language, or cognitive development, the matter requires prompt treatment and frequent follow-up visits and supportive training. For instance, a cleft palate problem invariably is accompanied by some otitis media. Such a child already is impaired to a degree by a communication deficit. The added illness hinders perceptual skill to the extent that loss of acuity affects perception. Therefore, particular attention must be paid to the status of the middle ear.

When conductive pathology is overlaid on a significant sensorineural hearing loss, the conductive components must be remedied so as to allow other habilitation training and amplification to be optimal. The fitting of hearing aids requires attention to the amount of gain, the intensity of sound to be allowed into the auditory system, the frequency range or spectrum to be admitted, and the varied patterns in the different portions of the frequency bands amplified. These specific differences in amplification properties are fitted to the patients' perceptions of clarity, intelligibility, pitch, quality, and sound comfort in search of a perfect union of person to machine. The compensation for conductive loss may be markedly different than that for sensorineural loss; thus additional or intermittent conductive impairment may be doubly disturbing to the basic sensorineural patient.

SENSORINEURAL HEARING LOSS

Medicine's best contribution to the area of sensorineural hearing loss is probably in its prevention. Immediate treatment of toxic conditions, conservative use of ototoxic medications, genetic counseling for parents who have already produced hearing-impaired offspring, and efficient treatment of upper respiratory infections or other diseases apt to produce damage to the cochlea or the auditory nervous system are the most productive for management of those at high risk.

Except for that caused by certain specific disease states (e.g., viral labyrinthitis) and certain medications (aspirin may produce ototoxic reactions that are reversible when use is discontinued), sensorineural hearing loss is permanent, irreversible, and frustrating.

Audiologic and Other Management

Audiologic evaluation, coupled with variously required other evaluations such as those performed by psychologists and speech/language pathologists, contributes to the diagnosis regarding site-of-lesion and, more importantly, regarding degree of impairment. An understanding of specific effects of patterns of hearing loss contributes more to habilitation and rehabilitation than any other single factor.

Once the basic diagnostic activity is under way, management plans may begin for infant stimulation, specifically of language. Later, stimulation for speech and consideration of cognitive development may be included in the management plan. Before the child is at the preschool level, treatment proceeds on several fronts, including any medical and surgical intervention that is necessary, fitting of hearing aids when appropriate, counseling of parents, plans for preschool educational programs, and general long-term plans.

In addition to hearing aids, specific activities may also take place in the area of auditory training, which teaches the child to differentiate specific warning sounds in the environment and later other alerting sounds and the various meanings of sounds that the child may be capable of heeding on both an uncompensated and a compensated basis. Other training forms take advantage of the visual modality for the benefit of communication and the other sensory modalities in training for speech production.

Training in sign language contributes to children's ability to develop symbolic behaviors, to increase their use of language, and to maintain other such linguistic shortcuts in categorizing their experience to the benefit of cognitive skills.

18

Infectious Diseases

Neonatal Septicemia, Meningitis, and Pneumonia

MOSES GROSSMAN, M.D.

NEONATAL SEPTICEMIA

Supportive therapy is vital for recovery of the infant. Thus attention to fluid and electrolyte balance, support of circulation and ventilation, and caloric intake are equally as important as the choice of antimicrobial agents. In nosocomially acquired infections, consideration must be given to removal of potentially infected catheters.

Initial *antimicrobial therapy* usually consists of ampicillin or penicillin and an aminoglycoside. We favor ampicillin because of its somewhat broader spectrum against the common newborn nursery pathogens, while, practically speaking, it is as effective against gram-positive bacteria as penicillin. Penicillin is more effective against anaerobic bacteria, but their role in neonatal sepsis seems to be of less importance. The choice of aminoglycoside is between gentamicin, tobramycin, kanamycin, and amikacin. We currently favor gentamicin or tobramycin; these antimicrobials are definitely preferable in nosocomial infections since they are effective against more strains of *Pseudomonas* and many strains of *Serratia*. We find it more convenient for the nursing staff and for the laboratory that performs the serum levels to use one aminoglycoside predominantly. Kanamycin is equally as effective for the vast majority of maternally acquired infections, offers no additional toxicity, and is used routinely in many nurseries. Gentamicin has had somewhat greater usage than tobramycin, but the effectiveness and pharmacokinetics of the two seem to be essentially identical with very similar potential for toxicity. We do not currently use amikacin for the initiation of therapy unless there is good reason to suspect gram-negative bacteria resistant to gentamicin and tobramycin.

For the sick infant whose circulation may be impaired, both ampicillin and aminoglycoside must be given intravenously to ensure good serum levels; the relatively well infant may receive these drugs intravenously or intramuscularly, depending on other considerations of care. The dosage guidelines are listed in Table 1. The penicillins have a wide enough efficacy versus safety ratio that one need not worry about obtaining blood levels in most infants. Aminoglycoside serum level determinations, on the other hand, are important in very sick infants, in very small infants, and in those with diminished kidney function. If chloramphenicol is used, frequent serum level determinations are imperative, since there is a great deal of individual variance in enzyme maturation, resulting in widely fluctuant serum levels. One must aim for an effective level and stay away from the potentially toxic zone (levels of 10 to 40 μg/ml are favored). If the blood culture is positive, it is always best to adjust the initial drugs selected so as to make the best possible therapeutic regimen based on the expected sensitivity of the organism, with a final adjustment when the actual sensitivity is determined. Treatment should continue for 7 to 10 days, depending on the organism and the initial site of infection, if known. Third generation cephalosporins appear to be safe and effective agents for gram-negative infections in the neonate. Moxalactam or cefotaxime can be used instead of or in addition to aminoglycosides.

If there is reason to believe that *Staphylococcus aureus* may be the causative organism, particularly in a nosocomial infection, methicillin should be included in the initial choice of drugs. Many institutions are experiencing a significant rise in methicillin-resistant strains of staphylococci. In that setting, vancomycin may be considered for the initia-

Table 1. ANTIMICROBIALS USED IN NEONATAL INFECTIONS*

| Drug | Route | Daily Dose (mg/kg/24 hr) (Doses per 24 hr) | |
		Infant 0–7 Days of Age	Infant 7–30 Days of Age
Penicillins			
Penicillin G	IV or IM	50,000–150,000 U (2–3)	100,000–200,000 U (3–4)
Ampicillin	IV or IM	50–100 (2)	100–200 (3–4)
Methicillin	IV or IM	50–150 (2–3)	100–200 (3–4)
Nafcillin	IV or IM	50–150 (2–3)	100–200 (3–4)
Ticarcillin	IV	200 (2–3)	250–350 (3–4)
Aminoglycosides			
Gentamicin	IV or IM	5 (2)	7.5 (3)
Tobramycin	IV or IM	4–5 (2)	7.5 (3)
Kanamycin	IV or IM	15–20 (2)§	20–25 (3)§
Amikacin	IV or IM	15 (2)	15 (3)
Cephalosporins			
Moxalactam	IV	100 (2)	150 (3)
Cefotaxime	IV	100 (2)	150 (3)
Others			
Chloramphenicol†	IV	25 (2)	50 (2)
Vancomycin	IV	30 (2)	45 (3)
Erythromycin	Oral	—	40 (3–4)
Amphotericin B‡	IV	0.1–1 (1)	0.1–1 (1)
Isonicotinic hydrazide	Oral	—	10–15 (1)

* The highest dose mentioned should be used for meningitis.
† These are initial dose guidelines. Frequent serum level determinations are essential to guide therapy.
‡ Given once a day over a period of 6 hours.
§ 20 to 25 mg/kg/24 hr may exceed the manufacturer's recommended dose.

tion of therapy, though its use is usually reserved until after the antimicrobial sensitivities have been determined. If *Pseudomonas* infection is suspected, ticarcillin might be added even before final identification. In the intensive care nursery, *Candida* species are significant pathogens. Amphotericin B is the drug used for the management of those infections. Group B beta-streptococci are the most common bacterial pathogens in the nursery at this time. While synergism between penicillin and aminoglycosides has been shown in dealing with the bacteria in the laboratory, clinically penicillin or ampicillin alone is adequate therapy for infections caused by this organism.

It is common to have negative blood cultures in an infant initially thought to have neonatal sepsis. After 72 hours almost all common bacteria should have grown, and it should be an exception, justified by special circumstances, to continue antimicrobial therapy beyond that period of time.

MENINGITIS

Septicemia during the neonatal period is frequently accompanied by meningitis. The goal of therapy is to ensure survival and to avoid neurologic sequelae and complications, which are found in more than a third of the survivors. The best strategy for this purpose is vigorous supportive therapy and early intervention with effective antimicrobials, resulting in early sterilization of the cerebrospinal fluid. This is more easily accomplished with streptococcal and listerial meningitis than when enteric organisms cause this infection. Antimicrobials used to initiate therapy are ampicillin and an aminoglycoside (in our hands, gentamicin), using the higher doses in the therapeutic range (Table 1). If the infection turns out to be due to Group B streptococci, penicillin alone is continued. In the case of *Listeria,* we continue ampicillin alone. In both instances one expects early sterilization of the cerebrospinal fluid; this should be confirmed by lumbar puncture a day or two after initiation of therapy; a final lumbar puncture is done at the end of therapy to ensure that CSF findings have returned to normal. In most instances 2 weeks of treatment are adequate for streptococcal and listerial meningitis.

Past experience in the management of meningitis due to gram-negative organisms with a combination of ampicillin and gentamicin has been dismal —it takes 3 to 4 days to sterilize the spinal fluid; and there is a 20% mortality and a 30% incidence of serious sequelae. There is some evidence that the addition of one of the third generation cephalosporins (moxalactam, cefotaxime or ceftriaxone) instead of using gentamicin may improve the outcome. Based on current evidence we recommend doing so, thus treating the infant with ampicillin and moxalactam. Antimicrobial sensitivity of the infecting organisms should guide the selection of the appropriate cephalosporin (only third generation cephalosporins adequately penetrate into the CSF). A lumbar puncture should be done daily or every other day to monitor the cerebrospinal fluid until it is sterile. Therapy should be continued for 2 weeks after the cerebrospinal fluid is sterile. We seldom treat gram-negative meningitis for less than 3 weeks.

We emphasized the importance of supportive therapy in assuring a favorable outcome in neonatal sepsis. Such vigorous support is particularly important in managing neonates with meningitis. Convulsive seizures are common; they are best stopped by diazepam initially, and then controlled using phenobarbital or phenytoin.

Fluid and electrolytes need to be monitored carefully since disturbances such as inappropriate secretion of ADH are common. Hydrocephalus (both communicating and noncommunicating) is a frequent complication. Thus head circumference must be followed carefully. We recommend a computed tomographic examination following neonatal meningitis. Hearing is commonly impaired and needs to be tested so as not to delay dealing with this important complication.

PNEUMONIA

Neonatal pneumonia may occur in one of three ways—as a result of intrauterine infection either by aspiration of infected amnionic fluid or through blood stream dissemination; more commonly as a result of aspirating infected material at birth; and, finally, by acquisition of infection in the nursery.

Therapy entails general supportive and specific antimicrobial therapy. Chest percussion, monitoring blood gases, provision of fluid and electrolytes, oxygen, and assisted ventilation when necessary are important aspects of supportive therapy. The most important antimicrobial for early-onset pneumonia is penicillin or ampicillin because of the high mortality, often associated with shock, in early-onset streptococcal pneumonia. Since the responsible pathogen is not known early, the initial antimicrobial regimen for pneumonia is the same as for sepsis—namely, penicillin or ampicillin and an aminoglycoside. Adjustments are made depending on the organism recovered. If *Pseudomonas* is suspected, ticarcillin or penicillin should be started at the onset; suspicion of staphylococcal pneumonia should lead one to include methicillin at the outset. Placement of chest tubes for drainage of empyema is essential in the case of staphylococcal pneumonia. It is also important to be certain that the staphylococci are methicillin-sensitive. The increasing prevalence of methicillin-resistant strains in hospital settings has led to greater reliance on vancomycin, the drug of choice in this situation.

Chlamydial pneumonia usually appears after the infant has left the nursery and is characterized by an afebrile course with staccato cough and eosinophilia. Erythromycin is the drug of choice for this infection but the infants usually are not very ill, and one can postpone initiating this more specific therapy until the diagnosis can be confirmed by cultural or serologic methods.

Most viral and bacterial pathogens may cause pneumonia in the infant, including some very treatable but uncommon etiologic agents—syphilis, tuberculosis, and so on. Successful therapy depends upon following clinical and epidemiologic clues and carrying out the requisite diagnostic procedures to come up with the definitive answer. At times this may include lung biopsy.

Bacterial Meningitis and Septicemia Beyond the Neonatal Period

RALPH D. FEIGIN, M.D.,
and JOSEPH P. NEGLIA, M.D.

Bacterial meningitis continues to be a significant problem. *Hemophilus influenzae, Streptococcus pneumoniae,* and *Neisseria meningitidis* are the most frequent pathogens in the normal child over one month of age and *H. influenzae* is responsible for more than 60% of cases.

Diagnosis is dependent upon careful examination of the cerebrospinal fluid (CSF), using Gram stain, culture, cell count, protein, and glucose (with simultaneous serum glucose for comparison). Countercurrent immunoelectrophoresis and latex particle agglutination tests of CSF, blood, and urine have been useful in rapid diagnosis of infection caused by these pathogens; results are not dependent upon the presence of viable organisms. These tests can be particularly valuable in patients who have received prior antibiotic therapy.

Initial Therapy

Ampicillin and chloramphenicol are recommended. Ampicillin is administered intravenously at 300 mg/kg/24 hr in six divided doses and chloramphenicol at 100 mg/kg/24 hr in four divided doses. Chloramphenicol may be discontinued once susceptibility to ampicillin has been established. Tube dilution sensitivity tests should be performed upon all isolates obtained from blood and CSF. Sensitivity of *H. influenzae,* type b, to ampicillin should not be inferred on the basis of beta-lactamase testing alone, as ampicillin resistance may be conferred by plasmids other than those that control beta-lactamase activity. Moxalactam (150 mg/kg/24 hr) in four divided doses also has been effective in treatment of meningitis due to *H. influenzae* (both ampicillin resistant and sensitive strains). Penicillin G (300,000 u/kg/24 hr) in six divided doses is the drug of choice for meningitis due to *S. pneumoniae* or *N. meningitidis*. In documented penicillin allergy, chloramphenicol may be used as a single drug for suspected or proven meningitis.

Intravenous antibiotics should be continued until the patient is afebrile for 5 days, but for at least 7 to 10 days in all cases. If clinical improvement is not noted within 24 hours or if the rate of improvement is slower than anticipated, repeat CSF examination is indicated. We favor re-examination of CSF at conclusion of therapy in all cases, since it permits the physician to document bacteriologic sterility at the time of discharge. This is not mandatory, however. At the end of treatment, CSF white blood cell counts and protein concentrations generally have not returned to normal and the CSF/serum glucose ratio may remain depressed. In all cases, CSF culture, Gram stain, and CIE should be negative. Retreatment is mandatory if they are not, and also may be suggested if more than 10% of CSF cells are polymorphonuclear or if the CSF glucose or CSF/blood glucose ratio is less than 20 mg/dl or 20%, respectively.

Supportive Care

The blood pressure, pulse rate, and respiratory rates of all children with suspected or proven bacterial meningitis should be monitored closely. Vital signs should be taken every 15 minutes until stable and then every 4 hours for the first several days. Temperature should be taken rectally every 4 hours.

A complete neurologic examination should be performed at admission and daily thereafter. A rapid neurologic examination to assess level of consciousness, pupillary response to light, extraocular motility, symmetry of movement, and activity of the deep tendon reflexes should be performed 6 to 12 times a day for the first several days.

The patient should be NPO for at least the first 24 hours, since vomiting may ensue and aspiration is best avoided. Also, careful measurement of intake and output can be achieved more readily if the child is receiving fluid intravenously.

Prospective studies have documented that almost 60% of children with bacterial meningitis develop the syndrome of inappropriate secretion of antidiuretic hormone (SIADH). In an attempt to determine the presence and severity of SIADH, body weight, serum electrolytes, and serum and urine osmolarities should be measured at the time of admission. The studies may be repeated several times during the first 24 to 36 hours in the hospital and daily for several days thereafter. Urine should be

obtained sequentially and careful measurement made of volume and specific gravity. The syndrome, when present, is best treated by fluid restriction. A multiple electrolyte solution containing 40 meq/l of Na^+ and Cl, 35 meq/l of K^+ and 20 meq/l of lactate or acetate should be administered initially at a rate of 800 to 1000 ml/m^2/24 hr. Fluid restriction is continued until the measurements detailed above prove that inappropriate secretion of ADH is not a factor or that its effect has dissipated. The best indication of fluid retention in excess of solute is an increase in body weight or decrease in serum sodium concentration. As the serum sodium increases toward normal, fluid administration may be liberalized progressively to normal maintenance levels of 1500 to 1700 ml/m^2/24 hr.

Head circumference should be measured and the head transilluminated at the time of admission and every day thereafter. This permits assessment of the development of subdural effusions or may suggest other causes of an enlarging head. Recent experience has shown transillumination to be a more reliable indicator of the presence of a small subdural effusion than is computed tomography (CT).

Computed tomography of the head may be recommended for children with bacterial meningitis in whom one or more of the following is documented: 1) focal or lateralizing neurologic signs; 2) focal seizures; 3) persistent increase in intracranial pressure with increasing head circumference that is unrelated to cerebral edema or to inappropriate secretion of antidiuretic hormone and does not respond to fluid restriction; or 4) suspicion of the presence of an intracranial process that antedated the meningitis or that appears to be concurrent with the meningitis.

Ultrasonography may be used to detect ventricular enlargement in children with open fontanels. This is less cumbersome and far less costly than CT scan and may be used to sequentially follow the course of ventricular enlargement.

The treatment of subdural effusions has been the subject of much debate. Recent studies suggest that treatment should consist of subdural paracentesis only, to curtail specific symptoms of increased intracranial pressure or when one suspects the effusion to be responsible for seizure activity or focal neurologic signs. In most cases of meningitis, subdural taps are not required. When vigorously sought, the frequency of subdural effusions in young children with bacterial meningitis is such that they can be considered part of the general disease process rather than a persistent or troublesome complication of meningeal infection.

Seizures occur before hospitalization or during the first several days of treatment in approximately 30% of afflicted children. When seizures are noted, a patent airway must be maintained and appropriate anticonvulsants administered. Initially, sodium phenobarbital, 7 to 10 mg/kg/dose, may be administered intravenously. Phenytoin, 5 mg/kg/24 hr, in two divided doses, may be used for seizure control. Phenytoin generally does not depress the respiratory center to the same extent as phenobarbital and may inhibit antidiuretic hormone release. If necessary, diazepam, 1 mg per year of age to a maximum of 10 mg, may be given intravenously as a bolus. Shock and/or disseminated intravascular coagulation may complicate meningitis and may necessitate vasopressor or heparin therapy.

Fifteen to 20% of children with bacterial meningitis will develop some auditory nerve function deficiency. Prior to discharge, total detailed neurologic, psychometric, and auditory evaluation is necessary to permit early corrective measures.

Children with invasive *H. influenzae* infection, including *H. influenzae* meningitis, frequently carry the organism in their nasopharynx after a course of systemic antibiotic therapy. Prior to discharge, those children who are returning to a home in which another child 4 years of age or less resides should be given rifampin, 20 mg/kg/dose, once daily (maximum 600 mg) for 4 days to avoid reinstitution of the organisms in the household.

Prophylaxis is indicated for household and day care center contacts of children with *H. influenzae* or *N. meningitidis* disease. Rifampin is the current drug of choice given as 20 mg/kg/24 hr in one daily dose for 4 days for contacts of the child with *H. influenzae* infection and as 20 mg/kg/24 hr in two divided doses for 2 days for contacts of the child with *N. meningitidis* infection. The dose for children under 1 month of age who are contacts of a patient with *N. meningitidis* infection is decreased to 10 mg/kg/24 hr (same schedule).

Four meningococcal vaccines are currently licensed in the United States: monovalent A, monovalent C, bivalent A and C and quadrivalent A, C, Y, and W135. Vaccine may be given to child contacts of patients with Type A, C, or W135 meningococcal disease in the doses recommended by the manufacturer. Group A vaccine is effective in children 3 months old and older; the other vaccines are effective in those 2 years of age and older. Safety of these vaccines in pregnant women has not been established. No highly immunogenic serogroup B vaccine has been prepared to date.

Septicemia

Septicemia beyond the neonatal period may be caused by any microorganism. In general, a careful history and physical examination will provide clues to a bacteriologic diagnosis. In the infant, the neonatal history may suggest specific infection with *S. agalactiae* (group B beta-hemolytic streptococci), *S. aureus*, *Pseudomonas*, or other enteric pathogens.

Sepsis in patients with impetiginous lesions or a history of recent surgery may be due to *S. aureus* or *S. pyogenes*. Infection with *S. pneumoniae*, *H. influenzae*, or other encapsulated pathogens is more likely in patients who have been splenectomized. Infection with *S. pneumoniae* or *Salmonella* is more frequent in children with sickle-cell disease or other hemoglobinopathies than in the normal population.

Whenever septicemia is suspected, two or three sets of blood cultures should be obtained over a period of several hours and antibiotic therapy should be initiated. A careful search should be made for the focus of infection. When, following careful physical examination, no source is discernible, a chest radiograph should be obtained and cultures of urine and CSF (if indicated) should be performed. Countercurrent immunoelectrophoresis on blood, CSF, and urine also may be helpful in establishing a specific bacteriologic diagnosis.

Until a bacteriologic diagnosis is established, ampicillin, 200 mg/kg/24 hours in six divided doses, and gentamicin, 5 to 7.5 mg/kg/24 hr in three divided doses, or kanamycin, 20–30 mg/kg/24 hr*in two or three divided doses, should be provided intramuscularly or intravenously to cover enteric microorganisms. Alternatively, penicillin G, 100,000 to 200,000 u/kg/24 hr intravenously in six divided doses, and chloramphenicol, 100 mg/kg/24 hr in four divided doses, may be utilized.

Shock and bleeding are common in septicemia, particularly when gram-negative organisms are recovered. In these patients, gentamicin or kanamycin should be given intravenously over a period of 30 minutes to 1 hour. If renal failure ensues, the usual first dose of aminoglycoside may be given but subsequent dosage must be altered. Subsequent adjustments are best made by measuring the concentration of the specific aminoglycoside in the blood. When this cannot be done, an appropriate dosage interval can be estimated by using the patient's serum creatinine concentration or calculated creatinine clearance.

When the cause of septicemia is due to *S. pneumoniae*, *S. pyogenes*, *S. agalactiae*, *N. gonorrhoeae*, *N. meningitidis*, or a penicillin sensitive *S. aureus*, generally penicillin may be utilized alone. Selected strains of *S. pneumoniae* have increased resistance to penicillin, and rare strains will not respond to clinical dosages. *Haemophilus influenzae* septicemia may be treated with ampicillin if the organism proves susceptible (see section on meningitis) or with chloramphenicol. Moxalactam has been shown to be effective in the treatment of both ampicillin sensitive and resistant *H. influenzae* infections (150 mg/

---

*This dose of kanamycin exceeds that recommended by the manufacturer.

kg/24 hr in four divided doses intravenously). The treatment of *Salmonella* septicemia must be guided by the sensitivity of the microorganism. In general, ampicillin or chloramphenicol may be utilized; chloramphenicol is preferred if *S. typhosa* is identified.

Penicillin resistant staphylococcal infection should be treated with methicillin administered intravenously in a dosage of 200 mg/kg/24 hr in six divided doses.* Oxacillin and nafcillin, 200 mg/kg/24 hr in six divided doses, are suitable alternatives. A cephalosporin or clindamycin will provide effective coverage for patients allergic to penicillin. Cephalosporins should not be given to patients who have had anaphylaxis or exfoliative dermatitis following exposure to penicillin. Peak serum concentrations of cefazolin generally are higher than concentrations of other cephalosporins when equivalent doses are employed. The drug can be provided in a dose of 50 mg/kg/24 hr in four divided doses intravenously. Cefotaxime, a new semisynthetic cephalosporin, also may prove useful in the treatment of septicemia. Cefotaxime (100 mg/kg/24 hr in four divided doses) provides better coverage against *Pseudomonas* and *Enterobacteriaceae* than other cephalosporins and reaches higher CSF concentrations. Clindamycin can be administered in a dose of 30 mg/kg/24 hr in three divided doses intravenously.

When *Pseudomonas* is identified, carbenicillin, 400 to 600 mg/kg/24 hr, in four divided doses intravenously, can be used alone *but preferably should be provided in combination with gentamicin.* Ticarcillin may be used instead of carbenicillin in a dose of 200 mg/kg/24 hr in four divided doses intravenously. Piperacillin†and mezlocillin, two new semisynthetic penicillins, also are effective in the treatment of *Pseudomonas* and *Klebsiella* infections and may be given intravenously in dosages of 300 mg/kg/24 hr in six divided doses.

A syndrome of pneumococcal bacteremia has been described in children between 6 and 24 months of age who do not appear to be seriously ill. These children frequently have temperatures in excess of 39.7°C (103.5°F) and white blood cell counts of 15,000 per mm³ or greater with no focus of infection discernible by history or physical examination. We recommend a blood culture in these children, as it is important to identify children who are truly bacteremic. Recent studies have shown that a skilled clinician can differentiate children who may have bacteremia from those who do not as effectively as any simple laboratory test. The deci-

---

*Manufacturer's note: The number of instances in which methicillin was administered intravenously to infants and children is not large enough to make specific recommendations.

†Manufacturer's note: Dosages in infants and children under 12 years of age have not been established.

sion to initiate outpatient treatment for suspected bacteremia should be made by the clinician on a case by case basis. When recall of patients is less than optimal or when a question of the necessity for antibiotics is entertained, we advocate initiation of penicillin or amoxicillin therapy.

Infective Endocarditis

JANE W. NEWBURGER, M.D.,
and ALEXANDER S. NADAS, M.D.

Infective endocarditis is one of the most serious complications of structural heart disease. It occurs primarily in children with pre-existing anatomic lesions of the heart, with an incidence that varies with the specific cardiac lesion, ranging from 0.2 cases/1000 patient-years in pulmonary stenosis to 23 cases/1000 patient-years in ventricular septal defect with aortic regurgitation. An identifiable potential source of bacteremia (e.g., dental manipulation, surgery) precedes infective endocarditis in approximately one fifth of cases in children. Streptococcal and staphylococcal species are responsible for most episodes in children; gram-negative and fungal organisms may also be found, most commonly following cardiac surgery or in debilitated patients. Despite its infrequent occurrence, the high mortality (19 to 25%), morbidity, and prolonged treatment course make its diagnosis, management, and prevention a matter of great importance to pediatricians and pediatric cardiologists.

GENERAL PRINCIPLES OF THERAPY

Spontaneous cure of infective endocarditis rarely if ever occurs; rather, cure requires prompt diagnosis and institution of antibiotic therapy. To select the appropriate antibiotic, the causative organism must be isolated and its sensitivity to antimicrobial agents determined by the tube dilution method. In general, bactericidal drugs are more effective than bacteriostatic drugs in eradicating infection. The effectiveness of antimicrobial therapy should be assessed by measuring the antibacterial activity of the patient's serum at various intervals after antibiotic administration against the infecting organism. Bactericidal effects should be seen at dilutions of 1 to 8 or higher for antibiotic therapy to be potentially effective. Serum drug levels, minimum inhibitory concentrations, and minimum bactericidal concentrations should also be obtained.

The duration of therapy necessary to effect cure is controversial. There is no conclusive evidence that a treatment course of 6 weeks is more effective than one of 4 weeks. We generally treat infective endocarditis caused by sensitive organisms such as

Streptococcus viridans for a minimum of 4 weeks, but extend the treatment course to 6 weeks or more when infection is caused by *Staphylococcus aureus,* gram-negative organisms, or organisms that are less sensitive to antimicrobial therapy. Although a treatment course of 2 weeks has been reported to effect cure of *S. viridans,* more data are needed before we would recommend this approach. Despite reports of success with oral antibiotics, we prefer to treat infective endocarditis with antibiotics administered intravenously.

SPECIFIC ORGANISMS

Streptococcus viridans is the most common organism causing bacterial endocarditis, accounting for approximately two thirds of cases in patients with underlying heart disease who have not undergone cardiac surgery. The drug of choice is penicillin G, 300,000 to 400,000 U/kg/24 hr (adult dose, 8 to 24 million U/24 hr) given IV in divided doses q 4 hr. In addition, some physicians use an aminoglycoside (e.g., gentamicin, 5 mg/kg/24 hr IV q 6 hr) for the first 2 weeks of treatment because of evidence of an in vitro synergistic effect of penicillin and streptomycin against *S. viridans.* In patients with proved hypersensitivity to penicillin, cephalothin (100 mg/kg/24 hr) or vancomycin (40 mg/kg/24 hr) may be used as alternatives.

Enterococci account for approximately 4% of cases of infective endocarditis in children. The treatment of choice is a combination of penicillin G, 400,000 U/kg/24 hr, and gentamicin, 5 mg/kg/24 hr, given IV q 6 hr. In patients sensitive to penicillin, effective therapy may be provided by vancomycin, (40 mg/kg/24 hr), sometimes in conjunction with gentamicin, 5 mg/kg/24 hr given IV q 6 hr.

Staphylococcus aureus causes approximately one third of cases of endocarditis in children. It most frequently presents as acute or early postoperative endocarditis, although it may occasionally present with a subacute course. The results of therapy in this group of patients are poorer than in those with *S. viridans* endocarditis. Early institution of antibiotic therapy is crucial; treatment should be initiated with penicillinase-resistant penicillin such as oxacillin or nafcillin, 200 mg/kg/24 hr, or cephalothin, 100 mg/kg/24 hr, given q 4 hr. If the organism is later proved to be susceptible to penicillin G, this agent may be substituted. During the first week of therapy, gentamicin (5 mg/kg/24 hr given IV q 6 hr) is often given in addition to the penicillinase-resistant penicillin. The necessity for continuing gentamicin should be determined by bactericidal levels. Vancomycin (40 mg/kg/24 hr) may be used in patients sensitized to penicillin and cephalosporin. Treatment should be continued for a minimum of 6 weeks even if the patient's response is prompt. Longer courses or a change in antibiotics may be necessary for resistant infections.

Staphylococcus epidermidis is an increasingly common cause of endocarditis, accounting for one fifth of cases following prosthetic valve replacement. Despite its low invasive capacity, the organism is often difficult to eradicate. Patients experience frequent relapses following completion of treatment courses with appropriate antibiotics, sometimes necessitating prosthetic valve replacement. The drug of choice for initial therapy is vancomcyin (40 mg/kg/24 hr). Addition of an aminoglycoside or rifampin, or both, may be necessary. Occasionally *S. epidermidis* is sensitive to penicillin G. Bactericidal levels are necessary to determine the optimal treatment regimen.

Gram-negative bacilli most often cause endocarditis early following cardiac surgery. The choice of antimicrobial agents must be guided by tube dilution studies. The newer B lactams (e.g. moxalactam) should be included among the antimicrobial agents tested. Antibiotic therapy probably should be continued for a minimum of 6 weeks.

Fungal infections of the heart, with the poorest prognosis of all types of endocarditis, fortunately are uncommon, occurring primarily following prosthetic valve surgery. Treatment with amphotericin B should be instituted promptly after diagnosis, usually followed by prosthetic valve replacement approximately 1 week after initiation of antimicrobial therapy. There are a variety of treatment regimens for intravenous therapy with amphotericin B. A standard regimen prescribes administration of 0.25 mg/kg the first day, followed by increases of 0.25 mg/kg each day to a final dose of 1 mg/kg/24 hr. No data exist on the optimal duration of treatment, which is commonly continued for 6 to 8 weeks following prosthetic valve replacement. When the organism is sensitive to 5-fluorocytosine, this drug may be used together with amphotericin B.

EMPIRIC THERAPY

Delay in institution of therapy of *acute* endocarditis may be costly; antibiotics should be started immediately after at least six cultures have been obtained in any child at risk who appears acutely ill and who has a compatible clinical picture. Examination of a buffy coat smear may reveal the etiologic organism before blood culture results are available. Since *S. aureus* is frequently the etiologic agent in acute endocarditis and in endocarditis occurring early after cardiac surgery, initial therapy should include a penicillinase-resistant penicillin, such as oxacillin or nafcillin, together with an aminoglycoside. Appropriate specific antimicrobial therapy should be started after identification of the causative organism.

In children with *subacute* or *chronic* illness compatible with infective endocarditis, one may legitimately delay the start of therapy for 2 or 3 days while awaiting results of blood cultures since, with few exceptions, initiation of antibiotic therapy commits the patients to a full treatment course. While awaiting culture results, one may document fever and other signs, symptoms, and laboratory findings of infective endocarditis. Once the etiologic organism has been identified, appropriate antibiotic therapy should be initiated.

In approximately 10 to 15% of cases of infective endocarditis, blood cultures never yield growth, but diagnosis is based on a highly suggestive clinical picture. Initial therapy for subacute infective endocarditis with negative blood cultures should include penicillin or ampicillin and an aminoglycoside to provide effective coverage against enterococcal species. Administration of these antibiotics should probably be continued for at least 4 weeks, during which time cultures and serologic tests may diagnose infection with fungi, *Brucella, Chlamydia,* or *Rickettsia.* If all studies are negative and there has been no clinical improvement at the end of a 4- to 6-week period, antibiotic treatment should be discontinued and the patient reassessed. In patients who have prosthetic material, an empiric trial of amphotericin B rarely may be warranted.

SURGICAL THERAPY

Although most cases of infective endocarditis can be treated successfully with antimicrobial agents alone, certain subgroups of patients continue to have high mortality rates, largely determined by the virulence of the etiologic organism, the site of intracardiac infection (e.g., prosthetic valve), and the degree of valve destruction. The leading cause of death in infective endocarditis is congestive heart failure, usually due to severe aortic or mitral incompetence. Surgical intervention has had a dramatic impact on survival, with survival rates of 73 to 86% for valve replacement even in the presence of ongoing infection.

The most frequent indications for surgery in the treatment of infective endocarditis include at least moderately severe or worsening congestive heart failure, infection uncontrolled by antibiotics (e.g., organism loculated in myocardial or valve ring abscess), and recurrent septic systemic emboli. Other less common indications include development of a mycotic aneurysm of the sinus of Valsalva or coronary artery, suppurative pericarditis, development of structural damage such as rupture of the ventricular or atrial septum, and perhaps visualization of very large vegetations on cardiac valves by echocardiography. Prompt surgical intervention is mandatory in critically ill patients, even when antibiotic therapy has been minimal.

PROSTHETIC VALVE ENDOCARDITIS

Infective endocarditis involving prosthetic material (e.g., valves, conduits, patches) presents partic-

ularly difficult problems in management. Patients with early (i.e., less than 2 months) infection of prosthetic valves following cardiac surgery have an exceedingly high mortality rate, ranging from 68 to 88% in series of adult patients. Causative organisms are often *S. aureus, S. epidermidis,* gram-negative bacilli, *Candida* species, and other opportunistic organisms. Mortality rate in late prosthetic valve endocarditis is somewhat lower (36 to 53%); the bacteriologic spectrum more closely resembles that occurring on native valves, with streptococci being the most commonly isolated species. Several investigators recommend combined early surgical and antimicrobial therapy for prosthetic valve endocarditis in general. Prompt and vigorous antibiotic treatment alone may sometimes be effective for prosthetic valve endocarditis, especially when it occurs late. However, if patients with late prosthetic valve endocarditis develop new regurgitant murmurs with congestive heart failure, prompt valve replacement is mandatory.

Whenever possible, prosthetic valve endocarditis should be managed in a tertiary care facility.

OTHER ASPECTS OF MANAGEMENT

All patients with infective endocarditis should have frequent physical examinations and continuity of care by at least one physician. Measures to relieve stress on the cardiovascular system include bed rest, fever control, erythrocyte transfusion for severe anemia, and maintenance of fluid and electrolyte balance. A complete dental examination and any necessary dental procedures should be performed as soon as the patient's condition permits and satisfactory antibiotic serum bactericidal levels have been achieved. Implications of the illness and prolonged hospitalization should be discussed with the child and parents at the time of admission; psychologic support is often helpful during the lengthy hospitalization.

COMPLICATIONS

Most children with infective endocarditis have defervescence within 1 week after initiation of antibiotic therapy. Fever occurring later during the course of therapy requires investigation of a variety of potential causes, including uncontrolled infection or metastatic suppuration, drug sensitivity, intercurrent infection, inflamed injection sites, thrombophlebitis (especially in adults), and arterial embolization. Persistence of low grade fever without positive blood cultures or any other signs of activity presents one of the most difficult problems in management of endocarditis, usually leaving the clinician to decide between the diagnoses of recurrent infection and drug sensitivity. Discontinuation of antibiotic therapy may occasionally be necessary and is a matter of clinical judgment.

Large arterial emboli arising from vegetations may be either suppurative or sterile; emboli do not necessarily indicate persistent infection. Symptoms and prognosis of embolization are related to the extent of infarction, the organ affected, and whether or not the embolus was suppurative.

Focal embolic and diffuse glomerulonephritis are the most frequent renal lesions associated with bacterial endocarditis. Diffuse glomerulonephritis is thought to originate from deposition of immune complexes and complement in a "lumpy-bumpy" manner throughout the glomerulus. This immune-complex glomerulonephritis usually improves as infection is controlled. When renal function is decreased, nephrotoxic antibiotics such as the aminoglycosides should be used cautiously, with monitoring of serum levels.

Congestive heart failure is usually associated with the development of hemodynamically significant valvar regurgitation, most often aortic. Other less common causes include rupture of a sinus of Valsalva into the cardiac chambers, perforation of the ventricular or atrial septum, formation of an aortopulmonary window, or development of myocarditis or myocardial abscesses. As noted earlier, the development of congestive heart failure during endocarditis often calls for prompt surgical intervention.

DISCHARGE AND FOLLOW-UP

We observe the patient for 48 hours following cessation of antibiotic therapy; at the end of this period, three sets of blood cultures are obtained and the patient is discharged from the hospital. At the time of a return appointment 2 to 4 weeks later, blood cultures are repeated. If the patient feels well and cultures are negative, all normal activities may be resumed. Elective surgery and catheterization should probably be deferred for 6 months following endocarditis.

PREVENTION

Since infective endocarditis cannot occur without a preceding bacteremia, attempts at prevention have focused on the use of antibiotic prophylaxis for those procedures following which a high frequency of bacteremia has been documented. The efficacy of the recommended antibiotic prophylaxis regimens has not been studied because of the rarity of the disease and the multiplicity of confounding factors. Nevertheless, we prescribe antimicrobial prophylaxis for all children with structural heart disease (with the exception of uncomplicated secundum atrial septal defect, proven surgically closed ventricular septal defect, and ligated and divided patent ductus arteriosus) who are subjected to dental procedures or manipulations of the respiratory, gastrointestinal, urinary, or genital tracts. Antibiotic prophylaxis should also be given to those patients who have had a previous episode of infective endocarditis, even in the absence of clinically detectable heart disease. Some physicians do not use prophylaxis in patients with pure pulmonic stenosis. Although the risk of endocarditis is low, physicians may choose to employ antibiotics in patients undergoing renal dialysis with implanted arteriovenous shunts and in patients with ventriculoatrial shunts placed to relieve hydrocephalus.

The most recent American Heart Association recommendations for antibiotic prophylaxis (Circulation 56:139A, 1977) are summarized below:

I. *For dental procedures and surgery of the upper respiratory tract* (e.g., tonsillectomy, bronchoscopy). Antibiotic prophylaxis is recommended for all dental procedures that may cause gingival bleeding, including professional cleaning, and is directed against alpha-hemolytic streptococci. In addition to antibiotic prophylaxis and probably even more important, children with structural heart disease should be strongly encouraged to maintain excellent oral hygiene practices and to keep routine dental appointments every 6 months to 1 year.

A. For most structural heart disease (excluding prosthetic valves or other high risk lesions):

1. *Penicillin regimens*

a. *Parenteral-oral combined:* Aqueous crystalline penicillin G, 30,000 U/kg (maximum, 1,000,000 U), mixed with procaine penicillin, 600,000 U given IM. *For children more than 60 pounds,* give penicillin V, 500 mg orally every 6 hours for 8 doses. *For children less than 60 pounds,* give penicillin V, 250 mg orally every 6 hours for 8 doses.

b. *Oral: For children more than 60 pounds,* give penicillin V, 2.0 gm orally 30 minutes to 1 hour prior to the procedure and then 500 mg orally every 6 hours for 8 doses. *For children less than 60 pounds,* give penicillin V, 1.0 gm orally 30 minutes to 1 hour prior to the procedure and then 250 mg orally every 6 hours for 8 doses.

2. *For patients allergic to penicillin,* give erythromycin, 20 mg/kg (maximum, 1 gm) orally 1.5 to 2 hours prior to the procedure and then 10 mg/kg (maximum, 500 mg) orally every 6 hours for 8 doses.

B. For patients with prosthetic valves or at very high risk:

1. *Penicillin Regimen*

Aqueous crystalline penicillin G, 30,000 U/kg (maximum, 1,000,000 U) mixed with procaine penicillin G, 600,000 U, given IM PLUS streptomycin, 20 mg/kg (maximum, 1 gram), given IM. Give 30 minutes to 1 hour prior to the procedure; then penicillin V, 500 mg (for children more than 60 pounds) or 250 mg (for children less than

60 pounds) orally every 6 hours for 8 doses.

2. *For patients allergic to penicillin,* give vancomycin, 20 mg/kg (maximum, 1 gram), IV over 1 hour; then erythromycin, 10 mg/kg (maximum, 500 mg) orally every 6 hours for 8 doses.

II. *For genitourinary and gastrointestinal tract surgery or instrumentation.* Antibiotic prophylaxis should be employed for surgery or instrumentation of the genitourinary tract (including urethral catheterization) and lower gastrointestinal tract, as well as for septic abortion or peripartum infection. The necessity for antibiotic prophylaxis has not been established for uncomplicated vaginal delivery, upper gastrointestinal tract endoscopy, percutaneous liver biopsy, sigmoidoscopy, barium enema, pelvic examination, uterine dilation and curettage, and uncomplicated insertion and removal of intrauterine devices. However, it may be wise to administer antibiotic prophylaxis for these procedures to those patients with prosthetic valves or otherwise at high risk.

1. *Penicillin regimens:* Aqueous crystalline penicillin G, 30,000 U/kg (maximum, 2,000,000 U) given IM or IV *or* ampicillin, 50 mg/kg (maximum, 1.0 gm) given IM or IV PLUS gentamicin, 1.5 mg/kg (maximum, 80 mg) given IM or IV *or* streptomycin, 20 mg/kg (maximum, 1.0 gm) given IM. Give initial doses 30 minutes to 1 hour prior to the procedure and repeat doses every 8 hours for two additional doses. Further doses may be necessary during prolonged procedures or in cases of delayed healing. One dose may be sufficient for brief procedures such as uncomplicated urethral catheterization.

2. *For patients allergic to penicillin:* Vancomycin, 20 mg/kg (maximum, 1.0 gram) given IV over 30 minutes to 1 hour PLUS streptomycin, 20 mg/kg (maximum, 1.0 gram) given IM.

A single dose of antibiotics begun 30 minutes to 1 hour prior to the procedure is probably sufficient, but the same dose may be repeated in 12 hours.

III. *For cardiac surgery:* Early postoperative endocarditis is most often due to *S. aureus* or, especially following prosthetic valve replacement, to *S. epidermidis.* Less common etiologic organisms include streptococci, gram-negative bacteria, and fungi. No single agent is effective against all these organisms and prolonged use of broad-spectrum antibiotics predisposes to superinfection with unusual or highly resistant organisms. For these reasons, antibiotic prophylaxis has been directed primarily against staphylococcus, using either a penicillinase-resistant penicillin (e.g., oxacillin, nafcillin) or cephalothin, which has the additional advantage of protecting against common gram-negative bacilli. In our institution, infants undergoing open heart surgery receive prophylaxis with oxacillin and gentamicin. Vancomycin may be used in patients who are sensitized to penicillins or cephalosporins. Antibiotic prophylaxis should be initiated shortly before surgery, with an additional dose given intraoperatively, and should be continued for no longer than 3 to 5 days postoperatively in order to reduce the likelihood of superinfection with resistant microorganisms.

Careful preoperative dental evaluation should be performed several weeks prior to elective cardiac surgery.

IV. *Other Considerations:* Antibiotic prophylaxis should be prescribed for surgical procedures on any infected or contaminated tissues (e.g., incision and drainage of abscesses). Prophylactic antibiotics are not required for diagnostic cardiac catheterization and angiography, following which infective endocarditis is extremely uncommon.

Clinicians should use their own judgment in determining the duration and choice of antibiotics under special circumstances, since it is not possible to make recommendations for all possible situations.

Staphylococcal Infections

HENRY R. SHINEFIELD, M.D.

The staphylococcus remains an important etiologic agent, both in community-acquired and nosocomial disease. The therapeutic approach to staphylococcal disease is conditioned by the capacity of *S. aureus* to form deep-seated abscesses and to persist in tissues for a long period of time.

In general, therapy for staphylococcal disease consists of a sound antimicrobial regimen coupled with surgery and general supportive therapy when indicated. Some staphylococcal infections (especially minor skin infections such as folliculitis) that occur occasionally in most people require no treatment. Established abscesses with localized collections of pus should be drained by methods ranging from incision and drainage of a skin abscess to closed underwater drainage of an empyema cavity.

The selection of a drug and the route of administration in the therapy of staphylococcal disease are conditioned by the age of the patient, the severity of the illness, and the probable antibiotic resistance of the staphylococcus (Table 1).

ANTIBIOTICS IN SERIOUS DISEASE

Almost every antibiotic has been evaluated for effectiveness in the treatment of disease caused by staphylococci. In general, bactericidal drugs administered parenterally should be used in the treatment of serious staphylococcal disease. At present most staphylococcal infections, whether community-acquired or hospital-acquired, are caused by organisms resistant to penicillin. Therefore initiation of therapy should be with a drug other than penicillin. If the organism is sensitive to benzyl penicillin (penicillin G), this is the drug of choice. When the disease is associated with a penicillin-resistant staphylococcus, the semisynthetic beta-lactamase-resistant (penicillinase-resistant) penicillins are the drugs of choice. The three beta-lactamase-resistant penicillin derivatives, methicillin, nafcillin, and oxacillin, are equal in clinical effectiveness despite some microbiologic differences in vitro.

Untoward reactions are also the same. In addition to toxic or hypersensitive reactions, such as fever, skin rash, and leukopenia, methicillin nephropathy is seen in about 0.1% of children treated with this antibiotic. Methicillin remains an important drug despite its well-documented association with renal reactions. These consist of hematuria or dysuria and usually do not appear until high-dose intravenous therapy has been continued for at least 10 days. In many cases these toxic or irritative reactions disappear when the dosage of the drug is reduced and the hydration of the patient improved. In a few cases hematuria represents a hypersensitivity reaction and persists until therapy is changed to a nonpenicillin drug. The other related antibiotics, nafcillin and oxacillin, also may cause nephropathy. Patients receiving any one of this group of antibiotics should be monitored with baseline and weekly or twice weekly urinalysis, BUN, creatinine, WBC, and differential count.

Cephalosporins are effective antistaphylococcal agents and can be used in most patients who are allergic to penicillin or one of its semisynthetic derivatives. However, there is cross-reactivity with penicillin in 5 to 15% of these patients. Therefore, care should be exercised when administering these drugs to a penicillin-sensitive patient. If the history reveals an immediate type of reaction to penicillin, such as anaphylaxis, urticaria, or diffuse pruritus, it is best to use some other antistaphylococcal agent. Of the available antistaphylococcal cephalosporins, cephalothin and cephapirin have almost identical pharmacokinetic properties and can be used interchangeably. Another cephalosporin, cefazolin, is excreted more slowly than cephalothin and cephapirin. This results in adequate therapeutic cefazolin serum levels even if the antibiotic is administered every 6 to 8 hours. It is also less irritating and therefore may be administered intramuscularly. On the other hand, cefazolin is more susceptible to staphylococcal beta-lactamase than are the other two cephalosporins. From the standpoint of clinical effectiveness there is no evidence that any one of the cephalosporins possesses greater antistaphylococcal activity than the others. The newer cephalosporin antimicrobials, cefamandole and cefotaxime sodium, as well as the semisynthetic cephamycin derivative cefoxitin are more expensive than the older cephalosporins and offer no advantage over the older ones in the treatment of staphylococcal diseases. Because of renal toxicity, another cephalosporin, cephaloridine, should not be used in pediatrics. Cephalosporins should not be used in central nervous system staphylococcal infections because they do not penetrate the blood barrier well nor do they diffuse well into the cerebrospinal fluid.

The aminoglycosides kanamycin and gentamicin are effective antistaphylococcal agents. Serious side effects of ototoxicity and nephrotoxicity restrict their use except in special situations. Gentamicin has been useful in some cases of ventriculitis associated with an infected ventricular shunt. In general, the use of multiple antimicrobial agents does not offer any advantage from the standpoint of either achieving a better therapeutic response or preventing the emergence of a resistant strain of *S. aureus.* However, in some cases synergism between gentamicin and a beta-lactamase-resistant penicillin or a cephalosporin has been demonstrated. It is recommended that two antimicrobials be used in clinical structures when this has been demonstrated and the patient fails to respond to a single agent.

Vancomycin is another antistaphylococcal agent. It is rarely used in pediatric patients because of the relative frequency of thrombophlebitis, hearing loss, and nephropathy. We have used vancomycin with success in patients with serious infection caused by an organism resistant to all other antistaphylococcal antibiotics or in patients allergic to both penicillin derivatives and cephalosporins. Oral vancomycin is the drug of choice in the treatment of pseudomembranous enterocolitis.

The proven toxicity of chloramphenicol, coupled with questionable therapeutic response, limits its usefulness in the treatment of staphylococcal disease. Oral administration of any antimicrobial agent in the treatment of serious staphylococcal disease is not recommended because of the unpredictable absorption, the care required to insure compliance, and the necessity of monitoring serum levels.

Antibiotics may be administered by the intravenous route, either continuously or intermittently. To insure delivery of medication and to avoid problems of antibiotic inactivation in intravenous solutions, we prefer to administer the antibiotic

Table 1. DOSAGE SCHEDULE OF DRUGS USEFUL IN TREATMENT
OF STAPHYLOCOCCAL INFECTIONS

Antibiotic	Oral (for mild to moderate infection)	
	1 Month to 50 kg	*>50 kg or Maximum*
PENICILLINS		
Benzyl (Penicillin G)	50,000–150,000 units/kg/24 hr (4)	1.6–4.8 million units/24 hr (4)
Phenoxymethyl (Penicillin V, V-Cillin, Pen-Vee K, others)	50–100 mg/kg/24 hr (4)	1–4 gm/24 hr (4)
Methicillin (Staphcillin)	—	—
Oxacillin (Prostaphlin)	50–100 mg/kg/24 hr (4)	1–2 gm/24 hr (4)
Nafcillin (Unipen)	50–100 mg/kg/24 hr (4)	1–2 gm/24 hr (4)
Cloxacillin (Tegopen)	25–50 mg/kg/24 hr (4)	1–4 gm/24 hr (4)
Dicloxacillin (Dynapen, Pathocil, Veracillin)	12.5–25 mg/kg/24 hr (4)	0.5–2 gm/24 hr (4)
CEPHALOSPORINS		
Cephalothin (Keflin)	—	—
Cephapirin (Cefadyl)	—	—
Cefazolin (Ancef, Kefzol)	—	—
Cephalexin (Keflex)	25–50 mg/kg/24 hr (4)	1–4 gm/24 hr (4)
Cephradine (Anspor, Velosef)	25–50 mg/kg/24 hr (4)	1–4 gm/24 hr (4)
OTHERS		
Erythromycin lactobionate (Erythrocin-Lactobionate-IV) *AND* Erythromycin gluceptate (Ilotycin Gluceptate)	—	—
Erythromycin stearate and estolate (Erythrocin, E-mycin, Ilosone, others)	25–50 mg/kg/24 hr (4)	1–2 gm/24 hr (4)
Clindamycin (Cleocin)	10–20 mg/kg/24 hr (4)	600–1200 mg/24 hr (4)
Vancomycin (Vancocin)	—	—
Gentamicin (Garamycin)	—	—
Kanamycin (Kantrex)	—	—

Note: Numbers in parentheses: Number of doses into which the daily dose should be equally divided.

intermittently over a 10- to 20-minute period at 4- to 6-hour intervals (Table 1).

ANTIBIOTICS IN MILD-TO-MODERATE STAPHYLOCOCCAL DISEASE

Here oral medications may be used. Because of better absorption, a phenoxy penicillin such as penicillin V is preferred over penicillin G if the organism is penicillin-sensitive. Cloxacillin or dicloxacillin is the drug of choice when treating penicillin-resistant staphylococcal disease. They are preferred over oral oxacillin because of higher serum levels attained with these antibiotics. Erythromycin can be used in allergic patients or if indicated by antibiotic sensitivities. An oral cephalosporin, cephalexin, can be used in individuals allergic to penicillin. The drug is well absorbed from the gastrointestinal tract. Again, caution should be exercised in its use in these patients because of possible cross-allergenicity with penicillin. Clindamycin is an effective antistaphylococcal agent. However, the frequent occurrence of colitis, particularly after oral administration, limits its usefulness.

The recommended duration of antibiotic therapy

Table 1. DOSAGE SCHEDULE OF DRUGS USEFUL IN TREATMENT
OF STAPHYLOCOCCAL INFECTIONS (Continued)

	Parenteral (for severe infection)		
<1 Week	*1 to 4 Weeks*	*1 Month to 50 kg*	*>50 kg or Maximum*
100,000 units/kg/24 hr IV every 12 hr	100,000–250,000 units/kg/24 hr hr IV every 6 hr	200,000–400,000 units/kg/24 hr IV every 4 hr	8–24 million units/24 hr IV every 4 hr
—	—	—	
50–100 mg/kg/24 hr IV every 12 hr	100–200 mg/kg/24 hr IV every 6 hr	200–300 mg/kg/24 hr IV every 4 hr	6–12 gm/24 hr IV every 4 hr
50–100 mg/kg/24 hr IV every 12 hr	100 to 200 mg/kg/24 hr IM or IV every 6 hr	100–200 mg/kg/24 hr IV every 4 hr	4–8 gm/24 hr IV every 4 hr
40–60 mg/kg/24 hr IV every 12 hr	60 to 100 mg/kg/24 hr IM or IV every 6 hr	100–200 mg/kg/24 hr IV every 4 hr	4–8 gm/24 hr IV every 4 hr
—	—	—	—
40 mg/kg/24 hr IV every 12 hr	60 mg/kg/24 hr IV every 6 hr	100 mg/kg/24 hr IV every 4 hr	6–12 gm/24 hr IV every 4 hr
40 mg/kg/24 hr IV every 12 hr	60 mg/kg/24 hr IV every 6 hr	100 mg/kg/24 hr IV every 4 hr	6–12 gm/24 hr IV every 4 hr
40 mg/kg/24 hr IV every 12 hr	50 mg/kg/24 hr IV every 8 hr	50 mg/kg/24 hr IV every 6 hr	3–6 gm/24 hr IV every 6 hr
—	—	—	—
Not recommended	10–20 mg/kg/24 hr IV every 8 hr, infuse over 0.5–1 hr	10–20 mg/kg/24 hr IV every 6 hr, infuse over 0.5–1 hr	1.5–4 gm/24 hr IV every 6 hr, 1 gm diluted in 100 ml
—	—	—	
Not recommended	20–40 mg/kg/24 hr IV every 6 hr, infuse over 30 min	20–40 mg/kg/24 hr IV every 6 hr, infuse over 30 min	1.2–2.4 gm/24 hr IV every 6 hr, 1 gm diluted in 100 ml
30 mg/kg/24 hr IV every 12 hr, infuse over 30 to 60 min	45 mg/kg/24 hr* IV every 8 hr, infuse over 1 hr	40–60 mg/kg/24 hr* IV every 6 hr, infuse over 1 hr	2 gm/24 hr IV every 6 hr, infuse over 1 hr
5 mg/kg/24 hr† IV every 12 hr	7.5 mg/kg/24 hr† IM every 8 hr	5 mg/kg/24 hr† IM every 8 hr	5 mg/kg/24 hr† IM every 8 hr
15 mg/kg/24 hr† IV every 12 hr	30 mg/kg/24 hr†‡ IM every 8 hr	15 mg/kg/24 hr† IM every 8 hr	1.5 gm/24 hr† IM every 8 hr

Note: Numbers in parentheses: Number of doses into which the daily dose should be equally divided.
*These doses may exceed the manufacturer's recommended dosage.
†May be given IV slowly over 20 to 30 minutes.
‡This dosage exceeds the manufacturer's recommended dosage.

as outlined is somewhat arbitrary and predicated on clinical experience and the established fact that eliminating *S. aureus* from infected or diseased sites is extremely difficult.

Nonspecific agents used in the therapy of disease associated with *S. aureus* include various vaccines, toxoids, gamma globulin, and bacteriophage. In controlled observations there is no good evidence that any of these substances is of significant value in the treatment of staphylococcal disease.

SPECIFIC STAPHYLOCOCCAL INFECTIONS

Bullous Impetigo and Staphylococcal Scalded Skin Syndrome (SSSS)

S. aureus may cause bullous impetigo. If only a few lesions are present, bullous impetigo usually responds to local treatment consisting of artificial rupture of the vesicles followed by cleansing with soap and water or alcohol. Since metastatic dissemination can occur, lack of response to local therapy is an indication for the use of antibiotics. In a patient not allergic to penicillin the drug of choice for oral therapy is a beta-lactamase-resistant antistaphylococcal agent such as cloxacillin or dicloxacillin, given in the dose described in Table 1. Emphasis is placed on the initial use of a semisynthetic beta-lactamase-resistant penicillin because a large number of S. aureus strains encountered today are not susceptible to penicillin. If the organism is found to be sensitive to penicillin, therapy should be changed to phenoxymethyl penicillin. Patients allergic to penicillin or one of its derivatives should receive oral erythromycin or an oral cephalosporin.

If the disease is extensive, denuding large areas of the body (SSSS), initially a parenteral antistaphylococcal agent such as methicillin or nafcillin should be given. Therapy should be changed to parenteral aqueous penicillin G if the organism is found to be penicillin-sensitive. For patients allergic to penicillin, parenteral erythromycin or a cephalosporin can be used. Therapy should continue 1 to 3 days after all evidence of infection has subsided.

These patients are generally febrile and may experience difficulty with fluid, electrolyte, and protein balance as well as temperature regulation. Heating or cooling blankets and appropriate fluids should be used when indicated. Hexachlorophene should not be used to cleanse the large denuded areas since it may be absorbed and produce convulsions.

Furuncle and Abscess

The furuncle and other skin afflictions are the most common lesions produced by the staphylococcus. They are frequently self-limited and heal spontaneously or may require simple drainage. If the lesions are accompanied by systemic symptoms or are surrounded by large areas of cellulitis, antibiotic therapy as well as incision and drainage is indicated. The choice of antibiotics is the same as for bullous impetigo. The decision in regard to the route of administration depends on the age of the patient, the extent of the disease, and the ability of the patient to tolerate oral medication.

A useful approach in the treatment of recurrent furunculosis that does not respond to local hygienic measures and appropriate antibiotic therapy utilizes the concept of bacterial interference. Individuals and families with chronic furunculosis may be protected from lesions by artificial nasal colonization with a strain of S. aureus of low virulence (strain 502 A).* This regimen includes the use of both a topical nasal antibiotic, such as neomycin or bacitracin, and an oral antistaphylococcal agent, such as

cloxacillin or dicloxacillin. The antibiotic is given until the nasal mucosa is cleared of the resident S. aureus, and then the patient is recolonized with S. aureus 502 A. About 80% of individuals with chronic recurrent furunculosis respond to such therapy. Those not likely to respond to this regimen include patients with underlying disease, such as diabetes, eczema, acne, or an underlying immunologic disorder. Antibiotics alone or efforts to increase host resistance with various toxoids and vaccines have not been consistently successful in curing this disease.

Metastasis of the staphylococcal infection to areas more vulnerable than the skin, such as the liver, lung, kidney, and brain, may occur. Deep abscesses may also occur as complications of an operative procedure or trauma. Deep abscesses require intensive therapy, which consists of drainage of accessible lesions after localization. Care must be taken to remove any associated foreign body to prevent chronic suppuration. Under these circumstances, parenteral antimicrobial therapy is mandatory and should be continued for 1 to 2 weeks after all clinical and laboratory evidence of infection has completely subsided. In brain or lung abscesses, this may mean the continuation of antibiotic therapy for as long as 6 to 12 weeks.

Septicemia and Endocarditis

Septicemia is symptomatic bacteremia. Staphylococcal septicemia may be secondary to an infection at a primary site in the skin, bone, joint, or deep abscess and in turn may be responsible for seeding these same sites, causing a secondary abscess. A concerted effort should be made to identify the primary focus of infection, since this must be eliminated to effect a cure. In children with deficiency in host resistance, septicemia may occur without any obvious primary site. Treatment consists of parenteral antibiotic therapy. Aqueous penicillin G is the drug of choice if the organism is sensitive to this agent; methicillin is given for treatment of a resistant S. aureus strain. Antibiotic treatment should continue for 1 week after all signs and symptoms of infection have abated.

Bacteremia may be secondary to staphylococcal endocarditis. Operative procedures on the heart and valves and "mainlining" drugs have increased the incidence of this disease. A high proportion of staphylococcal strains causing endocarditis are coagulase-negative. Staphylococcal endocarditis is treated by the parenteral administration of a bactericidal antibiotic. The treatment consists of aqueous penicillin G if the organism is highly sensitive to penicillin. If the organism is resistant to penicillin, methicillin should be used. It is important to start intensive therapy rapidly because the staphylococcus quickly destroys heart valves, with ensuing heart failure.

---

*May be obtained from the author on request.

Therapy should be initiated by the intravenous route and parenteral therapy should continue for at least 4 to 6 weeks. As in all serious staphylococcal diseases, oral medication should not be used. Some of the coagulase-negative staphylococci causing endocarditis are resistant both to penicillin and methicillin. Under these circumstances vancomycin should be used. If signs and symptoms persist or a relapse occurs in a patient with a prosthesis, it is likely that the only effective way of treating the infection and eradicating the bacteria is to remove the foreign body.

If the patient responds poorly to the beta-lactamase-resistant penicillin and the blood culture remains positive, it is possible that the causative organism is a "tolerant" S. aureus. These organisms are not killed at the same antibiotic concentration at which they are inhibited; the mean bactericidal concentration (MBC) is significantly greater than the mean inhibitory concentration (MIC). In these cases the specific S. aureus should be tested by the tube dilution technique and the MIC and MBC determined in order to select an appropriate antibiotic. Some of these organisms are not only tolerant to the beta-lactamase-resistant penicillins but are also cross-tolerant with other cell-wall active antibiotics, such as the cephalosporins and vancomycin. Under these circumstances, an antibiotic that acts by a mechanism other than cell-wall inhibition, such as gentamicin, should be substituted or added to the therapeutic regimen, if appropriate on the basis of MIC determinations.

Staphylococcal Enterocolitis

Staphylococci in small numbers can be recovered from the stool in about 10% of normal individuals. When staphylococci are present as the predominant aerobic bacteria in the stool, there may be symptoms of diarrhea, which may vary from mild to severe.

The severest clinical form of infection of the intestine is pseudomembranous enterocolitis. It has been demonstrated that this entity is caused by an overgrowth of the intestinal flora by *Clostridium difficile*, although conventional stool cultures may yield large amounts of S. aureus. In many cases this disease is precipitated by the use of an antimicrobial agent. In this disorder there is necrosis of the mucosa and formation of a pseudomembrane; fluid loss and shock is a common cause of death.

Treatment consists of 1) immediate discontinuation of the offending antimicrobial agent, 2) restoration of fluid and electrolyte balance, and 3) administration of oral vancomycin in a dose of 40 to 60 mg/kg/24 hr* for 7 to 10 days.

---

*This dose of vancomycin may exceed the manufacturer's recommended dose.

Infections of the Central Nervous System

Neurologic procedures using plastic tubes to relieve congenital or acquired obstructions to the flow of cerebrospinal fluid have resulted in a changing pattern of central nervous system staphylococcal disease; as much as 35% of central nervous system staphylococcal disease is secondary to such neurosurgical procedures. Occasionally, staphylococcal infection of the meninges or brain follows a primary infection about the face or at a distant site, such as the hip or foot.

Aqueous penicillin G is used if the organism is sensitive to penicillin, and methicillin is used for penicillin-resistant organisms. Therapy for meningitis that is not secondary to shunts should be continued for at least 1 week to 10 days after the patient is clinically well, and all laboratory data, including spinal fluid findings, have returned to normal. Average duration of therapy is about 3 weeks.

With high doses of methicillin, we have treated staphylococcal meningitis and brain abscesses successfully without the use of intrathecal medication. Some authorities suggest the routine use of intrathecal medication. In view of our results—lack of definitive evidence to support the usefulness of intrathecal therapy and possible untoward effects from the instillation of medication in the subarachnoid space—we do not recommend the routine intrathecal use of antimicrobial agents in the treatment of central nervous system staphylococcal disease until more data are available.

In cases that complicate neurosurgical procedures, the agent responsible for the infection may be a coagulase-negative staphylococcus rather than a coagulase-positive organism. It is important to determine the antibiotic sensitivity to the organism so that appropriate therapy can be instituted. Some of the coagulase-negative staphylococci are resistant to both penicillin and methicillin, and in these cases the drug of choice is vancomycin or gentamicin.

With infected shunts there is an associated cerebritis, with small collections of pus around the insertion of the tube. Therapy with antimicrobials alone usually is not sufficient to cure this type of infection; the foreign body must be removed by a second neurosurgical procedure before the staphylococci can be eradicated. Prior to removal of the shunt an attempt can be made to clear the infection without surgery. Some cases have been reported to respond to local instillation of gentamicin. One to 2 mg of gentamicin is placed in the shunt and flushed retrograde into the ventricle. This is repeated daily for 5 days or until the ventricular fluid is sterile, whichever is longer.

If the ventriculitis persists, the shunt must be removed. This is best done under cover of antibiotic therapy. To eliminate any nidus of infection in the central nervous system, the antibiotic is initiated before and continued for as long as possible following removal of the shunt. The duration of therapy before a new shunt is inserted depends on the clinical condition of the patient. A return of the signs and symptoms of increased intracranial pressure signals the time of surgery. This is usually 1 to 7 days after the infected shunt has been removed.

Diffuse glomerulonephritis may be a complication of coagulase-negative staphylococcal bacteremia that occurs in patients with a ventriculoatrial shunt. The renal disease probably is a result of an immunologic response to the staphylococcal infection rather than direct bacterial embolization of the kidney. Improvement in renal function is noted after removal of the shunt.

Toxic Shock Syndrome

This disease is caused by a toxin produced by *S. aureus.* It occurs most commonly but not exclusively in menstruating women and has been associated with the use of tampons. The disease is characterized by sudden onset of fever, diarrhea, shock, hyperemia of the mucous membranes, and a diffuse macular erythematous rash followed by desquamation of the hands and feet. Fluid loss and shock is a common cause of death in this disorder. Therefore primary attention should be paid to the replacement of fluid and electrolytes. Since most cases have been associated with resistant *S. aureus,* a beta-lactamase-resistant penicillin or cephalosporin should be used. The use of these antimicrobials during the initial episode has been shown to prevent recurrences in women during subsequent menses.

Prepubertal girls, postmenopausal women, and men have been reported with toxic shock syndrome. A diligent search for a focus of infection should be made and the infected site treated in these patients. Often the focus of infection is inconspicuous but represents a site for *S. aureus* organisms multiplying and elaborating a toxin that is widely disseminated by the bloodstream to multiple organs and is responsible for the systemic clinical syndrome.

Pyomyositis

Pyomyositis is an acute bacterial infection of the skeletal muscle, most frequently caused by *S. aureus.* In 5% of cases, the causative agent is *Escherichia coli, S. pneumoniae* or beta-hemolytic group A streptococci. In contrast to other staphylococcal infections, local erythema and heat are initially absent. Because of this and because of the minimal pain, the diagnosis may not be obvious unless the infection breaks through overlying muscle and fascia and involves the subcutaneous tissues. The term "tropical myositis" was applied to this condition because the first recognized cases occurred in the

tropics. Recently cases have been described in life-long residents of the United States, some of whom have been immunosuppressed.

The combination of swelling, minimal pain, absence of classic signs of inflammation, absence of a primary site of infection, and on occasion the history of trauma to the affected site has led to delay in definitive therapy in some of the cases. In these instances the muscle swelling was initially thought to be the result of trauma or tumor.

In all cases of pyomyositis, the infected site must be drained surgically. Because agents other than *S. aureus* may be involved, Gram stain and culture of the pus is essential for appropriate therapy. Beta-lactamase-resistant penicillin is the initial therapy recommended. Culture and sensitivity reports dictate the definitive therapy.

Blood cultures are rarely positive, therefore metastatic sites of infection are not frequently seen. However, persistent fever after appropriate antibiotic therapy and surgery should be a warning of the presence of other collections of pus.

Streptococcal Infections

RAM YOGEV, M.D.,
and STANFORD T. SHULMAN, M.D.

Group A β-hemolytic streptococci are responsible for a wide spectrum of human disease, which can be divided into acute (purulent) infections and nonpurulent sequelae. The acute infections include pharyngitis-tonsillitis, scarlet fever, otitis media, mastoiditis, sinusitis, pneumonia, arthritis, impetigo, erysipelas, and so on. The most common are pharyngitis and impetigo. The major nonpurulent sequelae are acute rheumatic fever and acute glomerulonephritis.

Because there are no reliable clinical findings, except for the presence of tender anterior cervical nodes, that enable one to diagnose streptococcal pharyngitis accurately, the throat culture is essential. For cost-effectiveness, routine throat cultures should be processed *only* for detection of group A streptococci; identification of other organisms or antibiotic sensitivity testing is not indicated. A major difficulty in the management of streptococcal pharyngitis is that a throat culture yielding group A streptococci does not differentiate active streptococcal infection from nonstreptococcal pharyngitis in a patient with chronic pharyngeal carriage of group A streptococci. At present, differentiation of bona fide streptococcal infection from chronic carriage with an intercurrent pharyngitis of other etiology may be extremely difficult.

Streptococcal pharyngitis is a self-limited illness that lasts for about 2 to 5 days without antibiotic treatment. Because antibiotic treatment of streptococcal pharyngitis has only a modest effect upon relief of symptoms—shortening the duration of symptoms by 12 to 24 hours—the justification for treatment is for prevention of a) acute rheumatic fever; b) suppurative complications such as peritonsillar abscess; and c) spread to others. Treatment has not been shown to prevent poststreptococcal glomerulonephritis. Because it is desirable to avoid the expense and risk of exposure to unnecessary antibiotics, we recommend treatment as soon as a definite diagnosis of streptococcal infection is made, that is, as soon as throat culture results are positive for group A streptococci.

The drug of choice for the treatment of streptococcal pharyngitis is a single intramuscular injection of benzathine penicillin G without shorter-acting penicillins (600,000 units for patients less than 60 pounds and 1.2 million units for those heavier than 60 pounds). Alternative therapy is oral penicillin G at a dose of 200,000 to 250,000 units three or four times daily for 10 full days for children and adults. Successful therapy implies not only the appropriate dose but also adequate duration, even though complete resolution of symptoms generally occurs long before completion of the treatment course. If one takes into consideration the low rates of compliance for a 10-day course of oral therapy (as low as 8% in a low socioeconomic population), our preference for intramuscular therapy becomes obvious. Failure to eradicate streptococci from the throat is more commonly associated with oral therapy but may also occur following intramuscular therapy. In general, follow-up throat cultures of asymptomatic patients are not recommended. If a culture is obtained and is positive, a second course of treatment should be considered. If the throat culture remains positive despite such therapy, the patient is probably a carrier who will not benefit from additional antibiotics.

Other antibiotics effective in vitro against group A streptococci should be used only in the penicillin-allergic patient. Erythromycin (40 mg/kg/24 hr not to exceed 1 gram) in three divided doses for 10 days is an acceptable alternative, although increasing numbers of strains of group A β-hemolytic streptococci resistant to this drug have been found. Clindamycin (10 to 20 mg/kg/24 hr given twice daily) may be as effective as penicillin or erythromycin, but should be restricted to situations in which less toxic antibiotics are contraindicated. Oral cephalosporins such as cephalexin or cefaclor (40 mg/kg/24 hr given three times daily) may be acceptable alternatives.

Certain antimicrobial agents have no place in the treatment of streptococcal pharyngitis. Because of the high prevalence of strains resistant to tetracycline, this drug cannot be recommended. Sulfonamides (which are effective as continuous prophylaxis for the *prevention* of streptococcal infection in rheumatic fever patients) do not eradicate strep-

tococci during an infection and should not be used. Penicillinase-resistant penicillins have no advantage over penicillin, even in patients who harbor penicillinase-producing staphylococci, and thus should not be used.

Several points regarding therapy require emphasis:

1. Studies have demonstrated that if appropriate therapy is instituted as late as 9 days after the onset of pharyngitis, rheumatic fever is preventable. Hence, delaying the onset of therapy until throat culture results are available incurs no significant risk to the patient and will greatly decrease inappropriate administration of antibiotics for viral illnesses.

2. Twenty-four to 48 hours after initiation of therapy, the patient can be considered not contagious and may return to school or to other activities.

3. Only symptomatic household contacts of patients with acute streptococcal pharyngitis should be cultured and, if positive, treated. The asymptomatic household member, even with a positive culture, has a very low risk of developing rheumatic fever or of disseminating streptococci and thus should not be cultured, unless there is previous history of rheumatic fever.

4. Scarlet fever represents streptococcal pharyngitis with rash. Therapy does not differ from that of routine streptococcal pharyngitis.

5. Special consideration should be given to patients who already have had acute rheumatic fever or rheumatic heart disease. These patients are at a high risk of developing recurrent rheumatic fever with symptomatic or asymptomatic streptococcal infection. To prevent recurrence, continuous lifelong prophylaxis is recommended by the American Heart Association. The drug of choice for continuous rheumatic fever prophylaxis is 1.2 million units of benzathine penicillin G intramuscularly every 4 weeks. This is preferred by many because it obviates the need for compliance with daily oral prophylaxis. Oral regimens include sulfadiazine* (500 mg bid) or penicillin G (250 mg bid), which appear equally effective. Sulfadiazine should not be used during the last months of pregnancy. Erythromycin (250 mg twice daily) should be used for prevention of streptococcal infection only in the exceptional patient who is allergic to both penicillin and sulfa agents.

The rare purulent complications of streptococcal pharyngitis of which the physician should be aware include peritonsillar or retropharyngeal abscesses, which are relatively infrequent; suppurative lym-

*Manufacturer's Note: Sulfadiazine is contraindicated in infants less than 2 months old, except in treatment of congenital toxoplasmosis.

phadenitis resulting from lymphatic spread; and paranasal sinusitis (usually maxillary). After drainage, if indicated, antibiotic treatment, preferably at least initially with parenteral penicillin, should continue for a minimum of 10 days in order to prevent the development of nonpurulent sequelae.

Streptococcal skin infections are either superficial (e.g., impetigo contagiosa and secondary infections of dermatologic conditions such as eczema and varicella) or deep (erysipelas and cellulitis). The major significance of streptococcal skin infections is their association with acute glomerulonephritis; however, there are no convincing data that even prompt appropriate antibiotic treatment prevents the development of nephritis. Treatment is recommended, however, to decrease spread of the infecting organism. Intramuscular benzathine penicillin is the drug of choice for impetigo in a dose of 1.2 million units for children over 60 pounds and 600,000 units for children under 60 pounds. Oral penicillin G or erythromycin appear as effective, and, if compliance is assured, are good alternatives. Additional local treatment, including scrubbing the lesions with hexachlorophene-containing soap or the use of topical antibiotics such as bacitracin may facilitate recovery. For very mild cases, local treatment alone is frequently sufficient. Improved hygiene with frequent bathing is most effective in preventing recurrences. Erysipelas requires longer parenteral penicillin therapy, particularly if the lesion is extensive or the host is debilitated or immunocompromised.

Streptococci other than group A are important causes of severe systemic infections. Group B streptococci play a major role in neonatal sepsis and meningitis (see Neonatal Infections). These bacteria are also major causes of urinary tract infections, bone and joint infections, and pneumonia in the first several months of life. Alphahemolytic streptococci (viridans streptococci) and enterococci (group D) play a major role in subacute bacterial endocarditis (see Infective Endocarditis). The former organisms are part of the normal flora of the mouth, while the latter are enteric bacteria. Therefore, it is recommended that patients with congenital or rheumatic heart disease who are undergoing dental or oropharyngeal procedures or genitourinary or gastrointestinal instrumentation should receive prophylaxis to prevent endocarditis, as emphasized by the American Heart Association.

Group B Streptococcal Infections

SAMUEL P. GOTOFF, M.D.

Group B streptococcal infections should be treated with penicillin in dosages from 100,000 to 300,000 U/kg/day, according to the severity of the illness and the immunologic status of the host. In patients allergic to penicillin, certain cephalosporins (but not moxalactam), chloramphenicol, or clindamycin may be substituted. Group B streptococcal infections occur predominantly in the perinatal period. Despite treatment with penicillin, the outcome is often unsatisfactory, and other approaches to therapy have been sought.

Synergism between penicillin and an aminoglycoside has been shown by killing kinetics in rabbits, but no clinical trials have been performed in humans. As almost all infants with suspected neonatal sepsis are treated with both agents until cultures are reported, it is impossible to compare the efficacy of penicillin alone. We discontinue the aminoglycoside when group B streptococci are identified. Meningitis, abscesses, and musculoskeletal infections are treated for 3 weeks. Bacteremic infections from other sources are treated from 7 to 10 days.

Immunity to group B streptococci depends on opsonophagocytosis mediated by antibody and, in most cases, by complement. Animal studies and uncontrolled clinical trials indicate that transusion of polymorphonuclear leukocytes improves the outcome. White blood cell transfusion should be considered as adjunctive therapy in patients with neutropenia, although further study is needed.

Deficiency of antibody to the type-specific polysaccharide antigen of group B streptococci is a risk factor in the development of neonatal group B streptococcal infection, and antibody has been shown to protect animals against experimental infections and to augment therapy with penicillin. Results with ISG and modified ISG depend on the level of specific antibody in these preparations, which is quite variable. A hyperimmune globulin containing antibody to the four type-specific polysaccharide antigens of group B streptococci might be worthy of a clinical trial but is not currently available. Most women lack protective levels of IgG antibody to the type-specific antigens of group B streptococci, and their offspring are therefore unprotected. Large amounts of serum or globulin would be necessary to provide transplacental immunity. Passive immunization of the newborn is theoretically possible. Active immunization of adult women has been demonstrated with some group B streptococcal vaccines, which are not available commercially.

Antibiotic prophylaxis of early-onset disease has been studied during pregnancy and labor and in the immediate neonatal period. Group B streptococci colonize the gastrointestinal and genitourinary tracts of adults. Administration of penicillin or ampicillin will generally suppress group B streptococci so that cultures are negative during therapy. Relapse or reinfection is frequent, and only one study has avoided recolonization by treating women from the 38th week of pregnancy to delivery. This approach is limited by the fact that many early-onset group B streptococcal infections occur in premature infants. Ampicillin administered to women in labor who are colonized blocks transmission of group B streptococci to the newborn infant. We limit prophylaxis to women with the following risk factors: prolonged ruptured membranes, prematurity, and amnionitis, as one of these risk factors is present in the majority of infants with early-onset group B streptococcal infection, who in turn have the highest mortality rate. Use of a selected obstetrical population minimizes the risk of reactions to ampicillin and alteration of bacterial flora in the nursery. Hospitals that incur more than one or two cases of early-onset disease annually might consider the following approach: identification of the colonized women by rectal and vaginal cultures at around 30 weeks' gestation and administration of ampicillin, 2 g stat followed by 1 g q 4 hr, during labor, to colonized women with prematurity (< 37 weeks), prolonged ruptured membranes (> 12 hrs), or amnionitis.

Administration of 50,000 units of aqueous penicillin G to newborn infants in the delivery room has been shown to diminish the incidence of group B streptococcal early-onset disease. The effect of universal penicillin prophylaxis on the gram-negative flora in the nursery has not been resolved, but more important is the failure of this approach in cases of group B streptococcal intrauterine infection. Because clinical studies of prophylaxis are limited, these recommendations must remain tentative and limited to situations where group B streptococcal infection becomes a special concern.

Listeria Monocytogenes Infection

ITZHAK BROOK, M.D.

Listeria monocytogenes represents a bacterial species consisting of gram-positive to gram-variable motile, asporogenous, acapsular aerobic to microaerophilic rods. The organism is widely spread in water and soil and causes diseases in various mammals, fish, and birds.

Although colonization with the organism is common, it causes disease in humans in a sporadic way, attacking primarily, although not exclusively, neonates, pregnant women, immunocompromised hosts, and older individuals.

Inapparent infections during pregnancy are transmitted transplacentally or during delivery. Listeriosis of the newborn can manifest itself in a serious generalized infection, in which respiratory distress and heart failure are the main symptoms, with appearance of miliary granulomatosis of almost all internal organs and skin.

Central nervous system infection, which can be purulent meningitis, encephalitis, and brain abscess, is another serious neonatal problem. Bacteremia usually accompanies central nervous infection; however, listerial endocarditis with embolization is rare.

Because of the severity of listerial disease, the pediatrician must suspect and diagnose the infection rapidly in susceptible hosts. Therapy of suspected sepsis in a neonate, as in the compromised host, is often initiated without knowledge of the etiology.

Listeria monocytogenes is susceptible in vitro to clinically attainable serum concentrations of a number of antimicrobial agents including penicillin, ampicillin, tetracycline, erythromycin, sulfonamides, cephalosporins, chloramphenicol, and aminoglycosides. Ampicillin and penicillin are the drugs of choice for the treatment of listeriosis. In vitro susceptibility to these drugs is usually below 1 μg/ml, and resistance to them is rare. Clinical failures in the treatment of listeriosis with penicillin can be partially ascribed to inadequate drug dosage or to its administration too late or for too short a time.

We must remember that an unusual gap exists between the minimal bactericidal concentration and minimal inhibitory concentration of both penicillin and ampicillin. Bactericidal concentrations are not attainable in the cerehospinal fluid. Additional evidence of the inefficacy of ampicillin alone is the high relapse rate in renal transplant patients with *Listeria* meningitis treated for 2 weeks with ampicillin.

Synergistic bactericidal activity between penicillin or ampicillin and streptomycin or gentamicin has been demonstrated in vitro, in vivo, and in clinical conditions. Combination therapy is thus recommended for patients with septicemic listeriosis, especially newborns, and patients with endocarditis or with immunosuppression for whom antimicrobial therapy must be bactericidal to be effective.

Initial therapy of listeriosis in the first week of life should be ampicillin 100–200 mg/kg/day IV or IM in two to three divided doses, and 200 mg/kg/day in three divided doses in the second through fourth week of life. The dose for older children and immunocompromised children should be 200 to 300 mg/kg/day in four to six divided doses. In severe cases of endocarditis or encephalitis a dose of 300 to 400 mg/kg/day in four to six divided doses may be needed. The treatment of all age groups should be maintained for a period of up to 4 weeks, depending on the patient's age and form of disease.

Addition of gentamicin 5 to 7.5 mg/kg/day in three divided doses is desirable early in the disease. Despite the low concentration of aminoglycosides in the cerebrospinal fluid, their use is indicated because of their synergism with penicillin or ampicillin. The patient's postnatal age and renal status may influence the route and dose of administration of the drugs, especially the aminoglycosides. Careful monitoring of serum levels may be required in certain cases. Two weeks of parenteral therapy are generally recommended for patients without meningitis. In meningitis, a longer course may be needed. The length of therapy should be decided after several lumbar punctures to ensure bacterial cure.

Combined therapy is warranted until all previously positive cultures become negative. Following that, ampicillin therapy can be continued alone for 2 weeks. In endocarditis or osteomyelitis, the ampicillin-gentamicin combination should be given for about 2 weeks; therafter, ampicillin alone should be continued for 4 weeks. Therapy should be continued for at least 1 week after defervescence. Listeriosis of the immunocompromised patients typically relapses; therefore, prolonged therapy for as long as 6 to 8 weeks may be indicated.

Other antimicrobial agents can be used in patients with penicillin allergy or penicillin resistant strains. Erythromycin, chloramphenicol, tetracycline, and sulfonamines have all been used successfully. However, these are bactericidal drugs and are less effective than penicillin or ampicillin. Recent in vitro work showed excellent activity of trimethoprim sulfa and rifampin against listeria. Chloramphenicol, because of its excellent penetration into the cerebrospinal fluid, is preferred for the therapy of intracranial infections. Tetracyclines can be used for children older than 8 years.

Supportive measures are important, particularly in listeriosis of the newborn. Patients with meningitis may also require respiratory assistance.

The ability to prevent fetal disease by antimicrobial therapy in the pregnant mother with positive endocervical cultures of listeria is unclear. Symptomatic maternal listeriosis may be treated with ampicillin or erythromycin.

Diphtheria

QUELLIN T. BOX, M.D.

The most important component in the treatment of diphtheria is the administration of specific antitoxin as promptly as possible following an adequately considered clinical diagnosis. The mortality rate in diphtheria is directly related to the duration of disease prior to antitoxin therapy. The doses of antitoxin in use have been empirically determined and are probably well in excess of maximally effective amounts. Ranges of 30,000 to 80,000 units are recommended, the higher doses being appropriate for patients with severe involvement and for those diagnosed late in the course of their disease. The entire dose is given initially; repeated doses are not given. Because of the relatively slow absorption of antitoxin from subcutaneous and intramuscular sites, early toxin neutralization is best assured by

the intravenous administration of at least half the dose of antitoxin. Although intramuscular antitoxin may be adequate in milder cases, I prefer to give the entire dose intravenously after the usual tests for serum sensitivity. Available antitoxin is of equine origin.

In case of a positive reaction to an intradermal test with 0.1 ml of a 1:1000 dilution of antitoxin, desensitization may be undertaken after appropriate preparation is made to ensure adequate management of adverse reactions, especially anaphylaxis. A facility such as a hospital emergency room or hospital ward treatment room fully equipped for conducting resuscitative measures should be used. A syringe is prepared for emergency use with 1 ml of 1:1000 aqueous epinephrine. A secure IV infusion is begun with 5% glucose solution, and baseline observations of blood pressure, pulse, and respiratory rate are made. Following is a typical schedule for a serum desensitization procedure, the test doses of antitoxin being given every 15 to 20 minutes:

0.25 ml	1:100 dilution	subcutaneously
0.5 ml	1:100 dilution	subcutaneously
0.1 ml	undiluted	subcutaneously
0.2 ml	undiluted	subcutaneously
0.5 ml	undiluted	intramuscularly

The entire dose of antitoxin diluted 1:20 in 5% glucose in water is then given intravenously, beginning with a slow drip for the first 20 minutes, the remainder then being given over a 30-minute period. A reaction occurring at any point in the serum testing or administration of the antitoxin requires that further administration be delayed pending appropriate management of the reaction and reevaluation of the indication for antitoxin therapy as weighed against the nature and severity of the reaction.

Antimicrobial therapy is never used in diphtheria as a substitute for specific antitoxin. Prior to antimicrobial therapy, paired nasopharyngeal and throat swabs are obtained to be cultured for toxicogenic *Corynebacterium diphtheriae*. Examination of stained direct smears is not advised. Crystalline penicillin G, 250,000 units/kg/24 hr divided every 6 hours IV, is given during the acute phase. After the involved mucous membranes are free of necrotic and purulent material, therapy is reduced to 600,000 units daily of aqueous procaine penicillin and continued to a total of 14 days. This therapy has been completely effective in the rapid elimination of infectivity (24 hours or less to achieve negative cultures) and in eventual bacteriologic cure. This regimen is also adequate for treatment of the frequently associated Group A streptococcal infections. For the patient allergic to penicillin, erythromycin lactobionate or erythromycin gluceptate, 20 mg/kg/24 hr divided every 6 hours IV, may be substituted for IV penicillin. Erythromycin, 40 mg/kg/24 hr divided every 6 hours orally, may be used in place of aqueous procaine penicillin. Cultures are repeated on 2 successive days after completion of antimicrobial therapy. For any individual with a persisting positive culture, a repeated course of oral antimicrobial agent is prescribed.

All patients with diphtheria should be hospitalized for treatment. Strict isolation procedures are indicated, especially for the acute period, during high-dose penicillin therapy, until the involved mucous membranes are free of necrotic and purulent material. Complete bed rest is indicated until the danger of severe complications is largely over, at least for 14 days. Fluid and electrolyte requirements are met by intravenous infusion until all danger of aspiration has passed and the patient can swallow without difficulty.

Close observation for complications is especially important. Palatal and pharyngeal paralysis may occur early and predispose to pulmonary complications from injudicious feeding attempts. Excessively vigorous or frequent nasopharyngeal or oropharyngeal suctioning may cause significant trauma or hemorrhage. Airway obstruction from desquamating pseudomembrane may require laryngoscopic or bronchoscopic removal. Tracheotomy should be done early for progressive airway obstruction, rather than being postponed until an emergency procedure is required.

Most current mortality in diphtheria is related to carditis. Appropriate cardiac monitoring is required for early detection of conduction disturbances and other manifestations of carditis. The presence of carditis requires intensive cardiac care, preferably in a unit specializing in such care. Emergency cardiac resuscitative equipment and medications, and personnel expert in their use, must be immediately available for the most successful management of severe carditis. Peripheral neuritis, a late-appearing complication, is usually benign and is self-limited, requiring no treatment. Occasional cases may progress in severity until respiratory support is necessary.

Treatment of diphtheria includes the evaluation of all household contacts. If further cases are diagnosed clinically, appropriate treatment is begun immediately. For all household contacts without evidence of diphtheria, erythromycin, 40 mg/kg/24 hr divided every 6 hours orally for 10 days, is prescribed. As with cases, contacts are cultured for toxicogenic *C. diphtheriae* before and after therapy, and treatment is repeated if positive cultures persist. For those who are determined to be adequately immunized, a booster dose of toxoid is also given. For those with inadequate or no immunization, a complete toxoid series is begun. Diphtheria antitoxin is never used prophylactically. Hospital personnel contacts should be adequately protected by routine toxoid immunization. Convalescents from diphtheria are also given a complete toxoid series, since they may not be immune.

Pertussis

JAMES W. BASS, M.P.H., M.D.

Pertussis or whooping cough is an acute infection of the respiratory tract caused by *Bordetella pertussis.* Illness indistinguishable from pertussis may be caused by *B. parapertussis* and *B. bronchiseptica.* Adenoviruses have also been implicated, alone or in association with *B. pertussis* infection. *Chlamydia trachomatis* infection in early infancy (< 4 months of age) has been shown to cause illness very similar to pertussis and is now probably more commonly seen in the United States. Patients with clinical pertussis should be isolated until it is determined if their illness is due to *B. pertussis* or *B. parapertussis.*

SUPPORTIVE CARE

Severe disease and a high incidence of complications are most often seen in young infants. Of children who die of pertussis, 75% are under 1 year of age, and most are only 2, 3, and 4 months old. Thus, it is wise to hospitalize children with pertussis who are less than 1 year of age. Older children with less serious disease can usually be managed as outpatients.

Patient care areas should be quiet and well ventilated with the air free of all irritants. There should be as little stimulation and manipulation of the patient as possible, since this often provokes cough paroxysms. Necessary procedures such as suctioning, feeding, administration of medications, diaper changing, examination, and laboratory tests are best done immediately after cough paroxysms when the patient is relatively refractory to further paroxysms. Adequate hydration and nutrition are essential. Younger infants should be given several small feedings daily of bland liquids or semi-solid nutrients. Foods that must be chewed and are difficult to swallow should be withheld. Children with frequent paroxysms requiring suctioning, and those with excessive vomiting and difficulty maintaining fluid and food intake may require parenteral fluids.

Infants under 6 months of age with severe pertussis frequently have bouts of prolonged paroxysmal cough followed by cyanosis and apnea without exhibiting the whoop characteristically heard in older children. These infants may die of asphyxia if immediate resuscitation is not available. When cough paroxysms occur, the infant should be positioned in a head-down position to prevent aspiration of the thick, tenacious secretions accumulating at the end of a paroxysm. Vomiting often occurs at the end of severe paroxysms, and aspiration of vomitus by the weak, exhausted, hypoxemic infant must be prevented. Suctioning and supplemental oxygen are indicated during and after severe coughing. Experienced and efficient nursing care is probably the most important factor in survival.

Mist therapy is not helpful. Continuous administration of well-humidified oxygen is necessary in patients who show sustained evidence of hypoxemia. Blood gas determinations are essential in patients with labored respirations, unstable vital signs, or altered mental status. Such patients usually have complications such as atelectasis or bronchopneumonia which result in hypoxia. Cough suppressants, expectorants, bronchodilators, and sedatives have not been shown to be of benefit.

SPECIFIC THERAPY

Recently, several well-designed controlled studies have failed to demonstrate any benefit of treatment with hyperimmune pertussis globulin. It is no longer recommended in the treatment of pertussis.

Antimicrobial agents have no effect upon the clinical course when given in the paroxysmal stage. Unfortunately, the diagnosis is seldom suspected before this stage except in those who have had known contact with pertussis patients. Erythromycin, tetracyclines, or chloramphenicol regularly eliminates pertussis organisms from patients with the disease within a few days and, in doing so, may render them noninfectious. Erythromycin is the most effective and least toxic. In addition, there is evidence that it may be of value in prophylaxis in exposed susceptible individuals, and that it may abort or attenuate the illness if administered in the early preparoxysmal stage. For this reason, all patients who have a positive smear for *B. pertussis* should be treated with erythromycin, 35 to 50 mg/kg/day orally in four divided doses for a period of 14 days. Treatment for less than 14 days is frequently complicated by bacteriological relapse.

Though ampicillin is known to be effective against *B. pertussis* in vitro, it is ineffective in producing bacteriological cures when compared with untreated controls. This discrepancy between its in vitro and in vivo effectiveness has been explained by its poor penetration into respiratory tract secretions. Erythromycin readily penetrates these secretions in effective concentrations. Ampicillin should not be used in treatment of patients with pertussis except for the management of certain complicating infections.

Corticosteroids significantly alter the severity and duration of pertussis, even when treatment is delayed until the paroxysmal stage. Two controlled studies substantiating this have been reported. In the first study betamethasone was given orally at a dose of 0.075 mg/kg/24 hr. In the second, hydrocortisone sodium succinate (Solu-Cortef) was given intramuscularly at a dose of 30 mg/kg/24 hr for 2 days; the dose was thereafter reduced gradually and discontinued by the seventh to eighth day. Significant reduction in the number, severity, and duration of paroxysms was noted in the corticosteroid-treated groups when compared with untreated controls. Corticosteroids are indicated in treating patients with severe pertussis. Either of the two regimens evaluated may be used; however, other corticosteroid preparations at comparable dosages should work equally well.

COMPLICATIONS

Bronchopneumonia develops in approximately 10% of hospitalized children with pertussis. The chest x-ray often reveals a characteristic "shaggy-heart" appearance with patchy infiltrates and atelectasis, most prominent along the borders of the heart. Pneumonia or other bacterial superinfections should be suspected in children who develop fever, since most patients with uncomplicated pertussis have normal temperature or only minimal elevations. Pertussis organisms are not invasive, and associated pneumonias are caused by the usual bacterial pathogens causing pneumonia in children. After cultures of the blood and sputum are obtained, specific antibiotic therapy should be given.

Atelectasis should be anticipated in most patients with severe disease. The tenacious secretions that accumulate in the distal bronchi and bronchioles cause inspissation with secondary patchy atelectasis, primarily in the area of the hilum and around the cardiac borders. Lobar or segmental atelectasis, also common, primarily affects the lower lobes, the right middle lobe, and the lingular segment of the left upper lobe.

Intermittent positive pressure breathing and other respiratory therapy procedures have not affected the incidence or degree of this atelectasis. Proper postural drainage by repositioning following cough paroxysms must be provided so that all pulmonary lobes may be drained effectively. Frappage or other vigorous chest physiotherapy maneuvers should not be instituted until the convalescent stage of the disease, as they frequently precipitate cough paroxysms during the paroxysmal stage of the illness. Nearly all atelectasis complicating pertussis clears spontaneously within 2 to 3 weeks following the paroxysmal stage of the disease. Bronchoscopy or resection for complications due to inspissated secretions or concretions is rarely indicated.

Otitis media is a frequent complication because the thick secretions may obstruct the eustachian tubes. Ascending infection into the middle ear develops from the mucous plug. The primary pathogens implicated by diagnostic tympanocentesis are the pneumonococcus, *Hemophilus influenzae,* and beta hemolytic streptococci. Although *Bordetella pertussis* is not an invasive pathogen and is not implicated etiologically in the pneumonias that complicate pertussis, studies have not excluded the pertussis organism as a significant cause of acute otitis media in these patients.

The acute otitis media should respond to erythromycin given for the primary infection* plus sulfisoxazole, 150 mg/kg/day in four divided doses.

A tympanocentesis should be performed so that the definitive cause of infection can be determined and specific therapy directed by antibiotic sensitivity testing.

Neurologic complications occur in 2 to 3% of patients. They may occur at any time during the course of the illness, but most often in the early paroxysmal stage. There may be a single, generalized convulsion, a series of convulsions, or status epilepticus. A child with a single convulsion or repeated convulsions with a normal neurologic examination between may recover without sequelae. Those who have repeated convulsions with coma between seizures or those who have coma following a prolonged episode of status epilepticus have a grave prognosis. If they survive, they frequently have severe neurologic handicaps.

A specific neurotoxin elaborated from pertussis organisms has been proposed as a possible etiology for pertussis encephalopathy, but none has been demonstrated. Patients dying with pertussis encephalopathy exhibit gross and microscopic histopathologic findings compatible with severe cerebral hypoxia. The incidence of pertussis encephalopathy might be lessened if the hypoxic episodes following severe cough paroxysms were better managed. Convulsions should be treated immediately with diazepam, 0.3 mg/kg intravenously or intramuscularly. If convulsions recur or are prolonged and protracted from the outset, phenobarbital, 5 to 8 mg/kg/day, in divided doses at 6 to 8 hour intervals intramuscularly, should be administered. The maintenance of a good airway and oxygenation is essential during convulsive episodes, since hypoxia may be the major cause of their precipitation and perpetuation.

Management of Exposed Susceptible Individuals. Patients with FA-positive whooping cough should be isolated until they have had at least three negative nasopharyngeal smears by FA studies done at intervals of 2 to 3 days each. Asymptomatic patients who have positive nasopharyngeal smears by FA examination may be incubating the disease. These patients and those in the catarrhal or paroxysmal stage of illness become culture-negative within 3 to 4 days after initiation of erythromycin therapy and are presumably noncontagious. As long as they continue to take erythromycin for a full 2 weeks and the nasopharyngeal smear remains FA-negative, isolation does not seem warranted. If FA or culture studies are not available, patients treated with erythromycin may be presumed noncontagious after 5 days of therapy, since culture and FA studies are regularly negative by this time.

Recent reports of pertussis outbreaks involving large numbers of newborn infants, other children, and even pediatric house officers in children's hospitals attest to the high degree to which patients with this disease are contagious. Vaccination after exposure is not protective. Controlled studies have shown pertussis hyperimmune globulin to be of no benefit in the prophylaxis of pertussis in exposed susceptible household contacts. Individuals who have had significant direct contact with pertussis patients and who cannot be followed by FA studies should probably be treated with erythromycin in the same manner as patients with the disease. This drug was apparently effective in helping control the spread of disease in the two hospital outbreaks of pertussis cited previously. Children under 6 years of age who have primary immunization with at least 3 or 4 DTP injections in infancy may be adequately protected after exposure if given a booster dose of 0.5 ml of DTP vaccine.

Bacterial Pneumonia

JEROME O. KLEIN, M.D.

Effective chemotherapy is now available for all forms of bacterial pneumonia encountered in the pediatric age group. Optimal treatment, however, requires definition of the etiologic agent. The physician must differentiate viral or mycoplasmal from bacterial pneumonia; if the agent is bacterial, the probable species must be decided. Clinical signs and laboratory values may help but are not definitive. A major effort must be made to obtain adequate materials for bacteriologic diagnosis; these include sputum, secretions from the posterior nasopharynx, and blood (bacteremia is frequent and a positive blood culture for a respiratory pathogen provides an unequivocal etiologic diagnosis). The physician also should consider the following: tracheal aspiration in young children unable to produce sputum; thoracocentesis when pleural fluid is present; and percutaneous lung aspiration in critically ill children who deteriorate while on therapy or are abnormal hosts with deficient immune mechanisms.

Therapy should be initiated promptly once bacterial pneumonia is diagnosed or strongly suspected. Initial therapy may be guided by the

---

*Contraindicated in infants under 2 months of age.

examination of the Gram-stained smear of sputum or tracheal aspirate. If these materials are unsatisfactory or unavailable, other criteria must be used. The relative frequency of respiratory pathogens in the various age groups may provide guidelines for initial therapy for the child with pneumonia who has no significant underlying pulmonary systemic illness or defect in immune function.

INITIAL CHOICE OF ANTIMICROBIAL AGENTS IN VARIOUS AGE GROUPS

Neonatal Pneumonia. The treatment of neonatal pneumonia is similar to that of other forms of severe neonatal infection, including sepsis and meningitis; initial therapy must include coverage for gram-positive cocci, particularly group B streptococcus, and gram-negative bacilli.

A penicillin is the drug of choice for the gram-positive organisms. If there is reason to suspect staphylococcal infection, a penicillinase-resistant penicillin is chosen. If there is no significant risk of such infection, penicillin G or ampicillin is used. The latter drug may provide a theoretic advantage because of greater in vitro activity against some enterococci and some gram-negative bacilli, particularly *Escherichia coli* and *Proteus mirabilis,* when used alone or in combination with an aminoglycoside.

Choice of therapy for suspected gram-negative bacillary infection depends on the antibiotic susceptibility pattern for recent isolates obtained from newborn infants. The patterns vary in different hospitals or communities and from time to time within the same institution. At present, a significant proportion of all gram-negative bacilli cultured from newborns at the Boston City Hospital are resistant to tetracycline, streptomycin, ampicillin, and cephalothin. Strains of *Pseudomonas aeruginosa* are resistant to all antibiotics except polymyxins, carbenicillin, gentamicin, tobramycin, and amikacin. Based on antibiotic susceptibility patterns of recent isolates of gram-negative enteric bacilli, we now use gentamicin to initiate therapy for severe neonatal infections.

Chloramphenicol has been used infrequently in newborn infants, owing to the association of the gray baby syndrome with high doses of this antibiotic. Perhaps becuase of the now minimal use in nurseries, chloramphenicol may be effective in vitro against gram-negative bacilli resistant to other antibiotics. Infants with neonatal sepsis due to a strain uniquely sensitive to chloramphenicol should be treated with this antibiotic in an appropriate dosage schedule (Table 1).

Because of the rapid changes in renal function during the first few weeks of life, different dosage schedules for selected antibiotics should be used for infants 6 days of age or younger and infants 1 to 4 weeks of age (Table 1).

Table 1. DAILY DOSAGE SCHEDULES FOR PARENTERAL ANTIBIOTICS OF VALUE IN TREATING BACTERIAL PNEUMONIA IN NEWBORN INFANTS*

Antibiotic	Dosage Schedule	
	≤6 Days of Age	1 to 4 Weeks of Age
Penicillin G	25,000 to 50,000 units/kg every 12 hours	35,000 to 70,000 units/kg every 8 hours
Ampicillin Methicillin Nafcillin Oxacillin	25 to 50 mg/kg every 12 hours	35 to 70 mg/kg every 8 hours
Carbenicillin	50 to 75 mg/kg every 6 hours	100 mg/kg every 6 hours
Kanamycin†	7.5 mg/kg every 12 hours	7.5 mg/kg every 12 hours
Gentamicin†	2.5 mg/kg every 12 hours	2.5 mg/kg every 8 hours
Tobramycin†	2 mg/kg every 12 hours	1.2 mg/kg every 8 hours
Amikacin†	7.5 mg/kg every 12 hours	7.5 mg/kg every 12 hours
Chloramphenicol‡ Premature	12.5 mg/kg every 12 hours	12.5 mg/kg every 12 hours
Full-term	12.5 mg/kg every 12 hours	25 mg/kg every 12 hours
Vancomycin	15 mg/kg every 12 hours	15 mg/kg every 8 hours

*IM or IV routes are satisfactory except where specifically noted.

†IM route usually used. IV administration over 30 to 60 minutes.

‡IV route only, inadequate absorption from IM sites.

The initial therapy should be re-evaluated when the results of cultures are available. Duration of therapy depends on the causative agent. Pneumonia due to gram-negative enteric bacilli or group B streptococcus is treated for 10 days; disease caused by *Staphylococcus aureus* requires 3 to 6 weeks of antimicrobial therapy according to the severity of the pneumonia.

Pneumonias in Children 1 Month to 5 Years of Age. The vast majority of bronchopneumonias at this age are caused by respiratory viruses. Therefore, if the initial clinical findings are consistent with viral infection and the child can be observed closely, specific therapy may be withheld pending the results of bacterial cultures. *Streptococcus pneumoniae* and *Hemophilus influenzae* are the major bacterial agents of concern. A penicillin is the drug of choice: penicillin G or V for pneumococcal pneumonia and ampicillin for *H. influenzae* infections. When the etiologic agent is unknown but a bacterial pneumonia seems likely, ampicillin should be used to provide coverage for both pathogens. However, about 20% of *H. influenzae* strains are currently resistant to ampicillin in the U.S. At present, ampicillin is still appropriate initial therapy for the young child with mild-to-moderately severe pneumonia. Chloramphenicol intravenously should be considered for the seriously ill child who has pneumonia that may be due to *H. influenzae*. Therapy must be re-evaluated when results of the cultures and antibiotic susceptibility tests are available (see Chemotherapy for Specific Pathogens to follow).

S. aureus has been an uncommon cause of acute pneumonia during the past 15 years. However, if clinical signs compatible with staphylococcal disease are present (such as empyema, abscess formation, or pneumatoceles), initial therapy should include a parenteral penicillinase-resistant penicillin (methicillin, nafcillin, or oxacillin).

Chlamydia trachomatis is a common cause of pneumonia in the first 6 months of life. Erythromycin or a sulfonamide appears to be effective in ameliorating signs of illness for infants who have pneumonia caused by this organism.

Pneumonia in the Child 5 Years of Age and Older. *S. pneumoniae* is the major bacterial cause of pneumonia in this age group. *H. influenzae* is uncommon and need not be considered in initial therapy.

Infection due to *Mycoplasma pneumoniae* is frequent in the school-age child, adolescent, and young adult. Erythromycin and the tetracyclines (for use in the child 8 years of age or older*) are effective in reducing the duration of illness; once the diagnosis is made or strongly suspected, treatment with one of these agents is appropriate.

CHEMOTHERAPY FOR SPECIFIC PATHOGENS

Pneumococcal Pneumonia. Penicillin G is the drug of choice for all children with pneumococcal pneumonia, except those considered to be allergic to that antibiotic.

For most children with mild-to-moderately severe disease, an oral penicillin is suitable. Phenoxymethyl penicillin (penicillin V) provides significant serum antibacterial activity (the peak is approximately 40% of an equivalent dose of IM aqueous penicillin G). Buffered oral penicillin G is less satisfactory, since the peak serum antibacterial activity is approximately one half that of the weight equivalent of penicillin V, and larger doses therefore are required.

Children who appear "toxic," or who have underlying disease or complications such as abscesses or empyema require the higher serum and tissue

---

*Manufacturer's note: The use of tetracyclines during tooth development (last half of pregnancy, infancy, and childhood to age 8 years) may cause permanent discoloration of teeth. This adverse reaction is more common during long-term use but has been observed following repeated short-term courses.

antibacterial activity provided by a parenteral form. Intramuscular aqueous sodium or potassium penicillin G is rapidly absorbed, high peak levels occurring within 30 minutes; the levels thus attained make this route optimal for treatment of severe pneumococcal disease. However, since the IM preparation is painful, the IV route should be used if therapy of any duration is anticipated.

Procaine penicillin G, IM, attains lower peak levels (approximately 10 to 30% of those achieved with the sodium or potassium salt), but activity is sustained for 6 or more hours. Since the level of antibacterial activity in the serum may be exceeded manyfold by oral penicillins, use of parenteral procaine penicillin G is restricted to patients who cannot tolerate the oral form (those who vomit or are comatose).

A single dose of benzathine penicillin G provides a low level of serum antibacterial activity for a period in excess of 14 days. Although this salt often has been effective in pneumococcal pneumonia, failures are frequent and it is not recommended.

The dosage schedule listed in Table 2 may be used to initiate therapy. The duration of therapy depends on the clinical response, but it should be continued for at least 3 days after defervescence and significant resolution of the radiologic and clinical signs.

Strains of *S. pneumoniae* resistant to penicillin G and other effective antimicrobial agents appeared in South Africa in 1977. To date, only one strain of *S. pneumoniae* highly resistant to penicillin G (although not resistant to other antibiotics that might be used as alternatives to penicillin) has been identified in the U.S.A. At present, no change in the use of penicillin G for treatment of pneumococcal disease is necessary, but physicians must be alert for the appearance of resistant strains.

Staphylococcal Pneumonia. The high incidence of penicillin G-resistant staphylococci in the hospital and the community requires the use of a penicillinase-resistant penicillin whenever staphylococcal pneumonia is diagnosed or suspected. Later, if the culture and sensitivity data indicate that the organism is sensitive to penicillin G, it should be used because of its efficacy and lesser expense.

There are differences among the various penicillinase-resistant penicillins in oral and parenteral absorption, in vitro activity, and enzyme degradation. However, clinical trials indicate that all are effective in treating staphylococcal disease when used in appropriate dosage schedules.

Since 1961, laboratories in Western Europe have reported varying proportions of strains of staphylococci resistant to methicillin and cross-resistant to the other penicillinase-resistant penicillins (and some of the cephalosporins). The incidence of these resistant strains has been low (approximately 1% or less) in the U.S.A. but outbreaks have oc-

Table 2. DAILY DOSAGE SCHEDULES FOR ANTIBIOTICS OF VALUE
IN BACTERIAL PNEUMONIAS OF INFANTS* AND CHILDREN

Antibiotic	Route	Recommended Dose Per Day	Schedule
Penicillin G	PO	100,000 units/kg	4 doses†
	IM or IV	100,000 to 200,000 units/kg	4 to 6 doses
Penicillin V	PO	100 mg/kg	4 doses
Methicillin	IM or IV	200 mg/kg	4 to 6 doses
Oxacillin } Nafcillin §	PO	100 mg/kg	4 doses†
	IM or IV	200 mg/kg	4 to 6 doses
Cloxacillin } Dicloxacillin	PO	50 mg/kg	4 doses†
Amoxicillin	PO	40 mg/kg	3 doses
Ampicillin	PO	100 mg/kg	4 doses†
	IM or IV	200 mg/kg	4 to 6 doses
Carbenicillin	IM or IV	200 to 600 mg/kg‡	4 doses
Cephalothin	IM or IV	200 mg/kg	4 to 6 doses
Cephalexin	PO	100 mg/kg	4 doses†
Cefazolin	IM or IV	50 to 100 mg/kg	4 doses
Cefamandole	IM or IV	50 to 150 mg/kg	4 doses
Cefaclor	PO	40 to 60 mg/kg¶	3 doses
Kanamycin	IM or IV‖	15 mg/kg	2 to 3 doses
Gentamicin	IM or IV‖	5 mg/kg	3 doses
Tobramycin	IM or IV‖	5 mg/kg	3 doses
Amikacin	IM or IV‖	15 mg/kg	2 doses
Chloramphenicol	PO	50 to 100 mg/kg	4 doses
	IV	50 to 100 mg/kg	4 doses
Clindamycin	PO	8 to 25 mg/kg	4 doses
	IM or IV	15 to 40 mg/kg	4 doses
Erythromycin	PO	20 to 50 mg/kg	4 doses
	IV	20 to 50 mg/kg	4 doses
Vancomycin	IV	15 to 50 mg/kg	4 doses

* 1 month of age and older.
† Schedule at least 1 hour before meals or 2 hours after meals.
‡ This dosage may exceed that recommended by the manufacturer.
§ Manufacturer's precaution: There is no clinical experience available on the IV use of nafcillin in neonates and infants.
‖ IV administration over 30 to 60 minutes.
¶ The manufacturer's schedule for serious infection is 40 mg/kg/24 hr, with a maximum daily dosage of 1 gram.

curred in hospitals including intensive care units. If a child with staphylococcal disease is given appropriate doses of one of these penicillins and does not respond as expected, resistance to the antibiotic must be suspected and sensitivity of the causative organism re-evaluated. Vancomycin is an effective antistaphylococcal agent and may be used for the patient with pneumonia due to methicillin-resistant *S. aureus.*

The rapid evolution of staphylococcal pneumonia and the frequent association of empyema, pneumatoceles, and abscesses demand close observation and meticulous nursing care. The duration of antibiotic therapy depends on the initial response, the presence of pulmonary and extrapulmonary complications, and the rapidity of resolution of the pneumonic process. A large parenteral dosage schedule should be used for 2 to 3 weeks, followed by an oral preparation for 1 to 3 weeks.

Hemophilus influenzae. This organism is sus-ceptible to a variety of antimicrobial agents, including the sulfonamides, tetracyclines, aminoglycosides, and ampicillin. All have been used with success in infections due to this agent. At present, ampicillin should be considered the drug of choice in young children with mild-to-moderate pulmonary disease. It provides coverage for both *S. pneumoniae* and *H. influenzae* when there is uncertainty as to the bacteriologic diagnosis, and the high dosage schedule needed for severe forms of disease can be given without concern for dose-related toxicity (Table 2).

Beginning in 1972, strains of *H. influenzae* (both type b and nontypable) resistant to ampicillin have been reported throughout the U.S.A. At present, approximately 20% of type b strains in the country are resistant to ampicillin. Because of these strains, recommendations for treatment of life-threatening disease that may be due to *H. influenzae* (meningitis, epiglottitis, or severe pneumonia) have been revised. Initial therapy for these patients includes IV chloramphenicol and penicillin G or ampicillin. The most appropriate regimen is chosen when results of cultures and antibacterial susceptibility tests are available.

The child with mild-to-moderate pulmonary disease is treated until a period without fever of at least 3 days and a minimum of 10 days ensues. The child with severe disease is treated for at least 2 to 3 weeks.

Pneumonia Due to Gram-Negative Bacilli. Initial therapy must be guided by the following factors: the source of infection, underlying disease process (burn, cystic fibrosis), host susceptibility (deficient immune mechanisms), and the antimicrobial susceptibility pattern for gram-negative organisms in the community and hospital. The basis for choice of antibiotic is similar to that outlined for suspected gram-negative bacillary pneumonia in the neonate. The regimen is modified if indicated by the results of the cultures and the susceptibility of the causative organism. Duration of therapy must be tailored to the clinical course and the response to therapy. Pneumonias with minimal pulmonary lesions and symptoms should be treated for at least 3 days after defervescence. Severe pneumonias should be treated for a period of 2 to 3 weeks.

THERAPY FOR THE PENICILLIN-SENSITIVE CHILD

Any patient with a significant history of allergic reaction to any of the penicillins must be considered sensitive to all of them; thus alternative antimicrobial agents should be considered.

Cephalosporins have been used with success in the treatment of staphylococcal and pneumococcal pneumonia and may be used as alternatives to penicillin. In contrast with previously available cephalosporins, the new agents cefamandole (for parenteral usage) and cefaclor (for oral administration) are active against *H. influenzae* (including ampicillin-resistant strains) and gram-positive cocci. Because of variable diffusion of cephalosporins into cerebrospinal fluid after parenteral or oral administration, they should not be used for patients with known or suspected meningitis.

Erythromycin and clindamycin are active in vitro against gram-positive cocci and are effective in the treatment of pneumococcal and staphylococcal pneumonias. Since some staphylococci may be resistant to these antibiotics, it is important to test the organism for susceptibility.

Vancomycin may be considered for use in the patient who is allergic to penicillin and who has severe staphylococcal disease.

Tetracycline should not be used in children under the age of 8 years because of the frequency of tooth staining. For those over the age of 8 years, it may be of value in infection due to *M. pneumoniae.* The small proportion of pneumococci and the significant number (approximately 30%) of strepto-

cocci resistant to tetracyclines limit their use in infections due to these agents.

ADJUNCTS TO CHEMOTHERAPY

Antibiotics are only part of the management of the pediatric patient with pneumonia; supportive measures, including the following, are also of the utmost importance:

1. Maintenance of fluid and electrolyte balance.
2. Humidification provided by "cool mist."
3. Oxygen for severe dyspnea or cyanosis.
4. Maintenance of mouth hygiene.
5. Antipyretics should be used sparingly, since the temperature course may provide a guideline for the therapeutic response.
6. Bronchoscopy is limited to instances in which a foreign body, tumor, or congenital anomaly is considered.
7. Tracheal intubation or tracheostomy may be considered when there is laryngeal obstruction, or when the patient is having difficulty clearing tracheal secretions and more efficient suctioning is warranted.
8. Drainage of pleural effusions may be necessary when the accumulation of fluid embarrasses respiration. Single or multiple thoracocenteses may be adequate when the volumes of fluid are small. If larger amounts are present, a closed drainage system with a chest tube under negative pressure should be placed. The tube should be removed as soon as its drainage function is completed, since delay may result in local tissue injury, secondary infection, and sinus formation.
9. Intrapleural instillation of antibiotic should be considered in early cases of empyema, particularly if the fluid is loculated and the presence of fibrous adhesions is a possibility. If a chest tube is in place, antibiotics are instilled following irrigation through the tube. In susceptible infections, aqueous crystalline penicillin G, 10,000 to 50,000 units; ampicillin, 10 to 50 mg; or a penicillinase-resistant penicillin or a cephalosporin, 10 to 50 mg, may be inoculated in 10 ml of diluent (sterile water or normal saline) after the tube is clamped. The clamp is maintained for 1 hour and then released for drainage. The instillations should be repeated 3 to 4 times each day that the tube remains in place. If thoracocenteses are done, antibiotic is introduced after pleural fluid is aspirated.

Meningococcal Disease

RALPH D. FEIGIN, M.D.,
and JOSEPH P. NEGLIA, M.D.

Acute meningococcemia may present as an influenza-like illness associated with fever, malaise, myalgia, and arthralgia. In a brief period of time, however, morbilliform, petechial, or purpuric lesions may be noted and profound hypotension may occur. The presence of hypotension, purpura, thrombocytopenia, and leukopenia frequently presages a fatal outcome.

Meningococcal meningitis follows blood stream dissemination and, in addition to the findings detailed above, vomiting, lethargy, seizures, and other signs of meningeal irritation may be observed. The ultimate survival of patients with meningococcal miningitis, in most series, is beter than that noted in patients with acute meningococcemia but without meningeal involvement.

Chronic meningococcemia is rare in children. It is characterized by chills, fever, maculopapular lesions, arthralgia, and/or arthritis. Erythema nodosum lesions may be observed in both acute and chronic meningococcal disease.

The patient should be isolated for 24 hours after the initiation of therapy.

THERAPY

Crystalline sodium penicillin G, 200,000 units/kg/24 hr should be provided intravenously in six divided doses. The total daily dosage should be increased to 300,000 units when there is evidence of meningitis. When the etiologic agent is in doubt, ampicillin should be given in a dosage of 300 mg/kg/24 hr in six divided dosages and chloramphenicol in a dosage of 100 mg/kg/24 hr in four divided doses. Chloramphenicol alone provides effective treatment for patients allergic to penicillin. Antibiotic treatment should be continued for 7 days in patients with meningococcemia and preferably for 10 days in patients with meningococcal meningitis. In some cases in which pericardial effusions, septic arthritis, or pneumonia complicates meningococcemia, prolonged therapy may be indicated.

Circulatory Failure. Shock frequently accompanies meningococcemia. When circulatory failure ensues, every effort must be made to ensure an adequate circulating blood volume. A central venous catheter should be placed and the urine output monitored. The latter may require catheterization of the bladder. The blood pressure, pulse rate and rhythm, and central venous pressure must be monitored frequently. The rapid infusion of osmotically active substances such as 5% dextrose in normal saline, 5% dextrose in lactated Ringer's, colloids, or reconstituted packed red blood cells may be required to maintain an adequate blood pressure and urine output. Fresh frozen plasma may be helpful in patients who also have disseminated intravascular coagulation. In patients with a high central venous pressure, cardiac decompensation may occur and digitalization may be necessary.

If circulatory failure persists, infusion of vaso-

pressors such as dopamine or dobutamine should be initiated. Dopamine infusion should begin at a rate of 5 μg/kg/min and may be increased to as high as 20 μ/kg/min as needed. The rate of dobutamine infusion may be adjusted from 5 to 10 μ/kg/min as needed to maintain blood pressure and urine output.

The use of steroids in the treatment of endotoxic shock is controversial. Controlled experiments in animals and selected studies in man suggest that benefit from their administration requires massive pharmacologic doses (250 times the normal cortisol secretory rate per day) administered as early as possible. Methylprednisolone, 15–20 mg/kg/dose can be infused intravenously every 6 hours and continued as needed. If given for 72 or more hours an appropriate weaning schedule will be required before discontinuing the drug.

In patients with meningococcal meningitis who develop hypotension, difficulty in the management of shock may be increased, for every effort must be made concomitantly to minimize the development of cerebral edema. The presence of cerebral edema may be suggested by an irregular respiratory effort, a falling pulse rate, hypertension, and persistent seizures. Fluid administration must be minimized where possible and colloid used in preference to crystalloid infusates. Severe cerebral edema also may be treated by use of a 20% solution of mannitol in distilled water. This should be administered in a dose of 1 to 2 gm/kg body weight given over 10 to 15 minutes. This may be repeated but attention to fluid and electrolyte balance is critical.

Seizures may be controlled with sodium phenobarbital, 7 to 10 mg/kg administered parenterally. Following this initial dose, anticonvulsant effect may be maintained with phenobarbital, 5 to 7 mg/kg/24 hr in two divided doses. Phenytoin may be provided in an initial dose of 5 to 10 mg/kg intravenously or intramuscularly and maintained with a dosage of 5 to 7 mg/kg/24 hr, also in two divided doses. When this drug is given intravenously, it is important that it be given into the injection post nearest to the patient and that this line be flushed with normal saline before, during, and after the infusion.

Disseminated Intravascular Coagulation. This complication is generally associated with hypotension. In addition to treatment of the basic disease with antibiotics and supporting the patient in shock as above, heparin, 100 units/kg, may be given by rapid infusion and repeated every 4 hours if necessary. The whole blood clotting time should be kept to 20 to 30 minutes prior to each infusion. While heparin may be given, it should be noted that heparin therapy has not been effective in the treatment of disseminated intravascular coagulation.

Prophylaxis

The rate of meningococcal disease among household and day care center contacts is greater than that in the community. For this reason, these contacts should be examined carefully and treated presumptively if early signs of meningococcal disease are present. A blood culture should be obtained prior to initiation of therapy with penicillin (as above) in these individuals. Apparently healthy contacts should be treated with rifampin. For adults, 600 mg twice daily for 2 days is recommended. For children between 1 month and 12 years of age, rifampin should be given in a dosage of 20 mg/kg/24 hr in two divided oral doses for 2 days. In infants less than 1 month of age the daily dose is decreased to 10 mg/kg/24 hr given by the same schedule.

In addition to chemoprophylaxis, consideration may be given to providing day care center and household contacts of patients with meningococcal disease due to serotypes A, C, Y, or W135 with the serotype-appropriate vaccine. Children less than 2 years of age should not be immunized with serogroup C, Y, or W135 vaccines. Children in contact with meningococcal serogroup A disease who are 3 months of age and older are candidates for receipt of monovalent serogroup A vaccine. The vaccine should be given as recommended by the manufacturer.

Close contacts also should be encouraged to seek medical attention if they develop malaise, myalgia, arthralgia, fever, or other signs that suggest the development of meningococcal disease. Prophylaxis is limited to household and day care center contacts of the patient and medical personnel with close personal exposure to the patient.

Infections Due to *Escherichia coli, Proteus, Klebsiella-Enterobacter-Serratia, Pseudomonas,* and Other Gram-Negative Bacilli

HARRIS D. RILEY, Jr., M.D.

Although the management of infections due to these organisms must be individualized, certain generalizations can be made.* Few infections that the physician is called upon to treat pose as difficult a problem as do those due to gram-negative coliform bacilli. Infections with these organisms are increasing in frequency, particularly as a hospital-associated phenomenon. Although new antibiotics have become available to which certain of these organisms are susceptible, the susceptibility of a given strain is unpredictable, and susceptible strains may develop resistance relatively rapidly. Furthermore, most of the antimicrobials that have activity against these organisms are accompanied by a significant risk of toxicity.

The fact that infections due to these organisms are particularly common in postoperative patients and in those debilitated by other disorders or therapies compounds the difficulties by limiting the choice of available therapeutic agents and makes evaluation of antibacterial treatment more perplexing. Because of the variability in response to therapy, careful bacteriologic study and in vitro susceptibility tests should precede initiation of therapy.

In general, comparatively large doses of the selected antimicrobial agent(s) should be utilized and should be continued for relatively long periods. Infection, especially bacteremia, due to these and other gram-negative bacteria, may be accompanied by clinical shock secondary to the elaboration of endotoxins. Appropriate supportive therapy for this complication is an important phase of the total management.

Antimicrobial agents of choice against the relatively common gram-negative bacilli are shown in Table 1. The most reliable guide to the choice of an antimicrobial agent is the results of in vitro antibiotic susceptibility tests. However, in many instances, particularly in infants and children, treatment must be initiated after appropriate cultures are obtained but before the results of these studies are known. Table 1 can be used as a general guide in such situations. The choice of a particular drug depends upon many different circumstances: epidemiologic information, particularly whether the infection is community- or hospital-acquired; the clinical picture, including the site of infection and presence of underlying disease; the frequency of resistance to various antimicrobials among various organisms in the local area; and others.

The dose, route of administration, and other details of therapeutic use of the various antimicrobial agents useful in the treatment of infections due to these organisms are listed in Table 2. Since these infections occur frequently in the neonatal and infancy periods, the difference in the pharmacology and metabolism of drugs in patients in these age groups, as well as in patients with impaired renal function, should be recalled. The dosage schedule for newborn and low birth weight infants is also included.

*The assistance of Chris Harrison, M.D. and Brenda L. Mings in preparation of the manuscript is acknowledged.

Text continued on page 527

Table 1. ANTIMICROBIAL AGENTS FOR INFECTIONS DUE TO GRAM-NEGATIVE
BACILLI OF RELATIVELY COMMON CLINICAL OCCURRENCE*

Organism	Drug	
Escherichia coli†		
Community-acquired	Ampicillin Kanamycin Tobramycin Gentamicin	Cephalosporin[1] Chloramphenicol Tetracycline
Hospital-acquired	Ampicillin Gentamicin Kanamycin Amikacin[3] Tetracycline	Tobramycin[3] Cephalosporin[1] Ticarcillin Chloramphenicol
Enterotoxigenic and enteroinvasive‡	Polymyxin (oral) Neomycin (oral) Kanamycin (oral)	Ampicillin Gentamicin (oral)
Enterobacter species	Gentamicin Tobramycin[3] Cephalosporins Carbenicillin or ticarcillin Nalidixic acid Kanamycin	Polymyxin or colistin Chloramphenicol Ticarcillin Amikacin[3] Tetracycline
Klebsiella pneumoniae	Gentamicin with or without a cephalosporin Tobramycin[3]	Tetracycline Cephalosporin[1] Chloramphenicol Amikacin[3]
Proteus mirabilis	Ampicillin Penicillin G Cephalosporin[1] Gentamicin	Kanamycin Tobramycin[3] Nalidixic acid
Indole-positive *Proteus* (*P. vulgaris, P. morganii,* *P. rettgeri*)	Gentamicin Kanamycin Tobramycin Chloramphenicol Carbenicillin or ticarcillin	Nalidixic acid Tetracycline Amikacin[3] Sisomicin[2, 3] Cephalosporin[4]
Pseudomonas aeruginosa†	Tobramycin[5] Polymyxin or colistin Ticarcillin Gentamicin	Pipercillin Azlocillin[2] Mezlocillin[2] M-formimidoyl Thienamycin[2] Tobramycin[3, 5] Sisomicin[2] Amikacin[3, 5, 6] Carbenicillin
Serratia marcescens	Amikacin[3] Gentamicin Kanamycin Trimethoprim-sulfamethoxazole	Chloramphenicol Nalidixic acid Carbenicillin

*In most instances, drug of first choice is listed first. Susceptibility tests are important in determining therapy for infections due to any of these organisms. However, in many instances, drug of choice depends on susceptibility results.

† For treatment of urinary tract infections, see text.

‡Indications tentative.

[1] Refers to one of the cephalosporins, administered parenterally or orally depending upon drug and nature of infection. See text and Table 2 for further details and information on new cephalosporins.

[2] Investigational drug.

[3] See text for discussion of indications and use.

[4] Cefoxitin appears to be the most effective cephalosporin.

[5] Combination of gentamicin or other aminoglycoside and carbenicillin or ticarcillin is usually synergistic. Both can be used in serious life-threatening infections. Use of carbenicillin or ticarcillin alone is associated with emergence of resistant *Pseudomonas* and super-infection with resistant *Klebsiella*.

[6] Synergistic with carbenicillin and ticarcillin against many strains.

Table 2. DAILY DOSAGE SCHEDULE FOR ANTIMICROBIAL AGENTS*

Drug	Oral	Intramuscular	Intravenous	Intrathecal	Adult or Maximum Dose
Penicillin G[1]	500,000–2,000,000 U in 5 doses ½ hr a.c.	20,000–50,000 U/kg in 4–6 doses	20,000–100,000 U/kg in 4–6 doses		20–100 million U/24 hr
Neonate & Prem.[2]	50,000 U/kg in 4 doses	20,000–50,000 U/kg in 2–4 doses	20,000–50,000 U/kg in 4 doses		
Chloramphenicol[3]	50–100 mg/kg in 4 doses[4]		50–100 mg/kg in 3–4 doses (10% solution)		3–4 gm/24 hr; maximum in child 2.0 gm/24 hr
Neonate & Prem.[2,4]	25[a]–50[b] mg/kg in 4 doses		15[a]–25[b] mg/kg in 2–4 doses (0.5 mg/ml)		
Tetracycline[5,e]	20–40 mg/kg in 4 doses	12 mg/kg in 2 doses	12 mg/kg in 2 doses (1 mg/ml)		2.0 gm/24 hr
Neonate & Prem.[2]	10–20 mg/kg in 4 doses	6 mg/kg in 2 doses	6 mg/kg in 2 doses (1 mg/ml)		
Kanamycin[6]	100 mg/kg in 4 doses	30 mg/kg in 3 doses	30 mg/kg in 3 doses (2.5 mg/ml)		Oral, 3–4 gm/24 hr IM, 1.0–1.5 gm/24 hr
Neonate & Prem.[2]	50 mg/kg in 4 doses	15–20 mg/kg in 2–3 doses (see text)	(see text)		
Neomycin[d]	100–150 mg/kg in 4 doses[f]				Oral, 6.0 gm/24 hr IM, 1.0 gm/24 hr
Neonate & Prem.[2]	50 mg/kg in 4 doses				
Streptomycin sulfate[7,d]		20–40 mg/kg in 2–3 doses		1.0 mg/kg or 20 mg/24 hr (5 mg/ml)	2.0 gm/24 hr
Neonate & Prem.[2]		10–20 mg/kg in 2 doses			
Sulfonamides[8]	120–150 mg/kg in 4 doses		120 mg/kg (24 mg/ml) in 2–4 doses		3–4 gm/24 hr
Neonate & Prem.[2,4]	50 mg/kg/day[e] in 2–3 doses				
Polymyxin B[9]	15–20 mg/kg in 4–6 doses	2.5–5.0 mg/kg in 4–6 doses	2.5–5.0 mg/kg in 3 doses (0.4 mg/ml 5% dextrose in endocarditis)	<2 yrs, 2 mg/24 hr or every other day >2 yrs, 5 mg/24 hr (0.5–1.0 mg/ml)	Oral, 500 mg/24 hr Parenteral, 200 mg/24 hr Intrathecal, 10 mg/24 hr
Neonate & Prem.[2]	10–15 mg/kg in 4 doses	3[a]–4[b] mg/kg in 4 doses			
Colistin[9]	15–30 mg/kg in 4 doses	5.0–8.0 mg/kg in 3 doses	1.5–5.0 mg/kg in 2–4 doses	<1 yr, 2 mg/24 hr[14] >1 yr, 5 mg/24 hr	5.0 mg/kg/24 hr IM
Neonate & Prem.[2]	10–20 mg/kg in 4 doses	1.0–2.0 mg/kg in 2–4 doses			
Novobiocin[10]	20–45 mg/kg in 4 doses				Oral, 2.0 gm/24 hr
Neonate & Prem.[2,4]	10–15 mg/kg in 2–3 doses				
Gentamicin[11]	5–10 mg/kg in 1 dose	3–7.5 mg/kg in 3 doses		1–2 mg/24 hr	IM, 5 mg/kg/24 hr[11]
Neonate & Prem.[2,12]		5 (3–7.5) mg/kg in 2–3 doses[18]			
Cephalothin[13]		80–160 mg/kg in 4–6 doses	80–160 mg/kg in 4–6 doses or in continuous infusion		Parenteral, 2–6 gm/24 hr
Neonate & Prem.[2]		50–100 mg/kg in 2–3 doses	50–100 mg/kg in 4 doses or in continuous infusion		

Table 2. DAILY DOSAGE SCHEDULE FOR ANTIMICROBIAL AGENTS* *(Continued)*

Drug	Oral	Intramuscular	Intravenous	Intrathecal	Adult or Maximum Dose
Ampicillin[15]	100–200 mg/kg in 4 doses	150–400 mg/kg in 4 doses	150–400 mg/kg in 4 doses		Oral, 2–6 gm/24 hr Parenteral, 2–4 gm/24 hr
Neonate & Prem.[2]	25–200 mg/kg in 4 doses	50–200 mg/kg in 2–3 doses[19]			
Paromomycin[9]	50–100 mg/kg in 4 doses[f]				2.0 gm/24 hr
Neonate & Prem.[2]					
Cephaloridine		50–100 mg/kg in 3 doses	30–100 mg/kg in 2–3 doses		4.0 gm/24 hr
Neonate & Prem.[2]					
Nystatin	1,000,000–2,000,000 U in 3–4 doses				
Neonate & Prem.[2]	400,000 U in 4 doses				
Amphotericin B[16]			1 mg/kg given over 6–8 hr period		1 mg/kg
Neonate & Prem.[2]					
Methenamine mandelate	100 mg/kg first dose; then 50 mg/kg/24 hr in 3 doses				4 gm/24 hr
Nitrofurantoin	5–7 mg/kg/24 hr; reduce dosage after 10–14 days to 2.5–5.0 mg/kg/24 hr				400 mg/24 hr
Neonate & Prem.[2]	Contraindicated				
Carbenicillin	100 mg/kg/day in 4 doses		400–600 mg/kg in 4–6 doses		40 gm/24 hr
Neonate & Prem.[2]			300 mg/kg/24 hr		
Carbenicillin indanyl sodium	30–50 mg/kg in 4 doses				2–3 gm (max)
Cephalexin	50–100 mg/kg/24 hr in 4 doses				12 gm/24 hr
Nalidixic acid[g]	12 mg/kg/24 hr				4.0 gm/24 hr
Cefazolin		50–100 mg/kg in 3 doses	50–100 mg/kg in 3 doses		6.0 gm/24 hr
Neonate & Prem.[2]		Not recommended	Not recommended		
Tobramycin		8–10 mg/kg in 3 doses	8–10 mg/kg in 3 doses		5 mg/kg/24 hr
Neonate & Prem.[2]		5 mg/kg in 2–3 doses	5 mg/kg in 2–3 doses		
Clindamycin	10–25 mg/kg in 4 doses	10–40 mg/kg in 4 doses	10–40 mg/kg in 4 doses		4.8 gm/24 hr
Neonate & Prem.[2]	Unknown	Unknown	Unknown		
Cloxacillin	50–100 mg/kg in 4 doses				4.0 gm/24 hr
Neonate & Prem.[2]	Not recommended				
Dicloxacillin	25–100 mg/kg in 4 doses				4.0 gm/24 hr
Neonate & Prem.[2]	Not recommended				
Methicillin		100–300 mg/kg in 4–6 doses	100–300 mg/kg in 4–6 doses		12.0 gm/24 hr
Neonate & Prem.[2]		50–200 mg/kg[20] in 2–3 doses	50–100 mg/kg[20] in 2–3 doses		
Nafcillin	50–100 mg/kg in 4 doses	100–200 mg/kg in 4–6 doses	100–200 mg/kg in 4–6 doses		12.0 gm/24 hr
Neonate & Prem.[2]		75–100 mg/kg in 2–4 doses[20]	75–100 mg/kg in 2–4 doses[20]		

Table 2. DAILY DOSAGE SCHEDULE FOR ANTIMICROBIAL AGENTS* *(Continued)*

Drug	Oral	Intramuscular	Intravenous	Intrathecal	Adult or Maximum Dose
Oxacillin	50–100 mg/kg in 4 doses	100–200 mg/kg in 4–6 doses	100–200 mg/kg in 4–6 doses		12.0 gm/24 hr
Neonate & Prem.[2]		50–200 mg/kg in 2–4 doses[20]	50–200 mg/kg in 2–4 doses[20]		
Penicillin V	25,000–400,000 U/ kg in 4 doses				6.4 million U/24 hr
Neonate & Prem.[2]	25,000–200,000 U/ kg in 3 doses				
Amoxicillin	40–100 mg/kg in 3 doses				3.0 gm/24 hr
Neonate & Prem.[2]	40–100 mg/kg in 3–4 doses				
Amikacin		20 mg/kg in 2–3 doses	20 mg/kg in 2–3 doses		
Neonate & Prem.[2]		Initial dose, 10 mg/kg[21]	Initial dose, 10 mg/kg[21]		
Ticarcillin			300 mg/kg in 4–6 doses		
Neonate & Prem.[2]			Initial dose, 100 mg/ kg[22]		
Lincomycin	30–60 mg/kg in 4 doses	20 mg/kg in 2 doses	20 mg/kg in 2 doses		Oral, 2 gm/24 hr IM, 8.0 gm/24 hr IV, 8.0 gm/24 hr
Cefaclor	40 mg/kg in 3 doses				2–3 gm/24 hr
Cefadroxil[h]	40 mg/kg in 2 doses				2 gm
Neonate & Prem.	Not recommended				
Cephradrine	40–60 mg/kg in 4 doses	50–100 mg/kg in 4 doses	50–100 mg/kg in 4 doses		2–3 gm
Neonate & Prem.	Not recommended	Not recommended			
Cephapirin		40–80 mg/kg in 4 doses	40–80 mg/kg in 4 doses		
Cefamandole		50–150 mg/kg in 4–6 doses	50–150 mg/kg in 4–6 doses		4–6 gm
Cefoxitin		50–150 mg/kg in 3–4 doses	50–150 mg/kg in 3–4 doses		12 gm
Neonate & Prem.		Not recommended	Not recommended		
Hetacillin	50–100 mg/kg in 4 doses				
Cyclacillin	0.5–1.0 gm in 4 doses				2 gm
Neonate & Prem.	Not recommended				
Bacampicillin	25–50 mg/kg in doses				3.2 gm
Cefotaxime		150–200 mg/kg in 4 doses	150–200 mg/kg in 4 doses		
Ceftriaxone		75 mg/kg in 2 doses	75 mg/kg in 2 doses		
Cefuroxime		75 mg/kg in 3 doses	75 mg/kg in 3 doses		
Cinoxacin for UTI only >12 y.o.	1000 mg in 2–4 doses				
Doxycycline	4–5 mg/kg in 2 doses				
Erythromycin	30–50 mg/kg in 4 doses		40–70 mg/kg in 4 doses		
Neonate & Prem.[2] and <4 mos	20–40 mg/kg in 3 doses				

Table 2. DAILY DOSAGE SCHEDULE FOR ANTIMICROBIAL AGENTS* *(Continued)*

Drug	Oral	Intramuscular	Intravenous	Intrathecal	Adult or Maximum Dose
Flucytosine	150 mg/kg in 4 doses				
Ketoconazole	5–15 mg/kg in 1 dose				
Metronidazole	20–30 mg/kg in 3 doses		20–30 mg/kg in 3 doses		
Neonate & Prem.[2]	Not recommended		15 mg/kg loading dose then 15 mg/kg in 2 doses		
Mezlocillin		300 mg/kg in 6 doses	300 mg/kg in 6 doses		24 gm
Neonate & Prem.[2]		≤2000 gm: <1 wk, 150 mg/kg in 2 doses; >1 wk, 225 mg/kg in 3 doses	<2000 gm: <1 wk, 150 mg/kg in 2 doses; >1 wk, 225 mg/kg in 3 doses		
		>2000 gm: <1 wk, 150 mg/kg in 2 doses; >1 wk, 300 mg/kg in 4 doses	>2000 gm: <1 wk, 150 mg/kg in 2 doses; >1 wk, 300 mg/kg in 4 doses		
Miconazole			30 mg/kg in 3 doses		
Minocycline	4–5 mg/kg in 2 doses				
Neonate & Prem.[2]	Not recommended				
Moxalactam		100–200 mg/kg in 4 doses	100–200 mg/kg in 4 doses		
Neonate & Prem.[2]		100 mg/kg in 2 doses, >1 wk, 150 mg/kg in 3 doses	100 mg/kg in 2 doses, >1 wk, 150 mg/kg in 3 doses		
Piperacillin ★Not recommended <12 y.o.		100–300 mg/kg in 4 doses			20 gm
Rifampin	15 mg/kg in 1 dose				
Meningococcal prophylaxis × 2 da	1200 mg in 2 doses; 1–12 y.o., 20 mg/kg in 2 doses; <1 y.o., 10 mg/kg in 2 doses				120 mg/kg
Hemophilus prophylaxis × 4 da	20 mg/kg/da in 1 dose				1200 mg/kg
Trimethoprim ★not <12 y.o.	200 mg/kg in 2 doses				
Trimethoprim (TMP)-sulfamethoxazole (SMX)	5–10 mg/kg TMP 25–50 mg/kg SMX in 2 doses		5–10 mg/kg TMP 25–50 mg/kg SMX in 3 doses		
Neonate & Prem.[2] and <2 mos			2 mg/kg TMP, 10 mg SMX loading dose, then 2 mg/kg TMP, 10 mg/kg SMX in 2 doses		
Pneumocystis prophylaxis	5 mg TMP/25, mg SMX/kg in 1 dose		5 mg TMP/25, mg SMX/kg in 1 dose		

Table 2. DAILY DOSAGE SCHEDULE FOR ANTIMICROBIAL AGENTS* (Continued)

Drug	Oral	Intramuscular	Intravenous	Intrathecal	Adult or Maximum Dose
Pneumocystis treatment	20 mg TMP/100, mg SMX/kg in 3 doses		20 mg TMP/100, mg SMX/kg in 3 doses		
Vancomycin Neonate & Prem.[2]	50 mg/kg in 4 doses		40 mg/kg in 2–3 doses 30 mg/kg in 2 doses		

*Some of these agents may be administered by other routes. For intrapleural, intra-articular, intraperitoneal, ocular, aerosol, and topical use, see Report of the Committee on the Control of Infectious Diseases, American Academy of Pediatrics, Evanston, Ill., 1964. Some, such as neomycin, are specifically contraindicated by the intrapleural and intraperitoneal routes.

[1] Phenoxymethyl penicillin or phenethicillin is preferred for oral therapy. Procaine penicillin should not be used in neonates. Sodium penicillin contains 1.5 meq. of sodium, and potassium penicillin G, 1.69 meq. of potassium per 1.0 million units. The latter should be avoided intravenously in neonates and in patients with impaired renal function.

[2] If renal output is reduced, decrease the dose still further.

[3] Should not be used for minor infections or when less hazardous agents are effective. Observe for bone marrow depression.

[4] Avoid during first week of life unless essential. Desirable to follow treatment with serial blood levels to avoid "gray" syndrome.

[5] Any of the tetracycline group of antibodies may be used.

[6] With parenteral administration, auditory nerve and renal injury may occur; frequent audiometric and renal tests are essential. Manufacturer's note: The intravenous dose of kanamycin should not exceed 15 mg/kg/24 hr.

[7] Auditory nerve damage can occur.

[8] A soluble sulfonamide should be used. Manufacturer's precaution: Systemic sulfonamides are contraindicated in infants under 2 months of age.

[9] Observe for renal and neural toxic effects.

[10] Severe skin and liver toxicity occasionally occurs. Manufacturer's warning: Use should be avoided in premature and newborn infants because it affects bilirubin adversely.

[11] In general, dose by the intramuscular route should not exceed 5 mg/kg/24 hr for no longer than 7 to 10 days except in serious or life-threatening situations. Observation for vestibular and renal toxicity should be carried out. Desirable to follow therapy with serial blood levels if renal function impaired. The intrathecal use of gentamicin is not mentioned in the manufacturer's instructions.

[12] For neonates, see No. 18.

[13] Doses up to 200 mg/kg/24 hr in infants and children have been utilized without untoward effect.

[14] For intrathecal use, colistin without dibucaine should be used.

[15] In severe infections, may be necessary to increase oral and intramuscular dose as much as 3 times that listed.

[16] Fever, thrombophlebitis and renal, hepatic, and bone marrow damage may occur.

[17] Infants <7 days, <2000 gm, 15 mg/kg in 2 doses; >2000 gm, 20 mg/kg in 2 doses. Infants >7 days, <2000 gm, 20 mg/kg in 2 doses; >2000 gm, 20 mg/kg in 3 doses.

[18] Dose should be given in 2 divided doses in infants <7 days and in 3 divided doses in infants >7 days.

[19] In infants <7 days, 50–100 mg/kg in 2 doses; >7 days, 100–200 mg/kg in 3 doses.

[20] In infants <7 days, 50–100 mg/kg in 2 doses; >7 days, 100–200 mg/kg in 3–4 doses. Pediatric IV doses not known due to rarity.

[21] After initial loading dose of 10 mg/kg, follow with 7.5 mg/kg dose every 12 hr. (Can be given IM or IV.)

[22] After initial loading dose of 100 mg/kg, dose is as follows: <2000 gm = 225 mg/kg in 3 doses during first week of life; 600 mg/kg in 6 doses after 7 days of age; >2000 gm, 300–400 mg/kg in 4–6 doses; 600 mg/kg in 6 doses after 2 weeks of age. Can be given IM or 15–20 minute IV infusion.

[a] Premature.

[b] Full-term.

[c] First dose should be doubled. Do not use sulfonamides in premature infants or infants under 2 months of age.

[d] In general, limit parenteral therapy to 10 days.

[e] Manufacturer's warning: The use of drugs of the tetracycline class during tooth development (last half of pregnancy, infancy, and childhood to the age of 8 years) may cause permanent discoloration of the teeth. This adverse reaction is more common during long-term usage of the drugs but has been observed following repeated short-term courses.

[f] May exceed manufacturer's recommended dose.

[g] Manufacturer's warning: Do not administer to children less than 3 months of age.

[h] Safety and dosage in children have not been established.

INFECTIONS

Escherichia coli Infections

Escherichia coli are gram-negative motile rods normally found as part of the bacterial flora of the gastrointestinal tract. They have the capacity to produce a powerful endotoxin, which enters the circulation and induces shock and the clinical pathologic picture of the Shwartzman phenomenon.

Infection in the Neonate. Gram-negative bacilli, particularly E. coli, are among the most common causes of septicemia and meningitis of the neonate. In most areas of the United States, E. coli and Klebsiella-Enterobacter-Serratia account for a large segment of the cases. E. coli bacilli also are a significant cause of pneumonia in this age group and have been shown along with other gram-negative enteric organisms to be a cause of otitis media in infants less than 6 weeks of age. E. coli also produces urinary infection often associated with jaundice in infants less than 2 months of age.

Supportive measures are critically important in the neonate with a systemic infection, irrespective of type or cause. In general, antimicrobials should be administered by the intravenous route because the depressed infant has decreased gastrointestinal absorption and microcirculatory changes in sepsis can lead to poor absorption of intramuscular drugs. Re-establishment and maintenance of body temperature in a heated environment are important, and urinary output should be monitored. Intravenous fluid and electrolyte therapy should be meticulously provided by standard methods. The complications of hyponatremia, hypoglycemia, or hypocalcemia may mimic or complicate septicemia. Thus, appropriate diagnostic biochemical determinations must be repetitively carried out and appropriate replacement therapy instituted. Lumbar punctures should be performed at frequent intervals in meningitis due to E. coli or other gram-negative enteric bacilli until sterilization of the cerebrospinal fluid has occurred, which is usually by the fourth or fifth day of therapy. Treatment should be continued for 3 total weeks or 2 weeks post-cerebrospinal fluid sterilization.

Antibiotic therapy is of cardinal importance in the management of infections due to E. coli. Because of changing patterns of resistance, in vitro susceptibility studies are essential. Kanamycin had been the drug of choice for E. coli infections in the neonate; however, in recent years kanamycin-resistant strains of E. coli have become more widespread. In many geographic areas, more than 40% of strains are resistant. In hospitals where the majority of E. coli strains remain susceptible to kanamycin, this drug may be used. The intramuscular or intravenous dosage is as follows: infants 1 to 7 days of age weighing less than 2000 gm, 7.5 mg/kg every 12 hours; infants 1 to 7 days of age weighing more than 2000 gm, 10.0 mg/kg every 12 hours; infants 8 to 30 days of age weighing less than 2000 gm, 10 mg/kg every 12 hours; infants 8 to 30 days of age weighing more than 2000 gm, 10 mg/kg every 8 hours.

In most areas, gentamicin plus ampicillin is currently the preferred combination of drugs for E. coli septicemia or meningitis of the neonate. For infants under 1 week of age, the dosage is 5 mg/kg/24 hr in equally divided doses every 12 hours. Beyond 1 week of age, the dosage is 5 to 7.5 mg/kg/24 hr in divided doses every 8 hours for both full-term and low birth weight infants. For intravenous administration, the dose is diluted in sterile normal saline and infused over a 1- to 2-hour period. If necessary, the drugs can be given intramuscularly except to infants with poor circulation. If renal function is impaired, the dosage of kanamycin or gentamicin must be reduced and serum levels monitored to avoid potential toxicity.

Ampicillin administered parenterally may be effective in infections caused by susceptible strains, especially those that are community-acquired. The daily dose administered intravenously for infants 1 to 7 days of age is 50 to 200 mg/kg in two doses, and for infants 8 to 30 days of age, 75 to 250 mg/kg divided into three doses. A combination of ampicillin and kanamycin or gentamicin is preferred initially because of possible synergism in action. Other drugs listed in Table 1 may be used if susceptibility studies show the organism to be sensitive. Amikacin and tobramycin are effective, but their use should be reserved for infection strains resistant to other antibiotics. Two of the newer cephalosporins, cefuroxine and cefamandole, show increased activity against E. coli, but CSF penetration is poor. Third generation cephalosporins such as moxalactam, cefotaxime, and ceftriaxone may be useful. General supportive care depends on the underlying problem. Serious E. coli infections in older infants and children should be treated with parenteral gentamicin. Ampicillin given intravenously in a dose of 200 mg/kg/24 hr at 4- to 6-hour intervals plus gentamicin, 3 to 7.5 mg/kg/24 hr in three divided doses is the initial treatment of choice. Other drugs may be used depending upon the results of susceptibility tests.

Urinary Tract Infection. E. coli remains the most common cause of primary uncomplicated urinary tract infection. The strains are usually quite susceptible to the sulfonamides or to ampicillin. Sulfisoxazole* 150 mg/kg/24 hr in four divided doses for a period of 2 weeks, affords effective therapy in most patients. Ampicillin, 50 to 100 mg/kg/24 hr orally in four divided doses, is equally effective but not superior. The sulfonamides are still preferred for urinary tract infection of this nature since they are usually effective, and the cost and incidence of associated untoward reactions are low.

Because these drugs are effectively concentrated in the renal parenchyma and urine, favorable treatment response may be observed even when in vitro susceptibility testing shows the organism to be resistant. For this reason, if a favorable clinical response has been achieved after 48 to 72 hours and pyuria has been diminished and the urine sterilized, treatment may be continued with the drug initiated. If this has not been accomplished by this time, it is likely that the organism is resistant.

In recurrent disease the infecting E. coli is likely to be sulfanamide-resistant, and antibiotic susceptibility data must be used as guidelines for selecting alternative drugs. However, the trimethoprim-sulfamethoxasole combination or cephalosporins administered orally are often useful in such situations.

---

*Manufacturer's Precaution: Sulfisoxazole is contraindicated in infants under 2 months of age.

It is most important to ensure that the patient demonstrates both a clinical and bacteriologic cure and that an asymptomatic bacteriologic relapse does not occur. If the repeat urine cultures at 48 to 72 hours are sterile, treatment should be presumed effective. After the 2-week course of therapy, repeat urinalysis and quantitative urine cultures should be performed within several days and repeated at monthly intervals thereafter for 3 months and again at 6 months and a year. Shorter courses of antimicrobial administration may be effective in uncomplicated lower urinary tract infections. Drugs for oral therapy of UTI in children over 12 years old include trimethoprim alone or cinoxacin,* a nalidixic acid derivative. If urinary tract infections recur, especially if polymicrobial in type, the presence of abnormalities of the urinary tract, especially those producing obstruction, should be suspected.

Diarrheal Disease. The association of E. coli with diarrheal disease has been known for years. Numerous outbreaks of diarrhea occurring in nurseries have been investigated, and certain antigenetically distinct strains of E. coli have been connected to these epidemics.

In recent years, the possible pathogenetic mechanisms for the diarrhea associated with E. coli have been elucidated by the demonstration of the toxigenic and invasive properties of some of the strains. Stool isolates of E. coli can be characterized as being 1) enteropathogenic; 2) enterotoxigenic (ETEC), by their ability to produce toxins; or 3) enteroinvasive (EIEC), by their capacity to penetrate mucosal cells. It is now known that strains may have none, one, two, or all three of these characteristics. Recent evidence also suggests that the intestinal mucosal adherence of some E. coli strains may be related to their pathogenicity.

E. coli has been shown to cause diarrhea by two separate mechanisms: enterotoxin production and mucosal invasion. Strains with invasive capacity produce the characteristic findings of bacterial dysentery, namely local inflammation with hyperemia, ulceration, and intraluminal exudate composed of polymorphonuclear leukocytes. Enterotoxigenic E. coli causes diarrhea by two means: (1) production of an antigenic heat-labile toxin that resembles cholera toxin, in that it activates cellular adenyl cyclase, thereby increasing intracellular cyclic adenosine monophosphate and promoting secretion of sodium and water; (2) production of a nonantigenic heat-stable toxin, the exact action of which is undefined. Heat-labile enterotoxin has been shown to cause diarrhea in humans; heat-stable enterotoxin, although known to be a major cause of diarrhea in animals, has also recently been shown to be associated with diarrheal disease in humans.

Supportive therapy for E. coli-mediated diarrhea, irrespective of pathogenesis, consists mainly of maintaining adequate fluid and electrolyte intake. Patients with evidence of dehydration should be hospitalized and managed with intravenous fluids and electrolyte therapy, details of which are described elsewhere. In these patients, it is important to determine serum electrolyte concentrations since hypo- and hypernatremia occur fairly commonly.

Infants who are not dehydrated can be managed as outpatients. The details of management are described in other sections but two points must be mentioned. Homemade salt solutions should *not* be prescribed because of the risk of inducing hypertonic dehydration. Evidence is accumulating that certain commercially available oral rehydration fluids can be used successfully in the outpatient treatment of mildly dehydrated children. Adsorptive agents that firm the stool or narcotic-containing agents that decrease bowel motility have *no* place for treatment of diarrheal disease in infants and young children. None of these agents is specifically directed toward the primary cause of the diarrhea. None has been shown to decrease the fluid and electrolyte loss across the bowel mucosa in E. coli diarrhea, but by decreasing bowel motility they may mask the amount of fluid accumulated in the bowel lumen. They may also allow heavier colonization of the offending organism with greater enterotoxin production in the jejunum. Deaths or severe central nervous system depression have occurred when atropine- or diphenyoxylate-containing antidiarrheals have been used in infants and children.

The effectiveness of antimicrobial therapy in E. coli diarrhea is open to some question. Specific antimicrobial therapy appears to shorten the severity and duration of diarrhea. Neomycin sulfate oral solution is the drug of choice in areas where neomycin resistance is not encountered frequently. It is administered in a dose of 100 mg/kg/24 hr divided into doses every 6 to 8 hours for 5 days. This dose is higher than that recommended by the manufacturer but has been found safe and effective. Continuation of therapy for more than 5 days is not advised because the bacteriologic cure rate is not improved and because neomycin may cause a malabsorptive state. Colistin sulfate oral suspension is the alternative drug of choice and is given in doses of 10 to 15 mg/kg/24 hr every 6 to 8 hours for 5 days. Antibiotic susceptibility testing should be performed because when resistant organisms are involved, treatment has resulted not only in failure but also spread of the infection, presumably by suppression of competing normal bacterial intestinal flora.

Controlled studies have not been performed to date evaluating the effectiveness of antibiotic therapy in the treatment of diarrhea due to en-

*Contraindicated in infants younger than 3 months of age.

terotoxigenic and enteroinvasive strains. Because the bacteria remain within the intestinal lumen in enterotoxigenic *E. coli* disease, it seems logical to speculate that nonabsorbable antibiotics might be useful in treatment. However, in an outbreak of diarrheal disease due to a strain of *E. coli* elaborating a heat-stable enterotoxin but which did not belong to an enteropathogenic serotype, oral colistin therapy was ineffective in eradicating the organisms from the stools of culture-positive infants and in preventing illness or shortening the carrier state. It is reasonable to presume that drugs effective against these strains in vitro might be beneficial in decreasing the severity and duration of diarrhea in those patients, as it has been shown to be with *Shigella* dysentery. If strains susceptible to ampicillin are involved, this drug should be administered at a dose of 100 mg/kg/24 hr in 4 to 8 divided doses, preferably intravenously.

It is not clear at this time whether older children with *E. coli* diarrhea should receive antimicrobial therapy.

Outbreaks of *E. coli* diarrhea in newborn nurseries can be catastrophic. Such outbreaks can be controlled by use of rapid fluorescent antibody techniques to detect the presence of organisms in the stool, and to follow such infants by segregation of colonized infants and treatment with oral neomycin or colistin in the dosages mentioned.

Other Infections. A variety of other infections, including pneumonia, peritonitis, and abscesses, may be caused by *E. coli.* The information in Tables 1 and 2 can be used for selection of antimicrobial therapy pending susceptibility test results. Surgical intervention and supportive measures depend upon the disease. *E. coli,* including nonenteropathogenic strains, has been causally linked to necrotizing enterocolitis in neonates. Therapy for *E. coli* infections, other than uncomplicated urinary tract infections, should be provided by the parenteral route.

Proteus-Providencia Infections

The variable, unpredictable response to antibacterial therapy of *Proteus* infections is striking, and prolonged therapy is often necessary. In addition to in vitro susceptibility studies, *Proteus* isolates should also be classified as to species because of the variability in the susceptibility of various species and strains to different antibacterial agents. For example, *P. mirabilis* is usually susceptible to ampicillin (or occasionally to large doses of penicillin G), and it is the drug of choice in most infections due to this species. Many strains of *P. mirabilis* are also susceptible to gentamicin, cephalosporins, ticarcillin, and kanamycin. Indole-positive species such as *P. vulgaris, P. rettgeri,* and *P. morganii,* for practical purposes, are always resistant to ampicillin and penicillin G. The drug of choice must be governed

by the results of in vitro susceptibility tests as well as the clinical condition of the patient. Many strains are susceptible to gentamicin, kanamycin, tobramycin, and nearly all to amikacin; these are usually the drugs of choice in infections due to these species. Some strains are susceptible to carbenicillin and ticarcillin and others to one of the cephalosporins, particularly the second and third generation agents.

Most strains of *P. vulgaris* are two- to four-fold more sensitive in vitro to tobramycin than to gentamicin. In vivo, however, strains resistant to gentamicin are likely to be resistant to tobramycin. Amikacin and sisomicin show increased activity against most strains of indole-positive *Proteus.* The use of these two agents should be reserved for infections due to organisms resistant to other available agents. Cefoxitin also shows activity against certain strains of indole-positive *Proteus.* Alternate drugs for infections due to susceptible strains are listed in Table 1. Some strains of *Proteus* are moderately susceptible to novobiocin, but this drug has a significant toxicity risk, and the response to therapy is often variable. Although in vitro the infecting organism is rarely susceptible, clinical results in certain refractory infections, especially of the urinary tract, with cycloserine* have been encouraging. This drug is potentially toxic and should be used with caution. The usual dose is 10 mg/kg/24 hr.

Organisms of the genus *Providencia* are closely related to *P. morganii* and *P. rettgeri,* and were formerly known as *P. inconstans* and included with "paracolon bacilli." They are easily differentiated from *Proteus* by their lack of urease. Members of the group have been isolated from human feces during outbreaks of diarrhea but also in normal individuals. They are primarily associated with urinary tract infections but may also cause sepsis and localized infections. *Providencia* organisms are highly resistant to antibiotics except for carbenicillin and the aminoglycosides; some strains are inhibited by cefamandole or cefoxitin and some by trimethoprim-sulfamethoxazole.

Providencia stuartii has recently emerged as a hospital pathogen in burned patients, appearing first in burn wounds but subsequently as a cause of pulmonary and urinary infection.

Klebsiella-Enterobacter-Serratia Infections

Klebsiella-Enterobacter-Serratia organisms have variable susceptibility to antimicrobial agents and must be tested in vitro. Frequently, however, antimicrobial therapy must be instituted before results of antibiotic susceptibility tests are available.

---

*Manufacturer's Precaution: Safety and dosage of cycloserine have not been established for pediatric use.

An aminoglycoside antibiotic, such as gentamicin, amikacin, or tobramycin (the choice depending upon the susceptibility patterns of organisms in the local area), is usually the drug of choice with certain exceptions. For example, many strains of *K. pneumoniae* are susceptible to cephalothin and some strains of *Enterobacter* are inhibited by carbenicillin and ticarcillin and by cefamandole, moxalactam and cefotaxime. Trimethoprim-sulfamethoxazole and second and third generation cephalosporins inhibit some strains of *Serratia.* In contrast to *Klebsiella* and *Enterobacter,* almost all strains of *Serratia* are resistant to the polymyxins. For serious *Klebsiella* infections, it is usually desirable to add a cephalosporin. Other drugs for treatment of infections due to members of the *Klebsiella-Enterobacter-Serratia* group, depending upon susceptibility results, are shown in Table 1.

Pseudomonas Infections

The *Pseudomonas* group is composed of gram-negative, motile rods, which are nonfermenters and occur widely in soil, water, sewage, and air. *P. aeruginosa* is the member of the genus most commonly pathogenic for human beings. *Pseudomonas* occurs in several antigenic types and several phage types that are equally pathogenic. Because of its ability to form a pigment that colors inflammatory exudate blue or green, the epidemic spread of *P. aeruginosa* in hospital wards has long been recognized. It is found in small numbers in the intestinal tract and on normal skin, particularly when other coliforms are suppressed.

P. aeruginosa is resistant to the more commonly used antimicrobial agents and therefore assumes prevalence and importance when more susceptible bacteria of the normal flora are suppressed. Although most strains of *P. aeruginosa* are susceptible to the polymyxins, these agents have been relatively ineffective in eradicating bacteremia and deep-seated tissue infections. Gentamicin and other aminoglycosides and carbenicillin or ticarcillin are usually more effective but the polymyxins still have a place in selected infections, particularly in urinary tract infections or in bacteremias arising from the urinary tract. In other instances, the organism may be eradicated but the ultimate results are often unsatisfactory because of the poor host defenses in debilitated patients.

Carbenicillin is effective against susceptible strains but some 30% of strains are resistant to it. It must be given in relatively large doses intravenously. During prolonged therapy with carbenicillin alone, organisms initially susceptible may become resistant. Most strains of *Pseudomonas* are inhibited by gentamicin but recently an increasing number of strains have been found to be resistant. Presumptive therapy for systemic *Pseudomonas* infection is a combination of tobramycin and ticarcil-

lin. The two drugs appear to act synergistically in vitro, and coadministration may delay emergence of *P. aeruginosa* resistant to ticarcillin.

Tobramycin has been found to be two to four times more active against *Pseudomonas* than is gentamicin. It is particularly valuable in treatment of infections due to gentamicin-resistant strains. When tobramycin is used in combination with ticarcillin, higher antibacterial serum titers are achieved than with either agent alone. See Table 2 for dosage. Pipercillin is now available but offers little advantage over ticarcillin except for its lower sodium content.

Ticarcillin, a new semisynthetic penicillin similar to carbenicillin, has activity against *Pseudomonas* organisms and, as further experience is gained, may prove to be a useful agent in treatment of such infections.

Amikacin inhibits many strains of *P. aeruginosa.* It may be used alone or in combination with carbenicillin. At the moment, its most valuable use is in the treatment of *Pseudomonas* infections due to strains resistant to gentamicin or to other agents.

Some of the newer, experimental agents (azlocillin, mezlocillin, and N-formimidoyl thienamycin) show activity against *Pseudomonas. Pseudomonas* is a preeminent opportunist, and the vast majority of infections caused by it occur in hospitals, particularly those housing patients with serious diseases. Since 1961 the incidence of *P. aeruginosa* bacteremia has increased and the respiratory tract has become an increasingly important source of infection. The use of gentamicin, carbenicillin, and colistin has not changed the outlook of *Pseudomonas* bacteremia. A polyvalent vaccine has proved useful in burned patients and further attention needs to be given to immunoprophylaxis. At the present time, control of the underlying disease condition contributes most toward survival of patients with bacteremia and other serious *Pseudomonas* infections.

The pseudomallei group of the genus *Pseudomonas* consists of *P. mallei* and *P. pseudomallei.* The former is the cause of glanders, a severe infectious disease of horses that can be transmitted to man. Human infections can usually be treated with sulfonamides.

Melioidosis due to *P. pseudomallei* is a disease resembling glanders in man and occurs chiefly in Southeast Asia but perhaps also in the Western hemisphere. *P. pseudomallei* is susceptible to many antibiotics in vitro. Tetracycline, chloramphenicol, or gentamicin, alone or in combination, may be the treatment of choice. Trimethoprim-sulfamethoxazole may be effective.

Outbreaks of nosocomial bacteremia due to *P. cepacia* secondary to contaminated antiseptics and disinfectants used in cleaning equipment or in skin asepsis for intravenous infusions have been described. Certain other pseudomonads may cause infections in humans. These include *P. fluorescens, P. maltophilia,* and *P. putida.* Less frequent are *P. acidovorans, P. alcaligenes, P. putrefaciens, P. pseudoalcaligenes, P. testosteroni, P. dimunita,* and *P. mendocina.* These organisms vary widely in their antimicrobial susceptibility, and treatment should be guided by in vitro susceptibility tests.

Aeromonas Infections

Organisms of the *Aeromonas* group are found in natural water sources and soil and are frequent pathogens for cold-blooded marine and fresh water animals. The most important members are *A. hydrophilia* and *A. shigelloides.* They may easily be mistaken in the laboratory for *E. coli.*

Aeromonads are resistant to penicillin and ampicillin. Most strains are susceptible to gentamicin, the tetracyclines, and colistin.

Noncholera Vibrio Infections

Noncholera vibrios are inhibited by a variety of antibiotics. Gentamicin is the drug of choice against infections due to *V. parahaemolyticus,* but ampicillin, tetracycline, chloramphenicol, cephalothin, and kanamycin are frequently effective. Most strains of *V. fetus* are inhibited by tetracycline, chloramphenicol, ampicillin, streptomycin, and kanamycin.

Infections Due to Other Gram-Negative Bacilli

Other Enterobacteriaceae. Certain other members of the Enterobacteriaceae sometimes cause infection in humans. *Arizona* organisms are coliform organisms which also belong to the Enterobacteriaceae family. As noted, these organisms more closely resemble *Salmonella.* However, nosocomial infections caused by members of this group, notably *Arizona hinshawii,* have been described.

Edwardsiella. *Edwardsiella* includes a group of motile, lactose-negative organisms that resemble salmonellae in some biochemical features and sometimes in pathogenicity for humans. They ferment only glucose and maltose. *E. tarda* has been isolated from a variety of mammals and reptiles. It is occasionally found in the human intestinal tract, especially in acute gastroenteritis, and it can produce serious septic infections. However, people are likely only accidental hosts. Tetracyclines, chloramphenicol, kanamycin,* and ampicillin are drugs of choice.

Citrobacter. The *Citrobacter* group is composed of Enterobacteriaceae previously designated as *Escherichia freundii* and the Bethesda-Ballerup of "paracolon" organisms. *Citrobacter* strains occur infrequently in normal feces. They have been recovered from urinary tract infections in various septic processes. Drugs of choice are aminoglycosides or third generation cephalosporins. Some strains are susceptible to chloramphenicol and tetracycline.

Other Gram-Negative Bacilli. *Acinetobacter.* *Acinetobacter lwoffi* (previously *Mimi polymorpha* and *Achromobacter lwoffi*) neither ferments nor oxidizes carbohydrates, whereas *Acinetobacter anitratus* (previously *Herellea vaginicola* and *Achromobacter anitratus*) utilizes glucose oxidatively and produces acid from 10% (but not from 1%) lactose-containing medium. These organisms are frequently antibiotic-resistant, and antibiotic susceptibility tests are required as a guide to therapy. Drugs likely to be effective are gentamicin, tobramycin, polymyxins, and new experimental agents azthreonam and N-formimidoyl thienamycin.

Moraxella. Moraxella[†] are similar to *Acinetobacter* but are oxidase-positive and highly susceptible to penicillin. They are primary animal parasites, most commonly present on the mucous membranes. Most of these organisms do not utilize carbohydrates.

Alcaligenes.[†] *A. faecalis* fails to ferment or oxidize any of the usual carbohydrates; it is usually motile. It may occasionally be confused on initial isolation with other nonlactose fermenters, chiefly *Salmonella* or *Shigella.* These organisms are not uniformly sensitive to any antibiotic; tetracycline and chloramphenicol are usually the most effective.

Flavobacterium. Flavobacteria[†] are widely distributed in soil and water and are encountered as opportunistic pathogens in humans. *F. meningosepticum,* which has high virulence for the neonate, has an unusual antibiotic susceptibility pattern for a gram-negative bacillus. It is usually susceptible in vitro to erythromycin, novobiocin, and rifampin, and to a lesser degree to chloramphenicol and streptomycin, but is resistant to gentamicin and polymyxins.

Streptobacillus moniliformis. *Streptobacillus moniliformis,* the cause of one type of rat-bite fever, is carried by many rats presumably as a saprophyte. Penicillin G is the treatment of choice, but streptomycin and tetracycline are also therapeutically effective. The wound should be immediately cleansed with soap and water. Tetanus prophylaxis should be carried out by standard methods.

Calymmatobacterium (Donovania) Granulomatis. Granuloma inguinale is an indolent, ulcerative disease, caused by a gram-negative bacillus that is antigenically similar to, but not identical with, *Klebsiella pneumoniae* and *K. rhinoscleromatis.* It can be

---

*Other aminoglycoside antibiotics may also be effective but clinical experience to date is limited.

†Also "nonfermenter."

treated successfully with tetracyclines, chloramphenicol, or streptomycin. Penicillin G is not effective.

Bartonella Bacilliformis. *Bartonella bacilliformis* is a gram-negative, very pleomorphic, motile organism which causes in humans two different clinical manifestations of the same geographically restricted bacterial disease.* The collective designation of the two syndromes is Carrión disease.

Penicillin, streptomycin, and chloramphenicol are dramatically effective in Oroya fever and greatly reduce the fatality rate, particularly if blood transfusions are also given. Control of the disease depends upon the elimination of the sand fly vectors. Insecticides, DDT, insect repellents, and elimination of breeding areas are of value. Prevention with antibiotics may be useful. Chloramphenicol should be used when the patient is also suffering from secondary *Salmonella* infection.

Others. There are a few other gram-negative bacilli which very rarely cause human infection but have been reported to do so. The type of infection they cause is variable but may be bacteremic or localized in various organ systems. Selection of antimicrobial therapy is based on in vitro susceptibility test results. The agents that are usually effective are listed here, but some of the newer agents mentioned, especially the newer aminoglycosides and cephalosporins, may prove useful with further experience.

Actinobacillus actinomycetemcomitans (HB group)	Tetracycline Streptomycin Chloramphenicol
Actinobacillus lignieresii	Kanamycin
Bordetella bronchiseptica	Tetracycline Polymyxins Chloramphenicol
Chromobacterium	Kanamycin or gentamicin Tetracycline Chloramphenicol
Comamonas terrigenia	Chloramphenicol Tetracycline
Erwinia (now classified as *Enterobacter agglomerans*)	Gentamicin Chloramphenicol Colistin Kanamycin
Hemophilus aphrodilus (HB group)	Penicillin G Gentamicin Cephalothin Chloramphenicol Tetracycline

---

*Recently cases of anemia with *Bartonella*-like bodies have been reported from Southeast Asia.

Infections Due to Anaerobic Cocci and Gram-Negative Bacilli

JOHN G. BARTLETT, M.D.

During the past decade there has been increasing interest in the role of anaerobic bacteria in a variety of infectious processes. This work has been accompanied by extensive progress in anaerobic bacteriologic techniques to recover, identify, and test antimicrobial susceptibility. Nevertheless, antimicrobial selection is often based on empiric decisions. This reflects difficulties encountered in recovering fastidious bacteria, problems with interpreting cultures yielding a polymicrobial flora, time delays in reporting, and the fact that most laboratories do not perform in vitro sensitivity testing. In many instances, surgery represents the most important therapeutic modality.

A commonly quoted adage is that anaerobic infections above the diaphragm generally involve penicillin-sensitive anaerobic bacteria, and this drug would be the agent of choice in the majority of cases (Table 1). Alternatives, depending to some extent on bacteriology results and the severity of the infection, include clindamycin, chloramphenicol, metronidazole, tetracyclines, and erythromycin. Anaerobic infections below the diaphragm often involve *Bacteroides fragilis,* requiring the use of an agent active against this specific microbe, such as clindamycin, chloramphenicol, metronidazole, carbenicillin, or cefoxitin.

Most authorities endorse these recommendations with certain noteworthy precautions. For example, *B. melaninogenicus* is a common anaerobic pathogen in orodental or pulmonary infections, and recent work shows that approximately 20 to 30% of strains are relatively resistant to penicillin. *B. fragilis,* while not a common isolate in these infections, has been found in up to 20% of anaerobic pulmonary infections. The clinical relevance of these observations is not readily apparent since clinical failures with penicillin therapy appear to be relatively infrequent. Patients who do fail to respond to penicillin generally require either surgical drainage or a change in antimicrobials to an alternative agent such as clindamycin.

With regard to subdiaphragmatic infections, attention is focused on *B. fragilis,* for which there are the several agents just noted. In vitro sensitivity tests show that the drugs most predictably active are metronidazole, chloramphenicol, clindamycin, and cefoxitin. Carbenicillin, ticarcillin, meslocillin, azlocillin, and piperacillin are somewhat less effective even at levels achieved with massive doses (Table 2). Clinical trials have shown no significant differences in response rates for the five agents listed in Table 2 when combined with an aminoglycoside for therapy of intra-abdominal sepsis. Moxalactam is more active than cefoperazone and cefotaxime versus *B. fragilis.* Nevertheless, the major advantage of these third generation cephalosporins is enhanced activity against *Enterobacteraceal* rather than anaerobes.

SPECIFIC AGENTS

Penicillins. Penicillin G is generally regarded as the drug of choice for anaerobic infections above the diaphragm, including orodental and pulmonary infections. Ampicillin, amoxicillin, carbenicillin, ticarcillin, and penicillin V show in vitro activity against anaerobes that is generally comparable to that noted with penicillin G. Semisynthetic penicillins that are resistant to penicillinase (oxacillin, nafcillin, methicillin, dicloxacillin, and cloxacillin) are inferior and should not be used for serious anaerobic infections. Carbenicillin and ticarcillin are often advocated for infections involving *B. fragilis,* based on the very high serum levels that are achieved with the usual doses, but these drugs are no more active in vitro against *B. fragilis* than is penicillin G, and 10 to 30% of strains are resistant at levels as high as 100 to 128 μg/ml.

Clindamycin. This drug is active against the vast majority of clinically significant anaerobes, including 95% of *B. fragilis,* and multiple clinical trials have documented efficacy in both patients and experimental animals. There are reports of high level resistance in up to 20% of strains in occasional locations, which appears to be chromosomal or plasmid conferred. Clindamycin is active against most anaerobic bacteria other than *B. fragilis,* with the exception of certain clostridia such as *C. ramosum, C. difficile,* and *C. tertium.* The most dreaded complication of clindamycin is pseudomembranous colitis, but the etiology of this disease is known and effective treatment is readily available.

Table 2. RELATIVE ACTIVITY OF ANTIMICROBIAL AGENTS AGAINST *BACTEROIDES FRAGILIS*

Agent	Median MIC (μg/ml)	Level (μg/ml)	Per Cent Strains Sensitive
Carbenicillin*	25	50	60–80
		100	70–96
Cefoxitin	8	16	70–90
		32	85–97
Chloramphenicol	4	8	98–99
		16	99–100
Clindamycin	0.5	4	96–98
		8	98–99
Metronidazole	1	8	99–100
		16	99–100

*Results apply to ticarcillin as well.

Chloramphenicol. Chloramphenicol is active against nearly all anaerobic bacteria, and there does not appear to be a problem with the emerging resistance. Many authorities regard this to be the agent of choice for anaerobic infections of the central nervous system, due to excellent in vitro activity as well as pharmacokinetic data indicating good penetration across the blood-brain barrier. Experimental animal studies indicate relatively poor activity in vivo against *B. fragilis,* and several clinical failures have been reported.

Cephalosporins. Most of these agents have a spectrum of activity quite comparable to that noted for penicillin G, although these drugs are somewhat less active on a weight basis. They are less active against clostridia and there are several case reports of patients who developed gas gangrene while receiving cephalosporins. In general, there is little difference between the first and second generation cephalosporins in terms of their activity in vitro,

Table 1. ACTIVITY OF ANTIMICROBIAL AGENTS AGAINST MAJOR ANAEROBIC BACTERIA

	Major Isolates: Intra-abdominal Sepsis		Major Isolates: Oral and Pulmonary Infections		
	B. fragilis	*Clostridia*	Anaerobic GPC	*Bacteroides melaninogenicus*	Fusobacteria
Penicillin G (8)*	5–15†	100	98–100	85–95	100
Cephalothin (8)	0–5	100	95–100	70–80	90–95
Clindamycin (4)	95–100	90–100	95–98	100	100
Chloramphenicol (8)	90–98	95–100	98–100	100	100
Tetracycline (2)	20–50	50–75	50–70	65–75	85–90
Erythromycin (2)	30–60	100	80–95	95–100	50–90
Metronidazole (8)	99–100	100	90–95	100	100

*Number in parentheses indicates arbitrarily selected concentration based on achievable serum levels with usual recommended doses in μg/ml.

†Results expressed as per cent susceptible, based on published data.

with the exception of cefoxitin, which is resistant to the cephalosporinase produced by *B. fragilis.* Most strains of this species are susceptible to 16 to 32 μg/ml, and clinical trials indicate good results in the treatment of patients with intra-abdominal infections. The levels used to indicate sensitivity are quite generous and require relatively high doses. The third generation cephalosporins are similar to cephalothin in their activity against anaerobes except for moxalactam, which is more active against *B. fragilis.*

Tetracyclines. These drugs have rather unpredictable activity against many anaerobic pathogens and should not be used for serious infections. With tetracycline, approximately 30 to 50% of anaerobic gram-positive cocci and 50 to 80% of *B. fragilis* are resistant at the levels readily achieved with the usual oral dosage. Doxycycline is somewhat more active against some *Bacteroides fragilis,* but 30 to 40% are resistant, and clinical trials have shown poor results.

Metronidazole. This drug is active against most obligate anaerobic bacteria, including virtually all strains of *B. fragilis.* Organisms usually resistant include microaerophilic cocci, *Propionibacterium,* the agents of actinomycosis, and virtually all aerobic and facultative anaerobes. An intravenous formulation is now available, although the drug is well absorbed when given orally and the parenteral preparation is considerably more expensive. Clinical trials have documented the efficacy of metronidazole in central nervous system infections, intra-abdominal sepsis, and infections of the female genital tract. However, it appears to be inferior to alternative agents for anaerobic pulmonary infections. The spectrum of this drug is rather strictly limited to obligate anaerobic bacteria so that the addition of another agent would be mandatory for patients with mixed infections in whom microaerophilic or aerobic bacteria are considered significant. In vitro studies indicate that metronidazole is the only drug that is consistently bactericidal against *B. fragilis,* and experimental animal models with infections involving this microbe show superior in vivo activity compared with alternative drugs. However, this benefit has not been demonstrated in clinical trials when compared with alternative agents such as clindamycin.

SURGERY

Anaerobic infections are frequently characterized by tissue necrosis and abscess formation. These suppurative complications usually occur relatively late in the course of the infections. Once present, however, surgical debridement or drainage is regarded as the most important facet of treatment. It is noteworthy that early institution of appropriate antimicrobials appears to be a critical factor in preventing these late complications.

The time from the onset of tissue invasion in which there is a readily demonstrable impact on the lesion is regarded as the "critical interval." Once abscesses have formed, most antimicrobial agents have minimal impact on bacteria at the infected site despite in vitro activity. The major justification for antimicrobials at this stage is to limit contiguous spread and bacteremia. These observations emphasize the importance of early institution of appropriate agents, often on the basis of empiric decisions or a gram-stained slide. They also call attention to the necessity for detection and drainage of possible loculated collections when infections fail to respond.

Hemophilus influenzae Infections

MARTHA L. LEPOW, M.D.

Hemophilus influenzae type b is the most common cause of systemic bacterial infection in childhood. Invasive disease caused by this organism is limited almost exclusively to children between 2 months and 6 years of age; approximately 50% of illnesses occur before 18 months. Guidelines for antibiotic therapy are given in Table 1 and are discussed individually for the more important organ systems.

Meningitis: Initial intravenous antibiotic therapy should consist of ampicillin 200 mg/kg/day, divided into four or six doses and chloramphenicol at 75 mg/kg/day, divided into four doses. This combination will adequately treat disease due to ampicillin-resistant strains, the prevalence of which is as high as 30% in some parts of the United States. Ampicillin is necessary for the rare chloramphenicol-resistant strains. Failure of a patient to respond clinically (temperature, peripheral blood leukocyte count, neurologic status) to this combination within 48 hours is an indication for repeat lumbar puncture. If the cerebrospinal fluid (CSF) does not show some resolution of inflammation and sterility, a multiply-resistant strain should be suspected. Third generation cephalosporins (actually cephamycin derivatives) moxalactam and cefotaxime penetrate the blood-brain barrier, and efficacy comparable to ampicillin and chloramphenicol has been demonstrated for both in the treatment of meningitis due to *H. influenzae* type b. They could be employed if a multiply-resistant organism is identified.

Initial fluid management should not exceed maintenance requirements, and osmolality of serum and urine should be monitored for evidence of inappropriate antidiuretic hormone effect.

Rarely, endotoxemia and septic shock may occur and is best treated by plasma expanders and O_2 administration. Nearly all of the ampicillin-resistant

H. influenzae type b strains produce beta-lactamase which can be detected as soon as colonies are available on solid media. Chloramphenicol can be discontinued if ampicillin sensitivity is demonstrated. If chloramphenicol is continued, peak and trough levels should be monitored to ensure a therapeutic level of 15 to 25 μg/ml and to avoid toxicity.

Acute Complications. In all children, the hazard of increased intracranial pressure should be recognized and its signs sought by repeated physical examination, monitoring head circumference and vital signs. Computed tomography (CT) scan can be employed for confirmation. Upon evidence of intracranial hypertension, therapy with mannitol should be instituted. Airway maintenance and O_2 administration are important. Anti-inflammatory steroids have been used, but there are no data to support any beneficial action. Seizures occurring early appear to be due to small areas of infarction secondary to cerebral vasculitis. Phenobarbital or phenytoin (Dilantin) can be used to control seizures and for maintenance anticonvulsive therapy. Inappropriate antidiuretic hormone effect should be managed with fluid restriction. Ventriculitis, especially in infants less than 6 months of age, may cause prolonged fever and hydrocephalus. The latter occasionally requires that ventricular drainage be instituted. Disseminated intravascular coagulation occurs uncommonly but is best managed with fresh frozen plasma and platelet transfusions, as necessary.

Monitoring Therapy. After the acute signs and symptoms of meningitis have subsided, the antibiotics should be continued at the same dose for 10 days (or at least 5 days after the temperature is less than 38°C rectally). As the meningitis resolves, the blood-brain barrier becomes less permeable to the antibiotics, so the dose may need to be increased with continuing therapy to maintain high CSF antibiotic concentrations throughout the course of therapy. With chloramphenicol, but not ampicillin, an adequate blood level can be obtained with oral administration. If the course is uncomplicated, a lumbar puncture is not necessary when treatment is terminated. Recurrences are rare and usually occur more than a few days after therapy is discontinued. If a lumbar puncture is done at 10 to 12 days after initiation of therapy, a lymphocytosis may be present with an elevated protein. A lower CSF sugar may persist for weeks.

Secondary Fevers. Secondary fevers occurring after initial defervescence with clinical improvement may be due to secondary foci such as subdural effusion. Although this process is common, drainage is not necessary unless there is increasing irritability, paresis, vomiting, or focal seizures. Transillumination can indicate the presence of subdural effusion. A CT scan will localize the effusion in most cases, but the diagnostic procedure of choice is subdural tap, if indicated. If the fluid contains bacteria, administration of an antibiotic that penetrates into such fluids well (chloramphenicol) should be considered. If the fluid is opaque (i.e., a subdural empyema), surgical drainage shortens the course

Table 1. ANTIBIOTIC THERAPY FOR INVASIVE HAEMOPHILUS INFLUENZAE INFECTIONS

	First Choice	Route	Duration	Alternative Drugs	Comments
Meningitis	Ampicillin 200 mg/kg/ 24 hr in 4–6 doses; Chloramphenicol 75 mg/kg/24 hr in 4 doses	IV IV or PO	Clinical improvement and afebrile 5 days	Moxalactam*, or cefotaxime, 100–150 mg/kg/ d in 4 doses; trimethoprim-sulfamethoxazole (TMP-SMZ) 8–20 mg/ kg/d of TMP in 4 doses†	Alternatives should be used when resistance present to primary drugs or they cannot be tolerated
Epiglottitis	As above	IV until extubated	7 days	Cefamandole, 100 mg/kg/ d in 3 doses	Alternative used only if there is no question of meningitis
Septic arthritis	As above	IV and PO	Parenteral until fever and local signs abate; then minimum of 21 days	Cefamandole, same dose as above	As epiglottitis
Osteomyelitis	As above	IV and PO	Parenteral until fever and local signs abate; then PO until ESR is normal	Cefamandole, same dose as above†	As epiglottitis
Pneumonia	As above	IV and PO	Until febrile 5 days	Cefamandole TMP-SMX	As epiglottitis
Cellulitis	As above	IV	7 days (longer if bacteremia demonstrated)	Cefamandole, same dose as above	As epiglottitis

*May be associated with prolonged prothrombin time and may effect platelet function.
†Not recommended for infants less than 2 months of age.

and the morbidity. Increasing head size may indicate subdural effusion, communicating hydrocephalus, or ventriculitis.

Persistent fever and focal signs may also indicate a brain abscess; this is rare but is more common with *Hemophilus* than with other meningotrophic organisms. Its diagnosis is usually apparent on CT scan (demonstrating enhancement of the vascular rim) or technetium brain scanning. Surgical drainage or prolonged antibiotic therapy, or both, may be required.

Cortical arterial or venous thrombosis may cause persistent fever. The optimal duration of therapy for *H. influenzae* meningitis with complications is unknown. In general, longer treatment regimens are used in infants with more severe disease, who most commonly are less than 6 months of age.

Epiglottitis. The most important factor in treatment of *H. influenzae* epiglottitis is to maintain a patent airway. This should be done at the time of diagnosis. Nasotracheal intubation, orotracheal intubation, and tracheostomy have been used successfully with comparable rates of morbidity. Use of a technique for which there is expertise and backup is more important than any specific procedure. Since bacteremia is common, initial antibiotic therapy for this illness is the same as for meningitis and should be continued for at least 7 days. In most instances, with successful therapy the signs and symptoms of acute infection abate and the child begins breathing around the tracheal cannula 2 to 3 days after initiation of antibiotic therapy. Local recurrence has not been reported. Secondary foci of infection are uncommon but include pneumonia and rarely meningitis.

Septic Arthritis. The mainstay of treatment is adequate drainage. The exact method of this varies with the joint involved and the age of the patient. Septic arthritis of the hip is a surgical emergency and should be externally drained at the time of diagnosis. Shoulders, knees, and elbows may require surgical drainage, particularly in young infants. Repeated needle aspirations along with appropriate antibiotic therapy have been used; however, surgical drainage may be necessary if fluid persists for more than a few days.

Initial antibiotic therapy, like that for other invasive *H. influenzae* illness, is ampicillin and chloramphenicol. A second generation parenteral cephalosporin (cefamandole) also has good anti-Hemophilus activity and may be used in ampicillin-resistant infections. It should be emphasized that this drug penetrates CSF poorly and meningitis has occurred after 3 to 5 days of therapy when this agent has been used for joint infection in young children. After the acute signs and symptoms have abated, including decrease in joint fluid and in polymorphonuclear leukocytes in the joint fluid and the child is afebrile for 5 days, therapy can be continued with oral amoxicillin for 2 to 3 weeks. Continued hospitalization of the child, adjusting the dose 100 mg/kg/24 hrs (and adding probenecid,* if necessary) to maintain a peak serum concentration of 20 μg/ml (a serum bactericidal titer of 1:8), is necessary for efficacious therapy. If the organism is ampicillin-resistant, the oral therapy can be continued with trimethoprim-sulfamethoxazole or chloramphenicol with monitoring of blood levels. A failure and ultimate relapse are inevitable if the joint fluid contains more than 50,000 polymorphonuclear leukocytes per microliter of joint fluid after treatment has been administered for 5 to 10 days. Fever and erythrocyte sedimentation rate can be used for guidelines for duration of therapy.

Osteomyelitis. In contrast to the treatment of staphylococcal osteomyelitis, drainage is usually not necessary or performed. *Hemophilus influenzae* type b osteomyelitis tends to be a less destructive disease than that caused by staphylococcus. In most instances, the infected extremity is put at rest, usually with casting. Initial antibiotic treatment is identical to that recommended for septic arthritis, with the same limitations. Parenteral administration should be continued until all focal signs and symptoms and constitutional indicators of infection have abated and the erythrocyte sedimentation rate (ESR) is decreasing (2–3 weeks); then oral therapy is continued until the ESR is normal. This is most commonly done with oral amoxicillin, maintaining a peak serum concentration of approximately 20 μg/ml (a bactericidal titer of 1:8).

Pneumonia. Pneumonia is commonly lobar with pleural effusion. Usually intravenous fluid and electrolyte therapy is also necessary in an infant with a combined metabolic and respiratory acidosis. Ampicillin and chloramphenicol should be used initially.

When antibiotic sensitivities do become available, the least toxic drug is continued, in most cases ampicillin. After the acute phase of the illness has abated and the child no longer requires supplemental oxygen, oral amoxicillin can be used. The infant's chest roentgenograms will not change appreciably over the next several weeks, which may be punctuated by intermittent temperature spikes of up to 38.3°C. However, the general trend is to a lower daily maximum temperature. The mean duration of treatment is 3 weeks but it may extend to 6 weeks. If the isolate was initially proven to be ampicillin-resistant, chloramphenicol, trimethaprim-sulfamethoxazole, or a second generation cephalosporin may be employed.

Cellulitis. The most common sites are facial and

---

*Manufacturer's note: Probenecid is contraindicated in children under 2 years of age.

periorbital. The seriousness of this illness lies with the associated bacteremia in 70 to 80% and secondary foci. The most common secondary foci are meningitis, followed by septic arthritis and pericarditis. Most infants defervesce within 18 hours of therapy; persistence of fever more than 48 hours after initiation of therapy should prompt questioning of bacteriologic sensitivity data, as well as a more studious search for secondary foci. In uncomplicated *H. influenzae* type b cellulitis the minimum duration of parenteral therapy is 7 days with the least toxic antibiotic.

Uncommon Systemic Infections. These may be complications of occult *H. influenzae* bacteremia and include the following:

Urinary Tract Infection. Since this infection is associated with bacteremia, parenteral therapy for a minimum of 7 days is indicated. The initial choice of antibiotics should be that used for bacteremic *H. influenzae* type b diseases—ampicillin and chloramphenicol. However, after initial treatment of the bacteremia (for 7 days), the therapy may be concluded with oral sulfisoxazole* (100 mg/kg/24 hr).

Epididymitis. These illnesses were recognized because of cultures yielding *Hemophilus* after scrotal exploration for presumed torsion of the testes. Therapy is the same as for the urinary tract infection.

Endocarditis. H. influenzae type b endocarditis may occur in children with cyanotic congenital disease with persistent *Hemophilus* bacteremia and low grade fever. Most case reports document successful therapy with 6 weeks of intravenous ampicillin or chloramphenicol if ampicillin resistance is encountered.

Neonatal Respiratory Distress Syndrome. H. influenzae type b can produce a clinical picture similar to group B streptococci in neonates—a premature or term infant who has apparent hyaline membrane disease in whom ventilation is accomplished easily but in whom shock intervenes within the first 24 hours. The antibiotics usually used are ampicillin (100 mg/kg/24 hr) and gentamicin (5 mg/kg/24 hr). Both antibiotics are usually active in vitro against the organisms from such cases, and the poor outcome seems to be related to the delay in recognition of the process. Moxalactam may be an alternative if meningitis is present and the isolate is β-lactamase positive, since chloramphenicol is contraindicated.

Occult Hemophilus Bacteremia. This illness occurs in infants under 2 years of age and is accompanied by a high temperature (39°C rectally) and leukocytosis. On examination, the child has no apparent focus of infection but has marked leukocytosis with a left shift. Approximately half of all cases of occult sepsis will have pneumonia (by chest x-ray) or otitis media. The remaining group of children, however, have no apparent focus. These children are at increased risk of an invasive infection, particularly meningitis, and should be treated as though they have this entity until CSF cultures prove otherwise, with admission to the hospital and initiation of therapy with ampicillin and chloramphenicol. Should the CSF cultures prove sterile and there is a clinical response, the antibiotics can be discontinued after 7 days. Throughout the course, however, a diligent search for secondary foci should be undertaken.

Otitis Media. One third of all otitis media is due to *H. influenzae,* with only 10% due to type b. Currently in the United States, as many as 30% of such organisms are ampicillin-resistant. Thus, one would predict that 10% of all otitis media patients should fail to respond when treated with ampicillin or amoxicillin.

Alternatives to ampicillin in otitis media of unknown etiology have consisted of sulfonamides (for the *Hemophilus* activity) and a drug active against gram-positive organisms. Penicillin G is preferred as the second antibiotic by some individuals, as it has some in vitro activity against unencapsulated *H. influenzae;* others prefer erythromycin. The trimethoprim-sulfamethoxazole combination has also been used for *H. influenzae* otitis. In uncontrolled trials, it has been found efficacious in children who failed to clear on amoxicillin or had ampicillin-resistant organisms. It is not clear, however, whether this is a significant improvement, as there was no comparative drug. Much of the same claim is made for cefaclor. This drug is costly, which precludes its routine use, and allergic reactions may occur. The role of decongestants and nasal drops and sprays is controversial. In most instances, the antibiotic is administered for 10 days, with a follow-up evaluation 4 days after conclusion of therapy. Prophylaxis with sulfisoxazole* during the winter months has been suggested for infants who have frequent bouts of otitis media.

SINUSITIS. Oral antibiotics, in addition to local treatment of the sinuses, usually are efficacious in this illness. Failure of antibiotic therapy is usually associated with persistent sinus ostium obstruction.

BRONCHIECTASIS. Long-term (6 weeks) administration of amoxicillin or trimethoprim-sulfisoxazole usually results in resolution of the exacerbation. In controlled studies, long-term sulfonamide administration has decreased the frequency of recurrences in individuals with *Hemophilus* bronchiectasis.

Prophylaxis of Contacts. A recent cooperative study under the auspices of the Centers for Disease Control indicated that rifampin was effective in de-

---

*Contraindicated in children less than 2 months of age.

*Contraindicated in infants under 2 months of age.

creasing the carrier state of *H. influenzae* type b and secondary attack rates in household contacts less than 4 years of age. There was indication of such effects in nursery schools and day care centers as well.

Accordingly, the Academy of Pediatrics Committee in Control of Infectious Diseases has recommended that rifampin be used at 20 mg/kg/day for 4 days in all household contacts of invasive *H. influenzae* type b disease if there is one under 4 years of age.

Prophylaxis of children in day care centers should be determined on an individual basis. Since rifampin is not a treatment for this disease, careful monitoring of contact illness will be very important so that treatment can be instituted, if necessary. There is no liquid preparation of rifampin, so that capsular contents will have to be administered with a suitable vehicle.

A capsular polysaccharide vaccine (PRP) is being proposed for licensure for administration to children over 18 months of age.

Tetanus Neonatorum

JAMES M. ADAMS, M.D.

Although neonatal tetanus is now rare in the United States, it is most prevalent among infants delivered at home and in segments of the population with inadequate maternal immunization. It must be differentiated primarily from neonatal seizures, but birth trauma, hypoxic injury, septicemia, and other diseases of the perinatal period are common in this group of patients and may coexist with neonatal tetanus.

General Supportive Care

Programs for outpatient management of tetanus have been implemented in developing nations, but the disease should be considered an indication for hospitalization of the newborn infant even if initial spasms are mild. The baby should be admitted to a neonatal intensive care unit or a unit able to provide electronic cardiac monitoring, a controlled thermal environment, skilled nursing care, and mechanical ventilatory support if necessary.

The infant should be placed initially in a servo or manually controlled incubator, protected from light and noise. This environment reduces the spasm-provoking external stimuli that reach the baby. Swaddling and minimized handling and disturbance of the infant further reduce the tendency of environmental stimuli to provoke self-perpetuating spasms. Such minimal intrusion into the environment of the infant requires close observation by trained personnel as well as careful electronic monitoring. Swaddling may result in overheating if the temperature of both the infant and its environment is not properly monitored and controlled.

Serum electrolytes, blood urea nitrogen, albumin, and urine specific gravity determinations aid in guiding metabolic and nutritional management. All infants should receive 1 mg of vitamin K_1 initially, and a VDRL specimen should be obtained. Prophylactic eye care should be administered with erythromycin ointment.

Intravenous fluids should be administered initially as 10% glucose in water with appropriate electrolytes at an infusion rate of 100 to 125 ml/kg/24 hr. Once spasms are controlled or if mechanical ventilation has been instituted and the condition stabilized, enteral feedings can be initiated by nasogastric tube if bowel sounds are present. A 24 calorie per ounce formula should be given initially at 25 ml/kg/24 hr by continuous nasogastric infusion and advanced progressively until intravenous fluids can be discontinued. For long-term growth and nutrition, formula intakes of 140 to 150 ml/kg/24 hr will be necessary. When the infant's course is stabilized on full milk drip feedings, intermittent gavage may be attempted. This feeding program is designed to avoid gastric distention, impairment of mobility of the diaphragm, and regurgitation. In term infants, if the formula utilized meets the recommendations of the American Academy of Pediatrics Committee on Nutrition, vitamin and mineral supplementation will not be required unless specific deficiencies are identified.

Bacteriologic Management

Because septicemia or meningoencephalitis cannot be ruled out during the initial hours of hospitalization, ampicillin (150 mg/kg/24 hr) and kanamycin (15 mg/kg/24 hr) should be administered parenterally following blood and cerebrospinal fluid cultures. When a diagnosis of tetanus has been confirmed, these antibiotics may be discontinued and 100,000 units/kg/24 hr of aqueous penicillin G given alone to finish a 10-day course of therapy.

Human tetanus immune globulin, 500 units, should be given in divided doses intramuscularly. All babies should receive an initial dose of diphtheria-tetanus (DT) vaccine prior to discharge as no permanent immunity results from *Clostridium tetani* infections treated with antitoxin. The initial immunization should be delayed, however, until 4 to 6 weeks after administration of antitoxin.

Positive cultures of *C. tetani* from the umbilicus are rarely obtained, even with anaerobic techniques. Antibody tests may confirm the diagnosis, but results are usually not available in the early days of the disease.

Control of Tetanic Spasms

Various tranquilizers and sedating agents have been utilized to control the violent spasms of tetanus. At best, these agents can be expected to modify the frequency or severity of the spasms rather than ablate them. In general, slightly better results can be expected from combination regimens and very high dosage ranges. The incidence of apnea, retention of pulmonary secretions, and other complications of CNS depression, however, is also increased. The potential for addiction with these drugs, particularly chloral hydrate, must be considered.

Phenobarbital 10–15 mg/kg/day may be given by nasogastric tube in two or three divided doses. Chloral hydrate, 40 to 60 mg/kg/day, may be added. Good results have been achieved abroad using a continuous infusion of diazepam, 20 to 40 mg/kg/day. This is combined with phenobarbital, 10 mg/kg/day. The safety of parenteral diazepam in the neonate has not been established, however, and respiratory depression requiring mechanical ventilation should be anticipated in some patients receiving this high dose regimen.

During the recovery phase of the disease, intermittent spasms, usually less severe, may require continuation of phenobarbital or diazepam 2 to 4 mg/kg/day per nasogastric tube for muscle relaxation.

Pulmonary Care

Virtually all deaths in tetanus neonatorum are respiratory. Specific pulmonary complications include apnea, hypoventilation, hypoxemia, pneumothorax, infection, and airway obstruction from retained secretions. Constant observation of color, respiratory rate, heart rate, and work of breathing is necessary. Arterial blood gases should be obtained as a guide to respiratory management and warm, humidified oxygen given as necessary to maintain PaO_2 at 60 to 80 torr. Transcutaneous oxygen monitoring is helpful in determining trends in oxygenation during spasms and at rest. Indications for mechanical ventilation are 1) apnea, 2) $PaCO_2$ persistently greater than 50 to 55 torr, 3) recurrent hypoxemia during spasms, and 4) continuous or rapidly recurrent spasms.

Infants should be ventilated through a nasotracheal tube in conjunction with neuromuscular blockade. Pancuronium bromide is given intravenously in an initial dose of 0.05 mg/kg. This may be increased to 0.1 mg/kg, given as frequently as needed to keep the infant quiet and immobile. Complete muscular paralysis is not necessary. As lung function in these babies is essentially normal but chest compliance and airway resistance subject to change throughout the course, we prefer a volume-controlled ventilator. As the infant receiving neuromuscular blockade is at the mercy of the environment, strict attention must be paid to suctioning, changes of position, chest percussion, and maintenance of sterile technique.

Infants should be maintained on mechanical ventilation until respiratory compromise is no longer produced by residual spasms. This may require 3 to 4 weeks. Tracheostomy should be the exception rather than the rule in neonatal tetanus. Modern neonatal intensive care has produced a low incidence of complications of prolonged endotracheal intubation, and tracheostomy itself is not without serious consequences in this age group.

Pulmonary infection is a constant threat, and the clinician should be alert to changes in temperature control, glucose metabolism, or pulmonary function as early warning signs. If changes in pulmonary function suggest pneumonia, complete blood count, blood culture, chest radiograph, and Gram stain and culture of tracheal secretions should be performed. Gram stain may aid in the initial choice of antibiotics, but in most instances appropriate therapy would include methicillin (200 mg/kg/24 hr) and gentamicin (7.5 mg/kg/24 hr).

Infant Botulism

STEPHEN S. ARNON, M.D.

Infant botulism, the recently recognized infectious form, occurs when ingested spores of *Clostridium botulinum* germinate, colonize the intestine, and produce in vivo the most potent poison known, botulinal toxin. The generalized flaccid paralysis produced by the toxin's blockade of peripheral cholinergic synapses, most notably the neuromuscular junction, constitutes the central challenge of management. Meticulous supportive care (nutritional, respiratory, nursing) is the basis of therapy. In the absence of complications, all hospitalized infants have recovered without residua.

In severely paralyzed patients the need for immediate hospitalization with intensive care will be obvious, even if the diagnosis is not. ("Suspected sepsis" remains the commonest admission diagnosis.) However, even the mildly weak and hypotonic infant should be observed where a respirator is immediately at hand, as the severity of paralysis may increase within hours, and aspiration, upper airway occlusion, or diaphragmatic paralysis may suddenly occur. Cardiac and respiratory monitoring should begin at admission, and prophylactic intubation is prudent.

The intensity of supportive care a patient requires will vary during the several weeks of hospitalization while the motoneurons regenerate new myoneural junctions and thereby restore movement. Some patients need total ventilatory and nutritional sustenance. Transcutaneous monitoring of blood oxygen tension is desirable because an affected infant will be unable to squirm or otherwise signal distress should the position of the endotracheal tube change. Similarly, cough and postural reflexes are generally absent, and if the patient is not carefully positioned after each handling, breathing difficulties may ensue. Few patients have needed tracheostomy despite prolonged intubation, and tracheostomy should not be considered a necessary part of management.

Gavage feeding permits easy supplying of fluid, electrolyte, and caloric needs, and may stimulate peristalsis, thereby hastening the elimination of *C. botulinum* toxin and organisms from the gut. The presence of gastric atony and of possible gastroesophageal reflux mandates close watch for residual volumes. However, with an infusion pump and crib blocks even quite paralyzed patients have been successfully fed by gavage. The patient should receive mother's milk if available; if not, a formula milk without added iron is the next choice. Intravenous feeding ("hyperalimentation") has been used as a last resort but brings with it the need for repeated phlebotomy (thus, nosocomial anemia) as well as the hazard of infection.

The presently available botulinal antitoxin is a horse serum product that is not used in infant botulism for several reasons. Most importantly, experience has shown that patients will recover completely without it. Also, evidence of its therapeutic efficacy is lacking. In addition, its use may induce lifelong hypersensitivity. Finally, serum sickness and anaphylaxis often occur when equine antitoxin is given to older children and adults. A human-derived botulism immune globulin, when developed, may have therapeutic benefit.

Antibiotics are used in infant botulism only to treat secondary infections, which occur most frequently in the lungs or urinary tract. Antibiotic therapy directed against *C. botulinum* organisms in the gut lumen has been tried but has failed to eradicate the bacteria or to stop excretion of toxin. Furthermore, it is possible that antibiotics effective against *C. botulinum* might be more effective against other gut anaerobes and may thereby create a larger ecologic space for *C. botulinum*. Also, clostridiocidal antibiotics may actually increase the pool of toxin in the gut available for absorption, as botulinal toxin is liberated with bacterial cell death and lysis. For this reason when antibiotics are needed to treat the common secondary infections of infant botulism, it may be desirable to use the combination drug trimethoprim-sulfamethoxazole (Bactrim, Septra), to which *C. botulinum* is resistant. This drug is approved for use in infants over 2 months of age. Aminoglycoside antibiotics, often begun at admission when infant botulism is mistaken for "sepsis," may exacerbate the paralysis by further blocking neuromuscular transmission.

During recovery, patients fatigue easily when muscular action is sustained, a consideration particularly important in deciding when to resume oral feeding, because of the hazard of aspiration. Patients should not be fed by mouth until they are fully able to gag and swallow. Tube feeding has been continued uneventfully at home by some parents. Patients are usually ready for discharge when gag reflex, swallowing, and coughing ability are adequate to protect the airway.

Some practical measures deserve mention. Bladder atony often is present, and the frequent emptying by Credé will reduce the risk of urinary tract infection. Since *C. botulinum* toxin and organisms remain present in patients' feces for weeks (and might be fecally–orally transmitted to other infants), scrupulous hand washing by all who handle the infant is mandatory. For the same reason, the patient's linen should be bagged separately and autoclaved. (Spores of *C. botulinum* are very heat-resistant.) Staff personnel with open lesions on their hands should not change the patient's diapers.

Normal bowel action may take weeks to return, and may be impeded by an inspissated bolus of feces, a possibility detectable by digital examination. During convalescence, a stool softener may be beneficial. Cathartics and enemas intended to reduce the quantity of intraluminal *C. botulinum* are ineffective, and repeated purgation is potentially dangerous. Once discharged, close contact with other infants (e.g., same crib) should be avoided for about 3 months or until excretion of organisms has ceased. The possibility of nosocomial infant botulism will exist as long as some hospital dietetic departments continue to use honey as the carbohydrate source in lactose-free ("CHO-Free") infant feeds.

Physicians who suspect infant botulism should contact their state health department to arrange for diagnostic testing of feces and serum.

Shigellosis

HEINZ F. EICHENWALD, M.D.

Shigellosis is an acute diarrheal disease caused by various species of the genus *Shigella;* in the United States, *S. sonnei* is most commonly involved. The illness may occur in diarrheic or dysenteric forms, which differ in presentation and clinical course: the former begins abruptly with high fever, toxicity, and prostration, often accompanied by seizures and the passage of large volume, watery stools. In the dysenteric form, onset of diarrhea is more gradual, increases in severity over 2 to 3 days, and is associated with abdominal pain, tenesmus, and moderate fever. The stool is characteristically small in volume but contains much blood and many polymorphonuclear leukocytes. On rare occasions, either form may progress to a subacute pseudo-membranous colitis.

The most important aspect of treatment of the diarrheic form is prompt replacement of water and electrolyte deficits, usually by parenteral administration of appropriate fluids; recently, orally administered electrolyte solutions* have been used successfully when intravenous fluids were unavailable. Severely toxic patients may rapidly progress to shock, which generally responds to appropriate parenteral crystalloids such as normal saline or Ringer's lactate solutions but may require the use of volume expanders, such as plasma.

Seizures, if present, are treated by intravenous diazepam (0.25 mg/kg). Should this fail to control the convulsions or should they recur, phenobarbital (10 mg/kg/IV) is used. Rarely is phenytoin (10 mg/kg/IV) needed. If the seizures respond poorly or only partially to anticonvulsant medication, a metabolic cause (hyponatremia, hypoglycemia) should be suspected.

In the dysenteric form of the infection, the child loses only moderate amounts of water and electrolytes, and rehydration can usually be accomplished with an oral maintenance solution.†

Once dehydration has been corrected, orally administered liquids can be used in most patients. The exact type is relatively unimportant as long as adequate free water is provided to allow excretion of excess amounts of electrolyte: weak teas, soups, or commercially available electrolyte solutions ("Lytren" or "Pedialyte") are all satisfactory. If the child accepts and tolerates these fluids well, his diet can be advanced over 3 or 4 days to more nutritious but lactose-free foods. Lactose is avoided because both forms of shigellosis may cause the patient to be unable to digest this as well as other disaccharides, a condition that may persist for several days or even longer.

Episodes of even moderately severe shigellosis are associated with extensive nitrogen losses, which continue well into convalescence. The condition of the child may therefore rapidly progress to a malnutrition syndrome which, in turn, renders the patient increasingly susceptible to other infections of the intestine, respiratory tract, and skin. Food provided during the convalescent period should therefore contain at least 5 to 6 gm of protein per kg each day.

Controlled studies have demonstrated that administration of appropriate antimicrobial medication results in two desirable effects: the duration of

diarrhea is reduced and the excretion of *Shigella* is terminated, rendering the child noninfectious to others. The results of these investigations also indicated that three requirements had to be met for an antimicrobial agent to be effective in the treatment of shigellosis: a) the organisms must be susceptible to the medication, b) adequate intraluminal levels of drug must be produced in both ileum and colon, and c) serum concentrations of the agent must exceed the minimum inhibitory levels for the organism. Because of these requirements, antibiotics such as streptomycin that are not absorbed following oral administratoin prove ineffective as do those that are absorbed sufficiently well in the upper intestinal tract that no drug reaches the colon, as is the case with amoxicillin.

The preferred antimicrobial agent varies with the geographic area where the infection was acquired. In most parts of North and Central America, a significant proportion of *Shigella* are resistant to sulfonamides and to ampicillin, so the preferred drug is trimethoprim-sulfamethoxazole (TMP-SMZ) in a dosage of 10 mg/kg/day (based on the TMP component) which is administered orally or intravenously twice a day for 5 days. For susceptible strains, ampicillin is equally effective in a daily dosage of 100 mg/kg/day divided into four doses administered intravenously, intramuscularly, or orally for 5 days.

Relatively limited data suggest that tetracyclines, chloramphenicol, or rifampin may be effective, but the toxicity of these drugs makes their use generally undesirable. Controlled studies have confirmed the efficacy of nalidixic and oxolinic acids, but these agents should not be routinely employed because of their neurotoxicity. Infectious complications of shigellosis are unusual; only very rarely do these bacteria gain access to the blood stream. Bacteremia caused by gram-negative enterobacteria occasionally occurs, generally late in the course of severe disease in malnourished children.

Efforts to treat diarrhea pharmacologically are either ineffective or dangerous, sometimes both. The administration of various adsorbents, such as refined clays or pectins, does not decrease the volume of fluid excreted in the stools, although stools may appear more solid. The use of diphenoxylate or tincture of opium increases the risk of toxic megacolon; use of these drugs must therefore be avoided.

---

*The World Health Organization *rehydrating* solution contains 90 mmol/L sodium, 20 mmol/L potassium, plus base and 2% glucose.

†A widely recommended *maintenance* solution for oral use consists of 50 mmol/L sodium, 20 mmol/L potassium, 30 to 50 mmol/L chloride, and base (citrate or bicarbonate 30 mmol/L). Intake is limited to 150 ml/kg/day; if the child still complains of thirst, water is offered.

Typhoid Fever

SANDOR FELDMAN, M.D.

Modern sanitation has dramatically reduced the incidence of typhoid fever in this country. In 1981 approximately 550 cases were reported in the U.S. However, worldwide, in underdeveloped countries

Salmonella typhi remains a significant health problem. Typhoid fever is still to be suspected in children with prolonged high fevers (39–41°C), headache, nausea, anorexia, malaise, irritability, cough, abdominal pain, leukopenia, splenomegaly, or rose spots. Constipation is common whereas diarrhea is relatively uncommon. *S. typhi* can be isolated from blood and bone marrow. Later in the course of infection the organism can be isolated from urine and stool. Elevated O-antigen agglutinating antibody ($\geq 1:320$) or rising O- and H-antigen agglutinating antibodies to *S. typhi* are suggestive of typhoid fever.

Therapy. Initial therapy should be intravenous chloramphenicol, 50 to 100 mg/kg/day (max. 2 gm/day) in four divided doses or ampicillin 100 to 200 mg/kg/day in four divided doses. Within 3 to 5 days there usually will be defervescence of fever and the symptoms will have begun to ameliorate. At that time, if the oral fluid intake is adequate, antibiotic therapy may be changed to the oral route. Amoxicillin 100 mg/kg/day in three divided doses may be substituted for ampicillin. Antibiotic therapy should be for 14 days. Alternatively, trimethoprim-sulfamethoxazole (TMP-SMZ);* trimethoprim, 10 to 12 mg/kg/day and sulfamethoxazole, 50 to 60 mg/kg/day in two divided doses has been found to be effective therapy for salmonellosis, including *S. typhi*. Intravenous TMP-SMZ requires 125 ml of diluting fluid for each 80 mg TMP. Children receiving this antibiotic intravenously should have careful monitoring of fluid intake. Although many of the cephalosporins have demonstrated in vitro activity against *S. typhi* and the other *Salmonella* serotypes, clinical studies to support their use are lacking. In some instances these antibiotics have been ineffective, despite in vitro activity.

Salmonellae, including *S. typhi*, have shown some resistance to ampicillin and chloramphenicol. Resistance to both antibiotics simultaneously is rare. Antibiotic resistant *Salmonellae* are imported from Southeast Asia, India, and Latin America. Antibiotic sensitivity to *Salmonella* isolates is required to ensure appropriate therapy.

Treatment for less than 14 days increases the risk of relapse, while treatment for more than 14 days does not decrease this risk. Relapse rates are reported to be from 10 to 20%. Relapse appears to be less following treatment with ampicillin (amoxicillin) or TMP-SMZ than with chloramphenicol.

Children with typhoid fever should be hospitalized for enteric isolation and nursing care. Careful handwashing measures are necessary to decrease the liklihood of intrafamily spread and spread to hospital personnel. During initial therapy, intravenous fluids may be required, with careful monitoring of fluid and electrolyte balance. The diet should be bland and well balanced, and include a generous amount of fluids.

Avoid antipyretic therapy with acetaminophen or salicylates, as they can produce hypothermia. Tepid sponge baths can be used to control fever. Physical activity should be markedly limited during the acute phase of the illness and curtailed during convalescence.

Prednisone, 2 mg/kg/day for 3 to 4 days, may be beneficial to the severely toxic and delirious patient. The routine use of steroids for fever and symptom control is not indicated.

Complications. Complications tend to occur during the third and fourth week of illness and are more frequent in the untreated and those whose therapy was started late. Recurrence of fever usually heralds onset of relapse or other complications. Gastrointestinal hemorrhage and intestinal perforation are the most severe life-threatening complications. Intensive supportive therapy, antibiotics, and blood products are administered as indicated. Failure of medical management to stabilize the patient may require surgical intervention. However, mortality rates after surgical intervention are high. Sound clinical judgment will be necessary to guide the medical and surgical management of this complication.

Acute cholecystitis with gallstones may require surgery. *S. typhi* involving the lungs, liver, bones, and joints will require prolonged antibiotic therapy.

Chronic Carriers. Chronic carriage is defined as fecal excretion of Salmonella for at least one year. Overall, the carriage rate of *S. typhi* is 2%; however, the rate is much lower in children. The most common source of the organism is the gallbladder with the presence of gallstones. Cholecystectomy should be considered.

Ampicillin, 100–200 mg/kg/day (amoxicillin, 100 mg/kg/day) or TMP-SMZ*(trimethoprim, 8 mg/kg/day—sulfamethoxazole, 40 mg/kg/day) for 3 to 4 weeks has been used successfully to treat *S. typhi* carriers. Failures are common.

Vaccination. In the U.S., typhoid vaccine is indicated for those persons exposed to documented typhoid carriers, such as household contacts, travelers to endemic areas, and laboratory workers with frequent contact with the organism. A heat-phenol inactivated vaccine is available commercially in the U.S. The acetone-inactivated vaccine is used by the military. An oral live-attenuated typhoid vaccine is presently under investigation and appears to confer immunity for at least 3 years.

---

*This use is not listed by the manufacturer. The combination is not recommended for infants less than 2 months of age.

*This use is not listed by the manufacturer. Also, it is not recommended for infants less than 2 months of age.

The heat-phenol inactivated vaccine is given subcutaneously in two doses, 0.5 ml/dose 3 weeks apart for children 10 years or older; children 6 months to 10 years old should receive two 0.25 ml doses 3 weeks apart. A booster dose of either 0.5 ml or 0.25 ml, depending on the child's age, should be given every 3 years for the child at high risk for typhoid fever. Adverse effects such as pain at the site of injection, fever, malaise, and headaches may require dose reduction.

Salmonellosis

SANDOR FELDMAN, M.D.

For the past several years there has been an increase in the occurrence of nontyphoidal salmonellosis in the U.S. Man usually acquires the infection through contact with infected domestic animals and pets or food such as poultry, meat, eggs, and milk products. Water-borne salmonellosis is uncommon in this country. There are three primary species: *S. typhi* (one serotype), *S. choleraesuis* (one serotype) and *S. enteritides* (over 1700 serotypes). In the latter group serotypes *S. typhimurium, S. enteritides,* and *S. heidelberg* are the most common isolates.

Children less than 5 years of age, particularly those under 1 year of age, have the highest incidence of salmonellosis. The immunosuppressed host, either from underlying disease or immunosuppressive therapy, appears to have an increased incidence, but not necessarily increased severity, of infection. Children with sickle cell anemia and other hemoglobinopathies are at increased risk for infection and severity of infection.

Gastroenteritis (Enterocolitis). This acute onset syndrome is the most common presentation of *Salmonella* infection. Within 4 to 48 hours of ingestion of the contaminated food there is nausea, vomiting, headache, malaise, and fever. These symptoms usually resolve and are followed by abdominal cramps and diarrhea. The latter may vary from a few loose stools to a fulminant diarrhea. The mainstay of therapy is fluid and electrolyte replacement either with oral (clear liquids) or intravenous fluids, depending on the child's clinical condition. Abdominal cramps may be treated with infrequent doses of paregoric. In general, antispasmodics and analgesics should be avoided, since overdose for this self-limiting symptom has been reported. Over-the-counter antidiarrheals play no role in the management of gastroenteritis. Usually the diarrhea resolves within a week. Once the child's appetite is regained and the stool frequency has decreased, a soft, bland diet can be instituted.

Antimicrobial therapy is not indicated in this self-limiting form of salmonellosis. However, ampicillin, TMP-SMZ,* or chloramphenicol should be considered in that order of preference and depending upon in vitro susceptibility tests of patients at increased risk for disseminated infections. Examples are newborns, infants during the first year of life, children with hemoglobinopathies such as sickle cell disease, or congenital immunodeficiencies, and children receiving prednisone, antimetabolites, and/or radiation therapy. Antibiotic therapy should be administered only during the acute phase of the infection.

Enteric Fever. The clinical features of nontyphoidal enteric fever are indistinguishable from those of typhoid fever. Antibiotic therapy and management is the same as that discussed under Typhoid Fever. Resistance of nontyphoidal *Salmonella* to ampicillin and chloramphenicol is increasing, particularly when the strain is imported from outside the U.S. Antibiotic sensitivities are required to ensure proper therapy for these infections. As with *S. typhi,* the cephalosporins are not indicated in treatment. Gastrointestinal hemorrhage and intestinal perforation are uncommon complications of non-typhoidal salmonellosis.

Bacteremia. This is characterized by a hectic fever pattern for days to weeks and chronic bacteremia without the constitutional symptoms of enteric fever or gastroenteritis. *S. choleraesuis* is frequently the causative serotype. Therapy is similar to that for typhoid fever and requires monitoring with blood cultures. Dissemination to other organ systems can be expected in about 10% of patients.

Local Infections. Localized infection of almost any organ system can occur following salmonellosis. Osteomyelitis in children with sickle cell anemia is well known. Surgical drainage of abscesses is indicated. Intravenous antibiotic therapy with ampicillin or chloramphenicol may be prolonged, depending on the infected organ. Antibiotic therapy should be continued for at least 1 week after the signs of infection have disappeared.

As in the treatment of all *Salmonella* infections, antibiotic sensitivities are required because of the increasing resistance. TMP-SMZ* is an alternative to ampicillin and chloramphenicol.

Salmonella meningitis, occurring chiefly in neonates and infants under 1 year of age, has a mortality rate of 85%, and relapses occur frequently. The duration of antibiotic therapy in children with meningitis should be at least 14 to 21 days with parenteral ampicillin, 200–300 mg/kg/day, or chloramphenicol, 100 mg/kg/day. Chloramphen-

---

*Manufacturer's precaution: Not recommended for infants less than 2 months of age.

icol should not be used in the newborn because of the high risk of the gray baby syndrome.

Chronic Carriers. Chronic carrying of nontyphoidal *Salmonella* occurs in less than 1% of infected children. Intrafamily spread can usually be prevented by hand-washing measures. Antibiotic therapy is not us__'y indicated.

Campylobacter Infections

MELVIN I. MARKS, M.D.

Campylobacter are vibrio-shaped gram-negative bacteria that commonly cause gastroenteritis (normally ss. *fetus*) in young children. Occasionally, the infection extends beyond the gastrointestinal tract, particularly in malnourished and immunocompromised hosts (usually ss. *intestinalis*). The major reservoirs are food, water, and domestic animals (dogs, cats, and fowl).

Gastroenteritis. By far the most common infections due to *Campylobacter* are confined to the gastrointestinal tract and are self-limited in most normal hosts. Nevertheless, carefully controlled prospective in vivo clinical studies indicate that treatment with erythromycin in dosages of 40 to 50 mg/kg/day, divided qid × 5 days, will rapidly eliminate *Campylobacter* from the stools of these patients. The patient should be free of diarrhea and fever for at least 48 hours before discontinuing therapy. Unfortunately, there is no effect on the course of diarrhea, fever, abdominal pain, or malaise that these patients experience. The problem with these studies is that therapy was initiated well into the course of diarrhea (usually 4 or 5 days after the onset of illness). It is possible that earlier therapy, (e.g., in a sibling of a known patient or in a day care center outbreak) might shorten the clinical course. Considering the low cost and minimal toxicity of erythromycin, it seems worthwhile to use this drug in confirmed and highly suspected cases of *Campylobacter* gastroenteritis. The bacteriologic effects of therapy might reduce spread; however, handwashing and hygienic precautions are also important control measures. In-hospital treatment should include careful disposal of excreta, doublebagging of bed clothes and bedding, and handwashing and excretion precautions.

The in vitro susceptibilities of *Campylobacter* are outlined in the accompanying table. Based on these data, and on clinical results, erythromycin is the drug of choice for treatment of gastrointestinal campylobacteriosis. In rare instances, organisms resistant to erythromycin have been reported. Thus, in vitro susceptibility tests are indicated in cases apparently resistant to antibacterial treatment.

Table 1. *CAMPYLOBACTER*—IN VITRO SUSCEPTIBILITIES

Highly susceptible to:	Thienamycin (investigational) Erythromycin Gentamicin, amikacin, tobramycin Tetracycline Furazolidine
Moderately (or variably) susceptible to:	Ampicillin Cefotaxime Chloramphenicol Moxalactam Clindamycin Trimethoprim/sulfamethoxazole
Resistant to:	Penicillins (including cloxacillin, carbenicillin, ticarcillin) Vancomycin Rifampin Cephalothin Cefamandole Metronidazole

Extragastrointestinal *Campylobacter* infections. When infection becomes bacteremic or involves joints or other extragastrointestinal foci, aminoglycosides should be used. Gentamicin in a dose of 5 to 7.5 mg/kg (divided q8h) intravenously is recommended. Therapy should be continued for at least a week after clinical defervescence and bacteriologic eradication in normal hosts, and 2 weeks in immunocompromised patients. Stool cultures should also be obtained in these patients and, should the stools be positive, appropriate hygiene and isolation procedures carried out. Drainage may also be necessary in certain localized infections.

In the rare case of *Campylobacter* meningitis, chloramphenicol, 75 mg/kg/day, or ampicillin, 400 mg/kg/day,* may be used. Even when high doses of these drugs are used, the cerebrospinal fluid concentrations may be inadequate to treat some cases of campylobacteriosis. If infection is persistent, therefore, combinations of ampicillin and gentamicin should be tried. Should thienamycin (currently investigational in the United States) prove clinically efficacious, it may become the drug of choice for extragastrointestinal campylobacteriosis.

Yersinia enterocolitica Infections

MELVIN I. MARKS, M.D.

Yersinia enterocolitica are gram-negative bacilli that frequently cause gastroenteritis in temperate climates in many countries of the world; however, these infections seem to be relatively infrequent in

---

*This dose may exceed that recommended by the manufacturer.

the United States. Several outbreaks in the U.S. have been associated with contaminated milk products, dogs, and cats. Invasion beyond the gastrointestinal tract is generally restricted to immunocompromised patients, although some normals may occasionally have bacteremia, septic arthritis, and focal abscesses. Rarely, deaths have been reported.

TREATMENT

Gastroenteritis. Guidelines for treatment of yersiniosis are gleaned from in vitro susceptibilities (Table 1) and clinical experience. However, a placebo-controlled prospective study showed no clinical or bacteriologic advantage of antibiotic therapy in children with *Yersinia* gastroenteritis. Therefore, as for *Salmonella* gastroenteritis, treatment is generally not recommended for *Y. enterocolitica* infections confined to the gastrointestinal tract. Exceptions are listed in Table 2. In such cases, treatment with trimethoprim-sulfamethoxazole* in a dose of 5 to 10 mg/kg/day (trimethoprim, 25–50 mg/kg/day; sulfamethoxazole, divided tid) is recommended. This treatment may shorten the course of fever and diarrhea if used early, but this is only theoretically possible, since the only controlled clinical study initiated therapy well into the course of illness. The intended function of the treatment in these cases is prevention of extragastrointestinal infection. Hence, treatment should be discontinued when diarrhea and fever subside.

Treatment of *Y. enterocolitica* gastroenteritis should include hygienic instructions about handwashing, particularly in relation to food-handling, bathing, and defecation. In hospital, excretion precautions and handwashing should be carried out.

Table 1. IN VITRO SUSCEPTIBILITIES OF *YERSINIA ENTEROCOLITICA*

Highly susceptible to:	Trimethoprim/sulfamethoxazole Aminoglycosides (gentamicin, amikacin, tobramycin) Cefotaxime Moxalactam
Moderately (or variably) susceptible to:	Kanamycin Tetracycline Chloramphenicol Rifampin
Resistant to:	Ampicillin Erythromycin Penicillin Cloxacillin Cephalothin Carbenicillin

*This use is not listed by the manufacturer. Not recommended for infants less than 2 months of age.

Table 2. INDICATIONS FOR ANTIBIOTIC THERAPY OF *YERSINIA ENTEROCOLITICA* GASTROENTERITIS

Under three months of age
Leukemia/lymphoma
Acquired or congenital immune deficiency disease
Moderate/severe malnutrition
Thalassemia
Appendicitis
Ulcerative colitis or other inflammatory bowel disease
Associated symptomatic intestinal parasitosis

Extragastrointestinal *Yersiniosis.* Extragastrointestinal *Y. enterocolitica* infections are rare, but can be life-threatening. When present, these should be treated aggressively with aminoglycosides or third generation cephalosporins. My choice is cefotaxime in a dose of 100–150 mg/kg/day divided qid. If the patient is able to take oral medication and therapy can be monitored by bacteriologic and microbiologic criteria, trimethoprim-sulfamethoxazole* should be used in the higher doses described above. Serum or other body fluid bactericidal activity should be followed to ensure adequate absorption and distribution of antibiotic. In most cases, therapy should be continued for a week after bacteriologic and clinical resolution, although 2 weeks are indicated in immunocompromised patients and in those with infections of the central nervous system. Surgical drainage of abscesses should also be carried out, if possible.

Like salmonellosis, infections in bones and meninges may relapse and recur weeks to months after therapy is discontinued. Thus, I treat these patients for long periods of time during their initial course of illness. For meningitis, this means at least 2 weeks after bacteriologic and clinical defervescence. In early bone infection, 6 weeks will usually suffice. When radiologic evidence of bone destruction is present at the time of initial therapy, at least 3 months of monitored antibiotic therapy are required. The Wintrobe erythrocyte sedimentation rate should be normal, and clinical and radiologic features favorable, before discontinuing antibiotics. Some detective work should also be carried out to ensure that repeated exposures to infection in animal or food reservoirs can be avoided for the patient and other contacts.

Brucellosis

ROBERT-GRAY CHOTO, M.D.

Brucellosis is a worldwide disease acquired primarily from domestic ungulates but also found in wild ungulates and other animals. Synonyms are undulant fever, Mediterranean fever, rock fever, Neapolitan fever, Cyprus fever, and mimic disease.

The infective organism is a gram-negative, non-capsulated, nonsporulating pleomorphic bacillus, *Brucella* sp. Person-to-person transmission is unknown except following transfusion of blood from infected donors. Because it is primarily an occupational disease (livestock farming, abattoir, veterinary, and laboratory workers), the 20 to 50 year age group is the most frequently infected.

The treatment choice for children includes tetracycline,* 20 to 40 mg/kg/24 hr orally in four divided doses; streptomycin, 25 to 40 mg/kg/24 hr IM in two divided doses; trimethoprim-sulfamethoxazole†, 5 to 10 mg/kg/24 hr orally in two to three divided doses; or triple sulfonamides,‡ 150 mg/kg/24 hr in four divided doses. For adults tetracycline is given, 2 gm/24 hr orally in four divided doses, or streptomycin, 1 to 2 gm/24 hr in 2 divided doses. All treatments are for 21 days.

In acutely ill patients, a 3-day course of glucocorticoids may avert a Herxheimer reaction. Relapses are less frequent with combination therapy with tetracycline and streptomycin. Repeat treatment is necessary if positive cultures persist or recur.

Tularemia

(Rabbit Fever; Deer Fly Fever)

CHRYSTIE C. HALSTED, M.D.

Tularemia is an uncommon and underdiagnosed infectious disease existing in nature as a zoonosis. In human beings, the spectrum of tularemia varies from asymptomatic infection to severe and fatal disease. The manifestations of illness are related in part to the type of exposure as well as to the type of the infecting organism.

The estimated 5% mortality in untreated ulceroglandular disease and 30% mortality with untreated pneumonic tularemia caused by the more virulent type A *Francisella tularensis* organisms can be eliminated by early, appropriate antibiotic therapy. Streptomycin, 30 mg/kg/24 hr, given IM in two divided doses for a 7- to 10-day course, is the treatment of choice. This regimen results in prompt defervescence of symptoms over 24 to 48 hours. Gentamicin in usual therapeutic doses has shown clinical efficacy in the treatment of tularemia in adults, a finding anticipated by its demonstrated in vitro bactericidal effect against *Francisella tularen-*

sis. Although gentamicin offers no therapeutic advantage over streptomycin in the treatment of tularemia, it has proved effective for the treatment of unsuspected tularemia when used empirically in the clinical setting of pneumonia and fever of unknown origin.

While other antibiotics, such as chloramphenicol and tetracycline, have been effective in treating the acute phase of tularemia, they have been associated with failure to eradicate the organisms, and relapse of disease may occur when they are discontinued. These relapses are not related to acquired antibiotic resistance by the organism, and thus a repeated course of treatment will again cause defervescence. Use of tetracycline and chloramphenicol for treatment of tularemia should be reserved for the unusual clinical setting in which streptomycin is contraindicated.

Plague

RUSSELL VAN DYKE, M.D., *and* JAMES D. CONNOR, M.D.

Plague is a bacterial disease caused by *Yersinia pestis.* It is usually contracted from the bite of a flea of an infected rodent, but can occur following direct contact with an infected rodent, rabbit, or carnivore. Person-to-person transmission can occur with pneumonic plague. Bubonic plague (plague lymphadenitis) is the usual form of the disease, with secondary septicemia, pneumonia, and meningitis as complications. Primary pneumonic plague, acquired by inhalation, is a fulminant disease, extremely contagious and with a high mortality.

Since plague carries a high mortality and a high risk of pneumonic transmission if treatment is delayed, specific therapy and isolation procedures must be initiated on clinical and epidemiologic grounds, prior to microbiologic confirmation.

Antibiotic Therapy

Streptomycin is the antibiotic of choice, given intramuscularly in a dose of 30 mg/kg/day in two to four divided doses for 10 days. Dividing the streptomycin into four daily doses early in the course may help prevent a Herxheimer-like reaction due to massive release of endotoxin from rapidly killed organisms. Since resistance to streptomycin can occur, the addition of a second antibiotic is suggested. Tetracycline, given orally (30–40 mg/kg/day) or intravenously if necessary (15–25 mg/kg/day) in four divided doses for 10 to 14 days is usually added. In children less than 8 years old, in pregnant women, and in patients with plague meningitis, chloramphenicol (75–100 mg/kg/day) should be substituted for tetracycline. Chloramphenicol levels should be monitored and the dose

---

*Use of tetracycline during infancy and childhood to age 8 years may cause permanent discoloration of the teeth.

†This specific use is not listed in the manufacturer's official directive. Also, not recommended for infants less than 2 months of age.

‡Manufacturer's Precaution: Not indicated in infants less than 2 months of age.

adjusted accordingly. Other antibiotics have unacceptable failure rates or inadequate clinical experience and are not recommended.

Supportive Therapy

Patients require close observation and therapy for complications including septic shock, disseminated intravascular coagulation, convulsions, pneumonia, and respiratory failure. Needle aspiration of a bubo is necessary for bacteriologic diagnosis. Incision and drainage are not warranted initially, but may become necessary if a fluctuant bubo persists despite antibiotic therapy. A bubo may take several weeks to resolve.

Isolation

Plague is a quarantinable disease and suspected cases should be reported to public health officials immediately. A case investigation, including identification of contacts, and initiation of rodent and vector control measures should follow. Strict isolation of all suspected cases of plague is necessary since pneumonic plague can present with little or no evidence of pulmonary involvement. Pneumonic plague poses a major hazard to contacts and health care workers. The use of scrub suits, cover gowns, face masks (including eye protection), and cover boots must be strictly enforced.

In patients without pneumonia or draining lesions, strict isolation can be discontinued following 72 hours of antibiotic therapy if sputum cultures are negative. The patient's clothing should be sterilized and the patient treated with an insecticide such as 2% carbaryl if fleas are present. All material leaving the patient's room, including laboratory specimens, should be handled with gloves and transported with caution. Laboratory personnel should be alerted to the possible hazard. All sheets, waste materials, instruments, urine, and feces should be autoclaved or incinerated.

Prophylaxis

Chemoprophylaxis is recommended for persons who have close contact with a patient with plague pneumonia or septicemic plague and for household contacts of patients with flea-borne plague of any clinical type. Oral tetracycline (15–30 mg/kg/day) or a sulfonamide (40–60 mg/kg/day) in four divided doses for 10 days may be used. All contacts, including medical personnel, should be under close surveillance and must have their temperature recorded twice daily for 10 days. Contacts who develop fever or other symptoms compatible with plague should be immediately hospitalized for antibiotic therapy and further evaluation.

Immunization

A formalin-killed plague vaccine available in the United States provides limited protection against illness and death. A history of plague immunization *does not* eliminate plague as a diagnostic possibility in a compatible case. Immunization should be considered for travelers to rural Vietnam, Cambodia, and Laos. Immunization is indicated for high risk individuals working in the field or laboratory with *Yersinia pestis* or with potentially infected rodents and fleas. The primary immunizing series consists of three doses of vaccine. In the adult, the first dose, 1.0 ml, is followed by the second dose, 0.2 ml, 4 weeks later. The third dose, 0.2 ml, is administered 6 months after the first dose. When required because of continuing exposure, three subsequent booster doses should be given at 6 month intervals. Thereafter, booster doses are given at 1 to 2 year intervals. For children less than 11 years of age, the dose of vaccine is reduced but the intervals between injections are the same as for adults (see Table 1). For more details regarding plague immunization, see *Morbidity and Mortality Weekly Report*, June 11, 1982, pp. 301–304.

Tuberculosis

EDWIN L. KENDIG, Jr., M.D.

Children and adolescents who show a positive reaction to tuberculin testing should receive antimicrobial therapy. Particular therapy is determined by the duration and extent of disease.

GENERAL THERAPY

Whenever a child has been found to be tuberculin-positive, location and removal of the tuberculosis contact must be accomplished as soon as possible. This search entails tuberculin testing and a chest roentgenogram of all adult contacts, including parents, grandparents, babysitters, household servants, and any others who may have been in contact with the child.

An adequate diet and the usual vitamin supplement for a growing child are necessary, but the question of bed rest varies with the type of disease. The child with asymptomatic primary tuberculosis requires no limitation of activity, and even those

Table 1.

Dose Number	Age (years)			
	Under 1	*1–4*	*5–10*	*Over 11*
1	0.2 ml	0.4 ml	0.6 ml	1.0 ml
2 and 3	0.04 ml	0.08 ml	0.12 ml	0.2 ml
Boosters*	0.02–0.04 ml	0.04–0.08 ml	0.06–0.12 ml	0.1–0.2 ml

*Smaller dose volume may be used if severe side effects are expected.

who are acutely ill should be allowed some activity as soon as possible, since it is recognized that complete bed rest may result in undesirable negative calcium and nitrogen deficiencies.

The child should be protected from intercurrent infection, since not only measles but also any acute infection or alteration in physiology, immunity, or metabolism, may lower resistance. The tuberculin-positive child who has measles while not then receiving therapy should be given isoniazid for a period of 8 weeks. The tuberculin-positive child who has not had measles should be protected by the use of measles vaccine, but should receive isoniazid therapy for a period of 8 weeks when the vaccine is administered. Other conditions requiring isoniazid prophylaxis include patients on adrenocorticosteroid therapy, surgical procedures requiring anesthesia, pertussis, and diabetes. Protection of the child from a source of tuberculous infection in the home is a necessity.

Chest roentgenograms at appropriate intervals are necessary.

Antimicrobial Agents

Isoniazid (INH). Isoniazid is the most effective antituberculosis agent yet available. It has a combined bactericidal and bacteriostatic action, penetrates the cell membrane, and moves freely into the cerebrospinal fluid and caseous tissue. After oral administration, a plasma concentration of 20 to 80 times the usual inhibiting concentration of the drug (0.05 μg/ml) may be attained within a few hours, and effective high concentrations persist for 6 to 8 hours. The drug may be found in the breast milk of mothers receiving INH therapy and may also cross the placental barrier. INH is excreted mainly in the urine.

The principal side effects of the drug are neurotoxic, manifested as convulsions or peripheral neuritis, and probably result from competitive inhibition of pyridoxine metabolism. Such side effects have been noted mainly in adults; however, a study of Pellock et al. (unpublished) suggests that pyridoxine deficiency in children is not unusual. At present, it is recommended only that precautions be exercised during adolescence. Pyridoxine, 25 to 50 mg daily, should be added to the treatment schedule during this period.

Rarely, isoniazid may be hepatotoxic. Since hepatic dysfunction is now reported more frequently (mainly in adults) than in previous years, the parent of the patient for whom INH is prescribed should be questioned carefully at monthly intervals for symptoms or signs of toxic effects of isoniazid. While studies appear to show that young children treated with INH show little tendency toward hepatotoxicity, the routine management at the Medical College of Virginia Child Chest Clinic includes serum bilirubin and serum glutamic ox-

aloacetic transaminase (SGOT) determination at the time of institution of treatment, again after 8 to 12 weeks of INH, and finally at the termination of therapy. If studies after 8 to 12 weeks show suspicious elevation of either serum bilirubin or SGOT levels, the patient is monitored closely until the levels return to normal values.

Other side effects are fever, gastrointestinal dysfunction, and many different types of skin rashes. When phenytoin (Dilantin) is given with isoniazid, interaction of the drugs may produce central nervous system symptoms, excessive sedation, and incoordination. Occasional reduction of the dose of phenytoin may be necessary. Patients receiving phenytoin or phenobarbital should be followed carefully.

The dosage of INH depends on the severity of the disease being treated. The drug is available for oral administration in tablets of 50, 100, and 300 mg, which may be crushed and administered in jam, preserves, or applesauce. A preparation for parenteral administration (intramuscular or intrathecal) is also available, but is seldom used. A chemical test for the presence of INH in the urine may help in determining patient compliance.

Although primary isoniazid-resistant tuberculosis has been reported in children, the significance has not yet been determined. Certainly the recommendation that initial therapy in children should be based on the drug-susceptibility pattern of the source case should be heeded.

Streptomycin (SM). Streptomycin was isolated from *Streptomyces griseus* in 1944 and became the first effective antibiotic agent against tuberculosis. The drug is bacteriostatic and bactericidal, acting to interfere with protein synthesis in tubercle bacilli. Intracellular penetration by the drug is relatively low. The drug usually inhibits growth of the tubercle bacillus in a concentration of 1.6 μg/ml. After parenteral administration, the drug rapidly appears in the blood stream, reaching a peak value in 2 hours. It diffuses into the pleural fluid, but does not pass the cerebrospinal fluid barrier to any appreciable extent unless there is inflammation of the meninges. Streptomycin is largely excreted in the urine, with an 80% recovery within 24 hours after administration.

The principal toxic effect of streptomycin is involvement of the eighth cranial nerve. Although loss of vestibular function may be permanent, children usually adjust without symptoms. Involvement of the auditory branch is a real danger, but this is much less frequent now than in the days of prolonged streptomycin therapy. Allergic manifestations such as fever and dermatitis may occur, and agranulocytosis has been reported.

The drug is never used as the sole therapeutic agent because of the rapid development of resistance. It is routinely given with at least one other tuberculostatic agent.

Streptomycin is administered by intramuscular injection in a suggested dosage of 20 mg/kg body weight/24 hr, with a maximal daily dosage of 1 gram. Streptomycin is supplied in crystalline form, usually as a sulfate, in vials containing 1 gram.

Para-Aminosalicylic Acid (PAS). Para-aminosalicylic acid has some bacteriostatic activity against the tubercle bacillus, suppressing growth and multiplication, and when used in conjunction with isoniazid or streptomycin acts to delay microbial resistance to these drugs. The chief value of PAS is that it apparently competes with isoniazid for acetylation in the liver, thereby increasing the amount of free isoniazid in the blood.

PAS is given orally and is readily absorbed. It diffuses into serous surfaces and reaches the cerebrospinal fluid in small amounts. PAS has no intracellular activity. It is rapidly excreted in the urine.

Gastrointestinal disturbances (nausea, abdominal distress, anorexia) are the principal toxic manifestations, but hypokalemia, goitrogenic effect, jaundice, and leukopenia may occur. PAS may also cause allergic reactions, including dermatoses and an otherwise unexplained fever.

Children usually have a much better tolerance for PAS than do adults. The drug should be prescribed in a dosage of 200 mg/kg body weight/24 hr in three divided doses. (Tolerance is increased in some patients when a smaller dose is used initially.) PAS is tolerated better after meals. When salts of para-aminosalicylic acid (sodium, potassium, calcium) are used, the dosage should be correspondingly higher: 250 to 300 mg/kg body weight/24 hr (maximum daily dose, 12 grams). PAS is supplied in 0.5-gram tablets, as a powder, or as a solution of the sodium salt. The solution is rarely used since it is stable for only 24 hours, and then only if kept in the dark and refrigerated.

Ethambutol (EMB). Ethambutol is an effective antimicrobial agent that acts by delaying the multiplication of bacteria through interference with RNA synthesis. It is rapidly excreted in the urine. Resistance to the drug develops slowly, and, like PAS, when given in combination with other antimicrobial agents it delays the onset of microbial resistance. It is also better tolerated and has less tendency to produce toxic effects than PAS. The drug is used mainly in adults, in whom it appears to have largely replaced PAS.

Retrobulbar neuritis, with resulting blindness, may occur but this is uncommon at recommended dosage levels. Monthly or bimonthly screening, including studies for visual acuity, color vision, and visual fields, is indicated, however. The drug should be discontinued if there is a 2-line loss of visual acuity as measured on the Snellen eye chart,

if there is contraction of the visual fields, or if there is loss of color vision. In view of this, ethambutol is rarely used in young children or when communication is difficult.

The dosage utilized for children at the Medical College of Virginia is 10 to 15 mg/kg body weight/24 hr.* The drug is supplied in 100-mg and 400-mg tablets and is administered in a single daily oral dose.

Rifampin (RIF). Rifampin is a derivative of *Streptomyces mediterranei.* The drug is bactericidal and inhibits DNA-dependent RNA polymerase. Rifampin is absorbed in all tissues but crosses the cerebrospinal fluid barrier only when there is infection. It crosses the placenta freely. Its teratogenic effect is not known.

Elimination is by way of the urine and bile, and the urine may appear orange to reddish brown in color. The same color may be noted in saliva, tears, sweat, sputum, and stool.

Rifampin thus far has been known to have few serious side effects. However, hepatotoxicity may occur, and, while this is usually transient, periodic monitoring by serum enzyme studies and serum bilirubin is indicated. Other side effects are gastrointestinal disturbances, dermatosis, thrombocytopenia, and reversible leukopenia. Particular care should be exercised when the patient is receiving both rifampin and isoniazid.† Pretreatment evaluation should include hematocrit, leukocyte and platelet counts, BUN, SGOT, and serum bilirubin determinations.

Rifampin may affect the pharmacologic action of other drugs given concurrently. It inhibits the action of coumarin. In adolescents receiving contraceptives, bleeding and pregnancy may occur. Other medications, such as para-aminosalicylic acid and barbiturates, inhibit the intestinal absorption of rifampin.

Rifampin is recommended for use in combination with at least one other antituberculosis drug. Although experience with children under 5 years of age is limited, dosage utilized at the Medical College of Virginia is 10 to 20 mg/kg body weight/24 hr, with a maximum daily dose of 600 mg.

Pyrazinamide. Pyrazinamide has so far been of little use in the treatment of tuberculosis in children. However, the drug is utilized in several of the short-course regimens for adult tuberculous disease and suggestion has been made that it be included in a similar short-course regimen for

---

*Manufacturer's Precaution: Not recommended for children under 13 years of age.

†When isoniazid and rifampin are used concurrently, the Center for Disease Control, Tuberculosis Division, recommends that the dosage of isoniazid should not exceed 10 mg/kg body weight/24 hr and the dosage of rifampin should not exceed 15 mg/kg body weight/24 hr.

children. It is bactericidal for intracellular bacilli within the macrophages but is not effective against extracellular bacilli. It may be hepatotoxic, and routine serum bilirubin and serum glutamic oxaloacetic transaminase (SGOT) determinations are indicated.

Other Drugs

Ethionamide, cycloserine, kanamycin, capreomycin, and viomycin are rarely used in the treatment of tuberculosis in children.

Adrenocorticosteroids

Apparently adrenocorticosteroids act to suppress the usual inflammatory response of the body with impairment of granulation tissue formation, macrophage activity, and fibroblastic repair. From this mechanism it appears likely that adrenocorticosteroids promote progression of tuberculous disease in the lung. This deleterious effect can be overcome, however, by specific, effective antimicrobial treatment. Indications for the use of adrenocorticosteroids in specific forms of tuberculosis will be presented under individual headings.

GENERAL PRINCIPLES OF ANTIMICROBIAL THERAPY

Isoniazid is at present the most effective antituberculosis drug known. Not only is it the most effective therapeutic agent but also it is the only drug proved to prevent complications of tuberculous disease. Thus, it must be included in every therapeutic regimen, unless contraindicated because of the patient's intolerance to the drug (allergy or hepatic dysfunction) or because the causative organism is isoniazid-resistant.

Isoniazid is used alone in the treatment of a positive tuberculin reaction and inactive primary tuberculosis (*Tuberculosis: no current disease*). However, there is some disagreement in regard to therapy of *active* primary tuberculosis. The use of two drugs is advised by some workers. While there is strong evidence that isoniazid *alone* is effective in preventing the vast majority of complications, certain instances of virulent infection or lowered host resistance may require the combined effect of two drugs, e.g., a young infant infected by a tuberculous mother.

In all other forms of tuberculosis, INH is used with at least one other drug: in such severe forms of tuberculosis as miliary tuberculosis and tuberculous meningitis. I favor a triple drug regimen. Therapy in children should be based on the drug-susceptibility pattern of the source case strain. If this information is unavailable, children with life-threatening forms of tuberculosis should be treated with three antimicrobial agents.

Positive Tuberculin Reaction (II Tuberculous infection, without disease). The Committee on Diagnostic Standards of the American Thoracic Society classifies the patient who has a positive tuberculin reaction with no other evidence of disease as *"Tuberculous infection, without disease."* However, it has been established that in more than 95% of cases the initial lesion of primary tuberculosis is in the lung parenchyma. If, therefore, a positive tuberculin reaction with no evidence of tuberculous disease elsewhere is found one must assume that there is a primary focus in the lung parenchyma, too small to be visible on roentgenogram, with associated regional gland involvement. However, *there is no clinical disease.*

All children and adolescents with a positive tuberculin reaction who have not previously had such treatment should receive INH, 10 to 15 mg/kg body weight/24 hr (maximum daily dosage, 300 mg), for a 1-year period. Periodic roentgenograms and the usual precautions (see Isoniazid) are advised.

For pregnant adolescents with a positive tuberculin reaction, it may be preferable to delay INH prophylaxis until after delivery.

Primary Pulmonary Tuberculosis (III Tuberculosis: current disease, lymphatic). The primary complex is composed of the primary focus, the involved regional lymph nodes, and the lymphatics between them. The most common form of primary tuberculosis (excluding the positive tuberculin reaction with no evidence of disease elsewhere) is the patient whose chest roentgenogram shows enlarged mediastinal lymph nodes with no demonstrable primary parenchymal focus.

The child with roentgenographic evidence of primary pulmonary tuberculosis should receive INH, 10 to 20 mg/kg body weight/24 hr (maximum daily dose, 400 mg) for a 1-year period. If the exposure to tuberculosis has been heavy or there is question as to host immunity (e.g., an infant exposed to a tuberculous mother), PAS, 200 mg/kg body weight/24 hr (maximum daily dose, 12 gm), or in certain instances, rifampin, 10 to 20 mg/kg/ body weight/24 hr (maximum daily dose, 600 mg), should be added to the regimen. Periodic roentgenograms and the usual precautions (see Isoniazid and Rifampin) are advised.

Progressive Primary Pulmonary Tuberculosis (III Tuberculosis: current disease, pulmonary). Local progression of the pulmonary components of the primary complex occasionally occurs and constitutes a more serious form of tuberculosis.

Treatment consists of INH, 10 to 20 mg/kg body weight/24 hr, with a maximum daily dose of 400 mg, and PAS, 200 mg/kg body weight/24 hr, with a maximum daily dose of 12 gm. Isoniazid is given in a single daily dose, and PAS is given in three divided doses. Rifampin may be necessary. Treatment should be continued for a 1-year period. The usual precautions are advised (see Isoniazid and Rifampin).

Obstructive Lesions of the Bronchus (Endobronchial Tuberculosis). Occasionally, endobronchial disease may result from penetration of the bronchus by caseous lymph nodes, resulting in caseous material or polypoid formation within the bronchus.

Bronchoscopy is desirable in such cases but should be carried out only if there are available an experienced bronchoscopist and an anesthesiologist, and the hospital is suitably equipped for the study of infants.

Treatment is the same as employed for progressive primary pulmonary tuberculosis, except that INH and rifampin are more often used. In addition, prednisone, 1 mg/kg body weight/24 hr for 6 to 12 weeks early in the course of the disease appears to give better results.

Pleurisy with Effusion. Any patient with a serous pleural effusion and a positive reaction to the tuberculin test must be assumed to have tuberculous pleurisy with effusion until proved otherwise. A diagnostic thoracentesis should always be done promptly. No more than 30 ml of fluid should be withdrawn unless the effusion is so massive that there is respiratory embarrassment. The fluid shows elevation of protein, and the cellular content, predominantly lymphocytes, except in the very early stage, varies from 200 to 10,000/ml³. Culture of the fluid should be done but will be useful only as a corroborative measure. Pleural biopsy may also be helpful.

Treatment consists of INH 15 to 20 mg/kg body weight/24 hr, and PAS, 200 mg/kg body weight/24 hr, and should be continued for at least 1 year. The addition of prednisone, 1 mg/kg body weight/24 hr, hastens the disappearance of pleural fluid. However, subsequent pulmonary function is not improved by the use of adrenocorticosteroids.

Miliary Tuberculosis. This is a generalized hematogenous disease, with multiple tubercle formation and manifestations that are more often pulmonary. Although recent studies in adults have shown that INH and rifampin are an effective mode of therapy in tuberculosis, I still prefer a three drug regimen in the treatment of such serious tuberculous disease.

The suggested treatment consists of INH, 20 mg/kg body weight/24 hr (maximum daily dose, 500 mg); rifampin, 10 to 20 mg/kg body weight/24 hr (maximum daily dose, 1 gm) and Streptomycin, 20 mg/kg body weight/24 hr. Streptomycin is continued for 1 month after satisfactory therapeutic response (usually 3 months), and INH and rifampin are continued for at least 1 year and often longer. Prednisone, 1 mg/kg body weight/24 hr, may be utilized in the management of occasional respiratory embarrassment. (See Isoniazid and Rifampin in regard to precautions.)

Chronic Pulmonary Tuberculosis (III Tuberculosis: current disease, pulmonary). This form of the disease usually occurs in adolescents. Since the lesions are extremely unstable in the adolescent, prompt therapy should be instituted and the patient carefully monitored. Antimicrobial therapy should consist of isoniazid, 10 mg/kg body weight/24 hr (maximum daily dose, 300 mg), and ethambutol,* 10 to 15 mg/kg body weight/24 hr, and should be continued for a period of 15 to 18 months. A short course treatment regimen with isoniazid and rifampin has been recommended for adults, and a recent study has demonstrated the effectiveness of such an approach in children. INH, 10–15 mg/kg body weight/24 hr (maximum daily dose, 300 mg), and rifampin, 10–15 mg/kg body weight/24 hr (maximum daily dose, 600 mg), is suggested for a 9 month period.

Extrapulmonary Tuberculosis.

TUBERCULOUS MENINGITIS. This is the most serious form of tuberculous disease. Before the advent of streptomycin it was presumably 100% fatal. At present, with the use of isoniazid and two other antituberculosis chemotherapeutic agents, the disease can almost always be cured if early diagnosis is established. Those treated early usually recover completely; if the diagnosis is delayed, there is more likelihood of neurologic sequelae or even a fatal outcome.

Therapy consists of isoniazid, 20 mg/kg body weight/24 hr (maximum daily dose, 500 mg); rifampin, 10 to 20 mg/kg body weight/24 hr (maximum daily dose, 600 mg); and streptomycin, 20 mg/kg body weight/24 hr (maximum daily dose, 1 gm).† The first two drugs are given for at least 1 year and streptomycin is given for 1 month after satisfactory clinical response, as determined by the general condition of the patient, disappearance of fever, and improvement in the cerebrospinal fluid picture. Antimicrobial agents appear to be effective in the treatment of tuberculous meningitis *if* they can reach the organism. Use of prednisone may decrease the likelihood of cerebrospinal fluid block, and, in addition, reduction of the inflammatory response may lessen the danger of irreversible thrombotic phenomena.

Promptness of response to antimicrobial therapy varies considerably. In general, the earlier the diagnosis, the more prompt will be the response. An affected child may lie in a stuporous, semicomatose, or even comatose state for months and finally effect an almost complete or even complete recovery.

TUBERCULOSIS OF THE SUPERFICIAL LYMPH NODES. A trigger mechanism is usually required for the activation of quiescent tubercle bacilli depos-

---

*Not recommended for children under 13 years of age.

†See Isoniazid and Rifampin discussions in regard to precautionary measures.

ited in foci throughout the body; this activation most often occurs in the superficial cervical lymph nodes. Obviously, lymphadenitis should be first treated with one of the wide-spectrum antibiotics or penicillin.

When a child has a positive tuberculin reaction and lymph nodes have been present for several weeks that measure 2 cm or more in diameter, are increasing in size, or showing early signs of suppuration, treatment is by excision and drug therapy. Isoniazid, 10 to 20 mg/kg body weight/24 hr (maximum daily dose, 400 mg), and PAS, 200 mg/kg body weight/24 hr (maximum daily dose, 12 gm), for a full year, are used. (Some workers favor rifampin instead of PAS.) If the mass of nodes is too great or if complete liquefaction of the nodes has already occurred and excision cannot be done, aspiration of the node (when liquefied) and the oral use of isoniazid and PAS may be effective. In my experience, medical treatment alone is usually not effective at this stage. Tonsillectomy is advised only if there are indications for it.

Infection with atypical mycobacteria may produce a picture identical to that caused by tuberculous infection. If the positive tuberculin reaction induration measures 5 to 9 mm in diameter, infection with one of the atypical mycobacteria probably exists.

RENAL TUBERCULOSIS. Tuberculosis of the kidney is blood-borne, and infection occurs either at the time of the early bacillemia or as part of generalized miliary tuberculosis. Symptoms and signs usually appear much later.

For renal tuberculosis, treatment should be carried out for 1 year. The therapeutic regimen should be INH, 10 to 20 mg/kg body weight/24 hr (maximum daily dose, 300 mg), and rifampin, 10 to 20 mg/kg body weight/24 hr (maximum daily dose, 600 mg).* Since there is a possibility that ureteral stricture may appear during therapy, an intravenous pyelogram and ureteral calibration every 4 to 6 months during treatment and annually thereafter for 10 years seem advisable.

TUBERCULOSIS OF THE BONES AND JOINTS. Most frequently involved are the head of the femur (hip), the vertebrae, and the fingers and toes. Treatment consists of INH, 10 to 20 mg/kg body weight/24 hr (maximum daily dose, 300 mg), and rifampin, 10 to 20 mg/kg body weight/24 hr (maximum daily dose, 600 mg), for 12 to 18 months. (See discussions in INH and Rifampin.)

All superficial and accessible abscesses should be drained. Immobilization of nonweight-bearing structures is not necessary; however, if weight-bearing structures (vertebrae, hip, and others) are involved, whatever means are necessary to prevent weight-bearing are carried out. The use of plaster casts and spinal fusion is seldom necessary.

INTRA-ABDOMINAL TUBERCULOSIS. This is rare in children. Tuberculous enteritis is usually secondary to a lung lesion and there is nearly always involvement of the mesenteric lymph nodes. In addition to INH and PAS therapy, as for progressive primary tuberculosis, the usual general measures for tuberculosis are necessary, and a low-residue diet of adequate caloric and vitamin content is also helpful. Therapy is otherwise symptomatic.

Tuberculosis of the mesenteric and retroperitoneal lymph nodes usually does not require local treatment. Rarely, excision of enlarged or calcified abdominal lymph nodes may be necessary for relief of pain.

Tuberculous peritonitis is treated as is progressive primary pulmonary tuberculosis. If exploratory laparotomy is required to establish the diagnosis, it is essential that suitable biopsy material be obtained for tissue section and bacteriologic study. If there is an associated enteritis, a low-residue diet provides some symptomatic relief. Adrenocorticosteroid therapy may also be helpful.

Other Indications for Antimicrobial Therapy. Any tuberculin-positive child who receives adrenocorticosteroid therapy for another disease should be given concurrent isoniazid therapy, 10 to 15 mg/kg body weight (maximum daily dose, 300 mg). The same treatment is necessary when there is any acute infection or alteration in physiology, immunity, or metabolism (see General Therapy).

Tuberculosis in the Neonate. Congenital tuberculosis rare (a few more than 300 cases have been reported) and the likelihood is almost nonexistent unless the mother has far-advanced pulmonary disease, generalized tuberculous infection, or genitourinary tract tuberculosis. Naturally, the placenta should be carefully examined. However, the infant may become infected at delivery or in early infancy.

The choice of prophylaxis for infants born of tuberculous mothers seems to lie between a single injection (BCG) and daily oral medication with isoniazid (10 to 15 mg/kg) for 1 year. The value of INH prophylaxis has been well demonstrated, and, properly administered, it probably constitutes the most efficacious approach. However, the problem of parent compliance makes BCG vaccination a logical choice for prevention of tuberculosis in infants of tuberculous mothers. Management of these infants varies with the severity of disease in the mother and the antimicrobial therapy received by her.

If the mother has noncavitary pulmonary tuberculosis for which she has been receiving antimicrobial therapy for at least 1 month, the infant should have a roentgenogram of the chest and a

---

*See Isoniazid and Rifampin discussions.

tuberculin skin test. If both roentgenogram and tuberculin reaction are negative, the infant should be given BCG vaccine and left with the mother. Decision as to the breastfeeding of infants born of tuberculous mothers must be individualized. However, if the mother has evidence of hematogenous tuberculosis or far-advanced pulmonary disease with sputum positive for tubercle bacilli, the infant should be isolated from the mother; since tuberculous infection may already have been acquired, although not demonstrable, the infant should receive INH, 15 to 20 mg/kg body weight for 3 months. At the end of that period the patient's chest roentgenogram and tuberculin reaction should be negative before the administration of BCG vaccine. The infant should then be isolated from the mother for an additional 6 weeks and until the mother is no longer considered to have active or infectious disease.

If the infant has already acquired tuberculous infection, isoniazid, 15 to 20 mg/kg body weight, and rifampin, 10 to 20 mg/kg body weight, should be administered for at least 1 year.

THE PREVENTION OF TUBERCULOSIS

Three methods have been shown to be reasonably effective in preventing tuberculosis: isolation of those adults with infectious tuberculosis, use of BCG vaccine, and administration of isoniazid to household contacts of tuberculous patients.

Studies by the United States Public Health Service have shown that the use of isoniazid in all household contacts results in less tuberculous disease during the year of prophylactic therapy and in a continuing good effect lasting at least 10 years following discontinuation of isoniazid therapy.

BCG vaccine has been conclusively shown to increase resistance to exogenous tuberculous infection and is mainly of use in this country to those children living in a home in which there is an adult with infectious tuberculous disease, or one with potentially infectious disease, such as a mother who has been discharged from a sanatorium with apparently arrested tuberculosis. It is also useful in population groups in which there is a high incidence of tuberculous infection. A main disadvantage of BCG vaccination is said to be the positive tuberculin reaction that results. In our experience with the vaccine *manufactured in the United States** the resultant positive tuberculin reaction induration nearly always measures 5 to 9 mm and rarely above 12 mm in diameter. If the reaction is 15 mm or more in diameter of induration, the physician can be reasonably assured that there has been infection with

virulent tubercle bacilli, and the patient should receive isoniazid therapy.

To be eligible for BCG vaccination, the patient must have a negative tuberculin reaction (PPD 5TU) and a negative chest roentgenogram within the previous 2 weeks. Eight to 12 weeks after vaccination, the same procedures should be carried out. At this time the tuberculin reaction should be, and practically always is, positive; if this is not the case, the vaccination is repeated.

Two methods of BCG vaccination are available: 1) multiple puncture disk method, and 2) intradermal injection. The former is the preferable procedure.

Leprosy

ROBERT R. JACOBSON, M.D., PH.D.

Leprosy (Hansen's disease) is a chronic infectious disease. It has been reported below age 1, but is very rare before age 2. Several different types occur, depending on the host's ability to generate a cell-mediated immune response to the causative agent, *Mycobacterium leprae.* The earliest form in all cases is referred to as indeterminate and if not treated may progress to one of the three common types: tuberculoid, borderline (dimorphous), or lepromatous. The borderline portion of the leprosy spectrum is further divided into borderline-tuberculoid, mid-borderline, and borderline-lepromatous. Treatment is relatively simple and straightforward unless reactive episodes develop. These occur in 40 to 50% of cases in the form of reversal (type 1) reactions in tuberculoid and borderline patients and erythema nodosum leprosum (ENL or type 2 reactions) in lepromatous patients. The aims of treatment, then, are to clear the infection and control reaction, thus preventing further neural, cutaneous, eye or renal damage.

The sulfones are the treatment of choice and the only approved therapy in the United States. Pretreatment evaluation should include a complete blood count, urinalysis, liver function tests, a G-6-PD screening test, skin scrapings and/or biopsy, and a complete physical examination. All adult cases are started immediately and maintained on 100 mg of dapsone daily (DDS, Avlosulfon). Typical pediatric doses: ages 12 to 18 years, 50 mg daily; ages 6 to 12 years, 25 mg daily; ages 2 to 5 years, 25 mg three times a week; ages 6 months to 23 months, 12 mg three times a week; and under 6 months, 6 mg three times a week. It is also recommended that all borderline and lepromatous cases also receive rifampin*(600 mg daily in adults) for at

---

*Manufactured by ITR Biomedical Research, University of Illinois at the Medical Center, 904 West Adams Street, Chicago, Illinois 60607, and distributed by Antigen Supply House, 8751 Shirley Avenue, Northridge, California 91324.

*This use is not listed by the manufacturer.

least the first 3 years of therapy to prevent the occasional emergence of sulfone resistant *M. leprae*.

Hemolysis is the only common side effect. Usually this is mild and rarely necessitates changing therapy except in some G-6-PD deficient patients and occasionally others. Other side effects are rare and include agranulocytosis, methemoglobinemia, exfoliative dermatitis, peripheral neuropathies, hypoalbuminemia, various gastrointestinal complaints, hepatitis, cholestatic jaundice, psychosis, headaches, and an infectious mononucleosis-like syndrome.

Sulfone resistant strains of *M. leprae* develop in some lepromatous and borderline cases, usually after prolonged irregular or low dose sulfone therapy, and cases of primary sulfone resistance are now being reported. Adult cases may be treated with 600 mg of rifampin plus 250 mg of ethionamide daily or 100 mg of clofazimine* (Lamprene, B663) daily plus either rifampin or ethionamide. All of these therapies are investigational in the United States. The major side effect of rifampin and ethionamide has been hepatotoxicy. Clofazimine produces a reversible skin pigmentation, decreased sweating and tearing and various gastrointestinal complaints.

Because of the rising problem with both primary and secondary sulfone resistance the World Health Organization's Study Group on the Chemotherapy of Leprosy for Control Programs in 1982 recommended that all new and relapsed borderline and lepromatous cases be treated with a combination drug regimen consisting of 100 mg of dapsone with 50 mg of clofazimine daily taken unsupervised plus 600 mg of rifampin with 300 mg of clofazimine given under supervision once monthly. This combination would be continued for at least 2 years and preferably to inactivity and then discontinued. Indeterminate and tuberculoid cases would be treated for only 6 months with just the dapsone plus rifampin. While this approach has much to recommend it, uncertainty as to the efficacy of only 6 months of therapy in mild cases and the advisability of discontinuing therapy in lepromatous patients together with the refusal of many patients to take clofazimine because of the resulting skin pigmentation have thus far limited its application in the United States.

Inactivity for a leprosy case is defined as negative (for bacilli) skin scrapings or biopsies for at least 1 year and no clinical evidence of activity, such as progressive neural deficits, reactions, or new skin lesions. This will usually take 1 to 2 years for indeterminate and tuberculoid cases, and therapy is then continued 3 more years. Borderline cases typically require 2 to 6 years of therapy to attain an inactive status and therapy is then continued 5 to 10 more years. Lepromatous and borderline-lepromatous cases will require 5 to 10 years before becoming inactive, but the patients should remain on therapy for life as a prophylactic measure to prevent reactivation, since total bacterial clearance is unlikely in spite of skin scrapings or biopsies negative for bacilli.

Isolation of patients is unnecessary since most people (95 + %) are apparently not susceptible, and close contacts generally have had maximal exposure prior to diagnosis of the index case. Various studies indicate that therapy renders the patient noncommunicable within about 3 months on dapsone or clofazimine and about 1 week on rifampin. When transmission occurs it is generally a result of contact with a multibacillary case (mid-borderline, borderline-lepromatous, or lepromatous) and case finding efforts in countries of low prevalence such as the United States are usually limited to the household. Following diagnosis of a new case, contact examinations are done at 6- to 12-month intervals for 5 to 10 years. It is recommended by some authorities that all household contacts of newly diagnosed multibacillary patients under the age of 25 be given 3 years of dapsone prophylactically in full therapeutic doses.

Mild reversal reactions or erythema nodosum leprosum (ENL) may require no therapy, or symptomatic measures such as aspirin often suffice. Severe reactions are controlled with high doses of corticosteroids—usually 60 mg or more of prednisone in an adult. If prolonged therapy is required, the dose usually can be tapered to an every-other-day schedule. Alternatives are clofazimine (200 to 300 mg daily for an adult) or thalidomide (100 mg four times daily, tapered to 100 mg daily). Both are investigational, and, while clofazimine may be useful in either type of reaction, thalidomide is useful only for control of ENL. Corticosteroids must be used when a neuritis develops to reduce the likelihood of permanent nerve injury. Ophthalmologic complications such as iridocyclitis require prompt therapy if permanent eye damage is to be avoided, and patients with a lagophthalmos and decreased lacrimation are treated with tear substitutes to avoid development of an exposure keratitis. These cases should be followed by an ophthalmologist if possible.

Other aspects of treatment are also important. Patient education to help the patient and his or her family understand this disease generally improves compliance and the likelihood of a satisfactory outcome. Physical therapy is often a great value, such as in prevention of permanent contractures when motor loss has occurred, thus simplifying any future reconstructive surgery. The patient must be taught how to avoid injuries to insensitive areas. Treatment of these patients is challenging but very

---

*Investigational drug.

rewarding. It can, however, sometimes be very difficult, especially when prolonged episodes of reaction occur. Thus it is advisable to seek the assistance of experts if complications arise.

Nontuberculous (Atypical) Mycobacterial Infections

ANDREW M. MARGILETH, M.D.,

Positive skin test reactions to nontuberculous mycobacterial (NTM) PPD antigens are common in school-age children, especially in the southern and mid-eastern Atlantic states. However, NTM disease represent < 5% of tuberculous granulomatous infections in infants and children. Although *Mycobacterium tuberculosis* (TB) as a cause of adenopathy has been recognized for centuries, lymphadenitis due to NTM has been reported for only 40 years. The natural history of NTM infections is still not clear and clinical diagnosis may be difficult.

CLINICAL FEATURES. The most common presentation of NTM infection in children is chronic cervical lymphadenopathy. Cutaneous (swimming-pool) granuloma and pulmonary disease occur less often. These patients appear healthy, and systemic symptoms are usually absent. Persistent cervical lymphadenopathy (> 3 weeks) in a healthy child with a mildly reactive (5 to 14 mm) tuberculin PPD-T, 5 TU, strongly suggests tuberculous adenitis. In our 13-year study of 112 children (17 infants) with NTM disease the nodes usually were mildly tender and at a single site, i.e., submandibular, anterior-superior, sub- or preauricular in 90%. Lymph nodes were unilateral in 85% and fluctuant in 32%. Of the 112 patients, 109 had cervical lymphadenitis; skin lesions (granuloma, abscess, or sinus) were noted in 18 (16%), fever in 20 (18%), and pharyngitis and/or upper respiratory infection in 22 (20%).

A presumptive distinction between TB and NTM disease prior to aspiration or biopsy can be made based on the history, physical findings, chest x-ray and results of differential PPD skin tests (Table 1). Of 836 infants and children PPD-tested for chronic adenopathy and/or a cutaneous mass during 13 years (1967 to January 1981), 134 (16%) had positive PPD tests. Based on further studies (repeat PPD tests and cultures of biopsied or aspirated nodes or abscess), 115 had NTM infections (112 with adenitis and 3 with skin granuloma). Of the remainder, 19 had adenitis due to TB.

Management

Lymphadenopathy. Treatment initially depends on the presumptive diagnosis. If atypical adenitis is suspected, we recommend excisional biopsy only.

Of 112 children, 93 (83%) had excisional biopsy, 6 (5%) had incisional biopsy and 9 (8%) were treated medically. In those treated by excisional biopsy results were excellent (84%); minor complications occurred in 15% (Table 2). Incisional biopsy and/or drainage (I & D) resulted in suppuration and sinus formation for 2 to 18 months in all 10 patients; this is not recommended.

Of nine patients treated medically during 4- to 9-year follow-up lymphadenopathy persisted for 6 months to 9 years, with gradual resolution in six children. Local intermittent sinus drainage and occasional extrusion of caseous material occurred for 2 to 12 months in two children. Two of the nine children received isoniazid (INH) for 3 to 6 months with no apparent effect. No chemotherapy was given to the other seven patients.

Chemotherapy: Specific Indications

In 41 (40%) of the 102 patients operated on, antituberculous medications were prescribed for periods of 3 weeks to 13 months: 1) INH, 15 to 20 mg/kg daily, alone in 12; 2) INH and PAS, 200 mg/kg daily, in 16; 3) INH and rifampin (RMP), 10 to 20 mg/kg daily, in 7 patients; 4) RMP alone in 6 patients. Most of the 41 patients were treated for several weeks to 9 months until culture results were known. Sensitivity studies in 18 of 42 positive atypical TB isolates showed that 16 strains were resistant to most of the antituberculous drugs tested; 5 were sensitive to rifampin (Table 3).

In our patients with NTM adenopathy the disease course was not modified by chemotherapy. Anti-TB chemotherapy is prescribed when 1) the family refuses surgical excision; 2) incisional drainage persists; 3) the TB contact and family history are positive; and 4) skin tests of the patient and/or family are PPD-T positive, especially if ≥ 15 mm, and/or are equal to or larger than the patient's NTM-PPD reactions. In these situations, INH and PAS or rifampin should be administered until cultures and antibiotic sensitivities are known, or until

---

Table 1. DIFFERENTIATION OF NONTUBERCULOUS MYCOBACTERIAL (NTM) INFECTIONS FROM HUMAN TUBERCULOSIS

	Mycobacterium Tuberculosis	*Atypical Mycobacteria*
History of contact*	Common	Rare
Lymphadenitis, cervical	Uncommon, bilateral	Common, unilateral
PPD-T skin test	15 mm or greater**	0 to 14 mm†
Chest roentgenogram	Pulmonary disease	Rarely abnormal
TBC chemotherapy	Effective	Ineffective, usually

*Person with active *M. tuberculosis* infection
**82% (18/22) patients initially tested, positive *M. tuberculosis* culture: PPD-T 100% positive (>15 mm) in 22/22 when retested
† 80% (39/49) patients retested with positive NTM cultures

Table 2. MANAGEMENT AND OUTCOME: 112 PATIENTS WITH CHRONIC LYMPHADENOPATHY
DUE TO NONTUBERCULOUS (ATYPICAL) MYCOBACTERIA (1967 TO JANUARY 1981)

Management	No. Patients	Percentage	Outcome	No. Patients	Percentage*
Aspiration and/or drainage incisional biopsy	10**	9	Suppuration and sinus formation (2–18 months)	10	100
No surgery or antimicrobial therapy	9†	8	Local drainage (2–12 months)	2	22
			Persistent lymphadenopathy (6 months to 9 years)	6	67
			Lost to follow-up	1	11
Surgical Excision	93‡	83	Excellent	79	85
			Local drainage (1–2 months)	4	4
			Local drainage (>2–6 months)	6	7
			Facial nerve paresis, transient	3	3
			Died (disseminated disease)	1	1
Totals	112	100		112	—

*Percentage of patients in each category.
**Nine patients had antituberculous chemotherapy, 6 had a poor or no response.
†Two patients had INH therapy, 3–6 months without effect.
‡Thirty patients had antituberculous chemotherapy with poor or no response.

Table 3. ANTIBIOTIC DOSAGE FOR NTM INFECTION OF LYMPH NODES,
SKIN OR PULMONARY DISEASE*

Drug	Dosage Daily kg/bw	Maximum Dosage Daily	Number of Doses Per Day	Duration of Therapy	Toxicity (Primary)
Isoniazid	15–20 mg	500 mg	1 or 2	≥12 months	Hepatic
PAS	200 mg	12 gm	3 or 4	≥12 months	Gastric
Rifampin**	10–20 mg	600 mg	1 or 2	6–12 months	Gastric
Ethambutol†	10–15 mg	—	1	≥12 months	Neuritis, optic
Minocycline	2.0 mg	400 mg	2	2–3 months	Dental, vertigo
Streptomycin‡ or	20–40 mg	1.0 gm	1 or 2	2–4 months	Oto/renal toxic
Kanamycin‡	10–15 mg	1.0 gm	1 or 2	2–4 months	Oto/renal toxic

*Rx to be continued if culture positive *M. tuberculosis:* excisional biopsy only is recommended for NTM adenopathy.
**Rifampin—when sputum negative for AFB, PAS or EMB may be substituted.
†Ethambutol (EMB) not recommended for children under age 6 years.
‡Streptomycin, kanamycin, single IM dose daily, then 3 × weekly after clinically improved.

healing is complete, which usually requires 2 to 6 months. Data are not available for determination of RMP dosage in children under age 5 years. If clinical response is satisfactory to the above drugs and/or cultures are positive for TB, treatment should be continued daily for 1 year or longer until healing is complete.

If NTM-PPD antigens are not available, a repeat PPD-T in 3 to 6 months that shows a larger reaction than before may help differentiate adenitis caused by NTM from that due to TB. Table 1 lists factors that may help direct initial management. A lack of response to antibiotics occurred in 76 of our 112 patients who had single or multiple antimicrobials, either alone or in combination (penicillin, ampicillin, cephalothin, tetracycline, sulfa preparations). However, some strains of *M. avium* (Group III) may be susceptible to erythromycin. *M. kansasii* (Group I) infections may respond to INH, rifampin, and ethambutol.

Skin

Cutaneous granulomas due to NTM infection are usually benign, self-limited, ulcerative or granulomatous lesions that develop several weeks after a minor abrasion incurred in fresh or salt water. If the lesions do not heal after several months' observation, excision is recommended. Minocycline, 2.0 mg/kg daily given orally for several months, may be effective. An 11-year-old took INH and PAS for 3 months after surgical excision of a knee granuloma. The lesion recurred in 2 months with a persistently positive culture of *M. marinum* (Group I). Minocycline, taken 4 months, was ineffective. Re-excision of the necrotizing granuloma and sinus tract was effective. An alternate plan in lieu of surgery is a combination of ethambutol,* 15 to 20 mg/kg

---

*Manufacturer's precaution: Ethambutol is not recommended for children under 13 years of age, since safe conditions for its use have not been established.

daily, and rifampin* orally for 6 to 12 months. Cultures of biopsy or aspirated material should be incubated at 30 to 33°C in a CO_2 atmosphere to enhance growth of *M. marinum.*

Pulmonary, Bone, or Disseminated Disease

Disseminated, bone, or pulmonary disease due to NTM is rare, and may be caused by *M. intracellularis, M. scrofulaceum, M. kansasii,* or *M. fortuitum. M. kansasii* infection usually responds to triple therapy: INH, ethambutol, and rifampin. One death due to disseminated *M. scrofulaceum* (Group II) occurred in our study. For severe infections due to the more drug-resistant NTM, a four-drug regimen is recommended: INH, ethambutol, rifampin, and daily IM streptomycin or kanamycin. Ethambutol, 25 mg/kg, is given daily for 2 months and then reduced to 15 mg/kg/day in one dose. Ethambutol is not recommended for children under 6 years of age. Monthly evaluation of visual acuity, visual fields, and tests for green color vision are essential. (See section on tuberculosis for toxicity and recommended tests for evaluation of liver, hepatic and urinary toxicity for INH, rifampin, and streptomycin.)

General Considerations

Isolation of patients is not necessary unless large amounts of caseous material are being discharged from the lesions. Atypical mycobacteria are difficult to grow. Since most are slow growers, it may take 2 to 5 months to ascertain the final type and antimicrobial sensitivities. These children should not be labeled "tuberculous." Careful follow-up, repeat PPD testing, and x-rays, if indicated, are necessary. Two of our patients had a relapse: one child with disseminated *M. scrofulaceum* infection subsequently died. The second child developed tuberculous tonsillitis following excision of a cervical NTM adenitis 2 years previously.

It is essential to distinguish these patients from those with TB infections in order to avoid unnecessary and prolonged courses of drugs as well as the stigma attached to a presumptive diagnosis of tuberculosis. Also, prophylactic INH therapy for healthy children who are positive NTM-PPD reactors is unnecessary. It must be hoped that NTM-PPD antigens will become available again in the near future.

For children with NTM disease we recommend surgical excision of the largest nodes or the skin granuloma. This is curative and provides material for histopathologic diagnosis and culture for mycobacteria. Alternatively, chemotherapy (INH, RMP, and/or ethambutol) may be effective for patients

with cervical adenopathy; minocycline may be effective for NTM skin granuloma. However, because of problems with compliance, parental concern, toxicity, and partial efficacy of these agents, the surgical approach is often most efficacious.

Syphilis

DAVID INGALL, M.D.

In the pediatric age group syphilis may be contracted via a congenital or acquired route. Infection from mother to fetus is more common than infection from person to person through contact with an infectious lesion during sexual activity (or abuse) in children. However, the teenage population appears to have an increasing incidence. In either circumstance, the etiologic agent, *Treponema pallidum,* continues to be sensitive to as little as 0.03 IU (0.018 ug/ml) of penicillin G. The essential goal of treatment is achievement of this treponemicidal level of antibiotic in the tissues that host the organism and maintenance of this concentration for a 10 day period during the spirochete's replication (once per 33 hours). This is accomplished best by parenteral administration of penicillin G.

Infection of the Fetus. Administration of parenteral penicillin G is the preferred drug in the gravid syphilitic just as it is in the nonpregnant adolescent or adult (vida infra). When administered in the first trimester, penicillin prevents fetal infection; thereafter it usually cures the disease. The alternative drug for penicillin allergic pregnant women is erythromycin, which crosses the placenta in an unpredictable fashion. Thus, the offspring of mothers treated prenatally with erythromycin should receive penicillin.

Congenital Syphilis. The infant at high risk for transplacental infection (positive cord blood VDRL) presents a perplexing diagnostic problem. A practical approach is to treat such patients at birth on the basis of certain frequent clinical occurrences: inability to document whether the mother has been treated or has received adequate therapy (penicillin and a falling VDRL titer): a low VDRL titer is consistent with latent maternal syphilis; the neonate may be infected and yet have no clinical manifestations at birth, and the mother-infant dyad may be noncompliant or lost to follow-up.

Prior to therapy, all infants with congenital syphilis should have a lumbar puncture to rule out neurosyphilis (positive VDRL in the cerebrospinal fluid [CSF]). Babies without clinical findings and with a negative CSF may be treated with 50,000 units/kg of benzathine penicillin G provided in a single dose. All other infants (those without clinical signs and with an abnormal CSF and those with clinical findings with or without an abnormal CSF)

---

*Manufacturer's precaution: Data are not available for determining dosage for children under 5 years of age.

should receive a 10 day course of either IM or IV aqueous penicillin G, twice a day, or IM procaine penicillin G, every day in a dose of 50,000 units/kg for at least 10 days. This conservative endorsement is based on the lack of proven efficacy of benzathene penicillin in congenital neurosyphilis plus the fact that the organism has been demonstrated in an otherwise normal CSF. Insufficient data do not permit recommendation of oral penicillin or alternative antibiotics in congenital syphilis.

After the first month of life, the same dose of penicillin is recommended as for congenital syphilis occurring during the neonatal period. In the young child, the total amount of penicillin should not exceed the dosage used for adolescents with syphilis of more than a year's duration (vida infra).

Erythromycin in the dose of 30 mg/kg/24 hours for 15 days is the only alternative agent for the penicillin allergic youngster less than 8 years of age. (Tetracycline is contraindicated below this age.) The dosage of erythromycin should not exceed the dose used for adolescents with syphilis of more than 1 year's duration (2 gm/day).

Adolescent Patient. Another sexually transmitted disease may coexist in a patient with syphilis and this should be kept in mind. Interviewing the patient in a positive interactional fashion for sexual contacts is an integral part of the management of the venereal disease patient. Such contacts may be unaware of their infection and thus not appreciate the need for diagnosis and treatment. Each physician should be cognizant of the law in his state concerning the treatment of venereal disease in this age group (minors) without parental consent.

The adolescent with early syphilis (primary, secondary, latent syphilis of less than 1 year's duration) should be treated with one injection of benzathene penicillin G, 2.4 million units total IM (1.2 million units in each buttock). For the patient who is allergic to penicillin, tetracycline is the recommended alternative antibiotic in a dose of 500 mg four times daily by mouth for 15 days. If the adolescent is intolerant of tetracycline, two options are available. Either erythromycin in a dose of 500 mg four times daily by mouth for 15 days may be substituted (treatment failures have been recorded) or, if compliance and serologic follow-up cannot be assured, the patient should be managed in a hospital with an expert consultant on desensitization to penicillin and its possible use as therapy.

For the teenager with syphilis of more than 1 year's duration, the same dose of benzathene penicillin G should be administered once a week for 3 consecutive weeks. The alternative drug is tetracycline except that with the same dosage the duration of therapy is at least 30 days. As in the treatment of early syphilis, if the patient is penicillin allergic, either of the two aforementioned options are applicable. But if erythromycin is used, the duration of therapy should be at least 30 days.

The extent to which treponemes persist after treatment of congenital syphilis is unknown. Also unknown is what happens to such patients in later life, particularly if they are subjected to immunosupressive therapy or illnesses.

The Jarisch-Herxheimer reaction is occasionally seen during the first few hours of treatment of congenital syphilis, just as in children and adolescents. This febrile response is usually benign and self-limited (12–48 hours) and may be treated symptomatically. Its occurrence is not a cause for discontinuation of penicillin.

Follow-up. Adequate follow-up is essential for all types of syphilis. Careful clinical and neurologic assessment is required, as are repeat quantitative determinations of the nontreponemal blood tests at 3, 6, and 12 months after therapy in patients with congenital or early syphilis. In these instances, the serologic tests will become nonreactive or reactive in a low titer within a year of adequate penicillin therapy. For the patients whose disease is of longer duration, the titers decline more slowly and should be repeated at the end of 24 months after therapy. Repeat serologic testing is of paramount importance in patients treated with antibiotics other than penicillin.

Retreatment should be considered when clinical signs persist (inadequate treatment) or recur (questionable reinfection). If the nontreponemal test fails to show a fourfold decrease within a year or demonstrates a fourfold increase in titer, retreatment is indicated using treatment schedules for syphilis of greater than 1 year's duration. Infants whose treatment is delayed or inadequate should be carefully followed for the stigmas of late congenital syphilis.

Leptospirosis

RALPH D. FEIGIN, M.D.

Leptospirosis is a disease caused by a single family of organisms of which there are multiple serogroups and serotypes. In the last decade, the dog has been incriminated as an important vector as well as a reservoir of this disease.

To be of maximum therapeutic benefit an antimicrobial agent must be administered before the invading organisms damage the endothelium of blood vessels and various organs or tissues. One problem in evaluating the efficacy of therapy to date has been that, generally, leptospirosis is a self-limited disease with a favorable prognosis. Even patients with severe icteric leptospirosis may recover without specific treatment.

Most claims of the beneficial value of antimicrobial agents in human leptospirosis are based on the response of individual patients rather than on controlled studies. However, when penicillin therapy was given to 28 patients prior to the fourth day of illness and compared with a control group of 33 patients who were given only supportive care, the duration of fever and the incidence of jaundice, meningismus, renal involvement, and hemorrhagic manifestations were diminished in the treated group. Therefore, when a diagnosis of leptospirosis is considered possible or probable and the patient has been ill for less than 1 week, treatment with penicillin or tetracycline (avoid the latter in children less than 8 years of age) should be initiated. Parenteral aqueous penicillin G (6 to 8 million units/m^2 of body surface/24 hr in six divided doses) provides optimal blood and tissue concentrations of penicillin. For patients who are sensitive to penicillin, tetracycline (20 to 40 mg/kg/24 hr) should be provided intravenously or orally in four divided doses for 1 week. Do not give tetracycline intravenously in excess of 1 gm total dose.

A sudden increase in body temperature, drop in systemic blood pressure, and exacerbation of other symptoms may accompany the initiation of penicillin therapy (a Herxheimer reaction). This reaction generally subsides spontaneously and is not a contraindication to continued treatment.

The management of leptospirosis requires careful attention to supportive care. Profound fluid and electrolyte changes may be noted, particularly significant hyponatremia. Thus, fluid and electrolyte balance must be accorded meticulous attention. Dehydration, cardiovascular collapse, and acute renal failure require prompt, specific treatment. In some cases, acute renal failure may be prevented by ensuring adequate renal perfusion and appropriate fluid administration early in the disease when prerenal azotemia and shock may be seen. If prerenal azotemia is suspected, diuresis may be attempted with the administration of a fluid or colloid load designed to expand extracellular volume and replace extracellular fluid deficits. In patients who do not respond to such therapy, acute tubular necrosis should be suspected, and appropriate fluid restriction should be initiated. Urine output, urine specific gravity, serum and urine osmolalities, and accurate measurement of body weight should be monitored sequentially. Children should receive sufficient fluid to replace insensible water loss plus their urine output. This may require adjustments of fluid intake on an hourly basis. Generally, a multiple electrolyte solution containing 5% or 10% glucose and 40 meq of sodium and chloride per liter, 35 meq of potassium per liter, and 20 meq of lactate or acetate per liter administered at a rate calculated as above is appropriate fluid therapy. If azotemia is severe or prolonged, peritoneal dialysis or hemodialysis should be instituted. Exchange transfusion has been suggested for patients with marked hyperbilirubinemia.

The use of corticosteroids in the treatment of severe cases has not been evaluated critically. Their use has been suggested in patients with impending hepatic coma. Anecdotal reports also suggest that they may be of value in patients with profound hypotension or shock.

Hemorrhagic manifestations of disease may be related to disseminated intravascular coagulation or thrombocytopenia without disseminated intravascular coagulation, or may merely reflect friability of blood vessels due to the severe vasculitis. Platelet transfusions have been used for patients with thrombocytopenia but generally the lifespan of the infused platelets is short. Heparin has been used for the treatment of disseminated intravascular coagulation, but there is little evidence to suggest that such therapy is beneficial.

When uveitis is present, ophthalmologic consultation should be sought. Conjunctival suffusion is common with leptospirosis and clears without specific topical therapy.

Rat-Bite Fever

GARY D. OVERTURF, M.D.

Two organisms may cause the clinical syndromes referred to as rat-bite fever: *Streptobacillus moniliformus* and *Spirillum minus*. *S. moniliformis* ("streptobacillary form") is characterized by a relatively short incubation period (usually less than 7 days), a morbilliform-petechial rash, septicemia, and arthritis (70%). *S. minus* ("spirillary form") is characterized by a longer incubation period (usually more than 7 days), eschar at the site of injury or bite, and a relapsing course. Occasionally these infections occur simultaneously. Accurate differentiation may be important, since streptobacillary forms may be more resistant to antibiotic treatment because of the occasional occurrence of penicillin-resistant L-forms (L$_1$ variant). *S. minus*, on the other hand, may be expected to respond to drugs that have proved effective in other spirochetal infections.

Penicillin is the drug of choice in both streptobacillary and spirillary rat-bite fever. In adults, uncomplicated infections due to *S. moniliformis* can be treated successfully with procaine penicillin, 300,000 to 600,000 units IM twice daily for 7 days. For pediatric patients an appropriate dosage could range from a lower dose of 10,000 units/kg/24 hours to doses up to 50,000 units/kg/24 hours. Duration of therapy for at least 7 days appears to be important, since relapse rates increase with lesser duration of therapy. Penicillin doses have traditionally been evaluated using intramuscular or intravenous preparations; although no controlled observations are available, it is probable that adequately administered oral penicillins with optimal bioavailability could probably be used in uncomplicated infections where compliance with therapy is assured. If the patient is allergic to penicillin, or if an isolated strain of *S. moniliformis* is resistant to penicillin, alternative drugs may be chosen based on susceptibility studies. However, empiric therapy with tetracycline (30–50 mg/kg/24 hr)*or streptomycin (20 mg/kg/day, divided in two doses) may be the most effective agents for both spirillary and streptobacillary forms. Erythromycin appears to be a third alternative and may be expected to be more effective in spirillary forms; little clinical experience exists with this agent in streptobacillary disease.

Treatment of endocarditis due to *S. moniliformis* is similar to that of streptococcal endocarditis. A suitable regimen for an adult is 12 to 20 million units of penicillin G daily for 3 to 4 weeks. Children should be treated with 100 to 150 mg (160,000 to 240,000 units) per kg/24 hr IV of potassium penicillin G for 3 to 4 weeks. Many physicians also recommend the use of streptomycin, 10 to 20 mg/kg daily, in combination with penicillin for part or all of the treatment course.

Although the spirillary form of rat-bite fever appears to be considerably more sensitive to penicillin therapy, treatment is usually instituted as for streptobacillary disease. Because of limited experience with spirillary rat-bite fever in this country, there are no specific guidelines in the literature for optimal dosages or duration of treatment.

Immediate wound care may help prevent infection. Tetanus prophylaxis or immunization should be administered when indicated. Many authorities recommend the routine use of penicillin prophylaxis (50 mg/kg/day) administered for 5 days after a rodent bite or alternatively, erythromycin (30–50 mg/kg/day) for children allergic to penicillin. No controlled data for such therapy exist, but its use is likely to be associated with few ill effects.

Prior to the advent of antimicrobial agents, mortality rate for these infections was about 10%. With the current use of effective antibiotics, the mortality rate approaches zero.

Pneumocystis carinii Pneumonitis

WALTER T. HUGHES, M.D.

Pneumonitis caused by *Pneumocystis carinii* is usually fatal if untreated. With specific antimicrobial therapy about 75% of patients can be expected to recover if treatment is begun early. Since the infection usually occurs in immunocompromised patients and a definitive diagnosis requires an invasive procedure, such as open lung biopsy or percutaneous needle aspiration, management requires close attention to complications from the underlying primary disease and the diagnostic procedures. Thus, associated or secondary viral, bacterial, or fungal infections may occur and pneumothorax or pneumomediastinum may complicate the diagnostic procedure. Hypoxia with low arterial oxygen tension (Pa_{O_2}) is regularly present, while carbon dioxide retention is unusual and the arterial pH is frequently increased. Unlike other infections in the immunosuppressed host, *P. carinii* infection remains localized entirely to the lungs.

When *P. carinii* pneumonitis is recognized as the first illness of an infant or child, careful search should be made for an underlying disease.

Specific Therapy. Trimethoprim-sulfamethoxazole (TMP-SMZ)* and pentamidine isethionate are equally effective in the treatment of *P. carinii* pneumonitis but TMP-SMZ is the drug of first choice because of its low toxicity and easy availability.

TMP-SMZ may be given orally or intravenously. The oral dose is 20 mg trimethoprim and 100 mg sulfamethoxazole per kg/day, divided into four parts at 6-hour intervals. It is advisable to give half of the calculated daily dose initially as a loading dose when the oral route is used. TMP-SMZ is available in tablet form ("regular size" with 80 mg trimethoprim, 400 mg sulfamethoxazole) and as a "double-strength" tablet with twice these amounts). An oral suspension contains 40 mg trimethoprim and 200 mg sulfamethoxazole per 5 ml. The intravenous preparation is available in 5.0 ml ampules containing 80 mg trimethoprim and 400 mg sulfamethoxazole. Each 5.0 ml ampule must be added to 125 ml of 5% dextrose in water. The dosage for intravenous use is 15.0 mg trimethoprim and 75.0 mg sulfamethoxazole per kg/day divided in three to four equal doses. Each dose is infused over a 60-minute period. From available data, peak serum levels of 3 to 5 μg/ml of trimethoprim and 100 to 150 μg/ml of sulfamethoxazole seem to be the optimal ranges.

The adverse and toxic side effects are essentially those of sulfonamides, and although uncommon they include transient maculopapular rash, nausea, vomiting, diarrhea, neutropenia, agranulocytosis, aplastic anemia, megaloblastic anemia, hemolytic anemia, methemoglobinemia, Stevens-Johnson syndrome, allergic reactions, toxic nephrosis, and drug fever. Folic acid deficiency has occurred rarely. It is reversible by folinic acid, 10 to 25 mg daily. Folinic acid does not interfere with the therapeutic effects of the drug.

---

*Manufacturer's warning: Tetracycline should not be used during tooth development (infancy and childhood to the age of 8 years) unless other drugs are not likely to be effective or are contraindicated.

*Manufacturer's precaution: Not recommended for infants less than 2 months of age.

Pentamidine is the drug of second choice because of its high frequency of adverse effects. Manufactured in England under the name Lomidine, it is investigational and available in the U.S. only through the Centers for Disease Control. Physicians may obtain the drug to treat specific cases by calling the Parasitic Disease Drug Service at 404–329–3311 or 404–329–3644.

Pentamidine is administered as a single daily dose of 4 mg/kg IM for 10 to 14 days. If improvement is apparent after 5 days of treatment, this may be reduced to 3 mg/kg/day. The total dosage should not exceed 56 mg/kg. IM injections should be given deeply into the anterolateral aspect of the thigh. Each 100 mg of the drug should be dissolved in 1 ml of sterile distilled water. Filtration of the drug in solution through a Millipore filter (0.22-micron pore size) immediately before injection is advisable to ensure sterility for the immunosuppressed host.

Adverse effects include induration, abscess formation, and necrosis at injection sites; nephrotoxicity; hypoglycemia or, rarely, hyperglycemia; hypotension; alteration in liver function; tachycardia; hypocalcemia; nausea and vomiting; skin rash; anemia; hyperkalemia; and thrombocytopenia.

Isolation. Recent studies indicate that *P. carinii* is transmitted by the airborne route. It is advisable to use respiratory isolation procedures to separate active cases of *P. carinii* pneumonitis from other compromised individuals at high risk for this infection.

Supportive Measures. Oxygen should be administered by mask as needed to maintain the PaO_2 above 70 mm Hg. The fraction of inspired oxygen (FIO_2) should be kept below 50 volumes % if possible, to avoid oxygen toxicity, since oxygen therapy usually is required for relatively long periods.

Assisted or controlled ventilation is indicated in patients with arterial oxygen tension less than 60 mm Hg at FIO_2 of 50% or greater. Those with acutely elevated $PaCO_2$, without pH changes and with or without hypoxemia, should be considered candidates for ventilatory therapy.

Patients receiving immunosuppressive drugs should have these discontinued if the status of the primary disease permits. Corticosteroids are of no benefit and may be deleterious to the course of the pneumonitis.

Fluid and electrolyte quantities are calculated by the patient's needs, but the solution should contain 5 or 10% glucose to help prevent hypoglycemia during pentamidine therapy. Metabolic acidosis must be corrected.

Bacterial pneumonia or sepsis may occur in association with *P. carinii* pneumonitis. In the seriously ill patient with marked neutropenia (absolute neutrophil count less than 500/cu mm) or evidence of bacterial infection, antibiotics should be given. Oxacillin, 200 mg/kg/day, and gentamicin, 5 to 7 mg/kg/day, are administered IV until the results of cultures are known.

Efforts should be made to improve the nutritional status of the patient by dietary means even during the acute stage of the disease. Multivitamins should be given empirically. The value of IV alimentation has not been determined.

Give blood transfusion if hemoglobin level is less than normal. The hemoglobin content must be sufficient to result in an arterial oxygen content of 15 to 20 ml/dl of blood at an arterial oxygen tension of 100 mm Hg.

Pneumothorax may be a complication of the diagnostic procedures. If it is less than 15% with no adverse effect on respiration, close observation is adequate. If it is more extensive, insertion of a thoracotomy tube with a water seal drainage system is necessary.

Parameters to Monitor. *Serum immunoglobulins:* At the onset of the illness, administer immune serum globulin (165 mg/ml) 0.66 ml/kg if the immunoglobulin G level is below 300 mg/dl.

Roentogenograms of chest should be done daily until there is clinical evidence of improvement. If needle aspiration of the lung, lung biopsy, or endotracheal brush catheter technique has been used as a diagnostic procedure, chest roentgenograms should be made at 30 minutes, 4 hours, and 12 hours after the procedure to detect pneumothorax.

Hemoglobin, WBC count and differential, and platelet estimate daily.

Measure body weight, intake and output daily.

Arterial blood gases: Measure pH, $PaCO_2$, PaO_2, and base excess or deficit initially and as often as necessary, based on severity of clinical course.

Serum electrolytes: Measure sodium, chloride, potassium, and carbon dioxide content every 3 days, or more frequently if indicated.

Total serum proteins, albumin, and globulin: Monitor every 3 days. Hypoalbuminemia may occur.

Blood pressure, pulse and respiratory rate: Monitor every 4 hours, or more often if the condition is critical.

For patients receiving pentamidine: Check *blood urea nitrogen (BUN), creatinine, and urinalysis* every 3 days. If the BUN exceeds 30 mg/dl, withhold pentamidine for 1 or 2 days; monitor *blood glucose* 4 to 6 hours after each injection of pentamidine. Administer glucose if blood glucose value is less than 40 mg/dl; monitor *serum glutamic oxaloacetic transaminase (SGOT)* every 3 days; withhold pentamidine for 1 to 2 days if evidence of hepatic toxicity exists; and monitor *serum calcium and phosphorus* every 3 days. If the serum inorganic phosphate level becomes increased and the calcium level becomes decreased from normal values on the basis of renal insufficiency, give calcium lactate, 15 to 20 gm/day, or calcium carbonate, 5 to 8 gm/day orally. The diet should be low in phosphate, and 25,000 to 50,000 units of vitamin D is given orally. For patients with renal impairment and receiving trimethoprim-sulfamethoxazole, the dosage should be regulated on the basis of serum drug levels. Measurement of serum levels of the sulfonamide is adequate. The level of free sulfonamide should be maintained with peak values between 100 and 150 μg/ml measured 2 hours after the oral dosage.

Expected Course. Fever, tachypnea, and pulmonary infiltrates usually persist with little change for 4 to 6 days. If no improvement is apparent after a week of therapy, concomitant or secondary infection most likely exists. These infections have included bacterial pneumonia or sepsis, systemic candidiasis, aspergillosis, cryptococcosis, histoplasmosis, and cytomegalovirus inclusion disease, as well as other viral infections. *P. carinii* pneumonitis may recur several months after apparent recovery in 10 to 15% of cases.

Prevention. Recent studies have shown that *P. carinii* pneumonitis can be prevented by chemoprophylaxis with TMP-SMZ.* Dosage is one fourth the therapeutic dose, 5 mg/kg of trimethoprim and 25 mg/kg of sulfamethoxazole per day in two divided doses. The protection is afforded only while the patient is receiving the drug.

Measles

H. CODY MEISSNER, M.D.

Since the introduction of an effective measles vaccine in 1963, the incidence of the disease has declined by more than 90%. In 1980, 14,000 cases of measles were reported in the United States. Disease presently occurs among individuals who either do not receive the vaccine, those who received the inactivated vaccine while it was available, and those who were unsuccessfully vaccinated with the attenuated strain. Associated with this decline has come a shift in the age distribution of people infected. At present, individuals 10 years or older account for more than 55% of reported cases.

Symptomatic Treatment. Because measles is generally a mild, self-limited disease, treatment is chiefly supportive. The measles cough is difficult to control and attempts at cough suppression with narcotics should be avoided. Because the coryza does not respond to oral antihistamines, it should be permitted to run its course. The conjunctivitis is usually self-limited; steroid or antibiotic containing ophthalmic preparations play no role in the resolution of a viral conjunctivitis. Corneal ulceration should be watched for and managed by an ophthalmologist when present. Severe headache or high fever should be managed with appropriate antipyretics and adequate fluid intake.

Complications

Respiratory Involvement. Because the upper respiratory tract is the primary portal of entry (the conjunctiva may be an alternate site), mild laryngitis or tracheobronchitis is invariably present during the course of uncomplicated measles. During the first year of life, respiratory involvement may be manifest as bronchiolitis. As a consequence of viral involvement of the respiratory tree, there may be localized tissue damage, increasing the risk of secondary bacterial infection. Secondary bacterial pneumonia is, in fact, the leading cause of death in measles. It should be emphasized, however, that prophylactic antibiotics are of no use and that indiscriminate use of antibiotics may be associated with an increased risk of superinfection by resistant bacteria. The frequently encountered bacterial agents in this setting are the staphylococcus, the pneumococcus, and *Hemophilus influenzae.* Direct extension of the measles virus to the lung parenchyma without bacteria involvement may also occur, presenting a difficult differential diagnosis. In either case, pneumonia should be suspected when there is increasing respiratory distress, leukocytosis, and persistence of fever beyond the third day of the rash. A late complication of respiratory involvement is obstructive laryngitis. Progressive hoarseness, inspiratory stridor, retractions, and restlessness point to respiratory obstruction and the immediate need for an adequate airway.

Central Nervous System Involvement. The tendency of the measles virus to involve the central nervous system has been documented by the detection of transient electroencephalographic abnormalities in up to 50% of patients with uncomplicated disease. Acute, symptomatic encephalitis occurs in approximately 0.1% of measles cases. There is no specific therapy and treatment is symptomatic. Corticosteroids have not been shown to be effective.

Subacute sclerosing panencephalitis, another form of encephalitis caused by the measles virus, is due to a persistent infection of the central nervous system established at the time of primary infection. This disease occurs several years after a measles infection and is almost invariably fatal.

Otic Involvement. Otitis media is one of the most frequently encountered complications of measles in both infants and older children. Persistence of fever beyond the third or fourth day of the rash is most frequently due to this problem. Evidence of an inflamed tympanic membrane should be promptly treated with appropriate antibiotics.

---

*This use is not listed by the manufacturer.

Miscellaneous Complications. A number of organ systems can be involved by the measles virus, resulting in myocarditis or pericarditis, thrombocytopenic purpura, corneal ulceration, and mesenteric adenopathy with nonspecific abdominal pain. These conditions are rare and should be managed as in any other patient. Hemorrhagic measles is a severe form of measles associated with hyperpyrexia, convulsions, coma, and at times, death.

Measles in the Compromised Host

Severe measles may occur in patients with abnormalities of cell-mediated immunity, such as patients with leukemia, lymphoma, or congenital immunodeficiencies. The major concern for these children is the development of giant cell pneumonia. Diagnosis may be made more difficult in these patients by the absence of a typical measles exanthem. Because severe disease may result from vaccination with the attenuated virus, use of the live vaccine is contraindicated in these patients.

Immunization

Passive. Measles can be modified or prevented by the administration of human gamma globulin. Administration of 0.25 ml/kg within 3 days of exposure will at least attenuate the illness in an unimmunized individual and may prevent a subclinical infection. Immunity is approximately of 4 weeks' duration. If a modified form of measles does occur in a person given gamma globulin, the incubation period may be delayed up to 3 weeks or longer. A person passively immunized with a preventive dose should receive the live vaccine 3 months after administration of gamma globulin. Any susceptible person older than 6 months who has been exposed to measles should receive passive immunization. Unimmunized individuals at high risk for severe disease, including children with malignant disease, children with abnormalities in cell-mediated immunity, and those receiving immunosuppressive therapy, should receive a dose of 0.5 ml/kg IM, to a maximum of 15 ml.

Active. Live and killed measles vaccines were licensed and distributed in the United States in 1963. Because of an association with atypical measles, the inactivated vaccine was taken off the market in 1968. The first live attenuated vaccine, the Edmondston B strain, was associated with reactions such as fever and rash so that a dose of gamma globulin was often administered with the vaccine. While this practice generally resulted in adequate antibody levels, further attenuation of the Edmondston strain led to the introduction of the presently available vaccines, which no longer necessitate the simultaneous administration of gamma globulin.

Despite the availability of effective, safe vaccines, outbreaks of measles continue to occur. Often, patients involved in outbreaks have received the attenuated vaccine. Explanations for an inadequate immune response to the live measles vaccine include improper refrigeration of the vaccine or exposure of the vaccine to heat or light, and vaccination of individuals who possess low levels of protective antibody. Because the measles vaccine is very sensitive to antibody inactivation, small amounts of transplacentally acquired maternal antibody can prevent an appropriate immune response. It is clear that vaccine administration at 12 months results in unacceptably low rates of seroconversion, and that the vaccine should be administered at 15 months of age, when all maternal antibody has been lost.

During a measles outbreak, live attenuated vaccine can be preventive if given before the day of exposure. At times it may be useful to vaccinate children under 12 months in such a setting, although reimmunization at 15 months is necessary. No untoward effects have been related to reimmunization. However, it is disturbing that some children immunized in the first year of life may fail to show an adequate immune response to a second immunization, even at 15 months.

Atypical Measles. Atypical measles is a syndrome primarily associated with administration of killed measles vaccine. After exposure to wild-type measles, such a person may develop a prodrome consisting of fever, cough, headache, and myalgias. This is usually followed by the development of pneumonia and a rash which begins on the extremities as maculopapular and converts to vesicular. Although the illness may be more severe than ordinary rubeola, there is no specific therapy.

Rubella and Congenital Rubella

ROBERT F. PASS, M.D.

Rubella (German measles) is a highly communicable acute viral infection that produces an exanthem and mild symptoms lasting a few days. The virus gains its importance as a pathogen by its ability to cross the placental barrier, infect the fetus, and damage developing vital organs. Prior to the widespread immunization of infants and children in the United States, epidemics occurred every 6 to 9 years and were accompanied by epidemics of the congenital infection.

Acute Rubella

Acquired rubella virus infection is characterized by a few days of malaise, low grade fever, posterior auricular, occipital, or cervical adenopathy, and a maculopapular rash that begins on the face and spreads to the trunk and extremities. Arthralgias or arthritis may accompany the acute infection, especially in adult females, and persist for up to 4 weeks. Since joint involvement is self-limited, steroids should be avoided. Encephalitis, a very infrequent complication, has been associated with fatalities. Thrombocytopenia often occurs transiently with rubella but is usually not associated with purpura or other evidence of a hemorrhagic diathesis.

Treatment. No specific antiviral drugs are available for treatment of rubella. Aspirin can be used to relieve constitutional symptoms and arthralgia. Encephalitis and thrombocytopenia should be treated with supportive care.

Congenital Rubella

Congenital rubella can cause a wide range of abnormalities, some of which are present in the newborn period and others that may not become detectable for months or years. Around two thirds of newborns with congenital rubella detected by virologic or serologic screening are asymptomatic at birth. Symptomatic newborns may have a great variety of abnormalities involving almost any organ; some of the more common are hepatomegaly, thrombocytopenia with or without petechiae, intrauterine growth retardation, encephalitis, interstitial pneumonitis, bony radiolucencies, retinopathy, deafness, cataracts, and cardiac abnormalities, notably pulmonic stenosis. The combination of the last three abnormalities is strong clinical evidence of congenital rubella. Fetal or neonatal death can occur, but most infected newborns survive to have chronic neurologic, sensory, developmental, or cardiovascular problems.

Management. The physician providing care for a congenital rubella patient must provide evaluation and supportive care for medical problems such as pneumonitis, seizures, or heart failure. The extent of impairment of hearing, vision, and developmental potential must be defined with age-appropriate assessments, and an effort must be made to prevent transmission of rubella from patient to hospital staff or community contacts. No specific antiviral drug is available and there is no known therapeutic agent that will change the course of the disease. Whenever congenital rubella is suspected because of clinical signs or history of maternal exposure, the diagnosis should be confirmed by isolation of virus from the newborn nasopharynx, conjunctiva, urine, or cerebrospinal fluid, or by serologic tests including detection of specific IgM antibody and demonstration of persistence of serum antibody to rubella.

Hearing loss is the most common associated defect; auditory evaluation should be performed within the first month of life, preferably using brain stem evoked response audiometry. It is very important to determine as early as possible whether hearing loss is present, so that steps can be taken to maximize the chances for development of speech. All patients with congenital rubella should also have ophthalmologic examinations in the newborn period. Extended management should be individualized; many patients will need periodic auditory, visual, psychometric, neurologic, or cardiovascular examination by specialists. Specific supportive therapy may be needed for motor deficits, speech or hearing difficulties, or developmental and learning disabilities. Most states have a division of crippled children's services that can fulfill these needs or identify other community agencies that can help.

Prevention of Congenital Rubella. IMMUNIZATION. To prevent congenital rubella, it is necessary to prevent acquisition of rubella by women in their childbearing years. Although identifying and immunizing susceptible women might seem the best way to accomplish this, European nations that adopted this approach are still experiencing epidemics of congenital rubella. In the United States, rubella immunization has been aimed at preschool children, with the goal of eliminating rubella epidemics. Although the proportion of young women who are susceptible has not changed since the prevaccine era, there has been a dramatic decrease in the incidence of rubella, an elimination of major epidemics, and more importantly, a parallel decline in the incidence of congenital rubella. In the United States, the number one goal for prevention remains the immunization of all healthy children with live rubella virus vaccine. It is recommended that this be accomplished by inoculation with the combined measles, mumps, and rubella vaccine at 15 months of age. Infants younger than a year should not be immunized, as persistent passively acquired maternal antibody may interfere with the development of lasting immunity. Children with unknown or questionable immunization records should be immunized at any age. Further reduction in the incidence of congenital rubella will require a more intensive effort to immunize all children as well as susceptible adolescents and young adults.

Immunization of postpubertal females is complicated by the theoretical risk of producing congenital rubella by inadvertently administering the vaccine during pregnancy. Although hundreds of such accidents have been studied, no cases of rubella syndrome have occurred. Vaccine virus can be transmitted to the fetus, and a few clinically normal children with laboratory evidence of congenital rubella have been born. It is important that women in their reproductive years be aware of the potential risk to the fetus, and be informed that they should not become pregnant for 3 months after vaccination. Women who are found to be susceptible at prenatal screening are an ideal group to immunize in the immediate postpartum period. Physicians serving adolescents and young adults should see that all of their female patients are protected against rubella; certain groups deserve particular attention, including health care workers and women who work with young children. Hospitals should require that all staff physicians and employees with any patient contact show proof of rubella immunity (seropositivity or previous immunization) or be immunized. Both male and female hospital workers should be included; hospital rubella outbreaks are costly and very difficult to contain. They can easily result in exposure of women receiving prenatal care and of unimmunized infants, who will further spread virus into the community.

Containment. Containment also has a role in prevention of rubella transmission. All rubella cases should be reported to appropriate local health department officials. Quarantine is of little use, since the incubation period may be as long as 21 days, infection is often asymptomatic, and viral shedding from the nasopharynx may persist for over 2 weeks. Containment is accomplished through identification and immunization of susceptible contacts. Infants with congenital rubella often shed virus for months, and thus can serve as a reservoir of rubella. When hospitalized, they should be in strict isolation for their first year of life; they should be cared for only by health workers with known rubella status. In addition, care should be taken to see that family and community contacts of these children have been immunized or are seropositive.

Exposure in Pregnant Women. Around 50% of first trimester maternal infections will be transmitted to the fetus; most of the survivors will have handicaps. The transmission rate and morbidity of congenital rubella decrease with advancing gestational age, but subtle sensory or learning deficits have followed infections after midgestation. A possible rubella exposure in a pregnant woman is clearly cause for concern.

This question is often raised when a pregnant woman has had contact with someone, usually a child, with an exanthem. It is important to determine whether the suspect index case actually has rubella. The immunization history should be defined and an acute serum sample obtained from the index case. If there is documentation of immunization or no rise in titer demonstrable when the convalescent serum is drawn 10 days later, it is very unlikely that rubella was the cause of the exanthem. Whether the pregnant woman has been exposed to a suspected or known case of rubella, an acute

serum should be obtained from her and her medical history reviewed for evidence of rubella immunity. This could include immunization or previous seropositivity. Many obstetricians screen for serum antibody to rubella at the first prenatal visit, so if there has been a previous pregnancy the results of such screening may be available. A history of clinically defined rubella (German measles or three day measles) is unacceptable; clinical diagnosis of rubella is notoriously inaccurate. If there is no proof of prior infection (immunization or seropositivity) then convalescent sera obtained 14 days after the earliest possible exposure and again 21 days after the latest possible exposure must be evaluated. If there is no demonstrable rise in titer, rubella infection is very unlikely. If an early serum sample has not been obtained, it can be impossible to detect a rise in titer; in this situation sera should be examined for rubella specific IgM antibody, the presence of which would indicate recent infection. For questions about the availability of antibody tests and to ensure speedy results one may wish to consult with the state health department or the Center for Disease Control in Atlanta. If evidence points to maternal rubella (significant rise in titer or presence of specific IgM antibody), the risk to the fetus and possibility of therapeutic abortion should be discussed with the mother.

Passive immunization has little place in the management of exposure during pregnancy. The use of human immune serum globulin will completely muddle the attempt to determine serologically whether infection has occurred, and should only be considered if the mother refuses to interrupt the pregnancy, knowing that she has rubella and that the fetus is likely to be severely handicapped. In this case a large dose, at least 20 ml, should be given as soon as possible after exposure, and the mother should be informed that there is no guarantee of efficacy.

Varicella and Herpes Zoster

JOHN A. ZAIA, M.D.

Varicella is the common childhood vesicular exanthem caused by primary infection with varicella-zoster virus (VZV). Herpes zoster is the clinical syndrome of segmental vesicular exanthem and pain associated with reactivation of latent VZV infection in a nerve ganglion. In the immunodeficient person, both primary and secondary VZV infection can produce progressive varicella and disseminated or chronic herpes zoster. Rarely, the clinical syndromes of VZV can be mimicked by herpes simplex virus.

VARICELLA (CHICKENPOX)

Symptomatic Treatment

As its vernacular name implies, itching is the major symptom of chickenpox (from Old English *gican,* to itch). Topical antipruritic agents, such as cold calamine lotion with benadryl, are helpful. Warm baths containing baking soda (one third cup per tub of water) can temporarily relieve pruritus and should be combined with oral antihistamines. For severe dysuria, a cold compress on the genital area during urination will ease the pain and minimize the likelihood of a functional bladder obstruction. Antipyretics should be used for fever.

Complications

Bacterial Infection. Bacterial superinfection involving the skin, the middle ear, or the lung is the most common complication of varicella. Pyoderma is the most frequently observed bacterial complication and can be minimized by attention to good hygiene, including daily bathing with a hexachlorophene-containing soap and close clipping of fingernails. Bacterial infection should be treated with appropriate oral antibiotics, usually erythromycin or a β-lactamase-resistant semisynthetic penicillin. Bacterial infection should be treated with soaks using Burow or Epsom salt solution; localized subcutaneous abscesses require incision and drainage. More serious bacterial infection can occur, such as scarlet fever, staphylococcal scalded-skin syndrome, and osteomyelitis, and should be appropriately treated.

Bacterial superinfection can involve the lower respiratory tract, producing pneumonia and bronchitis. Pneumonia in a normal child following varicella is usually bacterial and due to the usual respiratory pathogens—*Streptococcus pneumoniae, Hemophilus influenzae,* and *Staphylococcus aureus*—and should be treated with an appropriate parenteral antibiotic.

Thrombocytopenia. Bleeding disorders can occur during varicella and can be due to disseminated intravascular coagulation, vasculitis, or idiopathic thrombocytopenia. Purpura fulminans must be treated with supportive therapy and must include antibiotic therapy initially until sepsis is excluded. Anaphylactoid purpura can follow otherwise uncomplicated varicella and must be managed with appropriate attention to renal function and to occult hemorrhage. Idiopathic thrombocytopenic purpura can occur during active infection or during convalescence. Mild hemorrhage into vesicles during active infection does not require specific treatment, but excessive hemorrhage and profound thrombocytopenia should be treated with platelet support, judicious use of corticosteroids, and antiviral therapy.

Encephalitis. Cerebellar ataxia is the most common syndrome associated with varicella encephalitis and is generally a benign entity occurring before, during, or after the exanthem. Cerebral involvement with seizures and altered mental status has a grave prognosis. In the normal child, encephalitis is probably due to postinfection demyelination; there is no evidence to support active virus infection with hemorrhagic brain necrosis, as occurs in herpes simplex encephalitis. For this reason, specific antiviral therapy is not indicated, and management consists of anticonvulsant medication, sedation, and exclusion of other types of viral, bacterial, and toxic encephalopathy.

Hepatic Dysfunction and Reye's Syndrome. Hepatitis occurs in a majority of children with varicella and is usually manifested as asymptomatic elevation of transaminase. Rarely, symptomatic hepatitis occurs but should require no specific treatment. Reye's syndrome can occur in association with varicella and must be excluded in any child with varicella hepatitis.

Abdominal Pain and Mucositis. Varicella is a generalized infection involving all epithelial areas, including mucosal surfaces of respiratory, alimentary, and genitourinary systems. Laryngitis and laryngotracheobronchitis can occur in varicella and require symptomatic treatment with analgesics and humidification of air. Severe abdominal pain can be present due to inflammation of gut mucosa or to pancreatitis. Initial therapy should include cessation of oral intake intravenous fluid support, and adequate treatment of pain with morphine. Adrenal corticosteroids currently have no place in the management of normal inflammatory symptoms during varicella because of the unknown risk of progressive varicella.

Progressive Varicella

Varicella can progress to involve lungs, liver and other viscera, and brain in immunocompromised persons. Those at risk for this complication are children with primary immunodeficiency of T-cell function, children with neoplastic disease who are receiving cytotoxic chemotherapy, children with non-neoplastic disease receiving adrenal corticosteroids, and neonates whose mothers had varicella less than 5 days prior to delivery.

Chemotherapeutic Regimens Related to Progressive Varicella. The dose of corticosteroids that places a child in jeopardy of progressive varicella is not accurately known. Children with asthma, atopic dermatitis, nephrotic syndrome, and idiopathic thrombocytopenia, in whom the disease status is stable on low doses of corticosteroid (e.g., ≤ 0.25 mg/kg/24 hr of prednisone or alternate-day prednisone) usually do not have life-threatening varicella. Severe varicella has been described in children with such diseases only when the corticosteroid dose is high (1 to 2 mg/kg/24 hr of prednisone). It is important to maintain physiologic corticosteroid levels in the child who has relative adrenal insufficiency after corticosteroid therapy. Increasing the dose of corticosteroid may be necessary in such children during active varicella, but this should be done with caution. In the asthmatic child with varicella, inhalation of corticosteroids can be used without enhanced risk of pneumonia.

For the management of anticancer chemotherapy following chickenpox exposure, there are no good data regarding which drugs, if any, can be safely used during the incubation period. When possible, cancer chemotherapy should be temporarily interrupted; however, treatment of the malignancy must take precedence in patients receiving first-induction therapy or therapy for disease in relapse. Cancer chemotherapy is most safely deleted during maintenance therapy of disease remission and should be resumed 21 days after the exposure, or, if varicella should occur, 7 days after complete crusting of the varicella lesions.

Immunosuppressed persons who have had chickenpox (with the exception of bone marrow transplant recipients) are not at risk for developing severe chickenpox from re-exposure even when they remain on active immunosuppressive therapy.

Prevention of Progressive Varicella. GENERAL APPROACH. The approach to the child at risk for progressive varicella involves education of medical staff and parents to the need for prompt reporting of chickenpox exposure, adequate isolation of clinic patients, and passive immunization of appropriate patients. Medical facilities should provide for separate entrance and isolation of patients in any clinic that treats immunosuppressed pediatric patients. The medical staff personnel who have negative histories for chickenpox should be tested for immunity to varicella by a reliable method, such as immunofluorescence, radioimmunoassay, or enzyme-linked immunoassay.

PASSIVE IMMUNIZATION. This can be effective in preventing progressive varicella, using zoster immune plasma (ZIP), zoster immune globulin (ZIG), or varicella-zoster immune globulin (VZIG). VZIG is the only biologic material licensed for this purpose and can be obtained from several regional American Red Cross blood centers. The material should be used only for high-risk (see above) individuals who have no prior history of chickenpox and have had a close exposure to varicella or herpes zoster. In order to preserve its supply, VZIG is not recommended for use in normal children, in routine pregnancy, in immunosuppressed persons with a known history of chickenpox, or in the treatment of existing chickenpox. VZIG should be administered within 96 hours of exposure and is given IM at a dose of 1 vial/10 kg body weight (maximum, 5 vials). This therapy does not prevent infection but will modify the signs and symptoms of infection in most patients. Certain patients will still have unmodified varicella (>100 pox), and such patients remain at risk for progressive infection. Alternatively, ZIP, which is obtained from compatible volunteer blood donors during convalescence from herpes zoster, can be given IV at a dosage of 7 to 10 ml/kg. ZIP has the advantage of immediate availability to the circulation and should be used in the child in whom VZIG cannot be given within 96 hours after exposure.

Treatment of Progressive Varicella. GENERAL SUPPORTIVE THERAPY. Patients with progressive varicella can have involvement of single or multiple organ systems and can undergo rapid clinical deterioration and death. The patient should be hospitalized at a medical center that is adequately staffed and equipped with life-support systems. The initial evaluation requires monitoring of blood pH, P_{O_2}, and P_{CO_2}, documentation of extent of systemic involvement by serum chemistry evaluation of liver, renal, pancreatic, and cardiac function; assessment of the rate of progression of the viral infection by means of pox count, chest radiograph, and serial serum chemistry evaluation. Successful control of pain is of major importance because of the extent of epithelial surface involvement and usually requires intravenous opiates. In addition, bacterial superinfection must be assumed to exist, and, after appropriate blood, throat, and skin cultures are collected, broad-spectrum antibiotics, such as oxacillin and gentamicin, should be given intravenously until cultures are available.

ANTIVIRAL TREATMENT. Antibody to VZV in the form of ZIP, ZIG, VZIG, or normal immune serum globulin has not been demonstrated to be effective in treating progressive vericella. Similarly, the use of irradiated (3000 R) leukocyte transfusions of blood from herpes zoster–convalescent donors has not been demonstrated conclusively to treat this infection; however, in view of the defects of cellular immunity associated with progressive varicella, such treatment merits consideration.

There is no licensed chemotherapy for progressive varicella. Of the commercially available antiviral drugs, adenine arabinoside (Vira-A, 10 mg/kg/24 hr IV in a 12 hour infusion for 5 days) and acyclovir (Zovirax, 500 mg/M²/8 hr IV in a 1 hour infusion for 7 days) have been shown to prevent severe complications of varicella and herpes zoster in immunocompromised persons. For severe disseminated VZV infection in such patients, it is the opinion of the author that acyclovir is the drug of choice. Both of these antiviral agents are currently licensed only for the treatment of certain herpes simplex infections; their use for the treatment of VZV infection remains investigational and should require informed consent.

HERPES ZOSTER

Herpes zoster occurs in normal children, often those who have had chickenpox early in life. Compared with the adult-onset disease, herpes zoster in childhood has less severity of inflammation, pain, and postherpetic neuralgia. As with varicella, general supportive care is necessary, with attention to hygiene and to debridement of the crusted material with frequent Burow or Epsom salt soaking. Bacterial infection should be treated as in varicella. Inflammation can be intense and can mimic bacterial cellulitis. Nevertheless, there is no demonstrated need for treatment with adrenal corticosteroids in children. Ophthalmic zoster requires the assistance of an ophthalmologist for assessment of uveal inflammation. Uveitis should be treated with mydriatics and topical corticosteroids. Occasionally dendritic keratitis can occur and should be treated with Ara-A ointment.

In the immunosuppressed patient, herpes zoster can be more severe in terms of local inflammation and can progress to systemic involvement. Disseminated zoster should be followed for evidence of visceral involvement. If there is only cutaneous involvement, then prevention of bacterial superinfection and treatment of pain are the chief priorities. If there is visceral involvement, the patient must be treated as directed above for progressive varicella. Immunosuppressed patients can have severe postherpetic neuralgia, but in children this is usually temporary and responds to oral pain medication; regional nerve block is not indicated.

Herpes Simplex Virus Infections

JOSEPH W. ST. GEME, JR., M.D.

Herpes simplex virus (HSV) is one of the most prevalent of the human herpesviruses. The other members of this family of viruses are varicella-zoster virus, cytomegalovirus, and Epstein-Barr virus.

Primary Gingivostomatitis. This condition may last 1 week and be so painful that nutrition is impaired. Therapy is often unsatisfactory. Topical dental analgesic solutions, chilled fluids, soft foods, and systemic analgesic-antipyretic medications constitute the bulwark of symptomatic treatment for this ordinarily self-contained illness. Systemic dissemination may occur in immunodeficient individuals and require chemotherapy with adenine arabinoside or parenteral acyclovir, a highly specific anti-DNA virus purine analog.

Recurrent Herpes Labialis. Topical antiviral solutions, lotions, and ointments containing iodo-deoxyuridine and adenine arabinoside are of equivocal therapeutic value. Immediate treatment of recurrent lesions with acyclovir ointment at the first appearance of symptoms in nonimmunocompromised patients may ultimately prove beneficial. Immunocompromised children with limited infections should be treated swiftly with topical acyclovir. Topical application of acetone or alcohol may hasten the resolution and desiccation of vesicular lesions. These organic solvents may also diminish the quantity of HSV in these lesions because of the susceptibility of virions with abundant lipid envelopes to degradation by such chemicals.

Keratoconjunctivitis. Serious, destructive primary or secondary (reactivation) ophthalmic infections may occur due to HSV type 1. Occasionally, HSV type 2 may produce the same process in the newborn infant. Treatment of this illness marked the initial success with specific antiviral chemotherapy. Unless deep stromal tissues are affected, HSV keratoconjunctivitis responds nicely to therapy with topical 0.1% iododeoxyuridine ophthalmic solution. Occasional mutant strains of HSV, which do not elaborate the thymidine kinase enzyme necessary to activate this pyrimidine analog, are resistant to iododeoxyuridine and can be treated effectively with topical adenine arabinoside.

Vulvovaginitis, Cervicitis, and Prepucitis. Vulvar and vaginal lesions are particularly distressing. Unfortunately, topical therapy with iododeoxyuridine, adenine arabinoside, and adenine arabinoside 5'-monophosphate is ineffective. Initial results with topical acyclovir treatment of primary infections are promising. In general, HSV type 2 is less susceptible to these antiviral agents than is HSV type 1. Photodynamic inactivation of HSV with neutral red and other photoactive dyes, thought initially to be efficacious, has proved to be inadequate and, because of HSV mutagenic potential, may be hazardous. It is frustrating that genital HSV infections, so discomforting to women in particular and potentially threatening to the offspring of pregnant women, cannot be managed with any modality more salutary than sitz baths.

Meningoencephalitis. Following definitive diagnosis, therapy should be instituted for 10 days with parenteral adenine arabinoside at a dosage of 15 mg/kg body weight/24 hr over 12 hours in concentrations not exceeding 0.7 mg/ml of standard intravenous solution. Such treatment may reduce mortality from 70 to 30% and improve the quality of survival for those individuals who escape the lethality of this neurotropic virus.

Perinatal Infection. Recent collaborative study data indicate that the mortality and morbidity of these infections, particularly the moderately serious nondisseminated neonatal meningoencephalitis, can be attenuated by parenteral adenine arabinoside therapy at a dosage of 15 mg/kg body weight/24 hr over 12 hours, as described above. With localized meningoencephalitis, mortality was reduced from 50 to 10% and morbidity from 83 to 50% with adenine arabinoside therapy. Specific diagnosis is simpler in these perinatal infections because the predominant HSV type 2 can be isolated from the cutaneous vesicular lesions, conjunctiva, oropharynx, urine, and spinal fluid of these infants. The risk of transparturient transmission of this perinatal viral pathogen can be modified by cesarean section if the amniotic membranes remain intact. It is also comforting that the majority of the maternal infections seem to occur at some time other than the final few weeks of pregnancy.

Because so many of these genital infections during pregnancy represent reactivation of HSV type 2 in immune women, the duration of lesions is shorter and quantity of virus is less, and specific maternal IgG-neutralizing antibody is transferred to the infant across the placenta. Consequently, the risk of HSV transmission from women with primary lesions to their offspring, which is 50%, falls to 5% in women with secondary reactivated lesions.

Eczema Herpeticum. This unusual infection represents the topical inoculation of the eczematous skin of an infant or child with HSV type 1 as a result of contact with a person who has recurrent herpes labialis or is a silent virus shedder. The vesicular and vesiculoulcerative lesions may persist for a week or more. Infrequently, HSV disseminates to noneczematous skin and other somatic sites. Mortality and morbidity are very low unless the afflicted child is malnourished or immunodeficient. In these more precarious situations, one should consider treatment with large doses of standard gamma globulin, 0.5 ml/kg body weight, and parenteral adenine arabinoside,* in addition to wet-to-dry sterile saline dressings of the cutaneous lesions.

Mumps

JOSEPH W. St. GEME, Jr., M.D.

Mumps virus is a member of the paramyxovirus family, including the parainfluenza viruses, and spreads via the respiratory tract. Subclinical primary infection occurs in 30% or more of susceptible individuals. In contrast to measles and rubella, mumps virus infection is uncommon in the nonimmunized preschool child; the major occurrences of illness are noted in school-age children and young adolescents.

Uncomplicated mumps is managed very simply

---

*This use of adenine arabinoside is not listed by the manufacturer.

with rest, liquids, bland diet, and occasional analgesic-antipyretic therapy for general discomfort and high fever. The dose of aspirin is 60 mg/kg/24 hr, given in four to six divided oral doses. Acetaminophen can be given in a dose of 30 mg/kg/24 hr in three to four divided oral doses, although for salicylate-equivalent effect twice this dose may be required. There is no evidence that continued activity by adults with mumps increases the risk of orchitis. Most young children with mild disease continue on their regular diet without discomfort.

COMPLICATIONS

Meningitis and Encephalitis. In the past, mumps virus was the most common invader of the central nervous system. The widespread use of mumps vaccine has changed this statistic. Although the great majority of mumps virus infections of the CNS are benign episodes of aseptic meningitis, without immediate or long-term sequelae, perhaps 10 to 20% of cases are encephalitic, with convulsions and significant alteration of the sensorium. The term meningoencephalitis used to embrace all mumps virus infections of the CNS is misleading, since the encephalitic component is uncommon. Serious encephalitic disease is associated with diffuse vasculomyelinopathy and occasional ependymitis (see below).

Unique neurologic sequelae include acute cerebellar ataxia, transverse myelitis, transient paralysis that may mimic poliomyelitis, hemiplegia, diffuse infectious neuronitis (Guillain-Barré syndrome), sudden coma, diabetes insipidus, optic neuritis, and sensorineural deafness. Of these, deafness is the most common and may be sudden in onset; mumps virus has been recovered from the inner ear. Neurologic symptoms rarely may precede parotid gland swelling. Very frequently aseptic meningitis occurs without obvious parotitis. To confuse matters further, the rare occurrence of a morbilliform rash with mumps may challenge the differential diagnostic acumen of the physician confronted by a patient with aseptic meningitis during the summer season of enterovirus infections. Approximately half of all mumps patients have cerebrospinal fluid pleocytosis, and half of these individuals may manifest some evidence of mild neurologic illness. In some cases the CSF glucose content may be decreased, which is atypical for viral infections of the CNS.

Specific oligoclonal IgG mumps virus antibody can be detected in the CSF of children with aseptic meningitis, suggesting local antibody synthesis. The same observation has been made with some patients with multiple sclerosis. However, there are no clinical data at this juncture to suggest that mumps virus can produce a chronic, persistent CNS infection like measles and rubella viruses. In this vein, postnatal and perhaps transplacental fetal mumps virus infection can produce the chronic structural change of aqueductal stenosis and obstructive hydrocephalus.

Diagnostic lumbar puncture may relieve headache. More severe cases may require conservative parenteral fluid therapy, such as 1000 to 1200 ml/m²/24 hr, plus replacement of inordinate fluid loss due to persistent emesis. Otherwise rest, oral fluids, and analgesic-antipyretic therapy will suffice. Hospitalization is not mandatory if the CNS infection is unremarkable and one can be assured that the cause is mumps.

Orchitis. Approximately 10 to 20% of adolescent and postpubescent young men experience testicular swelling, usually unilateral. When orchitis occurs it is generally toward the end of the first week or the beginning of the second week and usually is accompanied by fever and chills. The swelling and inflammation may last from 4 to 7 days. Sterility is unusual although testicular atrophy may occur in 10 to 50% of patients. Despite the fact that 20 to 30% of all cases of orchitis have some element of bilaterality, the subsequent mild atrophy is insufficient to produce frank sterility. Just as aseptic meningitis and encephalitis may occur in the absence of parotitis, the same may be true of orchitis.

Large doses (20 ml) of mumps hyperimmune gamma globulin have been demonstrated to reduce the incidence of significant orchitis threefold. Currently, hyperimmune globulin is not recommended for prevention. The issue deserves further study. Although there are many anecdotal reports of dramatic therapeutic effect, controlled studies of steroid treatment of orchitis have demonstrated only the suppression of fever.

Bed rest, analgesics, ice packs, and gentle support of the engorged testis constitute the essential therapeutic strategem. Incision of the enveloping tunica albuginea represents extraordinary management of the most severely involved testis.

Pancreatitis. Mild, essentially asymptomatic pancreatitis may be more common than suspected, perhaps as frequent as 40% of all patients with mumps. Biochemical diagnosis may be made by the determination of elevated serum lipase and alpha-amylase values. Parotitis and generalized sialadenitis preclude the use of standard serum amylase determinations for the assessment of pancreatic disease. Pancreatitis may occur toward the end of the first week of mumps. Severe pancreatitis of sudden onset with marked abdominal pain and vomiting is unusual. Since this complication is transient, absolute bed rest, sedation, and parenteral fluids are adequate treatment. On rare occasions diabetes mellitus may follow mumps.

Myocarditis. Although the cause of myocarditis is seldom well identified, the group B coxsackieviruses, influenza virus, and mumps virus are important pathogens. Electrocardiographic abnormalities have been identified in 15% of mumps patients. There is some clinical and experimental support for the hypothesis that fetal mumps virus infection may result in myocarditis and, as an occasional consequence of the reparative process, the chronic congestive cardiomyopathy characterized by endocardial fibroelastosis. Significant myocarditis should be managed with bed rest, anticipation, cardiac monitoring, fluid and salt restriction, diuretics, and occasionally the careful use of digitalis. The role of steroid therapy remains controversial. Although the prognosis is usually favorable, on rare occasions well-documented mumps myocarditis in a child or adult has progressed to a congestive cardiomyopathy.

Other Complications. Hemolytic anemia, thrombocytopenic purpura, arthritis, thyroiditis, hepatitis, nephritis, and inflammation of the breasts, lacrimal glands, epididymis, and prostate are rare sequelae of mumps virus infection. Thyroiditis may be followed by hypothyroidism. In several reported cases of migratory arthritis, salicylate therapy has not been effective.

Congenital Infection

The risk of putative congenital anomalies and other embryopathic sequelae of mumps virus infection during pregnancy seems to be as low as 5%. The abnormalities observed in offspring of pregnant women with mumps include endocardial fibroelastosis, chorioretinitis, cataracts, mental retardation, and obstructive hydrocephalus due to stenosis of the aqueduct of Sylvius. Virus cannot be isolated from affected infants, but they and the great majority of infants spared any insult do exhibit cellular immunity to mumps virus antigen.

PREVENTION

Passive Immunization. Large doses of regular commercial gamma globulin (0.4 ml/lb) convert clinical illness into subclinical infection, very similar to the observations with measles and infectious hepatitis. Since the geometric mean titers of mumps virus neutralizing antibody in mumps hyperimmune gamma globulin are sixfold higher than that of regular gamma globulin, an equivalent modifying dose of hyperimmune globulin is 0.07 ml/lb. Lots of gamma globulin with high titers of neutralizing antibody, if administered early in the incubation of mumps, should modify or prevent mumps virus infection. There are insufficient data to confirm such a prediction. The primary target for this form of immunotherapy is the adult male. In this regard development of more satisfactory techniques for the rapid detection of the susceptible adult is needed.

Active Immunization. Parenteral administration of live attenuated mumps virus vaccine (the Jeryl Lyn strain) induces antibody in 95% of recipients and provides apparently complete and sustained immunity against natural mumps. With very few exceptions, even low levels of antibody seem to protect. Vaccine may be administered successfully alone or in combination with other live attenuated viruses, such as measles and rubella. Unfortunately, vaccine administered early in the incubation of mumps does not modify nor prevent subsequent natural infection. Live attenuated mumps virus infection suppresses tuberculin-delayed hypersensitivity, so tuberculin skin testing should be performed prior to or concurrent with the administration of vaccine. The vaccine induces both neutralizing antibody and cellular immunity to mumps virus, the latter ascertained by in vitro assays and skin testing with inactivated viral antigen. There is no place in current practice for the use of killed mumps virus vaccine.

Complications of immunization with live attenuated virus are very rare but include rash, pruritus, purpura, low-grade fever, parotitis, febrile seizures, unilateral nerve deafness, encephalitis, and the Guillain-Barré syndrome. The CNS illnesses have occurred approximately once per 1 million doses of vaccine. On only one occasion, a study of possible fetal infection, has vaccine virus been recovered from human specimens or tissues—in this instance the placentas of several pregnant women. Following widespread use of vaccine in the United States, the incidence of mumps has declined.

Influenza

PAUL F. WEHRLE, M.D.

The clinical symptoms and signs of influenza closely resemble those of many other acute respiratory infections. The specific diagnosis is suspected on epidemiologic grounds including season, prevalence of similar illnesses, and substantial increases in school absenteeism. Specific information regarding the virus type may be available through national, state, and local health departments.

In the older child complaints of aching, substernal discomfort, and frontal headache resembling that of acute sinusitis are helpful clinical symptoms, although bacterial causes should be excluded. Antimicrobial therapy is not indicated unless specific bacterial complications are recognized or suspected. Prophylactic immunization against influenza using currently available inactivated vaccines is recommended for infants and children more than 6 months of age, if chronic health problems or debilitating disease are present.

Treatment. Although uncomplicated influenza is a self-limited disease, some relief of symptoms will be appreciated. Bed rest, acetaminophen, sponging or tepid baths for fever relief, cough suppressants if cough is troublesome, and fluids to maintain hydration are usually sufficient. Although aspirin has been recommended previously, its use in influenza has been discouraged, since there is evidence that aspirin may be a factor in the association of at least some cases of Reye's syndrome with influenza.

Amantadine hydrochloride (Symmetrel) has been useful in the prophylaxis of influenza A infections among unimmunized individuals at risk. It also has been shown to shorten the course of illnesses resulting from influenza A virus if administered within the first 48 hours after onset of illness. It may be used in children at least 1 year of age in a dose of 4 to 6 mg/kg body weight/24 hours in two divided doses each for 5 days. The drug is available in both syrup and tablet form, and the total daily dose should be limited to 150 mg/day for children under 9 years of age. Older children may be given 100 mg twice daily.

Although not recommended for general use, prophylactic therapy with amantadine should be considered for high-risk children who have not been immunized, and dosage should be continued as long as influenza A remains prevalent among potential contacts.

Complications. Complications are primarily related to the respiratory tract. Tracheitis and laryngitis are common, and may be helped with steam or mist therapy. If fever persists, complications such as otitis media, sinusitis, or pneumonia must be suspected. The most likely pathogens are those bacteria normally found in the respiratory tract.

Convulsions sometimes occur, and a coexistent bacterial meningitis should be ruled out. Reye's syndrome, a serious complication, is found more frequently with influenza B infections; it occurs predominantly among school-age children. Intensive supportive therapy is required.

Immunization. Conditions for which influenza immunization may be indicated include 1) cardiac disease, especially with evidence of cardiac insufficiency; 2) chronic bronchopulmonary disease, such as cystic fibrosis, chronic asthma, chronic bronchitis, bronchiectasis, or limited respiratory function due to other causes; 3) severe metabolic disease; 4) chronic renal disease; and 5) chronic neurologic disorders, particularly those involving ventilatory function.

Two doses of inactivated, split-virus vaccine administered 4 weeks apart are required for primary immunization. Annual single doses during subsequent years are sufficient to maintain protection, unless major shifts in the antigenic structure of the virus occur. If such a shift should occur, this will be recognized by health authorities and information will be forthcoming. The vaccine is used in reduced dosage between 6 months and 3 years of age, while the split-virus product is preferred for children.

Although the Guillain-Barré syndrome appeared to follow use of the swine influenza vaccine, no evidence of this problem has been seen since 1978. Since the vaccine is prepared in embryonated eggs, it should not be administered to children with egg allergy.

Rabies

KENNETH W. BERNARD, M.D.

Rabies is a viral zoonosis that is most often transmitted to humans by contact with saliva from an infected animal. Rabies causes a multisystem infection that in humans almost invariably results in fatal encephalitis. Only 0–5 human rabies deaths are reported annually in the United States. Seventeen of 40 human cases (40%) from 1960 to 1982 were in persons < 18 years of age. Despite the reduction in the number of rabid dogs and cats in this country to approximately 200 per year for each species, 7211 documented rabid animals were reported in the U.S. in 1981—the highest number since 1954. This is primarily the result of an increase in skunk rabies. Although domestic dogs and cats account for only about 7% of rabid animals in the U.S., 55% of persons undergoing rabies postexposure prophylaxis report domestic pet exposures as the reason for treatment. Children ≤ 14 years of age account for 34% of all persons treated.

Once clinical manifestations appear, human rabies is almost universally fatal (Only three cases with survival have been documented; one was a 6-year-old boy). The mainstay of therapy therefore, is treatment of the individual after exposure but before the onset of clinical signs or symptoms.

RATIONALE OF POSTEXPOSURE TREATMENT

Species and Location of Animal. Different animal species are variably susceptible to rabies virus and, therefore, more or less likely to transmit the virus to humans. Local health authorities should be consulted to determine whether dogs, cats, and other animal species are potentially rabid in a specific geographic area. Bats and wild carnivores (especially skunks, foxes, and raccoons) are the most commonly reported rabid wild animals in the U.S. In most cases if a human has been exposed to one of these animals, and the animal is not available for rabies examination, postexposure prophylaxis should be instituted as soon as possible. Rodents (including squirrels, hamsters, guinea pigs, gerbils, chipmunks, rats, and mice) and lagomorphs (rabbits and hares) are rarely found to be infected

with rabies and have not been known to cause human rabies in the U.S. Thus rabies postexposure prophylaxis is rarely indicated for anyone bitten by these animals. Unusual exposures to these animals as well as to animals such as opossums, muskrats, and ferrets require consultation with local health authorities.

Type of Exposure. Rabies normally is transmitted to humans by introducing the virus into open cuts or wounds in the skin, or via mucous membranes. Intact skin is an effective barrier to the virus, and the virus is rapidly inactivated by desiccation, soap, and most common disinfectants. There are two categories of exposure: 1) bite: any penetration of the skin by teeth, and 2) nonbite: scratches, abrasions, open wounds, or mucous membranes contaminated with saliva or other potentially infectious material such as brain tissue from a rabid animal. Casual contact, such as petting a rabid animal (without a bite or nonbite exposure as described above), does not constitute an exposure and is not an indication for prophylaxis. An unprovoked attack is more likely to indicate that the animal is rabid than is a provoked attack. Unfortunately, what constitutes provocation is questionable, especially in the case of wild animals. Bites inflicted on a person attempting to handle or feed an apparently healthy animal can generally be regarded as provoked. In most other circumstances the distinction offers little help.

Evaluation of Animal. If a person is exposed to a potentially rabid animal, an attempt should be made to determine whether the animal was actually rabid before postexposure prophylaxis is begun. Because human rabies has been acquired from pets that have been vaccinated against rabies, the vaccination status of the animal should not ordinarily be used to determine whether postexposure prophylaxis should be given. If the source of the exposure is an apparently healthy domestic dog or cat, the animal should be confined, observed for 10 days, and evaluated by a veterinarian at the first sign of illness or just before release. Any illness should be reported immediately to the local health department. If the animal is ill when exposure occurs or if signs suggestive of rabies develop during the observation period, the animal should be humanely killed, its head removed and shipped intact, packed in ice (not frozen), for rabies examination by a qualified laboratory. Any stray dog or cat that bites a person should be killed immediately and the head submitted for rabies examination. Because signs of rabies in wild animals cannot be interpreted reliably, any wild animal that exposes a person to potentially infectious saliva should be killed at once and the brain submitted as described above. Quarantine is not recommended for any animals except domestic dogs and cats.

Fluorescent antibody testing of brain material from potentially rabid animals is, in expert hands, reliable and conclusive. If the brain is negative by fluorescent antibody examination, it can be assumed that the saliva contained no virus and the person bitten need not be treated.

POSTEXPOSURE PROPHYLAXIS

Because the incubation period in humans is long (usually 3 weeks to 3 months; mean 35 days), rabies prophylaxis given soon after exposure and before onset of clinical illness will prevent illness in virtually 100% of those treated with the optimal combination of local wound treatment, passive antibody administration, and human diploid cell rabies vaccine (HDCV). In one study in the U.S., no cases of human rabies developed in 374 persons bitten by laboratory-confirmed rabid animals who were given this optimal schedule of postexposure prophylaxis. Delay in instituting prophylaxis should be avoided. However, in the United States, the mean delay between exposure and treatment is 5 days, which suggests that there usually is time to completely evaluate the exposure incident before initiating specific therapy.

Local Wound Treatment. Thorough cleansing and mechanical scrubbing of the wound site with a 20% soap solution can reduce from 50 to 90% the risk of developing rabies in a wound contaminated with rabies virus. Quaternary ammonium compounds are no more effective than soap solution and their use has been associated with nosocomial infections related to bacterial contamination. A tetanus immunization history should be obtained and appropriate tetanus immunoprophylaxis given if necessary.

Passive Immunization. Once the decision is made to treat a person who may have been exposed to rabies, passive immunization with human rabies immune globulin (HRIG) should be given regardless of the age of the patient, species of animal, location or severity of bite, or whether the exposure was a bite or non-bite type. Passive immunization with HRIG is administered to provide protection for the initial 1 to 2 weeks before the vaccine elicits an active antibody response. Two cases of human rabies have developed in patients outside the United States who received HDCV *without* concomitant administration of passive antibody. Passive immunization with HRIG is not necessary only when the exposed person has previously received a recommended HDCV immunization regimen, or has been immunized for rabies with another rabies vaccine and developed an adequate rabies titer ($\geq 1:16$ by rapid fluorescent focus inhibition test). In these instances, only thorough wound cleansing and administration of rabies vaccine (HDCV) are necessary (see below).

HRIG is given as a single dose of 20 international units (IU)/kg or approximately 9 IU/lb. As much as 50% of the calculated dose should be infiltrated around the wound site; if the wound site is small, such as the nose or finger, the amount infiltrated must be reduced. The remainder of the calculated dose of HRIG should be given intramuscularly in the upper outer quadrant of the buttocks or the anterolateral aspect of the thigh. An excessive amount should not be given, because it can interfere with the development of active antibody; it should not be given in the same muscle as the vaccine.

If a significant delay of days or weeks has occurred between exposure and onset of treatment, it is still critical that HRIG be used at the time treatment is initiated, to provide immediate protection against rabies virus until antibody can be developed from the concurrent vaccine administration. If HRIG was omitted or was unavailable at the time that the vaccination series was begun, it can be given any time in the first 7 days after the initial vaccine dose; after 7 days, most persons receiving HDCV will have developed active antibody, and HRIG is not indicated.

HRIG is currently available from two sources in the U.S.: Hyperab, from Cutter Laboratories, Berkeley, California, and Imogam, from Merieux Institute, Miami, Florida.* Under unusual circumstances when HRIG is not available, equine antirabies serum (ARS) can be used as an effective substitute in a single dose of 40 IU/kg. Because anaphylaxis and serum sickness are frequent adverse reactions to horse serum, ARS should be used only if the risk of rabies is high and HRIG is unavailable.

Active Immunization. Two vaccines (HDCV) are currently licensed in the United States for human rabies immunization: Imovax, produced by the Merieux Institute, Miami, Florida, and Wyvac, produced by Wyeth Laboratories, Radnor, Pennsylvania.* Both are killed virus vaccines in which the virus has been grown in human diploid cells, but they differ in the method of viral inactivation. Both have been shown to produce adequate antibody titers in virtually 100% of persons given the recommended vaccine regimen. For postexposure prophylaxis, HDCV is administered as five 1-ml intramuscular doses given over 1 month. Infants and small children should receive the same dose as adults. The first dose should be given as soon as possible after exposure; an additional dose should be given on each of days 3, 7, 14, and 28 after the first dose. Other volumes or routes of

---

*The use of trade names is for identification only and does not imply endorsement by the Public Health Service or the U.S. Department of Health and Human Services.

administration (e.g., intradermal) have not been evaluated for postexposure use and should *not* be used for this purpose at this time. As previously stated, passive antibody consisting of a single dose of HRIG should be given with the first dose of vaccine or, if delay is unavoidable, any time during the first 7 days after the initial vaccine dose.

If a person previously received preexposure immunization with HDCV, postexposure prophylaxis consists only of thorough wound cleansing followed by two 1-ml intramuscular doses of HDCV given one each on days 0 and 3.

Rabies immunization is no longer a "painful series of 21 or 23 injections in the stomach." HDCV can be given intramuscularly in any appropriately sized muscle, such as the deltoid in an older child or the anterolateral aspect of the thigh in a small child. HDCV should not be given in the same muscle as the HRIG. Pain is no more frequent than with other more commonly used vaccines.

Duck embryo vaccine (DEV), the rabies vaccine used most frequently in the U.S. between 1958 and 1980, is no longer commercially available. Treatment failures using DEV have been described, and adverse reactions can be severe.

Because of the high immunologic potency of HDCV, routine serologic testing of persons who receive recommended pre-exposure or postexposure regimens is no longer recommended. Immunosuppressed persons may not develop an adequate antibody response to HDCV; in these individuals, serum should be collected at the time of the last dose of vaccine to assess antibody development. Occasionally, aberrant schedules of vaccine have been given, especially in persons whose treatment was begun in another country. In these persons a rabies antibody titer should also be determined. In such cases, local or state health officials or the Division of Viral Diseases, Centers for Disease Control, Atlanta, Georgia (404–329–3095 weekdays or 404–329–3644 after office hours) should be contacted for advice.

PRE-EXPOSURE IMMUNIZATION

Children living in or visiting countries where rabies is a constant threat should be given pre-exposure immunization. This protects persons at unusually high risk and those whose postexposure therapy might be delayed; it also provides the basis for a rapid anamnestic antibody response when booster doses of vaccine are given. In addition, it eliminates the need for passive immunization with HRIG and reduces the number of doses of vaccine needed should later postexposure treatment be necessary. The dose schedule for either the Wyeth or the Merieux vaccine consists of three 1.0-ml doses given intramuscularly, one each on days 0, 7, and 21 *or* 28. The Merieux vaccine is effective and safe for pre-exposure use when given as three

0.1-ml intradermal doses in the skin over the deltoid area, one each on days 0, 7, and 28. The Wyeth vaccine has not yet been evaluated for intradermal use. Neither vaccine should be used intradermally for postexposure prophylaxis. Determination of antibody titers following pre-exposure immunization, either intramuscular or intradermal, is unnecessary.

SPECIAL SITUATIONS AFFECTING IMMUNIZATION

Rabies Immunization During Pregnancy. A number of pregnant women in various stages of gestation have received pre-exposure or postexposure rabies prophylaxis with HDCV both with and without HRIG. No untoward effects have been reported for either mother or fetus.

Vaccination During a Febrile Illness. When a probable rabies exposure has occurred, postexposure prophylaxis should not be delayed while awaiting the resolution of a febrile illness.

Vaccination of Infants. Infants requiring rabies postexposure prophylaxis should receive the same quantity (1.0 ml) and number of vaccine doses (5) as an adult. HRIG should be given and the dose calculated on the same 20 IU/kg basis as in adults.

Vaccination of Immunosuppressed Persons. Immunosuppression markedly reduces the neutralizing antibody response of rabies vaccine recipients. Animal studies indicate that immunosuppression induced following an exposure may enhance the development of clinical rabies; thus it is essential that immunosuppressed patients receiving rabies prophylaxis be followed closely, with frequent determinations of antibody titers and additional doses of vaccine given if necessary.

Simultaneous Administration of Rabies Vaccine with Other Vaccines. There is no contraindication to the simultaneous administration of other vaccines during a course of rabies postexposure or pre-exposure prophylaxis. However, HRIG, being an immune globulin, may interfere with antibody production following vaccination with some live, attenuated virus vaccines such as measles.

ADVERSE REACTIONS TO RABIES IMMUNIZATION

HRIG is an immune globulin product concentrated by cold ethanol fractionation of plasma from rabies immunized human donors. Significant adverse reactions from this product are extremely rare, and none have been reported in the U.S. In the rare instance when ARS must be used because of the unavailability of HRIG, there is a 15% risk of serum sickness in children.

Adverse reactions such as encephalitis or death have not been reported following administration of

HDCV. Local reactions are common and usually consist of redness, swelling, slight induration, or local lymphadenopathy. Occasional systemic reactions consist of headache, nausea, fever, and rash. Occurrence is highly variable and cannot be predicted. Urticaria and anaphylaxis have been reported following administration of HDCV, especially in highly atopic individuals. Interestingly, when it has been necessary to continue the immunization schedule following severe systemic allergic reactions, the reaction did not always recur. Two cases of a transient Guillain-Barré–like illness in children have been temporally associated with HDCV. For most individuals, adverse reactions to HDCV are mild and not clinically significant. In one study, only 2 of 50 (4%) of children 1 to 13 years of age had mild systemic reactions. This is a lower reaction rate than observed in adults. Because of the suppression of antibody response by immunosuppressive drugs, steroids should not be used to treat adverse reactions to rabies vaccine unless the reaction is life-threatening.

TREATMENT OF HUMAN RABIES

The clinical course of human rabies is distinguished by five stages: incubation, prodrome, acute neurologic, coma, and recovery or death. Unconfirmed incubation periods have been reported to be as short as 9 days and as long as 19 years, but incubation periods less than 2 weeks or more than 1 year are distinctly unusual. In the prodromal stage the first symptoms are often nonspecific and may include headache, malaise, fever, gastrointestinal complaints, sore throat, and a feeling of apprehension or nervousness. A history of pain or paresthesias at the site of the bite can be elicited in approximately 50% of patients. In the acute neurologic phase, the patient may exhibit hallucinations, nuchal rigidity, bizarre behavior, and hyperactivity or obtundation. Attempts to drink during this period may result in severe spasms of the pharynx and larynx; these symptoms may result in a fear of water (hydrophobia). Similar spasms can often be seen when a jet of cool air is directed across the face of the patient and may result in a fear of drafts (aerophobia). Mental status deteriorates gradually and the acute neurologic phase may last from 2 to 10 days. Coma then results, which may last for hours or months, with death the almost inevitable outcome. Complications involve most organ systems and may include cerebral edema, inappropriate secretion of antidiuretic hormone, seizures, gastrointestinal bleeding, acute renal failure, hyperthermia or hypothermia, sepsis, hypoxia, respiratory arrest, cardiac arrhythmias, congestive heart failure, vascular thrombosis, and cardiac arrest.

It is essential that state and local health authorities be contacted whenever rabies is suspected, and

a physician with previous experience in the management of human rabies be consulted. The Centers for Disease Control (see telephone numbers on page 575) will provide expert assistance if necessary. It should be emphasized that the laboratory diagnosis of rabies cannot generally be made prior to 5 days after the onset of clinical symptoms, and may take as long as 2 or 3 weeks after the onset of clinical illness.

The expense in a hospital setting can approach $100,000. In addition to the medical cost of treating the patient, many health care providers have required postexposure prophylaxis because of possible contamination from ill patients. Because there have been no documented cases of human-to-human transmission except via corneal transplantation, the risk to attending health care workers is probably quite low. However, the virus has been isolated from saliva, urine sediment, cerebrospinal fluid, and numerous organ tissue specimens from human patients, and the patient should be placed in strict isolation as soon as rabies is suspected. Once clinical signs and symptoms have appeared, rabies vaccine and hyperimmune globulin will not ameliorate the course of illness and may, in fact, be detrimental. Treatment of clinical rabies with systemic and intrathecal interferon has been attempted, but results have not been encouraging.

During the last 10 years, 40% of those dying of rabies in the United States had no known animal exposure. It is recommended, therefore, that rabies be considered in any patient who presents with or without a bite exposure and who has the signs and symptoms of the early clinical disease.

Infectious Mononucleosis

NATHANIEL BROWN, M.D.,
and GEORGE MILLER, M.D.

Infectious mononucleosis is the common clinical syndrome resulting from primary infection with the Epstein-Barr virus (EBV) in the older child or young adult.

The clinical course is often moderately severe. Fever may persist for more than a week, and prostration may result from severe tonsillopharyngitis, malaise, fatigability, and anorexia. The latter manifestations often persist for several weeks. During this time, bed rest, aspirin or acetaminophen, saline gargles, and attention to fluid intake are appropriate. A few patients will have a secondary pharyngeal infection with group A beta-hemolytic streptococci and should be treated with penicillin or the equivalent in the usual doses. Ampicillin usually causes a skin eruption in mononucleosis patients and should not be used. When secondary infection is not present, antibiotics are not indicated and have no effect on the course of the disease. Patients with splenomegaly should be cautioned against vigorous activity and contact sports, until the condition resolves.

In the United States, there are perhaps 100,000 cases each year, and the outcome is almost always benign. However, several dozen deaths per year are attributed to this disease. The potentially serious complications fall into several categories, including splenic rupture; respiratory obstruction due to massive tonsils or paratracheal nodes; pneumonia; hematologic syndromes such as severe hemolytic anemia, leukopenia, thrombocytopenia, and aplasia; and neurologic syndromes such as meningoencephalitis, cerebellar ataxia, and Guillain-Barré syndrome. Many of these complications appear to result from excesses or aberrations in the cellular immune response to EBV infection. In such severe cases, steroids are often employed, particularly for respiratory obstruction or immune hemolytic anemia. A typical regimen would involve high-dose therapy initially (e.g., prednisone at 1 to 2 mg/kg/24 hr), with subsequent tapering. The use of steroids may entail an increased risk of secondary infection and should be discouraged except when strictly indicated. Finally, there are rare patients who appear to be unable to control the B-cell proliferation induced by EBV; these patients may succumb with a pathologic picture of fatal mononucleosis or acute lymphoma. Most appear to suffer from either a congenital immunodeficiency, which may be sporadic or X-linked recessive, or from profound immunosuppression induced for organ transplantation.

To date, viral DNA-polymerase inhibitors such as adenine arabinoside (Vidarabine) have not been shown to be effective in EBV infections. Newer agents, such as acyclovir, show promise in vitro, but clinical studies are still pending. There are few data on the use of interferon in EBV infection, but controlled trials may be undertaken, in certain clinical settings, as this substance becomes more available. In those rare and life-threatening cases in which the lymphoproliferation appears to be proceeding unchecked, careful consideration might be given to the use of cytotoxic agents, such as cyclophosphamide.

Acute Infectious Lymphocytosis

CHARLES GROSE, M.D.

Acute infectious lymphocytosis is a disease of young children characterized by an outpouring of normal-appearing, small, mature lymphocytes in the peripheral blood. The total white cell count ranges from 20,000 to over 100,000 per cu mm; recent studies indicate that the proliferating lymphocytes are T cells and null cells, whereas the absolute number of B cells remains unchanged. The etiology of the disorder remains obscure, although a coxsackievirus was cultured from several children during an institutional outbreak.

Usually the disease remains subclinical. When symptoms occur, they are nonspecific and include low-grade fever, cough, sore throat, and abdominal pain. Patients occasionally have skin rashes, but do not manifest generalized lymphadenopathy or hepatosplenomegaly. Since acute lymphocytosis is contagious, playmates of the affected child also may acquire the syndrome.

The disease is self-limited and abates within a few weeks without specific treatment. The more serious diagnoses of infectious mononucleosis and acute leukemia should always be entertained and excluded by careful examination of the peripheral blood smear and appropriate serologic assays, e.g., heterophile test or EB virus antibody titers. If the diagnosis remains in doubt, a bone marrow aspiration should be considered; the bone marrow in infectious lymphocytosis may show an increase in mature lymphocytes but is otherwise normal.

Cat-Scratch Disease

MARTIN L. SCHULKIND, M.D.

Cat-scratch disease (CSD) is presumed to be infectious; however, no bacterial or fungal agents have been implicated and a viral etiology is most likely. Thus antibiotics are not indicated in its therapy. Indeed, the reported clinical experience shows that antibiotics neither shorten the duration of the illness nor prevent suppuration of the lymph nodes. Despite the infectious nature of the disease, it is not transmitted from man to man; therefore, isolation of patients is not necessary. Similarly, although kittens are implicated in the transmission of CSD, they are not sick; neither is the nature, degree, nor duration of their infectivity known. Therefore, their disposal or isolation is not recommended.

Because of the self-limited nature of CSD most therapy is aimed toward making therapy comfortable and preventing disfigurement. Some patients have fever early in the course of the illness and should be treated with antipyretics. However, most are seen by their physicians when they have enlarged lymph nodes and at this stage rarely have fever. Some complain of pain in the area of lymphadenopathy, and mild analgesics are indicated in these situations. Parents should be cautioned about trauma to the area, and the application of warm soaks to the area may make the patient more comfortable. Patients need to be reminded that the lymphadenopathy may persist for weeks, as the natural course of the disease, and need only be observed for signs of suppuration or enlargement. In most situations, the lymphadenopathy resolves by itself.

In a small percentage of patients, the lymph node inflammation progresses to suppuration. When the suppuration becomes so painful that the patient cannot tolerate it, then aspiration, using a large bore hypodermic needle and aseptic technique, is indicated. Ethyl chloride spray is used as a topical anesthetic in these situations because the skin is so thin that the injection of local anesthetics would be impractical. Since the aspiration procedure will relieve much of the patient's pain, the use of systemic analgesics is often not necessary. Surgical excision of involved lymph nodes in CSD is not indicated unless one suspects some other etiology, such as a lymphoreticular malignancy. Aspiration of suppurant lymph nodes is very successful and obviates the need for surgical excision to achieve a good cosmetic result.

Eye care in patients with the oculoglandular form of CSD should only be symptomatic unless the rare complication of secondary infection occurs, in which case application of local antibiotics to the conjunctiva is justified. Surgical excision of granulomatous lesions of the conjunctiva in CSD is not necessary.

Patients who develop encephalopathy as a complication of CSD need only supportive care because of the self-limited nature of this complication. Invasive procedures should be avoided.

Lyme Disease

H. CODY MEISSNER, M.D.

Lyme disease is a newly described inflammatory disorder characterized by the presence of erythema chronicum migrans, recurrent attacks of arthritis, and occasional involvement of the nervous system and the heart. Epidemiologic observations first suggested that the principal vector of transmission is a tick. Transfer of a treponema-like spirochete during a bite from the adult tick *Ixodes dammini* now seems to be the major route of transmission of the disease.

One to 2 weeks after a bite from an infecting tick, erythema chronicum nigrans begins as a red macule, usually on the trunk or extremity at the site of tick attachment. Fever, chills, and malaise usually accompany the rash. Three to 4 weeks after the rash, arthritis or arthralgia may begin. Because of the variation in systemic involvement in Lyme disease, from minimal symptoms to prolonged or recurrent arthritis, the role of antibiotics has been difficult to define. There are some patients who receive antibiotics and who still develop the late complications of the disease, and there are others who do not receive antibiotics and who do not develop arthritis. However, it is likely that either penicillin or tetracycline may shorten the duration of the skin lesion by several days and at least moderate the development of arthritis. Thus, therapy should be started promptly with oral penicillin and continued for 7 to 10 days. Children allergic to penicillin should receive oral tetracycline, 250 mg four times a day for 7 to 10 days. Children less than 8 years of age should not receive tetracycline because of the danger of tooth discoloration. Salicylates may be prescribed while joint involvement is present; however, aspirin usually produces only minimal benefit. Salicylates are ineffective in preventing recurrent arthritis.

Involvement of the heart during Lyme disease generally produces distrubances of rhythm secondary to atrioventricular conduction abnormalities. Because of the possibility of cardiac disease, any patient suspected of having the disease should be carefully monitored with serial ECGs. Because some patients may develop third degree heart block, patients with conduction disturbances should be managed by personnel experienced in treating arrhythmias. In some instances pacemaker insertion has been necessary. Any evidence on chest x-ray or ECG of pericarditis or pericardial effusion should be evaluated with a cardiac ECHO. Some patients with first or second degree AV block have been satisfactorily treated with prednisone 1 mg/kg/day in 3 doses. Because of the similarity of many of the findings in rheumatic fever to Lyme disease, it is important to carefully exlude the possibility of rheumatic fever.

There are a number of manifestations of neurologic involvement. Generally, the earliest signs are those of aseptic meningitis. Headache and stiff neck may occur soon after onset of the rash or several weeks after its resolution. Encephalitis is nearly as common as meningitis. Therapy of CNS involvement is supportive and in most instances the outcome is good.

Cytomegalovirus Infections

ROBERT F. PASS, M.D.

Cytomegalovirus (CMV), a member of the herpesvirus family, is widely distributed in human populations and can remain latent in host tissues indefinitely. Reactivation of latent virus can result in intermittent viral shedding and in disease in profoundly immunosuppressed hosts. Cytomegalovirus is clinically important as a cause of mononucleosis, congenital infection, pneumonitis in young infants, post-transfusion illness, and febrile illness in immunosuppressed patients. A variety of therapeutic approaches are currently being studied but none is available outside experimental protocols.

CMV Mononucleosis. Although the vast majority of acquired CMV infections in normal children and adults are asymptomatic, CMV can produce a heterophil-negative mononucleosis characterized by fever, malaise, arthralgias, and atypical lymphocytosis. The disease is less likely to be accompanied by adenopathy and exudative pharyngitis than is the classic mononucleosis syndrome due to Epstein-Barr virus. Spontaneous remission in 1 to 2 weeks is the rule; rarely, the course can be complicated by encephalitis, Guillain-Barré syndrome, pneumonitis, or thrombocytopenic purpura.

Congenital CMV Infection. Cytomegalovirus is the leading cause of congenital viral infection. Approximately 1% of infants born in the United States have been infected in utero. Fortunately, over 90% of neonates with congenital CMV infection are asymptomatic at birth. The most common findings in symptomatic newborns are jaundice with direct hyperbilirubinemia, hepatosplenomegaly, microcephaly, thrombocytopenia, petechiae, and low birth weight. Both symptomatic and asymptomatic newborns are at risk for adverse sequelae affecting the CNS or organs of perception, but these problems are much more likely in the former group. Hearing loss is the most common handicap; mental retardation, seizures, motor deficits, poor school performance, chorioretinitis, optic atrophy, and defects in tooth structure have also been described. Congenital CMV infection can result in chronic illness, the full effects of which may take years to define.

Acquired CMV Infection. Premature newborns who receive multiple transfusions are at risk for acquiring CMV. Prematures who are born to seronegative mothers and thus have no passively acquired antibody can become seriously ill from this infection. They may develop interstitial pneumonitis, hepatosplenomegaly, jaundice, hepatitis, and thrombocytopenia. Older children and adults can acquire CMV through blood transfusions, but they are much less likely to suffer serious morbidity. The risk of acquiring CMV from blood products can be related to whether the recipient has antibody to CMV, to the number of units given and to the product used.

Around 20% of infants hospitalized with pneumonitis have been found to be CMV infected. These patients are often infected with other respiratory pathogens, notably *Chlamydia trachomatis* and *Pneumocystis carinii*. Respiratory symptoms and radiographic abnormalities can persist for months in these infants.

CMV Infection in Immunocompromised Hosts. Immunocompromised patients, especially those with impaired cell mediated immunity are particularly prone to CMV infection. These patients often shed CMV chronically in urine or saliva. Whether these infections remain silent or result in disease is a function of the underlying illness and the degree of immunosuppression. Clinical manifestations in these patients include elevated temperature, arthralgias, malaise, leukopenia, abnormal liver function tests, thrombocytopenia, and interstitial pneumonitis. Other pathogens often accompany CMV. The severity of illness ranges from a few days of fever to overwhelming multisystem disease which may be fatal.

Treatment

No therapeutic agent available for use in humans has been found to be effective in treating any of the above types of CMV infection. Adenine arabinoside and interferon reduce viral shedding in compromised hosts and children with congenital infection, but they have not significantly altered the course of illness. Management remains supportive. When CMV is recovered from immunosuppressed patients and young infants with pneumonitis, other pathogens should also be sought and treated with specific antimicrobial therapy if possible.

Children with congenital infection often need specialized assessments and services to identify and respond to handicaps. They should be managed much like patients with congenital rubella; auditory evaluations and eye examinations should be performed early in infancy and other services provided on an individual basis.

Prevention

Except for CMV transmitted with blood products and transplanted organs, the source of most acquired CMV infections is unknown. Cytomegalovirus does not spread in epidemics; most acquired infections are asymptomatic, and mechanisms of transmission are ill defined. Therefore, developing strategies for prevention of CMV infections in pregnant women is practically impossible. Young CMV infected children usually excrete virus for years and could thus provide a reservoir of infection. Susceptible women who have contact with children in hospitals, day nurseries, or schools could be at increased risk, but there is as yet no convincing evidence that this is the case.

Serious illness due to transfusion acquired CMV infections in premature newborns can be prevented by restricting seronegative babies to blood from seronegative donors. There is also evidence that use of frozen deglycerolized red blood cells is effective. Similar techniques could be used in older, normal hosts, but the expense and restrictions on availability of blood are difficult to justify, as transfusion acquired infections in these patients usually produce no symptoms or a self-limited heterophilnegative mononucleosis. In organ transplant recipients CMV infections can be due to reactivation of endogenous virus, to transfusions, or to the transplanted organ; there is no widely accepted means of preventing these infections.

Both active and passive immunization for CMV infections remain the subject of clinical investigations.

Mycoplasma Infections

JEROME O. KLEIN, M.D.

The mycoplasmas are a unique group of microorganisms that colonize mucosal surfaces, particularly those of the respiratory and genital tracts. *Mycoplasma pneumoniae,* the agent of primary atypical pneumonia, is the only mycoplasma found in the respiratory tract that is unequivocally associated with human disease. The genital mycoplasmas, including *Ureaplasma urealyticum* and *M. hominis,* are present in the genital tract of sexually active adults and have been associated with a variety of local and systemic infections. *M. hominis* may cause abscesses in newborn infants, usually as a result of impregnation into the skin and soft tissues of surface organisms by fetal monitors or forceps at delivery. *M. hominis* has also been a rare cause of neonatal meningitis.

M. pneumoniae and *U. urealyticum* are susceptible in vitro to erythromycin, tetracyclines, and chloramphenicol. *M. hominis* is resistant to erythromycin but susceptible to tetracyclines, chloramphenicol, and clindamycin.

Tetracyclines and erythromycin are effective agents for respiratory infections due to *M. pneumoniae.* Erythromycin (50 mg/kg/day in four doses for 7 days) shortens the clinical course of pneumonia due to *M. pneumoniae* and is the drug of choice for children younger than 9 years. Tetracyclines are effective, including tetracycline, chlortetracycline, and oxytetracycline (25 to 50 mg/kg/day in 4 doses for 7 days) or methacycline or demeclocycline (10 mg/kg/day in 2 doses for 7 days) and may be used for older children. Antimicrobial therapy may suppress but not eliminate the organism from the upper respiratory tract. The patient may relapse after conclusion of therapy and require a second course of the same drug.

Soft tissue abscesses due to *M. hominis* resolve with incision and drainage alone. The efficacy of specific antibiotics for neonatal meningitis due to *M. hominis* is difficult to determine, since many different regimens were used for each infant studied. Chloramphenicol is active against *M. hominis*

and achieves high concentrations in the cerebrospinal fluid. Tetracycline is more effective than chloramphenicol in vitro and may be of value in treatment of *M. hominis* meningitis, although bone and tooth toxicity limit use of tetracyclines in critically ill infants.

Viral Pneumonia

JOHN W. PAISLEY, M.D.

Viral pneumonia is a common pediatric problem, particularly in infants during the winter. Many mild cases probably remain undiagnosed.

Outpatient management of viral pneumonia includes fever control, adequate hydration, and avoidance of environmental pollutants (such as cigarette smoke) that may trigger bronchospasm during viral respiratory infections. Humidification may be helpful. Decongestants and sedatives should not be used. Most importantly, the caretaker should be able to recognize signs of clinical deterioration such as cyanosis, inability to feed, and respiratory fatigue.

Inpatient management includes both supportive and pharmacologic therapy. Respiratory isolation is important because of the high incidence of nosocomially transmitted respiratory viral infections. Ventilation is easier when the child is supine with elevation of the head of the bed. An intravenous line may be needed to correct dehydration and provide adequate maintenance fluid. Oral feedings in infants should be avoided when the respiratory rate is high (greater than 50 per minute) to minimize the risk of aspiration. Greater than homeostatic fluid intake has been standard therapy, presumably to help mobilize secretions. This is an undocumented assumption, however, and such therapy may even be harmful. Interstitial pulmonary fluid increases when intrapleural pressures decrease, as soon during an asthmatic attack. To the extent that airway narrowing occurs in viral pneumonitis, overhydration of the lung may already be present and could be exacerbated by overzealous fluid therapy.

A cardiorespiratory monitor may be needed, particularly if periodic breathing is observed in association with a viral infection. The respiratory rate and quality, skin color, degree of fatigue, and air exchange are important parameters to follow regarding impending respiratory failure. Arterial blood gases give more accurate information regarding the respiratory status. Depending on the clinical examination and the arterial Po_2, humidified oxygen delivered by hood or nasal cannula to young infants and by mask to older children may be necessary. Owing to transient changes in ventilation associated with obtaining a percutaneous arterial blood gas, the optimal FIO_2 can best be assessed with a transcutaneous oxygen monitor or ear oximeter. For seriously ill children, an indwelling arterial catheter may be needed. Excessive mist or continuous humidification by ultrasonic nebulizer should be avoided in infants owing to the potential for water intoxication. Intermittent suctioning of the nasopharynx and mouth may be helpful, especially in young infants. The need for postural drainage should be individualized. It is usually not very productive in viral pneumonia and may be stressful to the child.

Prophylactic antibiotics are of no benefit in viral respiratory infections. Antibiotics should not be used to treat organisms found in nasopharyngeal cultures (excluding group A streptococcus or *Bordetella pertussis*) or in other specimens such as nasotracheal aspirates or "sputum," both of which are invariably contaminated with oral flora when obtained from young children. A sudden deterioration in respiratory status may represent bacterial superinfection, but this complication must be evaluated when it arises.

Currently, only a few viruses are susceptible to specific chemotherapy. Herpes simplex and herpes zoster pneumonitis may occur, primarily in immunosuppressed children, and may be amenable to therapy with acyclovir or adenine arabinoside. Influenza A infections in adults and children over 2 years of age may be both prevented and treated, to some degree, with amantadine. The use of a rapid influenza diagnostic technique during a community influenza A outbreak might diagnose some children with influenza pneumonia early enough to achieve clinical benefit from amantadine therapy. Since influenza is an uncommon cause of pneumonia in young children, however, and since the value of this drug in infants has not been defined, blind therapy of viral pneumonia with amantadine is contraindicated. Recently, aerosolized ribavirin, an experimental agent, has shown promise as a specific therapy for lower respiratory infections caused by respiratory syncytial virus in infants.

Steroids have been shown to be of no benefit in the prototype of lower respiratory viral infections in children—bronchiolitis. Although they are occasionally used in life-threatening cases of viral pneumonia, they are probably no more than a physician placebo. If viral pneumonia is associated with an asthmatic exacerbation or perhaps croup, then steroid therapy may be a more appropriate consideration.

Despite the fact that viral respiratory infections have been associated with varying degrees of bronchial obstruction, bronchodilators have not been generally beneficial. If clinical evaluation suggests bronchoconstriction, a trial of a bronchodilator may be given. I prefer a rapid acting agent such as subcutaneous epinephrine or inhaled isoetharine.

If a beneficial effect is evident by substantial improvement in the respiratory rate, physical findings, or blood gas parameters, then maintenance bronchodilator therapy may be begun. If no benefit is apparent, then bronchodilators should not be continued. Although the rare child with both croup and lower respiratory tract infection may be a candidate for racemic epinephrine, it must be remembered that this drug is very irritating to the lower respiratory tract and can worsen underlying bronchospasm. The value of vagal blockers, e.g., atropine, has not been evaluated in viral pneumonitis.

Clinical and radiographic resolution of viral pneumonia may take weeks. Subsequent wheezing may be seen, particularly with viral pneumonitis or bronchiolitis occurring in infancy.

Viral Hepatitis

SAUL KRUGMAN, M.D.

Viral hepatitis is an infectious disease caused by hepatitis A virus (HAV), hepatitis B virus (HBV), and viral agents that are neither HAV nor HBV. So-called non-A, non-B (NANB) hepatitis is a temporary designation for diseases that may be caused by two or more additional hepatitis viruses.

The three types of hepatitis have features that may be similar or distinctive. The incubation period for type A is about 2 to 6 weeks; that for type B is 2 to 6 months; and that for NANB may be 2 weeks to 4 months. Type A usually is transmitted via the fecal-oral route. Therefore, infection is associated with close contact (household exposure) or the ingestion of fecally contaminated water or food such as shellfish. Types B and NANB may be transmitted by inoculation of contaminated blood or blood products, or by intimate physical contact. Hepatitis B is sexually transmitted.

The following specific markers of infection have been identified: hepatitis A antigen (HAAg) and antibody (anti-HAV); hepatitis B surface antigen (HBsAg) and antibody (anti-HBs); hepatitis B core antigen (HBcAg) and antibody (anti-HBc); and hepatitis B e antigen (HBeAg) and antibody (anti-HBe). These tests have made it possible to specifically diagnose types A and B hepatitis, to identify HBV-contaminated units of blood, and to identify NANB hepatitis by ruling out the other causes. Each type of hepatitis is followed by homologous but not heterologous immunity. In the U.S. about 25 to 50% of adults have serologic evidence of immunity to type A hepatitis (anti-HAV). In contrast, the prevalence of anti-HBs may range from 5% in healthy blood donors to 20% in health care workers with frequent blood contact, to 70% in such high-risk persons as immigrants from areas of high HBV endemicity, residents of institutions for mentally retarded, users of illicit parenteral drugs, homosexually active males, and household contracts of HBV carriers.

PREVENTION OF TYPE A HEPATITIS

General Measures. Procedures designed to block intestinal-oral pathways should be used for control; these include scrupulous handwashing, proper sterilization of food utensils, fly abatement, and exclusion of potentially infectious food handlers. Although close contact is the most common mode of transmission, common source epidemics stemming from contaminated food, milk, and water supplies may occur.

Passive Immunization. The efficacy of standard immune globulin (IG) for prevention has been well established. Postexposure prophylaxis is recommended for all who have had intimate exposure to a person with the disease. IG is also indicated for persons living in the same household because they are likely to have contact with the virus. However, routine use of IG in schools, offices, and factories is not warranted; spread of the disease is unlikely under the conditions existing in these open facilities. The recommended dose of IG (Table 1) should be given within 48 hours, if possible, but not later than 1 week after exposure.

Pre-exposure prophylaxis with standard IG is recommended for persons traveling to or working in areas where type A hepatitis is highly endemic. The recommended dose is shown in Table 1. A repeat dose should be given if exposure is continuous for more than 4 months. If the serologic test to detect anti-HAV is available, evaluation should be done to determine immune status of frequent travelers to areas where hepatitis A is prevalent. If antibody is present, IG should be discontinued.

Active Immunization. A licensed hepatitis A vaccine is not available. An experimental live attenuated hepatitis A vaccine is under study.

PREVENTION OF TYPE B HEPATITIS

General Measures. Contaminated blood, blood products, and needles are the most common sources of HBV infection. The most common mode of transmission is parenteral, but the virus can infect via the oral route. Blood obtained from commercial donors carries a 10- to 15-fold greater risk of causing hepatitis than blood obtained from volunteer donors. The indications for administering blood or blood products should be carefully assessed to be sure that the potential advantages warrant the risk.

The following precautions are indicated in screening blood donors: reject 1) persons whose blood contains HBsAg; 2) suspected narcotics addicts; 3) those who have received blood or who have had contact with a patient with hepatitis within the past 6 months; and 4) donors whose blood previously was suspected of causing hepatitis. The WHO Expert Committee on Viral Hepatitis has recommended that "volunteer blood donors need not be excluded on the basis of a previous history of hepatitis alone or on the finding of anti-HBs provided that   a) they have had no attack of hepatitis during at least the previous year and   b) their blood has been found negative for HBsAg by a very sensitive test."

Disposable equipment should be used if feasible. Equipment that cannot be discarded should be thoroughly cleaned and sterilized. The virus can be inactivated by boiling for at least 10 minutes, autoclaving at 15 lb pressure, or subjecting to dry heat at 170°C (338°F) for 30 minutes.

Passive Immunization. The efficacy of IG for the prevention of type B hepatitis depends on at least two factors: 1) the amount of anti-HBs present in the specific preparation; and 2) the dose of HBV present in the transfused units of blood or the accidental needle puncture. The higher the antibody content and the lower the dose of virus, the more likely are the chances for protection. The antibody content of hepatitis B immune serum globulin (HBIG) is 10,000-fold or more greater than that of standard IG.

HBIG is recommended for postexposure prophylaxis following 1) parenteral exposure, such as an accidental needle puncture; 2) direct mucous membrane contact, such as an accidental splash; and 3) oral ingestion, as in a pipetting accident, all involving HBsAg-positive blood or blood products. The incubation period following parenteral exposure may be very short (about 1 week between time of exposure and onset of viremia). Under these circumstances HBIG should be given within 48 hours, if possible. The incubation period following oral exposure is much longer (about 2 months).

Table 1. RECOMMENDED DOSE OF STANDARD IMMUNE SERUM GLOBULIN (ISG) AND HEPATITIS B IMMUNE SERUM GLOBULIN (HBIG)

Type of Exposure	Total Dose (ml)	
Type A hepatitis Single or short-term (<2 months)	0.5 (up to 50 lb) 1.0 (50 to 100 lb) 2.0 to 3.0 (over 100 lb)	ISG
Prolonged or continuous (>2 months)	1.0 to 2.0 (up to 50 lb) 2.0 to 3.0 (50 to 100 lb) 5.0 (over 100 lb)	ISG
Type B hepatitis	0.5 (newborn)** 0.5 to 1.5 (up to 50 lb) 1.5 to 3.0 (50 to 100 lb) 5.0 (over 100 lb)	HBIG

*Repeat once after 5 months if exposure continues.
**Infants born to HBV infected mothers should receive 0.5 ml at birth, 0.5 ml at 3 months, and 0.5 ml at 6 months.

It is important to test an exposed spouse for the presence of HBsAg and anti-HBs before administering HBIG. A study by Redeker et al.* involved 100 spouses exposed to type B hepatitis; 11% were HBsAg-positive and 16% anti-HBs-positive at the time of exposure. Thus, gamma globulin was not indicated for 27% of the spouses in this study. Occasionally, the so-called exposed spouse may be the index case because of an unrecognized carrier state.

The recommended dose of HBIG is shown in Table 1.

Active Immunization. An inactivated hepatitis B vaccine has been available since July 1982. Extensive studies have confirmed the safety, immunogenicity, and efficacy of the vaccine for prevention of acute type B hepatitis and the chronic hepatitis B carrier state.

The vaccine is recommended for immunization of all who are considered to be at increased risk of hepatitis B infection, including health professionals exposed to blood or potentially infectious secretions and to hemodialysis, thalassemia, and hemophilia patients; clients and staff of institutions for the mentally disabled; homosexually active males; intimate contacts of carriers; users of illicit drugs parenterally; infants who live in highly endemic areas; and other high-risk groups. The recommended dosage schedule is shown in Table 2.

Hepatitis B Infection during Pregnancy

Women who are HBsAg-positive may transmit hepatitis B to their newborn infants. If the HBsAg-positive mother is HBeAg-positive, her infant will have a 90% chance of acquiring hepatitis B infection. Most of these infants are infected at the time of birth, but about 5% may be infected in utero. HBIG, 0.5 ml, given shortly after birth and at 3 and 6 months, will prevent about 75% of the chronic infections.

The attack rate in infants whose HBsAg-positive mothers are anti-HBe-positive is less than 20%, and as a general rule, they recover completely and chronic hepatitis B is rare. However, very rarely the infection may be fulminant with a fatal outcome. Therefore, HBIG therapy is recommended for all infants of HBsAg-positive mothers regardless of HBeAg status.

Combined HBIG and hepatitis B vaccine given simultaneously at separate sites is immunogenic. HBIG does not inhibit the antibody response to the vaccine. Therefore, the combined HBIG and vaccine should confer immediate as well as long-term protection. Inactivated hepatitis B vaccine is now recommended for high-risk infants who are 3 months of age or older. When studies currently in progress are completed, it may be recommended for newborn infants.

It has been demonstrated that administration of HBIG and hepatitis B vaccine simultaneously at separately sites is immunogenic. HBIG does not inhibit the antibody response to the vaccine. Therefore, the combined use of HBIG and vaccine should provide immediate as well as long term protection. At the present time inactivated hepatitis B vaccine is recommended for high-risk infants, including newborns. Studies currently in progress indicate that administration of HBIG shortly after birth followed by immunization with hepatitis B vaccine is highly effective for the prevention of hepatitis B in infants born to hepatitis B carrier mothers. Therefore, the following guidelines are suggested for the care of HBsAg-positive mothers and their newborn infants:

1. Screen all high-risk pregnant women for HBsAg during the prenatal period, if possible, or soon after admission to the hospital. High-risk women of childbearing age are listed in Table 3. Screening of women who are not high-risk should be optional.

2. Newborn infants of HBsAg-positive mothers should receive 0.5 ml of HBIG intramuscularly within a few hours after birth, if possible.

3. At 3 months of age the infant's serum should be

Table 2. DOSAGE SCHEDULE OF INACTIVATED HEPATITIS B VACCINE

Group	Initial	1 Month	6 Months
Infants and children (3 months to 10 years of age)*	10 μg (0.5 ml)	10 μg (0.5 ml)	10 μg (0.5 ml)
Adults and older children	20 μg (1.0 ml)	20 μg (1.0 ml)	20 μg (1.0 ml)

*If the preliminary results of studies in newborn infants are confirmed, vaccine will be recommended for all age groups.

Table 3. HIGH-RISK PREGNANT WOMEN WHO SHOULD BE TESTED FOR HBsAg ROUTINELY

1. Immigrants from such highly endemic areas as Asia, Africa, Haiti, and various Pacific islands

2. Those with acute or chronic liver disease or contacts of persons with acute or chronic hepatitis B

3. Health professionals exposed to blood or to patients in institutions for the mentally retarded

4. Those who have been illicit injectable drug users

5. Those who have been rejected as blood donors

*N. Engl. J. Med. 293:1055, 1975.

tested for HBsAg to determine if HBV infection occurred.

   a. If HBsAg is detected, no additional therapy is necessary.

   b. If HBsAg is not detected in the infant's serum, give 0.5 ml HBIG and 0.5 ml (10 μg) of hepatitis B vaccine intramuscularly at separate sites.

4. At 4 months of age, give the second inoculation of hepatitis B vaccine (0.5 ml).

5. At 9 months of age, give the third (booster) dose of hepatitis B vaccine (0.5 ml).

6. At 12–15 months of age test for HBsAg, anti-HBc, and anti-HBs to determine the success or failure of treatment. The absence of HBsAg and the presence of anti-HBs with or without anti-HBc indicates success. The presence of HBsAg indicates failure.

Hepatitis B Carrier Mothers and Breast Feeding

Breast milk of hepatitis B carrier mothers may contain HBsAg. In addition, serum from cracked nipples may contain infectious hepatitis B virus. Thus, if a suitable substitute for breast milk is available, breast feeding should be discouraged. However, in many developing countries a suitable sterile substitute is not available and breast feeding should be encouraged in spite of the mother's carrier state.

TREATMENT

There is no specific treatment for children with types A or B viral hepatitis. The disease is generally so mild that bed rest is unnecessary after the acute stage. The child's diet and return to activity usually are gauged by the child's desire. When anorexia is present, food is rejected; broths and fruit juices should be offered. A normal diet is recommended when appetite returns. Corticosteroids and other drugs are not indicated for children with uncomplicated hepatitis.

Fulminant Hepatitis. Sudden onset of mental confusion, emotional instability, restlessness, coma, and hemorrhagic manifestations may progress to a fatal outcome within 10 days. Under these extraordinary conditions, the following measures should be considered: 1) corticosteroid therapy; 2) withdrawal of protein from the diet; 3) oral neomycin, 25 mg/kg every 6 hours, to suppress the bacterial flora of the intestinal tract; 4) laxatives and cleansing enemas; and 5) exchange transfusion.

Enteroviruses

JOHN F. MODLIN, M.D.

The enteroviruses are small (27 nm) RNA viruses that are common pathogens of man. The approximately 70 distinct serotypes thus far identified are classified as polioviruses, Coxsackie A viruses, Coxsackie B viruses, echoviruses, and, most recently, "enteroviruses," according to pathogenicity for laboratory animals. While virulent polioviruses have virtually been eliminated in advanced countries by mass immunization, the other classes are responsible for numerous common viral syndromes, including simple febrile illness with or without rash, herpangina, conjunctivitis, hand-foot-and-mouth syndrome, upper respiratory tract infection, pleurodynia, and aseptic meningitis. Virtually all of these syndromes are self-limited and require only general supportive care. The major task of the physician is to distinguish the enterovirus syndrome from a potentially more serious cause, that is, bacterial sepsis or meningitis.

However, some enterovirus infections have more serious consequences. Fortunately, these are less common, but, when they occur, they present a challenging therapeutic dilemma for the physician. Antiviral agents for enteroviruses do not exist, and there are no established methods for specific therapy for these serious infections. In some clinical situations (e.g., use of corticosteroids in myocarditis), pharmacologic therapy has been advocated by some on the basis of uncontrolled clinical observations. In other life-threatening enterovirus infections (e.g., neonatal infections), specific therapy may be attempted based on knowledge of the pathophysiology and the immune response of animals to experimental enterovirus infection. The basis of therapy of this nature is theoretical at best, for there has been little or no clinical experience. However, the dire prognosis of some overwhelming enterovirus infections may justify this approach in individual situations.

Neonatal Enterovirus Infections. Since severe neonatal infection occurs following exposure to infected nursery personnel, it is wise to exclude persons with known or suspected enterovirus infection from the newborn nursery and also to maintain good infection control techniques, such as handwashing, when enteroviruses are known to be prevalent in the community. However, the majority of neonatal coxsackievirus and echovirus infections are acquired vertically from the mother who becomes infected in the perinatal period. Recent data suggest that infants born to mothers who develop their infection within the last week of pregnancy are at greatest risk, perhaps because they lack transplacentally acquired maternal antibody to the infecting virus. Because of this, I would recommend delaying delivery, if possible, for 5 to 7 days in the woman who develops a known or suspected enterovirus infection late in pregnancy. I must emphasize however, that there are no clinical data to show that such a measure will prevent severe disease in the newborn infant.

The mechanism of enterovirus transmission from mother to infant is not well understood; it may well be that virus can infect the infant transplacentally prior to birth or during or after parturition. It appears however, that cesarean section delivery does not prevent infection.

There is no known effective therapy for the symptomatic, perinatally infected infant. Based on knowledge of the pathophysiology and the immune response of enterovirus infections in experimental animals, several therapeutic approaches might be considered. One is administration of human serum or plasma known to contain antibody to the specific enterovirus serotype. (The recently infected mother may be an appropriate donor.) The presence of antibody alone may not be sufficient to prevent continued virus replication, and other measures should be considered. Macrophage function is thought to play a role in experimental enterovirus infections, and, therefore, administration of a nonspecific macrophage-stimulating agent such as BCG may be tried. Finally, if one has access to human leukocyte interferon, this agent would also be worthy of consideration. Interferon has been shown to inhibit replication of enteroviruses in vitro, and there is evidence in laboratory animals that interferon may be important in the immune response to enterovirus infection.

Persistent Enterovirus Infections in Agammaglobulinemic Children. Several reports now document that children with agammaglobulinemia have unusually severe or persistent infection with enteroviruses. The majority of reported cases of paralysis resulting from administration of live, attenuated oral poliovirus vaccine (OPV) to infants occur in agammaglobulinemic children. In many cases, because of the young age at which OPV is generally given, the resulting paralytic disease may be the first manifestation of the congenital immune deficiency. Therefore, OPV should be withheld from any infant with a family history of congenital agammaglobulinemia until this disorder can be ruled out.

Older children with congenital agammaglobulinemia occasionally develop central nervous system enterovirus infections that may persist for months to years. So far, all reported cases have been caused by echoviruses. A wide spectrum of clinical disease occurs in these patients, ranging from few symptoms to progressive encephalitis and death. Some have had a dermatomyositis-like syndrome. Infusion of plasma containing specific antibody has met with variable success in the few reported patients in whom this mode of therapy has been attempted. Only plasma containing very high titers of specific antibody has succeeded in reducing or eliminating virus from the cerebrospinal fluid.

Myopericarditis. Acute inflammation of the myocardium, pericardium, or both is an occasional manifestation of systemic infection with several viral agents, most notably influenza A virus, Coxsackie B viruses, and echoviruses. Myopericarditis caused by the enteroviruses has a predilection for the hearts of physically active adolescents and young adults. Indeed, experimental animals infected with Coxsackie B virus develop more severe myopericarditis when forced to exercise. Until further clinical data are available, it is wise to caution patients with signs and symptoms of enterovirus disease against stressful exercise.

The treatment of myocarditis consists of bed rest and symptomatic relief of pain. If congestive heart failure is present, the judicious use of diuretics and cardiac glycosides (i.e., digoxin) is necessary.

The use of corticosteroids in viral myocarditis is highly controversial. Clinical studies in patients with acute myocarditis purport to show a beneficial effect of corticosteroids, sometimes in combination with azathioprine. These observations are flawed, however, by lack of control subjects and failure to make a specific viral diagnosis. Studies of myocarditis in animals, and in vitro studies of immune function in enteroviral infection, suggest that corticosteroids may enhance enterovirus replication and produce more extensive myocardial necrosis. Because of these data, I am hesitant to recommend use of corticosteroids or immunosuppressive agents in acute myocarditis until more definitive clinical data are available.

Aseptic Meningitis

H. CODY MEISSNER, M.D.

Aseptic meningitis is a syndrome consisting of fever, meningeal irritation, and mononuclear pleocytosis of the cerebrospinal fluid (CSF). This syndrome may be caused by a number of infectious or noninfectious etiologies. The critical point in the management of a patient with aseptic meningitis is the need for an accurate determination of etiology. In particular, the distinction between aseptic meningitis and encephalitis must be carefully considered. This is because of the increasing availability of antiviral agents that are effective for specific agents causing viral encephalitis but are generally not useful in the treatment of aseptic meningitis.

The majority of patients with aseptic meningitis will have a viral infection (mainly caused by coxsackie virus, echo virus, or mumps virus) and will require no specific form of therapy. For most patients, hospitalization is not necessary once the presence of a viral infection has been confirmed. An initial lumbar puncture is usually necessary to rule out a pyogenic process but once viruses are implicated, subsequent punctures are not necessary. As with most febrile patients, antipyretics are often helpful. Enteric precautions are indicated for any hospitalized patient with an enteroviral infection because the primary route of transmission is by fecal-oral spread. Virus may be detected in the feces for several weeks after the enteroviral infection.

The great majority of patients with aseptic meningitis recover without permanent sequelae, although fatigue and lethargy may persist for several weeks after the acute episode. In some instances of enteroviral meningitis, mild disturbances of motor function have been reported to last up to 1 year, but this is distinctly unusual. Recent data on enteroviral aseptic meningitis in children less than 1 year of age suggest that the prognosis is not always as good as it is with older children. Neurologic impairment such as delayed language and speech development may develop in a small number of very young children.

Encephalitis Infections— Postinfectious and Postvaccinal

DORIS SANDERS KELSEY, M.D.

Encephalitis of postinfectious or postvaccinal type may be evoked by a heterogeneous group of infections and both live and inactivated vaccinal products. It is believed to represent a hypersensitivity response to the inciting agent and occurs within 1 to 4 weeks of the event. The principal pathologic change is perivenous demyelination of white matter. The infecting agent is rarely recoverable. Thus, there is no need for specific antiviral or antibiotic therapy or patient isolation.

Treatment is totally symptomatic and supportive, requiring individualization according to the severity and complications of the illness. Milder cases may require only watchful observation. Seizure precautions should be observed, with utilization of anticonvulsants to achieve seizure control. Fluid and electrolyte balance must be carefully monitored. Respiratory care with proper suctioning, airway maintenance, and mechanical ventilatory support as clinically indicated is essential, as in any serious illness.

Management of increased intracranial pressure is extremely important. Dexamethasone given intramuscularly in a dosage of 0.2 to 0.5 mg/kg/24 hr is usually effective within 24 hours. There are no controlled studies indicating the efficacy of steroids in altering the basic course of the encephalitis. Utilization of a continuous intracranial pressure monitor in the seriously ill or comatose patient greatly facilitates optimal management regarding the dosage and frequency of osmotic agents needed to control cerebral edema. Mannitol may be given intravenously in a dosage of 0.25 gm/kg to 0.5 gm/kg. Maximum effectiveness is observed within the hour. Mannitol should be given in the smallest effective dosage and may be repeated at 4 to 6 hour intervals if indicated. Judicious monitoring of the state of hydration is required as changes in serum osmolarity and electrolyte disturbance occur commonly with repeated doses.

The prognosis of postinfectious and postvaccinal encephalitis is variable according to the specific inciting agent, but significant morbidity and mortality may occur even with intensive supportive care. In recent years a mortality rate of 8 to 9% has been reported with postinfectious encephalitis associated with the childhood infections of measles, mumps, rubella, and varicella. Fortunately, the incidence of postinfectious encephalitis associated with these childhood infections has declined since 1966, with effective immunization programs decreasing the frequency of occurrence of these diseases.

Psittacosis (Ornithosis)

CHIEN LIU, M.D.

Chlamydia psittaci is the etiologic agent for psittacosis and ornithosis. When the infection is contracted from pssitacine birds (parrots, parakeets, cockatoos, and budgerigars), the disease is often called psittacosis. Other avian species, such as pigeons and turkeys, are probably more common sources for the illness; therefore, the term ornithosis may be preferred. Since 1977, in the United States approximately 100 to 150 cases per year were reported to the Center for Disease Control. The cumulative cases reported in 1982 was 107. Pet shop employees, poultry workers, and pigeon handlers are at high risk; pediatric cases are relatively rare.

Psittacosis is a systemic infection with a sudden or insidious onset. Infected individuals usually have chills, fever, malaise, headaches, anorexia, sore throat, and photophobia. Nausea and vomiting are frequent. Cough is generally prominent, producing mucoid sputum that occasionally is blood streaked. Cyanosis may be present. In severe cases, mental confusion, delirium, or stupor may occur. In untreated cases, the fatality rate could reach 20%. Even with chemotherapy, up to 5% fatality may be expected.

The treatment of choice is tetracycline, in spite of the possibility of tooth staining in young children. Penicillin and sulfa drugs are not dependable. Chloramphenicol may be effective, but clinical experience is limited and it has obvious drawbacks. Aminoglycosides have no antichlamydial activities.

The dosage of tetracycline is 20 to 40 mg/kg/day divided into four oral doses. If the patient is unable to take oral medications, intravenous administration up to a maximum of 1 gm/day may be given. Long acting preparations such as doxycycline, 5 mg/kg/day, not to exceed 200 mg/day in two divided doses may also be used. The duration of therapy should be 3 weeks, as clinical relapse tends to occur in cases treated with a shorter course. Many treated patients have a relatively dramatic course with defervescence in 24 to 48 hours; others have a slower response. Even in successfully treated individuals, there may be a protracted recovery phase leaving the patient feeling weak and debilitated for months. For patients who cannot tolerate tetracycline, the recommended alternative is erythromycin at a dosage of 20 to 30 mg/kg/day in four divided doses.

Skillful supportive therapy is an integral part of good medical management. Adequate humidification of the patient's environment should be provided. If cough becomes distressing and interferes with the patient's sleep codeine at a dose of 0.5 mg/kg should be given at the time of sleep. When cough is excessive, affecting oral feedings and causing emesis during the child's waking hours, and traditional cough mixtures do not help, codeine should not be withheld. Other supportive therapeutic measures in terms of oxygen inhalation for relief of cyanosis, fluid and electrolytes replacement are important.

Rickettsial Disease

MICHAEL HATTWICK, M.D.

Five rickettsial diseases occur naturally in the U.S.: Rocky Mountain spotted fever (RMSF), endemic or murine typhus, epidemic typhus, rickettsial pox, and Q-fever. RMSF is the commonest and the only one with associated mortality. Treatment for all the rickettsioses generally is similar and includes appropriate antibiotic therapy, good supportive and nursing care, and appropriate treatment of complications.

Rocky Mountain Spotted Fever

Antibiotic Treatment. The mainstay of treatment is appropriate antibiotic therapy initiated as soon as the diagnosis is suspected or made. Mortality in untreated RMSF is 5 to 10%, and this appears not to be reduced unless appropriate antibiotic therapy is initiated within 5 days of clinical onset. Tetracycline and chloramphenicol are the only effective antibiotics.

Tetracycline is the drug of choice for most patients, with the exception of pregnant or lactating women, and of children under age 8 as discussed below. Tetracycline is given in a dose of 25 to 50 mg/kg/day orally with a maximum daily dose of 2 grams, in four divided doses. An initial loading dose equal to the usual total daily dose should be given when treatment is started. Tetracycline is rickettsiostatic, and final elimination of rickettsia

from the bone requires development of immune responses. To be effective, tetracycline must be started before irreversible tissue damage occurs, and continued for 3 to 5 days after fever has resolved. Treatment should therefore continue until fever and other symptoms resolve, and for no less than 12 to 14 days to allow adequate host immunity to develop.

Oral tetracycline absorption is interfered with by food and dairy products, and therefore should be given 1 hour before or 2 hours after meals. All oral preparations are equally effective. Doxycycline also may be used in a dose of 5 mg/kg/day in two equal doses.

In severely ill patients parenteral oxytetracycline hydrochloride may be given in a dose of 10 to 20 mg/kg for children over the age of 8 years. I prefer, however, to use chloramphenicol in severely ill patients of any age. Prolonged IV therapy with tetracycline may cause thrombophlebitis, so large-bore needles in large veins should be used. Parenteral tetracycline therapy has been associated with hepatic necrosis in some RMSF patients.

Treatment of children under age 8 with tetracycline may be complicated by staining of permanent teeth, but this should not be a problem after a single course of less than 15 days. The most frequent complication of tetracycline therapy is gastrointestinal irritation resulting in nausea, vomiting, abdominal pain, or, diarrhea. Less common complications are glossitis, photosensitivity, urticaria, moniliasis, intracranial hypertension, hemolytic anemia, anaphylaxis, and hepatic toxicity.

In severely ill patients, I prefer intravenous chloramphenicol in a total daily dose of 50 to 100 mg/kg. A maximum of 4 gm/day should be given, and the dosage reduced to 50 mg/kg/day as soon as clinical status improves. Higher doses increase the risk of bone marrow suppression. When the patient's clinical status improves and allows oral therapy, chloramphenicol may be continued in an oral dose of 50 mg/kg/day, in divided doses at 6 hour intervals, or oral tetracycline can be started in the doses noted above.

The major complication of chloramphenicol is dose related reversible depression of the bone marrow. Serial measurement of hemoglobin, reticulocytes, neutrophils, and platelets every 48 to 72 hours during therapy should be made. Neutropenia (less than 1500 neutrophils/mm^3), or thrombocytopenia (less than 150,000 platelets/mm^3), when due to bone marrow suppression, is an indication to discontinue chloramphenicol and switch to tetracycline. However thrombocytopenia and neutropenia can be due to RMSF itself. In the acute stage of RMSF (first 5 to 10 days) thrombocytopenia is more likely to be due to RMSF itself than to chloramphenicol induced marrow suppression, and chloramphenicol should be continued.

Early in the clinical course it may not be possible to distinguish RMSF from meningicoccemia, as both present with fever and petecchial rash. If the diagnosis is in doubt at the time the patient initially is seen, it is appropriate to combine therapy as indicated above for RMSF with therapy for meningococcal disease consisting of 20 million units of intravenous penicillin G daily. Penicillin, erythromycin, and cephalosporins are ineffective against rickettsia, but do not interfere with the effectiveness of tetracycline or chloramphenicol. Sulfonamides, including combination products such as trimethaprim-sulfamethoxazole, may make rickettsial infections worse and are contraindicated if RMSF is diagnosed or suspected.

Supportive Care and Treatment of Complications. Medical supportive care is based on treating the signs and symptoms of the disease and anticipating and promptly treating each possible complication. In mild cases outpatient treatment may be sufficient, but in most cases hospitalization with careful monitoring of vital signs is essential. The person seriously ill with RMSF will show a variety of physiologic problems including circulatory instability, abnormal mental status, oliguria, azotemia, hypoproteinemia, electrolyte imbalances, and edema. Supportive measures should be given to correct these abnormalities as they occur. Frequent feedings of a high protein, high calorie diet should be used to prevent significant protein depletion. Hypoproteinemia may require transfusions of serum albumin, which will be helpful in combating circulatory collapse and excessive edema. Significant anemia should be corrected with packed red cells. Whole blood or plasma generally should be avoided because of the possibility of intravascular clotting.

Coagulopathies occur frequently in RMSF. Half the patients will have thrombocytopenia and fulminant disease with extensive hemorrhagic rash. Some will also have associated disseminated intravascular coagulation (DIC) manifested by thrombocytopenia, prolonged prothrombin and partial thromboplastin times, hypofibrinogenemia, and an increase in serum fibrin split products. Platelet and coagulation factor transfusions are not helpful and should not be used. If thrombocytopenia is not associated with spontaneous hemorrhage, specific therapy is not indicated. If DIC develops and is accompanied by spontaneous bleeding not controllable readily by transfusions or local hemostasis, heparin may be required. If used, the initial dose of heparin is 100 units/kg by intravenous bolus, followed by continuous infusion at 100 units/kg/hr. If liver function abnormalities are present, vitamin K, 2 mg daily for 2 to 3 days may be beneficial.

RMSF is an infectious vasculitis, and circulatory collapse, hypotension, oliguria, and edema are usually secondary to primary vascular involvement. Adequate fluid balance is important and one third of intravenous fluids should consist of colloids because of the tendency for fluids to leak from the intravascular space through damaged capillaries. Hypovolemia may lead to shock and should be treated with volume repletion. Pulmonary edema has been observed and usually reflects vascular leakage rather than congestive heart failure. However, myocarditis is well recognized in RMSF and if pulmonary edema or abnormal chest x-ray are present, fluid therapy should be monitored carefully with serial evaluations of respiratory function to avoid fluid overload. Measurements of pulmonary artery and wedge pressure with a Swan-Ganz catheter can provide necessary information to determine the appropriate volume replacement in critically ill or hypotensive patients.

Use of adrenal corticosteroids has been advocated for the relief of toxicity in severely ill patients, but no controlled trials have clearly demonstrated their effectiveness. If used, large doses of methylprednisolone (Solu-Medrol), 30 mg/kg intravenously every 6 hours for 2 to 3 days are suggested. This treatment may benefit patients evidencing vascular collapse who are unresponsive to fluid replacement.

Central nervous system involvement is manifested by confusion, stupor, delirium, or coma and may be accompanied by seizures. If seizures occur, diazapam* in a dose of 0.3 mg/kg is given at a rate of 1 mg/min IV until seizures stop. Alternative medications include phenobarbital sodium (4–6 mg/kg IV) or phenytoin (5–7 mg/kg IV at a rate less than 50 mg/min). Avoiding excess use of fluids may help reduce cerebral edema, which is responsible for many of the neurologic complications.

Other complications include gastrointestinal hemorrhage due to vascular leakage, DIC, or stress ulcers. This should be treated with adequate blood replacement and gastric lavage if coming from the stomach. Renal insufficiency and failure are treated with fluid replacement and careful monitoring of fluid balance. Renal failure, when present, usually remits spontaneously as the clinical course improves. Congestive heart failure should be treated with cautious use of digitalis and diuretics. Necrosis of the fingertips, toes, ears, scrotum, or other skin sites may occur secondary to the severe vasculitis and are treated with local antibiotics and sterile dressings. If pulmonary function leads to hypoxia or cyanosis, oxygen should be given and fluid balance should be carefully monitored. Severe pain should be treated with codeine or meperidine. Aspirin should not be used because of the risk of bleeding, particularly in those with low platelet

---

*The safety of parenteral diazepam has not been established in the newborn.

counts, and acetominophen should be avoided in anyone with liver function abnormalities. Codeine, 0.5 to 1 mg/kg/dose every 4 to 6 hours for a total daily dose up to 3 mg/km should be adequate for pain control. Meticulous nursing care is required, with particular attention to skin care and intravenous sites to avoid superinfection or risk of bleeding.

Preventive Therapy. RMSF is transmitted by the bite of a tick, and the tick must remain attached to its host for approximately 2 hours to transmit adequate rickettsiae to the host for infection. Thus, preventive measures can effectively interrupt transmission from tick to man. The best prevention involves minimizing contact with ticks in endemic areas. This can be done by wearing long-sleeved garments, closed at the wrist and neck, tucking trouser bottoms into the tops of lace-up boots, inspecting the body, particularly the hair, groin, amillae, and beltline periodically, and removing any ticks found promptly. Tick repellents are only moderately effective. Precaution should be used in removing engorged ticks because infection through minor abrasions on the hands is possible. Once found, a tick can be removed by grasping it firmly from behind with tweezers or gauze-protected fingers and pulling slowly but firmly in the direction away from the head. The tweezers should be applied as close to the head as possible to encourage the tick to disengage. Touching the tick with hot matches, fingernail polish, gasoline, or alcohol may encourage the tick to disengage.

There is no evidence of need for prophylactic antibiotics following tick bites, and these generally should not be used, particularly for children, in whom prolonged or repetitive administration of tetracycline can result in staining of teeth and inhibition of growth. There is no commercially available RMSF vaccine, although efforts continue to develop cell culture based rickettsial vaccines.

Treatment of Other Rickettsial Illnesses. Both endemic and epidemic typhus are present in the United States, although not commonly recognized. The evidence of epidemic typhus is serologic and may represent either primary infection or late relapse of epidemic typhus known as Brill-Zinser disease. Clinical illness in endemic and epidemic typhus is similar to RMSF, although the rash is milder in typhus and occurs less commonly on the hands and feet in epidemic typhus than in RMSF. Therapy for these ilnesses is the same as for RMSF. Rickettsial pox is a self-limited benign illness that often requires no therapy and is characterized by an eschar at the site of a mite bite. Tetracycline or chloramphenicol treatment is effective.

Q-fever differs clinically from other rickettsial diseases, usually presenting as a nonspecific upper respiratory infection or atypical pneumonia. Q-fever does respond to tetracycline or chloram-phenicol, in doses noted above, but unlike other rickettsial disease, erythromycin, 40 mg/kg/24 hr in four divided doses, may also be effective. Since erythromycin is also effective against other atypical pneumonias, it is probably the antibiotic of choice in Q-fever presenting as atypical pneumonia. Hepatitis and endocarditis are complications of Q-fever. Endocarditis requires prolonged treatment with tetracycline until all signs of infection are resolved.

Rickettsial infections imported from other countries generally respond well to the standard antibiotic therapy described above for RMSF.

Chlamydia

MARC O. BEEM, M.D.

The *Chlamydia* indigenous to man are known by the species name of *Chlamydia trachomatis*. These organisms are uniformly sensitive to erythromycin, sulfonamides and tetracyclines, and the mainstay of the treatment of infections caused by *C. trachomatis* is the systemic administration of one of these antimicrobial agents. To achieve microbial cure and avoid clinical relapse, treatment should be continued in full dosages for a period of 2 weeks.

TYPICAL DRUG REGIMENS EMPLOYED

Erythromycin
Erythromycin ethylsuccinate:
Infants—40 mg/kg/day divided into 4 doses.
Adults—500 mg qid.
Sulfonamides
Sulfisoxazole*:
Infants—150 mg/kg/day divided into 4 doses.
Adults—1 gm qid.
Tetracyclines
Tetracycline HCl:
Infants—not recommended for treatment of infections.
Patients over 8 years of age weighing < 150 lbs —250 mg qid.
Patients over 8 years of age weighing ≥ 150 lbs —500 mg qid.

TREATMENT PROGRAMS FOR SPECIFIC CONDITIONS

Inclusion conjunctivitis
Neonatal
Erythromycin or sulfisoxazole, in dosages as outlined above, for 2 weeks.
Older child or adult
One of the above antimicrobial agents given for 2 weeks. This assures adequate treatment of the

---

*Manufacturer's Precaution: Not indicated in infants less than 2 months of age.

genital infection that may also be present. To prevent reinfection, sexual partners should also be treated.

Topical medications are not needed. Although this route of medication has long been employed in the treatment of chlamydial conjunctival disease, this often fails to bring about complete resolution of the conjunctival disorder and does not treat the respiratory or genital aspects of the infection.

Chlamydial Pneumonia of Infancy

Erythromycin or a sulfonamide, in dosages as outlined above, should be administered for 2 weeks.

These patients may have episodes of accentuated respiratory distress associated with increased lower respiratory tract secretions and paroxysms of staccato coughing. These aspects of illness are greatly helped by chest physical therapy. Occasional infants may have disease of a severity that requires supplemental oxygen; on rare occasions assisted ventilation may be necessary.

Nongonococcal Urethritis

Tetracycline in dosages as outlined above should be given for 2 weeks. If this cannot be used, erythromycin is the alternate drug of choice since this, like tetracycline, is also effective against the genital mycoplasma, *Ureaplasma urealyticum* (believed to be the likely cause of nonchlamydial, nongonococcal urethritis). Sexual partners also should receive this treatment for a period that overlaps the patient's treatment interval.

Legionella Sp. Infections

RICHARD D. MEYER, M.D.

Infections caused by *Legionella* sp. are being recognized with increasing frequency in both nosocomial and community settings. At least eight species have been implicated in human disease by immunofluorescent tests and/or cultures. *Legionella pneumophila*, the agent of legionnaires' disease, is the most commonly found; the others include *L. micadei* (Pittsburgh pneumonia agent), *L. bozemanii*, *L. dumoffi*, *L. gormanii*, *L. jordanis*, *L. longbeachae*, and *L. wadsworthii*. Multisystem disease, primarily manifested by pneumonia, is the commonly recognized presentation. *Legionella* infections occur in all age groups; immunosuppressed patients with T-cell dysfunction are at particular risk. Although more common in adults, legionnaires' disease has been documented in both immunosuppressed and apparently normal infants and children, and appears to account for a few percent of atypical pneumonias in previously healthy children.

Supportive Therapy

Supportive therapy with fluids and colloids for hypotension and ventilatory support for respiratory failure are sometimes needed in patients with *Legionella* infection. Antipyretics have little sustained effect on the temperature. Immunosuppressive agents should be omitted or the dosage reduced, if possible, but may be continued with effective antimicrobial chemotherapy if necessary for control of the primary disease. Corticosteroids have no role in treatment unless adrenal insufficiency is present. Pleural effusions are usually not a management problem but open drainage for empyema may be necessary. Isolation (respiratory guidelines) is recommended if organisms are seen in or grown from respiratory tract secretions, but no person-to-person transmission is known. Contacts do not require specific attention unless they may have been infected from the same source.

Chemotherapy

Although a minority of patients with *Legionella* pneumonia slowly recover after 6 to 8 days of illness, chemotherapy is indicated in all patients with pneumonia.

Erythromycin is the drug of choice, although no prospective comparative studies of chemotherapy have been performed. In various outbreaks, the case fatality rates were lowest with use of either erythromycin or tetracycline, and highest in patients treated with cephalothin or other cephalosporins. Use of erythromycin lowers the case fatality rate approximately fourfold over that of patients given no therapy.

Results of tetracycline therapy have been variable but most patients have responded. Penicillins, cephalosporins (including cefoxitin and the so-called third-generation cephalosporins) and aminoglycosides have no role in treatment of legionnaires' disease. Co-trimoxazole in high doses used for *Pneumocystis carinii* infections has apparently been used successfully in several cases, but it is not clearly effective.

Results of in vitro susceptibility testing do not necessarily predict clinical response. Many drugs active in vitro do not work clinically. Pharmacologic properties, including the ability of some antimicrobials to enter alveolar macrophages and monocytes where *Legionella* reside, are important. Erythromycin and tetracycline enter the alveolar macrophage well and are concentrated in it.

Erythromycin should be given as outlined in Table 1 for at least 3 weeks to prevent relapse. Administration of the drug (erythromycin lactobionate or gluceptate) is recommended for moderately or severely ill patients for the first several days of therapy or until a clinical response occurs. Then oral therapy can be given. Patients cannot always

Table 1. THERAPY FOR *LEGIONELLA* INFECTIONS

	Drug	Route	Number of Doses Per Day	Total Daily Dose
Mild illness with no respiratory compromise	Erythromycin	Oral	4	30–50 mg/kg/day
	Alternative— doxycycline*	Oral	1–2	5 mg/kg/day first day followed by 2.5 mg/kg/day daily
Moderately to severely ill	Erythromycin	IV	4	30–50 mg/kg/day for children under 50 kg; 3–4 gm/day for children over 50 kg
	Alternative— erythromycin with rifampin**	IV	4	As above
			1–2	10–20 mg/kg/day for children over 5 years not to exceed 600 mg/day†
	Alternative— doxycycline* with	IV	1–2	5 mg/kg first day, 2–4 mg/kg/day 12 hours later, and then daily for children under 50 kg; 200 mg first day and then 100–200 mg daily in children over 50 kg
	rifampin**	Oral	1–2	Doses as above

*Tetracyclines may not be effective in all cases; tetracyclines should not be used in children less than 8 years of age for even short courses unless clearly indicated.

**Rifampin should not be used as a single agent; erythromycin with rifampin preferred for pulmonary abscess.

†Not FDA-approved for children under 5 years of age.

tolerate high oral doses because of gastrointestinal side effects. Erythromycin base, stearate, ethylsuccinate, or estolate are the oral preparations. Use of rifampin orally in children should be considered in combination with erythromycin if the patient is critically ill, is heavily immunosuppressed, or has pulmonary cavities. Rifampin should not be given alone because of the possibility of emergence of resistance. Cavitary disease or empyema generally requires therapy of more than 3 weeks' duration.

If erythromycin cannot be given, doxycycline is the preferred tetracycline. Doxycycline is given in two doses the first day and then daily thereafter for 3 weeks. In moderately severe to severely ill patients, rifampin should be given with doxycycline for at least the first week of therapy.

The clinical response to erythromycin therapy is usually prompt with a return toward a sense of well-being and a decrease in temperature in a day or two. Pulmonary infiltrates may continue to progress, and clinical and radiographic evidence of pulmonary consolidation develop despite clinical response, as with other bacterial pneumonias. Other responses may be slower but it is unusual for fever, leukopenia, or confusion to persist for more than 3 or 4 days of erythromycin therapy.

A few patients may complain of persistent fatigue and weakness for several months after completion of effective therapy. In patients who develop respiratory failure and require ventilatory support, restrictive lung disease may develop. Otherwise, chest radiographs usually show resolution of infiltrates from 2 or 3 weeks to 3 months after initiation of therapy; a few patients are left with residual pulmonary scarring.

Systemic Mycoses

MARGARET A. KELLER, M.D.

The therapy of systemic fungal infection has long relied on the use of the fungicidal agent amphotericin B. Recent advances include newer agents as alternatives to amphotericin B and the use of combination therapy.

Since histoplasmosis and coccidioidomycosis are discussed separately, three other systemic mycoses encountered in children—systemic candidiasis, cryptococcosis, and aspergillosis—will be discussed here.

SYSTEMIC CANDIDIASIS

Although diagnosis of systemic candidiasis is often difficult, once it has been established amphotericin B is the drug of choice. Systemic candidiasis, by definition, should include all cases of *Candida* meningitis, osteomyelitis, endocarditis, arthritis, and endophthalmitis. An infected catheter or foreign body causing disseminated infection must be removed. Surgical intervention is usually needed in *Candida* endocarditis. Oral therapy with nystatin (800,000 units/24 hr divided q 6 hr for infants and 1.6 million to 2.4 million units/24 hr for children) is also used when gastrointestinal, esophageal, or oral infection is present. (Nystatin is not absorbed from the gastrointestinal tract.)

Amphotericin B

Amphotericin B is a polyene antifungal agent that binds to sterols in the cell membranes of both fungal and animal cells. Thus, toxicity is significant and usually limits administration. Therapy can be initiated with a test dose of 1 mg in adults or 0.1 mg/kg in children administered intravenously over 4 to 6 hours. This drug should be suspended in 5 per cent glucose in water, not saline, electrolyte solution, or hyperalimentation fluid, at a concentration less than 0.1 mg/ml. A standard regimen has been to increase the dose over a 7- to 10-day period to 1 mg/kg/24 hr. Such delay is frequently not feasible in an immunocompromised patient with severe infection. If the patient tolerates the test dose, 0.25 mg/kg can be given intravenously on the same day, 0.5 mg/kg on the second day, 0.75 mg/kg on the third, and 1 mg/kg (maximum 50 mg) on the fourth day. The patient's tolerance of the drug may necessitate a slower schedule. In acutely ill patients, 0.5 mg/kg has been administered following a test dose.

Acute toxicity related to drug administration is usually evidenced by fever, chills, nausea, vomiting, or headache. Premedication and medication during infusion can eliminate many of these drug effects. Aspirin (10 to 20 mg/kg) and diphenhydramine (1.25 mg/kg; adult dose, 50 mg) prior to infusion have been helpful. Intravenous hydrocortisone immediately prior to amphotericin B also has been effective. Cardiac arrhythmias can occur and dictate a peripheral site of administration.

Drug toxicity as manifested by azotemia usually limits the dosage and frequency of drug administration. Commonly, an alternate-day regimen is necessary. Although amphotericin B is nephrotoxic, it does not accumulate in serum in renal failure. Hypokalemia is a frequent complication that necessitates serum monitoring and oral potassium supplementation. Leukopenia, thrombocytopenia, and anemia occur, but transfusion is rarely necessary. Intrathecal administration is usually reserved for unresponsive cases of meningitis since complications can be severe. The total dose of amphotericin B varies with each patient and the clinical response. Approximately 30 to 35 mg/kg can usually be given over 6 weeks.

Flucytosine (5-Fluorocytosine)

Flucytosine (5-FC), a fungistatic agent, has been particularly useful in treating yeast infections. This drug achieves high levels in cerebrospinal fluid and urine and can be orally administered. The current recommended dose is 150 mg/kg/24 hr divided into four doses. Toxicity noted has been gastrointestinal (diarrhea, bloating), hepatic, and hematologic (leukopenia and thrombocytopenia). Fatal aplastic anemia has been reported. Since flucytosine is excreted mainly by the kidney, the dosage must be lowered in renal impairment.

Although de novo resistance can occur, emergence of resistance during therapy has been a particularly significant problem. Combination therapy may prevent this. When the causative organism is susceptible, treatment with flucytosine has been used in addition to amphotericin B for candidiasis. Firm guidelines for combination therapy are lacking, but flucytosine achieves much higher levels in cerebrospinal fluid, urine, and the eye than does amphotericin B, and this may be particularly useful in meningitis, pyelonephritis, and endophthalmitis. The accumulation of flucytosine during renal impairment necessitates close monitoring and dosage adjustment when amphotericin B-induced nephrotoxicity ensues. The combination of amphotericin B and flucytosine may result in increased hematologic toxicity, and close monitoring is necessary. Experience with a lower dose of amphotericin B in combination with flucytosine is not available in the treatment of candidiasis although such regimens have been successful in cryptococcal meningitis. (See discussion of cryptococcosis.) An initial flucytosine dose of 100 to 150 mg/kg/24 hr divided into four doses has been used.

Miconazole

Miconazole is an imidazole derivative that does not achieve significant levels in cerebrospinal fluid or urine. It has been used for patients with candidemia who cannot tolerate amphotericin B. Miconazole is metabolized by the liver and, therefore, dosage does not have to be adjusted in renal failure. The dosage in adults has ranged from 200 mg to 1200 mg per intravenous infusion every 8 hours. The pediatric intravenous doses suggested by the manufacturer are 20 to 40 mg/kg/24 hr divided into three doses.*

CRYPTOCOCCOSIS

Meningitis, disseminated disease in an immunocompromised host, osteomyelitis, and extensive pulmonary disease are treated with amphotericin B and flucytosine when the organism is sensitive.

Recent controlled treatment trials of cryptococcal meningitis have successfully used a lower dose of amphotericin B in combination with flucytosine. Amphotericin B (0.3 mg/kg/24 hr) and flucytosine (150 mg/kg/24 hr divided into four doses) were used for 6 weeks in the average patient. The amphotericin B prevents emergence of resistance to

---

*Safety and efficacy in children under 1 year of age have not been established.

the flucytosine. Cryptococcosis involving other sites could probably be treated similarly. The emergence of resistance to flucytosine during therapy is a significant problem when this agent is used alone and supports combination therapy. Intrathecal amphotericin B is usually not necessary. In unresponsive cases, intrathecal, ventricular, or cisternal amphotericin B is diluted in 10 per cent glucose in distilled water to a concentration not exceeding 0.25 mg/ml amphotericin B. Some authors have recommended 0.05 mg every third day in an infant; others have started with 0.01 mg. The initial adult dose is 0.025 mg. Complications include arachnoiditis, transient radiculitis, sensory loss, hearing loss, and other cranial nerve damage.

ASPERGILLOSIS

Disseminated aspergillosis is a fulminant illness, and many species of *Aspergillus* are resistant to amphotericin B and flucytosine. Yet the combination of these two agents may be synergistic. Rifampin has also been used in combination with amphotericin B. Amphotericin B damages the cell membrane and permits rifampin to enter the cell. Synergism has been demonstrated in vitro for rifampin and amphotericin B against *Aspergillus* strains. In vitro sensitivities and measurement of serum drug concentrations can be helpful in determining appropriate therapy.

Histoplasmosis

ABE R. FOSSON, M.D.

Two aspects of childhood infection by the soil fungus *Histoplasma capsulatum* are important when considering therapy. First, these infections are usually asymptomatic and benign. Second, administration of the standard proven chemotherapeutic agent, amphotericin B, has been regularly associated with undesirable side effects. For these reasons, even individuals symptomatic with infections of this fungus are often not treated. Chemotherapy should be limited to children with disseminated histoplasmosis and a compromised immune response, patients with compression of vital organs by histoplasmal lymphadenitis, or infants with acute progressive primary histoplasmosis with dissemination. When treatment is necessary, the total dosage utilized should be sufficient to tip the balance in the host's favor but small enough to avoid permanently damaging toxicity.

THERAPEUTIC REGIMEN

Amphotericin B is the drug of choice for the treatment of childhood infection with *H. capsulatum*. This drug should be given intravenously over a 6-hour period at a concentration of not more than 0.1 mg/ml in 5% dextrose solution buffered to pH 5.5. The dose used on the initial day of therapy has been 0.25 mg/kg; on the second day of therapy, 0.5 mg/kg; and on the third and subsequent days of therapy, 1 mg/kg/24 hr. The total cumulative dose should not exceed 50 mg/kg. Many children have chills and fever during administration of amphotericin B. These reactions can be prevented by giving 10 to 15 mg of intravenous hydrocortisone just prior to administering amphotericin B.

During the course of therapy renal function should be monitored twice weekly by blood urea nitrogen and creatinine determinations. If a prolonged course of amphotericin B therapy is necessary, these determinations will usually become abnormal. If so, the daily dose of amphotericin B should be adjusted to keep the blood urea nitrogen below 50 mg/dl and the serum creatinine below 3.5 mg/dl. Serum potassium levels also should be monitored and any hypokalemia corrected by oral or intravenous potassium supplements.

RESPONSE TO THERAPY

The child's progress should be monitored by repeated clinical assessments and peripheral blood counts. Early clinical signs of improvement in disseminated histoplasmosis in infants and immunologically compromised hosts are the appearance of a good mood, playfulness, improved appetite, weight gain, defervescence, and a reduction in hepatosplenomegaly. These changes are accompanied by a return of white blood counts, hematocrits, and platelet counts to normal levels. The optimal duration of therapy is not known. Clinical experience suggests that when these signs of patient well being and disease regression have been present for 1 week in an otherwise normal infant amphotericin B therapy may be discontinued. In the immunologically compromised individual, relapses are much more likely. In these patients the course of therapy should be extended until definite signs of clinical improvement have been evident for at least 2 weeks. Treatment of life-threatening histoplasmosal lymphadenitis with amphotericin B may be discontinued after clinical signs of improvement have been present for 1 week.

By using short courses of therapy and therefore small total doses of amphotericin B, as described, many children will not be treated longer than 2 weeks and major toxicity can be avoided. Relapses are unlikely with short courses of therapy. When relapses do occur the child may be successfully retreated with intravenous amphotericin B. The duration of retreatment courses may be based on the clinical response of the individual, but the period of well being before termination of therapy must be lengthened. Courses of therapy longer than 10 weeks should be avoided.

Improvements in therapy can be anticipated. Experimental data indicate that incorporation of amphotericin B into liposomes before intravenous administration may reduce toxicity and enhance efficacy. In addition, ketoconazole, a relatively safe orally administered drug, active against *H. capsulatum* has been approved for use in children. Until its place in the therapeutic regimen has been established, ketoconazole is not recommended for serious childhood histoplasmosis.

Coccidioidomycosis

ALLAN LAVETTER, M.D.

Coccidioides immitis resides endemically only in the soils of the three Americas. Infections with this fungus have been observed in Argentina, Paraguay, Bolivia, Venezuela, Colombia, Honduras, Guatemala, Mexico, and the United States.

There is as yet no consistently effective and benign therapy for coccidioidomycosis in humans. Fortunately, most symptomatic primary infections recover without therapy. However, because of the increased possibility of dissemination, patients with complement-fixation titers of greater than 1:16 should be considered for treatment. Other criteria that may be used to determine the need for treatment are persistent fever, prostration or debilitation, persisting or enlarging pulmonary involvement, and concurrent diseases likely to be adversely affected by coccidioidal infection or associated with compromised immunity.

Amphotericin B is the treatment of choice for disseminated coccidioidomycosis. There are almost no data regarding its use in neonates or older infants, and very few data from studies in older children. Thus, the guidelines for its usage in children are almost completely based on experience in adults. Its effectiveness and toxicity in children appear to be similar to those in adults.

The structure of amphotericin B resembles that of erythromycin except that erythromycin lacks the conjugated double bonds seen with amphotericin.

The probable mechanism of action of amphotericin B is that of binding to the sterol in the cell membrane, thus changing the permeability of the membrane. Cellular constituents are lost after exposure to the drug for brief periods of time, and the size of the constituents leaking from the cell increases as the dose of amphotericin increases.

The pharmacokinetics of amphotericin B suggest that the drug is taken up by some reservoir in the body from which it is later slowly released. Its serum half-life is 24 hours, and active drug can be detected in the serum up to 7 weeks after the last administered dose. With high doses of intravenous amphotericin B, therapeutic levels can be maintained in the serum even 48 hours after a dose.

The usual method of administering amphotericin B is to give a test dose of 0.5 to 1.0 mg intravenously. On succeeding days the dosage is gradually built up in 1- to 10-mg increments to a total dose of 0.5 to 1.5 mg/kg every day or every other day. In urgent situations it may be necessary to follow the small test dose with a larger therapeutic dose the same day, then increase the dosage on a daily basis more rapidly than just indicated.

The rapidity with which one can increase the dosage is largely determined by the toxic side effects of amphotericin, which are phlebitis, fever, chills, nausea, vomiting, azotemia, renal tubular acidosis, hypokalemia, hypomagnesemia, shock, and anemia. Other side effects include anaphylactic reactions, arrhythmias, coagulopathy, hemorrhagic enteritis, tinnitus, vertigo, pruritus, neuropathy, seizures, leukopenia, and thrombocytopenia. Patients receiving amphotericin B commonly also receive other medications to modify some of these toxic side effects, e.g., salicylates, antihistamines, antiemetics, and low doses of steroids.

Because of poor penetration into the cerebrospinal fluid, intrathecal (preferably cisternal) therapy is needed in the treatment of coccidioidal meningitis. Again, the initial dose is small (e.g., 0.025 mg) and subsequent doses are increased as tolerated to a maximum usually not exceeding 0.5 mg every 1 to 3 days.

The duration of amphotericin B therapy is not well established. Some authorities suggest treating until the complement-fixation titer has diminished to zero. Others suggest a total dose of 20 to 30 mg/kg. Development of drug toxicity, particularly renal toxicity, and the degree and rapidity of clinical improvement will influence the duration of amphotericin B therapy. The duration of therapy for coccidioidal meningitis is unknown. The decision to reduce or discontinue treatment is guided by the reduction of the complement-fixation titer to less than 1:32 and serial examination of the patient's cerebrospinal fluid. Some physicians favor continued periodic suppressive intrathecal amphotericin B indefinitely.

The methyl ester of amphotericin B is more soluble, and animal studies indicate it to be less toxic, than amphotericin B. However, it also appears to be less effective on a milligram-for-milligram basis. Thus its usefulness in human infections is not yet defined.

Combinations of amphotericin B with other antimicrobial agents have been tried experimentally to reduce the dose and therefore the toxicity of the amphotericin B. The combination of tetracycline with amphotericin B has been effective in mice and has allowed for a decrease in the dose of amphotericin B. In vitro polymyxin B reduced the minimum inhibitory concentration of amphotericin B against the spherule form of *Coccidioides immitis*. These combinations have not been evaluated in humans.

Miconazole and ketoconazole, both imidazoles, are antifungal agents with broad spectrums of activity. These drugs interfere with the biosynthesis of lipids in the fungal cell, especially with the synthesis of sterols, resulting in the increased permeability of the cell membrane and leakage of cytoplasmic contents, leading ultimately to the death of the fungal cell. Miconazole is administered intravenously while ketoconazole is well absorbed from the gastrointestinal tract. Neither drug penetrates well into the cerebrospinal fluid. Both drugs have been therapeutically effective in experimentally produced coccidioidomycosis in mice.

Miconazole has been administered to adults in doses of 200 mg three times a day initially. If well tolerated, the dose has been advanced in 200- to 400-mg increments per dose every 2 to 7 days to a maximum of 1200 mg three times a day. Pharmacokinetic data indicated that doses above 9 mg/kg or 350 mg/m^2 achieve blood levels above 1 μg/ml, the usual minimum inhibitory concentration of *Coccidioides immitis*. Patients have been treated for periods of up to 3 months.

Therapeutic results with miconazole therapy in humans were initially promising. Its relative lack of toxicity, compared with amphotericin B, represents a real advantage. However, as clinical experience with this therapy has increased, a significant number of patients have been noted either to fail to respond or to relapse shortly after miconazole treatment has been discontinued. At this time miconazole should be reserved for selected patients with disseminated coccidioidomycosis who cannot receive amphotericin B.

Ketoconazole has been administered to adults in initial doses of 200 mg once a day with frequent increases to 400 mg once a day. The larger doses seem to be needed in patients with skeletal infections and perhaps for others with more severe or isolated disease. Most patients who respond seem to require at least 3 months of treatment, and 6 to 12 months is currently the generally recommended treatment course. Adverse effects are uncommon and generally limited to transient nausea. Transient and continuous depression of testosterone levels have been reported with long-term ketoconozole therapy. Currently available clinical data are encouraging about the future usefulness of this drug.

Ambruticin is an antibiotic produced as a fermentation product of *Polyangium cellulosum*, var. *fulvum*. It has been effective orally in experimentally produced coccidioidomycosis in mice.

Human leukocyte transfer factor has provided temporary clinical improvement in a small number of human recipients.

Experimentation with a killed *Coccidioides immitis* spherule vaccine is in progress. It has been effective in protecting mice.

Cryptococcosis

RICHARD D. DIAMOND, M.D.

The most widely accepted regimen for the therapy of cryptococcal meningitis in adults is amphotericin B, 0.3 mg/kg body weight per day intravenously and flucytosine 37.5 mg/kg body weight every 6 hours orally for 6 weeks. This combination permits use of a lower than usual dose of the more toxic amphotericin B while preventing emergence of cryptococci resistant to flucytosine during therapy (a frequent problem when flucytosine is used alone). Unfortunately direct experience with this regimen in children is small. Thus, dosages and duration of courses may need to be adjusted empirically.

Monitoring of toxic effects of drugs is critical. Even with 0.3 mg/kg/day of amphotericin B, azotemia often occurs. Though amphotericin B is nephrotoxic, it does not accumulate in serum during renal failure. Therefore, doses should not be decreased unless it causes the serum creatinine to rise over 3.0 to 3.5 mg/dl or blood urea nitrogen exceeds 50 mg/dl. Likewise, patients with pre-existing renal failure require normal doses of amphotericin B. In contrast, flucytosine is cleared almost entirely by renal mechanisms, so that serum levels rise during azotemia. Complications of flucytosine therapy are usually mild (nausea, diarrhea, leukopenia, thrombocytopenia, anemia, and abnormalities of liver function parameters). However, continuation of the drug despite toxicity has resulted in cases of fatal agranulocytosis or diarrhea evolving to nonpseudomembranous colitis, with or without intestinal perforation. Recommendations for dosage adjustments during renal failure suggest lengthening intervals between doses of flucytosine according to changes in creatine clearance: 37.5 mg/kg every 12 hours for clearances of 20 to 40 ml/min, and every 24 hours for clearances of 10 to 20 ml/min. Estimates based upon serum levels of creatinine are especially likely to be inaccurate, particularly with early renal abnormalities were serum creatinine concentrations rise within the "normal" or near normal range but with more dramatic depression of clearances. Thus, calculated flucytosine doses are likely to be excessive if the above guidelines are used in early renal failure induced by amphotericin B, especially if creatinine clearances are estimated from serum creatinine levels. Thus, it is preferable to monitor serum flucytosine levels to maintain peak values below 100 to 125 μg/ml. This will usually reduce the incidence of flucytosine toxicity. When patients must be dialyzed, supplementary doses of flucytosine are needed, but no alteration in amphotericin B dosage should be made.

If combination therapy cannot be used, intravenous amphotericin B alone is effective but in somewhat higher doses (0.4–0.6 mg/kg/day). Amphotericin B must be administered in dextrose and water solutions without added electrolytes. This includes supplementary potassium chloride for amphotericin B-induced hypokalemia. Similarly, electrolyte solutions cannot be "piggy-backed" onto intravenous infusions of amphotericin B. However, amphotericin B can be mixed safely with 25–50 mg hydrocortisone and 1000 units heparin. Amphotericin B suspensions *are* light stable; therefore, infusions should not be covered because aggregation may be missed and unnecessary anxiety provoked those observing administration of an ensheathed, seldom-used, "mysterious" drug. First, a test dose of 0.1 mg/kg (up to a total dose of 1 mg/kg) is administered in 50 ml dextrose and water over 30 min, followed 3 to 4 hours later by an initial infusion of 0.3 mg/kg. Either the test or the initial infusion may provoke fever, chills, nausea, anorexia, or even hypotension. If these are troublesome, 25 to 50 mg of hydrocortisone for adults (lesser amounts for children) is given immediately by intravenous "push," and is included in subsequent infusions to ameliorate symptoms. Generally, acute toxicity becomes less of a problem after multiple doses of amphotericin B, so that hydrocortisone usually can be tapered and discontinued. Salicylates and antihistamines appear to be less effective in controlling amphotericin B reactions. Meperidine (administered separately) is effective if severe chills continue despite addition of hydrocortisone. Though disturbing, initial toxicity of amphotericin B is manageable and is not an acceptable reason for discontinuation of effective therapy for a life-threatening disease.

Amphotericin B is generally administered over 3 to 4 hours. Further prolongation of therapy does not decrease toxic effects, and some patients tolerate more rapid infusions. Daily doses can be increased in 5 mg increments at 1 to 3 day intervals until desired levels are reached. Phlebitis is common, usually as a chronic problem leading to sclerosis and disappearance of veins. Thus, it is desirable to begin administering amphotericin B via the smallest possible needle into the most distal, available veins, removing intravenous lines between infusions if they are not required for other reasons. Indwelling catheters are required in some patients. If possible, amphotericin B should not be administered through central intravenous lines; if this is necessary, flow regulating pumps should be used to control the rate of infusion, since evidences of cardiotoxicity may occur in occasional patients

receiving the drug by this route. During therapy, the patient may be switched from a daily dose of amphotericin B to a double dose given on alternate days. If acute reactions such as fever are not inordinately increased, anorexia and phlebitis are likely to be less severe, and outpatient therapy on a thrice weekly basis may be possible if prolonged treatment is required. Along with azotemia during therapy, some abnormalities in urinary sediments are common. Renal tubular acidosis may occur, and hypokalemia may require potassium chloride supplements, though clinically significant hypomagnesemia is rare. Permanent nephrotoxicity appears to be related more to the total dose of amphotericin B given, rather than to the severity of acute azotemia during therapy. Anemia due to suppression of erythrocyte production may be pronounced but is reversible after therapy and rarely necessitates transfusion.

Weekly cultures are made of specimens from any sites that were positive prior to therapy. When amphotericin B alone is used, therapy is continued for at least 6 weeks until weekly cultures are negative for 1 month during treatment. Titers of cryptococcal antigen change slowly, so may be followed at 2 to 4 week intervals. Though cultures of cerebrospinal fluid (CSF) become negative, some patients continue to have persistently positive India ink or nigrosin smears. Such patients usually are given more prolonged therapy (e.g., 2–3 months of amphotericin B), but are considered to be cured despite continued positive smears as long as cultures remain negative. At the conclusion of therapy with amphotericin B alone, most patients should have normal concentrations of CSF glucose, less than 15 to 20 leukocytes/mm^3, and a falling antigen titer which is approaching zero. Though improving, CSF protein concentrations may remain abnormal for years.

Follow-up examinations at 6 week to 3 month intervals after therapy should include CSF and serum antigen titers, in addition to cultures of blood, sputum and urine. Relapses may become evident initially with positive cultures outside the CNS. Almost all relapses occur within 1 year of completion of apparently successful initial therapy.

Addition of intrathecal therapy is seldom required; however it can be curative in a few patients, particularly those who relapse or fail to respond to usual courses of intravenous amphotericin B with or without flucytosine, or those who develop nephrotoxicity severe enough to preclude the use of intravenous amphotericin B. Amphotericin B may be administered intrathecally via the lumbar route, cisterna magna, or subcutaneous reservoir connected by catheter to a lateral cerebral ventricle. The last method is most widely used. However, despite the ease of administration of intraventricular drugs, insertion and usage of reservoirs may cause significant complications. Bacterial infections of functional reservoirs often can be cured with antibiotics alone, without removal of the foreign body. For intrathecal administration, amphotericin B is diluted to 0.25 mg/ml in sterile 5% dextrose in water, and 0.1 ml (0.025 mg) dilution in 10 to 25 ml of withdrawn CBF is given as the initial dose. Dosages can then be increased in 0.025 mg increments to 0.1 mg, then by 0.1 mg increments to the maximum dose tolerated, usually 0.5 mg in adolescents. Dosages in children must be individualized because the scanty data available provide no clear guidelines. Use-associated neurologic complications (common with the lumbar route) are unusual with reservoirs unless the catheter tip is malpositioned (e.g., in the third ventricle). However, headache, nausea, and vomiting may be severe but may be reduced by inclusion of 20 mg hydrocortisone with injections.

Increased intracranial pressure or a recrudescence of abnormalities after initial improvement signals a need for computed tomography to differentiate hydrocephalus from progressive cerebral edema due to ongoing meningoencephalitis. Especially when it is anticipated that a patient may require intraventricular therapy, use of ventricular drainage shunts must be avoided if possible because they divert amphotericin B out of CSF during therapy and lead to treatment failure or relapse.

Antifungal imidazole derivatives have been used in a few cases with mixed results. Accordingly, they cannot be recommended for therapy of potentially life-threatening cryptococcosis at this time.

In the absence of systemic data, therapy for extraneural, nonrespiratory cryptococcosis is assumed to be analogous to treatment of cryptococcal meningitis. Though isolated skin lesions rarely regress spontaneously, skin, bone, and visceral lesions are usually treated with combined amphotericin B and flucytosine for 6 weeks or amphotericin B intravenously (2–3 gm total dose in adults). Surgery generally is not required for therapy but may be necessary for diagnosis. When seemingly isolated lesions are totally removed, antifungal therapy usually is administered (even if briefly) because of the possibility of undetected lesions. Whenever extraneural lesions are detected, lumbar puncture (and cultures of other sites) is necessary to confirm that the disease is localized.

Management of isolated pulmonary cryptococcosis differs from that of extrapulmonary disease. First, it is critical to perform cultures of other sites (including CSF and urine) and antigen determinations to verify that the infection is restricted to the lungs. If so, and the patient has no predisposing factors such as lymphoreticular malignancy or corticosteroid therapy, most cases resolve without antifungal therapy. Excision of lesions may be curative but is not necessary, even if antifungal therapy is required. However, surgery is often necessary to establish the diagnosis because sputum cultures are often negative. Even so, the risk of postoperative meningitis is low, even if lesions are not entirely removed. Moreover, particularly in patients with other pulmonary disease (such as tumor), saprophytic colonization by cryptococci may induce positive sputum cultures that do not indicate invasive cryptococcosis. Thus, antifungal therapy usually can be postponed during a period of close observation for 2–3 months, as long as lesions remain stable or decrease in size, predisposing factors are inapparent, extrapulmonary cultures are negative, and cryptococcal antigen is undetectable in CSF.

Treated cryptococcal meningitis still has a case mortality rate of 25 to 30%, and another 20 to 25% of initially cured patients relapse. Most treatment failures occur in patients with predisposing factors that compromise immunologic host defense mechanisms and in those with more rapidly progressive infections or who show little improvement during treatment. Therefore, if corticosteroids are being given for other diseases, it is desirable to taper and discontinue them, if possible, prior to the conclusion of antifungal therapy. Even cured patients have about a 40% likelihood of significant residua, including blindness, cranial nerve palsies, motor impairment, personality change, and decreased mental function due to chronic brain syndrome or hydrocephalus. The last problem may cause late complications and death, even after the infection has been cleared, sometimes despite shunting procedures.

Visceral Larva Migrans

LEONARD C. MARCUS, V.M.D., M.D.

Visceral larval migrans (VLM) is caused by larval metazoan parasites, which normally infect lower animals, migrating in the deep tissues of humans. The most frequent cause of VLM is *Toxocara canis*, a common roundworm of dogs, and this discussion is limited to treatment of that nematode.

There is no generally accepted, safe, effective treatment. Thiabendazole (Mintezol, Merck Sharp and Dohme Co.) and diethylcarbamazine (Hetrazan, Lederle Laboratories)* have been used on a

---

*Diethylcarbamazine was discontinued by its manufacturer in early 1983. It may be available from the manufacturer or from C.D.C., Atlanta, Georgia.

relatively small number of children, with variable results. No statistically valid, controlled trial has been done with any therapeutic regimen.

The recommended dose of thiabendazole is 25 mg/kg after meals bid for 5 days. Symptomatic response to this treatment has varied from none or minimal to significant improvement. Side effects and toxicity include nausea, abdominal pain, diarrhea, headache, vertigo, drowsiness, skin rash, occasional bradycardia with hypotension, and hypoglycemia.

The recommended dosage for diethylcarbamazine is 2 to 4 mg/kg (2 mg/kg for adults) tid for 3 weeks. This drug can cause a severe allergic response if it is effective in killing the larvae, analogous to a Herxheimer reaction. For this reason, steroids should be given concurrently, especially if there is ocular involvement, to reduce local inflammation and systemic allergic response.

Some of the new benzimidazoles, e.g., fenbendazole, kill certain nematode larvae in tissue. They are currently being investigated for their effectiveness in treating visceral larva migrans.

Steroids are useful in reducing the inflammatory response to the worms. They can provide symptomatic relief for asthma-like attacks, seen in pulmonary involvement, and can save vision in ocular infections. Standard anti-inflammatory doses of steroids can be used and the dosage monitored and altered according to clinical response.

The use of photocoagulation and cryotherapy to control retinal lesions has had variable, poorly documented success but no documentation of this is cited.

The recent development of a fairly specific and sensitive serologic test, an enzyme-linked immunosorbent assay, permits more accurate diagnosis of VLM than previously available, and should allow better evaluation of therapeutic trials. It is questionable whether some of the reported treated cases really had *T. canis* infections.

Malaria

MOSHE A. EPHROS, M.D.

Malaria, among infections the greatest killer of children, is caused by *Plasmodium* protozoa, and is usually transmitted by the bite of an *Anopheles* mosquito. However, the parasite is imported to nonendemic areas by travelers and can be transmitted by blood: by transfusion, perinatally, and by the practices of drug abusers.

In children, the clinical manifestations of infection are nonspecific. Fever is usually present but is rarely periodic, and may not occur at all in infants.

Rigors are rare. Diarrhea, vomiting, and poor appetite are prominent. The child is dull, listless, and irritable. A febrile convulsion may occur. In infants, pallor and jaundice may be early signs. About 50% of children have splenomegaly. Hematologic abnormalities may include anemia, thrombocytopenia, and leukopenia.

Diagnosis is confirmed by demonstration of parasites in the peripheral blood. When parasitemia is very low, multiple examinations of thick smears at 6 hour intervals may be necessary.

In order to select appropriate therapy, certain questions must be answered:

1. *What species is responsible for the infection?* It is important to distinguish between relapsing malaria (*Plasmodium vivax, P. ovale,* and *P. malariae*) and *P. falciparum* malaria. Relapsing malaria is a self-limited illness that can relapse after months or years. In infants and immunocompromised hosts infections with *P. vivax, P. ovale,* and *P. malariae* can be life-threatening.

Mature forms of *P. falciparum* sequester in the microvasculature and cause sludging and obstruction, which result in tissue hypoxia that may lead to serious complications and even death.

Therapy of relapsing malaria that has been transmitted directly by the bite of a mosquito must be directed not only against the erythrocytic parasites but also against the exoerythrocytic parasites in order to prevent relapses.

2. *What is the geographic origin of the infection? Is this a region of drug-resistant malaria?* One should assume that any *P. falciparum* malaria acquired in Southeast Asia and localized areas of Central and South America is resistant to chloroquine. Sporadic chloroquine resistance is now being reported in East Africa.

3. *How sick is the patient?* A patient who is seriously ill with a relapsing malaria should be watched carefully until the clinical and laboratory (parasitemia) parameters have responded satisfactorily to therapy.

Any *P. falciparum* infection, regardless of whether the patient appears ill, and even if the parasitemia is low, should be treated immediately. Infection with *P. falciparum* can be rapidly fatal if not treated, and there can be multiple morbid complications. The patient should be observed in the hospital until clinical improvement and a decrease in parasitemia are evident for 48 hours.

The complications of falciparum malaria require intensive supportive measures. Transfusions with packed red blood cells are given in severe hemolytic anemia. Mannitol may be used in impending renal failure, and dialysis may be necessary. Careful attention to fluid and electrolyte balance is essential. Anticonvulsants are often required in cerebral malaria. Corticosteroids have not been helpful. Splenic rupture is a rare but life-threatening complication. Exchange transfusion should be considered in life-threatening infections.

4. *Was the infection acquired by mosquito or by blood?* Only the infective forms introduced by mosquito can establish the relapsing exoerythrocytic cycle. Therefore, if an infection is acquired by blood (e.g., by transfusion, perinatally, or by addict practices), only the erythrocytic cycle need be treated, since relapses cannot occur.

The details of treatment are outlined in the table on pages 600–607. The following comments are supplementary.

1. An overdose of chloroquine in children may be rapidly fatal.
2. Infants who are not acutely ill should receive chloroquine, 5 mg/kg/day for 5 days, because it is usually better tolerated than the 3-day course with an initial dose of 10 mg/kg.
3. An alternative dosage regimen for pyrimethamine is 1 mg/kg/day divided tid for 3 days.
4. For *P. falciparum* which is resistant to chloroquine, I recommend the following: a) Quinine for 3 days, with tetracycline for 10 (not 7) days (this limited course of tetracycline in young children should not be a cause for concern); or b) quinine for 5 days, in combination with clindamycin, 20 mg/kg/day, divided qid, also for 5 days, given po, IM, or IV (maximum: 600 mg every 6 hours); or c) quinine for 7 (not 3) days, in combination with pyrimethamine and sulfadiazine as outlined on page 603.

The prolonged duration of quinine therapy (often unpleasant for the patient), and the increasing resistance of *P. falciparum* to pyrimethamine/sulfadiazine (especially from Southeast Asia and more recently, Brazil) make regimen c less desirable than a or b.

For the most current information about areas where *P. falciparum* is resistant to chloroquine or other antimalarial drugs, call the C.D.C.

Babesiosis

MOSHE A. EPHROS, M.D.

Babesia species are intraerythrocytic protozoan parasites that are introduced into humans via tick bites. They are also transmitted by transfusion of blood.

Most of the babesiosis in the United States is found in the northeast: Nantucket, Martha's Vineyard, parts of Cape Cod, and islands of the Long Island complex.

Healthy children and adults who are infected are usually asymptomatic. In contrast, individuals with asplenia, premature babies, and other compromised hosts (including the aged) may have a severe illness that resembles malaria and is characterized by fever and hemolytic anemia. The diagnosis is made by seeing typical intraerythrocytic parasites on thick or thin blood films. Babesiosis is distinguished from malaria by morphologic, epidemiologic, and serologic criteria.

Chloroquine produces symptomatic improvement but does not reduce the parasitemia. Pentamidine isethionate, quinine, primaquine, pyrimethamine-sulfadoxine have also been used without clear benefit, as have exchange transfusions.

Recently, a premature baby infected with *Babesia* acquired from a blood transfusion, was cured with a combination of clindamycin and quinine. The curative efficacy of this combination is supported by experimental evidence in hamsters.

Therefore, any ill or immunocompromised patient with babesiosis should be treated with clindamycin, 20 mg/kg/day, po, IV, or IM, divided qid (maximum: 600 mg every 6 hours) and quinine sulfate, 25 mg/kg/day orally, divided tid (maximum 650 mg tid), both for 7 days.

Drugs for Parasitic Infections[*]

Parasitic infections are now encountered throughout the world. With increasing travel, and especially with the recent large emigration from Southeast Asia, the Caribbean, and Central and South America, physicians anywhere may see infections caused by previously unfamiliar parasites. The table that follows lists first-choice and alternative drugs with recommended dosages for most parasitic infections. In every case, the need for treatment must be weighed against the toxicity of the drug. A decision to withhold therapy may often be correct, particularly when the drugs can cause severe adverse effects. When the first-choice drug is initially ineffective and the alternative is more hazardous, it may be advisable to try a second course of treatment with the first drug before using the alternative. Several of the drugs recommended in the table have not been approved by the U.S. Food and Drug Administration. When a physician prescribes an unapproved drug, or an approved drug for an unapproved indication, it may be advisable to inform the patient of the investigational status and possible adverse effects of the drug. A second table on page 608 lists adverse effects of antiparasitic drugs.

[*]Reproduced, with permission from The Medical Letter, Vol. 24 (Issue 601), January 22, 1982.

amphotericin B — Fungizone (Squibb)

*antimony sodium dimercaptosuccinate (stibocaptate) — Astiban (Hoffmann-LaRoche, Switzerland)

benzyl benzoate — Scabanca (Canada); others

*bithionol — Bitin (Tanabe, Japan)

chloroquine — Aralen (Winthrop); others

copper oleate — Cuprex (Beecham)

crotamiton — Eurax (Geigy); Crotan (Alcon)

*dehydroemetine — Hoffmann-LaRoche, Switzerland

diethylcarbamazine — Hetrazan (Lederle)

diiodohydroxyquin (iodoquinol) — Glenwood Laboratories

*diloxanide furoate — Furamide (Boots, England)

furazolidone — Furoxone (Norwich-Eaton)

lindane (gamma benzene hexachloride) — Kwell (Reed and Carnrick); others

mebendazole — Vermox (Janssen)

*melarsoprol — Arsobal (Rhône Poulenc, France)

*metrifonate — Bilarcil (Bayer, Germany)

metronidazole — Flagyl (Searle)

*niclosamide — Yomesan (Bayer, Germany)

*nifurtimox — Lampit (Bayer, Germany)

*niridazole — Ambilhar (Ciba-Geigy, Switzerland)

oxamniquine — Vansil (Pfizer)

paromomycin — Humatin (Parke, Davis)

*pentamidine isethionate — Lomidine (Rhône Poulenc, France)

piperazine — Antepar (Burroughs Wellcome); others

†praziquantel — Biltricide (Miles Pharmaceuticals; EM Industries, Hawthorne, N.Y.)

primaquine phosphate — Primaquine (Winthrop)

pyrantel pamoate — Antiminth (Pfipharmecs)

pyrethrins and piperonyl butoxide — Rid (Pfipharmecs); others

pyrimethamine — Daraprim (Burroughs Wellcome)

pyrimethamine plus sulfadoxine — Fansidar (Roche)

pyrvinium pamoate — Povan (Parke, Davis)

quinacrine — Atabrine (Winthrop)

**spiramycin — Rovamycin (Poulenc, Canada)

*stibogluconate sodium (antimony sodium gluconate) — Pentostam (Burroughs Wellcome, England)

*suramin — Germanin (Bayer, Germany)

tetrachloroethylene — NEMA Worm Capsules, Vet (Parke, Davis)

thiabendazole — Mintezol (Merck Sharp & Dohme)

trimethoprim-sulfamethoxazole — Bactrim (Roche); Septra (Burroughs Wellcome)

**tryparsamide

---

*Available from the Parasitic Diseases Division, Center for Infectious Diseases, Centers for Disease Control, Atlanta, Georgia 30333; 404-329-3670.

**Not available in the USA.

†Available in USA only on investigational basis from manufacturers.

Reproduced, with permission, from The Medical Letter, Vol. 24 (Issue 601), January 22, 1982.

DRUGS FOR TREATMENT OF PARASITIC INFECTIONS

Infection	Drug	Adult Dose*	Pediatric Dose*
AMEBIASIS (Entamoeba histolytica)			
asymptomatic			
Drug of choice:	Diiodohydroxyquin[1]	650 mg tid × 20d	30–40 mg/kg/d in 3 doses × 20d†
Alternatives:	Diloxanide furoate[2]	500 mg tid × 10d	20 mg/kg/d in 3 doses × 10d
	Paromomycin	25–30 mg/kg/d in 3 doses × 7d	25–30 mg/kg/d in 3 doses × 7d
mild to moderate intestinal disease			
Drug of choice:	Metronidazole[3] **plus**	750 mg tid × 5–10d	35–50 mg/kg/d in 3 doses × 10d
	diiodohydroxyquin[1]	650 mg tid × 20d	30–40 mg/kg/d in 3 doses × 20d†
Alternative:	Paromomycin	25–30 mg/kg/d in 3 doses × 7d	25–30 mg/kg/d in 3 doses × 7d
severe intestinal disease			
Drug of choice:	Metronidazole[3] **plus**	750 mg tid × 5–10d	35–50 mg/kg/d in 3 doses × 10d
	diiodohydroxyquin[1]	650 mg tid × 20d	30–40 mg/kg/d in 3 doses × 20d†
Alternatives:	Dehydroemetine[2,4] **plus**	1 to 1.5 mg/kg/d IM (max. 90 mg/d) for up to 5d	1 to 1.5 mg/kg/d (max. 90 mg/d) IM in 2 doses for up to 5d
	diiodohydroxyquin[1]	650 mg tid × 20d	30–40 mg/kg/d in 3 doses × 20d†
OR			
	Emetine[4] **plus**	1 mg/kg/d (max. 60 mg/d) IM for up to 5d	1 mg/kg/d in 2 doses (max. 60 mg/d) IM for up to 5d
	diiodohydroxyquin[1]	650 mg tid × 20d	30–40 mg/kg/d in 3 doses N 20d†
hepatic abscess			
Drug of choice:	Metronidazole[3] **plus**	750 mg tid × 5–10d	35–50 mg/kg/d in 3 doses × 10d
	diiodohydroxyquin[1]	650 mg tid × 20d	30–40 mg/kg/d in 3 doses × 20d†
Alternatives:	Dehydroemetine[2,4] **followed by**	1 to 1.5 mg/kg/d (max. 90 mg/d) IM for up to 5d	1 to 1.5 mg/kg/d (max. 90 mg/d) IM in 2 doses for up to 5d
	chloroquine phosphate **plus**	600 mg base (1 gram) daily × 2d, then 300 mg base (500 mg) daily × 2–3 wks	10 mg base/kg/d (max. 300 mg base/d) × 2–3 wks
	diiodohydroxyquin[1]	650 mg tid × 20d	30–40 mg/kg/d in 3 doses × 20d†
OR			
	Emetine[4] **followed by**	1 mg/kg/d (max. 60 mg/d) IM for up to 5d	1 mg/kg/d in 2 doses (max. 60 mg/d) IM for up to 5d
	chloroquine phosphate	600 mg base (1 gram) daily × 2d, then 300 mg base (500 mg) daily × 2–3 wks	10 mg base/kg/d (max. 300 mg base/d) × 2–3 wks
	plus diiodohydroxyquin[1]	650 mg tid × 20d	30–40 mg/kg/d in 3 doses × 20d†

*The letter d indicates day.

†Maximum 2 grams per day.

Infection	Drug	Adult Dose*	Pediatric Dose*
AMEBIC MENINGOENCEPHALITIS, PRIMARY (Naegleria sp; Acanthamoeba sp)			
Drug of choice[5]:	Amphotericin B[6]	1 mg/kg/d IV, uncertain duration	1 mg/kg/d IV, uncertain duration
ANCYLOSTOMA duodenale (hookworm)			
Drug of choice:	Mebendazole	100 mg bid × 3d	100 mg bid × 3d for children >2 years
OR	Pyrantel pamoate[6]	A single dose of 11 mg/kg (max. 1 gram)	A single dose of 11 mg/kg (max. 1 gram)
ANISAKIASIS (Anisakis sp)			
Treatment of choice:	Surgical removal		
Alternative:	Thiabendazole[6,7]	25 mg/kg bid × 3d	25 mg/kg bid × 3d
ANGIOSTRONGYLUS CANTONENSIS			
Drug of choice:	Thiabendazole[6]	25 mg/kg bid × 3d	25 mg/kg bid × 3d
ASCARIS lumbricoides (roundworm)			
Drug of choice:	Mebendazole	100 mg bid × 3d	100 mg bid × 3d for children >2 years
OR	Pyrantel pamoate	A single dose of 11 mg/kg (max. 1 gram)	A single dose of 11 mg/kg (max. 1 gram)
Alternative:	Piperazine citrate	75 mg/kg (max. 3.5 grams)/d × 2d	75 mg/kg (max. 3.5 grams)/d × 2d
BABESIA, see Footnote 8			
BALANTIDIUM coli			
Drug of choice:	Tetracycline[6]	500 mg qid × 10d	10 mg/kg qid × 10d (max. 2 grams/d)
Alternative:	Diiodohydroxyquin[1,6]	650 mg tid × 20d	40 mg/kg/d in 3 doses × 20d†
Brugia malayi, see FILARIASIS			
CAPILLARIA philippinensis			
Drug of choice:	Mebendazole[6]	200 mg bid × 20d	200 mg bid × 20d
Alternative:	Thiabendazole[6]	25 mg/kg/d × 30d	25 mg/kg/d × 30d
Chagas' disease, see TRYPANOSOMIASIS			
Clonorchis sinensis, see FLUKES			
COCCIDIOSIS (Isospora belli)			
Drug of choice:	Furazolidone[6]	100 mg qid × 10d	1.5 mg/kg qid × 20d
Alternative:	Trimethoprim-sulfamethoxazole	160 mg trimethoprim, 800 mg sulfamethoxazole qid × 10d, then bid × 3 wks	
CUTANEOUS LARVA MIGRANS (creeping eruption)			
Drug of choice:	Thiabendazole	Topically and/or 25 mg/kg bid (max. 3 grams/d) × 2–5d	Topically and/or 25 mg/kg bid (max. 3 grams/d) × 2–5d
DIENTAMOEBA fragilis			
Drug of choice:	Diiodohydroxyquin[1]	650 mg tid × 20d	40 mg/kg/d in 3 doses × 20d†
OR	Tetracycline[6]	500 mg qid × 10d	10 mg/kg qid × 10d (max. 2 grams/d)
Diphyllobothrium latum, see TAPEWORMS			
DRACUNCULUS medinensis (guinea worm)			
Drug of choice:	Niridazole[2]	25 mg/kg (max. 1.5 grams)/d × 15d	12.5 mg/kg bid (max. 1.5 grams/d × 15d
Alternative:	Metronidazole[3,6]	250 mg tid × 10d	25 mg/kg/d (max. 750 mg/d) in 3 doses × 10d
Echinococcus, see TAPEWORMS			
Entamoeba histolytica, see AMEBIASIS			

*The letter d indicates day.
†Maximum 2 grams per day.

Infection	Drug	Adult Dose*	Pediatric Dose*
ENTEROBIUS vermicularis (pinworm)			
Drug of choice:	Pyrantel pamoate	A single dose of 11 mg/kg (max. 1 gram); repeat after 2 weeks	A single dose of 11 mg/kg (max. 1 gram); repeat after 2 weeks
OR	Mebendazole	A single dose of 100 mg; repeat after 2 weeks	A single dose of 100 mg for children >2 years; repeat after 2 weeks
Alternative:	Piperazine citrate	65 mg/kg (max. 2.5 grams)/d × 7d; repeat after 2 weeks	65 mg/kg (max. 2.5 grams)/d × 7d; repeat after 2 weeks
	Pyrvinium pamoate	5 mg/kg single dose (max. 350 mg); repeat after 2 weeks	5 mg/kg single dose (max. 350 mg); repeat after 2 weeks

Fasciola hepatica, see FLUKES

Infection	Drug	Adult Dose*	Pediatric Dose*
FILARIASIS			
Wuchereria bancrofti, Brugia (W.) malayi, Acanthocheilonema perstans, Loa loa			
Drug of choice:	Diethylcarbamazine[9]	Day 1: 50 mg Day 2: 50 mg tid Day 3: 100 mg tid Days 4 through 21: 2 mg/kg tid	Day 1: 25–50 mg Day 2: 25–50 mg tid Day 3: 50–100 mg tid Days 4 through 21: 2 mg/kg tid
Tropical eosinophilia			
Drug of choice:	Diethylcarbamazine[9]‡	2 mg/kg tid × 7–10d	2 mg/kg tid × 7–10d
Onchocerca volvulus			
Drug of choice:	Diethylcarbamazine[9]‡	25 mg/d × 3d, then 50 mg/d × 5d, then 100 mg/d × 3d, then 150 mg/d × 12d	0.5 mg/kg tid × 3d (max. 25 mg/d), then 1.0 mg/kg tid × 3–4d (max. 50 mg/d), then 1.5 mg/kg tid × 3–4d (max. 100 mg/d), then 2.0 mg/kg tid × 2–3 wks (max. 150 mg/d)
	followed by suramin[2,10]	100–200 mg (test dose) IV, then 1 gram IV at weekly intervals × 5 wks	10–20 mg (test dose) IV, then 20 mg/kg IV at weekly intervals × 5 wks
Alternative:	Mebendazole[11]	1 gram bid × 28d	

Infection	Drug	Adult Dose*	Pediatric Dose*
FLUKES, hermaphroditic			
Clonorchis sinensis (Chinese liver fluke)			
Drug of choice:	Praziquantel[12]	25 mg/kg tid × 1d	25 mg/kg tid × 1d
Fasciola hepatica (sheep liver fluke)			
Drug of choice:	Praziquantel[12,13]	25 mg/kg tid × 1d	25 mg/kg tid × 1d
Alternative:	Bithionol[2]	30–50 mg/kg on alternate days × 10–15 doses	30–50 mg/kg on alternate days × 10–15 doses
Fasciolopsis buski (intestinal fluke)			
Drug of choice:	Praziquantel[12,13]	25 mg/kg tid × 1d	25 mg/kg tid × 1d
Alternative:	Tetrachloroethylene[14]	0.1–0.12 ml/kg (max. 5 ml)	0.1 ml/kg (max. 5 ml)
Heterophyes heterophyes (intestinal fluke)			
Drug of choice:	Praziquantel[12,13]	25 mg/kg tid × 1d	25 mg/kg tid × 1d
Alternative:	Tetrachloroethylene[14]	0.1–0.12 ml/kg (max. 5 ml)	0.1 ml/kg (max. 5 ml)
Metagonimus yokogawai (intestinal fluke)			
Drug of choice:	Praziquantel[12,13]	25 mg/kg tid × 1d	25 mg/kg tid × 1d
OR	Tetrachloroethylene[14]	0.1–0.12 ml/kg (max. 5 ml)	0.1 ml/kg (max. 5 ml)
Opisthorchis viverrini (liver fluke)			
Drug of choice:	Praziquantel[12,13]	25 mg/kg tid × 1d	25 mg/kg tid × 1d
Paragonimus westermani (lung fluke)			
Drug of choice:	Praziquantel[12,13]	25 mg/kg tid × 1d	25 mg/kg tid × 1d
Alternative:	Bithionol[2]	30–50 mg/kg on alternate days × 10–15 doses	30–50 mg/kg on alternate days × 10–15 doses

Infection	Drug	Adult Dose*	Pediatric Dose*
GIARDIASIS (Giardia lamblia)			
Drug of choice:	Quinacrine HCl	100 mg tid p.c. × 5d	2 mg/kg tid p.c. × 5d (max. 300 mg/d)
Alternatives:	Metronidazole[3,6]	250 mg tid × 5d	5 mg/kg tid × 5d
	Furazolidone	100 mg qid × 7d	1.25 mg/kg qid × 7d

Infection	Drug	Adult Dose*	Pediatric Dose*
GNATHOSTOMIASIS (Gnathostoma spinigerum)			
Drug of choice:	Surgical removal		
OR	Mebendazole	200 mg PO q3h × 6d	

Hookworm, see ANCYLOSTOMA, NECATOR

Hymenolepis nana, see TAPEWORMS

Kala azar, see LEISHMANIASIS

*The letter d indicates day.
†Maximum 2 grams per day.
‡Discontinued by manufacturer.

Infection	Drug	Adult Dose*	Pediatric Dose*

LEISHMANIASIS

L. braziliensis (American mucocutaneous leishmaniasis) and L. mexicana (American cutaneous leishmaniasis)

Drug of choice:	Stibogluconate sodium[2]	Not certain, probably 600 mg IM or IV/d × 6–10d (may be repeated)	10 mg/kg/d IM or IV (max. 600 mg/d) × 6–10d
Alternative:	Amphotericin B	0.25 to 1 mg/kg by slow infusion daily or every 2d for up to 8 wks	0.25 to 1 mg/kg by slow infusion daily or every 2d for up to 8 wks

L. donovani (kala azar, visceral leishmaniasis)

Drug of choice:	Stibogluconate sodium[2,15,16]	600 mg/d IM or IV × 6–10d (may be repeated)	10 mg/kg/d IM or IV (max. 600 mg/d) × 6–10d
Alternative:	Pentamidine[2,15]	2–4 mg/kg/d IM for up to 15 doses	2–4 mg/kg/d IM for up to 15 doses

L. tropica (oriental sore, cutaneous leishmaniasis)

Drug of choice:	Stibogluconate sodium[2]	600 mg/d IM or IV × 6–10d (may be repeated)	10 mg/kg/d IM or IV (max. 600 mg/d × 6–10d
Alternatives:	Topical treatment[17]		

LICE (Pediculus humanus, capitis, Phthirus pubis)[18]

Drug of choice:	Pyrethrins with piperonyl butoxide	Topically[19]	Topically[19]
Alternatives:	Lindane	Topically[19]	Topically[19]
	0.03% copper oleate	Topically	Topically

Loa loa, see FILARIASIS

MALARIA (Plasmodium falciparum, P. ovale, P. vivax and P. malariae)
suppression or chemoprophylaxis of disease while in endemic area
(all Plasmodium except chloroquine-resistant P. falciparum)

Drug of choice:	Chloroquine phosphate[20]	300 mg base (500 mg) once weekly beginning 1 week before and continued for 6 wks after last exposure in endemic area	<50 kg: 5 mg base/kg once weekly beginning 1 week before and continued for 6 wks after last exposure in endemic area

prevention of attack after departure from areas where P. vivax and P. ovale are endemic[21]

Drug of choice:	Primaquine phosphate[22]	15 mg base (26.3 mg)/d × 14d (with last 2 wks of chloroquine prophylaxis)	0.3 mg base/kg/d × 14d (with last 2 wks of chloroquine prophylaxis)

treatment of uncomplicated attack (all Plasmodium except chloroquine-resistant P. falciparum)

Drug of choice:	Chloroquine phosphate[20,23]	600 mg base (1 gram), then 300 mg base (500 mg) in 6 hrs, then 300 mg base (500 mg)/d × 2d	10 mg base/kg (max. 600 mg base), then 5 mg base/kg 6 hrs later, then 5 mg base/kg/d × 2d

treatment of severe illness, parenteral dosage—only if oral dose cannot be administered (regardless of severity) (all Plasmodium except chloroquine-resistant P. falciparum)

Drug of choice:	Quinine dihydrochloride[2,24]	600 mg in 300 ml normal saline IV over at least 1 hr; repeat in 6–8 hrs if oral therapy still cannot be started (max. 1800 mg/d)	25 mg/kg/d; administer half of dose in 1 hr infusion, then other half 6–8 hrs later if oral therapy still cannot be started (max. 1800 mg/d)
OR	Chloroquine HCl[23]	200 mg base (250 mg) IM q6h	Not recommended

prevention of relapses ("radical" cure after "clinical" cure) (P. vivax and P. ovale only)

Drug of choice:	Primaquine phosphate[22]	15 mg base (26.3 mg)/d × 14d or 45 mg base (79 mg)/wk × 8 wks	0.3 mg base/kg/d × 14d

P. falciparum (chloroquine-resistant)[23,25] suppression or chemoprophylaxis

Drug of choice:	Pyrimethamine **plus** sulfadoxine[26,27]	1 tablet (25 mg pyrimethamine, 500 mg sulfadoxine) once weekly from one day before until 6 weeks after exposure	6–11 mos: 1/8 tablet; 1–3 yrs: 1/4 tablet; 4–8 yrs: 1/2 tablet; 9–14 yrs: 3/4 tablet once weekly from one day before until 6 weeks after exposure

treatment of uncomplicated attack[28] (chloroquine-resistant P. falciparum)

Drug of choice:	Quinine sulfate **plus**	650 mg tid × 3d	25 mg/kg/d in 3 doses × 3d
	pyrimethamine	25 mg bid × 3d	<10 kg: 6.25 mg/d; 10–20 kg: 12.5 mg/d; 20–40 kg: 25 mg/d
	plus sulfadiazine	500 mg qid × 5d	100–200 mg/kg/d in 4 doses × 5d (max. 2 grams/d)
Alternative:	Quinine sulfate **plus** tetracycline[6]	650 mg tid × 3d 250 mg qid × 7d	25 mg/kg/d in 3 doses × 3d 5 mg/kg qid × 7d

treatment of severe illness, parenteral dosage (chloroquine-resistant P. falciparum)

*The letter d indicates day.

Infection	Drug	Adult Dose*	Pediatric Dose*
MALARIA (Plasmodium falciparum, P. ovale, P. vivax and P. malariae) (continued)			
Drug of choice:	Quinine dihydro-chloride[2,24,28]	600 mg in 300 ml normal saline IV over at least 1 hr; repeat in 6–8 hrs if oral therapy still cannot be started (max. 1800 mg/d)	25 mg/kg/d; administer half of dose in 1-hr infusion, then other half 6–8 hrs later if oral therapy still cannot be started (max. 1800 mg/d)
MITES (Sarcoptes scabiei)			
Drug of choice:	10% crotamiton	Topically	Topically
Alternatives:	Lindane	Apply topically once	Apply topically once
	Benzyl benzoate	Topically	Topically
	Sulfur in petrolatum	Topically	Topically
Naegleria species, see AMEBIC MENINGOENCEPHALITIS, PRIMARY			
NECATOR americanus (hookworm)			
Drug of choice:	Mebendazole	100 mg bid × 3d	100 mg bid × 3d for children >2 yrs
OR	Pyrantel pamoate[6]	A single dose of 11 mg/kg (max. 1 gram)	A single dose of 11 mg/kg (max. 1 gram)
Alternative:	Thiabendazole	25 mg/kg bid (max. 3 grams/d) × 2d	25 mg/kg bid (max. 3 grams/d) × 2d
Onchocerca volvulus, see FILARIASIS			
Opisthorchis viverrini, see FLUKES			
Paragonimus westermani, see FLUKES			
Pediculus capitis, humanus, Phthirus pubis, see LICE			
Pinworm, see ENTEROBIUS			
PNEUMOCYSTIS carinii			
Drug of choice:	Trimethoprim-sulfamethoxazole	trimethoprim 20 mg/kg/d, sulfamethoxazole 100 mg/kg/d in 4 doses × 14d	trimethoprim 20 mg/kg/d, sulfamethoxazole 100 mg/kg/d in 4 doses × 14d
Alternative:	Pentamidine[2]	4 mg/kg/d IM × 12–14d	4 mg/kg/d IM × 12–14d
Roundworm, see ASCARIS			
Scabies, see MITES			
SCHISTOSOMIASIS[29]			
S. haematobium			
Drug of choice:	Metrifonate[2]	10 mg/kg every other wk × 3	10 mg/kg every other week × 3
Alternative:	Praziquantel[12,13]	40 mg/kg once	40 mg/kg once
S. japonicum			
Drug of choice:	Praziquantel[12,13]	30 mg/kg twice in one day	30 mg/kg twice in one day
Alternative:	Niridazole[30]	25 mg/kg/d PO (max. 1.5 grams) × 10d	25 mg/kg/d PO (max. 1.5 grams) × 10d
S. mansoni			
Drug of choice:	Oxamniquine	15 mg/kg once[31]	15 mg/kg once[31]
Alternative:	Praziquantel[12,13]	40 mg/kg once	40 mg/kg once
S. mekongi			
Drug of choice:	Praziquantel[12,13]	20 mg/kg three times in one day	20 mg/kg three times in one day
Sleeping sickness, see TRYPANOSOMIASIS			
STRONGYLOIDES stercoralis			
Drug of choice:	Thiabendazole	25 mg/kg bid (max. 3 grams/d) × 2d[32]	25 mg/kg bid (max. 3 grams/d) × 2d[32]
TAPEWORMS—Adult or intestinal stage			
Diphyllobothrium latum (fish tapeworm), Taenia saginata (beef tapeworm), Taenia solium (pork tapeworm),[33] Dipylidium caninum (dog tapeworm)			
Drug of choice:	Niclosamide[2]	A single dose of 4 tablets (2 grams) chewed thoroughly	**11–34 kg:** a single dose of 2 tablets (1 gram); **>34 kg:** a single dose of 3 tablets (1.5 grams)
Alternative:	Paromomycin[6]	1 gram q15min × 4 doses	11 mg/kg q15min × 4 doses
Hymenolepis nana (dwarf tapeworm)			
Drug of choice:	Niclosamide[2]	A single daily dose of 4 tablets (2 grams) chewed thoroughly × 5d	**11–34 kg:** a single daily dose of 2 tablets (1 gram) × 5d; **>34 kg:** A single daily dose of 3 tablets (1.5 grams) × 5d

*The letter d indicates day.

Infection	Drug	Adult Dose*	Pediatric Dose*
TAPEWORMS—Adult or intestinal stage (continued)			
OR	Praziquantel[12,13]	15–20 mg/kg once	15–20 mg/kg once
Alternative:	Paromomycin[6]	45 mg/kg once/d × 5–7d	45 mg/kg once/d × 5–7d
Larval or tissue stage			
Echinococcus granulosus (sheep, cattle, human, deer Hydatid cysts)			
Drug of choice: See footnote 34			
Cysticercus cellulosae (T. solium)			
Drug of choice: See footnote 35			

Toxocariasis, see VISCERAL LARVA MIGRANS

Infection	Drug	Adult Dose*	Pediatric Dose*
TOXOPLASMOSIS (Toxoplasma gondii)[36]			
Drug of choice:	Pyrimethamine[37]	25 mg/d × 3–4 wks	2 mg/kg/d × 3d (max. 25 mg/d), then 1 mg/kg/d[38] × 4 wks
	plus		
	trisulfapyrimidines	2–6 grams/d × 3–4 wks	100–200 mg/kg/d × 3–4 wks
Alternative:	Spiramycin[39]	2–4 grams/d × 3–4 wks	50–100 mg/kg/d × 3–4 wks
TRICHINOSIS (Trichinella spiralis)			
Drug of choice:	Steroids for severe symptoms		
	plus thiabendazole[40]	25 mg/kg bid × 5d	25 mg/kg bid × 5d
Alternative:	Mebendazole[6]	200–400 mg tid × 3d, then 400–500 mg tid × 10d	
TRICHOMONAS vaginalis[41]			
Drug of choice:	Metronidazole[3]	250 mg tid × 7d	15 mg/kg/d in 3 doses × 7d
TRICHOSTRONGYLUS species			
Drug of choice:	Thiabendazole[6]	25 mg/kg bid × 2d	25 mg/kg bid × 2d
Alternative:	Pyrantel pamoate[6]	A single dose of 11 mg/kg (max. 1 gram)	A single dose of 11 mg/kg (max. 1 gram)
TRICHURIS trichiura (whipworm)			
Drug of choice:	Mebendazole	100 mg bid × 3d	100 mg bid × 3d
TRYPANOSOMIASIS			
T. cruzi (South American trypanosomiasis, Chagas' disease)			
Drug of choice:	Nifurtimox[2]	5 mg/kg/d orally in 4 divided doses, increasing by 2 mg/kg/d every 2 wks until dose reaches 15–17 mg/kg/d	
T. gambiense; T. rhodesiense (African trypanosomiasis, sleeping sickness)			
hemolymphatic stage			
Drug of choice:	Suramin[2]	100–200 mg (test dose) IV, then 1 gram IV on days 1, 3, 7, 14, 21	20 mg/kg on days 1, 3, 7, 14 and 21
Alternative:	Pentamidine[2]	4 mg/kg/d IM × 10d	4 mg/kg/d IM × 10d
late disease with CNS involvement			
Drug of choice:	Melarsoprol[2,42]	2–3.6 mg/kg/d IV × 3 doses; after 1 wk 3.6 mg/kg/d IV × 3 doses; repeat again after 10–21 days	18–25 mg/kg total over 1 mo. Initial dose of 0.36 mg/kg IV, increasing gradually to max. 3.6 mg/kg at intervals of 1–5d for total of 9–10 doses
Alternatives:	Tryparsamide[39]	One injection of 30 mg/kg IV every 5d to total of 12 injections; may be repeated after 1 mo.	Unknown
	plus suramin[2]	One injection of 10 mg/kg IV every 5d to total of 12 injections; may be repeated after 1 mo.	Unknown
VISCERAL LARVA MIGRANS[43]			
Drug of choice:	Thiabendazole[6]	25 mg/kg bid × 5d	25 mg/kg bid × 5d

Whipworm, see TRICHURIS

Wuchereria bancrofti, see FILARIASIS

*The letter d indicates day.

FOOTNOTES TO TABLE OF DRUGS FOR TREATMENT OF PARASITIC INFECTIONS

1. Dosage and duration of administration should not be exceeded because of possibility of causing optic neuritis. Maximum dosage is 2 grams/day. Available from Glenwood Laboratories, Inc., 83 North Summit Street, Tenafly, New Jersey 07670.

2. In the USA, this drug is available from the Parasitic Diseases Division, Center for Infectious Diseases, Centers for Disease Control, Atlanta, Georgia 30333; telephone: 404–329–3670.

3. Metronidazole is carcinogenic in rodents and mutagenic in bacteria; it should generally not be given to pregnant women, particularly in the first trimester.

4. Dehydroemetine is probably as effective and probably less toxic than emetine. Because of the toxic effects on the heart, patients receiving emetine should have electrocardiographic monitoring and should remain sedentary during therapy.

5. One patient with a Naegleria infection was successfully treated with intrathecal administration of amphotericin B, miconazole, and rifampin (Morbid Mortal Weekly Rep, 27:343, Sept 15, 1978). Experimental infections with Acanthamoeba have been reported to respond to sulfadiazine.

6. Considered an investigational drug for this condition by the U.S. Food and Drug Administration.

7. Effectiveness documented only in animals.

8. There are no completely satisfactory drugs available for the therapy of Babesia infections in humans. Chloroquine has been used and produces symptomatic improvement but does not reduce parasitemia. Pentamidine isethionate has also been used. Recently one patient was successfully treated with clindamycin and quinine.

9. Diethylcarbamazine should be administered with special caution in heavy infections with Loa loa because it can provoke an encephalopathy. Antihistamines or corticosteroids may be required to reduce allergic reactions due to disintegration of microfilariae in treatment of all filarial infections, especially those caused by Onchocerca and Loa loa. Surgical excision of subcutaneous Onchocerca nodules is recommended by some authorities before starting drug therapy. (Diethylcarbamazine has been discontinued by manufacturer.)

10. Some Medical Letter consultants use suramin only if microfilaremia persists after diethylcarbamazine therapy and nodulectomy.

11. Limited data (AR Rivas-Alcala et al, Lancet, 2:485, 1981; 2:1043, 1981).

12. Available in USA only on investigational basis from manufacturers.

13. Limited data available on use of praziquantel for this indication.

14. Given on empty stomach. Although approved for human use, it is available currently only as a veterinary product. No alcoholic beverages should be consumed before or 12 hours after therapy.

15. Pentamidine should be used for failures with stibogluconate and sometimes for initial treatment in cases from Sudan (which are often resistant to antimonials). All solutions should be protected from light to avoid production of hepatotoxic compounds.

16. For the African form of visceral leishmaniasis therapy may have to be extended to at least 30 days and may have to be repeated.

17. Application of heat 39–42°C directly to the lesion for 20 to 32 hours over a period of 10 to 12 days has been reported to be effective.

18. For infestation of eyelashes with crab lice, use ophthalmic ointment containing 0.25% physostigmine or ophthalmic ointment of yellow oxide of mercury.

19. Some consultants recommend a second application 5 to 7 days later to kill hatching progeny.

20. Dosage is oral unless otherwise stated. If chloroquine phosphate is not available, hydroxychloroquine sulfate is as effective; 400 mg of hydroxychloroquine sulfate is equivalent to 500 mg of chloroquine phosphate.

21. For prevention of attack after departure from areas where P. vivax or P. ovale are endemic, which includes almost all areas where malaria is found, many experts prescribe primaquine phosphate. Others prefer to avoid the toxicity of primaquine and rely on surveillance to detect cases where they occur, particularly when exposure was limited or doubtful.

22. Primaquine phosphate can cause hemolytic anemia, especially in patients whose red cells are deficient in glucose-6-phosphate dehydrogenase. This deficiency is most common in Blacks, Asians, and Mediterranean peoples. Patients should be screened for G–6–PD deficiency before treatment.

23. In falciparum malaria, if the patient has not shown a prompt response to conventional doses of chloroquine, parasitic resistance to this drug must be considered.

24. Intravenous administration of quinine dihydrochloride can be hazardous, and it must be given slowly. Constant monitoring of the pulse and blood pressure is necessary to detect arrhythmia or hypotension. Oral drugs should be substituted as soon as possible. In an emergency, if quinine dihydrochloride is unavailable, quinidine gluconate has been used; 800 mg is diluted in 250 ml of 5% dextrose and administered *very slowly* IV under ECG monitoring; widening of the QRS interval requires discontinuation of this drug.

25. Chloroquine-resistant strains of P. falciparum have been reported from Bangladesh, Brazil, Burma, China, Colombia, Comoros, Ecuador, French Guiana, Guyana, India, Indonesia, Kampuchea, Kenya, Laos, Madagascar, Malaysia, Panama, Papua New Guinea, the Philippines, Solomon Islands, Surinam, Tanzania, Thailand, Venezuela, and Vietnam.

26. Chloroquine should be taken simultaneously because exposure to other species of malaria may also occur. Pyrimethamine plus sulfadoxine is available in a fixed-dose combined as *Fansidar* (Roche). Pyrimethamine is teratogenic in animals.

27. P. falciparum resistant to *Fansidar* have been reported in areas on the Thai-Kampuchean border, in Indonesia, Papua New Guinea, and in the Amazon region of Brazil; in these areas quinine, 325 mg bid, may be useful for prophylaxis for selected patients.

28. Quinine alone will control an acute attack of resistant P. falciparum but, in a substantial number of infections, particularly with strains from Southeast Asia, it fails to prevent recurrence. Addition of pyrimethamine and sulfadiazine lowers the rate of recurrence.

29. Not all patients with schistosomiasis need be treated. The decision to treat should be based upon such factors as the clinical status of the patient, viability of eggs, and concentration of eggs in urine and feces. An experienced clinician should be consulted before treatment is initiated. Hycanthone is widely used in some countries for treatment of S. mansoni and S. haematobium infections, but the drug can cause fatal hepatic necrosis and is suspected of being teratogenic and carcinogenic.

30. Niridazole is absolutely contraindicated in the presence of hepatocellular disease, portal hypertension, or mental disorders or seizures.

31. In East Africa, the dose should be increased to 30 mg/kg/d, and in Eqypt and South Africa, 30 mg/kg/d × 2d.

32. In disseminated strongyloidiasis, thiabendazole therapy should be continued for at least five days.

33. Niclosamide and paromomycin are effective for the treatment of T. solium but, since they cause disintegration of segments and release of viable eggs, their use creates a theoretical risk of causing cysticercosis. They should therefore be followed in 3 or 4 hours by a purge. Quinacrine is preferred by some clinicians because it expels T. solium intact.

34. Surgical resection of cysts is the treatment of choice. When surgery is contraindicated, or cysts rupture spontaneously during surgery, mebendazole (experimental for this purpose in the USA) can be tried (J.F. Wilson and R.L. Rausch, Amer J Trop Med Hyg, 29:1340, 1980).

35. Surgical resection is the treatment of choice. When contraindicated, especially in neurocysticercosis, praziquantel[12, 13] can be tried.

36. In ocular toxoplasmosis, corticosteroids should also be used for anti-inflammatory effect on the eyes.

37. To prevent hematologic toxicity from pyrimethamine, it is advisable to administer leucovorin (folinic acid), about 10 mg/day. Pyrimethamine is teratogenic in animals.

38. Every two to three days for infants.

39. Not available in the USA.

40. The efficacy of thiabendazole for trichinosis is not clearly established; it appears to be effective during the intestinal phase but its effect on larvae which have migrated is questionable.

41. Sexual partners should be treated simultaneously.

42. In frail patients, begin with as little as 18 mg and increase the dose progressively. Pretreatment with suramin has been advocated for debilitated patients.

43. Visceral larva migrans is usually a self-limited disease; treatment should be restricted to severe cases. For severe symptoms or eye involvement, corticosteroids can be used in addition.

BITHIONOL *(Bitin)*
Frequent: photosensitivity skin reactions; vomiting; diarrhea; abdominal pain; urticaria

CHLOROQUINE HCl and CHLORO-QUINE PHOSPHATE USP *(Aralen; and others)*
Occasional: pruitus; vomiting; headache; confusion; depigmentation of hair; skin eruptions; comeal opacity; irreversible retinal injury (especially when total dosage exceeds 100 grams); weight loss; partial alopecia; extraocular muscle palsies; exacerbation of psoriasis, eczema and other exfoliative dermatoses; myalgias
Rare: discoloration of nails and mucous membranes of mouth; nerve-type deafness; blood dyscrasias; photophobia

CROTAMITON *(Eurax; Crotan)*
Occasional: skin rash; conjunctivitis

DIETHYLCARBAMAZINE CITRATE USP *(Hetrazan)*
Frequent: severe allergic or febrile reactions due to the filarial infection; GI disturbances
Rare: encephalopathy; loss of vision

DIIODOHYDROXYQUIN *(Iodoquinol)*
Occasional: rash; acne; slight enlargement of the thyroid gland; nausea; diarrhea; cramps; anal pruritus
Rare: Optic atrophy and loss of vision after prolonged use in high dosage (for months)

DILOXANIDE FUROATE *(Furamide)*
Frequent: flatulence
Occasional: nausea; vomiting; diarrhea; urticaria; pruritus

EMETINE HCl USP
Frequent: cardiac arrhythmias; precordial pain; muscle weakness; cellulitis at site of injection
Occasional: diarrhea; vomiting; peripheral neuropathy; heart failure

FURAZOLIDONE *(Furoxone)*
Frequent: nausea, vomiting
Occasional: allergic reactions, including pulmonary infiltration; headache; orthostatic hypotension; hypoglycemia; polyneuritis; MAO inhibitor interactions
Rare: hemolytic anemia in G–6–PD deficiency and infants less than one month old

LINDANE *(Kwell; Gamene)*
Occasional: eczematous skin rash; conjunctivitis
Rare: convulsions; aplastic anemia

MEBENDAZOLE *(Vermox)*
Occasional: diarrhea; abdominal pain
Rare: leukopenia

MELARSOPROL *(Mel B; Arsobal)*
Frequent: myocardial damage; albuminuria; hypertension; colic; Herxheimer-type reaction; encephalopathy; vomiting; peripheral neuropathy
Rare: shock

METRIFONATE *(Bilarcil)*
Occasional: nausea; vomiting; bronchospasm; weakness; diarrhea; abdominal pain

METRONIDAZOLE *(Flagyl)*
Frequent: nausea, especially with single high dose; headache; dry mouth; metallic taste
Occasional: vomiting; diarrhea; insomnia; weakness; stomatitis; vertigo; paresthesia; rash; urethral burning; phlebitis at injection site
Rare: ataxia; encephalopathy; pseudomembranous colitis; neutropenia

NICLOSAMIDE *(Yomesan)*
Occasional: nausea; abdominal pain

NIFURTIMOX *(Bayer 2502; Lampit)*
Frequent: anorexia; vomiting; weight loss; loss of memory; sleep disorders; tremor; paresthesias; weakness; polyneuritis
Rare: convulsions

NIRIDAZOLE *(Ambilhar)*
Frequent: immunosuppression; vomiting; cramps; dizziness; headache
Occasional: diarrhea; slight ECG change; rash; insomnia; paresthesia
Rare: psychosis; hemolytic anemia in G–6–PD deficiency; convulsions

OXAMNIQUINE *(Vansil)*
Occasional: headache; fever; dizziness; somnolence; nausea; diarrhea; rash; insomnia; hepatic enzyme changes; ECG changes
Rare: convulsions

PAROMOMYCIN *(Humatin)*
Frequent: GI disturbance
Rare: eighth-nerve damage (mainly auditory); renal damage

PENTAMIDINE ISETHIONATE *(Lomidine)*
Frequent: hypotension; hypoglycemia; vomiting; blood dyscrasias; renal damage; pain at injection site
Occasional: may aggravate diabetes; shock; liver damage
Rare: Herxheimer-type reaction; acute pancreatitis

PIPERAZINE CITRATE USP *(Antepar; others)*
Occasional: dizziness; urticaria; GI disturbances
Rare: exacerbation of epilepsy; visual disturbances; ataxia; hypotonia

PRAZIQUANTEL *(Biltricide)*
Frequent: sedation; abdominal discomfort; fever; sweating; nausea; eosinophilia
Occasional: headache; dizziness

PRIMAQUINE PHOSPHATE USP
Frequent: hemolytic anemia in G–6–PD deficiency
Occasional: neutropenia; GI disturbances; methemoglobinemia in G–6–PD deficiency
Rare: CNS symptoms; hypertension; arrhythmias

PYRANTEL PAMOATE *(Antiminth)*
Occasional: GI disturbances; headache; dizziness; rash; fever

PYRIMETHAMINE USP *(Daraprim)*
Occasional: blood dyscrasias; folic acid deficiency
Rare: rash; vomiting; convulsions; shock

PYRVINIUM PAMOATE USP *(Povan)*
Frequent: turns stool red
Occasional: vomiting; diarrhea
Rare: photosensitivity skin reactions

QUINACRINE HCl USP *(Atabrine)*
Frequent: dizziness; headache; vomiting; diarrhea; yellow staining of skin
Occasional: toxic psychosis; insomnia; bizarre dreams; blood dyscrasias; urticaria; blue and black nail pigmentation; psoriasis-like rash
Rare: acute hepatic necrosis; convulsions; severe exfoliative dermatitis; ocular effects similar to those caused by chloroquine

QUININE DIHYDROCHLORIDE and QUININE SULFATE
Frequent: cinchonism (tinnitus, headache, nausea, abdominal pain, visual disturbance)
Occasional: hemolytic anemia; other blood dyscrasias; photosensitivity reactions; arrhythmias; hypotension
Rare: blindness; sudden death if injected too rapidly

SPIRAMYCIN *(Rovamycin)*
Occasional: GI disturbance
Rare: allergic reactions

STIBOGLUCONATE SODIUM *(Pentostam)*
Frequent: muscle pain and joint stiffness; bradycardia
Occasional: colic; diarrhea; rash; pruritus; myocardial damage
Rare: liver damage; hemolytic anemia; renal damage; shock; sudden death

SURAMIN SODIUM *(Germanin)*
Frequent: vomiting; pruritus; urticaria; paresthesia; hyperesthesia of hands and feet; photophobia; peripheral neuropathy
Occasional: kidney damage; blood dyscrasias; shock; optic atrophy

TETRACHLOROETHYLENE *(NEMA Worm Capsules, Vet)*
Frequent: epigastric burning; dizziness; headache
Occasional: drowsiness; Antabuse-like effect with alcohol
Rare: hepatic necrosis

THIABENDAZOLE *(Mintezol)*
Frequent: nausea; vomiting; vertigo
Occasional: leukopenia; crystalluria; rash; hallucinations; olfactory disturbance; Stevens-Johnson syndrome
Rare: shock; tinnitus

TRYPARSAMIDE
Frequent: nausea; vomiting
Occasional: impaired vision; optic atrophy; fever; exfoliative dermatitis; allergic reactions; tinnitus

Toxoplasmosis

JACK S. REMINGTON, M.D.,
and CHRISTOPHER B. WILSON, M.D.

Acquisition of useful data regarding therapy of *Toxoplasma* infection in humans has been hampered by several inherent problems. Acute cases available for careful study have been relatively few, and the diagnosis has often been made too late to institute treatment under controlled conditions. Evaluation of the efficacy of treatment is difficult because of variations in severity and outcome of the disease. Specific therapy acts primarily against the proliferative form of *Toxoplasma* but does not eradicate the encysted form of the parasite, which persists in the host, resulting in a chronic, usually asymptomatic, latent infection.

Specific Therapy. Pyrimethamine, a substituted phenylpyrimidine antimalarial drug (in the form of Daraprim), produces not only survival but also radical cure of animals given experimental infection. The suggested dosage of pyrimethamine in human patients is 1 mg/kg/24 hr in a single dose, with a maximum dose of 25 mg/24 hr. A dose of 2 mg/kg to a maximum of 50 mg/24 hr has been used, but with a proportional increase in toxicity. The dose is usually doubled (2 mg/kg) during the first day or two of treatment, however.* As the half-life of pyrimethamine is 4 to 5 days, a number of authorities administer the 1 mg/kg dosage only every 2 or 3 days. Trimethoprim, although chemically related, is substantially less active than pyrimethamine against *Toxoplasma*.

Pyrimethamine and sulfadiazine act synergistically against *Toxoplasma* with a combined activity eight times that which would be expected if their effects were merely additive. Comparative tests have shown that sulfapyrazine, sulfamethazine, and sulfamerazine are of a similar order of activity to sulfadiazine. All the other sulfonamides tested (sulfathiazole, sulfapyridine, sulfadimetine, sulfamethoxazole, sulfisoxazole) were much inferior. It appears logical to use multiple sulfonamides for treatment of toxoplasmosis, because additive effect with less toxicity would be expected. The usual dosage of sulfadiazine or triple sulfonamides is 100 to 150 mg/kg/24 hr in two or three equal doses by mouth in addition to pyrimethamine. The optimal duration of treatment has not been determined.

Both pyrimethamine and the sulfonamides are potentially toxic drugs. Most physicians are familiar with the untoward reactions to sulfonamides: crystalluria, hematuria, and hypersensitivity. Pyrimethamine is a folic acid antagonist, which produces

---

*This dosage of pyrimethamine is higher than that recommended by the manufacturer but has been found safe and effective.

reversible and usually gradual depression of the bone marrow. Although toxicity is dose-related, absorption of the drug is not uniform in all patients, and side effects are seen more frequently in patients who absorb the drug best. Platelet depression with its associated bleeding tendency is the most serious consequence of toxicity. Both leukopenia and anemia may occur as well. Less serious side effects are gastrointestinal distress, headaches, and a bad taste in the mouth. *All patients treated with pyrimethamine should have a peripheral blood cell and platelet count twice a week.*

Folinic acid (in the form of leucovorin-calcium) has been used to facilitate return of circulating platelets to normal. Precise data are not available on the dosage of leucovorin-calcium in young children. We usually employ 5 mg every other day in older children and adults. The parenteral form (Calcium Leucovoran Injection) may be ingested. This substance, which in contrast to folic acid does not appear to inhibit the action of pyrimethamine on the proliferative form of *Toxoplasma*, may be used in conjunction with this drug to allay toxicity.

Other agents, including spiramycin, clindamycin, and trimethoprim-sulfamethoxazole, are less active against *Toxoplasma* than the combination of pyrimethamine and sulfadiazine. Spiramycin, which is less toxic than pyrimethamine and sulfadiazine, has been used effectively in the treatment of pregnant women and may be effective in the treatment of infants with congenital infection. This agent is available in most countries except the United States. Clindamycin is concentrated in the ocular choroid and has been employed in the treatment of ocular disease. Because of insufficient data, the role of trimethoprim-sulfamethoxazole in the treatment of human toxoplasmosis is not clear.

Congenital Toxoplasmosis

If congenital toxoplasmosis is diagnosed, children should receive specific therapy whether the infection is clinically apparent or asymptomatic. Even in what often appears clinically to be an acute fulminant disease with multiple organ involvement, early instigation of therapy may prevent further tissue invasion and destruction by the proliferative form of the parasite, allowing regeneration and healing of tissues which have not been irreparably damaged. There are insufficient data to allow for proper evaluation of treatment in the asymptomatic infected infant; however, most investigators consider that treatment should be undertaken in the hope of preventing late untoward sequelae which develop in nearly all such infants. We recommend that therapy be continued for 6 months to one year.

Our knowledge of the treatment of congenital toxoplasmosis is meager. Because pyrimethamine has not been used extensively in young infants, the best course to follow is unknown. In the face of an extremely high mortality rate in cases of clinically apparent fulminant infection, and because of the serious sequelae that may develop in asymptomatic infants, it seems desirable to treat even very young infants.

In infants with the severe form of the congenital infection, corticosteroids have been recommended. Prednisone or methylprednisolone in a dose of 1 to 2 mg/kg/24 hr by the oral route may be given until the inflammatory process (such as chorioretinitis, high CSF protein) has subsided. If spiramycin can be obtained, a regimen using this drug has been recommended.

Acquired Toxoplasmosis

Whether the child with an active acquired infection should be treated depends on the nature of the clinical illness. This form of toxoplasmosis may range from acute fatal illness with meningoencephalitis and pneumonia to an essentially asymptomatic infection. Unfortunately, because the diagnosis is often made late in the disease, only a few patients have been studied extensively, and little is known of the efficacy of treatment of the acquired infection. Patients with the more severe form, and especially immunologically compromised patients, must be treated to prevent extensive tissue damage or a fatal outcome. We recommend treatment for a minimum of 6 weeks or until immune function improves. In asymptomatic infection and in the benign, lymphadenopathic form of the infection, specific treatment is rarely necessary. In most such cases which have been treated, it is not possible to distinguish between a therapeutic response and a spontaneous remission.

Ocular Toxoplasmosis

The greatest experience with chemotherapy has been obtained in cases of ocular toxoplasmosis. Since it is difficult to reach a definitive diagnosis of this disease, evaluation of the therapy must be based on statistical studies, which, in general, have been encouraging.

Hypersensitivity appears to play a predominant role in the pathogenesis of relapse of ocular toxoplasmosis, and in such cases corticosteroids should be used in addition to chemotherapy (at least sulfonamides). Because of the potential hazards associated with the use of corticosteroids, these drugs are best given only in cases of retinochoroiditis with involvement of the macula, maculopapillary bundle, or optic nerve. If the lesion appears in other areas of the retina, scarring usually occurs without significant loss of vision, and the potential toxicity of corticosteroids, as well as the possibility of their causing spread of organisms or breakdown of quiescent foci, probably contraindicates their use in this situation.

The daily dosage of prednisone in children is 1 to 2 mg/kg orally to a maximum of 75 mg/24 hr. The equivalent dosage of another corticosteroid may be given. Specific chemotherapy directed against the parasite is used concomitantly, as outlined. The dosage of corticosteroid may be tapered gradually when the lesion appears well demarcated and pigmentation has begun. Systemic or intraocular clindamycin has been used by some to treat patients who fail to respond to corticosteroids and pyrimethamine plus sulfadiazine; efficacy has not been proved in humans.

Cholera

MYRON M. LEVINE, M.D.

Cholera is an acute diarrheal disease caused by *Vibrio cholerae* serogroup O1. Cholera toxin, a potent enterotoxin elaborated by this bacteria, acts on the enterocytes of the proximal small intestine, leading to net secretion that culminates in diarrhea. As the world is presently experiencing a pandemic of cholera, this disease is encountered throughout much of Asia, Africa, and Oceania. However, it should not be regarded as an exotic tropical disease of no practical concern, for there exists an endemic focus of cholera along the Gulf of Mexico coast of the United States. More than two dozen confirmed cases have occurred in Louisiana and Texas since 1973 (most since 1978), with contaminated seafood being repeatedly incriminated as the vehicles of transmission. Although the cases have been confined to adults, it is conceivable that cholera may be seen in children who consume seafood. In less-developed endemic areas such as Bangladesh incidence rates are highest in children 2 to 4 years of age.

Clinical Presentation. Clinically what makes cholera special among diarrheal diseases is its exceptional purge rates, which can lead to rapid and severe dehydration and voluminous continuing stool losses. In severe cholera, stools rapidly progress to a rice-water consistency completely lacking in fecal qualities; severe nausea and repetitive vomiting often occur in this early stage. The clinical manifestations thus relate to the degree of diarrheal dehydration, as with other causes of diarrhea (Table 1). Treatment is essentially the same as treatment of other causes of diarrheal dehydration in children, with three provisos:

1. With severe cholera infection one must anticipate a continuing copious purge rate.
2. The mean sodium concentration of stool in pediatric cholera patients (circa 100 mmol/L) (Table 2) is notably higher than that (circa 50 mmol/L) found in diarrheal stool of children with non-cholera diarrhea.

Table 1.   CLINICAL ASSESSMENT OF THE DEGREE OF DEHYDRATION

Signs and Symptoms	Mild Dehydration	Moderate Dehydration	Severe Dehydration
General appearance	Alert, thirsty	Often lethargic, thirsty	Drowsy, apprehensive, cold extremities
Radial pulse	Normal rate and strength	Rapid and weak	Rapid, feeble, may be imperceptible
Anterior fontanel (infants)	Normal	Mildly sunken	Very sunken
Respiration	Normal	Deep	Deep and rapid
Elasticity (turgor) of skin	Normal	Pinched skin retracts slowly	Pinched skin remains tented, retracts
Eyes	Normal	Sunken	Deeply sunken
Mucous membranes	Slightly dry	Dry	Very dry
Urine flow	Normal	Reduced and concentrated	None
Percent loss of body weight	4–5	6–9	10 or more
Fluid deficit	40–50 ml/kg	60–90 ml/kg	$\geqslant 100$ ml/kg

Table 2.   CONCENTRATIONS OF ELECTROLYTES (mmol/L) IN STOOL OF CHILDREN AND ADULTS WITH CHOLERA AND IN ORAL AND INTRAVENOUS REHYDRATION SOLUTIONS

Fluid	Route of Administration	NA$^+$	K$^+$	Cl$^-$	Base*	Glucose
Cholera stool						
Pediatric	—	101	27	92	32	—
Teenagers and adults	—	135	15	90	30	—
Ringer's lactate	IV	128	4	109	28	—
Isotonic saline	IV	154	—	154	—	—
M/6 sodium lactate	IV	167	—	—	167	—
WHO glucose/electrolytes	Oral	90	20	80	30	111

*HCO_3^-, lactate or acetate.

3. Clinical cholera infection is a specific indication for antibiotic therapy, in contrast with most other infectious causes of watery diarrhea which usually do not require antibiotics.

THERAPY

Triage. The first step in therapy of the child with cholera is to rapidly but precisely estimate the extent of dehydration by means of medical history, physical examination, and documentation of weight loss (if a recent pre-illness weight is available). Patients in overt shock, and those with severe dehydration who show signs of impending shock or repetitive vomiting, should immediately receive intravenous isotonic fluids. Patients with mild and moderate dehydration should have rehydration initiated by the oral route with WHO glucose/electrolytes solution.

For the rapid expansion of the intravascular volume of children in shock, Ringer's lactate works well; if unavailable, isotonic saline or M/6 lactate can be successfully substituted. During the first hour of intravenous therapy patients should be given 30 ml/kg followed by an additional 40 ml/kg over the next two hours. Thereupon oral rehydration should be initiated with WHO glucose/electrolytes solution, 40 ml/kg being given over three hours. This oral solution provides considerable potassium (20 mmol/L).

Oral Rehydration. REPLACEMENT OF DEFICITS. In 95 to 98% of instances children with mild and moderate dehydration can be rehydrated and kept in maintenance fluid balance by oral rehydration alone. The success of this therapy rests on the fact that even while the small intestinal mucosa is in a state of net secretion due to the effects of cholera enterotoxin, glucose molecules (2% solution) are actively absorbed by active transport in the jejunum. Glucose-coupled transport of sodium occurs and molecules of water follow for osmotic reasons. HCO_3 and K^+ are also absorbed in this process.

Children with moderate dehydration should receive 100 ml/kg of WHO oral glucose/electrolytes solution over a period of 4 hours or less. The child should be re-evaluated clinically at that point. If the degree of dehydration is still moderate, another 4-hour course of WHO glucose/electrolytes solution should be given at 100 ml/kg. If the degree of dehydration is mild the child should receive 50 ml/kg of WHO glucose/electrolytes solution over 4 hours. In oral rehydration of children with cholera, WHO glucose/electrolytes solution, which contains 90 mmol/L sodium, should be given alone for replacement of fluid deficit.

Maintenance and Ongoing Losses. Once the fluid deficits have been successfully replaced (which usually requires 4–12 hours), as judged by clinical status, weight gain, and lowering of hematocrit and plasma protein concentration, the patients enter a maintenance phase of therapy. During maintenance ongoing stool losses are replaced on a volume-to-volume basis and plain water or low solute liquids (e.g., juices) are given to provide a source of free water for renal homeostasis.

Since copious continuing stool losses may be anticipated for up to 36 hours after hospital admission and since proper therapy is based on the volume of continued losses, the stool volume should be measured. Depending on the age of the child, the rice water stools can be collected in calibrated bed pans or in bucket-like receptacles in association with a cholera cot. The stool volume should be recorded every 4 hours on a simple intake-output worksheet. The volume of watery stool collected in the previous 4-hour period represents the volume of glucose/electrolytes solution that the child must drink during the next 4 hours to keep up with ongoing losses. This regimen is continued until diarrhea ceases or becomes minimal. In addition, children should receive low solute liquids or plain water (25–50 ml/kg/24 hr) to replace water losses that occur through the skin and respiration. Since the stool sodium concentration of children with cholera is 90 to 100 mmol/L at peak purge, a one-to-one volume oral replacement with WHO glucose/electrolytes solution is ideal. In teenagers and adults with cholera, stool sodium concentrations are much higher (135 mmol/L) (Table 2). Therefore older patients must ingest one and one-half volumes of WHO glucose/electrolytes solution for every volume of watery stool in order to successfully replace sodium losses.

If for any reason the child with cholera requires continued intravenous fluids to maintain hydration, K^+, 15 mmol/L in the form of KCl, should be added to the Ringer's lactate solution to replace the copious K^+ losses; in addition free water (25–50 ml/kg/24 hr) should be administered orally or by nasogastric tube.

Antibiotics. Cholera is an indication for antibiotic therapy, since appropriate antibiotics significantly curtail the duration and volume of diarrhea and rapidly eradicate stool excretion of *V. cholerae*, thereby diminishing the possibility of transmission. In general pediatric care, tetracycline is not favored for use in children because it can accumulate in developing teeth and bones. Nevertheless, it is the drug of choice in cholera because of its striking efficacy, short duration of therapy required (4 days, which precludes significant bone or dental accumulation of drug), low cost, and widespread availability. The recommended dosage of oral tetracycline for children is 50 mg/kg/day in 4 divided doses for 4 days.

In the case of known tetracycline resistance (which is generally rare but has occurred in outbreaks in East Africa and Bangladesh), alternative antibiotics that may be used include furazolidone (5 mg/kg/day in four divided doses × 5 days), erythromycin (30 mg/kg/day in four divided doses × 5 days) or trimethoprim/sulfamethoxazole (10 mg TMP and 50 mg SMZ/kg/day in two divided doses × 5 days).*

Complications. Approximately 1 to 4% of children with severe cholera manifest complications including neurologic signs due to hypoglycemia or effects of hypokalemia including paralytic ileus, muscular fibrillations, and, rarely, cardiac arrhythmias. The therapy regimen outlined above provides sources of glucose and K^+ to combat these clinical syndromes stemming from biochemical irregularities.

Immunization Practice

ANNE A. GERSHON, M.D.

Protection of children and adolescents against infectious diseases is a major task of the pediatrician. This is most often done by immunization with either live or inactivated viral agents or bacterial antigens (active immunization) or by administration of preformed antibody after exposure to a disease (passive immunization). This is a rapidly moving field, with frequent introduction of new products and changing recommendations for use of old ones. This discussion will focus on questions now most frequently asked by pediatricians and parents and the most up-to-date answers.

---

*Contraindicated in infants less than 2 months of age. This use is not listed by the manufacturer.

WHICH IMMUNIZATIONS ARE CONSIDERED "ROUTINE"?

The schedule for active immunization currently recommended by the Committee on Infectious Diseases of the American Academy of Pediatrics and the Advisory Committee on Immunization Practice of the U.S. Public Health Service is shown in Table 1. This table is meant to be a guideline and, while convenient, need not invariably be followed. For example, while trivalent oral polio vaccine (TOPV) and diphtheria tetanus pertussis (DTP) booster immunizations are to be given at 18 months of age, these may be delayed for a month or two if necessary without harm. In addition, if certain immunizations are delayed, the patient need not start again but the physician must be certain that the required amounts of immunizing agents are given. For example, 12 units of pertussis vaccine, the required amount for primary immunization, should eventually be administered. Whether the injections are 1 or several months apart does not seem to be important. Similarly, in an epidemic situation, measles vaccine may be given to infants over 6 months of age; however such infants should be reimmunized at 15 months to assure that they are protected.

Owing to space limitations, many details concerning immunization must be omitted from this discussion. The physician is referred to the "Report on the Committee on Infectious Diseases" (the so-called "Red Book"), published by the American Academy of Pediatrics for further discussion concerning individual vaccines.

Table 1. RECOMMENDED SCHEDULE FOR ACTIVE IMMUNIZATION OF NORMAL INFANTS AND CHILDREN

Age		
2 mo	DTP[1]	TOPV[2a]
4 mo	DTP	TOPV
6 mo	DTP	2b
1 yr		Tuberculin test[3]
15 mo	Measles, mumps, rubella vaccine	
18 mo	DTP	TOPV
4–6 yr	DTP	TOPV
14–16 yr	Td[4]—repeat every 10 years	

[1] Diphtheria and tetanus toxoids combined with pertussis vaccine.

[2a] Trivalent oral poliovirus vaccine.

[2b] A third dose of TOPV is optional but may be given in areas of high endemicity of poliomyelitis.

[3] Test should be done at the time of, or preceding, the measles immunization.

[4] Combined tetanus and diphtheria toxoids (adult type) for those more than 6 years of age, in contrast to diphtheria and tetanus (DT) toxoids which contain a larger amount of diphtheria antigen. Tetanus toxoid at time of injury; For clean minor wounds, no booster dose is needed by a fully immunized child unless more than 10 years have elapsed since the last dose. For contaminated wounds, a booster dose should be given if more than 5 years have elapsed since the last dose.

When Should Routine Immunizations Not Be Given?

The presence of fever, communicable disease, immunodeficiency (congenital or acquired), and pregnancy are contraindications to immunization. During an epidemic, however, pregnant women may be immunized against polio. Also, immunodeficient or immunosuppressed individuals may be given bacterial vaccines and inactivated viral vaccines (in contrast to live viral vaccines), although they may not respond immunologically to the immunizing agent.

Should Pertussis Vaccine Still Be Used?

In England and in the United States there has been controversy concerning the use of pertussis vaccine. Since many infants develop reactions to the vaccine, such as fever, crying spells, and sore arms, and since there has been a question about certain lots of vaccine causing sudden infant death (SIDS), some parents and physicians have questioned the utility of this vaccine. Pertussis, at this time, is not a very common disease in the U.S. It is important to recall however, that pertussis is potentially fatal in young infants. It is interesting to note that in England, when many infants were not being immunized against pertussis, the incidence of this disease began to increase. Thus while the vaccine is not without problems, it does appear to control spread of pertussis. Research on the development of an immunogenic but less toxic pertussis vaccine is ongoing. Fortunately, the proposed link to SIDS has not been substantiated, although it is rather difficult to rule out entirely. Most experts today agree that pertussis vaccine should be used according to the immunization schedule given. It is also accepted that unprotected adolescents and medical staff believed to be susceptible to pertussis may be immunized if exposure to the disease has taken place or is likely to. The dose for these individuals is 0.25 ml subcutaneously. Parenthetically, since doses smaller than 0.5 ml may not be expected to prevent reactions in young children, "splitting of doses" is probably of little use.

Pertussis vaccine should not be given to children with progressive neurologic disease. Those who had screaming spells lasting 3 hours or more, excessive somnolence, or temperature greater than 105°F should probably not be given further pertussis vaccine injections.

How Often Should Tetanus Boosters Be Given, and What Type of Material Should Be Used?

At one time it was recommended that tetanus boosters be administered every year, especially for children who would be outdoors for much of the summer. Because it was found that many children and young adults manifested hypersensitivity reactions to tetanus antigen and because the antibodies seemed to persist for many years, it is now recommended that tetanus boosters be administered only every 10 years, after completion of the primary series and first booster. It is recommended that tetanus boosters be administered as diphtheria-tetanus rather than tetanus alone, to protect against diphtheria as well. For children over age 6, adult-type vaccine (dT), which contains one tenth of the dose of diphtheria toxin, should be used. It is important to recall that these vaccines are toxoids, which protect against disease but not infection. In addition, the illnesses themselves do not confer immunity. Therefore children recovering from tetanus or diphtheria should be actively immunized.

For Whom is Live Polio Vaccine Dangerous?

Since the introduction of TOPV in the United States, the incidence of polio has fallen dramatically. Each year about 20 cases are reported; many occur in immunocompromised persons. Unlike most viral diseases, the ability to recover from polio seems to depend on humoral more than cellular immunity. For this reason TOPV should not be administered to persons with impaired immune function nor to persons who are likely to have close contact with such individuals. Live polio vaccination has been associated with serious sequelae, such as paralysis, in about 1 in 3 million vaccinees. Adults seem to be at somewhat greater risk than children. For this reason TOPV is usually not recommended for use in persons above age 18 years. This must be taken into consideration when the parents of an infant who needs polio vaccine have no recollection of being immunized themselves. Several courses of action are possible in this situation. Many pediatricians discuss the problem with the parents, and, assuming they agree, give no polio immunization to the parents on the grounds that they are very likely to be already immune. Since many close contacts of young infants are not only the parents but also babysitters, other relatives, and household help, this approach seems sensible. The risk is extremely low, and it is virtually impossible to protect everyone at risk. Another possible approach is to administer inactivated polio vaccine (IPV) to the parents. If this is done, two injections should be given to the parent prior to immunizing the child against polio with TOPV. Whichever course is taken, delay in immunizing the infant should be avoided.

What is the Best Way to Manage the Adolescent or Young Adult with No Previous Record of Immunizations?

It is obvious from this question that one extremely important aspect of immunization is meticulous record-keeping. The American Academy of Pediatrics (AAP) and Advisory Committee on Immunization Practice (ACIP) both recommend the use of a standard passport-sized immunization card to be filled in by the physician and kept by the parent. Unless this is done in our mobile society, it is very difficult to know who has been immunized against what. A very immediate and pragmatic reason for good record-keeping is that most states have begun to exclude children from school unless they have proof of adequate immunization. For those with no record or recollection, the only recourse is to immunize (and often this means reimmunization) with the standard vaccines listed in Table 1. At that point, the records should be kept.

It appears that it is not dangerous to administer viral vaccines to an individual who is already immune. Similarly, it has been found that young adults tolerate measles vaccine very well with no greater incidence of complications than infants or children have (fever, 5 to 15% and rarely rash: usually occurring 6 to 11 days after immunization).

Is Waning Immunity a Problem for Measles-Mumps-Rubella (MMR) Vaccine, and Are Booster Immunizations Necessary?

It is recognized that antibody titers following immunization are lower than those that follow the natural illness. At one time it was felt that eventually antiviral antibody might be lost. If this occurred, it was proposed that a booster immunization might then be necessary. Most experts agree, however, that waning immunity to measles, mumps, and rubella is not now a recognized problem. For this reason, among others, booster MMR immunization during the early school years has not been recommended by either the AAP or the ACIP. Experts who have recommended a booster MMR injection upon school entry have mainly wished to reach those children who escaped vaccination in infancy, plus the small percentage of children who did not have a "take" initially. Since most states now require proof of complete immunization prior to school entry, a second injection of MMR does not seem as crucial as it might have previously. About 5% of those immunized with viral vaccines may not experience a "take." This small number of vaccine failures is not thought to be a significant problem, as long as there are few cases of the illness in the community.

Perhaps the most convincing evidence for the success of MMR is the current incidence of measles and rubella. In 1982 there were less than 2000 reported cases of measles (500,000 cases per year in the pre-vaccine era) and less than 15 reports of congenital rubella.

Should Children Who Received MMR Before Their First Birthday Be Reimmunized?

It has been found that children immunized prior to their first birthday may not have developed active immunity to measles due to interference by persistence of maternally transmitted antibody. Such children should be reimmunized, although there may be a judgmental decision as to whether to do this. For example, children immunized several days before their first birthday probably do not require reimmunization. It has also been found that children immunized at age 12 months have, in general, a slightly lower "take" rate than those immunized after 13 months of age. For this reason, the suggested age for administering MMR is now 15 months. However, since 85 per cent of infants immunized at 12 months will have had a "take" for measles vaccine, and since there is very little measles in the United States at present, it is now not recommended that children immunized at 12 months of age be reimmunized.

Several reports of poor measles antibody responses in children immunized between 6 and 10 months of age have recently appeared in the literature. As many as 40% of these children failed to develop an antibody response after reimmunization. It is thought that these children may be tolerant to measles antigen, but the clinical significance, if any, is unknown. Until more information becomes available it would seem prudent to avoid immunizing children aged 6 to 10 months with MMR, if at all possible. Obviously in the midst of an epidemic, consideration of the potential risk of measles to young infants would have to be weighed against the theoretical risk of immunization. As an alternative, passive immunization could be administered.

Who Should Receive Rubella Vaccine in Addition To Infants?

Prepubertal girls who have never been vaccinated against rubella should be given the vaccine. For females past puberty, however, care must be taken to assure that the girl or woman is not pregnant. It is preferable to check for susceptibility to rubella prior to immunization although, if it is inconvenient or impossible, such persons may simply be immunized. Many experts suggest, however, that a serum sample be taken at the time of immunization and stored for 3 months. Should the girl or woman inadvertently become pregnant, she can then be tested for susceptibility. Should she have been immune at the time of immunization, an abortion might no longer have to be considered.

Sexually active women should be cautioned not to become pregnant for at least 3 months after receiving rubella vaccine. This is a precautionary measure; no cases of congenital rubella have been proved to be caused by rubella vaccine. The virus has been recovered on occasion from the products of conception when an abortion has been performed. A new rubella vaccine, RA 27/3, is now licensed and being used in the United States, so additional information concerning this point, however, will be necessary before it can be concluded that there are no risks associated with the use of this vaccine during pregnancy, because all previous information came from the formerly used vaccine, HPV-77. Over 100 infants have been born to rubella-susceptible women who were inadvertently immunized against rubella during early pregnancy. There have been no cases of congenital rubella among these infants. The estimated risk of developing congenital rebella from vaccine is now 3% or less.

The RA 27/3 vaccine that has now replaced HPV-77 appears to be somewhat more potent than the old vaccine. Despite this, however, it is unnecessary to reimmunize children who received HPV-77 with RA 27/3 vaccine, since children who received HPV-77 appear to maintain adequate immunity to rubella.

At this point it should also be mentioned that it is safe to immunize the child of a pregnant woman with no history of rubella immunization. This is because the vaccine virus does not appear to spread from one person to another. Since a susceptible child in the house is a potential hazard to the susceptible pregnant woman, many experts feel that this is an especially important time to immunize the child. Similarly, it is important that both male and female rubella-susceptible persons be immunized against rubella. This is because several instances of transmission of wild rubella virus from infected hospital employees to pregnant women have occurred. While rubella vaccine does not cause serious side effects when administered to adults, some minor discomforts may occur, especially in women over 25 years of age. These include transient arthritis of the small joints, lymphadenopathy, and fever. Adult women who are to be vaccinated should be told that such side effects may occur but that they are self-limited.

WHAT ARE THE INDICATIONS FOR THE USE OF LICENSED NONROUTINE IMMUNIZATIONS IN THE PEDIATRIC AGE GROUP?

Pneumococcal vaccine is now licensed for use. It provides protection against 14 of the 83 most common capsular types of pneumococci that cause pneumonia and meningitis. Its role in prevention of otitis media is unproved. It is therefore recommended for use in children over the age of 2 years (below that age there is a poor response) who are at high risk to develop severe pneumococcal infections. These include nephrotics and children with anatomic or functional asplenia. Booster injections of pneumococcal vaccine are not indicated and may cause hypersensitivity reactions.

It should be remembered that children for whom pneumococcal vaccine is indicated may have a poor antibody response to immunization, so vigilance for clinical disease must be maintained. Many pediatricians administer prophylactic antibiotics to such children in addition to immunizing them.

Influenza vaccine is recommended for children over 6 months of age with underlying heart, pulmonary, or other serious chronic disease for whom influenza may be a disastrous event. Since "whole" vaccines are associated with side effects, "split" (subvirion) products should be used for children less than 13 years of age. Two doses are required, 4 weeks apart. Since variations of influenza virus occur frequently, it is important to administer the currently recommended type of vaccine.

Meningococcal polysaccharide vaccines for groups A and C meningococci have been licensed and may be used in epidemic situations. Group A vaccine may be given to children over 6 months of age and Group C to children over 2 years of age. These vaccines may also be used after a close exposure has taken place, in conjunction with antibiotic prophylaxis, since half of secondary cases occur 5 days or more after the index case.

BCG vaccines are used in many countries where tuberculosis is common. These vaccines, of which there are many, vary in efficacy and reactogenicity. There is little use for BCG vaccine in the United States at present. Possible indications include young infants closely exposed to tuberculosis and older children and adults who are likely to be exposed due to travel or employment (certain health care workers).

An inactivated hepatitis B vaccine has recently been licensed in the U.S. This vaccine is prepared from plasma of hepatitis B carriers. Surface antigen particles are purified in the plasma and chemically inactivated, which results in a noninfectious and generally intact vaccine. The purified surface antigen particles are alum adsorbed and administered in a three dose schedule. The first injection is followed by boosters after 1 and 6 months. For children 3 months to 10 years of age, a 10 μg dose is given. Older children are given the adult dose, 20 μg.

The vaccine is well tolerated, with soreness and redness at the injection site being the only noted side effects. The vaccine induces an antibody response in over 90% of those immunized and confers protection to 80 to 95% of exposed susceptibles. It is not known at this time if further booster doses will be required.

The vaccine is extremely expensive and is therefore reserved for use in high risk groups. In the pediatric age group this might include institutionalized mentally retarded children, users of illicit injectable drugs, male homosexuals, frequent recipients of blood and blood products, household and sexual contacts of hepatitis B carriers, and certain populations of Alaskan Eskimos. Infants born to women who are hepatitis B carriers should be immunized as soon as possible after birth, even if they have received passive immunization. Passive immunization does not appear to interfere with the ability of hepatitis B vaccine to "take." Studies are now in progress to determine the efficacy of the vaccine when administered at birth to high risk infants. A line attenuated varicella vaccine is currently being tested in high risk groups in the U.S. Varicella-susceptible normal adults and children with acute leukemia in remission are being vaccinated because they are at risk of severe or fatal varicella. Results of studies thus far suggest that this vaccine is safe and effective in these high risk people. Continued study will be necessary to determine how protective the vaccine will be, although results to date are encouraging.

Additional experimental vaccines, as yet unlicensed and in varying stages of development, include *Hemophilus* B vaccine and groups A and B streptococcal vaccines. It is likely that these vaccines, if and when licensed, will be especially useful for high-risk exposed persons and the immunocompromised.

WHEN IS PASSIVE IMMUNIZATION INDICATED?

Many details concerning this subject must be omitted for lack of space. Newer approaches to passive immunization and the most frequently used approaches will, however, be discussed.

Passive immunization may be accomplished using immune serum globulin (ISG) for polio, measles, and hepatitis A. In general, the sooner passive immunization is given the more likely it is to be successful. Protection against hepatitis A is probably the most frequent indication for use of ISG. It should be administered in a dose of 0.02 ml/kg IM, to persons having close personal contact with individuals with hepatitis A. While it need not be given to children exposed casually at school, it should be used for day-care exposures, particularly where there are children in diapers.

For protection against certain other infections, special globulins are more efficacious than is ISG. Included are globulins against hepatitis B, rabies, tetanus, and varicella. All of these special globulins are now licensed, including varicella zoster immune globulin (VZIG), and all are available from human rather than equine sources. VZIG may now be obtained through the American Red Cross. VZIG should be used only for prevention or attenuation of varicella in high risk (e.g., immunocompromised) varicella susceptibles who have been closely exposed to vericella or zoster. This would include newborn infants whose mothers develop the rash of varicella 5 days or less prior to delivery or within 48 hours after delivery. A dose of 1.25 ml/10 kg of body weight is usually used. Passive immunization is probably not useful for treating established varicella or other infections (with the exceptions of diphtheria and tetanus) and should not be used for this purpose.

Hepatitis B immune globulin (HBIG) should be given to persons susceptible to hepatitis B who are intimately exposed by contaminated needles or close personal contact. A dose of 0.06 ml/kg (maximum, 5 ml) IM is given upon exposure and 4 weeks later. The risk of developing hepatitis after a needle stick with known contaminated blood is 1 in 20. If the source of blood is unknown it is 1 in 2000. In some cases, therefore, it may be advisable to administer ISG initially and then determine whether the source of blood contained hepatitis B. HBIG may be administered later, if indicated (within 7 days of the exposure). The cost of HBIG is 20 times that of ISG. Newborn infants born to women who are carriers of hepatitis B should receive HBIG as soon as possible after birth in conjunction with hepatitis B vaccine. Many experts suggest a dose of 0.5 ml HBIG at birth, and 0.5 ml (10 μg) of hepatitis B vaccine. At 6 months the child should be tested to determine if infection with hepatitis B virus has occurred. If it has not, a second dose of vaccine (0.5 ml) should be given. This sequence should be repeated when the infant is 12 to 15 months old. It is important to immunize such infants to try to prevent the chronic carrier stage from developing. Infants who are infected with hepatitis B virus at birth rarely develop severe hepatitis, but they are at high risk to become chronic carriers, particularly if the mother is not only positive for hepatitis B surface antigen but also the "e" antigen. With passive immunization alone, 25% of exposed infants will become carriers. Therefore, studies are currently in progress to determine whether active-passive immunization at birth will lower this rate. Until these studies are published, it seems reasonable to use active plus passive immunization as outlined above, since it is known that young infants can respond immediately to hepatitis B vaccine.

If a possible true exposure to rabies has taken place, both active and passive immunization should be given. It is now preferable to use the human diploid cell vaccine (5 doses) rather than the duck embryo vaccine (24 doses and a higher incidence of side effects). For further information, refer to the "Red Book."

Details concerning passive immunization against tetanus also may be found in the "Red Book." In general, for wound prophylaxis, 250 units of tetanus immune globulin should be used, in conjunction with tetanus toxoid. For treatment of tetanus, 3000 to 6000 units of tetanus antitoxin is used.

19

Allergy

Allergic Rhinitis

BERNARD A. BERMAN, M.D.

Although the disorders that compose allergic rhinitis are rarely fatal, they cause a significant adverse impact on the affected person's life style and on the stability of the family. For the uninitiated physician, it is often difficult to comprehend the extent of discomfort and misery caused by nasal allergy.

Seasonal allergic rhinitis (pollenosis, hay fever) is characterized by symptoms reappearing at the same time each year; perennial allergic rhinitis is associated with year-round symptoms. Perennial rhinitis produces a dryer nasal congestion than seasonal rhinitis. The mucus is thicker, and patients complain of a heavy postnasal drip. The older child may have frequent vacuum sinus headaches and morning sore throats. Patients also may have painful neck glands associated with low-grade fever. Parents of children with undiagnosed perennial allergic rhinitis frequently mention that their child has had "too many colds." These "colds," which often are allergic flare-ups, may last up to 14 days and are often accompanied by coughing and occasionally mild wheezing. Symptoms are almost identical to those caused by a viral infection. The most common allergens of seasonal allergic rhinitis are the pollens of grasses, weeds, and trees, while those of perennial allergic rhinitis are house dust, mold spores, animal danders, and occupational allergens (veterinarian, etc.)

Before one can develop a rational approach to management of allergic rhinitis, it is necessary to review briefly the various rhinitis categories. A precise classification is still not possible. We still do not understand the causes, pathophysiologies, biochemistries, and immune factors of the various types. However, based on current information, a working classification of rhinitis has been established:

Classification of Rhinitis

Seasonal Allergic Rhinitis. Characteristic symptoms of pollen sensitization; itching, sneezing, rhinorrhea, and nasal congestion; conjunctival injection; IgE-mediated; significant eosinophilia on nasal smear; possible increase in blood eosinophils. Most have onset of symptoms by 15 years of age or younger.

Perennial Allergic Rhinitis. Year-round nasal symptoms; more noticeable during heating season; IgE-mediated; nasal secretions more tenacious than seasonal rhinitis; sneezing and congestion are prominent, as are vacuum headaches. Significant eosinophilia on nasal smear. Sensitization to inhalant allergens, such as house dust, mold spores, and animal danders.

Non-Allergic Rhinitis with Eosinophilia (NARES). More common in adults. Marked congestion, rhinorrhea, and postnasal discharge; itching and sneezing common; many eosinophils on nasal smear. Commonly associated with aspirin sensitivity and nasal polyps; no identifiable IgE mechanism; possibly caused by autonomic imbalance.

Mastocytosis. Diagnosis by punch biopsy. Rare. Chronic congestion and rhinorrhea; itching and sneezing uncommon; cause undetermined; nonspecific mast cell degranulation with mediator release, but not IgE-mediated; more common in adults.

Vasomotor Rhinitis. Chronic nasal congestion with marked rhinorrhea; skin tests negative; non–IgE-mediated; no eosinophils; diagnosis by exclusion of other disorders causing rhinitis; poor response to treatment.

Infections. Chronic discolored rhinorrhea often associated with acute and chronic sinusitis; caused by various bacteria.

Miscellaneous. New growths, congenital anomalies, nasal septal abnormalities, hypothyroidism, immune complex disorders, nasal congestion from medications (e.g. reserpine), abuse of topical sympathomimetic agents, obstructive adenoids, atrophic rhinitis.

MANAGEMENT

Environmental Controls. The primary treatment of allergic rhinitis is to eliminate or reduce exposure to critical allergens. Any furred or feathered animal can be an allergen source, and should be excluded from the living quarters. In many cases, the presence of an animal in the home can convert a mild case of rhinitis into a severe allergic problem.

Plants that produce highly colored flowers can be important allergen sources when found in the home. Their pollens can exacerbate symptoms. House plants are a plentiful source of mold spores and should be removed from the home of the allergic child. Because of their high mold content, spruce or pine Christmas trees should be replaced by artificial ones.

Tables 1 and 2 provide environmental guidelines for patients with allergic rhinitis. These guidelines are flexible. Physician and parents together should select the ideas that will be most beneficial. Environmental controls are important but should not be permitted to become a greater restriction than the original symptoms. The child's physical comfort must be balanced with his or her social and psychological needs. Most patients benefit from the use of a home humidifier and purifier. Families with central heating and air conditioning may wish to add a central humidifier and an electrostatic precipitator to their climate control systems. In houses lacking central heating, a small window air conditioner helps reduce pollen, and an inexpensive cold-mist humidifier can provide sufficient moisture during the heating season.

For those with severe pollenosis or dust sensitivity, the physician may recommend a portable

---

Table 1. **WHAT THE PATIENT CAN DO TO REDUCE THE SYMPTOMS OF SEASONAL ALLERGIC RHINITIS**

1. During the height of the pollen season, avoid wooded areas and fields where the pollen concentration is highest.

2. Pollen concentrations are usually highest on hot, windy days. To minimize discomfort on these days, stay indoors in an air-conditioned room. Keep the air conditioner fresh air vent and the door closed.

3. Avoid tobacco smoke, perfumes, chemical vapors, and other noxious odors.

4. Keep the bedroom as dust-free as possible and remove all pets from the home.

5. Do not bring fresh flowers into the house.

Table 2. **WHAT THE PATIENT CAN DO TO REDUCE THE SYMPTOMS OF PERENNIAL ALLERGIC RHINITIS**

1. Keep the house as dust-free as possible. Dust at least three times a week with a damp mop or cloth.

2. Avoid contact with any pet that has fur or feathers.

3. Avoid tobacco smoke, perfumes, and rapid changes in temperature if they cause an increase in symptoms.

4. Replace feather pillows with Dacron or polyester pillows. Use synthetic fabrics for curtains, and make sure that the mattress does not contain horse hair. Avoid rug pads that contain Ozite, a mixture of cattle and hog dander. Remove all cotton-stuffed toys from the bedroom.

5. Discuss the use of air conditioners, air purifiers, and humidifiers with your physician. Some patients benefit a great deal from these devices but others do not find them helpful.

---

electrostatic precipitator or a high-efficiency particle accumulator (HEPA), which removes particles from the air by mechanical filtration. These appliances are quite expensive but dealers in many areas will rent them on a trial basis.

Pharmacologic Management. Most patients with allergic rhinitis require medication. Antihistaminics are prescribed most often to control sneezing, rhinorrhea, and itching. Antihistaminics do little to lessen congestion. They are most effective if begun early in the season (for patients with pollen allergy) and used on a regular basis. Chronic administration saturates many of the available H_1 receptors with the antihistaminic, blunting in part histamine's access to the receptor. More than 75% of patients with hay fever symptoms improve on this therapy.

H_1 antagonist antihistaminics are specific for allergic rhinitis; they compete with histamine at receptor sites. However, they also produce specific adverse effects, including personality changes, drowsiness, dryness of mouth and nose, irritability, anorexia, constipation, lack of coordination, and inability to concentrate. To eliminate these effects, the pediatrician should switch to an antihistaminic with a different chemical structure, reduce the dose, or withdraw the drug.

Although maximal response to antihistaminics is dose-related, the development of multiple side effects frequently limits the dose that can be given. Thus the dose prescribed by many physicians is less than optimal. Although all antihistaminics share similar pharmacologic properties, they differ in chemical structure, degree of potency, adverse effects, and cost. Antihistaminics have been grouped into six different classes according to chemical configuration (Table 3). With the exception of diphenhydramine (Benadryl), a Class I agent, and hydroxyzine (Atarax), a Class IV agent, well known for their sedative and antipruritic effects, the potency and side effects of an antihis-

Table 3. CLASSES OF ANTIHISTAMINES

Class	Generic Name	Trade Name	Average Dose for Child Under 12 Years of Age*	Comments
I Ethanolamines	Diphenhydramine	Benadryl	5 mg/kg/24 hours in 3–4 divided doses	Potent antipruritic Marked sedative effect
	Carbinoxamine maleate	Rondec	0.8 mg/kg/24 hours in 3–4 divided doses.	Very little sedative effect. Available only in combination
	Phenyltoloxamine	Naldecon Pediatric Syrup	Two teaspoonfuls 3–4 times a day.	Combination. Minimal seda- effect
II Ethylenediamine	Tripelennamine	Pyribenzamine	5 mg/kg/24 hours in 3–4 divided doses.	Give drug with meals
III Alkylamines	Brompheniramine maleate	Dimetane	0.5 mg/kg/24 hours in divided doses.	Most OTC preparations con- tain alkylamines
		Bromfed–PD Capsule	0.5 mg/kg/24 hours in divided doses.	Combination, excellent for bedtime use
IV Piperazine	Hydroxyzine hydrochloride	Atarax	2–5 mg/kg/24 hours in 3–4 divided doses.	Potent antipruritic. Strong sedative effect
V Phenothiazines	Promethazine	Phenergan	0.5 mg/kg/dose every 8 hours.	Not routinely recommended for allergic rhinitis
VI Piperidine	Azatadine maleate	Optimine	Orphan drug for children under 12.	
	Cyproheptadine	Periactin	0.25 mg/kg/24 hours in 3 divided doses	Excellent for cold urticaria. Increases appetite

*For very young child, dose may have to be titrated down. Consult package insert or PDR for complete prescribing information.

taminic are entirely unpredictable. The pediatrician should become familiar with at least one agent from each class since there is no evidence that other agents within the same class offer significant addi- tional benefits. Should a patient respond poorly to the optimal dose of an antihistaminic, one should prescribe an agent from a different class. Note that Class V agents (e.g., promethazine) are not rou- tinely recommended for the treatment of allergic rhinitis.

Physicians may choose from single-entity antihis- taminics, single-entity decongestants, combination antihistaminic with multiple drugs, combination antihistaminic with a decongestant, or immediate- or sustained-release preparations.

Oral sympathomimetics (decongestants), given alone or with an antihistaminic, lessen nasal con- gestion, although their effectiveness is not clear. Those most commonly employed are pseudo- ephedrine, phenylpropanolamine, and phenyleph- rine. Pseudoephedrine is the most commonly pre- scribed oral decongestant while phenylephrine is used mostly as a topical agent. Common side effects of oral decongestants are nervousness, insomnia, anorexia, personality change, and headache. Com- bination antihistaminic-decongestant preparations usually offer greater control of symptoms than ei- ther agent prescribed alone.

Many pediatricians still believe that antihistamin- ics are contraindicated in patients who have both allergic rhinitis and asthma.

Recent studies offer evidence that antihistaminics do not modify the course or severity of either mild or moderate asthma. If antihistaminics are effective, continue to use them when rhinitis coexists with asthma, but if the asthma becomes severe, withdraw the drug.

Remember that the patient's response to an an- tihistaminic cannot be predicted. Because of the sedative effects of antihistaminics, the drug should be started after school or on a weekend. At the outset, supply sufficient samples of several different classes to allow a comparison of clinical response and side effects, then initiate the following treat- ment plan: If the child is 6 to 12 years of age, a sustained-release, maximal-dose antihistaminic- decongestant is taken at bedtime. A smaller dose is given as a liquid or tablet during the day. A high- dose, sustained-release capsule is ideal for noctur- nal use when sedation is not a problem; also, the sustained action may prevent symptoms that usu- ally are prominent on arising. If the capsule cannot be swallowed the beaded pellets can be placed in apple sauce or a similar vehicle. Bromfed-PD (60 mg pseudoephedrine and 6 mg brompheniramine maleate) is a timed-release capsule that can be used at bedtime, while Rondec syrup (4 mg carbinoxa- mine maleate and 60 mg pseudoephedrine hydrochloride per 5 ml), ½ teaspoonful, is given morning and midafternoon. Tolerance to the sedative effect may develop within several weeks; thus, it may be possible to replace the low-dose, immediate-release syrup with large-dose bid timed-release Bromfed-PD. For a child under 6 years of age, Benadryl (12.5 mg diphenhydramine hydrochloride per 5 ml), 1 tablespoonful, is given at bedtime and during the day; Isoclor liquid (2 mg chlorpheniramine maleate and 30 mg pseudoephedrine hydrochloride per 5 ml), ½ teaspoonful, is offered morning and midafternoon.

Many antihistaminic-decongestant agents, previously available only by prescription, are now available over the counter (OTC). The media advertising associated with proliferation of these OTC drugs must be viewed with concern. The relative safety of antihistaminics is well documented; however, their side effects disrupt the child's quality of life. Furthermore, many OTC antihistaminics are orphan drugs; there are no data regarding their benefits and risks in children under 12 years of age. It is the pediatrician's responsibility to choose either a prescription or an OTC antihistaminic. The pediatrician is the person most qualified to recommend combinations that have the least number of unnecessary additional agents, and to determine, based on clinical response or side effects, whether to raise or lower the dose, or to withdraw the drug.

Intranasal Cromolyn. Cromolyn sodium is a prophylactic drug whose major effect is nonspecific mast cell protection from a variety of triggering mechanisms, including antigen-antibody reactions. Recent data indicate that cromolyn stabilizes the mast cell probably by interfering with calcium ion transport across the cell membrane, thus effectively preventing degranulation and liberation of the multiple mediators that provoke nasal congestion, rhinorrhea, itching and sneezing.

Cromolyn is effective in the treatment of allergic rhinitis when applied regularly in either a 2% or 4% solution topically to the nasal mucous membrane. In Europe and throughout the world cromolyn is available as a 2% nasal solution. In the United States, a 4% solution was recently approved for general use.

One recent study showed that frequent (four or five times a day) intranasal administration of 4% cromolyn solution was associated with markedly reduced symptoms and a decreased intake of antihistaminic agents. The authors concluded that intranasal use of cromolyn was efficacious and that side effects were minimal and transient.

A nasal syndrome that closely resembles allergic rhinitis is non-allergic rhinitis with eosinophilia (NARES) (sneezing, rhinorrhea, pruritus of the nasopharynx and conjunctiva, congestion, marked nasal eosinophilia, and negative skin tests). Cromolyn is of no benefit in the treatment of NARES.

There are no data to suggest that degranulation of nasal mast cells accounts for the symptoms of NARES. Thus, cromolyn's failure to help patients with this syndrome is strong evidence for the documented mechanism of cromolyn in the treatment of allergic rhinorrheas—IgE-mediated mast cell disorders such as allergic rhinitis and perennial allergic rhinitis.

Cromolyn, with its remarkable record of safety, administered with or without an antihistaminic agent, appears to be a first-line preventive agent for the treatment of allergic rhinitis.

Corticosteroid Hormones. Intranasally administered topical steroids are extremely effective when symptoms of nasal congestion respond poorly to optimal-dose conventional medications. Beclomethasone dipropionate and flunisolide are unique corticosteroids with enormous topical potency, rapid metabolic inactivation of the swallowed portion, and no demonstrable alteration of the hypothalamic-pituitary-adrenal axis when administered in recommended dosage. Occasional epistaxis or stinging of the nasal mucosa may necessitate brief withdrawal. For these agents to be effective, the nasal passageway must be patent. Beclomethasone dipropionate must be given regularly, initially two sprays in each nostril three times a day; then, when a favorable response is observed, usually in 10 days to 2 weeks, gradually taper to the lowest dose that maintains a good response, usually one or two sprays at bedtime. Topical corticosteroids are extremely helpful for the uncontrolled symptoms of seasonal and nonseasonal allergic rhinitis, nonallergic rhinitis with eosinophilia, and polyps associated with eosinophilic rhinitis.

Beclomethasone dipropionate (Vancenase and Beconase)*is available as a metered-dose nasal inhaler preparation, while flunisolide (Nasalide)†is dispensed by pump spray bottle.

Topical corticosteroid hormones should be considered second-line therapeutic agents, to be introduced only if the patient has an unsatisfactory response to antihistaminic-decongestant agents or intranasal cromolyn, or both. Whether they are used for seasonal or perennial allergic rhinitis, from time to time attempts should be made to wean the patient from this medication.

Systemic corticosteroids are the most potent agents available for treatment of severe, disabling allergic rhinitis. They are likely to be needed during brief peak periods of a pollen season. Orally administered prednisone, initially given as high-dose, 30 mg a day for 3 days, then as alternate-day therapy, 10 mg, for an additional 2 weeks, usually will re-

---

*Manufacturer's warning: Not recommended for children under 12 years of age.

†Manufacturer's warning: Not recommended for children under 6 years of age.

Table 4. THERAPY OF VARIOUS RHINITIDES

	Antihistamines	Decongestants	Cromolyn	Topical Steroids	Oral Steroids	Immunotherapy
Seasonal allergic rhinitis	Yes	Yes	Yes	Yes	Occasional	Yes
Perennial allergic rhinitis	Yes	Yes	Yes	Yes	Rarely needed	Yes
Non-allergic rhinitis with eosinophilia	? Yes	• Yes	No	Yes	Rarely needed	No
Vasomotor rhinitis	Occasional	Yes	No	Rare	No	No

verse the symptoms of patients temporarily disabled by severe rhinitis.

Corticosteroids should always be accompanied by decongestant-antihistaminic preparations.

General Measures

Irritated Nasal Mucosa. Older children with perennial allergic rhinitis, whose nasal discharge is thick and tenacious and who have a heavy, bothersome postnasal drip, often benefit significantly from instillation of warm, buffered saline solution. Saline douches help soothe and repair nasal mucosa, improve mucociliary flow, and promote liquefaction of the mucus. I recommend either Alkalol nasal irrigation, using a Birmingham applicator, or Salinex, delivered from a polyspray bottle. The young child is likely to reject intranasal instillation of any spray or liquid under pressure. Compliance is noticeably better in the older child.

Immunotherapy. Immunotherapy can be very helpful in treatment of specific IgE-mediated disorders such as seasonal or perennial allergic rhinitis. Immunotherapy should be considered an adjunct to holistic allergic management, not a substitute. Severity and duration of disease, response to environmental control, and conventional medication are key factors determining the need for immunotherapy. Patients who experience only several weeks of severe symptoms during the height of a pollen season will usually respond well to an antihistaminic-decongestant, intranasal cromolyn, intranasal topical steroids, or possibly a pulse dose of prednisone. These patients do not require immunotherapy. Patients with prolonged allergy,

Table 5. EXAMPLES OF USEFUL COMBINATION MEDICATIONS

	Contents	Antihistamine Class
Bromfed-PD Capsule	6 mg brompheniramine maleate, 60 mg pseudoephedrine hydrochloride	Alkylamine (III)
Bromfed Tablet (for children over 12 years)	4 mg brompheniramine maleate, 60 mg pseudoephedrine hydrochloride	Alkylamine (III)
Rondec Tablet (for children over 12 years)	4 mg carbinoxamine maleate, 60 mg pseudoephedrine hydrochloride	Ethanolamine (I)
Rondec Syrup (for children over 12 years)	each 5 ml contains 4 mg carbinoxamine maleate, 60 mg pseudoephedrine hydrochloride	Ethanolamine (I)
Deconamine Tablet	4 mg chlorpheniramine maleate, 60 mg d-pseudoephedrine hydrochloride	Alkylamine (III)
Deconamine Elixir	each 5 ml contains 2 mg chlorpheniramine maleate, 30 mg d-pseudoephedrine hydrochloride	Alkylamine (III)
Naldecon Pediatric Syrup	each 5 ml contains 2 mg phenyltoloxamine citrate, 0.5 mg chlorpheniramine maleate, 5 mg phenylpropanolamine hydrochloride, 1.25 mg phenylephrine hydrochloride	Ethanolamine (I) Alkylamine (III)
Extendryl Chewable Tablets or Syrup	each tablet or 5 ml syrup contains 2 mg chlorpheniramine maleate, 10 mg phenylephrine hydrochloride, 1.25 mg methscopolamine nitrate	Alkylamine (III)
Rynatan Pediatric Suspension	each 5 ml contains 12.5 mg pyrilamine tannate, 2 mg chlorpheniramine tannate, 5 mg phenylephrine tannate	Ethylenediamine (II) Alkylamine (III)
Trinalin Repetabs Tablets (for children over 12 years)	each tablet contains 1 mg azatadine maleate, 120 mg pseudoephedrine sulfate	Piperidine (VI)

whose symptoms emerge despite conventional management, or who develop complications, and whose quality of life is substantially reduced should be considered candidates for immunotherapy. The patient and/or parents must be informed of what immunotherapy can and cannot accomplish. They need to know that immunotherapy does not cure, but can in appropriately selected cases substantially reduce symptoms. Immunotherapy requires careful and regular supervision by both allergist and pediatrician to effect an optimal response.

Bronchial Asthma

HERBERT C. MANSMANN, JR., M.D.

PHILOSOPHY OF MANAGEMENT

When undertaking the care of the asthmatic patient, the clinician must first characterize the nature of the victim and establish the diagnosis while evaluating the extent of the physiologic and biochemical derangement. The recommended treatment measures are often seen as complex, leading to incomplete and confused interpretations of objectives. Initially the acute illness must be interrupted while implementing an approach to the long term implications. The primary care physician is able to appreciate at first hand the original developments as well as to see and prevent the continuum to more advanced disease. Yet, he or she must be able to classify patients, at whatever level they present themselves, so that appropriate intervention can be utilized. In order to accomplish this, a systematic approach will be presented.

Bronchial asthma is a reversible obstructive airflow disease that results in hyperinflation of both lungs. Therapy must be directed toward alleviating bronchospasm, mucosal edema, and inflammatory cell infiltration, as well as evacuating luminal contents and re-establishing mucociliary clearance. Patients often require several medications. Sustained control of each component of the disease process is mandatory.

Physicians need to become skilled in the application of behavioral strategies so that they can commit the patient to a regimen that will be adhered to. A positive approach is effective and necessary. Only when responsibility is shared by physician, patient, and parents will this be possible.

Therapeutic Objectives

Bronchial asthma is a smoldering disease process. If unchecked, illness will beget illness, and progressive pathologic involvement of the airways will lead to more severe physiologic derangements. The therapeutic objectives are presented in Table 1.

Severity Assessment

Classifications are essential to a systematic approach. Assessment of severity can initially be done by history, permitting the physician to identify the class of asthma the patient is likely to have. Frequency of acute breathlessness is the easiest method. Parents and patients can usually relate to this part of the disease and are very likely to accept specific therapeutic objectives. The physician can lay out a long-range plan that realistically includes events or responses to be expected if the patient's condition improves or progressively worsens. The physician's record should include frequency, duration, and severity of each episode, season of the year, amount of school missed, and emergency room visits. Optimally, the peak expiratory flow rate (PEFR) should be plotted on a normal curve each visit or bid at home in advanced situations. Memories are short, and such a data base facilitates consultation, as well as being very helpful to the consultant. Any patient with three or more episodes needs an *ongoing etiologic approach.* As children usually develop new specific IgE responses, optimally this assessment should be done semiannually, or at least annually if distance is a handicap. Once continuing asthma is evident, an aggressive physiologic and pharmacologic approach is essential. When a plan is evident, the physician can select a consultant, clearly at the secondary or tertiary level of care.

Pulmonary Function Tests. All asthmatic children old enough to cooperate, usually age 5 and older, should have PEFR done regularly, plotted on forms showing normal curves of rate verses height. Although the PEFR can be expected to be abnormally low when the patient is breathless, both the severity and the response to medication by injection, inhalation, or orally can be measured 30 to 60 minutes later. In more severe continuing and intractable asthma, response to therapy is best measured by PEFR performed and charted bid. If the PEFR is abnormal, the lung volumes are abnormal, but if the PEFR is normal, the lung volumes may or may not be normal. Therefore, complete pulmonary function tests (CPFT) are recommended regularly in Table 1.

PRINCIPLES OF THERAPY

Down and Up the Ladder. For many years the term has served as a way of systematically looking at therapy. As the patient becomes worse, he requires additional medications. The sequence of therapeutic measures (Table 2) represents going down the ladder, by *adding* a new agent as the disease progresses. As the patient improves, a therapeutic modality might no longer be necessary and the patient comes up the ladder. Table 3 lists the most logical order of discontinuation of modalities based on risk/benefit considerations. Environmental control and immunotherapy are placed at the bottom of Table 2 because there is not always an exact position for them; both should be implemented as soon as practical. They belong at the bottom of Table 3 because they should be the last therapies discontinued. Other differences in the tables should be noted.

PHARMACOLOGIC AGENTS

Antihistamines. For years antihistamines have been considered contraindicated in asthmatics. Allergen and specific IgE reactions release histamine, which causes increased capillary permeability leading to nasal and probably bronchial mucosal edema. Allergic rhinitis is commonly seen in asthmatic children, and mouth breathing is common.

Antihistamines with or without decongestants are usually essential to restore nasal breathing, which permits warm moist air to enter the lungs. Cold, dry air via the mouth can lead to cold induced asthma. Chlorpheniramine, an antihistamine H_1 blocker, also causes bronchodilatation when given intravenously. Therefore, antihistamines must be tried and evaluated for efficiency. One agent from each class as listed under therapy of allergic rhinitis should be systematically tried. Personal preferences include: Dimetapp, Benadryl, Pyribenzamine, Phenergan, and Atarax. During acute severe asthma, the dose due should be withheld. Antihistamines should be discontinued during the first 24 to 48 hours of status asthmaticus.

Theophylline. This is the most extensively stud-

Table 1. THERAPEUTIC OBJECTIVES BY CLASS OF ASTHMA

Class of Asthma	Identifying Characteristics	Therapeutic Objectives	Modalities of Therapy
CHRONIC FORMS			
1. Incipient asthma			
A. Allergic rhinitis (1/3 of patients)	Methacholine induced bronchospasm (MIB)	Prevent asthma Control rhinitis	E, I, A
B. Cough variant asthma	Exercise induced cough MIB	Control bronchospasm	E, T, CPFT/yr
2. Latent asthma	No asthma 5 yrs MIB	Prevent recurrence	E, CPFT/yr
3. Subclinical asthma	No asthma 1 yr MIB	Prevent recurrence	E, I, A, CPFT/6 mos
4. Mild episodic asthma	1–4 Attacks/yr FR & LV normal between attacks	Prevent continuing asthma Prevent bronchial hyper-reactivity	E, I, A, T—prn CPFT/6 mos between episodes
5. Continuing asthma	5–16 Attacks/yr FR normal between attacks LV increased between attacks Bronchial hyperreactivity Reaction to histamine Exercise induced asthma	Prevent intractable asthma Reverse bronchial hyper-reactivity and hyper-inflation Develop emotional growth, independence, and self-care	E, I, A, T, C, B—prn, SB—prn CPFT/6 mos FR each month/visit
6. Intractable asthma	Attacks q 2 wks to daily Constant wheeze FR—always low LV—always increased	Prevent irreversible asthma Reverse constant airflow obstruction	E, I, A, T, C, B, CS frequently, FR each visit or at home bid
7. Irreversible asthma	Incomplete response to bronchodilators Constant dyspnea	Prevent additional damage	All of above—intensively
ACUTE FORMS			
1. Acute severe asthma	Sudden increased dyspnea Hypocarbia	Prevent status asthmaticus	See Table 6
2. Early status asthmaticus	Unresponsive to epinephrine Normocarbia with dyspnea	Prevent advanced status asthmaticus	See Table 6 Aggressive pHa Control
3. Advanced status asthmaticus	Sustained hypercarbia	Prevent respiratory failure	See Table 6
4. Medically irreversible status asthmaticus	Hypercarbia Respiratory acidosis	Prevent death	Controlled ventilation

Adapted from Clin. Chest Med., *1*:339–360, 1980.

Glossary: A—antihistamine without or with decongestant; B—beta-adrenergic; C—cromolyn; CPFT—complete pulmonary function test—flow rates (FR) and lung volumes (LV); CS—corticosteroids; E—environmental control; I—immunotherapy; SB—steroid burst; T—theophylline.

Table 2. SEQUENCE OF "ADD ON" THERAPEUTIC MEASURES

1. Antihistamine without or with decongestant
2. Low dose theophylline—10–17 mg/kg/day
3. High dose theophylline—18–28 mg/kg/day
   a. Obtain serum levels when over 18 mg/kg/day
4. Beta-adrenergic agents, short term (prn) course
   a. Ephedrine sulfate—all ages
   b. Metaproterenol—over 5 years
   c. Terbutaline—over 11 years
   d. Albuterol—over 11 years
5. Cromolyn—20 mg qid
6. Beta-adrenergic agents, around-the-clock
7. Corticosteroids
   a. "Steroid burst"—5–10 days
   b. Long term prednisone—20–80 mg each a.m.
   c. Alternate day steroids
   d. Beclomethasone–inhaled
8. Environmental control
9. Immunotherapy

Table 3. ORDER OF DISCONTINUATION OF MODALITIES

1. Injectable medications
2. Reduce high-dose theophylline 20%
3. Corticosteroids
4. Beta-adrenergic agents
5. Theophylline
6. Antihistamine
7. Cromolyn
8. Immunotherapy
9. Environmental control

ied and used first-line bronchodilator. Even though most patients with mild episodic asthma and some patients with continuing asthma can be controlled with trough serum levels between 5 and 10 μg/ml, most severe continuing asthma and all intractable asthma patients require trough levels between 15 and 20 μg/ml for maximum control. Therapeutic level is often stated to be between 10 to 20 μg/ml; however, the maximum effective level must be highly individualized. Because of variable absorption, metabolism, and elimination characteristics, the oral dosing requirements vary from 400 to 2000 mg/day for adults and between 16 to 40 mg/kg/day in children under 9 years of age. This extremely wide range partly explains why serious theophylline toxicity occurred in the 1950s. Since this drug is so important, it is absolutely essential that we do not permit overdosing to occur.

THEOPHYLLINE TOXICITY. Although gradually increasing doses, with therapeutic drug monitoring, are the best preventives, the physician must recognize symptoms, so that the earliest temporary discontinuation or reduction of dose can be instituted. An increase in irritability, excitation, nausea, vomiting, hematemesis, headache, tremors, convulsions, coma, or shock must be suspected as being due to theophylline toxicity, and an immediate serum theophylline level must be obtained. Additional doses must be withheld until toxicity has been ruled out. Theophylline has not been reported to cause convulsions in children with serum levels under 30 μg/ml. Massive overdoses have been successfully treated with both charcoal and resin hemoperfusion. Physicians must, therefore, become aware of situations that decrease clearance, as this leads to accumulation and higher serum theophylline levels. Troleandomycin, erythromycin, cimetidine, influenza vaccine, and steroids increase theophylline

serum half-life. Since some viruses causing respiratory diseases have this potential, doses should be reduced 20% for 2 to 3 days to prevent toxicity if the serum level is near 20 μg/ml.

RECOMMENDED DOSING REGIMEN. The initial doses should be low with gradual increase over a period of days, just the same as with regular insulin, adjusting the dose to the patient's needs based on response. Ten to 16 mg/kg/day in four to six equal divided doses in an immediate release form, nonalcoholic liquid, or tablet of anhydrous theophylline is recommended. There is no role for aminophylline. By starting low, the low dose responder can be identified, providing considerable leeway when an occasional extra dose seems necessary. We usually start with 10 to 12 mg/kg/day, move to 14 after a few days, and then to 16 if necessary. During the next episode the dose can be more rapidly increased, once the physician has a feel for the patient's need. When high dose theophylline (HDT), i.e., over 18 mg/kg/day, is required, a trough serum level should be obtained periodically to keep it below 20 μg/ml. A dose of 24 mg/kg/day has been reported to present a 20% risk for those under 9 years of age, going over 20 μg/ml, a 40% risk for those between 9 and 12 years, and a 57% risk for those between 12 and 16 years. Table 4 lists guidelines for the use of theophylline serum levels.

SUSTAINED-RELEASE THEOPHYLLINE PREPARATIONS. Once the patient is stabilized and the dose requirement established, the slow release formulations (SRF) need to be considered. Since children often require every 4 hour around-the-clock dosing with plain theophylline, the author has added a SRF dose at bedtime for 20 years. As more experience and information have been obtained, around-the-clock SRF use has become popular. Because of the delayed absorption patterns seen, often for as long as 48 hours, the conversion dose should be reduced to 25 to 30% of the immediately available form. Give initially every 12 hours. Switch to every 8 hours if control is insufficient and HDT is indicated.

Each manufacturer details the merits of his product. Select only those containing anhydrous theophylline, with good published bioavailability (F), area under the curve ($AUC_{0-\gamma}$), and minimum peak to trough variation (ΔP-T) data. While much has been published in the pediatric literature, using

Table 4. GUIDELINES FOR THEOPHYLLINE SERUM LEVELS

GENERAL USE

1. Document adherence to therapeutic alliance—draw blood at any time poor control is observed
2. Toxic symptoms—draw blood immediately and also at 2, 4, and 6 hours to establish half-life
3. Evaluate suspected side effects—draw blood ½ to 1 hour after a dose taken on an empty stomach—peak level
4. Oral steady-state—do peak and trough level after 6 half-lives of maintenance therapy
5. Stat—serum level use to calculate intravenous dosing schedule
6. Intravenous steady-state is evaluated by obtaining several levels during continuous infusion
7. Document maximum bronchodilatation by doing pulmonary function tests at time of drawing peak level followed by aerosol bronchodilator and then a repeat pulmonary function test

USE WITH SOLUTION OR PLAIN TABLETS

1. Therapeutic level—lowest occurring level (trough) is obtained just before next oral dose
   a. Used when dose greater than 18 mg/kg/day—to prevent overdosing
2. Half-life—helpful to plan dosing regimen

USE WITH SUSTAINED RELEASE TABLETS

1. Trough level is obtained by drawing blood just before next dose
2. Peak level is obtained 4 to 8 hours after a dose, depending upon the preparation used

---

computer simulations to give a "Predictive Model" analysis of serum levels, there is no substitute for actual data. One study, often republished and cited, compared four patients studied for 20 hours with one product, while considerably more patients were studied for 28 hours with another SRF. Most studies are single dose analyses over 24 hours. Only three products have been studied for 48 hours after a single dose and also after multiple doses over 4 days (see Table 5). The mean F, AUC and ΔP-T data are practically identical. The F values of individuals varied a great deal, with one patient only

absorbing 57.4% over 48 hours. Therefore, individual response and serum levels should be evaluated. An acceptable ΔP-T value should not be greater than 5 μg/ml in order to obtain maximum control. Aerolate and Slo-Bid, capsules containing sustained-release beads, can be sprinkled over baby food, applesauce, or jelly, which is ideal for the small child. Theo-Dur tablets must not be crushed or the slow-release properties are lost. Three 100 mg tablets of Theo-Dur are not equal to one 300 mg tablet, since 50% and 35% of the theophylline are released more rapidly respectively.

Beta-Adrenergic Agents. These are excellent "add-on" prn medications to help control acute symptoms, if needed. Some patients with more severe continuing asthma and all with intractable asthma need such agents, in addition to theophylline, around the clock. Because of reported and personally documented cardiac irregularities, admittedly infrequent, a baseline electrocardiogram should be obtained. Moreover, because of this we have tried cromolyn in all patients requiring these drugs, in order to minimize their long-term use.

EPHEDRINE SULFATE. In spite of well publicized data, suggesting that there is no use for ephedrine and proving that fixed-drug combinations of theophylline and ephedrine should not be used to treat patients requiring HDT, data using adjusted ephedrine sulfate doses (49% less) have proven it to be efficacious and reasonably well tolerated. The mean dose was 0.84 mg/kg, with a range of 0.51 to 1.38 mg/kg every 8 hours. Ephedrine is the only oral bronchodilator other than theophylline approved for use in infants and children of all ages. It has been very effective over the past 25 years.

METAPROTERENOL. This drug is approved for use in children over 5 years of age. Although frequently used in younger children, it would seem prudent to prove that ephedrine sulfate is ineffective or produces too many side effects before using an unapproved drug in a child with a chronic disease with

Table 5. IDEAL EXAMPLES OF PHARMACOKINETIC MULTIPLE DOSE DATA

	ΔP-T (μg/ml) Mean ± SD	AUC$_{0-\gamma}$ (μg/hr/ml) Mean ± SD	F (%) Mean ± SD	Available Dosage Forms
A. Aerolate*	3.37 ± 1.38	108.84 ± 23.18	116.08 ± 26.03 (71.83–171.08)**	65, 130, 260 mg
B. Slo-Bid	2.63 ± 1.38	102.10 ± 35.99	103.02 ± 20.98 (62.00–129.10)**	100, 200, 300 mg
A. Theo-Dur	3.02 ± 0.93	107.87 ± 17.62	118.57 ± 18.66 (85.00–146.22)**	100, 200, 300 mg
B. Theo-Dur	3.51 ± 1.94	100.43 ± 34.30	101.43 ± 22.09 (57.40–141.80)**	100, 200, 300 mg

*Note two studies, A and B, were conducted on 15 normal nonsmoking adult males with a crossover between drugs.
**Range.

long-term medication needs, that is, requiring months, if not years, of therapy. A dose of 2.0 mg/kg/day is recommended. A dose of 10 to 20 mg qid has been proven effective in controlling asthma. It has also caused a significant increase in flow rates when added to the regimen of asthmatic children taking theophylline.

TERBUTALINE. This agent has been approved for those over 11 years of age. The same comment regarding use in younger patients applies. It is more β_2 selective than ephedrine and metaproterenol, and is effective up to 5 hours. Some patients develop hand tremor that often subsides with time. A dose of 2.5 to 5 mg every 6 hours is recommended.*

ALBUTEROL. The advantage to this preparation is that it is more β_2 selective than all others with virtually no cardiac effect. Its effect persists for 6 to 8 hours. Tremors are seen with this drug also. The dose is 2 to 8 mg every 8 hours.

Inhalation Therapy. Both metered dose inhalers and aerosolized solution of beta-adrenergic agents work very well in acutely ill patients with mild episodic asthma or early continuing asthma. In such cases oral bronchodilators are just as effective but take a longer time to work. Yet, many years of having to cope with patients who are psychologically dependent upon this modality have caused me to sharply restrict this delivery system. Some asthmatics with intractable asthma and some with chronic bronchitis are made more comfortable with these agents, especially if many medications are required and oral beta-adrenergic agents are poorly tolerated. Some patients with very irritable airways can take their inhaled cromolyn or steroids only if they are given 15 minutes after an inhaled beta-adrenergic agent. As the disease becomes better controlled, the inhaled medications are better tolerated, and pretreatment may not remain necessary.

It would appear prudent to reserve use of these agents for special situations because of the following factors: lack of a real need; inability of smaller children to cooperate; transient immediate relief of symptoms, which causes patients to use them more frequently; incorrect technique; lack of dosage control; drying and irritating effect resulting in coughing; and their documented placebo effect. In the past, abuses due to overusage because of the short duration of effect have resulted in toxic fatal complications. In spite of its long duration of effect, albuterol has also been reported to be abused. This might be due to its euphoric effect, which lasts less than 1 hour, and the patient's need for its excitation effect.

Cromolyn. Because of a considerable number of recent experimental evaluations, cromolyn is currently again undergoing extensive trial in the U.S. It has been shown to prevent allergen induced immediate and late-onset asthma, exercise induced asthma, hypothermic (cold) induced asthma, and irritant induced reflex bronchoconstriction. Cromolyn has the unique ability to ameliorate existing bronchial hyperreactivity, as well as to prevent its development during a pollen season. This prophylactic "umbrella" effect conceptually makes it the ideal drug, especially with its lack of significant side effects.

Effectiveness is extremely difficult to document. Occasionally the results are dramatic. It is most often now used in patients with predictable mild episodic asthma such as exercise induced and cold air induced asthma. A 20 mg dose 10 to 30 minutes before the precipitating event is usually sufficient. This is also true for rare breaks in environmental control, such as tobacco smoke exposure. Patients with pollen asthma should be treated 20 mg qid for 2 weeks before, during, and 1 or 2 months post season. Patients with continuing, intractable or irreversible asthma should receive an extensive trial, while on other medications, to control airflow obstruction and hyperinflation. Cromolyn 20 mg qid for 2 weeks should be increased to 40 mg qid for 2 weeks and then to 40 mg q 4 h for up to 12 weeks before failure is accepted. In the interim, it would be expected that the steroids and then the beta-adrenergic agent should be reduced or discontinued. Theophylline should not be reduced until lung volumes become and remain normal. The recent release of cromolyn nebulizer solution is an excellent advance for use in young children.

The individual dose should be withheld whenever acute breathlessness is present. If the symptom subsides, the next dose should be taken. During status asthmaticus, doses should be withheld for 12 to 24 hours. The maintenance dose can be restarted as a nebulized solution mixed with an aerosol β_2 agent as soon as tolerated. If the patient has been taking cromolyn bid or tid, the dose should be increased to qid until return to preattack baseline function.

Corticosteroids. Oral prednisone, 1 to 2 mg/kg/day, is the most frequently used preparation for "short bursts" lasting 5 to 10 days. If these become too frequent, such as two to three times a month, a short course of daily steroids should be considered. Withdrawal should be attempted a few times, with gradual reduction. Reduce the dose 10 mg per day until at 20 mg, then reduce by 5 mg every 3 to 4 days until at 10 mg, and then reduce by 2.5 mg every 3 to 4 days until no drug is being taken or symptoms recur. If symptoms return, alternate day steroids should be tried or a switch to inhaled beclomethasone, 2 puffs (84 μg) qid. Responsibility for patient care should be shared with a pediatric allergist when corticosteroids are required. The side effects demand that intensive

---

*Manufacturer's precaution: Not recommended for children under 12 years of age.

long-term care, including diagnostic, etiologic, physiologic, and pharmacologic approaches, be implemented. Institutions with such programs as at the Children's Heart Hospital of Philadelphia and the National Jewish Hospital should be considered. I believe that the need for corticosteroids represents a failure somewhere in the process of reversing this disease.

PREVENTION

As in pediatrics, prophylaxis is the essence of allergy and clinical immunology practice. Unfortunately, this very broad subject could be the subject of several complete chapters. The data are overwhelmingly convincing. Only the bare essentials of this subject can be addressed here.

Non-Specific Therapy

Environmental Control. The most potent allergens are derived from feathers, wool, mohair, horse dander and hair, cats, dogs, and other animals. Man-made chemicals also contribute, not always as allergens but as irritants. Access to most biologically produced substances must be limited to casual exposure. Even this is often inadequate to prevent continuation of symptoms. Children spend 8 to 12 hours in their bedrooms, so this is the place to start. Remove feather pillows, down comforters, and rugs; cover mattresses with airtight covers. The most difficult environmental problem is exposure to tobacco smoke, pets, and scented odors in the home.

Emotional Growth. It is absolutely essential that pediatricians and other primary-care physicians foster and explain the necessity of emotional growth and development, peer association, intellectual growth by regular school attendance, and self-care. Much too often, dependency grows as the disease becomes chronic. Parents must permit their children to live their own lives, in spite of continuing illness. Aggressive medical supervision and control of symptoms will encourage parents in this.

Specific Therapy

Immunotherapy. The scientific basis of immunotherapy, previously called desensitization and then hyposensitization, has been established in pollen induced allergic rhinitis and in cat induced mild episodic asthma. Its role in intractable asthma is in doubt, yet it offers the patient who is allergic to *unavoidable inhalants* a chance to change his immunologic nature. All patients with allergic rhinitis and mild episodic and continuing asthma should receive *only* this specific therapy.

TREATMENT OF DIFFERENT CLASSES OF ASTHMA

Incipient Asthma. Through the years the author has seen four groups of infants and children who could be considered as having a pre-asthma condition. The high proportion of infants with reversible bronchospastic component to their bronchopulmonary dysplasia should be evaluated for a family history of allergy and personal development of an elevated IgE. Such patients are often treated with around-the-clock theophylline. Follow-up for atopic diseases is encouraged.

"WET-BABY" SYNDROME. A small number of infants are profuse mucus producers and tend to have expiratory wheezing with viral infections. Most physicians would refer to such episodes as asthmatic bronchitis. Aside from evaluation and elimination of foods inducing symptoms, an environmental control program should be implemented. No dusting powder or scented disposable diapers should be permitted. Up to the age of 1.5 years, an effective oral mixture is equal parts of Elixir of Benadryl, syrup of ephedrine sulfate, N.F., and elixir of phenobarbital. The dose is 1 ml for each 3 months of age, every 3 to 4 hours. This often controls mucus production and bronchospasm. Theophylline may be added as a supplement, if necessary.

ALLERGIC RHINITIS WITH BRONCHIAL HYPERREACTIVITY. About one third of patients with seasonal allergic rhinitis have a positive methacholine bronchial challenge test. Whether they all end up with seasonal asthma is unknown. One half of patients treated with an immunotherapy placebo developed pollen asthma. Therefore, in such situations where allergic rhinitis is severe, immunotherapy is recommended in addition to symptomatic treatment.

COUGH VARIANT ASTHMA. These patients frequently have bouts of severe coughing that subside, leaving them apparently well. Yet, any exertion causes subclinical bronchospasm with cough as the sole clinical manifestation. They have methacholine bronchial hyperreactivity and exercise induced decrease in airflow. The latter can be prevented by around-the-clock theophylline, usually low dose. Environmental control and long-term observation are indicated.

LATENT ASTHMA. Patients who previously had a more severe, constant form of asthma, even though symptom-free for up to 5 years, still have methacholine bronchial hyperreactivity. Environmental control should be maintained for life. Immunotherapy is often discontinued after 2 years if there are no symptoms and no need for allergic medication during allergic seasons, and if injections are received monthly. One third have a recurrence of upper respiratory allergic symptoms due to unavoidable inhalant allergens, and will need to return to therapy for an indefinite period. Complete pulmonary function tests (flow rates and lung volumes) should be done annually.

SUBCLINICAL ASTHMA. The rare patient with only a few attacks 1 or 2 years apart and those with more frequent asthma but none for 1 year fit this class. They may or may not need around-the-clock medications to remain asymptomatic. Since symptoms are usually related to airflow obstruction, airflow rates should be normal for 1 year. Lung volumes ideally should be checked semiannually, but annually is probably satisfactory. There should be no hyperinflation. During this period medications should be gradually discontinued according to the previously described plan.

MILD EPISODIC ASTHMA. These patients have from one to six attacks per year and their flow rates and lung volumes return to normal within a few weeks of an acute episode. Therapy is continued,

---

Table 6. HOSPITAL MANAGEMENT OF PROGRESSING SEVERE ASTHMA

ACUTE SEVERE ASTHMA

1. *Epinephrine 1–100*, 0.01 ml/kg, subcutaneously, may be repeated two more times at 20 minute intervals. Maximum dose is 0.6 ml first hour, then every 4 hours. Third dose should be Sus-Phrine (Epinephrine suspension 1:200),

   or

   A. *Sus-Phrine*, 0.005 ml/kg, subcutaneously may be repeated at 6–12 hour intervals. Contains 20% in aqueous state for immediate effect. Maximum single dose 0.2 ml

   B. *Bronkephrine* (ethylnorepinephrine), 0.02 ml/kg, may be substituted if epinephrine pressor effect is excessive

EARLY STATUS ASTHMATICUS

2. *Stat studies*. Arterial blood gases, pH, serum electrolytes, CBC and diff, PA and lateral x-ray of chest, nose and throat cultures, and urinalysis
3. *Oxygen*, humidified, is given to maintain PaO_2 between 80 and 100 mm Hg
4. *Intravenous fluids* based on daily maintenance requirement, plus replacement of deficit should be calculated and divided into four equal 6 hour bottles. NPO
5. *Aminophylline*, loading dose of 5.0 mg/kg over 15 minutes, if none previous 6 hours, (otherwise give ½ dose), then add 5.0 mg/kg to *each* 6 hour IV bottle. If serum theophylline levels are available, the dose may be adjusted up to a 7.0 mg/kg loading dose and 1.56 mg/kg/hr, up to 28 mg/kg/day has been recommended
6. *Sodium bicarbonate*. If respiratory distress is severe or if acidosis proven, give 2 meq/kg of $NaHCO_3$ over a 5 minute period and repeat over next 45 minutes. If hourly pHa is less than 145 meq/L, repeat 4 meq/kg $NaHCO_3$ hourly
7. *Solu-Medrol* (paraben-free methylprednisolone sodium succinate) 2 mg/kg is given slowly over 10 minutes and 1 mg/kg is added to every 6-hour bottle.

ADVANCED STATUS ASTHMATICUS

A. *Solu-Medrol* dose is 4 mg/kg followed by 2 mg/kg every 6 hours for 24 to 48 hours
8. Record and evaluate BP, pulse, respiratory rate every 15 minutes, blood gases, pHa every 30 to 60 minutes, and Na, K, Cl every hour
9. *Antibiotics* as indicated for obvious clinical infection, WBC over 15,000 with or without fever and/or prolonged unresponsive asthma
10. Physician should evaluate patient *at least* hourly for several hours. Document that the medications and fluids being received on schedule. Assure staff physician that patient is adequately ventilating. Alert controlled ventilation team in event of impending ventilatory failure *Example:* If an increase in $PaCO_2$ of 5 mm Hg/hr over normal has occurred

Adapted from Clin. Rev. Allerg., *1*, in press, 1983.

---

with systematic reduction if the patient is improving from a more severe class. If the disease is progressing, an around-the-clock medication should be considered as the frequency increases, e.g., one or two per year to every other month.

CONTINUING ASTHMA. Progression from mild episodic asthma to every other month or every 2 to 3 weeks is a bad sign requiring more intensive intervention. A secondary level consultation should be obtained to maximize control and ensure reversibility. An aggressive program of evaluation and reevaluation at 6- to 12-month intervals is indicated. Between attacks, even when there is no airflow obstruction, hyperinflation is present. This must be reversed to prevent intractable and irreversible asthma.

INTRACTABLE ASTHMA. When there is constant significant airflow obstruction, the patient has intractable asthma. There is also chronic hyperinflation. The use of corticosteroids increases just to maintain any degree of normal life. Once this has occurred, aggressive therapy is essential. This may be possible only in a residential treatment center where emotional and intellectual growth is assured and where the reasons for previous failures can be more adequately addressed.

IRREVERSIBLE ASTHMA. The patient with constant, daily breathlessness at rest invariably has permanent lung damage. Every effort to prevent additional complications is mandatory. Frequent status asthmaticus and sudden unexplained death must be recognized as possibilities and thus be prevented.

ACUTE SEVERE ASTHMA. At any point in any of the classes described above, sudden breathlessness can occur. The vast majority of such patients respond to rest or additional oral bronchodilator, or both, in 1 or 2 hours. Persistence of symptoms suggests early or advanced status asthmaticus. Status asthmaticus is considered to occur when the patient is unresponsive to three injections of epinephrine. Table 6 outlines the therapy.

EARLY STATUS ASTHMATICUS. In acute severe asthma, hyperventilation leads to hypocarbia. If normocarbia occurs and the patient is still dyspneic, early status asthmaticus should be diagnosed.

Helpful predictive indices of severity include heart rate over 110/min, respiratory rate over 30/min, pulsus paradoxus over 18 mm Hg, peak expiratory flow rate less than 120 L/min, and moderate to severe dyspnea. Respiratory failure due to asthma is indicated by the presence of any three of the following: severe inspiratory retractions, absence of inspiratory breath sounds, generalized muscular weakness, decreased level of consciousness and pain response, cyanosis in 40% ambient oxygen, and/or a $PaCO_2$ of over 65 mm Hg. Intensive care is indicated when there is a rise over normal $Paco_2$ by 10 mm Hg/hour over 2 consecutive hours.

ADVANCED STATUS ASTHMATICUS. This diagnosis is evident when there is documented sustained hypercarbia. Acute respiratory failure is diagnosed when the $Paco_2$ is over 49 mm Hg and the Pao_2 is below 60 mm Hg. Therapy, as outlined in Table 6, must be aggressive. Once the presence of three of the above has been confirmed, controlled ventilation must be considered. Most patients with these signs will respond to intensive therapy in 1 to 12 hours. Our patients have not needed intravenous isoproterenol, having all responded to the above therapy, and controlled ventilation has usually not been necessary. One exception was a patient who did not adhere to the protocol and who required controlled ventilation on an emergency basis.

MEDICALLY IRREVERSIBLE STATUS ASTHMATICUS. When all else fails, intravenous isoproterenol infusion might be tried, yet even 20% of those so treated must receive controlled ventilation in order to prevent death. When ventilation cannot be accomplished, the physician must be prepared to try Halothane, bronchopulmonary lavage, or extracorporeal membrane oxygenation to buy time for the medical treatment to effectively reverse the process.

Serum Sickness

ROBERT C. STRUNK, M.D.

Serum sickness originally was defined as the systemic reaction that follows the injection of horse serum into human beings. Since horse antisera are used much less frequently than in the preantibiotic era, drugs are now the most common cause of this syndrome. The drugs most often mentioned as causing serum sickness are penicillins, cephalosporins, sulfonamides, hydralazine, phenylbutazone, and thiouracils.

The treatment of serum sickness consists of prevention, discontinuing the drug, and symptomatic therapy. Of these three, prevention is most obvious, but often is overlooked. Horse antisera are still required in the treatment of poisonous snake envenomation, poisonous spider bites, botulism and other clostridial infections, diphtheria, and transplant rejections with antilymphocyte globulin. Even in these settings the antisera should be used only when necessary, e.g., for a poisonous snake bite only if envenomation has occurred. Administration of antihistamines (cyproheptadine or hydroxyzine) from days 4 to 16 after antitoxin may prevent the manifestations of serum sickness. Another preventive measure is adequate immunization against diphtheria and tetanus toxins for all children. Human antisera should be used in place of horse anti-

sera when it is available, e.g., for treatment of tetanus and rabies. Obviously drugs should be used only when necessary.

Allergy testing probably should be performed before the administration of animal antisera. This is especially important when a patient has been previously exposed to the animal antisera or is atopic and sensitive to the dander. Scratch testing is done initially, using antigen diluted 1:20 with normal saline. If the scratch test is negative, an intradermal test is done using the smallest amount of antigen dilution that will produce a bleb (usually 0.02 ml), first with a 1:100 dilution and, if negative, a 1:10 dilution. If any of the skin tests are positive (after 15 minutes, a presence of a wheal 3 mm in diameter greater than the saline control), the patient should be considered at risk for anaphylaxis and rapid desensitization should be attempted. An IV infusion is started; aqueous epinephrine, injectable diphenhydramine, and a tourniquet are kept in readiness. An initial dose of 0.1 ml of 1:1000 dilution of the antiserum is injected subcutaneously into an extremity where a tourniquet can be placed proximally. If no reaction is observed, the dose is doubled every 15 to 20 minutes until the full dose is given. Larger volumes are given IM. If a reaction occurs and can be controlled with medication, desensitization is resumed with one half the dose that caused the reaction. Although this procedure reduces the risk of anaphylaxis, it does not alter the other manifestations of serum sickness.

Since serum sickness is almost always a self-limited disease, treatment should be conservative. Fever, malaise, tender lymphadenopathy, myalgia, and joint symptoms are treated with usual therapeutic doses of aspirin. Rarely, frank arthritis may require larger aspirin doses (approximately 80 mg/kg, to achieve a serum level of 25 mg/dl). Hydroxyzine is the most effective antipruritic agent (oral dose, 2 mg/kg/24 hr in four divided doses; this amount may be increased 2-fold if the patient is carefully observed for side effects). In addition to systemic therapy for pruritus, local application of cool, wet compresses or a tepid bath (possibly with the addition of a water-dispersible oil to help avoid drying) may be beneficial. Numerous local creams and ointments are often prescribed, but probably are no better than the cool water alone. Topical use of diphenhydramine or anesthetic agents should be avoided, as they can be sensitizing. Marked urticarial lesions or angioedema may require use of aqueous epinephrine 1:1000, 0.01 ml/kg subcutaneously (maximum 0.3 ml). Epinephrine aqueous suspension 1:200 (Sus-Phrine) in a dose of 0.005 ml/kg subcutaneously (maximum 0.2 ml) every six hours, may give more sustained relief.

If the above drugs fail to make the patient comfortable or if more severe symptoms are present, the use of oral corticosteroids should be considered. Prednisone, 1 to 2 mg/kg/24 hr orally (maximum 60 mg), is given in two to four divided doses. After 2 to 3 days, the symptoms should be relieved considerably. The dose should be reduced rapidly to a minimum that will control the symptoms, and then discontinued at the earliest possible time. If the patient is tuberculin-positive, isoniazid should be given concurrently with the prednisone.

Angioneurotic Edema

FRED S. ROSEN, M.D.,
and HARVEY R. COLTEN, M.D.

Angioneurotic edema is a symptom of circumscribed areas of swelling of the subcutaneous tissue. The swelling is never discolored or red, is never painful, and usually does not itch.

HEREDITARY ANGIONEUROTIC EDEMA

Affected individuals are prone to sudden, unheralded attacks of circumscribed subcutaneous edema. The swelling, which may be severe enough to cause remarkable disfigurement of the affected part, evolves very quickly and usually subsides within 72 hours. There is no discoloration, redness, pain, or itching. Despite the undistinguished appearance of the edema, involvement of the mucous membranes of the hypopharynx and larynx may result in untimely death from asphyxiation. Severe abdominal cramps may accompany angioedema.

The diagnosis is established by measuring the serum levels of C1 inhibitor and C4, which are low. Fifteen per cent of patients have normal levels of nonfunctional C1 inhibitor; the C4 level is nonetheless depressed.

Treatment. Daily administration of methyltestosterone Linguets* has prevented attacks of angioedema in approximately one third to one half of patients. It must be taken daily in a single dose of 10 to 25 mg. Methyltestosterone therapy is not recommended for children. Danazol* provides effective prophylaxis against attacks of angioedema when 100 to 200 mg are taken daily. Another impeded androgen, stanozolol,* is also effective in a dose of 2 mg a day. These impeded androgens are not recommended for long-term prophylaxis in children under 16 years of age. However, they may be taken for short periods (5 days) prior to surgery or dental work, circumstances that may provoke severe attacks of angioedema.

Epsilon-aminocaproic acid has been successful in halting attacks of angioedema.* However, the side effects with chronic administration of this agent are so annoying that its usage has been very limited. An analog, tranexamic acid, has been found to have fewer side effects, causing only occasional minor gastrointestinal distress. In doses of 1 to 3 gm/24 hr orally, it has proved effective in aborting attacks of angioedema. The drug has not yet been released by the Food and Drug Administration.

Infusions of plasma have been recommended in the therapy of attacks of angioedema. However, this approach is not recommended by us because it has been of questionable value and is not innocuous in the view of several observers who have attempted to use it. It is not possible to raise the level of C1 inhibitor (deficient in the inherited form of the disease) above 7 mg/dl, a level under which attacks of angioedema occur, except by infusing very large amounts of plasma. For instance, 100 ml of plasma would raise the inhibitor level by 1 mg/dl in a 40-kg child. Fresh plasma contains more substrate for C1 than inhibitor; consequently, its administration early in the course of an attack, prior to the onset of tachyphylaxis, might in fact exacerbate the symptoms. Such an event has been observed. Purified C1 inhibitor for infusion is available from the American Red Cross. It is useful in the treatment of attacks of angioedema.

Epinephrine is useful in controlling swelling in very few patients. Hydrocortisone also provides benefit very rarely in patients. Antihistamines are of no use. Intravenous administration of diuretics, such as meralluride or ethacrynic acid,† is helpful in halting the progression of life-threatening angioedema.

Tracheostomy should be performed without hesitation in patients with laryngeal obstruction. It is frequently life-saving.

NONHEREDITARY ANGIONEUROTIC EDEMA

Nonhereditary angioneurotic edema is generally a benign condition of diverse etiology. Food ingestion, drugs, insect stings in appropriately sensitive individuals, and psychic or physical factors may precipitate attacks of angioedema. The clinical consequences of angioedema are a function of the site involved; angioedema of the larynx may be fatal if prompt therapy is not instituted. Angioedema secondary to acute infection or to connective tissue disorder must be differentiated, since the diagnostic and therapeutic efforts must be specific for these primary diseases.

In the case of angioedema due to an obvious precipitating event (e.g., insect sting), an etiologic diagnosis by means of history and skin testing is not difficult but is of minimal value. Avoidance of expo-

---

*This use is not mentioned in the manufacturer's instructions.

†Manufacturer's precaution: Until further experience is accumulated in infants, therapy with the oral and parenteral forms of ethacrynic acid is contraindicated. (This use is not listed in the manufacturer's directive.)

sure, immunotherapy, and the availability of an emergency kit consisting of aqueous epinephrine, a tourniquet, ephedrine, and an antihistamine (such as diphenhydramine) are generally successful in preventing subsequent episodes of angioedema. The emergency kit should be carried by the patient at all times during periods when exposure to stinging insects is likely.

In angioedema due, for example, to food ingestion, skin testing is of doubtful value; and if the onset of clinical symptoms is delayed for several hours following ingestion of the offending agent, the history may not be helpful. In fact, it is estimated that in nearly 50% of all cases of nonhereditary angioedema, an etiologic diagnosis is not made.

Accordingly, although elimination of the offending agent is the most successful therapy, symptomatic therapy may be the only available measure. Aqueous epinephrine is of value, particularly in the more severe cases. Parenteral or oral antihistamines or oral sympathomimetics (ephedrine) are also indicated. Maintenance of adequate ventilation in instances of laryngeal edema may require intubation or tracheostomy if the response to epinephrine is not prompt. The role of corticosteroids in the treatment of angioedema has not been rigorously studied, though those agents are frequently employed. In no instance should corticosteroids be considered a substitute for epinephrine in the emergency treatment of severe cases of angioedema.

Allergic Gastrointestinal Disorders

S. ALLAN BOCK, M.D.

The term allergy has been badly abused over the last several decades, having been used by many to refer to any of a vast array of adverse reactions to environmental substances. The word allergy should be reserved for adverse reactions that can be shown to be associated with one or more immunologic reactions. These may involve humoral antibodies or cell-mediated immune reactions, or both.

Gastrointestinal allergy is most often due to ingested food proteins. While there may be associated skin or respiratory symptoms, gastrointestinal symptoms have been the most commonly evoked reactions during challenge studies with food in children. The commonest symptoms are diarrhea and vomiting; cramps, occult bleeding producing anemia, and failure to thrive also occur.

The pediatrician is the physician most often confronted by complaints about food allergy. The diet is blamed for most common symptoms that occur in the first few years of life (colic, diarrhea, constipation, frequent vomiting, and numerous skin rashes). Pediatricians need a systematic approach to the evaluation of these problems, which can often be very disruptive.

Before discussing treatment it is important to make a few comments about diagnosis so that the usual areas of confusion can be avoided. Several categories of adverse reactions to foods must be considered when children present with GI symptoms. These include enzyme deficiencies, toxic reactions (due to natural toxins or contaminants in the food supply), biochemical reactions involving mediators of inflammation or hormones (these are poorly defined), immunologically mediated reactions, and psychological reactions based upon acquired beliefs. The most important part of the evaluation of patients with putative adverse reactions to food is to prove unequivocally that the food is responsible for the symptoms. This is most objectively done by double blind food challenge, which in young children is easily accomplished by placing the suspect food in something the child consumes without problem. Prior to any challenge, the symptoms must have been resolved by using an elimination diet, which is described below. Once the adverse reaction has been objectively confirmed, the mechanism can be sought by using appropriate laboratory measurements. Small bowel biopsies are often required to confirm a diagnosis of gluten sensitive enteropathy and enteropathies to milk and soy proteins.

A brief comment about allergy skin tests in children is important. Contrary to most pediatric texts and many allergy books, skin testing can be quite useful in children, even young children. The biggest problem has been improper interpretation. Confusion always arises when a patient has a positive skin test but seems able to eat the food (or foods) without having symptoms. This is properly referred to as *asymptomatic sensitivity*. The antibodies detected have biologic significance but are clinically unimportant as long as the body's natural defenses (mucosal surfaces and skin) are intact. The presence of positive skin tests in the absence of symptoms when the food is ingested should *not* be referred to as "false positive" because in some conditions the antibodies may become clinically significant and then the term "false positive" might cause confusion. *Asymptomatic sensitivity* to the food in question is a better term.

Dietary Management. When a food has been shown to produce symptoms, the most important treatment is elimination of the food from the diet. Research in food allergy has found that most children with GI allergy react to one or perhaps two foods. Fortunately, the child who reacts to numerous foods is unusual. Thus, the elimination diet usually requires elimination of a single food. Consultation with a dietitian may be required to enable the parents to provide the child with a nutritious, appetizing diet. It may be necessary for the physician or dietitian to explain to parents the unfamiliar terms seen on labels, such as whey protein and casein from milk. There are numerous cook books that contain recipes for patients who have foods eliminated from their diets. Diets eliminating multiple foods are available but are most often useful during the diagnostic process, when the problem-causing foods are not yet identified.

Elemental diets are often important in the management of infants with adverse reactions to foods. These include nursing infants who may react to foods that the mother ingests that are transported through the breast milk. The three commonest elemental diets in current usage are Nutramigen, Pregestimil, and Vivonex. When using any of these formulas the physician must be concerned with adequate calorie and fluid intake. Each of these may be responsible for osmotic diarrhea, and if diarrhea is the symptom being evaluated, its persistence may be due to the solute concentration of the formula. Using diluted elemental formula for a few days may solve the problem.

When using elemental or elimination diets the pediatrician needs a plan for rechallenging the patient with the foods that had been eliminated from the diet. It is important to continue the diet long enough for the symptom to resolve. For some cases of diarrhea it has been our anecdotal experience that a number of symptom free weeks may be required before reintroduction of some foods is successful. Premature reintroduction of some foods seems to bring about a relapse even though the child can eventually be shown not to be sensitive to the food. This experience is not in accord with our current knowledge of turnover of GI mucosal epithelial cells and suggests an area for further research.

We have investigated the natural history of gastrointestinal food allergy in a number of our patients in whom the reaction was objectively confirmed and the mechanism was determined. The results of these studies indicate that the younger the child when the diagnosis is made, the more likely it is that he or she will "outgrow" the problem. In view of this prognosis we recommend a program of regular challenges at 3 to 6 month intervals, depending on the severity of the original reaction. Challenges must be started with small amounts and then increased over a period of time. The interval between challenges should not be less than time for the expected reaction to occur. For example, a 4-year-old has been found to exhibit vomiting and diarrhea from about 1 teaspoon of peanut butter 2 hours after ingestion, and it has been 6 months since the last challenge. The challenge should begin with about ¼ teaspoon. If there is no reaction, then the amount can be doubled and given 2 or more hours later until customary amounts are tolerated or a reaction occurs. For evaluation of gastroenteropathies from milk and soy, where the interval from ingestion to onset of symptoms may be days, the challenge process may take much longer but generally can be performed by introducing a modest quantity of food into the diet regularly and waiting for symptoms to appear or for the food to be tolerated. Milk and soy protein enteropathies seem to be uniformly "outgrown" by the third birthday. Much has been said about the effects of cooking and digestion on food allergy but we have not found these factors to be important in patients who truly have food allergy.

No discussion of this type would be complete without a comment concerning anaphylaxis from ingested food protein. Prostrating diarrhea is often more impressive than respiratory symptoms. Fortunately, anaphylaxis from foods is rare in children but it does occur. We have seen anaphylaxis from milk and peanut ingestion, and isolated cases have been reported from other foods. Some children with anaphylaxis to milk seem to "outgrow" the problem, but severe peanut reactions may persist. Children with anaphylaxis to foods should be challenged *only* in a hospital setting where emergency measures are available. The only reason to challenge these children is to determine whether the problem still exists. Unfortunately, no matter how careful one tries to be, children do get exposed to forbidden foods accidentally, and thus there is a degree of "wear and tear" on child and family in trying to perpetually avoid a food. In my opinion any child beyond infancy with anaphylactic sensitivity to a food should have a kit containing injectable epinephrine near at hand. The EpiPen is a convenient way to administer epinephrine in an emergency.

The following, suggested approach for patients with apparent GI allergy is based upon research studies, including an epidemiologic investigation currently in progress of 500 children followed from birth until their third birthday. When the child presents with a reported adverse reaction to a food (or foods) enough time should be allotted to take a history that will convince the physician that the observations are probably due to the suspected food. Unless the problem is anaphylaxis, a careful but deliberate open challenge should be used to confirm the reaction; it is highly desirable that this be done in the physician's office. If the reaction seems confirmed or highly probable after the challenge, then the food should be eliminated from the diet for 1 to 3 months, depending on the severity of the reaction. At this time the challenge is repeated. If the reaction is positive after three or more challenges in the first year following the diagnosis, I strongly recommend that double blind challenges be performed and, if positive, appropriate testing should be done to ascertain the mechanism. This approach may need to be altered for patients with suspected enteropathies in whom biopsy may be needed at the time of each challenge. The longer the reaction persists, the more strongly held will be the patient's (and parents') beliefs about the food. In this situation or if the symptoms are vague (abdominal pain or nausea without other reactions), then blind challenges become mandatory to reach an unequivocal diagnosis.

Pharmacologic Therapy. Unfortunately, there are few adequately controlled studies of medication in GI allergy. The three most commonly used medications are cromolyn, antihistamines, and corticosteroids. Cromolyn, a drug commonly used in asthma, apparently inhibits the release of inflammatory mediators from cells in the mucosa. In some studies administration of cromolyn prior to food ingestion does appear to eliminate GI symptoms. The problem with cromolyn as long-term therapy is that we do not know whether a deleterious immunologic reaction is occurring in the mucosa despite absence of symptoms. Therefore, the chronic use of cromolyn in children must be carefully weighed, with due concern about long-term effects of antigen exposure. I consider this therapy to be experimental in children and almost never use it except as part of a research protocol.

Antihistamines should be considered with the same reservations as cromolyn. Despite their widespread use, I know of no well controlled, blinded study of their effectiveness in GI allergy.

Corticosteroids should be reserved for cases of intractable and life-threatening diarrhea that do not resolve with the administration of elemental diets or parenteral nutrition. In these cases they may be life-saving but side effects must be attended to. Eosinophilic gastroenteritis is a rare condition that may not respond to any measures but steroids. Cromolyn requires further investigation in patients with this rare and challenging syndrome.

There are many places in this country where food allergens are injected or given orally or sublingually to children with GI allergy. Although the proponents of this therapy claim remarkable results they have yet to subject their theories to controlled investigation. Usually the children have not been shown by objective challenges to have adverse reactions to the food in question. The results are probably due to the power of suggestion rather than cause and effect. In my opinion children should not be subjected to this therapy until its efficacy is demonstrated.

A final comment about food allergy, elimination diets, and feelings. There is much confusion surrounding this field; this can only be alleviated by careful diagnostic testing. Prolonged elimination diets are difficult for mothers, and older children who are not convinced of the importance of their diet will violate it at every opportunity. Children dislike being on special diets and thus being labeled as different from their peers and perhaps being viewed as ill. When prolonged elimination diets are necessary, children need to be directly encouraged to express their feelings about the situation. The physician can help by providing guidance about how much "cheating" is allowable. Challenges should be used to shorten the length of time the diet is required by determining when symptoms have resolved. They should also be used to determine if a small amount of the food may be regularly tolerated. These measures will make the trials and tribulations of GI food allergy more tolerable to children.

Adverse Reactions to Drugs

H. JAMES WEDNER, M.D.

Adverse reactions to drugs are a major medical and economic problem in the U.S. Recent studies suggest that half of all hospital admissions are related to therapeutic agents. Thus, the physician must carefully weigh the therapeutic potential of any drug against the possibility of an untoward reaction, with an eye to minimizing adverse drug reactions, recognizing that any drug has a potential for undesirable side effects. I will not attempt to catalog the many side effects seen with drugs, as these are well documented; rather I will outline the types of adverse reactions that may be seen, with some emphasis on hypersensitivity reactions and an approach to their evaluation.

Adverse reactions may be classified into three broad groups: dose related toxic effects, idiosyncratic reactions, and hypersensitivity reactions. The toxic reactions are unwanted pharmacologic effects of the drug. They will occur to some extent in all patients if sufficient quantities are given. They are "normal" properties of the drug. Toxic reactions may be further subdivided into those that occur within the therapeutic dose range, commonly referred to as side effects, and those that occur when doses produce blood or tissue concentrations in excess of therapeutic levels. In some cases these two classifications will merge, since the sensitivity of individuals to side effects varies widely and one person may tolerate high levels of a drug with no observable side effects while others cannot tolerate the drug at all. Patient perception may also be of great significance, particularly where side effects are concerned. The same degree of a symptom, for example nausea, may severely compromise one patient and be overlooked by another. This is seen with many drug side effects and one is not hard pressed to list several. A good example is the somnolence associated with antihistaminics. Often this occurs within the therapeutic dose range. In some instances the somnolence is mild, while in others it may be overwhelming and necessitate discontinuing the drug. In this case, as with a number of drug groups, switching from one chemical class of antihistaminic to another may allow one to maximize the therapeutic potential while minimizing the side effect. Often if the drug is continued, the undesirable side effects will disappear, while therapeutic potential is maintained. In other cases it may be possible to minimize side effects by starting at relatively low doses and building up gradually over a period of time. This is true not only with antihistaminics but also with such diverse groups as beta-adrenergic agonists or antihypertensive agents. It is important to explain to all patients that a potential exists for an undesirable side effect and that this effect may disappear if they will persevere in taking the drug.

Toxic reactions to drugs occur at dosages that yield blood levels in excess of the therapeutic range. However, these are still intimately related to the chemical nature of the agent and the amount of drug given. Examples include cardiotoxicity with digitalis, postural hypotension with antihypertensive agents, and nausea, vomiting, and (with sufficient drug) convulsions with theophylline or its salts. One must remember that the gap between therapeutic and toxic levels of a given drug varies widely with the type of agent and may be quite broad, giving the physician a great deal of latitude in prescribing, or it may be narrow, requiring careful blood level monitoring to ensure maximum benefit with minimum chance of toxic side effect. A notable example of this occurs in the use of theophylline for the treatment of asthma. With theophylline, the therapeutic range is generally considered to be 10 to 20 μg/ml, while the toxic range, beginning with mild anorexia and progressing through nausea and vomiting, generally starts between 18 and 20 μg/ml and becomes progressively worse at higher blood levels. Because the ability to biotransform theophylline varies widely between patients it is impossible to predict with certainty the blood level that will be achieved by a given dose. Therefore, measuring the exact blood level is the only way to achieve maximum therapeutic benefit while minimizing side effects. It should also be noted that with theophylline, as with a number of other drugs, some patients may be uncomfortable at relatively low blood levels, in a small percentage of patients as low as 10 to 15 μg/ml. In this instance one can still achieve therapeutic benefit by carefully adjusting the dose to achieve a blood level that, while at the low end of the thera-

peutic range, reduces the majority of unwanted toxic effects to acceptable levels. Similar consideration should be given with any drug whose toxic and therapeutic ranges approximate one another.

One must remember that the toxic effects of some classes of drugs are related to the total amount given and not to the absolute blood level achieved. In these instances one must keep in mind the progressive amount of drug (dose X duration) and discontinue use before reaching the level associated with toxic side effects. Excellent examples are gold salt toxicity or the toxic effect of various antibiotics. The aminoglycoside antibiotics cause renal toxicity and ototoxicity based on the total amount of drug given; chloramphenicol also has a toxic effect, bone marrow depression, related to the total cumulative dose.

Idiosyncratic reactions to drugs are unrelated to the amount or duration of therapy. They may occur with the introduction of the drug or may occur after long periods on an adequate therapeutic dose. They are impossible to predict, with the exception that a patient who has had one idiosyncratic reaction to a drug is likely to have a second if the drug is reinstituted. Remember also that some idiosyncratic drug reactions may be relatively benign while others are life threatening. Fortunately, most idiosyncratic reactions fall into the former category. One must always be aware of the potential for an idiosyncratic reaction, and in instances where this reaction may be life threatening, one must balance the potential for idiosyncratic reactions with the potential for therapeutic benefit. This should take into account the frequency and severity of idiosyncratic reactions. For example, although chloramphenicol related aplastic anemia is disastrous, the percent of patients who actually experience this idiosyncratic reaction is very small. Thus, it would be inappropriate to withhold this drug in cases where it would be life saving for fear of an idiosyncratic reaction. On the other hand, use of this drug when another antibiotic, with significantly less potential toxicity, is available would be inappropriate.

Toxic effects and idiosyncratic reactions of drugs most probably have different underlying biochemical bases. However, in some instances toxic and idiosyncratic effects may be very similar. And if toxicity effects occur, such as bone marrow depression with chloramphenicol, it is important to differentiate these dose related toxic effects from the idiosyncratic reactions. A patient who has had an idiosyncratic reaction to a drug should not be given the drug again unless one is faced with dire consequences. On the other hand, overdosage related toxic effects can be corrected with appropriate dose regimens and the patient can receive that drug or a drug of the same class again.

Hypersensitivity reactions can occur with virtually any drug. These can be differentiated into three basic types: immediate hypersensitivity (Type I), delayed antibody mediated of the Arthus type (IgG Type II and III), and cell mediated (Type IV). Immediate type reactions may be further subdivided into anaphylactic and anaphylactoid reactions. Anaphylactic reactions are those in which the drug induces the production of IgE antibody directed against the drug; the reaction occurs on subsequent administration of the drug following interaction of the agent with specific IgE molecules bound to tissue mast cells circulating basophils. Anaphylactoid reactions occur when release of mast cell mediators is accomplished through a non-IgE mediated mechanism. This may be the result of direct interaction of the drug with the mast cell membrane (e.g., release of chemical mediators by the drug polymyxin B) or may occur secondarily (e.g., interaction of the drug with the complement system with generation of the anaphylotoxins C5a and C3a). These anaphylotoxins are capable of inducing the release of mediators from mast cells or basophils, or both. In either case the net result is the same since the mediators released are identical.

A complete discussion of the chemical mediators of anaphylaxis is beyond the scope of this review. It is important only to say that they include a broad diversity of chemical entities including histamine, the slow reacting substances of anaphylaxis (leukotriene C, D, and E), prostaglandin D_2, platelet activating factor, trypsin-like proteolytic enzymes, chemotactic factors for eosinophils and neutrophils, as well as heparin. These factors, alone or in combination, are responsible for the symptoms of immediate hypersensitivity reactions, pruritus, urticaria, angioedema, laryngeal edema, wheezing, and hypotension. The severity of the reaction will depend on the location of the activated mast cells and the number of mast cells activated. Hypersensitivity reactions may be extremely mild (hives or mild pruritus) or may be an overwhelmingly severe systemic allergic reaction (anaphylaxis).

Since anaphylactoid reactions do not require the IgE antibody, they may occur on initial use of a given drug, although they sometimes occur after prolonged exposure, an example being the severe reactions seen with radiocontrast dyes. Current evidence suggests that, in susceptible individuals, injection of radiocontrast media causes activation of complement with release of anaphylotoxins and subsequent stimulation of mediator release from mast cells. The reactions that are seen suggest two other major points concerning anaphylactoid reactions. First, not every person experiences this type of reaction when presented with the drug, and in most cases the factors that determine which patients will react to a given drug are unknown. Secondly, although not all individuals will have a reaction on initial exposure, in general, patients who have one anaphylactoid reaction to a given

agent will continue to have these reactions unless intervention is taken. In the case of radiocontrast materials, where necessary, pretreatment of patients with corticosteroids and an H_1 type antihistaminic will decrease the severity of or completely abolish the reaction in more than 90% of the cases.

Another group of agents that cause anaphylactoid type reactions, either local or systemic, with some frequency are local anesthetics. Although in a few cases reactions to local anesthetics are the result of true anaphylactic sensitivity, in most cases histamine and other mediator release appears to result from direct interaction of the drug with the plasma membrane of mast cells. In this and many other instances, it would appear that the reactivity to these drugs is highly class specific, and in this case it is possible by using appropriate skin testing and provocative dose challenge protocols to utilize a local anesthetic to which the patient does not react. There is also the fact that the patient may not be reacting to the drug per se but rather to some other constituent of the preparation. This is particularly true with preservatives such as metabisulfites or parabens. Indeed, a patient seen by the author for sensitivity to a number of local anesthetics turned out in fact to be highly sensitive to sodium metabisulfite and when tested with metabisulfite-free preparations of a number of local anesthetics had no reaction. This patient was subsequently able to undergo extensive dental work under local anesthesia using s preservative-free preparation.

A number of drugs cause immediate hypersensitivity reactions by mechanisms that involve neither IgE formation nor direct or indirect mediator release. The classic example is aspirin, which is second only to penicillin in the number of patients who exhibit hypersensitivity reactions, and which has been studied extensively. However, the mechanism for reactions to aspirin, especially aspirin sensitive asthma, remains obscure. Neither IgE mediated nor direct activation seems to be present. Since aspirin is a potent inhibitor of the enzyme fatty acid cyclooxygenase, thereby inhibiting prostaglandin synthesis, it has been suggested that individuals sensitive to aspirin have a marked inhibition of a necessary prostaglandin or enhanced secretion of detrimental lipoxygenase products such as the leukotrienes. However, efforts to identify these metabolites have been unsuccessful. There are many other drugs in which the differentiation between anaphylactic and anaphylactoid reactions is obscure.

Anaphylactic reactions, as pointed out above, are the result of the generation of IgE (and perhaps IgG_4) type antibodies. As such, the drug must serve as a hapten and be conjugated to tissue proteins to be immunogenic. For this reason the ability of any drug to cause anaphylactic reactions is related to its ability to bind covalently (or in some cases non-covalently) to appropriate tissue proteins. The classic example of this type of reaction is seen in penicillin-allergic individuals. Here the penicillin is coupled to protein via an amide bond forming a penicilloyl protein derivative, which in susceptible individuals is highly immunogenic. The great ability of penicillin to interact with protein probably makes reaction to this drug the number one allergic drug problem in the U.S. today. One must remember that the major offending agent is not the penicillin itself but rather the penicilloyl moiety generated by cleavage of the β-lactam ring. A significant percentage of individuals (15–18%) do not react to the penicilloyl moiety but to a group of "minor determinants," which can be detected by skin testing using penicilloic acid or penicillin G itself. The exact immunogen is not known and one relies on rapid conjugation of penicillin G or penicilloic acid to tissue proteins, which then interact with cell-bound IgE. Antibodies to penicillin are directed against the core of the molecule, that is, the sulfur-containing thiozolidone (5 membered) and the β-lactam (4 membered) rings. For this reason a patient sensitive to one penicillin should be considered sensitive to any penicillin derivative. There are some rare exceptions; at Washington University we have seen three patients sensitive to carbenicillin but to no other penicillin, but these are very unusual (also see below). The cephalosporins are also potential problems: a small proportion of individuals produce a true anticephalosporin IgE. A much larger percentage, between 5 and 15% of penicillin-allergic patients, have an antipenicillin IgE that cross reacts with cephalosporins. Thus, although some authors consider cephalosporins to be a suitable alternative in penicillin-sensitive individuals, we do not, and due care must be taken, such as provocative dose challenge (see below), when treating penicillin-sensitive individuals with cephalosporins.

The third generation cephalosporins and fourth generation penicillins are a special case. Anecdotal reports suggest low cross-reactivity of these two groups with antipenicillin IgE, as might be expected from an examination of their chemical structure, and our experience would confirm this. To date we have not had a positive skin test to piperacillin or moxalactam in either penicillin skin test positive or negative individuals. Whether susceptible individuals will produce IgE directed against these newer β-lactam antibiotics remains to be seen.

Because the appropriate immunogens have been elucidated, patients with suspected penicillin allergy can be skin tested. Studies by our group and others have shown that penicillin skin testing can determine with a high degree of confidence whether a patient is at risk for a severe systemic reaction upon receiving the drug. Unfortunately,

only the major determinant is available commercially (penicilloylpolylysine [Pre-Pen, Kremers-Urban]). This will still identify 85% or more of patients at risk for anaphylaxis to penicillins. We strongly recommend skin testing for all patients with suspected penicillin allergy where penicillin would be the drug of choice. Moreover, with penicillin (as demonstrated by our group) it is possible to desensitize highly sensitive individuals by using increasing amounts of oral followed by parenteral penicillin, and subsequently full therapeutic doses of the drug. This procedure allows acutely ill patients who require penicillin to receive the drug. Similar desensitization studies have not been carried out with other drugs except insulin, where desensitization is also of great value.

The exact chemistry of the penicillin immunogen has been elegantly described. However, with most drugs, although evidence suggests that an IgE antibody directed against the drug is present, the exact chemistry of the immunogen is largely unknown. As a result, one must rely almost solely on the historical evaluation of the patient to determine that this is indeed a drug related immediate hypersensitivity reaction, since adequate skin test reagents are not available and simple skin testing may yield spurious results. In situations where one suspects from the history that the patient has a true allergy, two procedures are available. The most logical is to find an alternative therapeutic modality. In our experience, when physicians are questioned carefully, it is possible to find an alternative noncross-reacting drug in most cases. If a second noncross-reacting drug is unavailable or would not provide sufficient therapeutic benefit, one can utilize a procedure similar to that described for penicillin—begin with extremely small doses of the drug and administer increasingly larger amounts until therapeutic levels are obtained. The patient should be monitored closely for signs of allergic reactions and the protocol modified or discontinued if they occur. If there is doubt as to the allergic nature of the reaction, one can use the "provocative dose challenge" technique, in which a subtherapeutic dose of the drug is given, preferably by the oral route, and the patient observed for allergic symptoms for 20 to 60 minutes. If no reaction occurs, a second and perhaps third and fourth challenge with increasingly larger doses can be given, and if no adverse reaction occurs, the drug can be given in full therapeutic doses.

The progressive desensitization and provocative dose challenge techniques are designed merely to circumvent or prevent a severe systemic allergic reaction (anaphylaxis). They are not designed to prevent every allergic reaction, and desensitized patients may still exhibit mild allergic reactions, usually evidenced by hives or generalized pruritus. These patients should be maintained on the drug as long as necessary and the minor allergic manifestations treated with an appropriate antihistamine in adequate doses. Once a patient with drug hypersensitivity has been adequately desensitized, it is important that the drug be maintained for as long as necessary. It is not clear how long the desensitized state remains; it may be as long as several days or it may be relatively short, 6 to 12 hours. In this case, stopping therapy would necessitate reinstitution of the desensitization protocol, which could be difficult since patients tend to be somewhat hyperreactive for a time after the desensitized state is lost.

In addition to inducing IgE type antibodies, drugs are capable of inducing IgG type antibodies. IgG type antibodies are often relatively innocuous and neither affect the bioavailability of the drug nor cause any significant side reaction. For example, more than 90% of patients who receive parenteral penicillin will develop IgG antipenicillin antibodies. This, however, does not mean that they will have difficulties when penicillin therapy is reinstituted. On the other hand, IgG antibodies may lead to a number of significant drug reactions. These generally result from antibodies directed to the drug itself haptenized on tissue proteins or antibodies, which are directed against tissue proteins that have been altered by interaction with the drug. Drug protein conjugates may interreact with antibody in the fluid phase, yielding significant amounts of antigen-antibody complexes. This results in a serum-sickness–like picture. In addition, if the complex is large, other organs may be affected; for example, kidneys in drug-induced lupus erythematosus or Henoch-Schönlein purpura. In addition, drugs may be bound only to a particular organ, yielding diseases that are organ specific. Perhaps the best example of such a drug reaction is the production of antibodies that react with quinine (quinidine) bound to platelets, resulting in quinine induced severe thrombocytopenia. Similarly, drugs may bind to the liver, yielding a drug induced hepatitis, or to a variety of other specific organs. Although these diseases may in many ways mimic other diseases (e.g., autoimmune type phenomenon), they are generally self-limited and respond well to simple removal of the drug. The use of corticosteroids in these drug reactions is controversial and in most cases there is rapid clearing of drug and drug protein conjugates by antibody, and the use of steroids neither hinders nor helps.

A variety of drugs are also associated with the development of delayed cell mediated or delayed immunity, in which case the drug-protein conjugate results in the production of "effector" or cytotoxic T cells. Delayed sensitivity has been associated with a large number of drugs. Whether given orally or parenterally or applied to the skin, the major organ affected is the skin. Where local application of the drug is the route of administration, the classic picture is a pruritic papulopustular eruption limited to the areas where the drug was applied. The most common systemic reaction is generalized eczematoid dermatitis. Others are erythema multiforme and in rare cases erythema nodosum. Although many drugs have been implicated in Type IV reactions, the actual proof in many cases has been difficult. Reapplication of a drug to the skin (patch testing) can be done to identify reactions; however, drugs given parenterally or orally may require more sophisticated studies, such as in vitro blast transformation. Simple incubation of the drug with white cells in vitro may be inappropriate since, as already discussed for Type I reactions, the true immunogen is a drug-protein conjugate. In "fixed drug eruption" (a skin reaction that occurs in the same limited area of the skin each time the drug is introduced), a serum factor that transforms lymphocytes has been described, suggesting that this is a Type IV reaction. Although patch testing or other laboratory studies can be performed, in most instances sophisticated laboratory studies are not necessary and sufficient information can be obtained from a careful history.

For all of the hypersensitivity states it is important to remember that immunogenicity or lack thereof, or the type of response stimulated, is related not only to the drug and its chemical properties but also to the route of administration. For example, many drugs when given orally are much less immunogenic than when given parenterally. A drug may induce a Type IV reaction when applied to the skin but be relatively nonimmunogenic in oral or parenteral form. A case in point is the antihistaminics, which are infrequent producers of hypersensitivity unless applied topically, where they commonly produce delayed hypersensitivity reactions. These considerations have practical benefit. Selection of the appropriate dosage form, avoiding those associated with the induction of hypersensitivity states, may help to prevent hypersensitivity reactions.

The list of drug-related adverse effects presented here, while not complete, does indicate the broad diversity of adverse reactions that can occur. Drugs may have side effects that represent pharmacologic actions other than those actually desired. These effects may occur at blood levels within the therapeutic range or at supratherapeutic levels, or may be related to a cumulative dose. The adverse reaction may be idiosyncratic or may result from hypersensitivity. Anaphylactoid hypersensitivity reactions may represent a pharmacologic effect of the drug on an unknown enzyme system (e.g., aspirin), interaction with complement system, or a direct action on the surface of the mast cell or basophil. In addition, drugs capable of conjugating to tissue proteins may generate an immune response against the drug protein complex. The immune response may be a Type I anaphylactic reaction due to production of specific IgE, a Type II or III response due to production of IgG and subsequent formation of either antigen-antibody complexes or cytotoxic antibodies, or a Type IV cell-mediated response.

The physician must be aware of the broad diversity of adverse reactions to drugs that can occur. In most cases a careful detailed drug history will alert the physician to the potential of an adverse reaction to a drug, and this can then be handled by use of an alternative therapeutic modality, by appropriate treatment of the patient to block the effects of mediator release, or by appropriate desensitization procedures. The patient as well as the physician must be apprised of the potential for side effects, the nature of these side effects, and the methods that will be utilized to decrease or circumvent them. In this way, one hopes, the problem of drug related adverse reactions can be minimized and, where they occur, treated appropriately. No drug is free of adverse effects and, as long as physicians continue to utilize drug therapy, adverse reactions will continue to be a major problem. This should not lead to therapeutic nihilism but to the use of measures to minimize or circumvent these reactions.

Physical Allergy

JOHN A. ANDERSON, M.D.

Physical factors, such as mechanical pressure, light, heat, cold, water, and exercise, may result in urticaria, angioedema, or systemic signs and symptoms usually associated with allergic reactions. As a group, these reactions are referred to as physical allergies. The exact incidence of physical factors resulting in "allergic" reactions in children is unknown, but urticaria caused by physical factors accounts for approximately 3% of all patients with urticaria and 10% of patients with chronic urticaria (mostly adults). Cold-induced urticaria followed by cholinergic urticaria is the most common physical urticaria seen in children.

The therapy used in physical allergy involves either avoidance of the physical agent or pharmacologic therapy designed to combat the effects of chemical mediators released by exposure to these agents.

GENERAL PRINCIPLES OF PHARMACOTHERAPY

Table 1 lists the antihistamines used for the treatment of physical allergy and the usual dose for children, beginning with the most commonly used drug. Table 2 lists the emergency and adjuvant drugs used in the treatment of these conditions.

The prime drug used in the emergency treatment

of urticaria and angioedema is Adrenalin. In the usual case of urticaria/angioedema and exercise-induced anaphylaxis seen in the emergency situation, a systemically administered antihistamine, such as IM Benadryl, is also given. Followup treatment could include Sus-Phrine, a long-acting form of epinephrine (4–6 hours), and antihistamines to be taken at home, such as Benadryl, 25 mg three times daily, or Chlor-Trimeton, 4 to 8 mg three times daily.

For prophylactic treatment of any of the physical urticaria/angioedema conditions or exercise-induced anaphylaxis, the use of a single antihistamine listed in Table 1 might be tried, but hydroxyzine (Atarax) usually is most effective. Because Benadryl and Atarax are likely to produce drowsiness, other antihistamines, such as either the chlorpheniramines or brompheniramines, might be tried. Cyproheptadine (Periactin) is most efficacious in the treatment of cold urticaria. In resistant cases of cold urticaria/angioedema, various combinations of antihistamines might be tried, including Benadryl, Atarax, or Chlor-Trimeton during the day, plus Phenergan or PBZ at night. Azatadine (Optimine*) and clemastine fumarate (Tavist*) are newer, longer-acting antihistamines usually used for the treatment of allergic rhinitis. However, in some cases of pruritus-urticaria/angioedema, these drugs might be tried if other antihistamines have failed to control the condition.

Recently, there have been reports of successful use of the combination of a new H-2 histamine receptor drug, cimetidine (Tagamet), with one of the H-1 antihistamines, such as hydroxyzine, in the treatment of chronic urticaria. Experience has shown the effect to be variable among patients.

In addition, terbutaline (Bricanyl) and theophylline compounds have been shown to decrease histamine release in hypersensitivity states. Both drugs decreased chronic urticaria/angioedema in some studies, in spite of the fact that neither drug has been shown to significantly alter the antigen-induced immediate-reacting skin test. From experience, we have found that some resistant cases of chronic urticaria/angioedema (physically induced or idiopathic) respond to the addition of either terbutaline† (2.5 mg three times a day) or a theophylline compound (enough Slo-Phyllin given three times a day to maintain a theophylline level between 10 and 20 μg/ml) with one of the single or multiple antihistamine regimens.

Corticosteroids may be used in the treatment of severe emergency urticaria/angioedema or anaphylaxis. These drugs may be helpful on a short-

---

*Safety and efficacy in children under 12 years of age have not been established.

†Manufacturer's Precaution: Not recommended for children under 12 years of age.

Table 1. ANTIHISTAMINES FOR TREATMENT OF PHYSICAL ALLERGY

Antihistamine Class (Histamine Receptor)	Drug (Common Name)	Usual Dose, 27-KG Child (Dose by Weight)
Ethanolamine (H–1)	Diphenhydramine (Benadryl) (more sedative)	12.5–50 mg 3 × daily (5 mg/kg/24 hr—not to exceed 300 mg/24 hr)
Ataractic (H–1)	Hydroxyzine (Atarax, Vistaril) (more sedative)	10–25 mg 3 × daily
Alkylamine (H–1)	1. Chlorpheniramine (Chlor-Trimeton, Teldrin) 2. Brompheniramine (Dimetane) (less sedative)	2–8 mg 3 × daily
Piperidine (H–1)	1. Cyproheptadine (Periactin)	2–4 mg 3–4 × daily (0.25 mg/kg/24 hr)
	2. Azatadine (Optimine)	1–2 mg 2 × daily; not recommended under 12 yr of age
Phenothiazine (H–1)	Promethazine (Phenergan)	6.25–12.5 mg 3 × daily
Ethylenediamine (H–1)	Tripelennamine (PBZ)	25–50 mg 3 × daily (5 mg/kg/24 hr—not to exceed 300 mg/24 hr)
Benzhydryl ether (H–1)	Clemastine fumarate (Tavist)	1.34 mg 2 × daily; not recommended under 12 yr of age
Thioguanidine (H–2)	Cimetidine (Tagamet)	20–40 mg/kg/24 hr; very limited experience in children under 16 yr of age

Table 2. EMERGENCY AND ADJUVANT DRUGS FOR TREATMENT OF PHYSICAL ALLERGY

Drug Type	Drug (Common Name)	Usual Children's Dosage
Sympathomimetics	Epinephrine HCL 1:1000 (Adrenalin)	0.1–0.3 ml/dose subQ (0.005–0.01 ml/kg/dose)
	Epinephrine 1:200 in thioglycolate (Sus-Phrine)	0.05–0.15 ml/dose subQ (0.005 ml/kg/dose)
	Epinephrine HCL 1:1000 (Adrenalin) in Ana-Kit (Hollister-Stier Labs.)	0.3 ml/dose; 2 doses possible
	Epinephrine HCL 1:100 (Adrenalin) in EpiPen (Center Labs.)	0.3 ml in automatic doser
	Metaproterenol (Alupent, Metaprel)	1–3 puffs by inhalation; not recommended under 12 yr of age
	Terbutaline (Bricanyl, Brethine)	2.5–5.0 mg 3 × daily; not recommended under 12 yr of age
	Albuterol (Proventil, Ventoline)	1–3 puffs by inhalation; not recommended under 12 yr of age
Methylxanthine	Theophylline (Slo-Phyllin 60, 125, 250 mg) (Theo-Dur 100, 200, 300 mg)	Therapeutic blood levels, 10–20 µg/ml
Corticosteroid	Prednisone (Prednisone 5 mg)	As needed
Other	Cromolyn Sodium (Intal)	20-mg powder by inhalation per dose; not recommended under 5 yr of age

term basis for exacerbation of the problem but are not a substitute for the antihistamines. Corticosteroids have not been helpful on a long-term basis in the routine treatment of physical allergies.

SPECIFIC THERAPY

Dermographia. Treatment of dermographia consists of avoiding trauma and, when necessary, the use of an antihistamine. Hydroxyzine (Atarax) is the most likely drug to be helpful in this condition (on an as needed basis), although other antihistamines and drug combinations may be tried.

Pressure Urticaria/Angioedema. Treatment consists of avoiding sustained pressures as much as possible. Antihistamines, and even corticosteroids, can be tried but are usually not helpful.

Vibratory Angioedema. Treatment consists of avoiding the vibrating stimulus. Usually the condition is mild and does not require medications.

Urticaria/Angioedema Secondary to Light Exposure. Drug ingestion combined with sunlight exposure may result in either a direct toxic rash (phototoxic reaction) or an immunologic contact dermatitis (photoallergic reaction). Drugs implicated in causing a phototoxic reaction include psoralens, topical coal tar, and dimethylchlortetracycline. Drugs implicated in photoallergic reactions include phenothiazines, sulfonamides, and griseofulvin. Bacteriostatic agents like bithionol and halogenated salicylamides, used in soaps and topical medications, can also induce reactions.

Light can also produce sunburn and exacerbate primary dermatologic and systemic diseases, including the polymorphic light eruption and systemic lupus erythematosus.

Management of this condition is often difficult and consists primarily of avoiding the reaction-producing light wavelength. In the case of drug sensitivity, the treatment consists of correctly identifying and then avoiding the causative drug or chemical.

Repeated exposure to small, increasing doses of sunlight may induce tolerance in some patients. It is advisable to wear protective garments whenever possible. Sunscreens or sun-blocking agents can be used to help protect skin exposed to sun in susceptible individuals.

Chemical sunscreens act by absorbing a specific portion of the ultraviolent light spectrum. Chemical sunscreens include agents such as paraaminobenzoic acid (PABA), esters of PABA, the benzophenones, digalloyl trioleate, the cinnamates, the anthranilates, the pyrones, and the salicylates. For an agent to be effective, it must have the ability to absorb ultraviolet light in the 290- to 320-nm range —the range at which virtually all sunburns occur. Five per cent PABA in 50 to 70% ethanol provides an excellent protection against sunburn. The benzophenones, unlike the other sunscreens, also absorb long-wave ultraviolet light in the 320- to 400-nm range. In a recent comparative study, a preparation of 7% octyl-dimethyl PABA ester and 3% oxybenzone (Improved Super Shade Lotion) proved superior as a chemical sunscreen to other agents, including 5% PABA (Pre-Sun Lotion).

Sensitivity to wavelengths of light above 320 nanometers may be avoided by the use of physical sunscreens or sun-blocking agents, even though they are less cosmetically acceptable than the chemical sunscreens. Some available agents include zinc oxide paste (RVPaque); titanium dioxide (A-Fil Cream or Solar Cream) and red veterinary petrolatum (RVP Cream or RV Plus).

The 280- to 320-nm UV light (sunburn range) is filtered by window glass. The higher wavelengths, which can still produce light sensitivity in some patients, are not filtered by ordinary glass.

Antihistamines and corticosteroids given orally may reduce the reactions to light. Although the antimalarial drug chloroquine has been used in resistant cases of light sensitivity, the results are disappointing.

Cholinergic Urticaria. "Keeping cool" is a good rule when one is considering the management of cholinergic urticaria. Antihistamines are usually helpful, beginning with hydroxyzine (Atarax) or diphenhydramine (Benadryl) and progressing to combination therapies. A trial on anticholinergic medications, such as Pro-Banthine,[†] 7.5 mg one to three mg one to three times daily, has been advised, but this drug has not been helpful in this condition in our experience.

Another method, that of deliberately producing the rash (such as taking a warm shower) in order to produce a short refractory period, is also not a helpful treatment method in our opinion.

Localized Heat Urticaria. This rare disorder can be confirmed by placing a carefully heated Erlenmeyer flask of water on an area of skin. The hive reaction usually occurs within minutes. Antihistamines have been reported to block the heat challenge.

Cold-Induced Urticaria/Angioedema. The mainstay of treatment in cold-induced conditions is to avoid chilling the body. During the summer, one should be careful about sudden changes in temperature, especially swimming in cold water. During the winter, one should be certain to wear good gloves and warm footgear since the skin of the extremities is already at a lower ambient temperature. A hat is important since the head is a major source of heat loss from the body. A mask can be helpful for protecting the exposed area of the face.

[†]Safety and efficacy in children have not been established.

In one study, cyproheptadine (Periactin) was the superior antihistamine in preventing cold reactions, but hydroxyzine (Atarax) and other antihistamines and antihistamine-theophylline or -terbutaline combinations should be tried in stubborn cases.

Gradual "desensitization" to cold by taking serial baths with increasingly cold water has been advocated as a therapy for this condition. In our opinion, the therapy is generally unsuccessful.

Exercise- and Cold-Induced Asthma. Most children with asthma have some degree of bronchoconstriction when they exercise; in some asthmatics, exercise is the major reason for wheezing. Children may also wheeze when exposed to cold air. Running is the exercise most likely to produce wheezing, and swimming is the exercise least likely to do so. The therapy in exercise-induced asthma involves avoidance of that type of exercise and the degree of exercise that produces significant difficulty—when possible. To restrict otherwise normal children, however, from all exercise, especially running, is not practical in our society.

In some cases, children can "run through" their exercise-induced asthma. Breathing through the nose rather than the mouth while exercising, thus allowing the inhaled air to become properly heated and humidified, reduces exercise-induced asthma. Recently, the use of a cheap, disposable, hard-paper surgical mask that fits over the nose and mouth has been found to reduce exercise-induced asthma significantly. The mask works by allowing the patient to "rebreathe" a reservoir of warm, humidified air when exercising.

Medication also can be used to reduce or prevent an exercise-induced asthma (Table 2). Cromolyn sodium‡ (Intal) by inhalation one half hour before exercise provides significant help in 60% of children up to 2 to 4 hours. Inhaled sympathomimetics taken immediately before exercising, such as the use of metaproterenol§ (Alupent) or albuterol (Proventil), are most efficacious in reducing the incidence of exercised-induced asthma, but there are some cardiovascular side effects with these drugs, as opposed to essentially no side effects with cromolyn sodium. Oral sympathomimetic agents and oral theophylline agents are helpful but not as efficacious as metaproterenol, albuterol, or cromolyn sodium. Inhaled atropine-like compounds, are helpful in this condition in about one third of the cases.

The treatment of cold-induced asthma is similar to that of exercise-induced asthma.

Exercise-Induced Anaphylaxis. Recently, a group of young adults have been described who develop symptoms of anaphylaxis, including pruritus, generalized urticaria, angioedema, nasal stuffiness, and, on occasion, abdominal colic, dizziness, and collapse while exercising, particularly jogging. These patients were found not to have exercise-induced asthma or cholinergic urticaria. The mechanism of action in this condition is not clear, although some patients are atopic and may be experiencing increased exposure during jogging to environmental allergens, such as pollen.

The therapy for this condition involves the avoidance of strenuous exercises like jogging. In some instances, this is not acceptable to the patients. The use of antihistamines, such as hydroxyzine (Atarax) or other drug combinations prior to exercise may be helpful. On an emergency basis, Adrenalin is the prime mode of therapy for anaphylaxis. Since some patients may have a history of a potential life-threatening episode of exercise-induced anaphylaxis and may refuse to discontinue the practice of strenuous exercise, they should be supplied with Adrenalin in a loaded syringe and taught to use this drug in an emergency situation. Ana-Kit (supplied primarily for patients allergic to stinging insects) contains such a conveniently loaded syringe of Adrenalin. The dose may be varied but usually is 0.3 ml, which is suitable for an older teenager and adult but not a young child. An automatically administered Adrenalin device that will penetrate clothing (i.e., of the thigh) is also available (EpiPen); the dose is fixed at 0.3 ml and is not suitable for young children. See Table 2 for recommended pediatric doses of epinephrine.

Anaphylaxis

IRVING W. BAILIT, M.D.

Anaphylaxis is the most frightening and potentially life-threatening allergic reaction in man. Clinical manifestations usually appear in 1 to 30 minutes. The rapidity of the reaction is directly related to its intensity. Deaths result from acute laryngeal edema, acute pulmonary emphysema, and cardiovascular collapse. Manifestations may affect different organ systems, which include skin (urticaria, angioedema), respiratory (acute wheezing, laryngeal stridor), cardiovascular (hypotension, shock), gastrointestinal (cramps, vomiting, diarrhea), and central nervous (seizures, loss of consciousness).

Atopic persons are more susceptible to anaphylaxis. Deaths are less common in children and are mostly caused by laryngeal edema. Classic anaphylaxis is the result of IgE mediated release of chemical mediators (histamine, leukotrienes, ECF-A, kinins, and prostaglandins) in previously

---

‡Cromolyn sodium is not recommended for children under 5 years of age.

§Inhalation form is not recommended for children under 5 years of age.

sensitized individuals. Anaphylactoid reactions are similar nonimmunologic responses resulting from direct release of mediators from tissue mast cells and basophils.

Numerous diverse agents can trigger anaphylactic reactions. The most common are drugs, especially penicillin and aspirin, and the stinging insects (yellow jacket, honeybee, hornet, wasp, and fire ant). Foods most likely to provoke an immediate allergic reaction include nuts, milk, egg, fish, shellfish, legumes, berries, and seeds. Radiographic contrast media will cause anaphylactoid reactions in 1 to 2% of those tested. Other causes are hormones, antisera, enzymes, exercise, and immunotherapy for venoms and environmental allergens.

TREATMENT

Anaphylactic reactions are sudden in onset and require immediate treatment. All medical personnel should be trained in the proper management of such reactions and have the needed medication and equipment readily available. They should also be trained in basic cardiopulmonary resuscitation. Initial management should be started in the office. Severe, unresponsive patients should be transferred to hospital intensive care units when transfer is feasible.

The most important drug is aqueous epinephrine (Adrenalin), 1:1000 (0.01 ml/kg). The usual pediatric dose is 0.3 ml (range 0.1–0.5 ml) given subcutaneously for mild reactions and intramuscularly for moderate reactions. Dose may be repeated three times at 15 to 20-minute intervals. Blood pressure should be monitored. In cases of cardiovascular collapse, epinephrine dose may be diluted in 10 ml of saline and given slowly over several minutes by intravenous injection.

If the antigen is introduced by an injection or sting on an extremity, apply a tourniquet proximal to the site and inject epinephrine 1:1000 (0.1–0.2 ml) subcutaneously at the injection/sting site to prevent antigen absorption.

Follow epinephrine therapy with diphenhydramine (Benadryl) given orally or IM (25–50 mg). Severe reactions should be treated intravenously (2 mg/kg) up to 50 mg per dose over 3 minutes. Continue this drug orally for 48 hours (5 mg/kg/24 hours).

In the presence of acute wheezing, administer aminophylline (5–7 mg/kg) in IV solution slowly over a 20-minute period. If necessary maintain by constant infusion (0.6–1.0 mg/kg/hr) and monitor theophylline levels.

Hypotensive patients should be placed in a recumbent position with the lower extremities elevated. Give IV normal saline rapidly (2000–3000 ml/m²/24 hrs.) Use volume expanders for hypovolemia. If IV saline and epinephrine do not main-

tain adequate blood pressure, use vasopressor drugs.

1. Metaraminol bitartrate (Aramine): Give 0.4 mg/kg in 500 ml of 5% D/W or saline slowly while monitoring the rate of infusion with the blood pressure response and possible cardiac arrhythmias.
2. Levarterenol bitartrate (Levophed) may be used as an alternative drug. Add 4 mg (4 ml) to 1000 ml of 5% D/W at a rate of 1 to 2 ml/min while monitoring the blood pressure. In children give 1 mg (1 ml) in 250 ml of 5% D/W at 0.5 ml/min.

Corticosteroids may be useful for control of persistent or recurrent symptoms. Since these drugs take up to several hours for significant effect they are not first line therapy for the acute episode. Start with 7 mg/kg of hydrocortisone (Solu-Cortef), 100 to 300 mg, followed by 7 ml/kg/24 hr at 4- to 6-hour intervals. Methylprednisolone (Solu-Medrol), 2 mg/kg/stat and 2 mg/kg/24 hr may also be used. Milder reactions can be treated with oral steroids.

Monitor vital signs and maintain a patent oral airway. Oxygen should be available and administered when there is evidence of hypoxia. In the presence of laryngeal edema a cricothyrotomy tube or a large (#12 or #14) needle should be available to establish a temporary airway until facilities and personnel are available to insert an endotracheal tube or perform a tracheostomy.

Measurement of central venous pressure, arterial blood gasses and electrocardiogram may be necessary for optimum management.

In addition to the above medications, necessary equipment includes a tourniquet, needles and syringes, parenteral fluids with intravenous tubing, oral airway, suction bulb, Ambu bag, and a cricothyrotomy tube or large needle (#12 or #14)

PREVENTION

Many anaphylactic reactions can be prevented by taking a comprehensive history of previous reactions to drugs, foods, immunizations, insect stings, and diagnostic agents. Avoid when possible drugs that have caused previous allergic responses.

A history of penicillin sensitivity is an indication to avoid penicillin and its analogs and the cephalothins to which they may cross react. Testing for reaction to penicillin using both the major and minor antigen determinants is a reliable method of determining the presence of penicillin hypersensitivity. Avoid penicillin positive skin test reactors and give penicillin orally in preference to parenteral administration. For life-threatening situations requiring penicillin (i.e., subacute bacterial endocarditis) in proven penicillin-sensitive patients, consider the newer methods of oral desensitization.

Remember that allergic children are more likely

to develop hypersensitivity to foods, drugs, and radiocontrast agents. Questionable food reactions may be skin tested by the scratch or prick method or by RAST testing. While many foods are tolerated with increasing age, some food anaphylaxis (nuts and fish) may persist for a lifetime.

Patients with previous anaphylactoid reactions to radiocontrast media in whom repeat study is mandatory should be pretreated with prednisone 50 mg orally every 6 hours for three doses prior to study and diphenhydramine (Benadryl) 50 mg IM 1 hour before the procedure.

Children who have had serious anaphylactic reactions to stinging insects and positive venom skin tests should be given protective immunotherapy to the offending venoms.

Known egg-sensitive children should be tested for reaction to vaccines grown from chick embryo tissue prior to administration of the vaccine.

Physicians who administer programs of immunotherapy to venoms or inhalant allergens must be prepared to treat systemic reactions. Local reactions can be used as a guideline in determining antigen dose. Seasonal allergens should be decreased during the active pollen season. Observe patients for at least 20 minutes after injection.

Children with a history of an anaphylactic reaction should have an emergency kit containing a loaded epinephrine syringe (AnaKit, EpiPen). Patient or parent must be instructed on the indications and technique for its use. A bracelet that identifies the patient and his hypersensitivity reaction may prove useful (MedicAlert Foundation, Turlock, California).

20

Accidents and Emergencies

Botulinal Food Poisoning

BARRY H. RUMACK, M.D.

Botulism is most frequently due to improperly home-processed foods such as vegetables, meats, fruits, pickles, and seafood. Rarely, commercial products are involved and recently these have been fish and meat products, especially in soups. Simple cooking for 6 to 10 minutes is capable of destroying the formed toxin.

Treatment. Empty the stomach, being careful to protect the airway. Administer activated charcoal and a cathartic. Hospitalize if there are *any* symptoms (paralysis, ptosis, blurred vision, diplopia, sore throat, other). Administration of antitoxin should be done under the supervision of the Centers for Disease Control or State health department. Guanidine therapy has been used in some cases, as has penicillin. The value of either of these drugs is questionable. Treatment consists primarily of antitoxin and respiratory support. Patients with minimal findings, usually mild neurologic, that do not progress will not require therapy. Treatment for the supportive and other needs of the patient is similar to treatment of any serious neurologic problem. Recovery is the rule with modern therapy.

Acute Poisoning

BARRY H. RUMACK, M.D.

The epidemiology of poisonings has been difficult to determine until recently because of previous poor case finding. The Rocky Mountain Poison Center, for example, reported 7545 cases in 1972

and 73,700 cases in 1982. This increase is well above the increase in population in the region served over this time and is probably due to increased visibility of the poison center and better case finding. Mortality had been reported at 1 or 2 cases a year since the poison center was opened in 1956 and jumped rapidly with modern data-collecting methods. A decline in mortality rate over the past 5 years is due to a number of factors, including advent of container closure safety laws; tremendous improvement in quality and availability of emergency physicians; earlier awareness of potential toxicity by parents and relatives; and rapidly available, high quality information concerning poison treatment. National statistics on poisoning are not readily available because of lack of sufficient case

Table 1. FORMS OF POISONING

	Per Cent
Drugs—Miscellaneous	15.4
Life Forms and Products	13.5
Central Nervous System Drugs	11.9
Household Products	11.8
CNS Drugs—Analgesics	9.5
Personal Products	8.4
Pesticides	6.3
Petroleum Products	5.7
Over-the-Counter Drugs	5.2
Dietary Supplements	2.8
Autonomic Drugs	1.9
Antiseptics	1.6
Local-Acting Agents	1.6
Gastrointestinal Products	1.5
Antimicrobials	1.1
Hormones	1.0
Cardiovascular Drugs	0.9

reports to the National Clearinghouse for Poison Control Centers.

Categories in which cases occur are presented in Table 1. The percentages have been rounded off and undoubtedly vary somewhat from community to community. Local poison centers should be consulted for area statistics and specific local problems.

While there are many poison prevention activities, one of the most effective is distribution of a poison checklist and a discussion of the problem by the pediatrician, nurse practitioner, or health associate at the 6-month checkup. Giving the mother a bottle of syrup of ipecac is probably the only way to make sure it actually will get into a home. Table 2 provides the checklist, which should be reproduced and distributed to parents.

MANAGEMENT OF THE INITIAL EVENT

Telephone

Most cases will initially come to attention over the telephone. If the parent or patient calls the

Table 2. CHECK LIST FOR POISON-PROOFING THE HOME

KITCHEN	☐ No household products under the sink ☐ No medicines on counters or open areas, refrigerator top, or window sills ☐ All cleaners, household products, and medications out of reach ☐ All cleaners, household products, and medications in original, safety top containers
BATHROOM	☐ Medicine chest cleaned out regularly ☐ Old medications flushed down toilet ☐ All medicines in original safety top containers ☐ All medicines, sprays, powders, cosmetics, fingernail preparations, hair care products, mouthwash, and so on out of reach
BEDROOM	☐ No medicines in or on dresser or bedside table ☐ All perfumes, cosmetics, powders, and sachets out of reach
LAUNDRY AREA	☐ All bleaches, soaps, detergents, fabric softeners, bluing agents, and sprays out of reach ☐ All products in original containers
GARAGE, BASEMENT	☐ Insect spray and weed killers in locked area ☐ Gasoline and car products in locked area ☐ Turpentine, paints, and paint products in locked area ☐ All in original containers
GENERAL HOUSEHOLD	☐ Alcoholic beverages out of reach ☐ Ashtrays empty and out of reach ☐ Plants out of reach ☐ Painted surfaces in good repair ☐ All household and personal products out of reach

physician rather then a poison information center, certain factors become imperative for providing quality care.

History Records. All poison calls must be noted, with time, name, address, phone number, substance, and amount ingested. Any advice provided should be written down. Some patients will become hysterical or comatose on the phone and will require the dispatch of emergency equipment. Follow-up calls may be necessary to change initial advice. In fact, it is considered inappropriate to manage a patient over the telephone without calling back at intervals (usually 1, 2, 4, and 24 hours) to make sure instructions have been followed and patients are responding appropriately.

Severity. Determination of the degree of the problem is important in order to make recommendations for care. No Danger—e.g., a patient who has eaten a crayon or sucked on a ball point pen. Potential Danger—e.g., a patient who has consumed a bottle of adult aspirins. Clearly the patient will have to be seen within a short time; the decision to be made is whether this should be at the office or hospital. Immediate Danger—e.g., a child who has ingested some strychnine-base rat poison. An emergency vehicle should usually be sent to the scene since it will have trained personnel, suction, and medications.

Prevention of Absorption

Eye. Rapid dilution with copious quantities of water is imperative. Any source of clean water should be used as gently as possible after an episode. A common error is to communicate to patients that they should go immediately to the emergency department. This should be done *after* initial dilution.

Skin. Many agents, such as organophosphate insecticides, are absorbed well through the skin. Warm soapy water with a soft cloth or sponge should be used to cleanse the skin following any chemical contact. Many patients have developed delayed symptoms because contaminated clothing was left in place. Medical personnel who come in contact with these chemicals also should clean off affected areas so they do not become patients.

Oral. The use of dilution should be reserved for the times and chemicals when a lowered concentration of the substance would decrease toxicity. Medication, for example, should not be diluted, since this might serve to enhance absorption. Water or milk is the safest agent for use. The use of dilution in such situations as caustic ingestion is particularly important within 30 seconds after ingestion if burns are to be prevented.

Emesis. Syrup of ipecac in appropriate doses (30 ml for adult dose; 10 to 15 ml for pediatric dose) has been shown to be a safe and effective means of producing emesis. While apomorphine has a more rapid onset of action than ipecac syrup has, the average percentage of recovery is the same. Apomorphine is notoriously toxic in children because of its narcotic depressant effects, which may persist past the reversal effects of naloxone administered to counteract the toxicity of this emetic. In addition, apomorphine may result in protracted vomiting, which is often unresponsive to narcotic antagonist intervention. Emesis 60 minutes after ingestion produces recovery of 30 per cent of gastric contents.

Emesis is generally contraindicated when the patient is comatose, convulsing, or without the gag reflex. Strong acid or base ingestion is another reason for not inducing emesis since this will re-expose the patient's esophagus to these agents, thus contributing to further damage.

Lavage. Gastric lavage with a large-bore tube is a rapid and effective way to empty the stomach. While there has been criticism in the past of this technique, most comparative studies were performed with ipecac emesis and a small-bore (No. 16 French) lavage tube. Proper lavage with large (No. 36 to 40 French) tubes utilizing 10 to 20 liters of warm tap water in an adult or 5 to 10 liters of warm saline in a child is the method of choice to empty the stomach if a contraindication to emesis exists, if the patient is symptomatic, or if an adult has ingested an unusually large or toxic amount of agent.

Cathartics. The rationale for the administration of cathartics in the poisoned patient is to hasten the toxin through the gastrointestinal tract to minimize its absorption. Although no controlled data are available for the use of cathartic agents, they are indicated in several situations: ingestion of enteric-coated tablets, when the lag time following ingestion is greater than 1 hour, and with hydrocarbons. Preferred agents are the saline cathartics (sodium sulfate, magnesium sulfate, citrate, or phosphates), which have a relatively prompt onset of action and lower toxicity than the oil-based cathartics, which have attendant aspiration risks.

Charcoal. It has been demonstrated that sufficient quantities of charcoal will bind many toxins that have not been removed by emesis or lavage. Charcoal can "catch up" with drugs and other agents once they have passed through the pylorus. Ample evidence shows that administration of charcoal following methods to empty the stomach will result in lower plasma levels than if emesis or lavage alone is used. Concomitant administration of activated charcoal with syrup of ipecac renders the ipecac ineffective. Hence, charcoal should not be administered until after emesis has occurred.

Enhancement of Excretion

Urinary excretion of certain toxins can be hastened by forced acid or alkaline diuresis or by dialysis (hemodialysis or peritoneal dialysis).

Diuresis. Forced diuresis is often useful in serious poisonings if the drug is excreted in the urine in active form. The technique should not be used unless it is specifically indicated, as it may increase the likelihood of cerebral edema, a common cause of death in poisonings.

Excretion of any of the following can be hastened by forced diuresis:

Alcohol
Amphetamines (acid)
Bromides
Isoniazid (big anion gaps; alkalinization needs will be massive)
Jequirity beans (alkaline diuresis)
Phencyclidine (acid diuresis)
Phenobarbital (alkaline diuresis)
Salicylates (alkaline diuresis)
Strychnine (acid diuresis)

Hypertonic or pharmacologic diuretics should be given, along with adequate fluids. The usual urine flow is 0.5 to 2 ml/kg/hr; with forced diuresis, urine flow should increase to 3 to 6 ml/kg/hr. Alkaline or acid diuresis should be chosen on the basis of the pK_a of the toxin, so that ionized drug will be trapped in the tubular lumen and not reabsorbed. (See Table 3.) Thus, if the pK_a is less than 7.0, alkaline diuresis is appropriate; if it is over 8.0, use acid diuresis. Osmotic load is also important, and either type of diuretic should be given at intervals. Caution: rhabdomyolysis may occur in some poisonings and is a contraindication to acid diuresis.

Alkaline Diuresis. This can usually be accomplished with bicarbonate. It is well to observe for potassium depletion, in which case it is necessary to administer potassium chloride or potassium citrate, which has both potassium and considerable alkalinizing ability. It is also available orally as K-Lyte effervescent tablets ("fizzies"), which are a quite palatable form. Follow serum K^+ deficiency carefully.

Acid Diuresis. This may be accomplished with ascorbic acid, arginine, or ammonium chloride, all of which may be given intravenously or orally. *Ascorbic acid* may be given in doses of 0.5 to 1 gm orally or intravenously as needed to obtain acid urine (pH of 4.5 to 5.5). *Ammonium chloride* may be given in a total dose of 2 to 6 gm/24 hr or 75 mg/kg/dose in 4 divided doses. It comes as a solution for intravenous use or as tablets or syrup for oral administration. *Mannitol* diuresis may accomplish an acid urine without any additional measures.

Dialysis. Hemodialysis (or peritoneal dialysis if hemodialysis is unavailable) is useful in the poisonings listed below. Dialysis should be considered part of supportive care if the patient satisfies any of the following criteria:
1. Clinical criteria
   a. Stage 3 or 4 coma or hyperactivity caused by

a dialyzable drug that cannot be treated by conservative means.

b. Hypotension threatening renal or hepatic function that cannot be corrected by adjusting circulating volume.

c. Apnea in a patient who cannot be ventilated.

d. Marked hyperosmolality that is not due to easily corrected fluid problems.

e. Severe acid-base disturbance not responding to therapy.

f. Severe electrolyte disturbance not responding to therapy.

g. Marked hypothermia or hyperthermia.

2. Immediate dialysis may be considered in ethylene glycol and methanol poisoning only if acidosis is refractory and blood levels of methanol of 100 mg/dl are consistently maintained.

3. Dialysis is indicated on basis of condition of patient—in general, dialyze if patient is in a coma deeper than level 3).

Alcohols	Fluorides
Ammonia	Iodides
Amphetamines	Isoniazid
Anilines	Meprobamate
Antibiotics	Paraldehyde
Barbiturates	Potassium
(long-acting)	Quinidine
Boric acid	Quinine
Bromides	Salicylates
Calcium	Strychnine
Chloral hydrate	Thiocyanates

(Other drugs may be dialyzable, but the information should be verified prior to institution of dialysis therapy.)

4. Dialysis not indicated except for support—therapy consists of intensive care.

Antidepressants (tricyclics and MAO inhibitors also)	Heroin and other opiates
Antihistamines	Methaqualone (Quaalude)
Barbiturates (short-acting)	Methyprylon (Noludar)
Chlordiazepoxide (Librium)	Oxazepam (Serax)
Diazepam (Valium)	Phenothiazines
Digitalis and related drugs	Phenytoin (Dilantin)
Diphenoxylate with atropine (Lomotil)	Synthetic anticholinergics and belladonna compounds

Amphetamines respond better to acid diuresis, but dialysis should be considered if the response is not adequate. While the long-acting barbiturates (cleared by the kidneys) are more readily dialyzable than the short-acting ones (cleared by the liver), dialysis may be helpful if the patient satisfies the criteria for supportive dialysis needs as outlined above. Salicylate poisoning generally responds very well to intensive alkaline diuretic therapy, but, if complications such as renal

failure or pulmonary edema develop, peritoneal dialysis with 5 per cent albumin or hemodialysis is indicated.

Peritoneal dialysis and exchange transfusion may be more useful in small children than hemodialysis. Again, the main purpose of these procedures may not be removal of the poison but restoration of fluid or acid-base balance. The infant who has been poisoned and whose serum sodium is rising because of excess bicarbonate administration may be helped considerably by an exchange transfusion even if little poison is removed.

Dialysis should *not* be performed as initial therapy but only when the criteria listed above are met.

Hemoperfusion

Perfusion of blood through charcoal- or resin-filled devices is gradually becoming more widely available in many centers. These techniques will probably allow rapid removal of many substances previously considered dialyzable but will not be likely to remove large quantities of agents with large volumes of distribution.

SPECIFIC POISONS OF MAJOR CONCERN TO PEDIATRICIANS

Acids

Products. Toilet bowl cleaners (such as bisulfate, which becomes sulfuric acid on contact with water), automobile batteries, swimming pool pH adjustment solutions, and acids in concentrated forms at hardware and paint stores.

Treatment. Emesis and lavage should be avoided to prevent re-exposure of mucous membranes. Dilution with simple solutions such as water or milk within the first 30 to 60 seconds may prevent or decrease future scarring and stricture formation. Unfortunately, most patients arrive in medical facilities at much longer intervals from ingestion, and dilution is probably ineffective. Dilution in the amount of 15 ml/kg to a maximum of 250 ml orally is adequate. For example, 150 ml of water in a 1 year old child who has swallowed some 28% acetic acid photographic stop bath will reduce the acid to a concentration well under that of vinegar used for salad dressing. Caution must be used with dilution to make sure that it is safe to give oral fluids. Steroids can be given in pharmacologic doses, although their value is unknown. Esophagoscopy should be reserved for concentrated acid ingestions or for those children salivating due to pain on swallowing. All children should be followed after 10 days to 3 weeks to be sure that pyloric stricture has not occurred.

Alkalies

Products. Contained in Clinitest tablets, drain cleaning crystals, and dishwasher soaps. Many new

Table 3. TOXICOKINETIC DATA OF DRUGS AND TOXINS
(NUMBERS EXPRESSED AS A MEAN OR AS A RANGE)

Agent	pK_a	Vd (l/kg)	Ther. T½ (hrs)	O.D. T½ (hrs)	Diuresis	Dialysis	Specific Therapy
Acetaminophen	9.5	0.75	2	4	No	No	N-Acetylcysteine
Amitriptyline	9.4	40+	36	72	No	No	Physostigmine
Amobarbital	7.9	2.4	16	36+	No	No	
Amphetamine	9.8	0.60	8–12	18–24	Acid	Yes	Chlorpromazine
Bromide	—	40+	300	300	Yes	Yes	
Caffeine	13	0.75	3.5	4–120	No	No	
Chloral hydrate	—	0.75	8	10–18	No	No	
Chlorpromazine	9.3	40+	16–24	24–36	No	No	
Codeine	8.2	3	2	2	No	No	Naloxone
Coumadin	5.7	0.1	36–48	36–48	No	No	Vitamin K
Desipramine	10.2	50+	18	72	No	No	Physostigmine
Diazepam	3.3	1–2	36–72	48–144	No	No	
Digoxin	—	7–10	36	13	No	No	
Diphenhydramine	8.3	—	4–6	4–8	No	No	Physostigmine
Ethanol	—	0.6	2–4	—	Yes (?)	No	
Ethchlorvynol	8.7	3–4	1–2	36–48	No	No	
Glutethimide	4.5	20–25	8–12	24+	No	No	
Isoniazid	3.5	0.60	2–4	6+	Alkaline	Yes	
Methadone	8.3	6–10	12–18	12–18	No	No	Naloxone
Methicillin	2.8	0.60	2–4	2–4	Yes	Yes	
Pentobarbital	8.11	2.0	10–20	50+	No	No	
Phencyclidine	8.5	—	—	12–48	Acid	Yes	
Phenobarbital	7.4	0.75	36–48	72–120	Alkaline	Yes	
Phenytoin	8.3	0.60	24–30	36–72	No	No	
Quinidine	4.3, 8.4	3	7–8	10	No	No	
Salicylate	3.2	0.1–0.3	2–4	25–30	Alkaline	Yes	
Tetracycline	7.7	3	6–10	6–10	No	No	
Theophylline	0.7	0.46	4.5	6+	No	Yes	

liquid drain cleaners contain little or no caustic agent. Those with less than 4% sodium or potassium hydroxide do not produce strictures, although they may produce burns. Industrial cleaners brought home in unlabeled containers may pose a significant hazard. Household bleaches (usually 5.4% sodium hypochloride) are not considered significant caustics.

Treatment. Immediate dilution with water or milk is the key treatment. All other therapy after the first 30 seconds simply treats sequelae. Vomiting should *not* be induced. Acid "neutralizers" (lemon juice, vinegar, and so on) should be avoided since they simply add to injury. A steroid in pharmacologic doses should be begun immediately and continued for 3 weeks if esophageal burns are discovered. Esophagoscopy is indicated in all patients with exposure to strong caustics, even in the absence of mouth burns. It is best performed 12 to 24 hours after exposure. This permits burns to develop to the point that they are readily seen but not to the point of necrosis. Patients are placed NPO immediately after dilution and observed for signs of mediastinitis (usually fever). Antibiotics are usually not given prophylactically. Dilatation of stricture may be attempted, but severe circumferential strictures may require surgical replacement of the esophagus.

Amphetamines and Related Drugs

Product. Numerous street drugs, such as "speed," STP, MDA, or DMT. While more closely regulated now, "diet pills" containing a variety of amphetamines and analogs are still found.

Treatment. In most cases nothing more is required than simple observation. Chlorpromazine has been used extensively to treat hyperactivity but should be avoided in the case of street drugs as it may result in synergistic hypotension. Diazepam is a safer choice. Forced acid diuresis should be considered in those patients in whom symptoms are severe and recur after initial diazepam treatment.

Anticholinergics

Products. Examples of medications: amitriptyline (Elavil, Triavil), anisotropine (Valpin), atropine, belladonna, benactyzine (Deprol), chlorpheniramine (Ornade, Teldrin, etc.), cyclopentolate (Cyclogel), desipramine (Norpramin, Pertofrane), dicyclomine (Bentyl), diphenhydramine

(Benadryl), doxepin (Sinequan), homatropine, hyoscine, hyoscyamus, imipramine (Tofranil, Presamine), isopropamide (Darbid), mepenzolate (Cantil), methantheline (Banthine), methapyrilene (Sominex, Compoz, Cope), nortriptyline (Aventyl), pipenzolate (Piptal), propantheline (Probanthine), protriptyline (Vivactil), pyrilamine, scopolamine, stramonium (Asthmador).

Examples of plants: *Amanita muscaria* (although muscarine is present in minute amounts, major toxic effects are anticholinergic), bittersweet (*Solanum dulcamara*), black henbane (*Hyoscyamus niger*), black nightshade (*Solanum nigrum*), *Lantana camara* (also known as red sage, wild sage), potato leaves, sprouts, tubers (*Solanum tuberosum*), wild tomato (*Solanum carolinense*).

Many antihistamines, antispasmodics, sleep aids, decongestants, analgesics, antiparkinsonism agents, and miscellaneous drugs, chemicals, and plants may produce clinically recognizable anticholinergic findings.

Treatment. In severe states, treatment will be necessary.

Convulsions	Diazepam
Myoclonic jerking	Physostigmine
Hallucinations	Physostigmine
Coma	Physostigmine
Hypertension	Physostigmine
Arrhythmias	Alkalinize blood to pH 7.50 and use physostigmine, lidocaine, or phenytoin

Physostigmine is a potentially dangerous drug and must be used with caution in asthmatics, diabetics, or those with gangrene. It must be given slowly (no more than 1 mg/min IV) or cholinergic overdrive may occur.

Benzodiazepines

Products. Valium, Librium, Dalmane, and a variety of minor tranquilizers.

Treatment. Patients with pure benzodiazepine overdoses rarely require more than observation. The use of naloxone, while not harmful, is probably not helpful. Physostigmine should not be used.

Cyanide

Products. Pesticides, metal polishes, photographic solutions, fumigating products, and some poisons. It is rarely seen and usually catastrophic.

Treatment. Creation of methemoglobin so as to provide an overwhelming supply of Fe^{+++} allows competition of the hemoglobin for cyanide with the cytochromes. TREATMENT CAN KILL. Pediatricians must be aware that the vial of sodium nitrite in the cyanide antidote kit is enough to kill most 1 to 2 year old children. Dosage of sodium nitrite in children is 0.3 ml/kg to a maximum of one vial.

Digitalis Glycosides

Products. Oleander, foxglove, digoxin, and digitoxin.

Treatment. Potassium must not be given unless depletion can be documented by measurements. Atropine may be useful initially. Phenytoin at low doses (1 mg/kg/dose) may be helpful. Cholestyramine orally may help lower levels. Kayexalate may be necessary to treat hyperkalemia. Pacemaker wires may be necessary. Specific antibodies—FAB fragments—are extremely effective but virtually unobtainable.

Ethanol

Products. Alcoholic beverages, cold remedies, perfumes, aftershave lotions, and fondue fuel.

Treatment. Intensive supportive care and correction of hypoglycemia. As numbers of young chronic alcoholics (ages 11 to 13 and older) increase, signs of withdrawal (delirium tremens, convulsions) must be expected and treated, usually with benzodiazepines. Extracorporeal techniques are not helpful in removing ethanol.

Hydrocarbons—Petroleum Distillates

Products. A wide variety of products contain natural (e.g., turpentine) and mineral (e.g., gasoline from petroleum cracking) hydrocarbons. The following divides these substances into toxicologic groups.

Group I—Heavy greases, oils, and petroleum jellies

Aspiration hazard	Slight
Systemic toxicity	Unusual

Group II—Gasoline, kerosene, and naphthas

Aspiration hazard	Moderate
Systemic toxicity	Moderate, and usually dependent upon aromatic content

Group III—Petroleum ether, benzine, and rapidly evaporating solvents

Aspiration hazard	Slight
Systemic toxicity	High, and usually due to anesthetic capacity

Group IV—Mineral seal oils (furniture polishes)

Aspiration hazard	High
Systemic toxicity	High, but only on secondary basis to aspiration since agents usually are not absorbed

Group V—Solvents containing toxic constituents or halogenated solvents

Aspiration hazard	Moderate
Systemic toxicity	Very high, and dependent upon the toxic constituent Most commonly pesticides heavy metals, benzene, 1,1,1-trichloroethane

Treatment. Recommended treatment, while considered controversial in the middle 1970s, is straightforward if each group is considered for its own toxicity rather than lumping all hydrocarbons together. Induction of emesis was the most controversial recommendation. Data from the National Clearinghouse demonstrate no increase of aspiration when ipecac emesis is utilized. This is because most patients who have aspirated have done so in the act of swallowing rather than vomiting. Induction of emesis should, however, be reserved for those situations when large quantities of hydrocarbons with risk of systemic toxicity have been consumed. Estimates of volume consumed are extremely difficult in children.

Examples of agents which may be useful to vomit are cleaning solvents with 1,1,1-trichloroethane, benzene, and pesticides with hydrocarbon solvents.

Examples of agents which do not need to be vomited are mineral seal oils, heavy greases, and petroleum jellies.

Steroids should not be administered, as they decrease the mononuclear cell response, and simultaneous antibiotics do not protect from an enhanced infection rate. Antibiotics should be used only on indication, such as increasing infiltrate size or positive tracheal aspirate. Fever per se is not an indicator for antibiotics. Administration of oils to "thicken" the hydrocarbons is no longer considered appropriate as lipoid pneumonitis may occur. Lavage should be avoided because of the increased risk of emesis and lack of control of the emetic stream with a tube in the pharynx. Generally, most children will have a benign course and do not need hospitalization. Observation for 24 hours or until cessation of symptoms is necessary in 2 to 5% of cases.

Iron

Products. As a medication in various concentrations, as an additive to multiple vitamins, and in soluble form in garden supplies. Elemental iron does not equal the weight of the tablet and must be calculated for each preparation as a percentage of weight after subtraction of other elements and rates of hydration. The usual 300-mg tablet contains about 60 mg of elemental iron.

Treatment. If the patient is not yet vomiting, then induction of emesis or lavage with a large-bore tube should be performed. Lavage is gener-ally performed with 5% sodium bicarbonate or a similar solution. The use of oral or lavage deferoxamine has been abandoned because of the poor stoichiometry and expense. Production of iron carbonate or iron phosphate is most likely equally effective. Fleet's phosphate solution diluted 1:4 has the dual advantage of a cathartic effect. When used in excess, this solution has resulted in the death of a child.

Total iron and total iron binding capacity together will provide an accurate estimate of free (unbound) iron. Treatment with deferoxamine intravenously is usually instituted if free iron is greater than 50 or total iron is in excess of 500. Stage I is best treated without regard to the iron poisoning but rather with an eye toward correction of hypotension and acidosis. Severe Stage III may not respond to standard treatment because of iron deposition in vascular structures. Exchange transfusion has been used from time to time in this situation with some good response. Extracorporeal techniques such as dialysis are of no benefit.

Lomotil

A combination of opiate and atropine is particularly toxic even in "therapeutic" doses to children. The drug is contraindicated under all circumstances under age 6.

Treatment. Naloxone (Narcan) is an effective antidote for the diphenoxylate and should be used in sufficient doses. Discharge from care should not occur until the patient has been symptom-free for 12 to 24 hours without naloxone administration.

Should arrest or hypoxia occur, the standard treatment for such a state, with the addition of naloxone, is appropriate.

Metals—Arsenic, Lead, and Mercury

Products. A wide variety of products ranging from old paint and plaster to ant poisons may contain these metals. Frequently the source of the metal is unknown, and because of some neurologic or other problem, the physician wishes to "rule out" this possibility.

Treatment. Dilution is the major therapeutic step for all these metals. Arsenic and mercury can be effectively removed with British anti-lewisite (BAL) (dimercaprol). BAL, unfortunately, is painful and produces a serum-like reaction in 70 to 80% of patients. BAL, therefore, should be used only in patients unable to take oral drugs or who are acutely ill. D-penicillamine is the drug of choice in these patients if they can take it orally and are not penicillin-allergic. For diagnostic and therapeutic purposes, a D-penicillamine mobilization test should be done. It allows significantly greater accuracy than a single urine test for heavy metals. The test and followup treatment are performed as follows:

Day 1—Collect a 24-hour urine specimen.

Day 2—250 mg of D-penicillamine at 0, 6, 12, and 18 hours and collect a 24-hour urine specimen. Comparison of these two urine specimens will indicate whether there are significant body burdens of lead, arsenic, or mercury. If the result of day 2 is more than three times that of day 1 (in μg per 24 hours total) and over 150 μg, it is considered a positive test.

Days 3–7—250 mg D-penicillamine qid.

Days 8–12—No drug.

Day 13—Begin cycle again and continue until the initial 2-day mobilization is normal. If more than three cycles are needed, then pause for 1 month after day 7.

Children under 10 kg should have 100 mg/kg periodically in four divided doses (to a maximum of 1 gm per day) rather than 250 mg qid.

Organophosphate and Carbamate Insecticides

Products. Chlorthion, Co-Ral, DFP, Diazinon, Malathion, Para-oxon, Parathion, Phosdrin, TEPP, Thio-TEPP, Carbaryl.

Treatment. Atropine plus a cholinesterase reactivator, pralidoxime (Protopam), is a chemical antidote for organophosphate insecticide poisoning. After establishing a clear airway and eliminating any cyanosis, large doses of atropine should be given and repeated every few minutes until signs of atropinism are present. An appropriate starting dose of atropine is 2 to 4 mg intravenously in an adult and 0.05 mg/kg in a child. The patient should receive enough atropine to stop secretions (approximately 10 times the normal dose). As much as 1 gm of atropine per 24 hours may be needed in an adult.

Because atropine antagonizes the parasympathetic effects of the organophosphates but does not alter the muscular weakness, pralidoxime should also be given immediately in more severe cases and repeated every 8 to 12 hours as needed (1 gm IV for older children and 250 mg intravenously for infants at a rate of no more than 500 mg/min). Pralidoxime should be used in addition to—not in place of—atropine if red cell cholinesterase is less than 25% of normal. Pralidoxime is probably not useful later than 36 hours after the exposure. Morphine, theophylline, aminophylline, succinylcholine, and tranquilizers of the reserpine and phenothiazine types are contraindicated. Hyperglycemia is common.

Decontamination of the skin (including nails and hair) and clothing with soapy water is extremely important. Decontamination of the skin must be done carefully to avoid abrasions, which increase organophosphate absorption significantly.

Phencyclidine

Products. Sold only as an illicit drug, e.g., angel dust, PCP, and peace pill.

Treatment. An adequate supportive environment is all that is required in most instances. Serious cases may require haloperidol to control behavior. Forced acid diuresis may be effective; however, recent reports of rhabdomyolysis and renal failure indicate care should be taken before diuresis is induced.

Narcotics and Synthetic Congeners

Products. Propoxyphene (Darvon), heroin, Talwin, Demerol, codeine, and so on.

Treatment. Children receiving an overdose of opiates can develop respiratory depression, stridor, coma, increased oropharyngeal secretions, sinus bradycardia, and urinary retention. Methadone is less likely to cause miosis than other narcotics. Pulmonary edema rarely occurs in children; deaths usually result from respiratory arrest and cerebral edema. Convulsions may occur with propoxyphene overdosage. Patients are usually in a coma on admission. If seizures are seen, then Darvon must be considered. Small pupils, absent bowel sounds, and bradycardia are common.

The treatment of choice is naloxone (Narcan), 0.4 mg intravenously, which rapidly produces a marked improvement without causing respiratory depression. The dose can be safely repeated and increased as needed. Nalorphine (Nalline) is an older drug with a respiratory depressant effect of its own. It should no longer be used. An improvement in respiratory status may be followed by respiratory depression, since the depressant action of narcotics may last 24 to 48 hours while the antagonist's duration of action is only 2 to 3 hours. Give intravenous fluids cautiously, since narcotics exert an antidiuretic effect and may precipitate cerebral or pulmonary edema.

Withdrawal in the Addict. The severity of withdrawal signs should be evaluated as explained in Table 4. Diazepam (Valium), 10 mg every 6 hours orally, has been recommended for the treatment of mild narcotic withdrawal in ambulatory adolescents. Ambulatory or hospitalized patients with moderate or severe withdrawal signs can be given the same dose of diazepam intramuscularly. Diazepam is recommended because it is nonhepatotoxic, nonmutagenic, is not known to affect the fetus when given to pregnant women, and is a good anticonvulsant. Diazepam therapy can be discontinued when the withdrawal score falls below 2. Diphenoxylate with atropine (Lomotil) is used to treat severe diarrhea and abdominal cramps.

Methadone maintenance is not usually recommended for adolescents, although it may be used for withdrawal purposes. One method of administration is to give methadone orally every 12 hours, starting with a 25-mg dose and decreasing the amounts by 5 mg every 12 hours. When the dose of methadone is 10 mg, add 3 tablets of diphenoxylate

Table 4. SCORING SYSTEMS FOR COMA, HYPERACTIVITY, AND WITHDRAWAL

Classification of Coma
0	Asleep, but can be aroused and can answer questions.
1	Comatose, does withdraw from painful stimuli, reflexes intact.
2	Comatose, does not withdraw from painful stimuli, most reflexes intact, no respiratory or circulatory depression.
3	Comatose, most or all reflexes are absent but without depression of respiration or circulation.
4	Comatose, reflexes absent, respiratory depression with cyanosis, circulatory failure, or shock.

Classification of Hyperactivity
1+	Restlessness, irritability, insomnia, tremor, hyperreflexia, sweating, mydriasis, flushing.
2+	Confusion, hyperactivity, hypertension, tachypnea, tachycardia, extrasystoles, sweating, mydriasis, flushing, mild hyperpyrexia.
3+	Delirium, mania, self-injury, marked hypertension, tachycardia, arrhythmias, hyperpyrexia.
4+	Above plus: convulsions, coma, circulatory collapse.

Classification of Withdrawal
Score the following finding on a 0-, 1-, 2-point basis:

Diarrhea	Hypertension	Restlessness
Dilated pupils	Insomnia	Tachycardia
Gooseflesh	Lacrimation	Yawning
Hyperactive bowel sounds	Muscle cramps	

1 to 5	mild
6 to 10	moderate
11 to 15	severe

Seizures indicate severe withdrawal regardless of the rest of the score.

(From Frederick H. Lovejoy, Jr., M.D., in Gellis and Kagan, Current Pediatric Therapy 9, W. B. Saunders Co., 1980.)

with atropine (Lomotil) three times daily for 1 day, followed by 2 tablets three times daily for 2 days. If signs of withdrawal recur, 10 mg of methadone orally or diazepam (orally or intramuscularly) is given.

The abrupt discontinuation of narcotics (cold turkey method) is not recommended and may cause severe physical withdrawal signs.

Withdrawal in the Neonate. A newborn infant in narcotic withdrawal is small for gestational age and demonstrates yawning, sneezing, decreased Moro reflex, hunger but uncoordinated sucking action, jitteriness, tremor, constant movement, a shrill and protracted cry, increased tendon reflexes, convulsions, vomiting, fever, watery diarrhea, cyanosis, dehydration, vasomotor instability, and collapse. The onset of symptoms commonly begins in the first 48 hours but may be delayed as long as 8 days, depending upon the timing of the mother's last "fix" and her predelivery medication. The diagnosis can be easily confirmed by identifying the narcotic in the urine of the mother and baby.

Several methods of treatment have been suggested for narcotic withdrawal in the neonate. Phe-

nobarbital, 8 mg/kg/24 hr intramuscularly or orally in four doses for 4 days and then reduced by one third every 2 days as signs decrease, may be continued for as long as 3 weeks. Methadone may be necessary in those infants with congenital methadone addiction who are not controlled in their withdrawal by large doses of phenobarbital. Dosage should be 0.5 mg/kg/24 hr in two divided doses but can be gradually increased as needed. Slow tapering off may be necessary over 4 weeks for methadone addiction.

It is not clear whether prophylactic treatment with these drugs decreases the complication rate. The mortality rate of untreated narcotic withdrawal in the neonate may be as high as 45%.

Nitrites

Products. Nitrite and nitrate compounds found in the home include amyl nitrite, nitroglycerin, pentaerythritol tetranitrate (Peritrate), sodium nitrite, nitrobenzene, and pyridium. High concentrations of nitrites in water or spinach have been the most common cause of nitrite-induced methemoglobinemia.

Treatment. After administering activated charcoal, induce vomiting and follow with a saline cathartic. Decontaminate any affected skin with soap and water. Oxygen and artificial respiration may be needed. If the blood methemoglobin level exceeds 40% or if levels cannot be obtained, give 0.2 ml/kg of 1% solution of methylene blue intravenously over 5 to 10 minutes. Avoid perivascular infiltration, since it causes necrosis of the skin and subcutaneous tissues. A dramatic change in the degree of cyanosis should occur. Transfusion is occasionally necessary. Epinephrine and other vasoconstrictors are contraindicated. If reflex bradycardia occurs, atropine can be used to block it.

Phenothiazines

Products. Chlorpromazine (Thorazine), prochlorperazine (Compazine), trifluoperazine (Stelazine), and so on.

Treatment. Extrapyramidal signs are dramatically alleviated within minutes by the slow intravenous administration of 1 to 5 mg/kg of diphenhydramine (Benadryl). No other treatment is usually indicated. Dialysis is contraindicated. Patients with overdoses should be treated conservatively. An attempt should be made to induce vomiting with apomorphine after administration of activated charcoal. Charcoal absorbs chlorpromazine and probably other phenothiazines very well. Emetics are often unsuccessful in this situation because phenothiazines are potent antiemetics; gastric lavage, therefore, may be the only practical way to remove gastric contents. A large amount of intravenous fluid without vasopressor agents is the preferred method of treating tranquilizer-induced

Table 5. DRUG FORMULARY IN TOXICOLOGY

Substance	Indications	Adolescent Dose	Pediatric Dose
Activated charcoal	Gastrointestinal decontamination	5 to 10 times the estimated amount ingested or 15 to 30 gm in 60 to 120 ml of water. Mix well before use. Give orally or by nasogastric tube	5 to 10 times the estimated amount ingested or 0.5 to 1 gm/kg mixed with 30 to 60 ml of water mixed with 5 to 10 ml of cherry syrup before use. Mix well before use. Given orally or by nasogastric tube
Ammonium chloride	Enhanced urinary excretion of basic compounds by acidification of urine	1.5 gm IV every 6 hours up to a maximum of 6 gm/24 hr. Oral dose 8 to 10 gm daily	75 mg/kg/dose IV or orally every 6 hours up to maximum of 2 to 6 gm/24 hr
Amyl nitrite pearls (kit from Eli Lilly and Company)	Cyanide poisoning	Inhalation for 30 seconds out of every min. New ampule every 3 mins	Same as adolescent dose
Atropine sulfate	Organophosphate and carbamate insecticides	2 to 3 mg/dose of IV solution (0.4 mg/ml) every 2 to 5 min until fully atropinized and then as necessary to maintain atropinization	0.05 mg/kg of IV solution (0.4 mg/ml) every 2 to 5 min until fully atropinized and then as necessary to maintain atropinization
Calcium disodium ethylene diamine tetra-acetate (calcium disodium versenate) (CaEDTA)	Heavy metal (lead) poisoning	1 gm IM or IV over 1 hour twice a day for 5 to 7 days. Repeat course after rest period. Add procaine for IM use	50 to 75 mg/kg/24 hr IM or IV divided into 2 to 3 doses for 5 to 7 days. Repeat course at 50 mg/kg/ 24 hr after rest period. Add procaine for IM use
Chlorpromazine (Thorazine)	Amphetamine-induced hyperactivity and psychosis	25 mg/dose IV every 6 hours. Reduce dose if barbiturate ingested. Titrate subsequent doses to desired response	1 mg/kg/dose IV every 6 hours. Reduce dose if barbiturate ingested. Titrate subsequent doses to desired response
Deferoxamine (Desferal)	Iron poisoning	1 to 2 gm IM every 6 to 8 hours. For severe intoxication IV dose at a rate not to exceed 15 mg/kg/hr. Do not exceed 6 gm in 24 hours	50 mg/kg not to exceed 1 to 2 gm IM every 6 hours. For severe intoxication IV dose at a rate not to exceed 15 mg/kg/hr. Do not exceed 6 gm in 24 hours
Dexamethasone (Decadron)	Cerebral edema	10 mg IV as an initial dose followed by 4 mg every 6 hours IV	0.4 mg/kg IV as an initial dose followed by 0.1 mg/ kg/dose IV every 4 to 6 hours
Diazepam (Valium)	Control of seizures	5 to 10 mg/dose IV titrated to control seizures	0.1 to 0.25 mg/kg/dose IV titrated to control seizures*
Dimercaprol (BAL)	Heavy metal (arsenic, mercury, lead, gold) poisoning	3 mg/kg/dose IM at 4- to 6-hour intervals for first 5 days, then 3 mg/kg/dose every 12 hours for next 5 to 9 days	3 to 4 mg/kg/dose IM at 4- to 6-hour intervals for first 5 days, then 3 to 4 mg/kg every 12 hours for next 5 to 9 days
Diphenhydramine (Benadryl)	Phenothiazine extrapyramidal reaction	25 to 50 mg/dose IV slowly, then every 6 hours orally or IV for maintenance	1 to 2 mg/kg/dose IV slowly, then every 6 hours orally or IV for maintenance
Ethacrynic acid (Edecrin)	Enhanced urinary excretion	50 mg/dose or 0.5 to 1.0 mg/kg/dose IV every 8 hours	0.5 to 1.0 mg/kg/dose IV every 8 hours†

Table 5. DRUG FORMULARY IN TOXICOLOGY (Continued)

Substance	Indications	Adolescent Dose	Pediatric Dose
Ethanol	Methanol and ethylene glycol poisoning	Ethanol given as a 50 per cent solution IV at a dose of 0.5 to 1.5 ml/kg every 2 to 4 hours to maintain a blood level between 100 and 150 mg/dl. In mild cases, 3 to 4 ounces of whiskey every 4 hours orally	Same as adolescent dose.
Furosemide (Lasix)	Enhanced urinary excretion	20 to 40 mg/dose IM or slowly IV (over 1 to 2 minutes) every 8 to 12 hours	1 to 3 mg/kg/dose IM or slowly IV (over 1 to 2 minutes) every 8 to 12 hours
Glycerol	Cerebral edema	2 gm/kg/24 hr in 4 divided doses orally	3 gm/kg/24 hr in 4 divided doses orally
Ipecac syrup	Induction of emesis	30 ml orally with fluids followed by motion	15 ml orally repeated in 15 min if not effective. Given with fluids followed by motion
Isoproterenol (Isuprel)	Hypotension	2 mg in 1000 ml of 5 per cent dextrose in water (conc. of 2 μg/ml), IV at rate of 0.1 μg/kg/min and increased slowly as needed	Same as adolescent dose.
Levarterenol (Levophed)	Hypotension	4 ml vial added to 1000 ml of 5 per cent dextrose in water (conc. of 4 μg/ml), IV at rate of 0.1 to 0.2 μg/kg/min and increased slowly as needed	Same as adolescent dose.
Magnesium sulfate (Epsom salt)	Gastrointestinal catharsis	5 gm or 50 ml of a 10 per cent solution orally and repeat every 4 hours until productive of stool	250 mg/kg/dose orally and repeat every 3 hours until productive of stool
Mannitol	Enhanced urinary excretion Cerebral edema	25 to 50 gm in a 20 per cent solution IV over 30 min every 4 to 6 hours (max. 200 gm/24 hr)	1 to 2 mg/kg in 20 per cent solution IV over 30 min every 4 to 6 hours (max. 100 mg/24 hr)‡
Metaraminol (Aramine)	Hypotension	10 mg/ml in a 10-ml vial. Add 100 mg to 1000 ml of 5 per cent dextrose in water (conc. of 100 μg/ml). Given IV at rate of 5 μg/kg/min and increased slowly as needed	Same as adolescent dose.
Methylene blue	Methemoglobinemia	1 per cent solution given IV slowly over 5 to 10 min at a dose of 10 mg, repeated in 4 hours if needed	1 per cent solution at a dose of 1 to 2 mg/kg given IV slowly over 5 to 10 min, repeated in 4 hours if needed

Naloxone hydrochloride (Narcan)	Reversal of narcotic depression	0.4 mg IV repeated every 2 to 3 min for 2 or 3 doses for initial effect. Continue therapy until narcotic effect no longer present	0.01 mg/kg/dose IV repeated every 2 to 3 min for 2 or 3 doses for initial effect. Continue therapy until narcotic effect no longer present
Oxygen	Carbon monoxide poisoning	100 per cent oxygen by inhalation	Same as adolescent dose.
D-Penicillamine (Cuprimine)	Heavy metal (lead, mercury) poisoning	250 to 500 mg orally every 6 to 8 hours, depending on severity	For acute therapy 25 to 50 mg/kg/24 hr in 4 divided doses orally for 5 days. For chronic therapy 25 mg/kg/24 hr in 4 divided doses orally (max. 1 gm/24 hr)
Physostigmine salicylate (Antilirium)	Anticholinergic poisoning	2 mg slowly over 2 to 3 min IV with repeat in 2 to 5 min if no effect. Once effect accomplished, give lowest effective dose slowly every 30 to 60 min with recurrence of symptoms	0.5 mg slowly over 2 to 3 min IV with repeat in 2 to 5 min if no effect. Once effect accomplished, give lowest effective dose slowly every 30 to 60 min with recurrence of symptoms
Pralidoxime chloride (2PAM)	Organophosphate insecticide	0.5 to 1.0 gm IV after initial treatment with atropine, given slowly at a rate of 500 mg/min and repeated every 8 to 12 hours as needed	250 mg/dose given slowly IV after initial treatment with atropine and repeated every 8 to 12 hours as needed
Prednisone	Caustic injury to esophagus	10 to 20 mg/dose IV, IM, or orally every 6 hours for 2 to 3 weeks with dosage tapering at end of therapy	2 to 3 mg/kg/24 hr IM, IV, or orally every 6 hours for 3 weeks with dosage tapering at end of therapy
Sodium bicarbonate	Enhanced urinary excretion of acid compounds by alkalinization of urine	2 meq/kg/dose IV during first hour followed by sufficient $NaHCO_3$ to keep urinary pH>7.5 (generally 2 meq/kg every 6 to 8 hours). Additional potassium necessary to accomplish alkalinization	2 to 4 meq/kg/dose IV during hour followed by sufficient $NaHCO_3$ to keep urinary pH>7.5 (generally 2 meq/kg every 6 hours). Additional potassium (3 to 4 meq/kg day) necessary to accomplish alkalinization
Sodium thiosulfate (kit from Eli Lilly and Company)	Cyanide poisoning	50 ml of 25 per cent solution at a rate of 2.5 to 5.0 ml/min IV 15 min after sodium nitrite. May be repeated once	1.65 ml/kg of 25 per cent solution at a rate of 2.5 to 5.0 ml/min IV 15 min after sodium nitrite. May be repeated once
Sodium nitrite (kit from Eli Lilly and Company)	Cyanide poisoning	10 to 20 ml of 3 per cent solution at a rate of 2.5 to 5.0 ml/min IV. May be repeated once with persistence or recurrence of symptoms	0.33 ml/kg of 3 per cent solution at a rate of 2.5 to 5.0 ml/min IV. May be repeated once with persistence or recurrence of symptoms
Vitamin K1	Hypoprothrombinemia	5 mg/dose IV	2 to 5 mg/dose IV

*Manufacturer's Warning: Safety not established in the neonate.
†Manufacturer's Precaution: Until further experience in infants is accumulated, therapy with ethacrynic acid is contraindicated.
‡Manufacturer's Warning: Dosage requirements for patients 12 years of age and under have not been established.

neurogenic hypotension. If a pressor agent is required, norepinephrine (levarterenol) should be used. Epinephrine should not be used because phenothiazines reverse epinephrine's effects.

Plants

Many common ornamental, garden, and wild plants are potentially toxic. Small amounts of a plant that are ingested may cause severe illness or death. These effects usually involve the cardiovascular, gastrointestinal, and central nervous systems and the skin.

Autumn Crocus (Colchicine). Monitor fluids and electrolytes. Abdominal cramps may be relieved with meperidine or atropine.

Caladium (Arum Family) (Dieffenbachia, Calla Lily, Dumb Cane (Oxalic Acid). Accessible areas should be washed thoroughly. Corticosteroids relieve airway obstruction. Apply cold packs to affected mucous membranes.

Castor Bean Plant (Ricin-a Toxalbumin). Fluid and electrolyte monitoring. Saline cathartic. Forced alkaline diuresis will prevent complications due to hemagglutination and hemolysis.

Foxglove and Cardiac Glycosides. If vomiting has not occurred, induce emesis or provide lavage followed by charcoal cathartics. Potassium should not be given in acute overdosage unless there is laboratory evidence of hypokalemia. In acute overdosage, hyperkalemia is more common.

The patient must be monitored carefully for electrocardiographic changes. The correction of acidosis will better demonstrate the degree of potassium deficiency present. In some cases, phenytoin (Dilantin), beta-adrenergic blocking agents such as propranolol (Inderal), or procainamide (Pronestyl) is necessary to correct arrhythmias. A pacemaker may be needed.

It has recently been noted that digoxin has an enterohepatic circulation. The use of oral binding agents such as cholestyramine resin (Cuemid, Questran) has been suggested in massive digitalis overdoses.

Jequirity Bean (Abrin-a Toxalbumin). Symptomatic. Renal failure can be prevented by alkalinizing the urine. Gastric lavage or emetics are contraindicated because the toxin is necrotizing. Saline cathartics are indicated.

Jimsonweed. Emesis or lavage should be followed by activated charcoal and cathartics. Physostigmine, 0.5 to 2 mg intravenously (can be repeated every 30 minutes as needed) dramatically reverses the central and peripheral signs of atropinism. Neostigmine is ineffective because it does not enter the central nervous system. High fever must be controlled. Catheterization may be needed if the patient cannot void.

Larkspur (*Delphinium ajacine,* Delphinine). Symptomatic. Atropine may be helpful.

Monkshood (Aconite). Activated charcoal, oxygen. Atropine is probably helpful.

Oleander (Dogbane Family) (Oleandrin). If vomiting has not occurred, induce emesis or provide lavage followed by charcoal cathartics. Potassium should not be given in acute overdosage unless there is laboratory evidence of hypokalemia. In acute overdosage, hyperkalemia is more common.

The patient must be monitored carefully for electrocardiographic changes. The correction of acidosis will better demonstrate the degree of potassium deficiency present. In some cases, phenytoin (Dilantin), beta-adrenergic blocking agents such as propranolol (Inderal), or procainamide (Pronestyl) is necessary to correct arrhythmias. A pacemaker may be needed.

Poison Hemlock (Coniine). Symptomatic treatment. Oxygen and cardiac monitoring equipment are desirable. Assisted respiration is often necessary. Give anticonvulsants if needed.

Rhododendron (Andromedotoxin). Atropine can prevent bradycardia. Epinephrine is contraindicated. Antihypertensives may be needed.

Yellow Jessamine. (The active ingredient, gelsemine, is related to strychnine.) Symptomatic treatment. Because of the relation to strychnine, forced acid diuresis and diazepam (Valium) for seizures would be worth trying.

Strychnine

Products. Rodenticides, tonics, and cathartics. It is also occasionally added to hallucinogenic drugs.

Treatment. If the patient is seen before the onset of symptoms, vomiting should be induced, followed by administration of activated charcoal, which is a very efficient adsorber of strychnine. Since ipecac is also adsorbed by activated charcoal emesis must be induced before charcoal is given. Convulsions can be controlled with diazepam (Valium), 0.1 to 0.3 mg/kg to a maximum of 10 mg. External stimulation should be minimized. Forced acid diuresis is very helpful, since strychnine is not significantly protein-bound and is present in large concentration in the serum. It is rapidly cleared in the urine. The hyperacute nature of strychnine intoxication makes hemodialysis impractical.

Tricyclic Antidepressants

Products. Amitriptyline, imipramine, doxepin, trimipramine, nortriptyline, desipramine, protriptyline, and so on.

Treatment. Treatment of the five major problems of arrhythmias, coma, convulsions, hypertension (and, later, hypotension), and hallucinations consists of intensive supportive measures followed by administration of physostigmine in the following doses: child under 12 years of age—0.5 mg intravenously over 60 seconds. If there is no effect, the dose may be repeated at 5-minute intervals to a maximum of 2 mg. Repeat as necessary only for life-threatening situations. Adult and adolescent— 2 mg intravenously over 60 seconds. If there is no effect, repeat in 10 minutes to a maximum dose of 4 mg. Repeat for life-threatening situations.

Physostigmine is a dangerous drug that must be given slowly to avoid iatrogenic convulsions. It is contraindicated in asthma, vascular gangrene, or urinary tract obstruction. Propranolol or phenytoin may be used if physostigmine is ineffective for treatment of arrhythmias. Alkalinization with sodium bicarbonate, 0.5 meq/kg intravenously, may dramatically reverse ventricular arrhythmias. Bicarbonate should be administered with physostigmine to all patients with significant arrhythmias to achieve a plasma pH of 7.5 to 7.6. Forced diuresis is contraindicated. A QRS interval greater than 100 milliseconds specifically identifies patients with major tricyclic antidepressant overdosage.

Hypotension is a major problem, since tricyclic antidepressants block the reuptake of catecholamines. This may produce a rebound hypotension following initial hypertension. Treatment with physostigmine is not effective. Infusion of sodium bicarbonate, 0.5 meq/kg, to produce a plasma pH of 7.5 or 7.6 will help avert hypotension. Vasopressors are generally ineffective, and the mortality rate is 60% in patients with hypotension who prove unresponsive to initial fluids. Orogastric charcoal, 0.5 gm/kg every 4 to 6 hours during the first 24 hours following ingestion, appears to interrupt an enterohepatic recirculation of tricyclics and shorten the plasma half-life.

DRUG FORMULARY

Table 5 lists the most commonly used drugs for treatment of poisoned patients. These drugs all should be available in a hospital intending to treat poisoned patients.

Salicylate Poisoning

ALAN K. DONE, M.D.

SEVERITY ASSESSMENT

Both the need for and the nature of treatment depend on the severity of poisoning, which is influenced by a number of factors. Among patients poisoned with a single acute dose of salicylate, the serum salicylate level and, less so, the dose are the most reliable indicators of severity and the need for hospitalization and treatment. Clinical assessment should always prevail if it suggests greater severity, but in such acute cases it is more likely that the level or dose will portend a serious prognosis before the clinical manifestations do and before problems

become irreversible. Dosage data are notoriously inaccurate, but if a believable estimate can be made (e.g., by counting the remaining pills and subtracting from the number originally present) the *single* dose of aspirin likely to produce problems that require treatment is about 1.5 to 2 grains per lb (200 to 280 mg/kg). All salicylates produce the same type of poisoning and relationships of dose and blood levels to severity, but oil of wintergreen (methyl salicylate) deserves special mention because of its potency: it provides about 3 gm of salicylate per average (4-ml) child's swallow, or the equivalent of 10 adult-sized (5-grain) aspirin tablets.

Meaningful interpretation of serum salicylate levels requires consideration of the time since ingestion, because the severity of salicylate poisoning is determined by the magnitude of the level at its peak and its duration, rather than its height at the moment. The approximate levels that dictate the clear need for hospitalization and/or dialysis for potentially fatal poisoning in cases in which salicylate was ingested in a single dose only are:

Hours:	4	8	12	18	24
Admission	80	70	60	50	40
Dialysis	100	90	80	70	60

unless clinical signs indicate more serious poisoning.*

In chronic poisoning resulting from repetitive administration of excessive aspirin, there is little or no correlation between serum salicylate (unless very high) and severity. Unfortunately, such instances account for the majority of very severe and fatal aspirin poisonings at present, especially in sick infants, and are characterized by accentuation of all the manifestations, particularly the CNS ones, possibly because of relatively greater entry of salicylate into the brain and a greater likelihood and severity of acidosis. These patients may continue to exhibit severe symptoms and acidosis even after the serum salicylate level has fallen to low or undetectable levels, and there is at least suggestive evidence than an additional determinant of such a course is cerebral glucose deprivation, even in the absence of systemic hypoglycemia.

Aside from chronic poisoning, the principal determinant of the nature and necessary treatment of salicylate poisoning—along, of course, with the degree of salicylemia—is age. Young children tend to develop metabolic acidosis quickly, superimposed on a usually fleeting respiratory alkalosis (the

---

*Graphs providing more detailed assessment of salicylate levels can be found in Pediatrics 26:800, 1960 and in Done's *The Toxic Emergency*, or many pediatric or clinical toxicology texts.

younger the child, the greater the likelihood and severity of the acidosis), and uncompensated acidosis is the rule in children under about 4 years of age who have been intoxicated for about 12 hours or longer. In contrast, adults frequently present with persisting respiratory alkalosis, and frank acidosis is uncommon, being confined either to debilitated, starved, or chronically or very severely poisoned individuals. Illness with relative dehydration and possibly diminished capacity to excrete the drug also may predispose to the occurrence and increased severity of salicylate poisoning and its accompanying acidosis. Persistence of acidosis, for whatever reason, greatly increases the amount of salicylate in the CNS. All these predisposing factors should be kept in mind when deciding on treatment and should weigh heavily in favor of dialysis if other indications for it are equivocal.

Findings of hyperpnea, lethargy, vomiting, and fever may be present even in mild poisoning requiring no treatment, but their combination with excitability, coma or convulsions, and severe electrolyte or acid-base disturbances suggests more serious poisoning that demands intensive treatment. Laboratory measurements of value in assessing severity include blood pH, P_{CO_2}, carbon dioxide or bicarbonate content, glucose (because life-threatening hypoglycemia occurs uncommonly), sodium and potassium, and urine pH and specific gravity. In addition to the aforementioned acid-base disturbances, both hypernatremia and hyponatremia requiring treatment may occur, and at least some degree of potassium depletion is inevitably present. Correction of the latter is extremely important not only for its own sake, but because it may worsen during the administration of the sodium bicarbonate needed for treatment, and it will prevent the excretion of the alkaline urine that can accelerate salicylate elimination (see below). The serum potassium level must be interpreted, however, in relation to the blood pH in this type of variable or mixed acid-base disturbance; the lower limits of acceptable serum potassium levels (meq/l) are, respectively, about 4.7 in the presence of acidosis, 3.7 with a normal blood pH, and 2.7 with alkalosis. Lower levels than these suggest the need for more intensive potassium therapy than otherwise would be required, and a more cautious approach to sodium bicarbonate administration until potassium depletion is corrected.

Serum salicylate measurements are essential and should be repeated every few hours to ascertain that the level is declining at an acceptable rate. Further, in no case should judgments about hospitalization and treatment be rendered until one is certain that the level has reached its peak (e.g., by showing a decline on repeat measurement or by the passage of sufficient time). In this regard it is important to note that salicylate absorption may continue for as long as 12 hours or more, particularly from methyl salicylate or poorly dissolved aspirin preparations. The latter occasionally may form an undissolved aspirin bolus in the stomach, from which salicylate absorption can continue for periods even of days.

MINIMIZING ABSORPTION

Because of the potentially variable duration of salicylate absorption, it is difficult to set a time limit after which gastric emptying is no longer productive. Certainly, after ingestion of a potentially toxic or uncertain dose, the stomach should be evacuated via emesis induction or gastric lavage if the patient is seen within about 4 hours in the case of aspirin and 6 hours in the case of oil of wintergreen. Although it is true that the most patients will have absorbed nearly all that they are destined to within those times, prolonged absorption occurs often enough for us to draw no time limit on gastric emptying unless it can be proved through repeat serum salicylate measurements that appreciable absorption is not still taking place. This is particularly important when there is involved either a cheap brand of aspirin that may have a slow dissolution, delayed-absorption capsules, or massive aspirin ingestions such as may be encountered in serious adult suicide attempts. Patients seen within the aforementioned time intervals should have their stomachs evacuated at the earliest possible moment, without awaiting salicylate measurements. In those seen later, in whom continued absorption is less likely and slower if present, it may be reasonable to await the measurement of one or more salicylate levels to determine whether gastric evacuation or other interventions are indicated, unless, of course, they already are symptomatic.

Emesis is best induced by giving syrup of ipecac in a dose of 20 to 30 ml followed by a glass of water; half or more of the dose can be repeated if vomiting has not occurred within about 15 minutes. Emesis should not be induced in patients who are comatose, convulsing, or severely obtunded. In these circumstances, or otherwise in lieu of emesis induction, gastric lavage can be performed, and in the small child should be done with half isotonic saline in a volume of about 500 ml, using as large a tube as can be passed through the mouth (never the nose, because the tube then necessarily is too small) to best ensure that intact tablets can be recovered. Lavage should be performed with adequate precautions to prevent aspiration (e.g., patient in Trendelenburg position on the left side or prone, with suctioning facilities immediately available, and including use of a cuffed endotracheal tube if the patient is comatose or severely obtunded). If for any reason (see above) the continued presence of undissolved tablets or a bolus of the aspirin is suspected, lavage should be performed employing a similar concentration of sodium bicarbonate. The latter usually will help to ensure dissolution of the material so that it can be recovered, but also renders it more capable of ready absorption, so the solution should be removed from the stomach as rapidly as possible. Failure of this procedure to dissolve a large aspirin bolus could be confirmed by a barium swallow and abdominal x-ray and may require that endoscopy be used as an approach through which the mass can be broken up so as to be more readily dissolved.

Salicylate remaining in the GI tract should have its passage hastened by a saline cathartic such as sodium or magnesium sulfate, and/or its absorption retarded by activated charcoal in a dose of about 10 times the estimated dose of salicylate. Charcoal should not be given before ipecac, however, as it may retard the emetic effect.

FLUID THERAPY

The aims should be to minimize salicylate entry into the brain while also hastening its elimination and correcting any life-threatening fluid-electrolyte or acid-base disturbances that may be present. The earlier practice, still recommended by many, of intermittently administering alkali specifically to raise the urine pH and/or blood pH or bicarbonate was based on (1) the undisputed fact that salicylate excretion is much greater in an alkaline urine, and (2) the notion that the acid-base disturbance per se was the greatest threat. On the basis of current knowledge, such practices should be replaced by *constant* buffering of blood pH in the normal or slightly alkaline range by continuous infusions of sodium bicarbonate.

Patients with salicylate poisoning sufficiently severe to require parenteral fluid therapy inevitably will be potassium-depleted; until this is corrected, excretion of an alkaline urine cannot be forced with alkali, and infusions of sodium bicarbonate with urine pH as the end-point may result in sodium or alkali overload and worsening of potassium deficit effects. Further, evidence now suggests that the central nervous system effects of salicylate are principal determinants of lethality, and acidosis (through effects on salicylate ionization and therefore penetrability) may owe much of its deleterious effects to increased salicylate entry into the brain. The success of attempts to reverse this trend depends not only on buffering of blood, but also on constant maintenance of an extra-cellular-intracellular pH gradient that favors ion-trapping of salicylate in blood and its being non-ionized in the cell (brain). Thus, only an extracellular alkalinizer such as sodium bicarbonate should be used, and ones such as tromethamine that buffer intracellularly as well should be avoided, as should intermittent alkali administration that produces only fleeting correction of acidosis.

Thus, it is important that continuous bicarbonate solutions be given and that potassium deficits be replaced simultaneously in amounts as nearly equivalent as possible to those of sodium. Except in rare cases of life-threatening excesses or deficiencies of sodium or potassium, the above aims are best met in severe cases by maintenance IV infusions of hypotonic solutions containing compatible quantities of sodium, potassium, glucose, and water, once initial hydration to restore and ensure kidney function has been achieved. In patients with minor symptoms, oral fluids may suffice; in those with severe poisoning, IV fluid administration is recommended as follows:

1. Initial hydration with a potassium-free "voiding" solution, which should be at a rate and osmolality sufficient to achieve plasma volume expansion persistent enough to promote urine production. It should be a 5% dextrose in water solution that is also at least one third isotonic with regard to sodium. Most or all of the sodium can be in the form of bicarbonate, particularly if acidosis is known or suspected to be present. In any event, as a routine it is satisfactory to use a solution containing 50 meq/l sodium bicarbonate. The infusion rate is 400 ml per m^2 in 1 hour or less. If urine flow then is not yet established, the same solution can be continued at one half to two thirds the stated rate. In the presence of shock, plasma, plasma volume expanders, or blood should be given initially in a dose of 10 to 15 ml/kg infused as rapidly as it will flow.

2. After adequate urine flow is established, the correction fluid should contain potassium in concentration as high as can be safely infused—but not in excess of 40 meq/l except in the presence of severe hypokalemia (see below)—and approaching as closely as possible the concentration of sodium. Sodium should be present in an amount of about 50 to 55 meq/l; the greater the severity or likelihood of acidosis (see above), the more sodium should be provided in the form of bicarbonate, and the ability to maintain the desired buffering of blood pH is facilitated if sodium is present somewhat in excess of chloride. The recommended amounts of sodium are based on the estimation that the tolerance limit for sodium, except in the presence of severe hyponatremia (see below), is about 250 meq/m^2/24 hr. When the suggested solutions are infused at the IV rate recommended for moderate to severe salicylate poisoning, 3 to 5 l/m^2/24 hr, it is possible to remain below this limit. Appropriate solutions can be prepared conveniently either by adding 15 meq sodium bicarbonate (17 ml of 7.5%) to each liter of "electrolyte 75," "Isolyte M" or "Butler-Talbot solution" (ones that contain 40 meq/l sodium and 35 meq/l potassium), or by adding 40 meq of potassium chloride and 50 meq of sodium bicarbonate (57 ml of 7.5%) per liter of 5% dextrose in water.

These two solutions would contain the following concentrations of electrolytes (in meq/l):

Solution	Na	K	Cl	HCO3
E75 + 15 meq NaHCO3/l	55	35	40	35
40 meq KCl + 50 meq NaHCO3/l	50	40	40	50

There is no strong basis for selecting one over the other; the former solution would be more appropriate for mild than for severe acidosis because of its lesser content of bicarbonate, but it also contains slightly more sodium and less potassium. Within the limits noted above, the volume and rate of administration depend on the severity of poisoning and any evidences there may be of dehydration. With severe symptoms and/or dehydration, the higher quantities are used, and it may be desirable to give one half of the total day's fluid in the first 8 hours. The figures given here are average ones, and the actual approach to fluid therapy ought to be individualized, with the composition and rate of administration of the fluid regulated by careful observation of urine output, body weight, and blood electrolytes, pH and gases.

3. Rare patients, usually infants with chronic poisoning, may have blood pH so low (less than 7.15) that the acidosis itself requires more rapid buffering than the above would give. This should be done only with sodium bicarbonate, for reasons detailed elsewhere (Pediatrics 62:890, 1978), which can be given by slow IV push in doses of 3 to 5 meq/kg. Such buffering will only be fleeting at best, and so should be followed by continuous infusions of the type noted above. The alkalosis of salicylate poisoning, when present, requires no measures except avoidance of its aggravation by undue alkali therapy.

4. Either hyper- or hyponatremia of dangerous proportions occasionally may be seen. Hypernatremia rarely would require any modification of the fluid therapy noted above, the greatest threat in such cases being excessively rapid reduction of the elevated serum sodium level. The latter, however, would require careful monitoring. Severe hyponatremia if symptomatic calls for the infusion of hypertonic (3%) saline in amounts based on the calculated sodium deficit below a completely tolerable level of 130 meq/l of serum: Deficit (meq/kg) = meq/l below 130 × 0.6 × weight in kg; since each ml of 3% saline contains about 0.5 meq sodium, the amount of 3% sodium chloride needed is twice this figure. It is important that this be given rapidly (i.e., within 1 to 1.5 hours). Again, careful monitoring of serum sodium level is crucial.

5. Oliguria calls for different measures, depending on its cause. Inadequate replacement of fluid losses is suggested by persisting signs of dehydration, the excretion of a concentrated urine, and sometimes an elevation of the BUN or creatinine, and calls for increasing the rate of fluid administration. Fluid retention, possibly due to inappropriate ADH secretion, is suggested by hyponatremia with corresponding reduction of serum osmolality, absence of clinical evidence of dehydration, and concentrated urine, sometimes with peripheral or pulmonary edema. It calls for treatment similar to that noted above for the correction of hyponatremia, or else for fluid deprivation for a sufficient period to allow serum osmolality to increase to the point at which diuresis can occur. If symptoms are sufficiently severe and fluid restriction does not result in resumption of urine output readily, it may be advisable to give a slow IV infusion of 20% mannitol, 1 gm/kg, in addition to fluid restriction. Primary renal failure is suggested by dilute urine, progressive azotemia, and possibly rising serum potassium and/or the development of edema, and it calls for judicious restriction of fluid intake. All three situations call for no, or very careful, potassium administration until urine flow again becomes adequate. If the origin is renal failure, dialysis (see below) may be indicated in order that salicylate elimination can proceed.

SYMPTOMATIC/SUPPORTIVE CARE

Attempts to modify the hyperpnea or its immediate effects have uniformly been valueless. In deeply comatose or convulsing patients, respiratory insufficiency may occur and require assisted ventilation. It must be remembered that the hypermetabolism entails increased oxygen demand, and so respirations may be inadequate even with severe hyperpnea. For this reason, in addition to the disturbances mentioned above, serial evaluations of acid-base status are important, and here particularly one would be concerned about a rise in Pco_2.

Convulsions portend such a poor prognosis that they themselves are indications for measures to remove salicylate artificially (see below). In addition, it is important to rule out the possibility that they are caused by complications that require correction: severe hyponatremia or water intoxication may require administration of hypertonic saline and/or mannitol (see above); with any suspicion of hypoglycemia it is important to administer glucose IV, although the amounts advocated in the fluids noted above should be sufficient to prevent its occurrence; a reduction in the level of ionized calcium may take place, particularly during intensive alkali administration, and will require the administration of calcium (2 to 5 ml of 10% calcium gluconate slowly IV) and curtailment of the administration of alkali. Convulsions not due or responsive to the above may require diazepam, paraldehyde, or a short-acting barbiturate to terminate seizures, and phenobarbital or, rarely, phenytoin to prevent their recurrence.

Hemorrhagic phenomena may result from a variety of coagulation defects that are rarely seen except in chronic or the very most severe acute cases. However, since at least some such events are preventable (especially those due to hypoprothrombinemia), it is worthwhile to administer vitamin K_1 oxide in a dose of 50 mg IV in very severe or chronic cases.

Acute pulmonary edema is a rare complication and may require the use of oxygen, bronchodilators, possibly rapid digitalization, and/or positive pressure alcohol vapor inhalation. Hyperpyrexia is sometimes of sufficient severity to require specific treatment, and for this purpose cautious sponging with tepid water is the safest procedure, although occasional patients may require carefully monitored measures similar to those used for the intentional production of hypothermia.

Renal failure is rare but is an absolute indication for artificial salicylate removal (see below) in patients who still have dangerous salicylate levels. Other causes of oliguria noted above are sometimes correctable by the measures mentioned but occasionally also may be indications for the same approach. In any event, the development of absolute or relative renal insufficiency may be insidious, and in terms of one of the major goals of therapy of salicylate poisoning (reduction of the salicylate load available to the brain) it is important to utilize serial measurements of serum salicylate level, because its failure to fall rapidly enough may be the single most important indicator of need for the interventions described below.

ARTIFICIAL REMOVAL OF SALICYLATE

Forced diuresis, as by administration of diuretics, osmotics, or fluid volumes in excess of those required, is of little value because salicylate excretion is far more dependent on the pH of urine than on its volume. Because of the aforementioned difficulties of achieving urine alkalinization in very severe cases, rapid reduction of salicylate levels through artificial means becomes the only hope for occasional patients. In either acute or chronic poisonings, indications may be renal failure and an inadequate rate of decline of the salicylate level. In patients with single-dose acute poisoning, the use of the serum salicylate level is of great value in determining when such procedures are indicated; in fact, the early finding of a salicylate level that suggests a fatal outcome is a compelling indication for not awaiting the development of symptoms that by then may be irreversible. In chronic poisoning, where the salicylate level does not correlate well with severity unless it is very high, these decisions must be made on the basis of symptoms and progress alone. The persisting presence of severe acidosis not readily responsive to fluid-electrolyte therapy after salicylate has disappeared from the circulation in an infant with chronic poisoning is an indication for such intervention. The occurrence and persistence of such severe symptoms as convulsions, particularly when rapid improvement does not follow other treatment, may be an indication in any patient. In those with chronic poisoning in whom the decision is a difficult one to make on the basis of serum salicylate levels, their measurement on CSF may be helpful; the finding there of a level more than about 50% of that in blood, particularly in the presence of severe CNS symptoms, may be adequate indication.

The principal means available for artificially reducing the salicylate level include dialysis, hemoperfusion, and exchange transfusion. Hemodialysis is by far the most efficient but is more difficult and risky in very young children and may require some time to get under way. It may be worthwhile instead, or while awaiting the implementation of hemodialysis, to utilize peritoneal dialysis because of the ease with which it can be performed immediately in almost any medical setting. The efficiency of peritoneal dialysis in removing salicylate is greatly increased when 5% salt-poor human albumin is used, because salicylate is avidly protein-bound; however, this is both difficult to obtain and costly, and so alternating protein-containing and conventional dialysis solutions may be worthwhile. It should be pointed out that some patients, particularly infants with chronic poisoning and persisting acidosis, will improve with peritoneal dialysis or hemodialysis to a degree out of proportion to the amount of salicylate removed, suggesting that the procedure provides removal of additional materials (e.g., organic acid metabolites, and so on) or provides a reservoir from which unidentified needs can be met (e.g., for fluids, electrolytes, and so on). Exchange transfusion is most practical in very young children or infants and may be the most efficient procedure in some settings.

Acetaminophen Overdose

BARRY H. RUMACK, M.D.

PRINCIPLES OF THERAPY

Charcoal has been shown to bind acetaminophen, but owing to the rapid absorption of this drug (peak levels at 30 minutes for liquid preparations; 60 minutes for tablets) its practical usefulness is limited. In addition, while the time to peak levels may be prolonged with overdose, charcoal may interfere significantly with the absorption of the oral antagonist to acetaminophen, N-acetylcysteine.

Emesis frequently is a spontaneous event following acetaminophen overdose, particularly in children, but ipecac syrup is known to produce more complete evacuation of gastric contents and should be used.

The first 24 hours following overdose is characterized by the nondiagnostic findings of malaise, nausea, and mild diaphoresis. A high index of suspicion must be present and careful history elicited if adequate therapy is to be provided.

In adults 140 mg/kg (14 times the therapeutic dose) of acetaminophen in an acute ingestion has been associated with hepatic injury. Based on current data, this quantity will not be smaller, and may be larger in the young child. The quantity of available glutathione for in situ liver detoxification of toxic intermediates from the minor pathway of acetaminophen determines the extent of potential hepatic injury. Therapy is designed to supply glutathione surrogates (cysteamine, N-acetylcysteine) to provide adequate substrates for detoxification. Drugs that stimulate the minor metabolic pathway, e.g., phenobarbital and Dilantin, will contribute to the occurrence of hepatotoxicity at a lower overdose quantity.

TREATMENT PROTOCOL

N-acetylcysteine (Mucomyst 20% solution) has been used under an investigational new drug license since 1976. At present, the IND license applies to all age groups. In adolescents and young adults, in whom suicidal ingestions have led to severe hepatotoxicity (75 to 100%) and death (5 to 10%) in untreated cases of more than 140 mg/kg, N-acetylcysteine has been used as follows:

1. 20% Mucomyst solution diluted into 4 volumes of carbonated beverage to decrease gastrointestinal irritation and disguise odor and taste.

2. 140 mg/kg loading dose within 24 hours of ingestion given orally or by gastric tube.

3. 70 mg/kg every 4 hours thereafter for a total of 18 oral doses.

Intravenous use of Mucomyst, as reported in Great Britain, is not appropriate in the United States. Solutions are not nonpyrogenic and the drug is not licensed for this route.

Preliminary data indicate that therapy should be continued for the full 3 days as stipulated. Daily laboratory monitoring of liver function, clotting parameters, and renal function is indicated. Liver enzymes peak on days 3 to 4 and should rapidly return to normal unless an additional underlying hepatic process is present. The progression to hepatic encephalopathy, as judged by constructional apraxia, should be accompanied by steps toward support of impending hepatic failure and should include neomycin and cleansing enemas, protein-free diet, vitamin K, and perhaps lactulose.

Support through the acute illness should lead to complete return of normal liver function. Followup liver biopsies in adults reveal complete absence of any lesion and no evidence of a progressive condition.

Cysteamine, an antagonist utilized in the United Kingdom in adults, must be given IV and is accompanied by a number of unpleasant side effects. The IV use of N-acetylcysteine in Great Britain has been reported to be efficacious and without these side effects, but it has not been necessary to use it other than by the highly effective oral route in the United States.

Increased Lead Absorption and Acute Lead Poisoning

HERBERT L. NEEDLEMAN, M.D.

Prompt recognition of excess lead exposure followed by direct and appropriate management will result in markedly improved neuropsychologic outcome. Theoretically, since excess lead exposure is wholly a product of human activities, lead poisoning is a completely preventable disease. But, until removal of lead from the human environment (mainly in paint, air, and food) has taken place, screening of children at risk, followed by diagnosis and treatment, will continue to be essential hygienic activities.

Frank lead poisoning should be treated with urgency. Lead poisoning is defined by the Centers for Disease Control as existing when a child has two successive venous blood lead levels equal to or greater than 70 μg/dl, or a venous blood level greater than 50 μg/dl and a free erythrocyte porphyrin (FEP) determination greater than 250 μg/dl, or an elevated FEP ($>$ 109 μg/dl) with an elevated blood lead level ($>$ 30 μg/dl) and symptoms (headache; lethargy; abdominal pain; intellectual, behavioral, or motor impairment).

Treatment of Symptomatic Lead Intoxication

Treatment rests upon these principles: (1) removal from source; (2) maintenance of adequate urine output while avoiding overhydration; (3) reducing soft tissue lead by administration of chelating agents; (4) prevention of seizures and increased intracranial pressure; (5) detection and abatement of source; and (6) followup for detection of neuropsychologic deficit.

Children with symptomatic poisoning should be admitted to the hospital. Intravenous fluids are given to maintain urine output at 350 to 500 ml/m^2/24 hr. Since these patients are at risk for cerebral edema, care must be taken not to overhydrate them.

Once urinary flow has been established, chelation therapy is begun. Therapy is begun with British anti-lewisite (BAL), 4 mg/kg IM. This is repeated every 8 hours. Following the initial dose of BAL, calcium disodium edathamil (EDTA) is given by IV drip or deep IM injection with procaine. The dose of EDTA is 15 mg/kg every 8 hours. The use of calcium disodium edathamil is necessary to prevent calcium depletion.

If patients do not have encephalopathy and respond to therapy, BAL may be discontinued after 48 hours. If encephalopathic signs are present, BAL is administered for 5 days. EDTA is administered for 5 days. A repeat course is given after a 48-hour rest if the lead level in blood is greater than 40 μg/dl or if 24-hour urinary lead excretion is greater than 750 μg on the fifth treatment day. It may be necessary to repeat EDTA in 5-day courses a number of times, alternated with rest periods, if body stores are very high.

Increased intracranial pressure is a serious sign that requires close observation and management. Twenty per cent mannitol IV and dexamethasone, 3 mg q 6 hr IV, should be administered. Surgical decompression has no place in the management of lead encephalopathy. Seizures are best managed with IV Valium.

At the time a child is diagnosed, the public health authorities should be notified and the sources of lead identified and removed. If a symptomatic child is re-exposed to lead at high dose, the outlook for central nervous system function is bleak. All children in the family should be screened for lead. If the cause of the exposure was scraping and sanding wooden trim in the house, all adults should be screened also.

Management of Asymptomatic Cases

If the venous blood lead level is greater than 70 μg/dl, a course of BAL-EDTA should be instituted. If the blood lead level is between 60 and 69 μg/dl and the FEP is greater than 100 μg/dl, a 5-day course of EDTA should be started. If the blood lead level is between 40 and 59 μg/dl, a provocative chelation test should be done. A single dose of EDTA, 50 mg/kg IM, is administered, and a 24-hour urine collection begun. If the urine contains more than 1 μg of lead/mg EDTA given, an elevated soft tissue lead level has been demonstrated. The patient should then receive a 5-day course of EDTA.

Toxicity of Chelating Agents

BAL frequently may produce toxic side effects in a number of patients. Commonest is a febrile reaction. Other side effects are transient granulocytopenia, hypertension, and sterile abscesses.

EDTA most commonly produces a lower nephron nephrosis. Renal effects are generally reversible and disappear with the cessation of therapy. Other side effects include a febrile reaction 4 to 8 hours after infusion of the drug, sometimes accompanied by myalgia, headache, nausea, and vomiting. Patients receiving EDTA should be monitored for depletion of calcium, zinc, and iron.

Long-Term Management

Children without symptoms who have venous blood lead levels greater than 30 μg/dl but less than 60 μg/dl may be treated with oral D-penicillamine provided two conditions are met: (1) continued contact with the source has definitely been eliminated, and (2) no history of penicillin allergy has been obtained. Oral penicillamine in the face of continued ingestion of lead is dangerous and should not be used.

Adjunctive Management

Lead absorption and toxicity are enhanced by low calcium intake, protein depletion, and iron deficiency. Disadvantaged children are exposed to more lead in general, and their diets are generally less than optimal. Therapeutic diets, with restitution of deficits, are an essential part of the management of lead intoxication. This requires contined monitoring and supervision.

Educational Rehabilitation

Children who recover from lead exposure tend to be more distractible and less organized and do less well on psycholinguistic tasks. Early psychoeducational diagnosis and remedy may prevent school failure and its attendant sequelae. It is a part of the total management of the child.

Prevention of Lead Exposure and Intoxication

Lead in the environment is largely a residuum of human activity. Primary prevention depends upon its removal from the surroundings of children and women of childbearing age, rather than its removal from the body by pharmacologic means. The chief sources of lead are automobile emissions, food, paint, and, in some circumstances, factory emissions. All of these are subject to regulation, but the enforcement of legislation is often sporadic. Physicians should support appropriate regulatory activity with vigor and serve as advocates for the patients who are their charge.

Iron Poisoning

CAROL B. HYMAN, M.D.

Iron intoxication from ingestion of medicinal iron is one of the most common causes of poisoning in childhood. Since it can result in serious morbidity, or be fatal, all parents should be advised on *Prevention:* 1) Keep all medicinal iron hidden and out of the reach of small children. 2) Do not take iron or iron-containing medications or vitamins in a child's presence. 3) Keep in childproof bottle with cap tightly closed at all times. 4) Always know the amount of medication left in the bottle. 5) Have syrup of ipecac available in the home, with the dose clearly marked on the label: for a child less than 1 year, two teaspoons; for children one year of age and up to a weight of 90 pounds, one measured tablespoon; for children greater than 90 to 100 pounds and adults, two measured tablespoons.

Assessment of the Severity of poisoning depends on the following: 1) *The amount of elemental iron ingested.* Ferrous sulfate contains 20% iron, ferrous gluconate, 12.5% and ferrous fumerate, 33%. 2) *The maximum serum iron level.* This occurs 2 to 4 hours after ingestion. Less than 100 μg/dl is normal; between 100 and 350 μg/dl, mild iron poisoning may occur, depending on the serum transferrin level, as it is the unbound iron which is toxic; between 350 and 500 μg/dl, iron poisoning is present and may be serious; between 500 and 1000 μg/dl, serious toxicity is present; and greater than 1000 μg/dl may be lethal. 3) *Symptoms.* These are a) gastrointestinal, owing to the caustic effect of iron on the mucosa; b) cardiovascular, from the effects of free or unbound iron in the circulation; and c) central nervous system (CNS) depression. 4) *Time from iron ingestion or stage of iron toxicity.* The *acute stage* occurs from 0 to 6 hours after iron ingestion. Gastrointestinal symptoms may include nausea, vomiting, abdominal pain, and melena; cardiovascular symptoms may include pallor, tachycardia, and hypotension and, in the CNS, lethargy and coma. *Stage II* is quiescent, and occurs 6 to 24 hours after ingestion. There may be periods of lethargy or no symptoms. The physician must be wary of this phase, as it precedes *stage III,* in which there may be a *recurrence of symptoms* 12 to 48 hours after iron ingestion. Symptoms may be severe and include hematemesis, melena, cyanosis, vasomotor collapse, pulmonary edema, lethargy, and coma. In addition, metabolic acidosis, leukocytosis, coagulation defects, liver disease, and oliguria may be present. With severe poisoning, a *fourth* stage may manifest 4 to 6 weeks later, with gastric scarring and pyloric obstruction.

MANAGEMENT

Treatment is based on the factors discussed above. On the first patient contact, by phone or in the hospital, the physician should take a brief history to include age of the child, type of iron ingested (pills, liquid, name of product), amount, and time ingested. In addition, the physician should determine if the child is asymptomatic, symptomatic but alert, in shock, or unconscious. The parent should be advised to bring the child to the hospital without delay and not to forget the "empty" bottle of iron preparation.

If the child is conscious, and the general condition is good, the following steps should be taken: 1) *induce vomiting* with ipecac. The child must first drink, preferably tea or chocolate milk, as they bind iron, although plain milk or water can be used. Avoid juices or vitamin C-containing liquids, as they increase iron absorption. Immediately after drinking, give syrup of ipecac (see above for dose). *Examine vomitus* to determine the amount of iron (number of tablets, etc.) removed. Consideration may be given to having a parent induce vomiting at home prior to bringing the child to the hospital. 2) *Gastric lavage,* using a large bore tube and a 3% to 5% sodium bicarbonate solution (1 ampoule containing 44 meq bicarbonate to 3 to 5 parts of saline), will form a relatively nonabsorbable ferrous carbonate complex. 50 to 100 ml of this solution may safely be left in the stomach, as it is not toxic. Do not use disodium phosphate (Fleet enema) for a lavage solution, as it may be toxic. 3) *X-ray the abdomen,* as iron tablets are radiopaque. Repeat x-ray to determine the effectiveness of vomiting and lavage in removal of iron. If iron tablets remain, depending on the amount, *emergency surgery* may be necessary. Once dissolved, iron tablets may not be visible by x-ray. 4) *Intravenous fluids* must be started immediately, and should include Desferal and plasma, as these bind iron. Desferal is compatible with all commonly used intravenous fluids, including plasma and red cells. Since preparation of a Desferal-containing fluid takes time, the initial IV should be started without delay, using whatever fluid is available. The dose of IV Desferal for mildly affected patients is 2 to 5 mg/kg per hour. With serious toxicity, the dose can be increased to a maximum of 10 to 15 mg/kg per hour. Both chelated iron (ferrioxamine) and free iron can cause serious hypotension. 5) *Intramuscular Desferal,* 40 mg/kg, should be given to all patients when first seen. The urine should be collected and observed to determine if it becomes pink-orange, as this indicates iron toxicity. 6) *Chelation therapy* may be stopped when discolored urine and free iron in the serum are no longer present.

Patients who are in shock or comatose, or in whom the serum iron is greater than 1000 μg/dl, require emergency treatment. No effort should be made to induce vomiting, but gastric lavage may be tried. Intravenous fluids to maintain blood pressure must be started immediately, and oxygen and vasopressors used as necessary. Consideration should be given to an *immediate exchange transfusion* or *plasmapheresis* to remove iron while it is still in the blood stream. These procedures may be life saving.

In mild cases, the child may be discharged after 6 to 24 hours of observation if he or she remains asymptomatic and in good condition, there is no pink-orange urine after Desferal, the serum iron is less than 500 μg/dl and the x-ray of the abdomen does not show the presence of iron tablets. If there is any doubt about the degree of iron poisoning, the patient should remain longer under observation.

Long term follow-up of children with severe iron toxicity is necessary to observe for the development of gastric or pyloric scarring. These may require dilatation and management by a gastroenterologist.

Insect Stings and Arthropod Bites and Stings

PHILIP C. ANDERSON, M.D.

ARACHNIDS

Scorpions. In Arizona and nearby states, most stings of the scorpion (Centuroides) can be treated simply, and only a few require antivenoms or hospitalization. In the more northern United States, most scorpion stings are rarely worse than stings of hornets. Exotic scorpions imported from Africa or India may be extremely venomous and should be treated cautiously, according to regional experts. The more severe cases in the United States may respond to atropine, phenobarbital, and specific antivenom secured by calling the Poison Control Center. Antihistamines, morphine, or nonspecific antivenoms are contraindicated. Tourniquets and ice packs must be used with caution.

Spiders. Only two species of spiders in the United States present important risks for children, the brown recluse spider *(Loxosceles reclusa)* and the black widow spider *(Latrodactus mactans)*. Recluse spider bites occur mostly within homes in mid-America, geographically from the eastern mountains, to the arid plains to the west, and roughly south to the Gulf from about I–80 and the Ohio turnpike. Bites are accidental, often when the spider is trapped in clothing as the child dresses in the morning. At first not usually tender, the bite quickly (2 hours ± a few minutes) becomes extremely tender, and the center appears to be a sinking blue infarct in the skin with hemorrhage at the edges. Prompt evaluation by a physician is needed to anticipate systemic loxoscelism. The history of "seeing a spider" is not useful to the diagnosis because spiders are so plentiful and imagination is strong. Careful differential diagnosis must include infection, all trauma, injected chemicals, artifacts, vascular disorders, and drug effects. Rarely, the venom is able to provoke systemic hemolysis and coagulation disorders, which may lead to renal failure and coma. Treatment of brown recluse bites centers on splinting, padding, and resting the injured site while watching out for hemolysis by sequential urinalysis. In the event of systemic dysfunction, precise hydration must be ensured to optimize renal function. Methods of managing coagulopathy must

be considered, and prompt consultation is valuable, in the most severe cases.

The black widow is mainly a southern spider but it occurs throughout the United States. The venom is neurotoxic and in large amounts can cause a neurotransmitter overdose (acetylcholine). Acute symptoms (in 10 to 30 minutes) include salivation, sweating, cardiac dysrhythmia, hypotension, muscle cramping, and waves of severe abdominal pain. In small children or the elderly, the bite may become threatening and, if so, bed rest, a calcium gluconate intravenous solution, diazepam, and blood pressure regulation are usually sufficient to allow recovery in 48 hours. However antivenin *(Latrodectus mactans)* may be needed in the most severe bites. The more rapid and severe the onset of symptoms after envenomation, the more the risk, and deaths are reported.

Ticks. Trivial tick bites are extremely common, and most people are well aware of how to remove ticks entirely from skin without leaving the head or mouth parts imbedded. Regular checking of children twice daily to remove all ticks is wise when they play in infested areas. The principal adverse effect of the tick bite is a secondary bacterial infection or foreign body reaction at the site, which may require a physician's aid. Rickettsia infections (erythema chronicum migrans), tick paralysis, and the spirochetal disease Lyme disease are all uncommon. Antibiotic therapy may be useful in certain complications. Proper clothing and repellents can prevent tick bites.

Mites. Scabies is epidemic in the United States and the only parasite commonly invading the epidermis. About 6 weeks after infestation, a child develops an extremely pruritic papular eruption, especially on fingers, wrists, elbows, axillae, nipples, waist, buttocks, genitalia, waist, knees, and feet. The disease spreads vigorously through the family. Correct diagnosis relies on scraping mites from the skin, microscopic identification, and close follow-up examinations. Assurances that all infested family members and other close contacts are well treated are essential to curing the disease. Recurrences are common in families where all are not treated.

Applications of lindane (Kwell) will eradicate scabies, but lindane must be used very carefully on the very young, those with chronically damaged skin, and children with latent atopic dermatitis. Proper diagnosis and treatment of all family members at one time will prevent unnecessary overtreatment. Lotion or creams (1% lindane) are best applied carefully on the skin and in every crease from chin to toes and left for about 8 hours, but somewhat longer or shorter times appear safe and effective. A more conservative therapy is the application of 6 to 10% powdered sulfur in petrolatum applied twice a day for four days.

Chiggers. Grassy fields are commonly infested with chiggers (larval trombiculae), which attach briefly to skin and bite along the lines of the tight fitting clothing of children. Nothing benefits the itching or improves healing after the bites, but correct use of repellents and treated clothing will prevent trouble. Traditional remedies, including fingernail polish, have no therapeutic worth. Adverse effects are occasional hypersensitivity reactions, and pyodermas, mostly due to scratching. In extreme cases, sedation with antihistamines may be needed to assure sleep for a night or two.

INSECTS

Bees, Wasps, Hornets. Bees, wasps, and hornets (Hymenoptera) are the most threatening of all the arthropods because severe allergy to the venom is widespread. Modern diagnosis of potential severe allergy is accurate, and desensitization is needed, using the purified antigens. Swarms of "bee-wasp-hornets" may be frightening, and their stings induce a severe and acute but temporary illness with urticaria, edema, and hypotension, which is not a systemic hypersensitivity reaction. Cool compresses and antihistamine medications are simple therapy for common stings.

Lice. Lice are common parasites of humans. Blood meals are obtained by regular biting, and eggs are attached to hairs. Lice are easily visible to the unaided eye and can be precisely identified under the microscope. Head lice, pubic lice, and body lice are closely related types. Lindane lotions and creams, used just as for the therapy of scabies, in a single dose, will reliably destroy all lice and the eggs. Shampoo can be worked into scalp or other well-wetted hairy areas and left to soak for about 4 minutes before thorough rinsing. One shampoo is adequate if all members of the group are cured together.

Fleas. Probably more humans are bitten by fleas than by any other arthropod. Many persons have developed immunity to flea venom and are wholly unreactive, while others develop numerous hives and pruritic papules, often with tiny vesicles. Eradication of fleas from the home is almost impossible, but some limitation in numbers is possible and temporary control can be achieved. Steroid creams are effective for reducing itching from flea bites. In some tropical areas, in arid regions, and on beaches, fleas may be unbearable, in which case rigorous use of repellents may help.

Gnats, Flies, and Mosquitoes (Diptera). Blood-sucking flies and mosquitoes are common in the United States, including such vicious types as sand flies, gnats, "punkies," "no-see-ums," midges, pine flies, black flies, buffalo gnats, stable flies, horse flies, and others. Their bites may cause blood to run, large ecchymoses to remain in the skin, and painful or pruritic nodules to last for many days. In small children, astonishing edema of the face and generalized urticaria may arise quickly after inapparent bites and cause the family to dash for the emergency room. In the United States, only a few flies implant larvae or transmit diseases. Treatment consists of prompt escape from infested areas, cool packs, and antihistamine medications. Repellents are valuable.

Animal and Human Bites and Bite-Related Infections

WILLIS A. WINGERT, M.D.

NON-VENOMOUS ANIMAL BITES

Domestic and Wild Animal Bites

Dogs are responsible for 85% of all reported animal bites. About 50% of dog and cat bites are provoked or occur following teasing, feeding, or playing with the animal.

In the management of domestic or wild animal bites, there are three major considerations: 1) the care of lacerations, puncture wounds, scratches, or crushed necrotic tissue; 2) the inoculation of infectious bacterial organisms from the animal's mouth; and 3) the risk of transmission of rabies virus from animal to man.

Carry out the following steps:

1. Anesthetize the wound appropriately.
2. Wash all lacerations and puncture wounds for at least 15 minutes with 20% soap solution. Benzalkonium chloride (Zephiran), aqueous solution, is an alternative.
3. Since dog bites tend to produce crushing injuries (the jaws exert a pressure of 400 lb/sq inch during a bite), meticulously and aseptically debride all traumatized or potentially nonviable tissue, making sure to remove all foreign particles.
4. Obtain complete hemostasis.
5. Irrigate the wounds thoroughly with at least 1000 ml normal saline solution. This is a major deterrent to secondary infection.
6. Large lacerations and facial wounds may require sutures. If so, provide adequate drainage. Do not suture puncture wounds, which are difficult to irrigate thoroughly and which have high incidence of secondary infection.
7. If the wound is on the hand or arm or if the animal's teeth penetrated to the bone or to a tendon sheath, administer prophylactic penicillin G or a cephalosporin. Initial cultures are not helpful; they rarely correlate well with subsequent infection.
8. Observe all wounds, especially those caused by cats, for secondary or generalized infection. Recheck the wound no later than 48 hours, and

sooner if the area becomes painful or inflamed. The most common secondary infections from dog and cat bites result from the gram-negative organism *Pasteurella multocida* and from gram-positive *Staphylococcus aureus* and *S. epidermidis*. *P. multocida* characteristically causes local pain, swelling, inflammation, local abscesses, and lymphangitis with regional lymphadenopathy manifested as early as 4 hours and as late as 48 hours after the bite.

9. Observe selected patients for at least 21 days. Bites by rats, mice, and cats may transmit two pathogenic organisms causing systemic disease: *Spirillum minus:* After an incubation period of 14 to 18 days, an indurated lesion appears at the bite site, accompanied by marked regional adenopathy, a purple or red macular body rash, prolonged relapsing fever, and myalgia. *Streptobacillus moniliformis:* After an incubation period of 7 to 10 days, fever, chills, and severe headache occur, followed by a dull red maculopapular rash on the extremities and a persistent polyarthritis. Both organisms are susceptible to penicillin. If symptoms develop, hospitalize the patient, obtain a blood culture and administer vigorous penicillin therapy (100,000 U/kg/day) IV or IM. Tetracycline 50 mg/kg/day PO (maximum 2 gm/day) is effective in penicillin-allergic patients. Notify parents of children under 8 years of age of possible dental defects if tetracycline is required.

Cat bites and scratches also may transmit tularemia, either in ulceroglandular or typhoidal form, and cat-scratch disease, the causative agent of which has not been isolated.

Monkey bites may transmit Herpes virus simiae, which causes a potentially fatal encephalitis or myelitis in humans after a 1- to 3-week incubation period.

10. Splint extremities which are extensively lacerated until the wounds have healed—7 to 10 days.

11. Capture, isolate, and observe domestic animals for 10 days. Determine the vaccination status of the animal if possible. If the animal does not become ill or die during this period, rabies prophylaxis is unnecessary. Animals that have received rabies immunization within 2 years are unlikely to transmit rabies, but require observation.

If the animal becomes ill during the period of observation, a veterinarian should evaluate the animal and may sacrifice it and ship the head under refrigeration to a qualified laboratory for examination of the brain by fluorescent antibody technique.

12. Immunize all patients meeting the following criteria:
   a. Bitten by an escaped wild animal, whether the animal appears sick or well. This is especially important if the animal was behaving aberrantly. The prevalence of rabies in wild animals has doubled in the past 3 years. The major animals involved are skunks, foxes, bats, and raccoons. These species should be considered rabid until proved otherwise. A normally shy and nocturnal wild animal that appears aberrantly near human habitation in the daytime and displays aggressive behavior or partial paralysis, must be considered rabid. Rabies in small rodents and lagomorphs (rabbits and hares) is extremely rare, and bites by these animals usually do not not require prophylactic treatment.
   b. Bitten by a domestic animal that is ill or behaving aberrantly. Rabies is manifested by two types of aberrant behavior: "Furious," i.e., highly excitable; unpredictable; unusually aggressive, anorexic, or displaying pica; drooling. "Paralytic": Dogs and cats may run away and hide in secluded places, and cattle may stand immobile and drooling as though a foreign body were lodged in their throat. In some geographic areas, rabies may occur more frequently in cats than in dogs, possibly due to exposure to rabid skunks (feral cats) and to lack of rabies immunization.
   c. Bitten by a stray domestic animal that is not captured in a community in which the incidence of rabies is high, either in that domestic species or in the local wild fauna. Contact the local public health department for information. A captured stray animal should be evaluated by a veterinarian and held for examination or killed immediately for examination of the brain.
   d. Bitten by a wild animal, sick or well, that is kept as a pet. Rabies virus may be present in saliva for a variable period before the onset of clinical symptoms. The duration of this period depends upon the species. Asymptomatic rabid dogs may secrete the virus up to 3 days, cats for 2 days. However, asymptomatic skunks may secrete the virus for 18 days and bats for several months.

13. Prophylactic treatment:
   Administer human rabies immune globulin (RIG), 20 IU/kg as a single dose, for rapid passive immune protection (half-life about 21 days). Infiltrate half the dose around the wound site if such infiltration does not compromise circulation to the area (e.g., finger or toe).
   Administer human diploid cell strain (HDVC) rabies vaccine, (Merieux Institute or Wyeth), 1 ml intramuscularly, immediately, and repeat on days 3, 7, 14, and 28 after the first dose. (The World Health Organization currently recommends a sixth dose 90 days after the first).
   Do not mix the vaccine and the serum together

in the same syringe and do not inject at the same site.

RIG is administered once, at the beginning of prophylaxis, but may be administered up to the eighth day after the first dose of HDVC. Thereafter an active antibody response to HDVC has occurred, and RIG is not necessary.

In patients who are receiving corticosteroids and immunosuppressive agents, measure the rabies serum antibody titer at least by day 28, since response may be inadequate. If the titer is less than 1:20, give additional booster doses at 14-day intervals until repeat antibody testing indicates a titer of > 1:20. State or local health departments may be contacted for serological testing.

14. Prevent tetanus by administering a tetanus toxoid booster or 250 units of human immune tetanus globulin if unimmunized.

15. Educate parents regarding suitability of pets for children.
    a. Use judgment in timing, purchase, and choice of a pet: Large breeds and guard dogs (e.g., German shepherds) are more dangerous than small breeds and working dogs (e.g., beagles, spaniels). Children under 5 years of age seldom exercise good judgment around pets and often provoke animals to bite.
    b. Always supervise small children when around dogs and cats, either strange animals or family pets.
    c. Keep aggressive animals under strict control, especially guard dogs.
    d. Completely immunize all pets, both dogs and cats, and keep immunizations current.
    e. Wild animals are dangerous, unpredictable pets.

16. Pre-exposure rabies treatment: For those likely to be exposed to rabies, by occupation or recreation (e.g., veterinarians or spelunkers), consider pre-exposure immunization. Three 1 ml doses of rabies HDCV at 0, 7 and 28 days are required, with booster doses or antibody determinations at 2-year intervals thereafter.

HUMAN BITES

Human dental plaques and gingivae harbor at least 42 different species of organisms, and human saliva contains 10^8 bacteria per ml. Pathogenic organisms include *S. aureus* (frequently penicillinase-producing strains), group A and viridans streptococci, *Eikenella corrodens* (which causes indolent ulceration), *Bacteroides melaninogenicus*, *Proteus* sp., *Escherichia coli*, *Neisseria* sp., *Klebsiella* sp., *Aerobacter* sp., *Mycobacterium tuberculosis*, *Actinomycetes* sp., spirochetes, and hepatitis B virus. Atypical strains of *Pasteurella multocida* have been isolated from human bite wounds.

A blow by the clenched fist with stretched exten-sor tendons may strike the incisor teeth of an adversary, resulting in a serious penetrating wound. As the hand opens, the tendons retract, lie proximally to the laceration and tend to seal pathogenic bacteria within a closed tendon sheath. The infection then spreads through various compartments of the hand, resulting in tenosynovitis, septic arthritis, osteomyelitis, and immobile joints.

Treatment

1. Culture the wound for both aerobes and anaerobes, even though the results are seldom helpful in guiding early therapy.
2. Anesthetize the area appropriately. For extensive wounds, a general anesthetic may be required.
3. Irrigate the area with at least 1000 ml normal saline solution.
4. Debride meticulously, removing crushed, devitalized tissue and visible foreign bodies.
5. X-ray the area for foreign bodies not grossly visible.
6. Except for facial wounds, do not suture. Apply dry, sterile dressings daily.
7. Immobilize extremities that have sustained lacerations.
8. Administer tetanus prophylaxis either by a tetanus toxoid booster or by human tetanus antitoxin, 250 units IM.
9. Administer a broad spectrum antibiotic: Cephalexin, 50 mg/kg/day, or cefaclor, 40 mg/kg/day PO.
10. Suture facial wounds: Eliminate dead space by closing with absorbable 3-0 or 4-0 suture. Close facial skin with 4-0 or 6-0 nylon sutures. Examine the wound at 24 and 48 hours for infection or inflammation.
11. Hospitalize all patients with extensive wounds, wounds that involve joints and bones (fractures), lacerations involving the hand or foot, or inflammation developing in a minor wound. Administer penicillin G, 200,000 U/kg/day (or ampicillin, 100–150 mg/kg/day), and methicillin, 250 mg/kg/day, intravenously. If the patient is allergic to penicillin, administer cefamandole naftate, 10 mg/kg/day or cefazolin 100 mg/kg/day. Evaluate the wound daily and obtain appropriate cultures to identify specific organisms. The type and duration of further intravenous therapy are guided by the clinical response. Continue all antibiotic therapy for at least 10 days.
12. If seen 12 hours after the bite, 60% of all wounds will be seriously secondarily infected by *S. aureus*, *E. corrodens*, or related bacteria. Hospitalize the patient. Administer penicillin G or ampicillin plus methicillin plus an aminoglycoside (Amikacin, 20 mg/kg/day or gentamicin, 5 mg/kg/day), intravenously until a pathogen is isolated by culture. Vancomycin or

a cephalosporin is an alternative drug for penicillin-sensitive patients.

13. Inspect all wounds at at least 12-hour intervals for the first 48 hours. Suppurative tenosynovitis is a surgical emergency.

14. Biting is a common form of child abuse. If the child is less than 5 years of age or if circumstances of the trauma are uncertain, photograph the bitten areas. Consult a forensic pathologist for identification of the assailant either by pattern and measurement of the tooth marks or by three-dimensional scanning electron microscopy. Examine the patient carefully for other signs of injury or neglect, including x-rays of long bones and chest for old or new fractures. Report suspected cases promptly to local authorities as required by state law.

VENOMOUS ANIMAL BITES

Poisonous Snakes

Nineteen species of venomous snakes occur in the United States: Seventeen species of the family Crotalidae, or pit vipers, including rattlesnakes (genera *Crotalus* and *Sistrurus*) and the copperheads and moccasins or cottonmouths *(Agkistrodon)*; and two species of the family Elapidae, or coral snakes, which are limited to southern and southwestern states.

Pit viper venoms are complex poisons containing, depending on species, 3 to 12 small lethal proteins and peptides and 5 to 15 digestive enzymes. The pharmacologic actions of these components include the following:

1. Local tissue necrosis.
2. Capillary endothelial cell injury resulting in altered permeability and transudation of erythrocytes and plasma into tissues and pulmonary alveoli.
3. Local progressive swelling.
4. Hypovolemia.
5. Pulmonary edema.
6. Coagulation defects.
7. Hemolysis.
8. Renal shutdown.
9. Disturbance in neuromuscular transmission by venoms of the coral snakes and the Mojave rattlesnake *(C. scutulatus)*.
10. Probable liberation of histamine, bradykinin, adenosine, and prostaglandins with specific pharmacologic actions.

Envenomation, therefore, produces complex poisoning involving almost all organ systems either primarily or secondarily.

Management

First Aid in the Field

1. Avoid panic. Studies on experimental animals indicate that the median lethal dose (LD_{50}) of venom is increased significantly by increasing muscular activity.

2. Identify the species and size of the snake, if possible. If not possible, using a long stick, kill the snake with sharp blows on the neck. Do not mutilate the head, since the scale pattern is a major method of species identification. Transport the dead snake in a cloth bag or at the end of a long stick to the closest person capable of identifying the species. Never handle an allegedly dead snake.

3. Immobilize the extremity by splinting as if for a fracture.

4. Transport the victim to the nearest medical facility without delay.

5. *Do not:* a) excise the bitten area; b) apply a tourniquet; c) use cryotherapy; d) make incisions over the fang marks and apply suction. These measures have *never* been demonstrated to be effective in humans and both traumatize the envenomated areas with introduction of secondary infection and interfere with subsequent clinical estimation of severity of envenomation.

Hospital Management

1. Establish a physiologic baseline:

   a. Verify that the snake was poisonous. Pit vipers: indentation or pit between but below level of eye and nostril on each side of head; vertical elliptical pupils; triangular head with definite neck area; moveable maxillary fangs; single row of subcaudal plates just below anal plate at tail (harmless snakes have a double row); rattles (Crotalus species). Coral snakes: round pupils; Small, fixed maxillary fangs; a black snout; a species-specific sequential pattern of color bands completely encircling the body—red-yellow (or white)-black (mimics have other sequences).

   b. Record vital signs.

   c. Rapidly evaluate signs and symptoms: One or more distinct fang punctures, usually somewhat irregular; local progressive swelling; ecchymosis; hemorrhagic blebs at or near bite site; fasciculations of face and extremities; paresthesias of face, mouth, and tongue: numbness, tingling, metallic taste; history of known sensitivity to horse serum and antibiotics.

   d. Obtain blood for the following determinations: complete blood count and erythrocyte morphology; platelet count; type and cross-match; coagulation screen—prothrombin time, PTT, fibrinogen level, fibrin split products (if available), bleeding time (template). If severely envenomated, BUN, serum electrolytes, serum protein, blood gases and pH.

   e. Urinalysis with particular attention to hematuria.

   f. Measure and record the circumference of the

injured extremity at proximal point of edema and approximately 4 inches proximal to this level.

2. In case of pit viper bites, determine the severity of envenomation. Grade the reaction as follows: No envenomation: No local or systemic reaction although fang marks are present.*

   Minimal: Local swelling but no systemic reaction.

   Moderate: Swelling that progresses beyond the site of the bite with a systemic reaction, paresthesias, and/or laboratory changes such as a decrease in platelets or fibrinogen level, fall in hematocrit, or hematuria.

   Severe: Marked local swelling and ecchymosis, progressing rapidly up the extremity; severe general symptoms such as bleeding or shock; marked laboratory changes.

3. Perform a skin test for sensitivity to horse serum.

   Inject intradermally 0.02 ml of a 1:10 dilution of antivenin.

   Inject 0.02 ml normal saline at another site as a control.

   Note: This skin test is neither highly reliable nor sensitive.

4. Start intravenous infusions in two extremities: One line for life support if needed: Administration of blood, plasma, epinephrine or measurement of central venous pressure. A second line to administer antivenin.

5. Administer an adequate amount of antivenin intravenously: Antivenin (*Crotalidae*) Polyvalent, North and South American anti-snake serum (Wyeth Laboratories). Initial dose, based on grade of envenomation:

   No envenomation: 0 antivenin
   Minimal: 5 vials (50 ml)
   Moderate: 10 vials (100 ml)
   Severe: 15 vials (150 ml)

   Exceptions: Small children require 1½ times the recommended dose. Patients known to be bitten by *C. scutulatus* should receive an initial dose of 10 vials.

   Dilute the antivenin in 250 ml 0.25 normal saline and administer intravenously as rapidly as possible, preferably over 1 to 2 hours. Rate of administration depends upon the child's weight (20 ml/kg/hr) and appearance of a systemic reaction to the antivenin. Verified bites by coral snakes require five vials of *Micrurus fulvius* antivenin (Wyeth) administered intravenously in 250 ml 0.25 normal saline as rapidly as possible, preferably within 2 hours.

6. Monitor and support the physiological status of the circulatory, respiratory, and renal systems.

   a. Monitor the vital signs, especially the blood pressure. Insert a central venous catheter in severely envenomated patients. Treat hypovolemic shock by administering 10 to 20 ml/kg of a plasma expander (*not* a crystalloid solution).

   b. Repeat hemoglobin, hematocrit and platelet levels every 1 to 2 hours. Transfuse with 10 ml/kg packed red cells or whole blood if levels are falling.

   c. Obtain serial electrolyte determinations and correct abnormalities in fluid and electrolyte balance as indicated.

   d. Monitor intake and output as an index of renal function. Repeat the urinalysis periodically for evidence of hematuria or proteinuria.

   e. Administer oxygen by mask as needed. In case of coral snake or Mohave rattlesnake envenomation, prepare to insert an endotracheal tube and ventilate mechanically.

   f. Every 20 minutes, measure the circumference of the affected extremity and compare with the initial determinations. Mark the progress of swelling with a timed line. Note development of any systemic reactions (shock, hemorrhages). Repeat the initial dose of antivenin intravenously every 1 to 2 hours until no further progression of swelling occurs and no general symptoms appear.

7. If envenomation is severe or if incision and suction has been applied, administer a broad spectrum antibiotic (ampicillin or amoxicillin) prophylactically for secondary infection for 7 to 10 days. Later cultures of the wound will guide the choice of antibiotic.

8. Prevent tetanus by administering tetanus toxoid as a booster for previously immunized patients or 250 units of human immune tetanus globulin if unimmunized.

9. Immobilize the extremity in a position of function on a well-padded splint. Maintain at or slightly below heart level. Debride hemorrhagic blebs, vesicles, and superficial necrotic tissue aseptically between the third and fifth days, provided coagulation studies are within normal limits. Cleanse daily and cover with dry sterile dressings.

10. Begin rehabilitation therapy within 5 days to prevent contractures and deformities.

11. Observe for serum sickness developing after 7 to 14 days. Administer prednisone 2 mg/kg/day in 4 divided doses or an equivalent amount of dexamethasone. Continue until all signs and symptoms have subsided. Antihistamines are of little value except for sedation or to alleviate pruritus.

---

*Bites by the Mojave rattlesnake (*C. scutulatus*) require careful evaluation since the venom, while very lethal neurologically, may cause only slight local reaction.

12. Notify police or the State Department of Fish and Game if the patient was bitten by a captive venomous snake. Most states require a license to collect or maintain a venomous animal.

ARTHROPODS

Spiders

Spider venoms cause two major types of reactions: neurotoxic reactions due to black widow (*Latrodectus mactans*) bites; and local tissue necrosis due to bites of at least 24 species, including the notorious brown recluse (*Loxosceles* sp.), jumping spiders (*Phidippus*), wolf spiders (*Lycosa* sp.), orb weavers (*Argiope* and *Neascona* sp.), and others. Tarantulas inflict painful but rarely toxic bites.

Latrodectus venom blocks neuromuscular transmission, probably due to excess release of transmitter substance (acetylcholine) from nerve terminals with subsequent depolarization and exhaustion.

Other spider venoms cause necrosis of the dermis by several mechanisms: Cellular damage to the endothelium of capillaries and venules with subsequent thrombosis and infarction; and interaction with complement, causing localized lysis of polymorphonuclear leukocytes and mast cells and releasing kinins and other proteolytic enzymes and histamine.

Black Widow (*Latrodectus mactans*) Envenomation

1. Identify the offending spider, if possible:
   a. *L. mactans* female is shiny, coal black, with a 1 to 1.5 cm long body and a leg span up to 5 cm. A red marking, characteristically shaped like an hourglass *but* with several variations, is present on the ventral abdomen. Note: In southern states, this genus also has red and brown species.
   b. Determine the situation in which the bite occurred: *Latrodectus* builds disorganized webs in dark recesses, cracks in walls, outdoor privies, rarely in open areas.
   c. The bite is usually moderately painful.
   d. Examine the bite site with a magnifying lens for fang marks: two small puncture wounds about 1 mm apart.
2. Hospitalize all children who develop symptoms or signs, usually within 2 hours after the bite: severe local and radiating pain; muscle fasciculation, spasm, or rigidity; hypertension.
3. Relieve muscle spasm by careful intravenous administration of 10% calcium gluconate, 200 mg/kg, or diazepam (Valium), 0.3 mg/kg (this drug also relieves nausea and vomiting).
4. Administer one ampoule (2.5 ml) of *Latrodectus mactans* antivenin IV in 60 ml 0.5 normal saline after appropriate skin tests for horse serum sensitivity.
5. Serially monitor vital signs and symptoms for 48 hours. Control hypertension with appropriate medication (propranolol) as required.
6. A second dose of antivenin may be administered if symptoms persist. This is very unusual.

All Other Spider Bites

1. Identify the etiology of the bite, if possible.
   a. Spider bites usually cause little or no initial pain and often are not felt by the patient. Severe pain would indicate some other offender.
   b. Spiders rarely bite more than once. Multiple lesions rule out arachnidism.
   c. The appearance of the bite varies from local erythema and edema to a wheal or a vesicle, which may ulcerate. Severe envenomation, especially by *Loxosceles,* results in a "target lesion": A small bleb surrounded by an ischemic ring, later outlined by an erythematous ring of extravasated erythrocytes.
2. Identify the offending spider if possible. The highly poisonous recluse spiders live indoors in closets, trunks, and attics, and outdoors in woodpiles and under rocks. The web is irregular. *Loxosceles* sp. range from 9 to 12 mm in size and are fawn or brown in color with a dark brown mark on the dorsal cephalothorax (often resembling a violin). Using a magnifying glass, count the eyes: small, black dots on head. *Loxosceles* sp. have six eyes (all others have eight).
3. Hospitalize the patient if a typical target lesion appears or if a lesion increases rapidly in size within 12 hours.
4. Administer dexamethasone, 0.10 mg/kg, intramuscularly every 6 hours. When the lesion no longer progresses, give dexamethasone, 0.05 mg/kg, or prednisone, 0.25 mg/kg, orally every 6 hours for 5 days.
5. Obtain serial blood and platelet counts and urinalyses for 48 hours from small children suspected of being bitten by *Loxosceles* sp. The venom causes intravascular hemolysis, hemolytic anemia, hemoglobinuria, thrombocytopenia, and coagulation defects.
6. Administer a systemic antibiotic to all patients with ulcerating lesions or lymphangitis. Drugs of choice are dicloxacillin 25 mg/kg/day or a cephalosporin (cephradine) 100 mg/kg/day intravenously or cefaclor 40 mg/kg/day by mouth.
7. Administer appropriate tetanus prophylaxis.
8. Cleanse ulcerating lesions daily with an antiseptic solution (e.g., betadine) and cover with a dry sterile dressing. After the eschar sloughs, surgically debride the entire area and repair by plastic surgery.
9. Apply a topical steroid ointment such as triamcinolone ointment 0.1% qid to minor lesions that show no evidence of progression or ischemia. However, observe the lesion at 24-hour intervals for secondary infection.

Scorpion Stings

Two lethal scorpions, *Centruroides sculpturatus* and *C. gertschii*, are found in the Southwest from Arizona to California and in Texas and northern Mexico. Other scorpion stings produce a painful local but not severe systemic reaction, probably by local release of kinins.

Centruroides venom increases release of acetylcholine at the presynoptic terminal of the neuromuscular junction, causing depolarization and subsequent muscle twitching, fibrillation, and excessive continuous muscular activity. The venom stimulates sympathetic nerves directly and may cause a "sympathetic storm" with marked central nervous system stimulation leading to convulsions and to hypertension. Direct cardiotoxicity with myocardial edema and necrosis has been observed.

Treatment

1. Identify the offending scorpion. The potentially dangerous *C. sculpturatus* is a small (2 to 7.5 cm) uniformly yellow scorpion without stripes and with few tactile hairs. Examine the stinger with a magnifying glass (handle the animal with tweezers). A small tubercle (spine or tooth) occurs on the last segment of the tail, just below the sting. Observe and tap the area which has been stung. Since *Centruroides* venom is low in digestive enzymes, swelling and bleeding are rare. However, the area is extremely sensitive to touch and tapping may cause excruciating pain.
2. Stings by scorpions other than *Centruroides* require only relief of pain: Cold compresses over the wound, injection of a local anesthetic, e.g., lidocaine directly into the wound site, or acetaminophin orally. *Do not* administer narcotics. These drugs potentiate the action of scorpion venom.
3. Administer tetanus prophylaxis as indicated.
4. Hospitalize patients stung by *C. sculpturatus*. Monitor vital signs, especially blood pressure. Obtain an electrocardiogram. Control CNS symptoms by sedation with phenobarbital, 5 to 10 mg/kg IM, repeated every 6 to 8 hours as required. Administer propranolol as a sympathetic blocking agent for marked hypertension not responding to sedation.

Scorpion antivenin is available only in Arizona from the Poisonous Animals Research Laboratory, Arizona State University, Tempe. Call the Regional Poison Control Center: 602-253-3334.

This antivenin has not yet been approved by the Food and Drug Administration.

Other Arthropods

Centipede bites cause pain, local swelling and tenderness, lymphangitis, lymphadenopathy, and rarely local necrosis. Treatment consists of relief of pain by analgesics, cold compresses, or injection of local anesthetic such as lidocaine.

Triatoma protracta, the western conenose, kissing or assassin bug, is 10 to 20 mm long and black or dark brown in color. The bug's long proboscis breaks the skin of children (often around the lips), injects a lytic saliva, and ingests the victim's blood. An unidentified protein component in the saliva causes an allergic response in children. The area swells and itches, and the patient may develop nausea, faintness, chills, or anaphylactic shock.

If the reaction is mild, apply a topical steroid and administer an antihistamine by mouth, such as chlortrimeton, 2 to 4 mg, every 6 hours.

For severe reactions, administer prednisone 2 mg/kg/day PO in four divided doses until the reaction subsides.

Burns

BONNY H. BOWSER, M.H.S.A.,
and FRED T. CALDWELL, Jr., M.D.

Burn injury is the third most common cause of accidental death in children. As a general rule, children with burns of less than 10% of the body surface may be handled as outpatients.

The most common cause of thermal injury in young children is scalding (33%). Scald injury usually produces a partial thickness burn which will heal in 7 to 21 days. Scald injury produces deeper skin destruction in infants because they have thinner skin. Full thickness burn injury usually results from clothing flame burn.

Assessment of the Patient

A history of sustaining burn injury in an enclosed space should alert the clinician to the possibility of inhalation injury. Examination of the upper airway should be performed. Singed vibrissae, carbonaceous material in the mouth and upper airway, or edema and inflammatory changes are not reliable indicators of inhalation injury. Bronchoscopy with a 3 mm fiberoptic bronchoscope is the most useful early examination for predicting inhalation injury. Erythema, edema, and carbonaceous material in the lower tracheobronchial tree correlate with significant inhalation injury. If signs of inhalation injury are noted, 40% humidified oxygen should be administered by mask. Maintenance of an adequate airway may require early endotracheal intubation. The indications for intubation are: 1) impending or partial airway obstruction secondary to edema; 2) inability to handle copious secretions; and 3) inability to adequately ventilate without assistance. Mechanical ventilation will usually be needed for the intubated patient. Tracheostomy is rarely indicated and should be avoided if possible. Indications for tracheostomy in burn patients are the same as for any other patient. Establishing and maintaining an adequate airway is the number one priority.

A large bore IV should be placed and at the same time blood drawn for clinical analysis including hematocrit, electrolytes, osmolality and arterial blood gases. Blood levels of carbon monoxide should be obtained if smoke inhalation or asphyxia is suspected. Once intravenous fluids are running, all residual clothing should be cut away and jewelry removed. At this point an accurate body weight should be obtained and the area and depth of injury estimated. An accurate assessment of burn area may be obtained using the Lund and Browder chart, which makes adjustments for age.

Visual inspection is the most common method of estimating depth of injury. Very superficial and very deep injury can be accurately determined. The intermediate depths, including deep dermal injury, are difficult to determine in a single examination. Partial thickness burn wounds are usually pink to red in color and may be covered with blisters. Such areas are sensitive to pin prick and touch. Full thickness burn areas are usually dry and are pearly white or gray in color. Deeper injury may have a brown leather appearance with visible coagulated vessels. Such areas are anesthetic.

Early Wound Care

Early wound care should follow simple surgical principles. Using sterile technique, all debris, loose tissue, and blisters should be gently removed. If pain medication is required, small doses of morphine should be administered intravenously.

When debridement is complete, wounds should be cultured and dressed with silver sulfadiazine cream and occlusive sterile dressings.

Transport Considerations

All life-threatening thermal burns are best treated in a burn center. Before transport, a secure IV should be obtained and a balanced salt solution administered according to plan. In addition, a Foley catheter should be placed and adequacy of the patient's airway reviewed. Wounds should be dressed for transport. Wet dressings should not be applied for transport, for severe whole body hypothermia may result.

Triage Criteria

These criteria should be modified according to the experience of the attending physician and the burn care resources that are readily available.

All burn patients should be admitted to a hospital if 1) the total burn area is greater than 15% of the body surface area (BSA); 2) the total area of third degree burn is greater than 2%; 3) the age is less than 2 years; 4) there is evidence of airway or inhalation injury; 5) there is electrical injury; 6) there is any associated injury or pre-existing disease; 7) the burns involve hands, face, feet, or perineum; 8) child abuse is suspected.

The patient should be transported to a specialized burn treatment facility if 1) the total area of injury is greater than 20% of the BSA; 2) the total area of full thickness injury is greater than 10% BSA; 3) there is severe airway or inhalation injury; 4) severe electrical injury is present; 5) there is significant associated injury or pre-existent disease; 6) deep burns of the hands, face, feet, or perineum are present.

Intravenous Therapy

Burn injury results in generalized increased capillary permeability, resulting in a decrement in plasma volume directly proportional to the size of the injury. This results in the rapid development of burn shock if appropriate treatment is not promptly started. The reduced plasma volume is reflected by a rise in hematocrit and an increase in blood viscosity, with impaired peripheral tissue perfusion. Both peripheral and pulmonary vascular resistance are increased, accompanied by a sinus tachycardia, with the result that initially blood pressure is maintained in spite of the massive plasma loss. The cardiac index decreases immediately following injury, as does the rate of urine formation.

Intravenous fluid replacement is indicated for all burns greater than 20% of body surface area. The rate of urine output, vital signs, and blood pH are major determinants of the rate of fluid administration. Blood pressure and pulses are of little help in evaluating the response to treatment. Subclavian catheters are indicated for large burns, and in critical burn injuries, placement of a Swan-Ganz catheter permits sequential measurement of the pulmonary artery wedge pressure and cardiac index.

Placement of IV sites through burn wounds should be avoided if possible. All catheter sites need daily care to minimize the risk of infection. All invasive lines should be removed as soon as the patient's condition will allow, usually by 48 hours postburn.

Fluid needs for the first 24 hours postburn are estimated as 2 ml/kg·% BSA burn of lactated Ringer's solution. One half of the calculated volume is given during the first 8 hours postburn and one quarter in each of the next two 8-hour periods. These are only guidelines for rate of fluid administration, as the patient's response and condition determine the actual rate. Urine output, sensorium, acid base status, and vital signs are the best indicators for adequate resuscitation. Volumes of fluid administered should be guided by urine output if all other indicators remain within acceptable extreme limits. Acceptable rates of urine formation are based on 1 ml of urine per hour per kilogram of body weight in patients weighing less than 30 kg and 30 to 50 ml of urine per hour for patients weighing more than 30 kilograms.

Colloid administration is not indicated during the first 24 hours postburn but may be added during the second 24-hour period. The colloid may be administered as 0.5 ml colloid/kg·% BSA burned. The calculated insensible fluid loss and the desired urine output are also replaced as 5% dextrose in water. (The insensible fluid loss is calculated by subtracting the output from the input and correcting for weight changes over the corresponding 24-hour period.)

Burns of 20% or less of the body surface area can usually be resuscitated with dilute salt solutions given by mouth.

Normal daily fluid requirements for small burns resuscitated orally may be increased 1% for each percent body surface burned.

After resuscitation is complete, caution must be applied when the patient returns to ad lib oral intake. There is a prodigious water and salt loss through the burn wound that may lead to dehydration and/or hyponatremia if not carefully replaced. The fluid loss is usually replaced as the previous day's insensible fluid loss plus the desired urine output. Salt losses are usually adequately replaced by the normal dietary intake of sodium and other electrolytes.

Nasogastric Tube

Ileus is commonly observed during the first several days in burns involving more than 30% BSA. These individuals as well as any patient with nausea, vomiting, or abdominal distention should have a nasogastric tube inserted to reduce the risk of aspiration pneumonitis. The nasogastric tube is a convenient route for administration of antacid preparations, which should be administered to the patients with large burns during resuscitation. Oral antacid administration should continue for several weeks after the patient resumes normal food intake. Antacids are used to help control the known increase in the incidence of stress ulceration following burning.

Nutrition

Nutrition is vital to wound healing and the patient's immunologic status. The body responds to burn injury with an increased metabolic rate that is related to burn size, a negative nitrogen balance, and weight loss. There is a rapid rate of tissue breakdown and loss of protein; therefore, the patient's caloric needs must be met to achieve a positive nitrogen balance. The physician should counsel the patient regarding diet and the need for increased intake of protein, carbohydrate, and fat. Many patients do not understand these terms and

need to have a detailed description of the foods that constitute these major categories. Serious weight loss must be avoided. A 10% loss of weight may lead to an impaired immune response, loss of muscle strength, loss of body cell mass, and delayed wound healing.

Patients with burns of less than 30% BSA should begin eating almost immediately following admission. Patients with burns greater than 30% BSA should begin eating as early as 48 hours and rapidly progress to a full diet with an emphasis on high protein and calorie intake. Daily calorie counts should be kept for each patient in danger of nutritional compromise. Oral alimentation is the first line of defense; however, the energy requirements may be so great in some patients with large burns that the patient cannot realistically reach his caloric goals and will require enteral support. Patients who continue to lose weight on a regular diet will usually stabilize their weight if supplemented with continuous nasogastric tube feedings.

Intravenous hyperalimentation is not recommended for the burn patient with a functioning bowel because of the high risk of infection associated with central lines in burn patients.

The hypermetabolic response may be aggravated by fear, pain, fever, and a cold environment. Therefore, every attempt should be made to minimize these factors. The fear of a dressing change and the pain involved may be lessened by counseling, supplemented with medication. Procedures should be carefully explained, consistent, and carried out as rapidly as possible. The dressing room should be kept warm and exposure time kept to a minimum.

A chronic anemia usually accompanies burn injury and is refractory to iron therapy. Periodic transfusions of whole blood are usually required to correct the anemia. This anemia persists during the course of hospitalization until the burn wounds are healed.

Fever

Burn patients are routinely febrile, and the magnitude of this response is directly related to the size of the burn wound. It is common for the body temperature of burn patients to reach 39°C (102°F) daily, and the increment in body temperature is refractory to acetaminophen (Tylenol) and/or aspirin. Antipyretics are best reserved for elevations above 39°C and should alert one to the possibility that the fever may be of bacterial origin. Blood cultures should be obtained for any temperature in excess of 40°C (104°F).

Analgesia

Burn patients treated with occlusive dressings require analgesia only during dressing changes and manipulations of the burn wounds. The intravenous route with small doses, repeated as needed is the preferred method of narcotic administration for both the acute and chronic burn patients.

Minor burn pain may usually be controlled with Tylenol or aspirin administration. Other drugs in common use for dressing changes include cath mix, meperidine (Demerol), hydroxyzine (Vistaril), diazepam (Valium), and codeine. Methoxyfluorane, administered utilizing the penthrane whistle setup, is approved for pediatric use. This type of analgesia provides amnesia of the dressing change.

Tetanus Prophylaxis

Tetanus toxoid is administered as indicated by the patient's immunologic status. It is always given for large or deep burn wounds.

Escharotomy

Escharotomies are indicated for cases in which there is a constricting band of eschar, as in a circumferential full thickness injury. A constricting eschar produces a tourniquet effect, and, as edema becomes progressively more pronounced, circulation may become compromised in areas distal to the band. The necessity for escharotomy is best assessed by examination of the peripheral pulses with the Doppler device. A full thickness burn of the entire trunk will often impede the full excursion of the thorax, thereby resulting in alveolar hypoventilation and respiratory embarrassment.

Escharotomy may be performed without anesthesia in areas of full thickness injury. A dilute local anesthetic solution can be injected along the line of the planned escharotomy site if pain sensation is present. Using the cutting cautery or a scalpel, an incision is made in the midlateral and/or midmedial line of the limb. The incision should cross all the involved joints and penetrate only to a depth that allows the cut edges of the eschar to spontaneously spread. This will lessen the subeschar tissue pressure.

A fasciostomy will rarely be needed unless the injury involves the subfacial tissues.

Wound Care

Superficial burn wounds (first degree) resulting from excessive sun or heat lamp exposure or flash burns are best managed with qid applications of a commercial sun tan preparation or cocoa butter cream. Bandages are not indicated for this type of injury.

The second and third degree burn injury should ideally be managed employing occlusive dressings and a topical antimicrobial agent. Silver sulfadiazine cream is the standard topical agent for the treatment of most major burn wounds. Topical antimicrobials commonly used as a second line of defense are cerium nitrate cream, silver nitrate soaks, and mafenide acetate cream. Small partial thickness burns that are managed on an outpatient basis may

be treated with a commercial tribiotic ointment preparation that is available without prescription.

After the wound is initially debrided of loose, nonviable tissue, cleansed with warm sterile saline and blotted dry, silver sulfadiazine cream is applied. A thick layer of absorbent coarse mesh gauze is applied over the cream, and this dressing is held in place with Kerlex or a flexible net dressing.

Burned limbs should be elevated continuously above the level of the heart during the immediate postburn period and until the subsequent edema subsides. Upper extremity burns should be elevated by suspension. A sleeve of stockinette is a convenient method to facilitate hand elevation. Elevate the head of the bed for facial burns. Pillow elevation is usually adequate for burns of the feet. Burned limbs should be actively exercised during the first 48 hours to facilitate mobilization of edema fluid.

Inpatient burn dressings should be changed at least once daily. Dressings are not soaked off but rather used as a method of gentle debridement of necrotic tissue. After the wound begins to epithelialize, the outer layer of dressing is removed each day and the layer of dressing next to the wound is soaked with warm saline and gently removed. When only patchy areas of nonhealed wound remain, a layer of petrolatum gauze is applied to prevent adherence of the fragile healed epithelium to the bandage. Unless grafting is required, the wound may be managed entirely with silver sulfadiazine cream and occlusive dressings.

If grafting is required to effect closure of full thickness defects, the graft is affixed with staples or Steri-Strips and the grafted area and donor sites are covered with fine mesh gauze soaked with tribiotic solution. On the first postgraft day, the first layer of fine mesh gauze is left in place and the upper layers of dressing are changed. It is possible to inspect the integrity of the graft through the fine mesh gauze. Tribiotic soaked gauze is placed over the fine mesh gauze and the dressings are reapplied. At 48 hours post graft, the fine mesh gauze on the grafted area is soaked with tribiotic solution and removed. A new layer of tribiotic soaked gauze is applied daily and covered with occlusive dressings.

The graft donor site is initially treated with tribiotic soaked fine mesh gauze and occlusive dressings. At 24 hours, the outer layer of dressing is removed and the dry fine mesh gauze is left in place. The donor site is left dry and treated with heatlamps. As re-epithelization of the donor site occurs, the gauze lifts and is trimmed daily.

Small outpatient burn dressings need not be changed daily. These wounds should be inspected daily by the physician for the first 2 days and then cleansed, medicated, and bandaged every other day at home. Parents should observe the burn wound and dressing procedure at the physician's office to gain confidence and learn the bandaging technique. These patients should return to the physician's office weekly for follow-up care, until wound closure is complete. Superficial partial thickness burn injuries should heal within 7 to 21 days if kept free of infection.

Infection may prolong the healing process or convert the partial thickness burn to a full thickness injury and require skin grafting for closure.

Burns involving joints and extremities require physical therapy and active range of motion exercises to prevent contractures, deformity and loss of function and mobility.

Very deep burns of extremities and joints will require splinting and exercise to preserve function and prevent contractures. Exercises are performed daily when the burn dressings are changed and throughout the day for nonsplinted areas.

Early ambulation is encouraged unless the plantar surface of the feet is burned. Ambulation prevents muscular atrophy and increases joint range of motion.

Burn injury often produces hypertrophic scarring. Pressure gradient garments are now available for use in scar control. These garments are custom fitted and constructed for each individual patient. The physical therapist measures the patient and orders the garments, which are worn for 8 to 12 months following wound closure while the scars are maturing. Diligent use of these garments improves cosmetic results and minimizes subsequent contractures and deformity.

Patients ready for discharge are instructed to keep the burn scars well lubricated with lanolin or cocoa butter and to protect the scar from sun exposure for at least a year.

Sepsis

Sepsis is the major cause of death in burn patients; however, it rarely occurs in patients with small burns or larger partial thickness injuries.

Surveillance of wound flora is necessary. Wound cultures are obtained upon admission and at frequent intervals thereafter until wound closure is complete. Quantitative surface wound cultures monitor the levels of bacteria and warn the clinician of impending sepsis prior to the appearance of visual changes in the wound. Colonization of the burn wound with pathogenic organisms usually occurs in larger burns by the second week. Patients with wound cultures that exceed danger levels (10^5 organisms/cm^2 wound surface) for possible necrotizing wound infection or systemic sepsis should be switched to bid dressing changes, using a topical antibacteral preparation that is bactericidal for the offending organism. However, if bacterial counts persist at a danger level indicative of necrotizing infection, systemic antibiotics should be administered, based on culture sensitivity reports. Otherwise, prophylactic antibiotics are not used. The most common pathogenic organism recovered from burn wounds is coagulase positive staphylococcus; however, *Pseudomonas aeruginosa* is more invasive and leads to most septic complications and deaths.

Psychosocial Aspects

Children are usually comfortable when the burn wound is treated with an occlusive dressing. Apart from the daily dressing change, they usually remain relatively pain free. However, many patients, even those with small injuries, do not adjust well to the fear and pain associated with dressing changes. After prolonged hospitalization, aggression, regression, and combative and manipulative behavior may be manifest. This type of pediatric patient may also suffer from a separation anxiety. These problems should be anticipated and psychologic and sociologic support given.

Family involvement during the patient's inpatient stay is important for the child's psychosocial adjustment to hospitalization. The family will usually be successful in promoting food intake, reassuring the child, explaining daily procedures, and assisting with ambulation and exercise regimens.

Activities that promote self-help should be encouraged. Play therapy is important for psychosocial adjustment, and also promotes physical recovery. Activities that divert the patient's concerns of treatment and self-image are encouraged. The continuation of inpatient schooling is encouraged and serves to reduce the stress associated with return to society following discharge.

For these reasons, skilled, experienced, and consistent nursing care is required to provide the type of psychosocial support needed by the burn patient.

Near-Drowning: An Update

RALPH C. FRATES, Jr., M.D.

A near-drowned person is one who has been submerged in a fluid medium, almost always water, and has suffered cessation of respiration and alteration of consciousness. Only patients who survive the first 24 hours following their initial insult are considered near-drowned; those who die within the first 24 hours are drowned. I think this complicated nosology gives physicians some idea of our difficulty in dealing with this common form of childhood trauma.

Remarkable progress has been made in our understanding and treatment of near-drowning over the last 30 years. Widespread adoption of an effective means of cardiopulmonary resuscitation

(CPR), mechanical ventilation with positive end-expiratory pressure (PEEP), and the more recent introduction of the possibility of cerebral resuscitation are saving lives that would have been lost in past years. Whatever the means, it is clear that tissue hypoxia is what kills or cripples the near-drowned. Therefore, the management priority is correction of tissue hypoxia.

Immediate Treatment. Prompt CPR is by far the most effective therapy. If at all possible, mouth-to-mouth resuscitation should be instituted even before the patient is pulled from the water. Every patient deserves a chance at all-out CPR no matter how lifeless his appearance. This is especially true for patients immersed in cold water (20°C [68°F] or less). The child's diving reflex may be activated by cold water. This reflex shunts warmed, oxygenated blood from extremities, skin, and viscera to a slowly pulsing heart-brain circuit. Because of the child's relatively large surface to volume ratio, core heat loss is swift and the rapid induction of immersion hypothermia may reduce the patient's cerebral oxygen demands in a protective manner. Prolonged CPR and rewarming of cold-water near-drowning victims has resulted in total recovery of several patients, one of whom was trapped underwater by ice for 40 minutes.

Treatment in the Emergency Room. Here, the most important therapy is ventilation and oxygenation. Immediate and forceful ventilation with pure oxygen using a self-inflating resuscitation bag and tightly fitted mask is essential unless the patient is alert and breathing comfortably. This approach may eliminate the need for endotracheal intubation, pressor agents, intravascular volume expansion, or bicarbonate infusion. Should the patient fail to wake up and breathe spontaneously after a few minutes of bagging, however, he should receive 2 meq of sodium bicarbonate by vein for each kilogram of estimated body weight. Nasotracheal and nasogastric tubes should be inserted and carefully checked for position and function. The nasogastric tube is worthwhile because 1) occasionally a patient will ingest enough fresh water to cause severe hyponatremia with subsequent seizure, and 2) gastric distention from oxygen or air pushed in during resuscitation can cause bradycardia from vagal nerve stimulation, at least in babies. Once the patient is intubated and normotensive (shock almost always responds to ventilation and oxygenation), 10 cm H_2O of PEEP should be added to a ventilator already delivering 100% oxygen.

Victims of diving accidents and comatose patients should be managed as though they had post-traumatic brain and spine injuries until proved otherwise. The patient's cervical spine should be stabilized with sand bags when on a table or stretcher, all turns and body transfers should insure little or no spinal movement, and expert tracheal intubation with the least neck extension possible should be employed. Computed tomography of the brain and careful roentgenographic evaluation of the spine should follow these patients' resuscitation and stabilization.

Treatment in the Hospital. All near-drowning patients should be admitted to the hospital for 24 hours. The caveat includes even patients who are alert and have normal physical examinations, chest roentgenograms, and laboratory studies. The rationale for admission of well-appearing patients is that they may develop "secondary drowning" (pulmonary edema or aspiration pneumonitis) or cerebral edema. For patients with minimal distress, enough supplemental oxygen by mask or nasal prongs to keep their PaO_2 at 70 torr or better is administered. Maintenance intravenous fluids, adjusted to correct any electrolyte imbalance, should be given while the child is kept NPO. Febrile patients need cultures of blood and any sputum, and treatment with intravenous ampicillin 200 mg/kg/day is usually started (although this practice is somewhat controversial). Careful observation of the child's vital signs, urine output, and respiratory and neurological findings should be serially recorded every few hours. Most children can be discharged safely the next day, to be re-evaluated as an outpatient in a week or less.

Patients in obvious respiratory distress or who are obtunded or comatose should be admitted to the intensive care unit. Alert patients who require a FiO_2 of 0.6 or greater to maintain a PaO_2 of 60 torr or more should be intubated, as should all obtunded or comatose patients. PEEP of 10 cm H_2O or more should be used to insure adequate oxygenation. Pulmonary oxygen toxicity seems to be associated with prolonged exposure to FiO_2 of 0.6 or greater, and so should be avoided where possible. However, it is also important to remember that "the brain gets soft before the lungs get hard," so PEEP and the FiO_2 should be increased as much as necessary to maintain the PaO_2 at 70 torr. Insertion of a bladder catheter, nasogastric tube, central venous line in the right atrium, and a radial arterial catheter are all recommended at this point, as is electronic surveillance of the patient's cardiogram. Regular tracheal suctioning should be started through an adapter so that PEEP is not lost. Begin chest percussion and bronchial drainage following in-line inhalation of bronchodilator (i.e., 0.3 ml metaproterenol in 2 or 3 ml saline) every 4 hours and turn the patient in a side-back-side rotation every 2 hours to avoid stasis of bronchial secretions. A tracheal aspirate for Gram stain and culture is sent daily.

To prevent gastrointestinal bleeding, the gastric pH needs to be kept above 3.5 by means of one to two ounces of antacid hourly per nasogastric tube. Most near-drowned patients who are being ventilated seem to have better arterial blood gases when they are sedated (morphine, 0.1 mg/kg to 0.5 mg/kg, subcutaneously every hour or as needed) and paralyzed (pancuronium, beginning with 0.1 mg/kg but often requiring 0.4 mg/kg every hour and as needed). Intravenous fluids are given at approximately 60% of maintenance requirements, and furosemide, 0.5 mg/kg to 1.0 mg/kg, may need to be given to initiate and maintain urine output of 1 ml/kg/hour. The reason for keeping the patient somewhat dry is to prevent further leakage from already-damaged capillary beds in the lung (pulmonary edema) and brain (cerebral edema) and hence, to prevent further tissue hypoxia or anoxia.

The obtunded patient whose neurological status is deteriorating and the comatose patient need insertion of an intracranial pressure (ICP) monitor such as a Richmond Bolt. Pupillary changes follow rather than precede brain swelling. Therefore, pupillary changes cannot be relied upon as indicators for emergency treatment of intracranial pressure increases. The goal of therapy is to keep the patient's ICP less than 15 torr. Dean and McComb* reported complete recovery in 3 of 20 comatose, near-drowned children whose ICP never exceeded 20 torr. This is a truly remarkable result. In my experience, warm-water near-drowned children in coma who present with fixed and dilated pupils and require CPR either die or survive in a vegetative state.**

The methods of controlling ICP vary from center to center. Dr. Alan W. Conn and associates have advocated their HYPER therapy approach.† In their experience, comatose near-drowned patients are "hyper*h*ydrated and hyper*v*entilating, with hyper*p*yrexia, hyper*e*xcitability, and hyper*r*igidity." Their recommendations for treatment are incorporated in my previous discussion, but with three principal differences. First, I prefer to keep the patient normothermic or somewhat chilled by means of a cooling blanket (rectal temperature 36°C to 37°C), rather than the 30°C ± 1°C Dr. Conn uses. My rationale is that both experimental and clinical work suggest that prolonged and profound hypothermia may lead to septicemia because of inactivation of white blood cells. Secondly, HYPER therapy now calls for phenobarbital injections to achieve serum levels between 50 to 75 mg/liter. The efficacy of barbiturate coma in the therapy of severe hypoxic encephalopathy is questionable. Large doses of shorter-acting barbiturates such as pentobarbital may drop cerebral perfusion pressure (CPP) below the critical 50 torr point by decreasing cardiac output, even while decreasing ICP. It is important to remember that mean arterial pressure (MAP) minus intracranial pressure equals cerebral perfusion pressure, or MAP − ICP = CPP.

I prefer not to use barbiturates to induce coma but to use as small a dose as possible and then only to abort an intractable pressure spike. Finally, the use of dexamethasone or other steroids to prevent brain swelling from hypoxia probably does not work. Several days of steroid therapy is enough to increase the likelihood of gastrointestinal bleeding.

What does work in controlling ICP, I believe, is as follows: 1) elevation of the head of the bed to about 60 degrees; 2) maintenance of P_{CO_2} from 25 to 30 torr; 3) keeping the patient in a dark, quiet area; and 4) sedation, fluid restriction, normothermia, and paralysis as previously outlined. In an emergency, vigorous bagging of the tracheal tube with 100% oxygen and 1 mg/kg mannitol by rapid IV infusion or furosemide 0.5 to 1.0 mg/kg by IV push seem to work as well as anything else. Those patients who are going to return to normal ICP usually do so by their fourth to sixth day of treatment.

---

*Dean J. M., McComb, J. G.: Intracranial pressure monitoring in severe pediatric near-drowning. Neurosurgery 9:627, 1981.

**Frates, R. C., Jr.: Analysis of predictive factors in the assessment of warm weather near-drowning in children. Am J. Dis Child 135:1007, 1981.

†Conn, A. W., Barker, G. A., Edmonds, J. F.: Near-drowning: A neurologic approach. *In* Gellis, S. S., Kagan, B. M.: Current Pediatric Therapy. 10th ed., Philadelphia, W. B. Saunders Co., 1982, pp. 658–660.

21

Unclassified Diseases

The Histiocytosis Syndromes

JEFFREY M. LIPTON, M.D. PH.D.

The histiocytosis syndromes were originally categorized by many as malignant neoplasms, and have been treated as such with aggressive chemotherapy and radiation therapy. Although these modalities are still used, significant differences between the histiocytosis syndromes and true malignant disease suggest conservative management for many patients. The clinical course of malignant neoplasia is relentlessly progressive with virtually no survival in nontreated patients. The histiocytosis syndromes are characterized by frequent spontaneous remissions and exacerbations, with varying morbidity and survival in untreated patients, depending upon the extent of the disease. Pathologically, the lesions of histiocytosis appear as reactive infiltrates, possessing little of the cellular atypicality and homogeneity characteristic of malignancy. Although the etiology of these phenomena is unknown, histiocytosis syndromes appear to represent a reactive autoimmune disorder triggered by unknown stimuli.

Historically, the histiocytosis syndromes comprise eosinophilic granuloma, localized lesion(s) confined to bone; Hand-Schüller-Christian syndrome, protracted multiple site involvement with the classic but rare triad of skull defects, diabetes insipidus, and exophthalmos; and Letterer-Siwe syndrome, visceral lesions involving skin, liver, lungs, bone marrow, lymph nodes, spleen, and other reticuloendothelial organs. Since there is a continuum of disease that frequently does not fit these rigid and arbitrary criteria, it is important to individually group each patient. Therefore, the initial evaluation of patients with histiocytosis should determine the site and extent of disease to identify cosmetically and functionally significant lesions.

Once this is accomplished the patient is grouped according to the criteria outlined in Table 1. The grouping helps determine both therapy and prognosis. Patients in groups 0 to 11 do quite well, with little morbidity and no mortality. They frequently need little or no systemic therapy. Patients in group III require systemic therapy and generally do well, while significant morbidity and mortality are encountered in group IV.

Optimal management for patients with histiocytosis balances therapeutic intervention, utilized to minimize both short and long term disease-related morbidities, with a relative therapeutic nihilism in order to reduce treatment-associated morbidity.

Supportive Care

The primary caretaker should coordinate the care of these patients. Subspecialty consultation should be sought from dentists, orthopedists, and otolaryngologists experienced in treating histiocytosis patients. The goal of therapy must be to minimize loss of function and cosmetic deformity.

Severely ill patients are hospitalized and given maximal antibiotic ventilatory, nutritional (including hyperalimentation), blood product, skin care, physical therapy, and medical and nursing support as required in each individual case. Scrupulous hygiene is quite effective in limiting auditory canal, cutaneous, and dental lesions.

Local Therapy (Surgery and Radiation Therapy)

After exhaustive work-up, those patients with disease involving a single bone and some patients with disease involving multiple lesions and multiple bones can be managed with local therapy. This involves surgical curettage for patients whose lesions are in easily accessible, noncritical locations. Complete "cancer operation" resections are not neces-

679

Table 1. GROUPING SYSTEM FOR HISTIOCYTOSIS*

Factor	Points
Age	
>2	0
<2	1
Extent of disease	
<4 organs	0
>4 organs	1
Dysfunction* (1, 2 or 3 systems)	
No	0
Yes	1

Group	Total Points
0	monostotic eosinophilic granuloma
I	0
II	1
III	2
IV	3

1. Liver dysfunction*
hypoproteinemia (TP <5.5 gm/dl and/or albumin <2.5), edema, ascites, hyperbilirubinemia (>1.5 mg/dl).

2. Pulmonary dysfunction*
tachypnea, dyspnea, cyanosis, cough, pneumothorax, pleural effusion

3. Hemopoietic dysfunction*
anemia (<10 gm/dl hemoglobin), leukopenia (<4,000/mm^3), thrombocytopenia (<100,000)

*By arbitrarily assigning either 0 or 1 point for absence or presence of one of the three important prognostic variables we can use the grouping system.

sary. Surgical restraint *must* be exercised to avoid drastic cosmetic and orthopedic deformities and loss of function. Localized radiation therapy (450–900 rad and up to 1500 rad for large lesions) in 200 rad fractions utilizing only megavoltage equipment is currently employed. Care should be taken to avoid irradiating potentially sensitive normal structures such as the lens of the eye or the thyroid, if at all possible. Patients at risk of skeletal deformity, visual loss secondary to exophthalmos, pathologic fractures, vertebral collapse, or diabetes insipidus and those suffering from severe pain or symptomatic adenopathy even when multiple lesions exist should receive radiation therapy to those areas. Lesions in poorly accessible sites or those recurring after curettage should also be irradiated.

Chemotherapy

Patients in groups I and II can be observed for signs of spontaneous improvement. If there are symptomatic lesions or failure to thrive, treatment should be pursued. Patients in group III will benefit dramatically from chemotherapy, while those in group IV will frequently die despite chemotherapy.

Experimental modalities are being pursued at specialized centers for group IV patients.

The basic principle of systemic therapy is to begin with the most benign treatment and then add increasingly toxic agents, never worse than the disease while trying to prevent permanent disability. Table 2 outlines our current chemotherapeutic treatment program.

Careful monitoring of blood counts and clinical status is maintained, since chemotherapeutic toxicity can cause severe complications in these already compromised patients. We recommend treatment by physicians experienced in the administration of these agents. Alkylating agents, chlorambucil in particular, should be avoided because of the substantial risk of chemotherapy induced malignancy.

Sarcoidosis

D. GERAINT JAMES, M.D.

Sarcoidosis is a multisystem granulomatous disorder of unknown etiology, predominantly affecting lungs, eyes, skin, and the reticuloendothelial

Table 2. CURRENT DANA-FARBER CANCER INSTITUTE CHEMOTHERAPEUTIC TREATMENT PROGRAM FOR HISTIOCYTOSIS

PROGRAM I
1. Vinblastine—0.15 mg/kg/week intravenously as a single weekly dose. If the patient is not improved after 2 weeks, increase the dose by 0.025 to 0.05 mg/kg/wk. The highest nonmyelosuppressive dose is used. In addition if there is no or slow improvement add:

2. Prednisone—2 mg/kg/day orally. With improvement, taper to the smallest effective dose on an alternate day schedule. With continued improvement or satisfactory control, a slow taper of prednisone is undertaken but prednisone should be discontinued prior to the vinblastine taper. Vinblastine is tapered from weekly to every other week to every 3 weeks and then the dosage is reduced to 0.15 mg/kg/every 3 weeks prior to discontinuation. Reinstate lowest effective dose for disease rebound

PROGRAM II—*if program I fails*
1. Methotrexate—10 mg/m^2/week intramuscularly or intravenously, and

2. 6-mercaptopurine (6 MP)—20 mg/m^2/day for 14 days of 21 day cycle.

The highest nontoxic dose is used (toxicity: myelosuppression, mouth sores, hepatotoxicity). Upon improvement both drugs slowly tapered. Methotrexate is tapered from weekly to every other week to every 3 weeks. The 6 MP schedule is maintained while the dose is reduced 10–15% per cycle. Reinstitute lowest effective dose for disease rebound

PROGRAM III—*if programs I and II fail*
1. Nitrogen mustard—3 mg/m^2/week intravenously on days 1 and 8 of a 28 day cycle. The dose may be increased the following cycle by 10%. The highest nonmyelosuppressive dose used. Taper by reducing frequency of cycle by 1 week. Reinstitute lowest effective dose for disease rebound

system. It is rarely recognized in childhood. A recent international comparison of two large series suggests that in the U.S.A. the child is most likely to be black and symptomatic, with a high incidence of reticuloendothelial involvement, hyperglobulinemia, and hypercalcemia. In contrast, the Japanese patient is detected by routine chest radiography, is symptom-free, and has few abnormal physical signs. In Hungary, one half of a large series was symptom-free, and bilateral hilar lymphadenopathy was detected in 22 of 31 children. Indications for treatment depend upon whether the patient has symptoms or is suffering.

Prednisolone constitutes the sheet-anchor of the treatment for sarcoidosis. Since prolonged systemic treatment is undesirable in children, it is important to recognize (a) precise indications for prednisolone, (b) alternative routes of administration, and (c) alternative treatments.

INDICATIONS FOR PREDNISOLONE

Ocular Involvement. Topical corticosteroids should always be administered for iridocyclitis, in eye drops applied frequently during the day, reinforced with a corticosteroid eye ointment at night. If there is no substantial and continuing improvement for the first 10 days, then the concentration of corticosteroid in the anterior segment of the eye may be increased by a local subconjunctival depot of cortisone. Oral corticosteroids are indicated if local treatment does not lead to a rapid response or if ophthalmoscopy reveals posterior uveitis. In addition, the inflamed iris should be rested by local atropine eye drops to maintain a dilated pupil.

An Abnormal Chest Radiograph that does not show spontaneous improvement in the course of 3 months. Bilateral hilar lymphadenopathy is likely to subside without treatment, particularly if it is associated with erythema nodosum. On the contrary, pulmonary infiltration that remains static or worsens during the course of 6 months is an indication for oral steroids in an effort to prevent the development of irreversible pulmonary fibrosis.

Breathlessness. If this symptom is present, the disease has already reached a stage of irreversible pulmonary fibrosis or disturbed gas transfer. Steroid treatment provides symptomatic relief but does not influence the already grave prognosis.

Persistent Hypercalciuria. Steroids will prevent excess gastrointestinal absorption and excessive urinary excretion of calcium. Calcium metabolism usually reverts to normal within 10 days.

Disfiguring Skin Lesions. When lupus pernio or other unsightly lesions distress patients, oral and local corticosteroids may correct the deformity. Unfortunately, small doses of steroids must be continued indefinitely if the cosmetic improvement is to be maintained. In order to minimize the side effects of oral corticosteroids, local intralesional steroids or chloroquine or both are helpful alternatives.

Neurologic Involvement. The more acute the presentation, the more likely it is to respond to systemic corticosteroids, which should be administered as soon as the diagnosis has been established.

Glandular Involvement, particularly if there is disordered function, e.g., dry eyes due to lacrimal gland involvement, dry mouth due to salivary gland enlargement, hypersplenism due to sarcoidosis of the spleen.

Myocardial Involvement. It is easy to include involvement of the heart in a theoretic list of indications for corticosteroid therapy, but much more difficult, in practice, to recognize myocardial sarcoidosis. It is, of course, suspected and treated when a patient with multisystem sarcoidosis develops cardiac arrhythmia or bundle branch block.

Alternative Routes of Administration

Oral prednisolone may cause fluid retention and a cushingoid facies. This is least likely to occur with prednisolone-21-stearoyl-glycolate. Triamcinolone acetonide, alone or in combination with chloroquine, may be injected directly into disfiguring skin plaques with benefit. Prednisolone eye drops may be reinforced by subconjunctival or retro-orbital hydrocortisone.

OTHER DRUGS

Treatment may be necessary when there are contraindications to corticosteroid therapy, or it has proved fruitless. Under these circumstances it is worth considering treatment with oxyphenbutazone or indomethacin, chloroquine, or potassium para-aminobenzoate.

Oxyphenbutazone.* In a controlled trial comparing oxyphenbutazone, prednisolone, and a placebo in the management of pulmonary sarcoidosis, both active drugs were significantly better than the placebo. Prednisolone and oxyphenbutazone were equally effective. Whereas one in six patients showed spontaneous regression of pulmonary sarcoidosis in 6 months, this trial showed the number is increased by oxyphenbutazone or prednisolone to one in two patients. Not only does oxyphenbutazone influence the radiologic picture but also, like corticosteroids, it can prevent the development of sarcoid tisssue, for it may suppress the evolution of sarcoid tissue in the Kveim-Siltzbach nodule. Oxyphenbutazone and also indomethacin†‡ are of value in acute sarcoidosis but not in the chronic fibrotic form of the disease.

---

*Manufacturer's Warning: Oxyphenbutazone is contraindicated in children less than 14 years of age. (This usage is not listed by the manufacturer.)

†Safety of indomethacin in children has not been established.

‡This usage is not listed by the manufacturer.

Chloroquine. The way in which chloroquine acts is unknown, but it is helpful in the management of sarcoidosis with pulmonary fibrosis.* It is of no value in acute sarcoidosis; it is antifibrotic rather than anti-inflammatory.

Potaba. Potassium para-aminobenzoate (Potaba)* is known to have an antifibrotic effect and is worth considering in pulmonary fibrosis and lupus pernio due to sarcoidosis. Three-gram Envules, at a dosage of 1 gm/10 lb body weight to a maximum of 3 gm/24 hr, should be taken by mouth daily for several months. This form of treatment is an effective alternative to corticosteroids and chloroquine; giving all three in rotation helps to overcome the undesirable long-term complications of steroids and chloroquine.

Immunosuppression

Azathioprine* and chlorambucil* have met with mixed success, possibly because patients for such treatments have been incorrectly selected. They have usually been patients with hard-core chronic fibrotic sarcoidosis who have already resisted all other forms of treatment. Azathioprine can be used with advantage in combination with long-term steroids, allowing the dose of the latter to be reduced and thereby minimizing the adverse effects of steroids.

Immunostimulation

We have prepared transfer factor from patients with cured sarcoidosis and used it to reconstitute impaired cellular immunity in sarcoidosis. It was occasionally helpful. Levamisole also reconstitutes impairment of cellular immunity but does not have a worthwhile effect on the clinical features of sarcoidosis. (Levamisole is an investigational drug in the United States.)

Persistent Hypercalciuria

Hypercalciuria is swiftly brought under control by oral corticosteroids. If they are contraindicated, then sodium phytate or an oral phosphate preparation is an alternative means of preventing overabsorption of calcium. An effective and palatable effervescent phosphate preparation containing 500 mg of elemental phosphate and also sodium cellulose phosphate is recommended in a 5-gram dose three times daily with meals. A high chapati diet may also be considered because of its phytate content.

AGENTS THAT SHOULD NOT BE USED

Calciferol. Patients with sarcoidosis are peculiarly sensitive to vitamin D, which causes unpleasant symptoms associated with hypercalcemia, hypercalciuria, and elevated blood urea levels. In pre-corticosteroid days, calciferol was often given in sarcoidosis. It is useless, toxic, and obsolete. Vitamin D preparations should be withheld during pregnancy.

Antituberculous Drugs. They have no influence on the course of sarcoidosis and should not be used for the treatment of sarcoidosis. An argument could be made out for prophylactic isoniazid along with corticosteroids in countries where there is considerable tuberculosis. Tuberculin injections had a vogue, especially for sarcoid uveitis, but they are no longer indicated.

Radiotherapy. Radiotherapy is no longer used, even for the lymphoproliferative forms of sarcoidosis.

Familial Mediterranean Fever

ARTHUR D. SCHWABE, M.D.

Familial Mediterranean fever (benign paroxysmal peritonitis, familial paroxysmal polyserositis, recurrent polyserositis Armenian disease) is an inherited disorder of unknown etiology characterized by irregularly recurring attacks of fever and pain in the abdomen, chest, or joints. The disease most commonly afflicts individuals of Armenian, Jewish, or Arabic ethnic origin. The painful, febrile paroxysms, which are caused by inflammatory reactions of the peritoneal, pleural, or synovial membranes, usually begin in early childhood and continue throughout life. Attacks of peritonitis and pleuritis begin suddenly and subside spontaneously within 72 hours. Symptoms of joint inflammation tend to persist longer, sometimes for several months, but rarely leave residual damage. As a rule, single joints, most commonly a knee or an ankle, are involved. Chronic, irreversible changes are almost exclusively confined to the hip and sacroiliac joints. Laboratory abnormalities are nonspecific, reflecting only the presence of inflammation.

Principles of Treatment. Because the precise etiology is unknown, management consists of symptomatic treatment of the acute attack and prophylactic measures designed to prevent or reduce the frequency of the recurring paroxysms. In selecting any therapeutic regimen for this disease, the following observations must be borne in mind:

1. Most attacks are self-limited and may be followed by prolonged, asymptomatic intervals, sometimes lasting several years.

2. Patients who have frequent attacks are particularly prone to become addicted to narcotics.

3. Acute appendicitis may be difficult, if not impossible, to differentiate from the peritonitis of familial Mediterranean fever manifested solely by right lower quadrant pain.

---

*This usage is not listed by the manufacturer.

4. There is a high incidence of amyloidosis, principally involving the kidneys, in non-Ashkenazi Jews and Arabs with this disease.

Treatment of the Acute Attack. Bed rest is recommended during the febrile period of each severe attack, but it is not obligatory for many mild episodes. The fever, which may rise to 40°C (104°F), and the pain usually respond to oral aspirin, 10 mg/kg every 4 to 6 hours. When nausea, vomiting, or paralytic ileus is present, the drug should be administered in suppository form.

Narcotics should be avoided unless absolutely necessary for relief of pain from severe peritoneal inflammation. Under such circumstances, a single IM dose of meperidine hydrochloride (Demerol), 1.5 mg/kg, may be given. Pleural effusions accompanying attacks of pleuritis are transient and require no specific therapy.

Prevention of Attacks. Colchicine,* 0.6 mg twice or three times daily, is effective in preventing the attacks in approximately 70% of patients. In affected children with retarded growth and development, the administration of this drug may induce a spurt in growth and weight. There is also a suggestion that daily administration of this drug may prevent the development of amyloidosis in those ethnic groups at high risk. At the present time it is suggested that the use of colchicine be reserved for those children who are incapacitated by frequent and severe attacks and who have not responded to dietary restriction of fat. Corticosteroids are not effective in preventing attacks.

---

*This use is not listed in the manufacturer's official directive.

22

Special Problems in the Neonate

Intrauterine Growth Disturbance

M. DOUGLAS CUNNINGHAM, M.D.

Normal fetal growth may be impaired at any point in gestation by adverse maternal, placental, or fetal conditions. Three specific and readily identified conditions are frequently seen in populations of infants delivered of high-risk pregnancies. Each form of fetal growth disturbance is of different etiologic origin but with similar complications and therapeutic requirements.

Small for Gestational Age (SGA). Undergrown infants of this category weigh at or below the tenth percentile for gestational age at birth. Likewise, their length will reflect impaired linear growth by being less than the tenth percentile. The distinguishing feature is a greater occipital-frontal head circumference; usually at or slightly above the 25th percentile. Poor placental nutrition is implied, and the pattern of growth suggests "brain-sparing." Activity and neurologic development of the SGA newborn may be advanced beyond the assessed gestational age.

Serum glucose levels may fluctuate soon after birth and require close monitoring with Dextrostix at a minimum of 30-minute intervals. Readings of less than 45 mg/dl should prompt initiation of intravenous glucose administration. Confirmation of glucose levels by a clinical chemistry laboratory is suggested. Abnormal neurologic signs such as eye-rolling, facial twitching, jitteriness, or seizure-like movements are consistent with hypoglycemia and should preclude any attempts at oral feeding. However, if intravenous glucose is to be delayed because of difficulties in starting an infusion of glucose, a nasogastric tube can be passed and glucose water given.

Intravenous glucose for neonatal hypoglycemia should be given continuously by a regulated infusion pump. Glucose as a 10% solution in water given at 100 to 120 ml/kg/24 hr will deliver glucose at a rate of 6 to 8 mg/kg/minute and will correct most newborn hypoglycemia. Continued frequent Dextrostix monitoring is suggested. Occasionally, gradual increases of the glucose infusion to 10 mg/kg/minute will be necessary. Glucocorticosteroids are rarely needed to augment therapy if glucose is infused in this manner. Attempts to rapidly decrease a glucose infusion are to be avoided. Gradual decreases supplemented by simultaneously increased oral intake will allow a smooth transition of nutritional intake and maintenance of normal serum glucose levels.

Routine administration of glucose to SGA infants without first monitoring glucose levels is not advised. Albeit rare, transient diabetes mellitus of the neonate can present as a SGA infant with hyperglycemia and ketoacidosis.

Serum calcium levels may be low (less than 6 mg/dl) in SGA infants, necessitating supplemental intravenous calcium. Calcium gluconate at 200 to 400 mg/kg/24 hr can be given in intravenous fluids to maintain normal serum levels. Acute management of hypocalcemia is by a single intravenous infusion of 75 mg/kg of calcium chloride or 100 to 200 mg/kg of calcium gluconate. Any calcium solution must be administered slowly and with continuous cardiac monitoring to avoid bradycardia and arrhythmia.

Body temperature must be closely monitored and normal body temperatures (axillary, 32°C) carefully preserved. A radiant warmer with a servo-control mechanism for constant warming is essential in caring for SGA infants. They have little subcutaneous fat for insulation and a large surface area per body mass. Heat losses may be considerable, even in incubators with servo-control convection heating.

Placental dysfunction may include chronic hypoxia with resultant polycythemia. Hematocrit determinations of 60% or greater raise the threat of hyperviscosity. Hematocrit values must be venous to avoid an incorrect value reflecting capillary stasis. Specific hematocrit levels of polycythemia dictating partial plasma exchange transfusion are without consensus. Any level of 60% or greater associated with signs of central nervous system irritability, demarcation of digits, hypoglycemia, early jaundice, or priapism in males is an indication to readjust the hematocrit by plasma exchange. Generally, asymptomatic polycythemia of 65% is treated expectantly in the newborn period by partial plasma exchange using the following formula:

$$\text{Volume of exchange} = \frac{(\text{observed Hct} - \text{desired Hct})}{\text{Observed Hct}}$$

$$\times \text{ blood volume (80 ml)} \times \text{weight (kg)}$$

Small for gestational age infants have increased nutritional needs in the neonatal period. Once complications have been cleared and regular oral feedings are established, caloric intake can be increased to 120 cal/kg/24 hr. By 2 weeks of age, many SGA infants will require 130 to 140 cal/kg/24 hr to sustain a daily growth pattern of 20 to 30 grams of weight gain. Isotonic 24 cal/oz formulas have been particularly useful for feeding these infants once regular alimentation on 20 cal/oz formula has been achieved. These feeding guides are not meant to preclude breastfeeding. If initiation of breast feeding is successful, the mother is encouraged to nurse as often as the infant demands, even if seemingly continuous suckling is at times desired. For some mothers this will be too trying, and supplemental bottle feedings will be required. To deny accelerated caloric intake in SGA infants for the sake of "successful" breastfeeding seems ill-advised.

The long-term neurologic outcome of SGA infants is unclear. Multiple maternal and neonatal factors and many complications confound follow-up studies. A greater number of neurologic limitations are generally attributed to SGA infants as a group, but specific identifying factors and predicting circumstances are lacking.

Intrauterine Growth Retardation (IUGR). This term specifically applies to fetal circumstances of intrauterine blighting intrinsic to the fetus and is infectious or genetic in origin. Irrespective of maternal and placental support of the fetus, growth is impaired. Infectious agents such as *Toxoplasma,* cytomegalovirus, or rubella virus are specific examples of intrauterine infection resulting in small fetuses. Genetic conditions such as Bloom syndrome, Seckel bird-headed dwarfs, trisomy 18, or Silver syndrome are typically marked by retarded intrauterine growth. Maternal conditions of alcoholism, severe undernutrition, and heart disease are also responsible for IUGR. Hypertensive cardiovascular disease, as seen in advanced maternal diabetes mellitus, toxemia, or chronic renal disease, generally gives rise to SGA infants rather than IUGR infants.

Infants designated IUGR differ from SGA infants by being disproportionately undergrown and below the tenth percentile for head circumference, length, and weight. Limited head growth throughout the neonatal period further distinguishes the IUGR infant. Careful examination of such undergrown infants should lead to signs of congenital abnormalities or infection. Appropriate cytogenetic studies are warranted. Likewise, long bone survey roentgenograms for lucencies, skull roentgenograms for intracranial calcifications, and immunoglobulin levels may lead to the diagnosis of intrauterine infection. By definition, major and minor birth defects are more common to IUGR infants in contrast to SGA infants, although birth anomalies are more frequent in SGA infants than the normal neonatal population as a whole.

Postmaturity. Extended gestation, usually 42 to 44 weeks, may result in altered fetal growth. The neonate may appear long, thin, and wasted and be covered by loose squamating skin. The fingernails are strikingly long and yellow stained, as is the umbilical cord. The placenta is of normal size but is firm and filled with sandlike calcifications. The head circumference is normal for term to slightly increased, and the length is usually greater than the 50th percentile. Conversely, the weight is between the tenth and 50th percentile.

Frequently, these infants have been documented to have fetal distress and birth asphyxia manifested by low Apgar scores. Anticipation of birth asphyxia and providing supportive measures at the time of birth is the key to precluding complications of cold stress, acidosis, and meconium aspiration.

Because of limited placental nutrition during the extended gestation, subcutaneous wasting takes place. Like the SGA infant, temperature instability and excessive heat loss can take place. Immediate drying and servo-control radiant warming are necessary.

Intrauterine distress, presumably due to chronic hypoxia secondary to advanced placental aging and involution, leads to meconium passage into the amniotic fluid. At birth steps must be taken to suction the upper airway before the first breath is taken. Examination of the hypopharynx for meconium by Laryngoscopy is recommended. If meconium resides at the level of the vocal cords, endotracheal suctioning is recommended. Meconium aspiration and pneumothorax are accompanying complications of the postmaturity syndrome. Management of both conditions should follow recommendations noted specifically for each elsewhere in the text.

Birth injuries are common to postmature infants as in large for gestational age infants. In part, this is related to their greater size (length) and advanced bone age. The extended intrauterine age leads to increased bone mineralization and hardness. Skull fractures, clavicle fractures, and long bone fractures have been noted more frequently in these infants with difficult vaginal deliveries.

Hypoglycemia is encountered in postmature infants; it is less frequent and somewhat less pronounced than for SGA infants. Frequent Dextrostix monitoring is required. Because of the frequency of birth asphyxia and uncertain neurologic status, oral feedings for hypoglycemia should be approached with caution in the first 24 hours. Glucose replacement would follow the guidelines noted for SGA infants.

Hypocalcemia may complicate postmaturity, especially in the face of birth asphyxia and/or meconium aspiration. Calcium replacement and maintenance would follow those guidelines already mentioned for SGA infants.

Polycythemia and hyperviscosity are of special concern in postmature infants with central nervous system compromise and pulmonary disease following meconium aspiration. Prompt documentation of the central venous hematocrit is important. In the compromised infant early plasma exchange to adjust the hematocrit to a level between 50 and 55 is recommended. Serial hematocrit determinations at 4-hour intervals following the first exchange transfusion are suggested because some infants show a tendency to rebound polycythemia.

Birth Injuries

JOSEPH L. KENNEDY, JR., M.D.

The introduction of fetal monitoring techniques and the more common use of cesarean section, particularly in breech birth, have combined in recent years to make serious birth injury less common. The newer techniques have in themselves contributed some problems. Pediatricians must be intimately familiar with the marks of the normal birth process so that they may offer a worried parent justified reassurance. Attempts at treatment of minor birth injuries are often interfering and may in fact foster undue parental concern.

Superficial Injuries. *Caput succedaneum and molding* are to be expected in most deliveries. The shape of the infant's head is often of deep concern to the parents. Molding may be marked when the infant is large, the labor long, the mother primigravid, or the membranes ruptured prior to the onset of labor. Parents should be reassured that the head will look normal in a matter of days and that molding is normal and not associated with brain damage. The edema, suffusion, and localized intradermal hemorrhage of the presenting part begins to regress within 12 to 24 hours. Within the caput may be found localized abrasions, lacerations from intrauterine scalp sampling, and the puncture marks, sometimes with localized hemorrhage, of the monitoring electrode. These breaks in the skin represent a potential portal of entry for bacteria, particularly when there has been premature rupture of membranes or a long labor. Local treatment with a topical antibiotic cream or powder may prevent abscess or cellulitis.

The caput associated with the use of vacuum extraction may be more marked. Lesions similar to the caput occur not uncommonly with breech delivery. Bruising and edema of the genitalia worry parents; reassurance is usually warranted. Severe intratesticular hemorrhage may, however, produce late fibrotic changes. Hemorrhagic necrosis of portions of the labial or perianal areas results in localized sloughing with healing in 10 to 14 days. No treatment is needed other than careful cleaning of the affected areas. Unusual presentations such as that of face, arm, or leg result in similar localized changes. Extensive enclosed hemorrhage, particularly in the premature infant, may be a significant extravascular source of bilirubin and, rarely, a significant source of blood loss. Muscle crush injury with shock, disseminated intravascular coagulation, and renal damage has been described.

Lacerations may be caused by amniotomy, episiotomy, fetal blood sampling, fetal incision at cesarean section, or by the edge of a forceps blade. Sutures are sometimes required. Topical antibiotic cream or powder may be used to prevent infection. These wounds do well without a dressing.

Superficial forceps injury consisting of erythema with abrasion, superficial drainage, and crusting will heal rapidly and without scarring. Dressings are contraindicated. *Deep forceps injury* (subcutaneous fat necrosis) becomes evident between the fourth and eighth days. It heals spontaneously in a matter of weeks. Progression to an abscess is seen rarely. As with other neonatal skin injuries, warm soaks are contraindicated because of the susceptibility of the neonate to waterborne bacterial infection and of the newborn skin to thermal injury. Subcutaneous fat necrosis presumably from trauma attendant to delivery is occasionally seen elsewhere on the body, where it may be confused with a local cellulitis.

Scalp abscess occurs in 5% of infants who have had intrauterine monitoring. Most lesions are small and self-limited. A few have required incision and drainage. Careful cultures always reveal bacteria, usually those of the vaginal flora. Systemic antibiotics are not indicated unless signs of septicemia are present, nor is continued hospitalization required. Large or enlarging lesions should be followed weekly until resolution begins, because there have been a few reports of osteomyelitis and subgaleal abscess. Biparietal scalp necrosis with abscess formation occurs when the widest part of a large fetal head is pressed against the ischial spines during labor. Management is similar.

Tight nuchal cord causes localized cyanosis, edema, suffusion, and petechiae above the neck. Similar changes may be seen with face presentation, nuchal encirclement during breech delivery or during vertex delivery with shoulder dystocia, or when ergotrate has been given to the mother before the trunk has been delivered. Localized facial cyanosis alone may be seen in severe congenital hypothyroidism, and in a rare infant who responds to a cold environment primarily by vasoconstriction of the face. The soft tissue lesions require no treatment. Infants with nuchal cord should be watched for respiratory distress, which may occur because of nasal mucosal edema in an infant who is an obligate nasal breather. Nasal obstruction is relieved with an oral airway. Some infants born after partial cord compression become hypovolemic because of sequestration of the infant's blood in the placenta, when flow in the umbilical vein is impeded. Serial monitoring of blood pressure, pulse, respiratory rate, and hematocrit should be done in infants with a history of cord compression.

Cephalhematoma is usually unilateral and parietal in location. It is initiated during the birth process and hence is rarely demonstrable within the first few hours of life. Associated linear skull fractures are not rare, but skull radiographs are unnecessary since depressed fractures do not occur in the absence of other trauma, and since the expectant treatment is the same whether or not a linear fracture is present. Resolution of the lesion may take 4 to 10 weeks. It is sometimes accompanied by calcification of the lesion, new bone formation, and occasionally, a partial collapse of the swelling. Initially the periosteal stretching may produce local tenderness; it has become customary for this reason to lay the infant's head on the unaffected side. Parents are often very anxious and need a great deal of reassurance that healing will occur without untoward effects. The breakdown of hemoglobin in a large cephalhematoma may cause the serum bilirubin to rise by 3 to 5 mg/dl but can never be the sole explanation for marked neonatal jaundice. Cephal-

hematoma should never be aspirated because of the danger of introducing infection.

Subaponeurotic hemorrhage occurs rarely after difficult deliveries and vacuum extraction. The premature infant is somewhat more susceptible. Diagnosis is made by the appearance of increasing scalp swelling crossing suture lines, often fluctuant or crepitant, associated with pitting edema. Hemorrhage may be severe enough to cause death in hypovolemic shock. Prompt diagnosis and treatment with blood and plasma expanders may be lifesaving. The milder lesions will regress spontaneously, but, like other enclosed hemorrhages in the neonate, may be associated with some rise in serum bilirubin, and rarely with disseminated intravascular coagulation.

Intracranial Hemorrhage. The exact diagnosis of a neonatal intracranial hemorrhage (*subdural hemorrhage, intraventricular hemorrhage, intracerebral hemorrhage,* or *subarachnoid hemorrhage*) is less important than the immediate management of the affected infant. Diagnosis of hemorrhage is suspected when there is lethargy, hypotonia, seizures, focal neurologic signs, irregular respiration, apnea, fall in hematocrit, metabolic acidosis, bloody spinal fluid, full fontanel, or irritability. The maternal history is usually one of abnormal presentation, prolonged second stage of labor, or difficult delivery, often with oxytocin augmentation. Intraventricular hemorrhage, common in the small sick premature infant in whom it may not represent a true birth injury, is rare as a solitary finding in the term infant. Computer tomography (CT scan) is the best way of ascertaining the location and extent of the hemorrhage, but echoventriculography offers a more convenient way of obtaining almost as much information.

Routine tapping of the subdural space in an infant without skull fracture, localizing signs, or evidence of increased intracranial pressure is contraindicated since it may in itself cause subdural bleeding. Neurosurgical consultation is advisable if the diagnosis is suspected. In most infants, careful observation and symptomatic treatment are preferable to overvigorous diagnostic measures.

Seizures should be controlled with phenobarbital, 10 mg/kg IV or IM followed by 6 mg/kg/24 hr parenterally in two divided doses. The initial 10 mg/kg dose may be repeated if necessary. Serum phenobarbital levels should be kept in the range of 10 to 25 μg/ml. Phenytoin (10 mg/kg IV) is of little additional help and has a 24-hour delayed onset of action. It should be used only when seizures are severe, prolonged, and refractory to treatment. Intravenous diazepam is synergistic with the barbiturates, and the combination of the two drugs has been reported to cause severe respiratory depression. Diazepam should not be used unless artificial ventilatory support is immediately available. Hypoglycemia, hypocalcemia and hyponatremia are common in these infants; a search for these metabolic abnormalities should be made in every infant and appropriate treatment undertaken.

Supportive therapy of the infant with intracranial hemorrhage should include IV nutrition, treatment of associated hypoglycemia, monitoring for hypovolemia and appropriate replacement of blood or plasma, and careful attention to fluid balance to prevent aggravation of a seizure disorder by overhydration.

As recovery ensues, electroencephalography may sometimes give helpful prognostic information. CT scan, serial echoventriculograms, and monitoring of head circumference daily for 10 days, then twice weekly, will give early indication of the need for neurosurgical intervention for hydrocephalus.

Skeletal Injuries. *Clavicular fracture* occurs with shoulder dystocia, particularly with large infants and with breech delivery. Diagnosis is made by the obstetric history and by finding pain, crepitus, or angulation on palpation. There is usually only little displacement; healing with palpable callus is evident at 2 to 3 weeks. A figure-eight bandage is unnecessary; simple pinning of the shirtsleeve to the shirt with gentle handling suffices. A follow-up examination should be done at 2 to 6 weeks to identify the rare fracture that goes on to nonunion.

Fractures of the humerus, femur, or other long bones are usually associated with difficult breech delivery. Simple fractures of the humerus in good alignment require only immobilization and splinting, and the arm adducted and the forearm flexed at 90°. Poor alignment will require casting. Fractures of the femur do best with immobilization by splint or cast, together with traction. Prognosis for birth fractures is good.

Separation of an epiphysis of the humerus (usually proximal) or *femur* (usually distal) is suspected when there is pain and lack of movement of the affected extremity after a difficult delivery. Diagnosis is confirmed by x-ray studies at 10 to 14 days, when callus formation will be evident. Treatment is similar to that for fracture. Brachial plexus injury can be associated and should be looked for.

Neuromuscular Injuries. *Brachial plexus injury* is caused by lateral traction of the neck during difficult breech extraction or vertex delivery with shoulder dystocia. When injury is severe or extensive, chest fluoroscopy (or inspiratory and expiratory films) should be done to identify diaphragmatic paralysis. Immediate treatment consists of pinning the arm in abduction, external rotation and supination for 10 to 14 days. After this time physiotherapy is begun with careful passive exercising several times daily. Careful neurologic follow-up is mandatory. The prognosis is generally good except when the damage extends to the lower nerve roots. Diaphragmatic paralysis requires chest physiotherapy during the immediate neonatal period, follow-up

x-ray films, and careful observation during any intercurrent respiratory infection.

Facial palsy, sometimes associated with brachial palsy but more commonly an isolated finding, is usually resolved in several weeks. It requires no treatment except when the eye is involved. In this instance instillation of 0.5% methylcellulose drops should be made four times daily to prevent corneal ulceration.

Paralysis of the radial, obturator, or external popliteal nerves is uncommon, requires no treatment, and resolves spontaneously.

Sixth nerve palsy, usually unilateral, is found not uncommonly at birth. Its cause is unknown and it disappears spontaneously by age 1 month.

Spinal cord injury occurs with severe anoxia or with difficult breech deliveries, particularly when the fetal neck is hyperextended. The injury is therefore preventable by cesarean section. The management of the woman in labor with a breech presentation should include an x-ray film to identify the 5% of infants at risk. Early diagnosis and supportive care should help minimize problems in the infant who is to survive. Diagnosis is suggested by flaccid paralysis with areflexia of arms and legs, diaphragmatic breathing, and urinary retention. Four-hourly Credé maneuver of the bladder will help prevent bladder damage and urinary tract infection. Chest physiotherapy and positioning is useful in the infant with thoracic involvement to prevent atelectasis and pneumonia. X-ray films of the spine will occasionally show a fracture or dislocation. The prognosis in general is poor, but an occasional, severely affected infant has survived with only minimal residual damage.

Internal Thoracic Injuries. Attempt at amniocentesis may puncture the lung causing *pneumothorax* and sometimes subcutaneous emphysema after birth. Treatment is immediate tube thoracostomy with underwater drainage. Prognosis is good. Some cases of *chylothorax* are thought to be due to injury to the thoracic duct during delivery. Treatment of chylothorax causing respiratory embarrassment consists of repeated needle aspirations.

Internal Abdominal Injuries. Intra-abdominal bleeding may occur from rupture of the liver or spleen, the latter usually only when it is enlarged, as with erythroblastosis. Shock, abdominal distention, and occasionally a bluish discoloration of the abdomen warrant immediate surgical intervention, with concurrent replacement of intravascular volume with blood, plasma, or albumin. More commonly rupture of the liver results in a *subcapsular hematoma* with gradual deterioration over several days. Infants at risk because of birth history should have careful monitoring of pulse, blood pressure, and hematocrit, together with daily gentle palpation of the surface of the liver. The liver or spleen also may be injured by amniocentesis, intrauterine blood transfusion, or vigorous resuscitative efforts at birth.

Injury of the adrenal glands may be hypoxic rather than traumatic in origin. Blood transfusion to restore volume together with prompt surgical intervention may be lifesaving in the infant with massive hemorrhage. Milder lesions may be followed carefully. There is no need to administer corticosteroids.

Rupture of the bladder at delivery, presenting as ascites, is almost totally confined to male infants with bladder neck obstruction. Treatment is of the underlying condition.

Other Birth Injuries. Serious eye injuries are rare. Subconjunctival and retinal hemorrhages are common, unassociated with other bleeding, and require no treatment. Discoloration of the nasal septal cartilage has been recently suggested as a cause of deviation of the tip of the nose. When the deviation is made more marked on depression of the nasal tip, otorhinolaryngologic consultation may be indicated. Skull fractures are rare and are usually of little clinical significance. Small linear fractures are not uncommonly found when multiple serial x-ray films are done on infants with cephalhematoma (cf. supra). Linear fractures require no treatment; followup should be done at 2 months, however, to rule out the development of a leptomeningeal cyst. Depressed "fractures" are usually intrauterine spontaneous skull depressions. Neurosurgical repair is indicated for cosmetic reasons since many do not resolve spontaneously. Attempts to elevate the depressed area by applying pressure or suction are contraindicated since further damage may result.

Neonatal Resuscitation

ROBERTA A. BALLARD, M.D.

Resuscitation of the newborn infant is one of the most essential skills to be acquired by any pediatrician. These skills will generally be applied in resuscitation of term infants who develop difficulty during labor or at the time of birth. However, occasionally most pediatricians are called upon to resuscitate and stabilize a more seriously ill, smaller preterm infant. They therefore must also have the essential information and skills for initial resuscitation of these infants.

PREPARATION

Preparation is the most essential part of neonatal resuscitation. Very little can be done for an asphyxiated newborn by someone who is untrained and has no equipment. Therefore, wherever an infant is to be born there must be someone in attendance with the necessary skills and proper apparatus to carry out effective resuscitation. Secondly, an excel-

Table 1. EQUIPMENT FOR NEONATAL RESUSCITATION

LOW-RISK/TERM INFANT

Radiant warmer to maintain temperature control
Stethoscope
Source of warm, humidified oxygen
Suction source
Nasogastric tube and syringe
Apparatus for bagging infant, either anesthesia bag or Ambu bag with masks for different size infants
Suction catheters and DeLee trap
Endotracheal tubes (Portex), sizes 2.4, 3, and 3.5
Fluids (D_5W, $D_{10}W$, normal saline)
Medications (Narcan, sodium bicarbonate, atropine, calcium gluconate, epinephrine)
Clock or stopwatch
Tubes for obtaining blood gases, other samples
Equipment for placing umbilical arterial catheter
Equipment for micro technique blood gases
Portable x-ray equipment

EQUIPMENT FOR HIGH-RISK/PRETERM INFANT

All of above, plus

Manometer for gauging pressure being used in ventilation
Blender for delivering oxygen in concentrations ranging from room air to 100%
Heart-rate monitoring equipment
Blood-pressure monitoring equipment
Transcutaneous oxygen-monitoring equipment (if possible)
Blood-gas syringes heparinized and ready to use
Blood-gas laboratory immediately available (10-min turnaround time)
Volume expander (25% human albumin) and/or blood available on emergency basis
Umbilical artery catheter set-up and ready to insert

---

lent cooperative understanding between pediatrician and obstetrician is essential, so that infants who are likely to require resuscitation can be managed in a cooperative fashion with both the pediatrician and the appropriate additional staff present at the birth. Table 1 lists the basic equipment required for resuscitation of a low-risk or high-risk preterm infant.

The final step in preparation to resuscitate a newborn is to think through while awaiting the delivery what the infant's set of problems are likely to be and to prepare specifically for that infant (e.g., if the mother is hemorrhaging, the infant is more likely to need a volume expander; for the infant who is being born through thick meconium, suctioning will be the most important planned activity). In addition, it is important to identify who is available to help with resuscitation and what their skills are.

Ventilatory Resuscitation/Low-Risk Term Infant

Meconium. Careful obstetric management with minimal drug administration and avoidance of birth asphyxia is the most desirable (although not always possible) preventive approach. However, many infants will pass meconium before or during their labor process, thus complicating resuscitative measures. Infants born through meconium may be completely normal or be among the most severely ill infants in neonatal intensive care units. Resuscitation is the critical pivot upon which the outcome depends. A tinge of color in the amniotic fluid indicates that the infant has been in trouble at some time; however, it is unlikely to result in airway obstruction. Therefore, although the infant's nasopharynx should be well suctioned prior to delivery of the chest, this type of infant does not require intubation at the time of birth. The infant born through thick particulate material must have this material removed from the trachea as well as nasopharynx. In addition to suctioning prior to delivery of the chest, this infant requires intubation and then deep suctioning done, either with a large-bore catheter or by using the endotracheal tube itself as a "straw" and pulling the meconium out into a gauze or mask, with repetition of this maneuver until thick material is no longer obtained. Oxygen should then be administered by mask or endotracheal tube. Since meconium indicates that an infant may have experienced borderline hypoxia in utero and may have pulmonary vascular constriction, and since term infants are not at particular risk of retrolental fibroplasia, administration of 100% oxygen should be generous in these first few minutes after birth.

Asphyxia. Immediately upon receiving the infant, the pediatrician should quickly clear the nasopharynx of any blood or thick mucus. Assessment of both high-risk and low-risk infants is then begun, usually by assigning an Apgar score at 1 and 5 and sometimes at 10 minutes of life. The Apgar score is arrived at by the assignment of a score value of 0, 1, or 2 for each of the following: heart rate, color, respiration, response to stimulation, and spontaneous activity. Obviously, Apgar scores vary with the observer; however, the habit of assigning Apgar scores is good discipline for assessing the condition of an infant and making further treatment evaluations.

The following is an outline of appropriate responses to different Apgar scores:

SCORE 0. A live-born infant should virtually never be assigned this score. Resuscitation of an infant with a true Apgar score of zero is probably a subject for ethical discussion. However, often, in the excitement around the birth of an asphyxiated infant, it is impossible to spend the time to determine whether an infant truly has an Apgar score of zero. Therefore, it is appropriate to give the infant a single thump on the chest and immediately proceed to intubation and support of respiration and then turn to assessment of cardiac status.

SCORE 1 to 3. Infants with scores in this range need immediate intubation and expansion of the lung as part of resuscitation; however, if the equipment is not immediately available or no one with skill is available, a bag or mask is often adequate to

begin ventilation. Initially the chest should be slowly expanded five to ten times with pressures of 25 to 30 cm H_2O to stimulate breathing; if this is not successful, proceed to ventilate at a rate of 60/minute at pressures adequate to expand the lungs, usually 20 to 30 cm H_2O.

SCORE 4 to 6. These infants require stimulation with 100% oxygen blown across the face and some expansion of the lungs with use of a bag and mask apparatus. Ordinarily, most will respond and begin inflating their lungs rapidly. It is important to empty the stomach of any infant receiving bag and mask ventilation.

SCORE 7. Initially these infants are generally grunting or somewhat pale and will respond to a brief period of 100% oxygen blown over the face.

There are two important points to remember in resuscitation of the term infant: 1) that pulmonary vascular resistance is decreased and pulmonary blood flow increased by administration of oxygen (these infants are not at significant risk for retrolental fibroplasia), and 2) that the newborn infant's lung is normally full of fluid at the time of birth, and that the normal pathway for reabsorption of this fluid is into the pulmonary arterial system. Excessive suctioning of clear fluid from the nasopharynx only causes atelectasis.

Preterm/High-Risk Infant. Successful resuscitation of the preterm infant of less than 32 weeks' gestation requires as much notification as possible and at least two skilled team members to participate. For infants weighing less than 1250 grams, it is appropriate to intubate and at least briefly inflate the lungs to assist reabsorption of lung fluid and to expand alveoli and enhance release of surfactant. Ventilatory measures for other preterm infants should be those described above for the respective Apgar scores. However, in resuscitation of the preterm infant the desirability of administering lower concentrations of oxygen must be kept in mind.

Ordinarily, resuscitation of a preterm infant, particularly one weighing less than 1500 gm, should begin with use of 40% oxygen, since these infants are at high risk for retrolental fibroplasia; it is easy to increase the oxygen concentration if rapid improvement in the infant's color is not observed. Initial ventilation should be done with warm, humidified gas to avoid cooling and drying of the airway. Most infants who require intubation will need a brief period of hand ventilation with pressures sufficient to cause chest wall movement and to enable auscultation of good breath sounds bilaterally. These pressures may vary from 20 to 30 cm H_2O or occasionally even more to expand the chest initially. Ventilation should be carried out at a rate of approximately 60 per minute, and an end-expiratory pressure of 2 to 4 cm H_2O should be applied.

Cardiac Resuscitation. The myocardium of the newborn infant is exceedingly strong, and, as a general rule, it can be assumed that a newborn requiring resuscitation is having problems with ventilation rather than with cardiac function. Therefore, activity should be concentrated on ventilation, and heart rate will usually adjust accordingly. Occasionally an infant requires external cardiac massage if the heart rate falls to less than 60 per minute and remains there for more than one minute. This can be done by placing the hands over the chest with both thumbs over the midsternum and the fingers supporting the back. The sternum is then compressed approximately two thirds of the distance to the vertebral column at a rate of 120 to 150 per minutes and a ratio of three to four compressions per breath.

General Support Measures

It is important to maintain temperature control during any resuscitation. The specific measures for doing this will vary with individual units but should be included in the resuscitation plan. In a preterm infant of less than 30 to 32 weeks' gestation, or in any infant who does not respond rapidly to the respiratory support measures described above, a cardiac monitor should be connected and an umbilical arterial catheter should be placed to permit measurement of blood pressure and monitoring of acid-base status. If an umbilical arterial catheter cannot be placed, it may occasionally be necessary to insert an umbilical venous catheter to approximately 7 to 9 cm for administration of fluids or drugs.

Sodium Bicarbonate Therapy. Sodium bicarbonate should never be administered to an asphyxiated newborn before ventilatory control has been established. Whenever possible, an arterial blood gas should be obtained before administration of sodium bicarbonate; however, when this is impossible and when the infant has not responded with spontaneous respiration and improved color to adequate ventilation, sodium bicarbonate diluted 1:1 with water may be administered at a dose of 1 to 2 meq/kg over a period of 5 to 6 minutes. When blood gases are obtained, sodium bicarbonate should never be administered if the P_{CO_2} is greater than 45, and should be given only in the case of an infant with an arterial pH of less than 7.2, with a base excess of greater than –10.

Volume Expanders. If the history indicates possible maternal hemorrhage prior to delivery, and if the infant's hematocrit is less than 40% or falling rapidly in the face of poor perfusion of the skin and low arterial blood pressure (usually less than 35 mm Hg for a term infant or less than 25 mm Hg for a small preterm infant), it may be necessary to give volume expanders *very slowly.* In the anemic infant, packed red blood cells are the expander of choice, given at 5 ml/kg over a period of 10 to 15 minutes, repeating as necessary. Other volume expanders that may be used are fresh frozen plasma, albumin diluted with saline at 1:4, or normal saline if none of the above is available. An infant who needs a volume expander will ordinarily have a very brief increase in arterial blood pressure, followed by drifting downward again after administration of 5 ml/kg. In these infants, one usually observes improved peripheral perfusion and often improved respiratory status as volume is given.

Administration of Other Agents. Administration of narcotics to the mother during labor should always be noted, and, if depression secondary to these agents is possible, naloxone (Narcan) should be given in a dose of 0.01 mg/kg. Dextrostix should be checked on asphyxiated and preterm infants, and fluid administration begun with 5 or 10% dextrose at a rate of 50 to 65 ml/kg through the umbilical arterial line as soon as the infant is stabilized. Rapid pushes of high concentration of glucose should be avoided, since they produce a rebound hypoglycemia and, in addition, may contribute to worsening of asphyxial damage to the brain. Infants who have experienced severe antepartum asphyxia and who do not respond to ventilation and bicarbonate may occasionally respond with improved myocardial contractility to the administration of calcium gluconate, which may be given 100 mg/kg by slow IV push. In rare circumstances, administration of other agents, such as atropine at a dose of 0.01 mg/kg may be necessary. Intracardiac administration of epinephrine to an infant at the time of birth is rarely indicated and should be used only as a measure of last resort. This measure has implications for ethical thinking as to whether this infant was in truth a stillborn, rather than a liveborn, infant. The dosage of intracardiac epinephrine is 0.1 mg/kg per dose of 1:10,000 solution. I personally have never found it necessary to administer this drug during neonatal resuscitation (as opposed to situations in which cardiac arrest occurs later in an infant's course).

Things to Avoid In Resuscitation

Successful resuscitation avoids producing iatrogenic damage to newborn infants. The important *don'ts* of resuscitation are as follows: 1) Don't panic if an endotracheal tube cannot be immediately placed—rely on bag amd mask ventilation and call for help. 2) Don't do excessive suctioning of clear fluid—the normal process is for reabsorption of fluid through the lung. 3) Don't use oxygen concentrations greater than 40% to resuscitate a premature infant unless the infant clearly requires it. 4) Don't use excessive end-expiratory pressure during resuscitation. The infant's lungs may be normal and excessive pressure may decrease venous return to the heart. 5) Don't administer excess volume or sodium bicarbonate, since each of these agents has been associated with the production of intraventricular hemorrhage in animal models. 6) Don't rely heavily on cardiac resuscitation and thus neglect ventilatory resuscitation. 7) Don't withhold oxygen from the term or post-term infant who may need it to reduce pulmonary vascular constriction.

Ethical Considerations

The eventual outcome of infants who have been asphyxiated at birth is a product of the length and severity of their intrapartum asphyxia as well as the experience of asphyxia at birth. Mentioned above was the case of the true Apgar 0 infant, with no cardiac activity at birth, who does not respond to a thump on the chest plus adequate ventilation. This infant should ordinarily be considered a stillbirth because asphyxia severe enough to actually stop the heart has probably produced severe and irreversible neurologic damage. Resuscitation of these infants at 20- or 30-minutes of age with cardiac stimulants virtually always results in severely damaged outcomes. The outcome infants with low Apgar scores requires repeated evaluations over the first hours to days after birth. Frequently, even then, it is impossible to predict infants who will become normal or who will have either mild or severe problems later.

Respiratory Distress Syndrome

WILLIAM OH, M.D.

The management of respiratory distress syndrome (RDS) will be divided into three components: prevention, supportive therapy, and assisted ventilation.

PREVENTION OR AMELIORATION OF RDS

Since RDS is primarily a disease of developmental delay in lung maturation, the most logical way of preventing or minimizing the severity of this disease is to prevent premature onset of labor and delivery of a premature infant. However, the state of the art is such that while some premature labors are secondary to complications of pregnancy, such as premature rupture of membrane, multiple pregnancy, incompetent cervix, and so on, a large proportion of premature labors are still unexplained. Therefore, the approach to prevention of RDS is twofold: (1) to delay the delivery of a premature infant as long as possible until the incidence of RDS would be the lowest. This goal can be achieved by the use of a tocolytic agent to stop premature uterine contraction and by identification of the risk of RDS by amniocentesis and assessment of surfactant levels in the amniotic fluid; and (2) when the delivery of a premature infant is inevitable because of the maternal and fetal risks involved in prolonging the pregnancy, pharmacologic intervention to reduce the incidence and severity of RDS is feasible under certain circumstances.

In regard to the use of tocolytic agents, several drugs have been tried clinically with variable degrees of success. The currently approved tocolytic agent (by the Food and Drug Administration) is ritodrine hydrochloride, a beta-mimetic agent. This drug is given intravenously at first until the uterine contraction is successfully stopped; thereafter it can be continued in the oral form. As with other tocolytic agents that have been tried previously (intravenous alcohol, diazoxide, terbutaline), the effectiveness of this drug is variable, but it is most effective under the following circumstances: intact membranes, early stage of labor, and absence of complications such as third trimester bleeding and chorioamnionitis. Ritodrine hydrochloride is also not without potential risk both to the mother and to the infant. In the mother, pulmonary edema may occur when a large fluid load is given along with ritodrine hydrochloride. In the infant, hyperglycemia during the first hours of life also has been documented as a result of the maternal transfer of ritodrine hydrochloride into the fetus prior to delivery. These potential complications should be considered whenever this drug is used.

Several pharmacologic agents or hormones have been shown to accelerate fetal pulmonary surfactant production. These include glucocorticoid, thyroxine, xanthine derivatives (aminophylline, theophylline), tocolytic agents (intravenous alcohol), heroin, estrogen, prolactin, and epidermal growth factor. To date, administration of glucocorticoid to the mother has been found to be beneficial in several clinical trials. However, this drug is not without potential maternal and fetal risks; therefore, its usage should be individually justified and the risk-benefit ratio carefully assessed. The known risks for glucocorticoid include potential increase in the incidence and severity of maternal and neonatal infections, particularly in the presence of high-risk factors such as prolonged rupture of amniotic membranes with chorioamnionitis. It has also been shown that administration of glucocorticoid to a severely toxemic mother may increase the risk of intrauterine fetal death. Since chorioamnionitis, along with prolonged rupture of membranes, and toxemia of pregnancy concurrent with intrauterine growth retardation are associated with advancement of fetal lung maturity, these two maternal complications would generally preclude the administration of glucocorticoid for the purpose of preventing RDS.

Another important factor that should be considered in the issue of antenatal prevention of RDS with glucocorticoid administration to the mother is the fact that it would require a minimum of 24 hours of treatment time for significant clinical effectiveness. On this basis, it is important to point out that unless there are adequate clinical parameters to assure that the delay in the delivery of the fetus for at least 24 hours is achievable, glucocorticoid should not be administered to the mother.

The two most commonly used synthetic glucocorticoids for maternal administration are betamethasone (6 mg/dose for 2 doses IM at 12-hour intervals) and dexamethasone at the same dose. Once again, it is emphasized that the indication for maternal glucocorticoid administration to prevent RDS should be individually determined, with careful assessment of the risk-benefit ratio. Although a number of obstetricians from various perinatal centers still frown on the use of maternal glucocorticoid therapy for the prevention of RDS, the consensus is that with proper clinical determinations of indications, this drug may be used under the following circumstances: (1) when fetal lung immaturity is evident by a low lecithin:sphingomyelin ratio (less than 2:1) in the amniotic fluid, or a negative foam stability test (a semi-quantitative test for the presence of surfactant in the amniotic fluid), (2) in the absence of clinical complications such as severe toxemia and maternal infections, and (3) if there are assurances that the delivery can be delayed for at least 24 hours following the administration of the glucocorticoid to the mother.

SUPPORTIVE THERAPY FOR RDS

It is well known that RDS is a self-limiting disease, starting generally at birth and lasting for 3 to 5 days. The duration and severity of the disease as well as the occurrence of complications depend on the effectiveness of the supportive therapy. It is also known that the recovery from RDS depends on the ability of the neonatal lung to generate adequate surfactant during the first 3 to 5 days of life. The ability to generate surfactant in turn depends on the level of lung maturity, the cellular injury that may occur during the course of therapy, and the maintenance of optimal oxygenation, perfusion, acid-base balance, fluid and electrolyte balance, and thermal control. The goals of supportive therapy are to maintain these physiologic conditions without iatrogenic complications.

Oxygen Therapy

Oxygen treatment is one of the most important components of the supportive therapy for RDS. The goal of oxygen therapy is to achieve adequate tissue oxygenation without producing oxygen toxicity in the retina (retrolental fibroplasia) and in the lung (bronchopulmonary dysplasia or chronic lung disease). To achieve adequate tissue oxygenation, the following parameters must be attained: arterial blood PO_2 between 50 and 70 mm Hg, hemoglobin oxygen saturation of $\geq 95\%$, and an adequate perfusion to assure delivery of a normal amount of oxygen into the tissue. The latter can be achieved by maintaining normal hemoglobin mass as well as arterial blood pressure and blood flow.

The oxygen can be administered to infants placed in the incubator. If a higher concentration is desirable without frequent fluctuation, a plastic hood may be used as a chamber in which the infant's head can be placed and oxygen administered into it. This method of oxygen delivery is particularly helpful and desirable when nursing procedures require frequent entry into the incubator. It is also essential that the oxygen be delivered in a warm and humidified form to prevent local damage to the mucous membranes of the respiratory tract. The ambient oxygen concentration should be monitored at frequent intervals and recorded; the oxygen tension should be monitored in the arterial blood or by the use of a transcutaneous PO_2 monitor. The latter is a noninvasive instrument that has been developed recently to continuously record the cutaneous oxygen tension; the accuracy has been verified by a good correlation with the simultaneously obtained arterial blood PO_2. The frequency of its use is increasing in various perinatal centers, particularly in the management of very severely ill infants with respiratory distress.

The source of arterial blood samples and the frequency of the monitoring of arterial PO_2 will depend on the severity of the disease and the risk of oxygen toxicity in the infants being treated. In general, infants with higher gestational age and larger birth weight having lower risk for retrolental fibroplasia, and having less severe disease probably require less intensive arterial blood PO_2 monitoring. In these circumstances, it may be feasible to monitor the oxygen therapy by sampling from a peripheral artery (temporal, radial, or brachial arteries), at 4-to 6-hour intervals. In these circumstances one is often tempted to use arterialized capillary samples of PO_2 measurement; however, it is emphasized that this manner of PO_2 measurement is notoriously difficult to rely upon, particularly in acutely ill, hypoperfused, and young infants.

In severely ill infants, samples obtained from an indwelling umbilical arterial catheter placed in the descending aorta are preferred, and the frequency of blood sampling can be adjusted according to the clinical severity of the disease. Utilizing infants' color as a way of monitoring the adequacy of oxygenation may carry a significant risk of oxygen toxicity since a "clinically pink" infant may have a PaO_2 in the range that may result in retrolental fibroplasia. Therefore, in those infants who are at high risk for retrolental fibroplasia, the PaO_2 should be monitored while oxygen is being administered under whatever concentration the infant may require.

Acid-Base Balance

RDS is associated with respiratory and metabolic acidosis. The respiratory acidosis is due to retention of CO_2, while the metabolic acidosis is a result of anaerobic metabolism with accumulation of lactic acid. The respiratory acidosis can be monitored closely with periodic blood gas analysis, as previously described; intervention with assisted ventilation is necessary if the CO_2 retention is significant enough to cause secondary apnea or impending apnea. That level is generally in the range of 60 to 70 mm Hg of Pa_{CO_2}, which is generally associated with a pH of less than 7.20.

Infants with RDS often may have fetal distress prior to delivery, which in turn may be associated with significant metabolic acidosis at birth. If the degree of metabolic acidosis is significant (pH $\leq$ 7.20), sodium bicarbonate may be given in an appropriate manner to correct the acidosis. Since inappropriately large doses of sodium bicarbonate administration may increase the incidence of intracranial hemorrhage, it is important that the dosage, form, and route, as well as the speed of administration, are correct. It is mandatory that an acid-base determination be done prior to the use of alkali so that the actual base deficit as well as the degree of acidosis can be estimated and the appropriate dose of bicarbonate calculated. The formula used is: Dose of sodium bicarbonate (meq/kg body weight) = base deficit $\times$ 0.3 $\times$ body weight. The sodium bicarbonate should be given in the form of half-strength sodium bicarbonate solution (0.9 M sodium bicarbonate mixed with sterile water in a 1:1 proportion), and the drug may be given intravenously (not umbilical vein) over a period of 1 meq per 3 to 5 minutes.

The subsequent development of metabolic acidosis indicates that the infant's treatment in regard to correction of hypoxemia is not optimal. Therefore, when the clinician has to repeatedly utilize sodium bicarbonate to treat metabolic acidosis, the oxygen therapy and maintenance of tissue perfusion should be reassessed.

Treatment of Hypotension and Hypovolemia

Hypotension may occur during the course of treatment of RDS. This complication can be detected by continuous monitoring of the arterial blood pressure, either by direct measurement of arterial blood pressure through an indwelling umbilical arterial catheter or by use of the noninvasive ultrasound blood pressure device DINAMAT* if the direct measurement of blood pressure is not feasible. A nomogram for normal arterial blood pressure for neonates of various birth weights and postnatal ages should be available in the intensive care nursery, and the diagnosis of hypotension can be made if the blood pressure of the infant falls below two standard deviations of the mean. The initial approach to treatment of hypotension is to

provide intravascular infusion of a volume expander in the form of Plasmanate at a dose of 10 ml per kilogram body weight. If the volume depletion and shock are associated with anemia, suggesting hemorrhage, blood transfusion should be given at the dose appropriate to correct the estimated amount of blood loss.

If hypotension persists following volume expansion, one may use vasoactive drugs such as dopamine.† The dose is 5 to 10 μg/kg/min initially, and the dose should be titrated subsequently according to the infant's arterial blood pressure.

Temperature Control

It is well known that temperature control in very small infants, particularly those with RDS, is of prime importance for optimal survival. The goal of temperature management is to maintain the normal core body temperature of the sick infant at an ambient thermal environment that will entail the lowest metabolic rate. This ambient temperature is defined as neutral thermal environment and is variable depending on the infant's body weight and postnatal age. Such a nomogram has been devised, and it should be made available to the clinicians caring for infants with RDS in the nursery. As noted, another important maneuver for maintaining normal body temperature is to assure that the oxygen delivered to the infant is properly warmed and humidified to minimize heat loss via the respiratory tract.

Fluid and Electrolyte Management

During the course of management of RDS, appropriate maintenance of fluid and electrolyte balance is important to assure a normal metabolic milieu and prevent cardiopulmonary complications. It has been shown that fluid overload in low birth weight infants, and particularly those with RDS, may lead to increased incidence of symptomatic patent ductus arteriosus. Therefore, the amount of fluid given to these infants should be limited to what is required for maintenance, which amount of fluid given to these infants should be limited to what is required for maintenance, which amounts to approximately 90 to 120 ml/kg/24 hr for infants weighing between 1000 and 1500 grams; in infants weighing below 1000 grams, the fluid requirement is higher, but the amount should be individually determined because of variability in their requirements, particularly in the area of normal fluid loss via the route of insensible water loss. Sodium requirement of these infants is 2 meq/kg/24 hr. A system of monitoring the fluid and electrolyte balance should also be instituted by measuring the urine volume, urine specific gravity

---

*DINAMAT (No. 847), manufactured by Applied Medical Research, 5041 West Cypress Street, Tampa, Florida 33607.

†Manufacturer's Warning: Safety and efficacy of dopamine in children have not been established.

or osmolarity, changes in body weight, and serum electrolytes. These parameters should be determined and recorded on a daily basis; the status of fluid and electrolyte balance can be interpreted on the basis of these data.

Application of Continuous Positive Airway Pressure

Continuous positive airway pressure (CPAP) is a useful mode of treatment for moderately severe RDS. This mode of treatment is based on the principle that by applying a certain amount of positive pressure (2 to 6 mm Hg) during the expiratory phase, one can mechanically maintain alveolar stability, thus improving ventilation. It is necessary to determine the arterial blood gases for proper institution of this treatment. In general, during the first 24 hours of life, infants with RDS requiring oxygen up to 60% to maintain a PaO$_2$ of 50 mm Hg would be appropriate candidates for the institution of CPAP. It has been shown that by starting CPAP early (not waiting for the oxygen concentration to reach 100% to maintain PaO$_2$ at 50 mm Hg), the clinical course of RDS can be modified to a less severe form. The institution of CPAP can be done noninvasively by nasal prongs to avoid intubation.

ASSISTED VENTILATION

In infants with severe RDS, assisted ventilation is necessary to increase the survival rate. The usual indications for the use of respirators are as follows: (1) PaO$_2$ $\leq$ 50 mm Hg at an FIO$_2$ of 1.0; (2) PaCO$_2$ $\geq$ 70 mm Hg; (3) pH $\leq$ 7.20; and (4) persistent apnea. Positive pressure respirators are used, which would require intubation. The endotracheal tube is introduced either through the nasal cavity or the oral cavity. The choice of respirator and route of intubation depends on the expertise of the medical, nursing, and respiratory therapy personnel in the intensive care unit. The amount of peak inspiratory pressure applied initally depends on the size of the infant and the compliance of the lung. One may start with an arbitrary number of pressures and judge the effectiveness of ventilation by the chest expansion, breath sounds, and color of the infant. It is essential that blood gas determinations be done to judge the effectiveness of ventilation. The inspiratory-expiratory ratio (IE ratio) of the respirator setting should be maintained at approximately 1 to 1.5. The frequency of blood gas determinations will depend on the severity of the disease and the progress of therapy. Positive end expiratory pressure (PEEP) is generally used to improve the alveolar stability. Complications such as extrapulmonary air leak, infection, and symptomatic patent ductus arteriosus should be watched for and promptly treated.

When the infant's condition improves, the weaning process may begin by lowering the peak inspiratory pressure, followed by lowering the oxygen concentration. The weaning process should always be monitored closely by the blood gas determinations, either by arterial blood sampling through the umbilical arterial catheter or by the use of a transcutaneous PO$_2$ monitoring device.

Neonatal Pneumomediastinum and Pneumothorax

STEPHEN L. GANS, M.D.,
and EDWARD AUSTIN, M.D.

Pneumomediastinum. The treatment of pneumomediastinum is the treatment of its underlying cause. Direct mediastinal drainage is rarely indicated or effective. This space is not bounded at its upper and lower extremities and therefore does not build up pressure; in addition, it is filled with areolar tissue much like a sponge, which makes it difficult to remove trapped air.

In the neonate the most frequent causes of pneumomediastinum are positive pressure therapy for resuscitation and the treatment of respiratory distress syndrome. Its main significance is that it provides a warning of the possible development of pneumothorax or pneumopericardium, both potentially lethal and necessitating prompt therapy.

Other causes in the infant and child are bronchial rupture from cough or trauma, bronchiolitis, acute asthma, cystic fibrosis, and pertussis. Esophageal perforation by penetration, trauma, or ingested foreign body must also be considered. Treatment for these conditions is detailed elsewhere in this book.

Pneumothorax. The same conditions that cause pneumomediastinum may cause pneumothorax. However, in addition to treating the primary problem, prompt attention and care must be provided for this potentially lethal complication.

Asymptomatic pneumothorax of less than 20 per cent, usually discovered by chest radiographs, should be carefully observed.

Symptomatic pneumothorax or any pneumothorax greater than 20% requires chest aspiration and drainage. In an emergency, aspiration with a 23-gauge needle connected to a three-way stopcock and 20 ml syringe may be temporarily helpful. The use of an intravenous catheter instead of a needle may lessen the risk of lung puncture.

When adequate equipment and trained personnel are available, a chest tube should be inserted *without* prior aspiration of air. The air acts as a protective cushion to prevent lung injury when introducing the chest tube. A convenient and effective thoracostomy tube for infants is the No. 12 French Argyle catheter with stylet. It has an end hole, three side holes, and a radiopaque stripe so that the position of the last hold and catheter can be checked by chest x-ray film. A similar larger catheter is available for older patients.

We usually choose a site low in the axilla, but the pneumothorax can be drained from any lateral position where the presence of air is verified by roentgenography. The skin is widely prepared with an appropriate antiseptic, and sterile drapes are applied. After infiltration with ¼ per cent lidocaine, a nick is made in the skin, just large enough to accommodate the catheter, overlying the rib just below the anticipated chest entrance. The tube with stylet is then introduced into the pleural cavity by firm pressure and a slight drilling motion, over the rib and through the intercostal space, using the other hand to grasp the tube and prevent overinsertion and lung damage when the pleural cavity is entered.

The trocar is slightly withdrawn so that its point is covered and the catheter is advanced just beyond the last hole and immediately connected to water seal drainage, where bubbling will be observed. The tube is secured to adjacent skin with a silk suture and a small firm dressing is applied. The catheter is further secured to the chest wall with adhesive tape, and all tube connections are reinforced with tape to prevent accidental disconnection. A chest radiograph is obtained immediately to check the position and effectiveness of the tube, and appropriate adjustments are made if necessary.

Because there is concern in some quarters about perforation of the lung with the pointed trocar, an alternate method of tube placement is described here. After infiltration anesthesia, a 3–0 silk pursestring suture is placed at the introduction site, and a small skin nick is made with a pointed blade. A hemostat is used to spread the underlying tissues of the intercostal space and enter the pleural cavity. There will be an audible escape of air, and the chest tube is introduced and advanced through this hole with the trochar withdrawn into the end of the tube. After proper placement, the pursestring suture is tied and a secure dressing is applied. The tube is connected with water seal drainage as before, and chest x-ray films are taken.

Water seal drainage is usually adequate to expand the lung completely. Continued bubbling of air and failure of expansion is unusual but mandates the use of suction up to – 15 cm/H_2O to inflate the lung and seal the pleura. Failure to accomplish expansion of the lung with this maneuver, particularly when associated with deterioration in the patient's condition, may indicate thoracotomy to close a large unsealed lung perforation.

In the older child, pneumothorax may be caused by trauma, asthmatic attacks, bronchiolitis, cystic fibrosis, or staphylococcal pneumonia or may occur spontaneously. Tube thoracostomy is usually required, and appropriate treatment is instituted for the primary condition. Recurrent spontaneous pneumothorax should be treated by resecting or oversewing portions of the lung with blebs, or by pleurodesis obtained by injecting quinacrine or tetracycline through a chest catheter.

Bronchopulmonary Dysplasia

M. DOUGLAS CUNNINGHAM, M.D.

Protracted mechanical ventilation during and beyond the neonatal period has resulted in the recognition of bronchopulmonary dysplasia (BPD) as a form of chronic pulmonary disease of infancy. The small airways and alveoli are damaged by prolonged exposure to increased oxygen concentrations and the repeated barotrauma of the ventilator cycles. The dysplastic changes of the infant lung cause impaired ventilation/perfusion, decreased tracheobronchial toilet, cystic and emphysematous changes, and altered pulmonary vascular and lymphatic flow. Clinical management of BPD aims toward minimizing respiratory tract insult, compensating for complications, and maintaining nutritional support during recovery.

Paramount to recovery from BPD is to successfully wean an infant, first from mechanical ventilatory support, and second from increased concentrations of inspired oxygen. Decreased mechanical support requires aggressive and persistent withdrawal of ventilator rate, pressure, and distending airway pressure settings. Plotting of mean airway pressures allows the clinician to view the effect of decreasing the several respirator settings. Once mean airway pressure has been decreased to 5 cm H_2O or less and oxygen concentration to 30% or less, success in weaning completely from the respirator is nearly complete.

Continued withdrawal of mechanical support and supplemental oxygen over days or weeks must be persistently attempted. Converting ventilatory support to continuous positive airway pressure is an intermediary step to final extubation and oxygen by hood. Discontinuance of all supplemental oxygen usually requires a further 2 to 6 weeks beyond stopping mechanical support in moderate-to-moderately severe cases. Transcutaneous oxygen monitoring is a useful aid in the weaning process. Infants with BPD are extremely sensitive to oxygen levels, and transcutaneous monitoring allows for gradual weaning without undue hypoxic stress. Maintaining arterial PaO_2 levels of 45 to 55 torr will suffice and be well tolerated in most cases of BPD. The blood hemoglobin must be supported during this time of weaning. Success at weaning BPD patients from respirators and oxygen is limited if hemoglobin levels are allowed to decline to 13 mg/dl or lower.

Arterial $PaCO_2$ levels may safely rise to 50 to 60

torr provided pH values remain at 7.28 or greater. Usually renal compensation with bicarbonate retention will buffer the decreased pH with base excess values of +4 to +6 meq/l. Excessive ventilation to relieve $PaCO_2$ retention will increase mean airway pressure and heighten the barotrauma. Aminophylline therapy may be helpful in some cases of respirator weaning by acting as a bronchodilator. A loading dose of 5 mg/kg over 20 minutes intravenously followed by 2 mg/kg every 8 hours should maintain a blood level of 8 to 12 mg/l. Persistent tachycardia or gastric distention may require discontinuance of the aminophylline.

Chest physiotherapy that is provided gently and persistently is helpful to BPD patients. Chest physiotherapy, as described in the following article on Neonatal Atelectasis, should be applied regularly for BPD patients, but with vibration substituted for percussion. Secretions lead to atelectasis and further ventilatory compromise, but excessive and forceful therapy tires the infant and produces bouts of hypoxemia. Rehospitalization for intercurrent infections is more common in BPD patients. Appropriate antibiotics and chest physiotherapy are indicated.

The dysplastic changes of the lungs severely disturb the ability of the pulmonary vascular and lymphatic beds to handle fluid. Specific retention of fluid in BPD-affected lungs is frequently seen in the weaning and convalescent stages. Increased and unexpected weight gain with increased ventilatory effort usually heralds BPD fluid retention. Fluid intake limited to 150 mg/kg/24 hr is helpful. Utilizing a humidified oxygen-air mix decreases insensible fluid losses. Fluid management should point toward a serum osmolality of 285 to 290 mOsm. With fluid retention and respiratory compromise, diuretic therapy is beneficial. Furosemide, 1 to 2 mg/kg/dose, is used to initiate diuresis. Some patients require only occasional doses. Still others, more severely affected, will require daily or alternate-day treatment. Regular furosemide therapy is best augmented by daily spironolactone (1.5 to 1.7 mg/kg/24 hr) to minimize potassium losses. Prolonged furosemide usage may lead to hypercalciuria and hypochloremia. Doses of furosemide in small infants beyond 2 mg/kg/24 hr increase the risk for ototoxicity.

The nutritional status of the BPD patient is very important for recovery. Successful weaning and convalescence require progressive weight gain. Infants weighing less than 1200 grams are less likely to be weaned. Increased caloric intake up to 150 cal/kg/24 hr is required to meet growth demands and the work of increased respiratory effort. Hypercaloric formulas (24 to 30 cal/oz) will allow for increased nutrition without excessive water intake. Careful monitoring of gut tolerance is advisable when hypertonic formulas are given. Early in recovery nipple feeding is not advised as it increases the work of breathing and risks aspiration. Nasogastric feedings will be required for prolonged periods, and deep line hyperalimentation may be required in more severe cases. A balanced caloric intake is sought.

Special vitamin or mineral additives are not recommended as adjuncts to prevention of BPD or enhancement of recovery. The role of vitamin E as an antioxidant in BPD is unproved. Excessive doses of vitamin E are to be discouraged until appropriate clinical trials confirm efficacy; fatty changes in the liver with hepatomegaly may result.

Lipid emulsions for augmenting hyperalimentation in low birth weight infants are well established. However, hypoxemia and hypercapnia may result when lipid emulsions are given to some BPD patients. Lipid deposition in the lung capillary and lymphatic beds leads to an alveolar-capillary block. At doses of less than 2 gm/kg/24 hr the effect can be seen, and the frequency and severity increase with dosages reaching 4 gm/kg/24 hr. Caution and close blood gas monitoring must be applied when giving BPD patients lipid emulsions. Long-term complications of severe BPD include: lobar emphysema (see elsewhere in this text), cor pulmonale, sudden infant death, and abnormal pulmonary function with exercise limitations. Cor pulmonale is associated with increased pulmonary artery pressure and usually leads to progressive decline and death of the patient. It is only seen in the most severe and advanced forms of BPD. Digoxin is of little benefit.

Pulmonary function studies suggest limited exercise tolerance in the 2 to 3 years after recovery from BPD. However, lung growth and remodeling continue through 7 to 8 years of age. Complete recovery is now being documented by pulmonary function testing in some cases.

Some BPD patients may be able to go home and be maintained on nasal oxygen and chest physiotherapy. Home care teams of visiting nurse, social worker, and respiratory therapist are needed to assist parents in adequately supporting a child with advanced BPD in the home. However, improved mechanical ventilation and disappearance of the advanced cystic changes of BPD should lessen the need for home care. An increasing number of BPD victims are being cleared of their disease by the time adequate weight gain for discharge has been reached.

Neonatal Atelectasis

M. DOUGLAS CUNNINGHAM, M.D.

Postnatal collapse of segments or lobes of the infant lung results in nonaerated lung parenchyma, or atelectasis. Extrinsic pressure must be relieved if it is the cause of collapsed lung tissue. Aberrant thoracic masses or accumulations of intrapleural blood, air, or fluid may be the sources of difficulty. Intrinsic lung collapse resulting from endobronchial occlusion results from thickened or copious secretions and poor tracheobronchial toilet. Inflammatory lung disease is the most common cause of occluding secretions. Occasionally, premature infants requiring prolonged mechanical ventilation and endotracheal intubation will experience lobar atelectasis, particularly of the right upper lobe. Infants with bronchopulmonary dysplasia (BPD) have a migrating or recurrent atelectasis because of the inability of the damaged airways to expel secretions effectively.

Bronchial secretions are most easily managed by initiating vigorous chest physiotherapy. Frequent and persistent chest percussion, vibration, and postural drainage of affected lobes are effective in most cases. Moderately forceful percussion of the neonate over the affected lobes by a nurse trained in the care of newborn and small infants is essential. Percussion can be performed by using a soft rubber infant oxygen face mask. The air-filled rubber seal of the mask protects the infant's chest from bruising. Vibration following percussion, and while postural drainage is taking place, is another effective means of loosening tenacious bronchial secretions. Propping the infant continuously in a position to effect selective lobar postural drainage is necessary, as more effective clearing by cough is not possible in infants. Frequent turning of infants assures continued bronchial drainage. Right upper lobe atelectasis following extubation in premature infants can be relieved by keeping the infant in the prone position. Moreover, the use of a water flotation mattress with continuous oscillation has been helpful in treating some cases of protracted atelectasis.

Adequate hydration of infants to insure fluidity of secretions must be maintained. Urine output of 3 to 5 ml/kg/hr with a specific gravity of 1.006 to 1.012 and a serum osmolality of less than 290 mOsm should signify adequate hydration. Fluid administration of 120 to 150 ml/kg/24 hr will attain these parameters of good hydration in most infants. Humidification of air by plastic head hood or face mask will decrease insensible fluid losses of the respiratory tract, decrease drying of secretions, and aid the effusion of airway secretions. The mist should be warmed to 32°C to avoid chilling the infants. The use of mucolytic agents is discouraged.

Failure of chest physiotherapy, hydration, and humidification to relieve segmental or lobar atelectasis after 48 hours warrants consideration of endotracheal intubation for initiation of regular tracheal lavage and suction. Endotracheal tubes smaller than 3.5 mm internal diameter rarely lend themselves to effective suctioning. Inserting as large an endotracheal tube as anatomically allowable (3.5 or 4.0 mm) should be considered. Sterile normal saline is used for lavage. Instilling 0.5 to 1.0 ml and disseminating it by brief bag-to-endotracheal tube hand ventilation carries it into the lower airways. Lavage is followed by sterile endotracheal suctioning. Regular chest physiotherapy with the endotracheal tube in place should continue on an every 2- to 3-hour basis, with lavage and suctioning immediately afterward. The neonate should be managed in an infant intensive care seting, with ongoing cardiorespiratory monitoring. Careful attention should be paid to thermoregulation during the procedures. The avoidance of tiring the infant with excessively long chest physiotherapy is important. Chest physiotherapy and endotracheal suction and lavage procedures should not exceed 8 to 10 minutes at 2- to 3-hour intervals.

The application of 3 to 4 cm H_2O pressure as continuous distending airway pressure (CDAP) by way of the endotracheal tube may be helpful in some instances of stubborn atelectasis. Monitoring of arterial Pa_{CO_2} for retention is advised. Lowering of CDAP by 1 cm of water pressure should be done if Pa_{CO_2} values increase or if chest roentgenograms show hyperexpansion of nonatelectatic lobes. Prolonged intubation is to be discouraged as this step may aggravate the existing atelectasis.

Nearly all neonatal atelectasis resolves following the above procedures. Some particularly difficult right upper lobe postextubation atelectasis may require several periods of reintubation and lavage (1 to 6 hours in duration) over 1 to 2 weeks before resolving entirely. Only after an extended effort should direct visualization and suction with fiberoptic bronchoscope be considered for neonatal segmental or lobar atelectasis. Direct laryngoscopy and blind suctioning of the lower airway are discouraged because suction collapse of noninvolved lung may occur, and undue suction excoriation of tracheal or bronchial mucosa can lead to bleeding and further endobronchial occlusion. Vagal stimulation and profound bradycardia or laryngospasm may also occur.

Lobar Emphysema

M. DOUGLAS CUNNINGHAM, M.D.

Progressive newborn respiratory distress secondary to congenital lobar emphysema is an emergency calling for prompt surgical evaluation. Continued expansion of the affected lobe (usually right or left upper) can result in further compression of adjacent lung, shift of the mediastinum and cardiovascular compromise, impaired cerebral venous drainage, and possibly herniation of the emphysematous lung across the anterior mediastinum with compression of the contralateral lung. An expeditious lobectomy is curative.

Preoperative and intraoperative management

call for close attention to intravascular blood volume, arterial blood pressure monitoring, and careful fluid management. If the enphysematous lobe is detected within 72 hours of birth, umbilical vein catheterization affords central venous pressure (CVP) monitoring with a No. 3.5 or 5.0 French catheter positioned above the diaphragm in the inferior vena cava. The normal range for CVP should be 6 to 8 cm H_2O pressure. Umbilical artery catheterization with the catheter tip at the level of the third or fourth lumbar vertebra and attached to a transducer will allow close monitoring of pulse pressure. Decreased arterial blood pressure or narrowing of the pulse pressure indicates significant mediastinal shift.

Fluid management to maintain an adequate urine output (3 to 5 ml/kg/hr) with a specific gravity of 1.006 to 1.012 is recommended. The tachypnea of respiratory distress heightens insensible water loss, as does exposure of the lung and pleural cavity during thoracotomy. Fluid administration of 5 or 10% dextrose in water at a rate of 120 to 150 ml/kg/24 hr can be initiated and modified through patient monitoring. Electrolytes should be added to intravenous fluids if urine output is satisfactory and normal serum electrolytes have been documented.

Airway management should include supplemental oxygen, as indicated by arterial blood gases drawn from the umbilical artery line. Endotracheal intubation prior to anesthesia may be required for control of increased secretions, CO_2 retention, or ineffective ventilatory effort. Mechanical ventilation by respirator or hand bag is to be avoided unless respiratory insufficiency is pronounced or apnea ensues. Positive pressure ventilation may increase the displacement of intrathoracic structures by the emphysematous lobe. Constant distending airway pressures should be avoided until surgical control of the distended lobe is attained.

Congenital lobar emphysema with mild respiratory distress detected beyond 1 month of age may be managed without surgical intervention. Some cases have shown a gradual decrease of hyperinflation and result in a functional lung. Supportive therapy includes treatment of any underlying pneumonia, chest physiotherapy for secretions, and supplemental oxygen. Needle aspiration should never be considered, and positive pressure by face mask ventilation is to be avoided. Recurrent bouts of respiratory distress and intercurrent lower respiratory infections suggest the need for surgical intervention, as just discussed.

Acquired lobar emphysema in the neonate is seen in association with advanced bronchopulmonary dysplasia (BPD) following a long-standing need for continuous mechanical ventilation. Hyperexpansion of the scarred and fibrotic lung tissue of Grade IV BPD results from the loss of elasticity and continued positive pressure ventilation. Additionally, patients with BPD have decreased tracheo-

bronchial toilet with decreased secretions occluding lung segments. Marked lobar emphysema complicating the extensive cystic changes of Grade IV BPD requires a prompt decrease of as much positive pressure ventilation as possible and a lessening of any continuous distending airway pressure. Gentle chest physiotherapy and humidification of the air-oxygen mixture will assist in the management of acquired lobar emphysema. Before surgical intervention is attempted, selective intubation of the contralateral main-stem bronchus is recommended. This is best accomplished under fluoroscopy using a Portex (TM) endotracheal tube.

Some cases of acquired lobar emphysema secondary to BPD have resolved after 24 to 72 hours of by-pass intubation and ventilation of the contralateral lung. The by-passed lung is allowed to become atelectatic and the emphysematous lobe to completely decompress. Extubation and assumption of bilateral ventilation allow for gradual reexpansion. If the acquired lobar emphysema has resolved completely, it will most likely not recur, and the usual respiratory management of BPD can continue. If the emphysematous lobe fails to decompress or reappears with progressive ventilatory compromise, lobectomy is advised.

Other acquired emphysematous lobes in the neonatal period are usually secondary to bronchial obstruction. Bronchial secretions or aspirated material creates a ball-valve effect and hyperexpansion of the distal lung. Usually vigorous chest physiotherapy will suffice to relieve the obstructing secretions, but bronchoscopy may be required in acute situations.

Meconium Aspiration

WILLIAM OH, M.D.

Meconium staining of the amniotic fluid occurs in approximately 10% of all deliveries. In this population, combined obstetric and pediatric management in the removal of the meconium from the upper airway at birth will reduce the incidence of meconium aspiration syndrome from 2% to less than 0.1%. This strongly suggests that the most important aspect in the management of meconium aspiration is recognition of infants at risk (meconium staining of amniotic fluid) and perinatal approach in the removal of the meconium from the airway at the time of delivery. This is accomplished as follows: As soon as the head of the infant is delivered, the obstetrician should aspirate the nasopharyngeal and oropharyngeal area with a DeLee suction catheter. As soon as the baby is delivered, the pediatrician should suction the oropharyngeal cavities with the rubber bulb syringe. If meconium is present, the vocal cords should be inspected by laryngoscopy to see if it is present in the vocal cords. If meconium is present, a DeLee suction catheter or an endotracheal tube is used to remove it from the trachea. The infant should then be handled in the same manner as in the chapter on resuscitation in the newborn. There has been considerable controversy regarding the need of laryngoscopy and visualization of the cord in an infant who has meconium staining but has already taken the first few breaths and is vigorously crying and breathing. The reason for this concern is that in infants who already have initiated their respiration soon after birth, the meconium is likely to be aspirated already, and that attempts to remove this material by laryngoscopy and passing the tracheal tube would probably be futile. Furthermore, in inexperienced hands, the attempt to intubate and pass the DeLee suction or endotracheal tube may cause a vagovagal response resulting in bradycardia and apnea. Because of the beneficial results of vigorous aspiration of meconium, it seems prudent to recommend that in the presence of severe asphyxia in an infant who does not take the first breath and is depressed during the first minute of life, the physician should make all attempts to laryngoscope the infant and aspirate the meconium from the trachea. In infants who take the first breath but continue to be somewhat depressed within the first minute of life, laryngoscope and trachea aspiration should also be done. However, it seems inappropriate to insist that laryngoscopy be done for removal of meconium in infants who vigorously breathe and cry soon after birth, particularly if the operator is not experienced in performing such a procedure.

All infants born with meconium staining of the amniotic fluid should be observed closely during the first 6 hours of life. Since the presence of meconium in the amniotic fluid (in a vertex presentation) generally indicates intrauterine fetal asphyxia, the infant should be observed not only for evidence of meconium aspiration but also for other clinical complications of asphyxia. These complications include hypoglycemia, polycythemia, and hyperviscosity, renal complications such as acute tubular necrosis, and postasphyxia encephalopathy. Therefore, during the first 6 hours of life, blood glucose should be monitored for hypoglycemia by screening with Dextrostix (Ames Laboratories), a semiquantitative assessment of the blood glucose, using one drop of blood obtained by heel puncture. If this assessment indicates that the blood glucose value is less than 40 mg/dl, a quantitative blood glucose analysis should be done to confirm the hypoglycemia. In the meantime, intravenous glucose infusion should begin, giving a dose of 6 mg/kg/min; if the hypoglycemia is confirmed, treatment should be continued with the glucose infusion, otherwise the infusion can be reduced and discontinued if the infants can tolerate oral feeding.

Because of the high incidence of polycythemia in infants with meconium aspiration venous blood should be obtained for hematocrit measurement. If the hematocrit exceeds 65%, the diagnosis can be entertained, and if the infant is symptomatic, treatment with partial exchange transfusion can be instituted. The latter is performed generally by removal of 10 to 15% of the estimated blood volume (80 ml/kg) and replacement with equal volume of a colloid solution such as Plasmanate. For instance, in a 3 kg infant, 25 to 35 ml of blood is removed and the same amount of Plasmanate infused.

In anticipation of potential oliguria and anuria due to renal injury resulting from asphyxia, infants with meconium aspiration should be maintained on a low intravenous fluid regimen (no more than 40 ml/kg/day) to replace insensible water loss and some potential stool water loss. If the infant begins to urinate during the first 12 to 24 hours of life, the fluid rate can be increased accordingly.

Another common metabolic complication in infants with meconium aspiration is hypocalcemia, which can be diagnosed by serum calcium determinations during the first 24 hours of life. If hypocalcemia occurs (serum calcium less than 7 mg/dl in preterm and 8 mg/dl in full term infants), intravenous calcium gluconate can be given at a dose of 50 mg/kg every 6 hours.

The clinical manifestations of postasphyxia encephalopathy are increased muscle tone, jitteriness, and at times, seizure. Hypotonia may also occur. The treatment of choice for seizure is sodium phenobarbital, IM or IV at a loading dose of 15 to 20 mg/kg body weight and a maintenance dose of 5 to 6 mg/kg/day given every 12 hours.

During the first 3 hours of life, the cardiorespiratory manifestations are the most important parameters for observation in infants with meconium staining. Monitoring of the cardiorespiratory status is best done in the Special Care Nursery or in a designated area in a nursery where constant observation by experienced medical and/or nursing personnel are available. At the end of the 6-hour period, if the infant is symptom free with reference to cardiorespiratory status, he or she can be cared for in the normal nursery. If respiratory distress develops, a chest roentgenogram should be performed to establish the diagnosis and rule out the possibility of other causes of respiratory distress such as pneumothorax, pneumonia, or congenital cardiac anomalies. Treatment for respiratory distress is supportive, including oxygen administration to maintain arterial Po_2 between 50 and 70 torr; if hypotension develops, volume expansion with Plasmanate at a dose of 10 ml/kg body weight should be administered intravenously. Metabolic acidosis is not uncommon in these infants; if the acidosis is mild (pH $\geq$ 7.20), supportive treatment to ensure appropriate tissue oxygenation with oxygen therapy and maintenance of tissue perfusion are often adequate. Sodium bicarbonate infusion should be avoided in these instances. However, in very severe metabolic acidosis (pH $\leq$ 7.20), particularly if this occurs in spite of appropriate oxygen and volume therapy, sodium bicarbonate can be used cautiously; the dose can be calculated on the basis of blood gas data.

Meconium itself is sterile, so that in most instances antibiotic therapy is not necessary. However, when risk factors are involved, such as prolonged ruptured membranes with evidence of chorioamnionitis, or if there is definite radiologic evidence of pneumonia, antibiotics can be instituted. The antibiotic treatment of choice is usually ampicillin, in a dose of 100 mg/kg/day intravenously given every 12 hours, and one of the aminoglycosides (either kanamycin at 15 mg/kg/day given twice a day or gentamicin at a dose of 6 mg/kg/day given twice a day). Both aminoglycosides can be given intravenously.

Pneumothorax is a common complication; therefore, close observation of the respiratory status should be done to specifically detect pneumothorax if the infant's clinical condition deteriorates. If pneumothorax occurs, emergency placement of a chest tube for decompression of the pleural cavity should be done.

Disorders of the Umbilicus

WILLIAM OH, M.D.

The umbilical cord, through its vessels, serves as the lifeline for the fetus in utero. This structure contains the umbilical artery, umbilical vein, urachus, the remnants of omphalomesenteric vessels and Wharton jelly. Various pathologic conditions ranging from congenital malformations to bleeding may affect many of the structures contained in the umbilical cord and may require treatment during the neonatal period. Most of the abnormalities are relatively benign, with the exception of an inflammatory process (omphalitis) that may lead to sepsis, and congenital anomalies such as a large omphalocele that may require immediate surgery.

CLAMPING OF THE UMBILICAL CORD

At the time of birth a certain amount of placental transfusion occurs when the umbilical cord is left intact during the first minute of life. If the infant is delivered by cesarean section, the amount of placental transfusion depends on timing. If the cord is clamped before the fetus is removed from the uter-

ine cavity, the infant will not receive a significant amount of placental blood and the blood volume will be equivalent to what the fetus had in utero. If the cord is not clamped when the fetus is being removed from the uterus, a significant amount of blood may be transfused from the fetus into the placenta, resulting in hypovolemia. Therefore, the preferred method in a cesarean section birth is to clamp the umbilical cord either before or immediately after the fetus is delivered.

In vaginal delivery, the amount of placental transfusion depends on the residual uterine contractility following delivery, the position of the infant in relation to the birth canal, the timing of the closure of the umbilical artery, and the timing of the umbilical cord clamping. Assuming that the infant is held approximately 10 to 15 cm below the birth canal, the amount of blood transfusion from the placenta to the fetus is approximately 20 to 25 ml/kg during the first minute of life. Therefore, a 15- to 30-second interval between the delivery of the infant's buttock and the clamping of the umbilical cord will allow an amount of placental transfusion giving the neonate a blood volume of approximately 90 ml/kg of body weight. This blood volume is appropriate for subsequent cardiopulmonary adjustment. Allowing a greater amount of placental transfusion by prolonging the timing of cord-clamping or by milking the umbilical cord toward the infant may lead to hypervolemia and polycythemia. If the cord is clamped immediately after delivery of the infant's buttock, no placental transfusion will occur and the infant's blood volume will be approximately 80 ml/kg. In most full-term infants this amount of blood volume is adequate for achieving appropriate neonatal circulatory adaptation; however, in some instances, particularly in infants with low birth weight, hypovolemia may ensue, and in the presence of hyaline membrane disease morbidity may be increased.

In vaginal delivery, therefore, the umbilical cord should be clamped between 30 seconds to 1 minute following the delivery of the infant's buttock. This will allow appropriate time for the physician to dry the infant's skin, clear the respiratory airway, and in the meantime give the infant the appropriate amount of blood transfusion. If the cord is tightly wound around the infant's neck, or if there is some other indication for immediate separation of the fetus from the placenta, the umbilical cord may be clamped sooner; in such instances the blood volume status of the infant should be assessed closely.

CONGENITAL ANOMALIES OF THE UMBILICAL CORD

Single Umbilical Artery. This occurs in 1 per 1000 singleton live births and 5 to 6 times more often in twin births. The condition is associated with a higher frequency of other congenital malformations, particularly those involving the genitourinary tract and the cardiovascular, skeletal and gastrointestinal systems. Because of this association, the number of umbilical vessels should be counted immediately after cord cutting, and the information registered in the medical record for future reference. Since the umbilical artery tends to retract soon after birth, a count of vessels on the umbilical cord several hours after birth may be inaccurate and give a falsely high incidence of single umbilical artery. Since in most instances congenital single umbilical artery is an isolated malformation, an in-depth diagnostic investigation probably is not necessary. However, its presence should raise the index of suspicion. If other clinical findings are noted, a thorough diagnostic workup should be performed to identify other congenital anomalies.

Congenital Omphalocele. In this congenital defect of the umbilicus, abdominal contents protrude into its base. The contents are covered only by peritoneal sac, which may become infected or ruptured. Immediate surgical repair before rupture or infection occurs is the key to successful management. If the sac of the omphalocele has ruptured, a synthetic material such as Silastic may be used until the abdominal content is gradually contained. If the omphalocele is too large for surgical closure, one may attempt therapy with the direct application of 2% merthiolate on the omphalocele sac, two or three times a day, with the aim of achieving gradual epithelialization of the sac over a 2- to 3-month period. During this time, gradual containment of the abdominal contents also may be achieved.

Patent Urachus. This is a rare anomaly in which the allantoic duct failed to close and remained as the patent urachus in the umbilicus. One should suspect this condition if there is a persistent drainage of yellowish fluid from the umbilicus. Surgical closure may be indicated.

INFECTION, HEMORRHAGE, AND OTHER CONDITIONS

Omphalitis. This is a local inflammatory process of the umbilicus due to one of the pyogenic bacteria; it usually occurs during the first week of life. The condition usually is benign but potentially may serve as the initial focus of infection, leading to systemic spread and sepsis. Prevention can be achieved by appropriate cord care to minimize the heavy contamination of the cord with pyogenic organisms, particularly *Staphylococcus aureus*. Local treatment of omphalitis consists of cleansing with 3% hexachlorophene solution three times a day, application of local antibiotic ointment (such as 1% bacitracin-polymyxin-neomycin ointment) and systemic antibiotics in the form of ampicillin and an aminoglycoside initially, and by appropriate antibiotics as determined by culture and sensitivity studies of the cord specimen. If abscesses are present,

incision and drainage should be performed. Isolation procedure should be instructed to prevent nursery spread of the infection.

Hemorrhage of the Umbilicus. This generally is due to one of the following causes: inappropriate clamping of the cord; hemorrhagic disease of the newborn; failure of the cord vessels to thrombose; and, in some instances, mechanical irritation and premature separation of the dried cord stump. Treatment consists of pressure dressing and assessment for the systemic causes of the hemorrhage.

Granuloma. In this common disorder of the umbilicus, soft red granulation tissue is located at its base. The lesion often is accompanied by serosanguineous discharge, frequently foul-smelling, and can be prevented by appropriate cleansing of the umbilicus at the time the cord falls off. The actual treatment of the granuloma consists of cauterization with silver nitrate at frequent intervals over a period of several days until the granuloma dries and heals. The condition is benign and generally responds to cauterization.

Neonatal Ascites

DENIS M. MURPHY, M.B., B.Ch.

Because of the diversity of conditions giving rise to ascites in the neonatal period, it is necessary to divide this discussion into two sections. In the first part, principles of management of the ascites and its complications are described. In the second section, the management of the underlying conditions causing ascites will be discussed individually. It should be borne in mind that neonatal ascites is a rare condition and, consequently, opinion on the management of the underlying causes is based for the most part on reviews of reports of single cases or very small series. Although ascites is seen in infants with severe forms of erythroblastosis fetalis, its treatment will not be discussed here because the complexity of the problem is beyond the scope of this brief review.

GENERAL MANAGEMENT

Delivery. Although dystocia is common, most infants with neonatal ascites can be delivered successfully by conservative means. A minority of reported cases have required delivery by cesarean section. Fetal paroxysmal supraventricular tachycardia (PST) is not an indication for section unless the accompanying ascites is severe enough to obstruct delivery. However, fetal PST is often mistakenly diagnosed as fetal distress, resulting in an unnecessary section.

Ventilation. If ascites is severe at delivery, the abdominal distention may result in respiratory embarrassment. Assisted ventilation is then required and should be delivered through an endotracheal tube, to prevent gaseous distention of the stomach. Ventilation can then be effected using an Ambu bag or a mechanical ventilator.

Paracentesis. Once ventilation is secured, attention should turn to paracentesis. There are two reasons for this procedure: 1) to relieve abdominal distention and respiratory embarrassment, and 2) for diagnostic evaluation of the ascitic fluid. The infant is placed in the supine position. The site of paracentesis is selected in the right or left lower abdominal quadrant, lateral to the rectus muscle. A sandbag may be placed under the opposite side, displacing the coils of intestine away from the site of paracentesis. The abdomen is prepared with antiseptic swabs and draped. An 18-gauge lumbar puncture needle with stylet in place is introduced into the peritoneal cavity. A slight "give" is felt as the peritoneum is penetrated. The needle is advanced 1 to 2 cm into the peritoneal cavity and the stylet removed. Enough fluid is withdrawn to relieve respiratory embarrassment, then the needle is removed. (After resuscitation is completed, a second paracentesis can be performed to more effectively decompress the peritoneal cavity.) In most cases spontaneous respiration is at once restored by this maneuver, and the infant than can be moved to an oxygen-enriched atmosphere under a hood.

Fluid and Electrolyte Management. The disturbance requiring correction is usually hypotonic dehydration accompanied by metabolic acidosis and hyperkalemia. If circulatory collapse has occurred, colloid plasma expanders should be infused rapidly to a volume of 20 ml/kg body weight. Dehydration in the absence of circulatory collapse may be corrected more slowly over the ensuing 24 hours. Even in those infants not in shock, serum albumin is usually depleted and intravenous replacement necessary during the course of rehydration. Massive loss of protein in one reported case resulted in severe deficiencies of all clotting factors, with the exception of Factor VIII. There was no evidence of circulating anticoagulants. Administration of fresh frozen plasma appears to be the treatment of choice in this very rare situation.

Electrolyte deficiencies are corrected by replacing sodium, chloride, and bicarbonate while correcting dehydration. The total deficit for each electrolyte is calculated on the basis that the infant's body water represents 70% of its weight. One half of the calculated deficit together with the calculated maintenance dose is administered over a period of 12 hours. The electrolyte status is then rechecked and half the remaining deficit again administered. Hyperkalemia is not often a problem because of the infant's toleration of higher potassium levels (up to 9 meq/l), and because sodium replacement tends to reduce potassium excess. If necessary, sodium polystyrene sulfonate (Kayexa-

late) may be given by enema or nasogastric tube in a dose of 1 gm/kg every 4 to 8 hours.

Repeat Paracentesis. Following stabilization of the infant's general condition, repeat paracentesis should be performed to further decompress the peritoneal cavity.

MANAGEMENT OF UNDERLYING ANOMALY

Urinary Ascites. Early and adequate urinary drainage is the first prerequisite for the successful management of neonatal urinary ascites. Initially, a No. 5 F. urethral catheter is passed in order to obtain a cystogram. Vesical decompression may then be maintained by means of the urethral catheter. However, because of the risk of urethral stricture inherent in the prolonged use of a urethral catheter in small boys and the tendency of small catheters to block, many authorities advocate suprapubic drainage in this age group. When extravasation occurs at bladder level, catheter drainage alone may result in cure. However, if ascitic fluid reaccumulates, laparotomy and closure of the bladder perforation may become necessary.

In most cases extravasation occurs from the renal pelvis, and bladder drainage then will fail to provide adequate decompression. The marked improvement in survival of these infants recorded over the past few years has been due mainly to the recognition of the need for prompt upper tract diversion. In most cases this has been achieved by nephrostomy. Loop cutaneous ureterostomy may be preferable in that the infant is free of tubes, which may act as a nidus for infection. When the site of extravasation can be localized with certainty to one kidney, decompression of that kidney alone will suffice. However, in many cases, bilateral decompression is necessary because of failure to localize the leak.

Following stabilization of the infant's general condition, sooner or later one comes to the treatment of the underlying lesion itself. In the majority of neonates with urinary ascites the obstruction is caused by posterior urethral valves, for which numerous methods of treatment have been described.

OPEN SURGICAL PROCEDURES. 1. Excision of the valves through an incision in the prostatic urethra, which is approached retropubically. 2. Disruption of the valves by a sound, which is passed downward from the bladder. 3. Fulguration of the valves through an otoscope introduced through a perineal urethrostomy.

These open methods have been accompanied by considerable blood loss and a high incidence of postoperative incontinence.

ENDOSCOPIC PROCEDURES. Endoscopic resection, incision, or fulguration of the valves is now the treatment of choice. The determining factor in the method used is the caliber of the urethra. Careful calibration using Otis bougies is the first step. If the urethra is of adequate diameter, the infant resectoscope may be used to incise or excise the valves. If the urethra is not of adequate caliber, the resectoscope may be passed through a perineal urethrostomy. An infant urethroscope and electrode may be used to fulgurate the valves in place of a resectoscope. After operation, an indwelling catheter is left in place for 48 hours. Prophylactic antibiotics should be administered before operation and continued until after removal of the catheter.

FLUOROSCOPIC FULGURATION. A nonendoscopic method of fulguration of the valves has been described in which an insulated hooked electrode is passed under fluoroscopic control and made to engage the valves. They are then destroyed by short bursts of current. Again, an indwelling catheter is left in place for 48 hours.

NONOPERATIVE TREATMENT. Treatment of urethral valves by leaving a Foley catheter indwelling for 4 weeks in the hope of eroding the valves is mentioned here only to condemn it because of the likelihood of post-treatment stricture formation.

Less common causes of urinary ascites and their treatment are outlined below:

1. A single orthotopic ureterocele was the obstructive lesion in one reported case. Optimum treatment would appear to consist of upper tract diversion by nephrostomy. Subsequent transurethral resection of the ureterocele may allow delay of the ureteroneocystostomy, which is always necessary in the management of the large orthotopic ureterocele.

2. Ureteral stenosis at the ureterovesical junction has been treated by excision of the narrowed segment and ureteroneocystostomy.

3. The only recorded case of ascites due to urethral atresia was in a stillborn infant.

4. Rupture of a neurogenic bladder with urinary ascites has been reported. The preferred treatment, after closure of the perforation has been demonstrated by cystogram, is intermittent catheterization. The medical literature contains reports of four cases of urinary ascites in which urinary obstruction did not occur. The patients have required no further treatment.

Chylous Ascites. Most cases of chylous ascites subside on conservative management. Following paracentesis, the infant should be given a diuretic. In all probability, reaccumulation of ascitic fluid will occur, necessitating repeated paracentesis. The infant should be placed on a fat-free high-protein diet—the fat being replaced by medium- and short-chain fatty acids, which are absorbed directly from the intestine into the portal circulation.

The repeated paracentesis necessary in this condition can result in hypoproteinemia and malnutrition. Intravenous reinfusion of the unaltered ascitic fluid has been practiced, but, while this is a safe procedure, its benefits have not been universally accepted. When malnutrition occurs, intravenous hyperalimentation is indicated.

A small minority of infants require surgical intervention because of persistent ascites despite dietary modification. It seems worthwhile to attempt intraoperative identification of a leaking lacteal by administration of lipophilic dye preoperatively. Sudan black, 25 grams in 200 ml of cream may be administered orally 8 hours preoperatively. Ligation of such a leaking lacteal has been successful. Chylous cysts have also been excised successfully at laparotomy. Other conditions that have been identified as causing chylous ascites include mesenteric lymphadenitis, intestinal obstruction, and mesenteric compression by umbilical vein remnants.

A high incidence of abnormal electroencephalographic findings in children who had chylous ascites at birth is found.

Ascites Due to Ruptured Ovarian Cyst. Ruptured ovarian cyst is a rare cause of neonatal ascites. The identification of bloodstained fluid at paracentesis requires immediate laparotomy to exclude trauma to an intraabdominal viscus. Of the six cases reported in the literature, two were diagnosed only at autopsy. The other four were cured by laparotomy and resection of the cyst. It should be stressed that such follicular ovarian cysts are often bilateral, consequently as much ovarian tissue as possible should be conserved during removal of the cyst.

Paroxysmal Supraventricular Tachycardia (PSVT). Digitalis is the accepted mode of therapy for PSVT and usually abolishes the arrhythmia in 6 to 12 hours. Vagal stimulation by unilateral eyeball or carotid pressure rarely works and should be avoided in the sick infant. The total digitalizing dose for a premature infant is 0.04 mg/kg, and for a full-term infant is 0.05 mg/kg. Half the digitalizing dose is given initally, and the remainder is divided in two doses and given 4 and 12 hours, respectively, after the first. The daily maintenance dose is 0.01 mg/kg. Digitalization must be carried out under electrocardiographic monitoring.

Digitalization causes a very significant diuresis in these infants. This may result in a sudden reduction in the infant's weight, necessitating a reduction in the digoxin dose in order to avoid digitalis toxicity. The maintenance dose should be adjusted daily until the weight is stable. Serum levels should be kept below 3.0 ng/ml. Signs of digitalis toxicity include severe slowing of the sinus rate, ventricular ectopic beats, and supraventricular tachycardia with AV nodal block. Digitalis toxicity usually responds to withdrawal of digoxin and correction of potassium deficiency, if it exists. If digoxin fails to control the PSVT, propranolol, 0.01 mg/kg intravenously over 5-10 minutes repeated at 6-hour intervals, should be substituted until the arrhythmia has stopped, the weight is stable, and the edema has cleared. Recurrence of PSVT can be most simply prevented by using digitalis therapy for 6 to 12 months after the arrhythmia has cleared.

Ascites Due to Neonatal Liver Disease. Acites occurs in neonatal liver disorders such as congenital bile duct atresia, giant cell hepatitis, and neonatal cirrhosis. However, in most cases the ascites develops slowly and represents only a minor complication of a very complex underlying problem. It rarely demands the same urgency in treatment as indicated in the other forms of ascites discussed here. In the case of bile duct atresia, early operation to bypass the site of obstruction offers the only hope of successful treatment. In the past, laparotomy was delayed in these infants because of the ill effects on infants who turned out not to have atresia. However, improved anesthesia as well as better postoperative care has reduced the risk to the infants with hepatitis. When bypass of the atresia is not possible, and in those infants with giant cell hepatitis or cirrhosis, general supportive measures should be employed.

Gross ascites was present at birth in only one reported neonate with giant cell hepatitis. This infant responded to exchange transfusion, repeated paracentesis, and administration of albumin, diuretics, vitamins, and iron.

Toxoplasmosis. Toxoplasmosis has been reported as the cause of four cases of ascites. Three infants were stillborn and the fourth survived only 1.5 days. Although treatment will not reverse existing tissue damage, it may prevent further progress of the disease. Pyrimethamine, 2 mg/kg, is given daily for 3 days as a loading dose and 1 mg/kg daily thereafter for a total course of 4 weeks.* Sulfadiazine, 100 mg/kg/24 hr, is administered concurrently with the pyrimethamine. Red blood cell, leukocyte, and platelet counts should be performed twice weekly and the pyrimethamine discontinued if there is any significant decrease. Administration of folinic acid during the course of treatment provides protection against myelosuppression. Spiramycin (an investigational drug) (2 to 3 gm/24 hr for 3 weeks) is an alternative though less effective form of therapy.

Iatrogenic Ascites. Iatrogenic ascites in association with retroperitoneal extravasation and hydrothorax has been reported in neonates undergoing intravenous hyperalimentation. Such extravasations have been shown to clear spontaneously following discontinuation of hyperalimentation.

Infants of Drug-Dependent Mothers

ROSITA S. PILDES, M.D.,
and GOPAL SRINIVASAN, M.D.

Drug withdrawal is the final insult to the neonate who has been exposed in utero to pharmacologic agents that may adversely affect total development as well as development of individual organ systems. Treatment, therefore, should be instituted as early in pregnancy as possible.

INTRAPARTUM CARE

A detailed history of drug intake must be taken on all pregnant women at the time of admission, keeping in mind that not all neonatal withdrawal syndromes are due to narcotics and not all women taking drugs are drug dependent. This information must then be relayed to the pediatrician to facilitate therapeutic intervention in the neonate without excessive investigation because of inadequate information. Drugs that have been reported to cause neonatal withdrawal symptoms are listed in Table 1.

The intrapartum period is the most inopportune time for withdrawal of drugs from the mother, who is already undergoing the additional stress from labor and delivery. Methadone and meperidine are commonly used to prevent intrapartum withdrawal. Excessive fetal movements and increased oxygen requirements secondary to withdrawal may cause fetal distress; fetal monitoring is therefore essential and a physician well versed in resuscitation should be present in the delivery room. Respiratory depression at birth may result from excessive use of drugs prior to delivery but can usually be overcome by prompt attention to the airway. Naloxone (Narcan) is not recommended, because the drug may precipitate acute withdrawal symptoms, including seizures.

Most drug-dependent mothers do not take a single drug, and the presence of other drugs may alter or potentiate the withdrawal response of the infant. A very careful history of additional drugs must be

Table 1. **DRUGS ASSOCIATED WITH NEONATAL WITHDRAWAL SYNDROME**

Narcotics
  Heroin
  Methadone
  Codeine
Barbiturates
Analgesics
  Pentazocine (Talwin)
  Propoxyphene hydrochloride (Darvon)
Tranquilizers and Sedatives
  Bromides
  Chlordiazepoxide (Librium)
  Desipramine hydrochloride (Pertofrane)
  Diazepam (Valium)
  Ethchlorvynol (Placidyl)
  Glutethimide (Doriden)
  Hydroxyzine hydrochloride (Atarax)
Combination of Drugs
  Ts and blues (Talwin and Pyribenzamine)
Alcohol
Sympathomimetics
  Amphetamines
Phencyclidine (PCP)

---

*This dose may exceed that recommended by the manufacturer.

obtained, and a toxicology screening of cord blood and urine collected during the first day of postnatal life should be performed.

NEONATAL CARE

Treatment in the neonatal period is directed not only at therapy of the withdrawal syndrome but also at problems secondary to prematurity and intrauterine growth retardation. Supportive therapy includes correction of hypoxemia, hypoglycemia, and polycythemia and provision of adequate fluid calories. Respiratory alkalosis secondary to tachypnea rarely requires therapy. The increased incidence of syphilis, gonorrhea, and hepatitis in drug-dependent mothers must be kept in mind and the infant checked accordingly.

Therapeutic intervention is not always necessary since symptoms, when present, are often self-limited. A quiet, comforting environment with gentle handling, swaddling, and frequent feedings may be sufficient. Therapy is indicated when the symptoms interfere with adequate weight gain and well-being. These include 1) vomiting or diarrhea, 2) marked irritability and tremors that interfere with sleep or feeding, and 3) seizures.

Therapeutic regimens vary considerably among centers, and a number of scoring systems have been developed in an attempt to standardize evaluation of symptoms and treatment responses. Most of the pharmacologic agents used have been successful in controlling the acute withdrawal syndrome. Although narcotic withdrawal symptoms are relieved most specifically by the use of a narcotic, most pediatricians are reluctant to use a narcotic for fear of promoting drug dependence in the infant.

The various pharmacologic agents that have been used for therapy of drug withdrawal are outlined in Table 2. The choice of drugs is arbitrary; we prefer phenobarbital or chlorpromazine, but paregoric is often used in infants with diarrhea. In general, the drug is titrated starting with the smallest recommended dose until the desired effect is achieved. Once the infant is asymptomatic for 2 to 3 days, the drug is tapered until it is completely discontinued. Infants whose symptoms are controlled for only short periods of time may need more frequent administration. Tapering should be started by first gradually lowering the dose and then increasing the length of time between administrations. The tapering process may proceed every 48 hours as long as withdrawal symptoms do not reappear. Tremors, however, may persist for months.

Phenobarbital has been used extensively since 1947 and appears to provide adequate control of symptoms. Suppression of withdrawal signs is accomplished by a generalized, nonspecific central nervous system depression. Side effects include excessive sedation, which may lead to inadequate fluid and caloric intake. Diarrhea may remain uncontrolled. The duration of phenobarbital therapy ranges from 4 to 14 days in our nursery. The potential for withdrawal symptoms from phenobarbital therapy must be kept in mind; usually, infants requiring treatment for 2 weeks or less have not shown signs of barbiturate dependence.

Chlorpromazine was introduced in 1959 and is effective in controlling symptoms within hours after it has been initiated. The drug may be given orally or intramuscularly if vomiting or diarrhea is present. Side effects include extrapyramidal signs in infants who have received more than 2.8 mg/kg/24 hr. In our nursery, the mean duration of therapy with chlorpromazine has been 9 days, with a range of 3 to 17 days.

Paregoric (camphorated tincture of opium) has been used since the nineteenth century. Paregoric appears to control symptoms, with restoration of normal central nervous system function as measured by sucking behavior, whereas central nervous system depression may be observed with phenobarbital or diazepam therapy. The usual dose of paregoric is 0.05 to 0.1 ml/kg every 4 hours before feeding. If at the end of the 4-hour period symptoms have not decreased, the dose may be increased. Once the symptoms are controlled for at least 48 hours, tapering may begin. One of the drawbacks in the use of paregoric is the prolonged period often required for the tapering process (20 to 45 days). In addition, paregoric contains camphor, a known central nervous system stimulant. Camphor is absorbed rapidly and excreted slowly in the urine because it is lipid soluble and requires glucuronide conjugation. For this reason, tincture of opium (laudanum) is preferable whenever a narcotic is used. Care must be exercised in using the correct dilution since laudanum comes in a 10 percent solution equivalent to 1% morphine whereas paregoric contains 0.04% morphine. Laudanum must be diluted 25-fold to obtain the same dilution and can then be used similarly to paregoric.

Diazepam is effective in suppressing withdrawal signs but does not appear to offer any advantages over the other drugs. Diazepam is usually given intramuscularly at the onset but may be continued orally. Once symptoms are controlled, the initial dose is cut in half; the time interval between doses is then increased to 12 hours, then the dose is cut

Table 2. DRUGS USED FOR TREATMENT OF NEONATAL WITHDRAWAL SYNDROME

	Dose/KG	Route	Interval Between Doses
Phenobarbital	1–2 mg	IM or PO	q 6 hr
Chlorpromazine	0.5–0.7 mg	IM or PO	q 6 hr
Paregoric	0.05–0.1 ml	PO	q 4–6 hr
Diazepam	0.3–0.5 mg	IM or PO	q 8 hr

in half again. The drug is usually administered for only a few days since it is poorly metabolized and excreted and has a prolonged half-life. Moreover, the parenteral preparation contains sodium benzoate, which competes with bilirubin for albumin-binding sites.

Methadone has been introduced more recently because of its wide use in therapy of heroin addiction in adults. Theoretically, methadone is the drug of choice in infants of methadone dependent mothers.* However, methadone is not easily available, the dose is not standardized, and there is greater difficulty in weaning the infant. Moreover, withdrawal symptoms from methadone respond to the same drugs used for heroin withdrawal.

The variety in therapeutic approaches indicates that the optimal regimen has yet to be demonstrated. Further studies based on clinical as well as biochemical observations are necessary to compare the effects of the various drugs. Unfortunately, long-term effects are difficult to obtain since followup of infants of addict mothers is fraught with numerous problems.

Management of the neonate also requires sensitivity toward the needs of the mother. Support, encouragement, and teaching are necessary to improve the mother's self-esteem. The infant should not be transferred to the high-risk nursery except when therapeutic intervention is necessary. Since the mother will frequently be discharged prior to the infant, these hours of early contact may be the most important in promoting maternal-infant bonding and possibly preventing the high incidence of child abuse.

Breastfeeding by drug-addicted mothers should be undertaken cautiously, with careful monitoring of the infant. The advantage of promoting maternal-infant bonding must be weighed against the potential risk to the neonate. For example, methadone is excreted in breast milk; yet, breastfeeding should be encouraged in mothers enrolled in methadone programs and the dose of methadone cut down to minimum levels. Drugs such as heroin have been known for years to be excreted in breast milk and at one time withdrawal symptoms were treated by breastfeeding with gradual weaning. Almost all analgesics (codeine, Demerol, Darvon, Talwin, Valium, barbiturates) appear in breast milk in low levels but may accumulate in the neonate. Individual variation on drug excretion will determine whether the neonate will be sleepy, hypotonic, or depressed or have poor sucking. Thus, breastfeeding recommendations must be individualized and should be based on the risk to benefit ratio to the infant.

*The use of methadone in infants is not listed by the manufacturer.

POSTNEONATAL CARE

Exacerbation or recurrence of withdrawal symptoms may be present for 3 to 6 months after birth and include restlessness, agitation, tremors, and brief periods of sleep. Medication should be avoided if at all possible. Additional problems that arise after discharge are thrombocytosis and an increased incidence of the sudden infant death syndrome (SIDS).

DISCHARGE PLANNING

The social service department should be involved with the family, and the infant can be discharged to the mother if there are adequate support systems in the home. Many addicted mothers appear anxious to keep their babies but do not have a realistic view of their own ability to care for the infant. Good prognostic signs include a stable marital relationship, successful raising of other children, addiction to a single drug, enrollment in a drug program, and a short duration of the addiction. The caretakers should be aware of the expected behavior of the infant, such as increased sensitivity to auditory stimuli, decreased visual orientation, excessive crying, and increased sucking needs. The infants often respond to a soft soothing voice, gentle rocking, holding, and use of a pacifier. Followup visits by a visiting nurse, social worker, or ex-addict counselor may be helpful. A great deal of time and energy is invested in each case to insure supervision of the child's care, but, despite all efforts, approximately 15 to 20% of the infants require placement in foster homes.

LONG-TERM PROGNOSIS

Early withdrawal symptoms of irritability, hyperactivity, sleep and feeding problems, and hypertonicity may persist for several months.

Longitudinal studies are scarce because a large percentage of the patients are lost to followup. In one study, behavioral disturbances, brief attention span, and temper tantrums were identified in 7 of 14 infants of heroin addict mothers. Growth parameters followed to 1 year of age may be impaired, and a high correlation has been reported between the hyperexcitable state in the neonate and neurologic and behavioral dysfunction at 1.5 to 4 years of age.

Maternal Alcohol Ingestion Effects on the Developing Child

SALLY E. SHAYWITZ, M.D.

Maternal drinking during pregnancy is associated with a broad range of effects on the developing fetus; generally, the more severe outcomes reflecting increased consumption of alcohol by the mother. Thus, the teratogenic effects of ethanol may be reflected by the full blown syndrome referred to as the fetal alcohol syndrome or by less severe outcomes termed fetal alcohol effects. Fetal alcohol syndrome is characterized by pre- and postnatal growth deficiency: facial abnormalities including small palpebral fissures, flat nasal bridge with anteverted nostrils, hypoplastic philtrum and thin upper vermilion border, and central nervous system dysfunction. When the effects are less pronounced and more subtle, for example, central nervous system dysfunction manifest as disturbances of attention and activity regulation rather than mental retardation, the term fetal alcohol effects is utilized. The manifestations of the teratogenicity of alcohol in any child will vary depending on dose, duration, and timing of exposure to alcohol, presence of other risk factors (smoking, age, drug abuse), and metabolic factors unique to the mother and fetus.

With an estimated incidence ranging from 1 to 2 per 500 live births, fetal alcohol syndrome is not a rare disorder and currently is the third most frequent cause of mental retardation (following Down syndrome and spina bifida). The disorder is entirely preventable, although controversy exists concerning precise ceiling or threshold levels of alcohol ingestion during pregnancy. A risk is established with ingestion of the equivalent of 3 ounces of absolute alcohol per day or about 6 drinks a day. In 1977, the National Institutes on Alcohol Abuse and Alcoholism recommended that a pregnant woman not exceed two drinks per day; more recently, in July 1981, the Surgeon General's Advisory on Alcohol and Pregnancy advised "women who are pregnant or considering pregnancy not to drink alcoholic beverages ...".

Although the effects of alcohol on embryogenesis are irreversible, steps may be taken to mitigate their consequences. The first step in treatment must be recognition and diagnosis. Recognition requires awareness of the clinical presentation and willingness of the pediatrician and other health professionals to seriously inquire about the mother's drinking habits during pregnancy. Worldwide investigations have now shown that no social class or ethnic or professional group is immune to alcohol abuse. Inquiry about drinking habits should be incorporated into the routine questions asked mothers at office visits. These women may be nursing or pregnant. Conversely, knowledge of increased maternal alcohol ingestion may offer an explanation of developmental or other difficulties the child is experiencing or prompt closer scrutiny of the child for possible fetal alcohol effects.

The untoward effects of ethanol may affect the child throughout development; infants born to alcoholic mothers present the pediatrician with a unique set of potential management difficulties.

Unless, as is true on rare occasions, the gravid woman presents with alcohol on her breath or is a known alcoholic, diagnosis may be difficult in the neonatal period. The neonate with severe fetal alcohol syndrome manifested by microcephaly and growth retardation is predisposed to a variety of problems, including asphyxia, hypoglycemia, hypothermia, polycythemia, and feeding difficulties that respond to the usual supportive therapies including provision of adequate calories, fluid, and electrolytes and correction of metabolic aberrations. The neonate is also susceptible to an alcohol withdrawal syndrome which, if it occurs, presents within the first 24 hours of life. Onset of symptoms of jitteriness and unusual cry in a child with features of fetal alcohol syndrome warrant suspicion of incipient alcohol withdrawal, and are an indication for careful monitoring, a process facilitated by using score sheets adapted from those used to monitor other neonatal withdrawal syndromes. Symptoms, including high pitched or continuous cry, tremors, jitteriness, increased tone, loose stools, regurgitation, sweating, and irritability, are similar to those observed in narcotic withdrawal syndrome; seizures and opisthotonic posturing are more constant findings in alcohol withdrawal. Nevertheless, the presentation is typically mild, and it is unusual for the symptoms to require treatment.

The decision to begin therapy is arbitrary and usually reflects signs of increasing jitteriness or onset of seizures. The drug of choice is phenobarbital, usually administered as a loading dose of 10 mg/kg intravenously and then at 5 mg/kg/day to maintain phenobarbital blood levels at 20 to 30 μg/dl. In the rare event that seizures continue, phenytoin should be added at an intravenous loading dose of 15 mg/kg and a daily maintenance dose of 5 to 7 mg/kg, calculated to maintain blood levels at a range between 10 and 20 μg/dl. Pharmacotherapy is continued for a 4 to 6 week period. Current trends of multidrug abuse may further complicate management; thus, alcohol may intensify the central nervous system depressant effects of narcotic analgesics and potentiate the hypotensive effects of benzodiazepines.

Clearly, while initial therapeutic decisions are concerned with stabilizing the infant and management of acute symptoms as they arise; these problems will respond to medical management and the pediatrician will be concerned with evolving a long-term management protocol that will reflect psychosocial as well as biomedical concerns. The treatment of the child with fetal alcohol syndrome is that of a child with a complex, chronic handicapping condition in which not only the child but his mother and the entire family are also in need of intervention, treatment, and ongoing supportive services. The mother's ability to function as the primary caregiver may be jeopardized by multiple factors including physical debility secondary to chronic alcoholism, incapacity reflecting continuing alcohol abuse, and her own complex reactions to a damaged child and to the knowledge of her own role in the etiology of the child's difficulties. The mother's coping abilities are undermined not only by maternal factors but also by the infant's own characteristics. A propensity to feeding difficulties and sleep disturbances and to exhibit poor habituation predict that the infant will be difficult to care for and will make more than the usual demands on the mother. Birth of an impaired baby may place further stress and lead to increasing deterioration or complete disintegration of an already tenuous marital situation. The child may have to be placed with relatives or foster parents until the mother is able to provide care. Placing the affected infant with an optimal surrogate does not appear to significantly improve the ultimate outcome, as reflected by cognitive and behavioral functioning.

The initial stage of the long-term management plan must be directed at the mother-infant dyad and facilitation of the bonding process. A critical first step in allowing the mother to acknowledge her problem, while at the same time developing confidence in her maternal abilities, is to share the diagnosis and its implications with her. This process must be handled with great sensitivity so that the mother is not so overwhelmed by feelings of guilt that she either rejects or is unrealistically solicitous toward the infant. When we inform the mother of the possible etiologic role played by alcohol, we also emphasize the complexity of the genesis of the child's problems, indicating that there are usually multiple determinants for many of the problems that the child is experiencing. Thus, the mother is not burdened with sole responsibility for every adversity that befalls her child. The prognosis must be realistically presented, indicating that the infant may be difficult to care for and that, as the child develops, the demands placed on the parents will likely be greater than usual.

Awareness of the diagnosis and its implications at this early stage will foster realistic planning and may strongly motivate the mother to seek and accept help. The mother's knowledge of the detrimental effects of alcohol during pregnancy should also help prevent recurrences. She should also be made aware that the alcohol is present in breast milk and that nursing is contraindicated if she is drinking at all. Discussions should not be restricted to the difficulties and problems the child will encounter; the more salutary aspects of the syndrome and the therapeutic possibilities should be stressed as well. The complex problems faced by both child and family can best be addressed by a team of health professionals, including in addition to the pediatrician, a social worker, a nurse, and a developmentalist. Optimally, the members of the team meet the new mother while the infant is still in the nursery and make her aware of the availability of their services for the infant, the family, and herself.

Newborns exposed to alcohol in utero may appear normal at birth or exhibit only a few subtle indications of such exposure; however, it should not be inferred that problems reflecting alcohol teratogenicity will not develop later in such children. The effects of alcohol abuse during pregnancy may not become apparent for months or even years. Children with milder facial and growth abnormalities and normal intelligence may not present difficulties until the time of school entry (see below), emphasizing the importance of long-term follow-up for all children whose mothers drank during pregnancy.

Discharge plans must consider the special needs of the infant, the mother, and the mother-infant dyad. The infant should be followed closely, with special attention to growth and nutrition. Infants who have received oral feedings through the use of nasogastric tubes are prone to delays in oral feeding development and may require nutritional supplementation by nasogastric tube until age 18 months. Techniques establishing the association between oral feeding and satisfaction of hunger, together with frequent removal of nasogastric tubes prior to oral feeding, facilitate more normal feeding patterns. Home visits are beneficial in assessing the specific needs of the infant and his family and in providing specific, concrete suggestions for child care. Constant reassurance that the baby's feeding and state difficulties do not reflect poor mothering, together with guidance to enhance parenting skills, will foster bonding and diminish the possibility of rejection or child neglect and child abuse. The pediatrician should become aware of alcohol treatment resources including alcohol counselors, individual and family therapists, alcohol rehabilitation centers, and family service agencies in the community. The pediatrician plays a pivotal role as intercessor between the mother and the agency working with her. By encouraging her to utilize these services initially and inquiring about her own status on a continuing basis, the pediatrician will enhance the mother's (and family's) willingness to accept professional help and to continue to participate in a treatment program.

There exists an ever-increasing list of abnormalities that are thought to reflect the teratogenic effects of alcohol. Generally, they may be classified into central nervous system effects producing developmental disturbances affecting behavior, learning, and intelligence and malformations of other organ systems producing a range of aberrations with minor congenital anomalies at one extreme and life-threatening neoplasms at the other.

Treatment of the developmental disabilities is enhanced when diagnosis is made early and the

Table 1. ORGAN INVOLVEMENT AND SYNDROMES ASSOCIATED
WITH ALCOHOL TERATOGENICITY

Organ Systems	Disorder	Special Features
CNS	Mental retardation Learning disabilities Psychosis	Mild to moderate attentional problems, hyperactivity, language disability Schizophrenia
Ophthalmologic	Malformation of retinal vessels, hypoplasia, atrophy of optic discs Blepharophimosis Strabismus	Tortuosity of arteries and veins Esotropia
Renal	Renal hypoplasia	Unilateral or bilateral
Endocrine	Adrenal neoplasm	Ganglioneuroblastoma—reported in fetal hydantoin-fetal alcohol syndrome
Hepatic	Hepatoblastoma Extrahepatic biliary atresia	
Cardiac	Ventricular septal defect Secundum atrial defect Tetralogy of Fallot Aortic arch interruption Patent ductus arteriosus	Often associated with hypoplastic pulmonary artery With type A aortopulmonary fenestration
Skeletal	Retarded bone age Abnormal limb development	Bone fusion in the upper limb, clinodac- tyly, camptodactyly, radioulnar synos- tosis, carpal fusion, pseudoepiphysis of metacarpals, hypoplastic toe nails
Muscular	Hernias	Diaphragm, umbilicus, groin, diastasis recti
Immunological	Defects in host defense Propensity to infection	Hypogammaglobulinemia Dysgammaglobulinemia Decreased E-rosette forming lymphocytes Low EAC rosette forming lymphocytes

child referred for appropriate services. In infancy, referral is made to a rehabilitation center or developmental disabilities clinic, where a range of services, including OT, PT, social work, and most importantly support and counseling for the mother are available. Participation in an infant stimulation program allows the mother to feel that she is making an active, positive contribution to her child's treatment and actually provides her with constructive techniques to utilize with the infant. As the child gets older, it is likely that the child will require special education services. The pediatrician can make the mother aware of these services even at the preschool level and can monitor the child's educational program. At times, when the mother is known to be an alcoholic, a child's school difficulties are almost reflexly attributed to a difficult home situation without considering the possibility of a learning problem. The pediatrician must ensure that each child with fetal alcohol effects who is experiencing school problems be given an evaluation for a possible learning disability. Hyperactivity and inattention have frequently been described in fetal alcohol syndrome and may be responsible for the school difficulties experienced by affected children who have normal intelligence. These symptoms respond well to stimulant therapy, as discussed elsewhere in this volume. As the child enters preadolescence or adolescence, participation in an Alateen program allows him to share and work through his own feeling and problems with others who are or have been in similar situations.

A comprehensive, current listing of organ system involvement with particular syndromes reported and associated with fetal alcohol syndrome is provided (Table 1). It is not yet clear how aggressive the pediatrician should be in working up the child with fetal alcohol syndrome for the possibility of any of these problems. In most reports, the incidence of these findings increases with the severity of the fetal alcohol features in a particular child. However, the actual incidence of these associated findings is not known, some having been described in only a very few patients with fetal alcohol syndrome. At this time, it appears most prudent to closely follow those affected patients who are having the more severe involvement, and to be increasingly vigilant for the development of symptoms relating to these problems. At the earliest suspicion, further evaluation specific to the symptomatology is initiated. Awareness of the wide range of possible abnormalities associated with alcohol abuse during pregnancy emphasizes the need for thorough physical examinations both in response to symptoms and as part of a routine well child examination.

Preparation of the Neonate for Transfer

JEFFREY B. GOULD, M.D. M.P.H.

Successful infant *transport* is dependent upon 1) anticipating the need for transport before the infant critically deteriorates, 2) stabilizing the infant to minimize stress and hypoxemia, and 3) preparing the parents.

When to Transport

The decision to transfer an infant to a more specialized facility is ideally made when the patient's diagnostic and therapeutic requirements are expected to exceed those available in the hospital of birth. The key to success is to initiate transfer before the patient's condition seriously deteriorates, thus avoiding many possible complications and greatly improving the outcome. Lists of conditions "requiring transport" usually include such categories as very low birth weight (<1500 gm), severe asphyxia, respiratory distress, sepsis/meningitis, metabolic abnormality, multiple congenital anomalies, and surgical emergencies. As hospitals become more experienced members of perinatal transport networks, there has been local refinement of these lists by multidisciplinary newborn committees consisting of physicians, nurses, and administrative and technical staff. This local refinement based on an assessment of the local facilities, medical, nursing, and support capabilities; past experience caring for "transport infants"; and past experience with the time and difficulties of transports serves to fine tune the transport decision. It is often difficult to decide if an infant really needs transport or should be observed for "a few more hours." When in doubt, a call to the senior transport physician on call will be useful.

The Initial Transport Call

The initial transport call sets into motion a course of collaborative care that begins in the local hospital (stabilization phase), continues in the tertiary care center (intensive care phase), and often terminates with transport of the infant back to the local hospital (growth and preparation for discharge to home phase). This initial call must contain information that will identify the patient's immediate and projected needs. Such factors as perinatal history, condition at birth, subsequent course, and current status are critical, as they allow the transport consultant to evaluate the working diagnosis, assess the ongoing treatment, and suggest steps to further stabilize the infant. The initial call also helps the team set their operational priorities; establish the composition of the transport team (need for respiratory therapist, senior neonatologist, etc.); assess the need for special or extra equipment (e.g., extra heat devices for a very small premature, extra supplies of saline for a large gastroschisis), and in some cases recommend the tertiary care facility that can best meet the infant's specific needs.

Another important aspect is the determination not to transport an infant. Such decisions are usually reserved for moribund infants whose likelihood for survival would not be improved by transport to a more specialized facility. It is often helpful to make this decision in consultation with the "transport neonatologist."

Stabilization Prior to Transport

Regardless of the illness, the more stable the infant at the time of transport, the greater is the likelihood of a favorable outcome. The stabilized infant has 1) a normal temperature (37°C rectal, 36.3°–36.5°C skin); 2) an arterial oxygen level that is neither brain damaging (<40 mm Hg) or eye damaging (>80 mm Hg); 3) a pH that is not severely acidotic (<7.3); 4) a hematocrit and blood volume that provide for good tissue perfusion; 5) fluid status that avoids dehydration and water intoxication; and 6) no metabolic derangement such as hypoglycemia or hypocalcemia.

Temperature. Infants who are hypothermic have increased oxygen consumption, a tendency toward acidosis and hypoglycemia, and tolerate stress poorly. One of the most important aspects of stabilization is to keep the patient from getting hypothermic. The typical transport infant is a premature who has required extensive resuscitation in the delivery room. These infants are usually cold when they reach the nursery. While their physiologic needs are being attended to (e.g., intubation, starting IV, placing catheters) their temperature and chances for intact survival will continue to fall unless special equipment (such as radiant warmers) is used and special precautions taken. Even though a small premature is on a radiant heat bed, a prolonged period under sterile drapes while a catheter is being placed can lead to a serious drop in temperature. Also, an infant will rapidly cool when removed from a warm incubator for emergency intubation. An adequate number of devices to supply heat to exposed infants is a sound investment for even the smallest nursery. A hypothermic infant's temperature should be checked every 15 minutes until normal.

Oxygenation. Central cyanosis, and an oxygen level below 50 to 60 mm of Hg should be treated by increasing the percent oxygen. The persistence of poor color, low oxygen levels, and high levels of CO_2 (>60 mm Hg) suggests that ventilation is inadequate, especially when the cardiac rate falls to less than 100. The patient should be treated with artificial ventilation by bag and mask or bag and endotracheal tube. The adequacy of ventilation and the specific treatment of a persistently low heart rate may be treated using the guidelines for neonatal resuscitation (see section on Resuscitation).

Acidosis. The Ph may be determined from a warmed heel stick or even a venous sample. When the pH is <7.3, acidosis should be treated. If the CO_2 is >50, this respiratory acidosis should be treated by increasing the depth (watch the chest for adequate movement) or rate of ventilation. If the base deficit is greater than 10, correct this metabolic acidosis by giving a slow infusion of sodium bicarbonate (as described in section on Resuscitation).

Hypovolemic Shock. Shock due to low blood volume may present as pallor, cool skin, poor capillary filling, poor urine output, and persistence of low oxygen and a metabolic acidosis. This should be treated with whole blood or blood products as described in section on Resuscitation.

Dehydration. The signs of dehydration are similar to those of hypovolemic shock. While the hematocrit is usually low in hypovolemia, it is often high in dehydration. Treatment involves expansion of the blood volume with 10 ml/kg of fresh frozen plasma or 5% albumin followed by the infusion of D-5-W.

Metabolic Considerations. The blood sugar should be followed with Dextrostix. Hypoglycemia may be treated with 2 to 4 ml/kg of D-25-W IV stat followed by an infusion of D-10-W. Be sure to continue following Dextrostix.

In addition to the major steps to stabilize infants, some acute processes will require medical intervention prior to the arrival of the transport team. Suspected sepsis as evidenced by hypo- or hyperthermia, lethargy or irritability, vomiting, unexplained deterioration, or pneumonia, especially in an infant born to a mother with prolonged rupture of membranes or a temperature must be immediately treated using standard guidelines. A gastric aspirate for smear and culture, blood culture, L.P., suprapubic tap, one surface culture, and a culture of the placenta should be obtained. In many instances these specimens are sent with the infant to the tertiary center.

Seizures will also require immediate treatment following standard guidelines.

A pneumothorax is often diagnosed following sudden and unexplained pulmonary deterioration. This must be immediately aspirated if symptomatic. However, one need not use a chest tube as the introduction of "INTRACATH" type needle at the anterior axillary line at the level of the nipple will often suffice as a temporary measure. The needle should be attached to a syringe or vacuum and water trap set up for continuous evacuation.

Intestinal obstruction at esophageal, duodenal, or lower levels should always be treated with an indwelling catheter attached to an intermittent suction device. Intermittent suctioning by staff using a syringe is usually not very effective and poses a serious risk of aspiration.

Certain surgical conditions also require immediate therapy. Myelomeningocele, gastroschisis, and omphaloceles should be kept moist and clean by covering with moist, warm saline packs. The infant must be positioned to take the stress off the mass, and evaporative heat loss must be avoided.

There are two common pitfalls to be avoided in caring for a critically ill infant prior to transport: 1) not giving standard neonatal care such as eye prophylaxis, vitamin K, or identification prints and 2) not recording the time and quantity of all medications and fluids given the infant and all urine and stool output.

While it is impossible to discuss all the problems and their immediate treatments here, this is precisely the goal of the initial transport call—to assess the patient's needs and to develop therapies to be followed prior to the arrival of the transport team.

Preparation of Parents

To most parents transport of their infant is devastating. The period of maternal-infant separation increases their anxiety and despair. It is helpful to explain to both parents the reason for transport and the greatly improved outlook for the majority of transported infants. Prior to transport, the transport physician should also speak with the parents. The father or another central family member should be encouraged to visit the infant as soon after admission as possible. Firsthand experience with the neonatal intensive care unit (NICU) and its staff can then be carried back and serve as a source of support to the mother. The NICU should contact the referring hospital several hours after admission so that a report of the infant's current status and prognosis can be relayed to the mother.

Although a great deal of time may have been spent with the mother or parents prior to transport, during this initial shock period it is unlikely that many of the details will be remembered. It is helpful to meet with the mother or parents 12 hours after transport. I have found the question, "Things were pretty hectic after the birth of your baby. I wonder if you could tell me what you understand about his/her condition and its treatment?" to be extremely useful.

Final Preparation for Transport

Prior to the arrival of the transport team one should collect copies of the mother's and infant's charts, 10 ml of clotted maternal blood, 10 ml of clotted cord blood, copies of x-rays and EKG's, culture specimens, and the placenta. With the arrival of the transport team, the status of the patient's stabilization will be re-evaluated, as will the need to institute further therapy prior to transport. Attempts will be made to ensure optimal stabilization and decisions will be made as to whether the infant should have a more stable peripheral IV, an umbilical artery catheter, or perhaps intubation for marginal respiratory status, if these were not already required during the period of pretransport stabilization; as a last step the team will contact the tertiary center for a final consultation. The patient's course, needs, and expected time of arrival will be discussed. At this point it is important that the route from nursery to ambulance be cleared by holding elevators, clearing corridors, and positioning the vehicle.

Breastfeeding

LEWIS A. BARNESS, M.D.

Breastfeeding is recognized as the preferred feeding for term infants. Breast milk provides essential nutrients as well as immunologic benefits for the infant, and may be less allergenic than cow's milk formulas.

Preparation

The decision to nurse is usually, and should be, made before delivery. The physician should meet with the mother and father several months before delivery, not only to support the decision to nurse but also to advise on the preparation for nursing. The advantages of nursing should be explained to the couple. These include immunologic factors, easy digestibility, possible prevention of allergies, convenience, and possible psychologic advantages. When these are enumerated, many elect to breastfeed.

The breasts should be examined for protractibility of the nipples. Inverted nipples can be improved either by drawing the thumbs away from the nipple (Hoffman technique) or by wearing a milk cup with the bra. Breast tissue should be palpated for tumors or cysts. Texture should be estimated in the third trimester by picking up the superficial tissue. If the tissue is not elastic, massage should be recommended. Massage of the breasts for several minutes three or four times per day is performed after the hands are lubricated. The hands are placed well above the breasts. Pressure is exerted with the thumbs across the top and fingers underneath, until the breasts are slightly flushed. Massage may prevent engorgement or nipple soreness. Soap, alcohol, or other drying agents should not be used on the nipple. A comfortable, supportive nursing bra without a plastic liner prevents distortion of the shape of the breast and will not macerate the nipple.

First Feedings

The baby should be put to the breast as soon as the mother is sufficiently awake after delivery. Nursing at frequent intervals for 5- or 10-minute periods helps prevent soreness of the nipples and breast engorgement. The baby may first lick the breast before learning to latch-on and suck. The mother may not experience a let-down reflex in the breast related to oxytoxin release for the first feedings. The let-down is felt as a "pins and needles" sensation and may be produced by sucking or by other stimuli such as the baby's cry or touch or by intercourse.

The baby may not be able to grasp the nipple easily because the breast is distended. Breast massage may release the milk sufficiently to allow nursing. The mother should be comfortable, with the baby's whole body rotated toward her, and the baby's and mother's eyes should face each other. The mother guides the nipple to the baby's cheek and mouth to stimulate rooting. At the end of the nursing if the baby is still sucking, suction should be broken before the baby is removed from the breast; this is done by inserting the mother's fifth finger into the corner of the baby's mouth.

Occasional Problems

A phone call from the physician several days after discharge from the hospital obviates many subsequent problems and questions.

Failure to Thrive. The mother and baby should be examined at about 2 weeks. The baby should have started to gain. Overconfidence in the omnipotence of breastfeeding may lead to a too casual approach to illness in the infant. Failure to gain usually is due to insufficient intake and may be associated with hypo- or hyperelectrolytemia, hypoglycemia, or debility. A trial period of 2 or 3 days or more frequent feedings may suffice. If milk production is inadequate, a 2 or 3 day trial of a substance to decrease prolactin inhibition, such as chlorpromazine 10 to 25 mg once daily in the morning, usually increases milk supply. Supplemental feedings should be avoided for this trial period, as bottle feeding requires a different sucking mechanism than nursing and may result in insufficient emptying of the breast. If milk supply remains inadequate, a Lact-aid (Box 6861, Denver CO 80206) may be used to provide the supplement.

Engorgement. Engorgement results from increased vascularity of the breast as well as from accumulation of milk. Manually expressing milk before nursing, as well as more frequent nursing, usually is effective. Warming for 5 to 10 minutes before feeding dilates ductules and encourages let-down and relaxation. Breast massage and a supportive brassiere may make the mother more comfortable.

Sleeping-Crying. The baby may cry frequently when young during the learning period. Frequent nursing for the first 2 weeks usually suffices. If the infant is sleepy during feeding, gently raising the feet toward the head arouses the baby sufficiently to nurse.

Sore, Cracked Nipples. Engorgement is one of the chief causes of sore or cracked nipples. Nipple soreness usually disappears when nursing is established. Feeding more frequently for short periods, manually expressing a little milk before nursing so that the baby does not need to suck as hard, offering the less sore breast first, and using different positions during nursing may relieve the pain. Emollient cream such as lanolin over the sore nipple may be helpful but otherwise the nipple should be kept dry and exposed to air as much as possible. The baby should not be allowed to sleep at the breast.

If monilia infection is present, nystatin cream 3 or 4 times daily over the nipples and nystatin drops in the baby's mouth usually are effective.

Mastitis. Mastitis is a breast infection that usually occurs following engorgement. If not treated, breast abscess may follow. The breast is tender, red, and hot, and staphylococcus, streptococcus, or other organisms may be present. The baby should nurse every 2 to 2½ hours, usually first from the less sore breast. Treatment is as for engorgement, plus antibiotics that are safe for the infant. Antibiotics should continue for 10 days. Increased fluid intake, bed rest, and mild analgesics help. If an abscess forms, nursing is usually not possible until the pain lessens.

Lumps. Breast lumps are common during the nursing period, and usually are caused by clogged ducts. Nursing from the lumpy breast first helps to drain the duct. I recommend moist heat, showers, massage during nursing, and change of position during nursing. The brassiere should be checked for constriction.

Leaking. Leaking may be due to any stimulus of the let-down reflex. This may be stopped by pressing the heel of the hand firmly against the breast. Plastic liners in the brassiere should be avoided if possible.

Breast Milk Jaundice. Breast milk jaundice is due to factors in human milk that cause an increase in unconjugated bilirubin; it is usually first noted at 4 to 5 days and peaks at 2 to 3 weeks. While no adverse effects have been documented, serum bilirubin can be lowered by ceasing nursing for 24 to 72 hours. The baby is given a supplementary formula and the mother is advised to use a breast pump or manually empty the breasts several times daily.

Supplemental Vitamins. The well-nourished mother produces a milk with adequate vitamins. However, supplemental vitamin D should be given to infants exposed to little sunlight. Iron should be added at 6 months. Fluoride should be given to infants who live in areas where the water contains little fluoride.

Drugs. Most drugs can be given in therapeutic doses to the mother without noticeable adverse effects in the infant. The following drugs should not be used by the nursing mother: atropine, meprobamate, ergot, bromides, iodides, antineoplastic agents, and oral antidiabetic agents.

Feeding the Low Birth Weight Infant

WILLIAM C. HEIRD, M.D.

Although there is widespread agreement that improved nutritional management of the low birth weight (LBW) infant may lessen morbidity and may even improve overall survival, the goals of nutritional management remain undefined. Some feel that the growth rate achieved with human milk fed at 180 to 200 ml/kg/24 hr is sufficient. Others, however, feel that the goal should be continuation of the intrauterine growth rate. The fact that human milk contains insufficient amounts of protein, calcium, sodium, and perhaps zinc to allow accumulation of these nutrients at the intrauterine rate, even if absorption of each is complete, prevents consolidation of these two views. Thus, discussions of the nutritional requirements of low birth weight infants are often heated and, to date, have resolved few questions.

In reality, neither goal is achieved very often until after the first 2 to 4 weeks of life. Even then, the intrauterine growth rate is rarely achieved. Moreover, data to support the obviously logical concept that continuation of the intrauterine growth rate during extrauterine life is either necessary or efficacious are lacking. Until such data are available, however, the possibility that failure to maintain the intrauterine growth rate may result in delayed growth and development of maturing organ systems, thus contributing to the handicaps of LBW infants, cannot be discounted. On the other hand, some data suggest that the amount of protein required to assure continuation of the intrauterine growth rate may exceed the low birth weight infant's metabolic tolerance. If so, the resulting metabolic derangements (e.g., acidosis, hyperaminoacidemia) may exert deleterious effects on growth and development of various organ systems that are equal to or even greater than those of a slower growth rate.

Most reported studies comparing the growth rates of infants fed human milk or isocaloric amounts of formulas containing greater amounts of protein and minerals have demonstrated the superiority of the formulas. Thus, the poorer growth rate of infants fed human milk cannot be disputed. Nor can the possibility that the nonnutritional components of human milk (i.e., macrophages, lymphocytes, immunoglobulins, complement factors, factors that either inhibit or stimulate growth of various bacteria) may enhance the infant's defense mechanisms against infection. If so, human milk feeding may be more efficacious with respect to the infant's intact survival than the greater somatic growth achieved with an alternate regimen. However, there is little reason to believe that treated human milk (i.e., frozen or heated), which is commonly used for feeding LBW infants, in fact will exert these alleged benefits. Freezing destroys the cellular elements while heating destroys, or inactivates, both the cellular and protein components. Since untreated milk is likely to be contaminated with various microorganisms, its use cannot be recommended.

The adequacy of the protein content of human milk for low birth weight infants has been questioned since the demonstration, some 40 years ago, that low birth weight infants fed artificial formulas of high protein content had greater weight gains than those fed human milk. However, this study did not address the possibility that all or part of the greater weight gain might be due to water retention secondary to the greater electrolyte and mineral intake of infants fed the high protein formula. Subsequent studies demonstrated that at least part of the weight gain attributed solely to the greater protein intake probably was due to water retention. However, clinical studies designed to differentiate between the effects of protein and mineral intake indicate a direct relationship between either greater weight gains or greater increases in length and protein intake.

Despite better growth, protein intakes greater than 4 gm/kg/24 hr result in both acute and long-term complications. Fever, hyperbilirubinemia, lethargy, and high blood concentrations of urea nitrogen result acutely from protein intakes in the range of 4 to 6 gm/kg/24 hr. Also, low birth weight infants who receive protein intakes of this magnitude have a higher incidence of strabismus and also lower IQ scores at 4 to 8 years of age than those who receive more moderate protein intakes. Acute metabolic problems associated with protein intake

are a function of the quality as well as the quantity of protein intake. Metabolic acidosis and hyperammonemia are more common in infants fed formulas containing unmodified cow milk protein (80% caseins; 20% whey proteins) than in those fed formulas providing an identical quantity of modified ("humanized") cow milk protein (40% caseins; 60% whey proteins). Elevated blood urea nitrogen concentrations and elevated plasma amino acid concentrations are common in both groups of infants.

In addition to lower growth rates, infants fed banked human milk (protein intake, approximately 2 gm/kg/24 hr) have lower plasma albumin concentrations than those fed protein intakes of either 2.25 or 4.5 gm/kg/24 hr. However, they do not exhibit clinical signs of hypoalbuminemia. Since the protein content of milk produced by mothers who deliver prematurely is some 20% higher than that of mothers who deliver at term, low birth weight infants who are fed their own mother's milk (or banked milk of mothers who deliver prematurely), in fact, may grow as well as those who are fed artificial formulas. However, data to substantiate this possibility are lacking.

Recent clinical experience confirms the theoretic predictions that the sodium and calcium content of banked human milk is inadequate for the low birth weight infant. Hyponatremia is a frequently encountered problem in low birth weight infants, particularly in those fed with human milk and formulas of low sodium content. Hypocalcemia, inadequate bone mineralization, and even fractures secondary to inadequate skeletal mineralization also are being reported with greater frequency. Some of the latter problems, of course, might be due to inadequate vitamin D intake or the inability of the low birth weight infant to convert dietary vitamin D to the active form. However, inadequate calcium intake is just as likely a possibility. Some data suggest that the milk of mothers who deliver prematurely also may contain higher concentrations of sodium and calcium than banked human milk. Thus, it is possible that these problems would not occur in low birth weight infants fed their own mother's milk, but clinical studies to support this possibility are lacking.

Theoretic calculations suggest also that the zinc content of human milk is inadequate to allow its accumulation at the intrauterine rate. Despite these calculations, clinical zinc deficiency apparently is an infrequent problem in infants fed solely with human milk. However, the fact that overt clinical signs of zinc deficiency are not common does not rule out the possibility of inadequate zinc stores.

The foregoing discussion illustrates the general lack of concrete information concerning the goals of nutritional management, and therefore, the nutrient requirements of the low birth weight infant.

Table 1. RECOMMENDED NUTRIENT INTAKES
FOR LOW BIRTH WEIGHT INFANTS*

Nutrient	Recommended Intake†
Protein	1.8 gm
Fat	3.3 gm
	(300 mg essential fatty acids)
Carbohydrate	—
Sodium	20 mg
Potassium	80 mg
Calcium	50 mg
Magnesium	6 mg
Phosphorus	25 mg
Chloride	55 mg
Iron	0.15 mg
Zinc	0.5 mg
Copper	60 μg
Manganese	5 μg
Iodine	5 μg
Vitamins:	
Vitamin A	250 IU
Vitamin D	40 IU
Vitamin E	0.7 IU
	(1.0 IU/gm linoleic acid)
Vitamin K	4 μg
Vitamin C	8 mg
Thiamin	40 μg
Riboflavin	60 μg
Niacin	250 μg
Vitamin B_6	35 μg
	(15 μg/gm protein)
Folic acid	4 μg
Pantothenic acid	300 μg
Vitamin B_{12}	0.15 μg
Biotin	1.5 μg
Inositol	4 mg
Choline	7 mg

*Committee on Nutrition, American Academy of Pediatrics.
†Minimum levels of intake recommended per 100 Cal. Recommended caloric intake is 100–150 Cal/kg/24 hr.

The Committee on Nutrition of the American Academy of Pediatrics, however, has made tentative recommendations based on the existing information (Table 1). Until further information is available, these recommendations provide useful guidelines for judging the adequacy of any nutritional regimen. Human milk fed in reasonable volumes (up to 200 ml/kg/24 hr) does not provide the recommended intakes of a number of nutrients, viz., protein, sodium, calcium, and possibly zinc. Some who prefer to provide the potential nonnutritional advantages of human milk routinely provide supplemental sodium and calcium. Another approach is to be aware of the potential inadequacies of human milk and institute adequate monitoring to detect hyponatremia, hypocalcemia, and/or inadequate skeletal mineralization; should any occur, supplementation obviously is indicated.

For most low birth weight infants, the foregoing discussion is largely academic. The infants' underlying illness as well as a number of neurophysiologic deficiencies (i.e., poor or unsustained suck, uncoordinated swallowing mechanism, delayed gastric emptying, and poor intestinal motility) makes delivery of any enteral nutritional regimen within the first several days of life difficult, if not impossible. For these infants, many feel that a nutritional regimen that prevents catabolism and allows some increment in lean body mass is satisfactory. This more realistic goal for the first several days of life can be achieved in sick low birth weight infants with a parenteral regimen that provides 60 Cal/kg/24 hr, an amino acid intake of 2.5 g/kg/24 hr, and necessary electroytes, minerals, and vitamins. A similar regimen delivered enterally, of course, should produce the same results. Whether such a regimen adequately maintains growth and development of various organ systems and vital physiologic mechanisms remains to be demonstrated.

Various methods of delivering nutrients by the intravenous route (total parenteral nutrition) as well as methods of delivering feedings by the gastrointestinal tract (e.g., continuous nosagastric or transpyloric infusions) have been proposed as alternatives to more conventional feeding techniques. While no one method is likely to be ideal for all situations, utilization of a combination of these methods of nutrient delivery, allowing the particular clinical problem(s) of an individual infant to be the basis for selecting the method of delivery, should result in improved nutritional management. In many infants, in fact, utilization of a combination of conventional as well as these less conventional methods of feeding permits delivery of sufficient nutrients to achieve intrauterine growth rates. This practical approach may even permit delivery of the controlled nutritional intakes necessary to conduct the nutritional studies required to provide needed information concerning the nutrient requirements of the low birth weight infant as well as the relative advantages and disadvantages of human milk.

Within reason, every infant should be given a trial at conventional feeding—i.e., tolerated nipple or gavage feedings of human milk or a standard formula plus intravenous supplementation with 5 to 10% glucose solutions. If adequate nutrients cannot be delivered in this way, a trial of continuous nasogastric or transpyloric infusion seems warranted. Tolerated enteral feedings delivered conventionally or by continuous infusion also can be supplemented by intravenous infusions of appropriate mixtures of glucose, amino acids, and lipid. In the event that enteral feedings are not tolerated, parenteral administration of a balanced nutritional mixture deserves serious consideration. A regimen that provides 75 Cal/kg/24 hr plus amino acids, electrolytes, minerals, and vitamins can be delivered by peripheral vein infusion without imposing an unreasonable fluid load. Since such a regimen almost certainly maintains existing body composition, it is particularly applicable for infants who are likely to tolerate enteral intake within a brief period of time. Total parenteral nutrition using a central vein catheter allows delivery of a more concentrated nutrient mixture. This technique is particularly useful in situations associated with prolonged intolerance of enteral feedings, i.e., longer than peripheral intravenous infusion sites can be maintained or in patients with preexisting malnutrition.

Neonatal Intestinal Obstruction

THOMAS S. MORSE, M.D.

Congenital intestinal obstruction is the most frequent indication for major surgery in the first week of life. The vast majority of neonates with this common affliction can look forward to completely normal lives provided the obstruction is recognized and treated immediately.

Esophageal atresia is treated by end-to-end anastomosis after division of the tracheoesophageal fistula that usually accompanies it. If this is not possible, the upper end of the esophagus is exteriorized in the neck, the fistula divided, and a gastrostomy placed. Later the gap is bridged by a loop of colon or a gastric tube.

Antral and duodenal webs can usually be excised, but bypass is sometimes needed as in the case of duodenal atresia, stenosis, and annular pancreas, which are treated by duodenojejunostomy. Jejunal and ileal atresias are treated by resecting the atretic ends and anastomosis. Meconium ileus is treated by Gastrografin enemas, and when this is unsuccessful by resection and anastomosis. Meconium plugs are washed out with barium enemas.

Hirschsprung's disease is treated by colostomy or ileostomy, followed later by resection of the aganglionic segment and abdominoperineal anastomosis. Colon atresias usually require ileostomy and later repair. Malrotation is treated by untwisting the volvulus and dividing the retroperitoneal bands that compress the duodenum. Imperforate anus in girls can usually be treated by perineal anoplasty without colostomy, but in boys colostomy is almost always necessary in the newborn period, followed later by abdominoperineal or sacroperineal anoplasty.

Provided the baby is not extremely premature or afflicted by multiple anomalies, the prognosis is excellent when the primary operation, whether immediate or delayed, can be accomplished. If colon interposition is necessary, the results are good but not excellent. Meconium ileus has a high mortality because it occurs only in infants with fibrocystic disease of the pancreas. The results in Hirschsprung's disease and imperforate anus depend on the care with which the primary operation is done, and even more on the meticulous followup the surgeon gives the patient. Unless the *surgeon* follows the child all the way to adulthood, the results of operations for imperforate anus and Hirschsprung's disease are usually substandard.

Hemolytic Diseases of the Neonate

ROBERT R. CHILCOTE, M.D., *and* LAWRENCE M. GARTNER, M.D.

When presented with evidence of hemolysis, the clinician must rapidly consider the possible causes of red cell destruction and the potential impact of anemia on oxygen delivery and increased bilirubin production. Should hemolysis continue at a rate that threatens the neonate, the clinician must rapidly institute measures to alleviate this process— most often by exchange transfusion.

CLINICAL PRESENTATION

A carefully taken family history of an expectant mother may warn of impending fetal and neonatal hemolysis and allow the obstetrician and pediatrician to formulate a plan to monitor the fetus, possibly with amniocentesis. Particular attention should be given to previous obstetrical events and transfusions that could have sensitized the mother to Rh or other blood group antigens. Likewise, a history of familial icterus, early gallbladder disease, or splenectomy should alert the physician to inquire further about inherited red cell abnormalities. If the fetus is at risk, appropriate consultation should be obtained well before the time of delivery. This allows time to obtain diagnostic studies on maternal, paternal, and sibling blood specimens. Narrowing the range of diagnostic possibilities may allow the team to obtain definitive studies on infant cord blood.

Conditions that shorten fetal red cell life-span induce increased red cell synthesis; anemia develops when production fails to compensate for destruction. Severe anemia causes a hydropic fetus, a condition attended by high fetal and neonatal mortality and characterized by pallor, edema, hepatomegaly, and anemia at birth. The birth of a hydropic infant without diagnosis is an indication for further hematologic investigation, even if the infant is born dead. Small amounts of fetal or neonatal blood can be examined and used to classify the abnormalities so that the family may be counseled about the risk of recurrence, possible prevention, and management of future pregnancies.

Toxic levels of indirect bilirubin are not found in utero because of the placenta's capacity to transfer unconjugated bilirubin into the maternal circulation. However, after birth, hemolytic rates that may reduce the hemoglobin concentration by only a few grams per deciliter and thereby escape detection on routine hematologic screening may produce bilirubin loads that quickly exceed the newborn's capacity to conjugate the newly formed bilirubin and excrete it into bile. In the presence of severe hemolysis, the pale, anicteric neonate may become visibly yellow within 30 minutes after delivery. Unconjugated bilirubin is a lipophilic substance that may, under circumstances as yet incompletely understood, cross the blood-brain barrier and poison neuronal cells. When the concentration of indirect bilirubin rises above 20 mg/dl in the healthy full-term infant, the infant becomes at risk for bilirubin encephalopathy. This risk is markedly increased even at much lower serum bilirubin concentrations when there is or has been poor tissue perfusion, acidosis, hypoxemia, hypoalbuminemia, bacterial infection, or hypoglycemia, especially in the preterm infant.

Newborns with ongoing hemolysis will usually become icteric in the first 24 hours of life, often within 6 hours of birth. Destruction of less than 10% of circulating red cells may not necessarily lead to a clinically detectable change in hemoglobin concentration, hematocrit, or reticulocyte count, but may raise the bilirubin concentration to a level greater than expected for physiologic jaundice of the newborn. An indirect bilirubin in excess of 12 to 14 mg/dl in the full-term infant suggests that hemolysis is contributing to the bilirubin load; if the child is anemic, an elevated bilirubin value is even more significant. One must consider the hematocrit of the bilirubinemic child, since the source of bilirubin is dependent on the red cell mass. Thus, a child with a hematocrit of 30% as opposed to 60% will produce only half as much bilirubin and have a lower serum concentration. In contrast, however, enhanced enteric bilirubin absorption due to intestinal obstruction, absence of feeding, or caloric deprivation may increase serum bilirubin concentrations without increase in red cell destruction. The factors that control serum bilirubin levels are complex; nevertheless, changes in indirect bilirubin concentrations provide a better clinical guide to changes in the rate of red cell destruction than changes in hemoglobin or reticulocyte levels.

Severe and persistent hemolysis rarely elevates the direct-reacting serum bilirubin concentrations. An exception to this rule is seen in infants with severe Rh erythroblastosis requiring multiple intrauterine transfusions. In these cases, elevation of the direct fraction may be seen in the cord blood, reflecting the inability of the placenta to transfer the water-soluble conjugated (direct-reacting) pigment. Transient elevations of the direct fraction may also be seen during recovery from severe hemolytic disease. Cholestasis resulting from severe hemolysis in the neonate has been proposed as a cause for the "inspissated bile" syndromes, although this diagnosis is difficult to substantiate.

In the face of anemia, the cardiovascular system increases red cell delivery to maintain tissue oxygenation while the marrow releases increased numbers of immature cells, particularly nucleated red cells and reticulocytes. The initial workup of infants with hemolysis depends heavily on laboratory parameters. Serial hemoglobin levels, bilirubin values, and determinations of the proportion of reticulocytes and nucleated red cells in cord blood help separate infants with clinically significant brisk hemolysis from those with less severe hemolysis. A cord blood hemoglobin concentration of less than 14 gm/dl is evidence of anemia. It should be noted that anemia, even when severe, does not appreciably change the neonatal heart rate, respiratory pattern, or blood gases; one must follow the hemoglobin level.

DIFFERENTIAL DIAGNOSIS

Diseases that destroy the red cell can be either intrinsic, such as abnormalities of red cell metabolism, membrane function, or hemoglobin, or extrinsic, such as isoimmunization. A list of causes of hemolysis in the neonate is given in Table 1.

Rh-negative mothers sensitized to the Rh antigen by a previous pregnancy, abortion, or transfusion of Rh-positive red cells or blood products containing Rh-positive cells will, when the conceptus is Rh-positive, develop antibody titers that rise with pregnancy. Polyclonal anti-D antibodies belonging to the IgG fraction cross the placenta and attach to fetal red cells, causing their destruction. Anemia may develop and when severe may cause hydrops fetalis. The direct Coombs' test is positive and erythrocyte precursors as immature as erythroblasts are released into the circulation.

ABO blood group and other minor antigens may also induce hemolysis but the impact is generally less severe than in Rh disease—though there are occasional dramatic exceptions. Mild to moderate hyperbilirubinemia develops more often in ABO incompatibility but does not require exchange

Table 1. HEMOLYSIS IN THE NEONATE

Extrinsic abnormalities
  Rh(D) erythroblastosis
  ABO incompatibility (generally blood group O mothers)
  Minor blood group incompatibilities
  "DIC" (secondary to poor tissue perfusion, hemorrhagic shock, infection, cavernous hemangioma, etc)
  Large hematomas, swallowed blood
  Congenital infection (herpes, toxoplasmosis, CMV, rubella, syphilis, malaria)
  Bacterial sepsis

Intrinsic abnormalities of red cell
  Hereditary spherocytosis, elliptocytosis, pyropoikilocytosis
  Hexose shunt abnormality (G6PD deficiency)
  Glycolytic enzyme deficiency (deficiency of PK, GPI, TPI, PGK, HK)
  Galactosemia
  Hereditary 5' nucleotidase deficiency
  Stomatocytosis
  Abnormal fetal hemolglobin (alpha or gamma chain)

transfusion. The hemoglobin may fall in the first weeks of life, occasionally to levels as low as 5 to 6 gm/dl. Although these infants should be followed closely for the development of feeding difficulties (the neonatal equivalent of exercise intolerance), transfusion is rarely necessary. "Spherocytes" are present on the peripheral smear, a result of membrane loss to reticuloendothelial cells. The osmotic fragility test is positive and it may be difficult to distinguish this disorder from hereditary spherocytosis. However, with ABO incompatibility, the Coombs' test is positive and with time becomes negative. In hereditary spherocytosis the abnormally fragile cells persist and family screening with the osmotic fragility test will often diagnose an affected asymptomatic parent.

Mothers who have autoimmune diseases with IgG antibodies against the red cell may, even when splenectomized, give birth to infants with immune hemolytic anemia. In these situations, the Coombs' test is positive but evidence of blood group incompatibility is lacking.

As the incidence of Rh disease declines, intrinsic abnormalities of red cell function are becoming increasingly important causes of hyperbilirubinemia and anemia. Hereditary spherocytosis ("congenital icterus"), an autosomal dominant disorder, is one of the more common hemolytic anemias of man and can present with severe hemolysis in the neonatal period; this may occur even if other affected family members have not experienced this complication, since the severity of the clinical disease may differ dramatically among those with the same genotype. In this disorder and several others to be discussed below, an experienced laboratory can make the diagnosis on cord blood. Knowledge of the diagnosis alerts the pediatrician to potential problems in the first months of life, such as life-threatening splenic sequestration or aplastic crisis. Failure to obtain samples for study before transfusion may unnecessarily delay diagnosis.

Recently, an extremely severe type of spherocytosis with bizarre poikilocytes due to unstable red cell membrane structure has been described. The red cells are characterized by deficiencies of cytoskeletal membrane proteins and thermal instability occasioning the name "pyro"-poikilocytosis.

Abnormalities of alpha or gamma chain structure are probably underdiagnosed in the newborn, but in non-Oriental populations do not cause hydrops or severe neonatal hemolytic anemia. Sickle cell disease, a beta chain abnormality, does not cause hemolysis until 4 to 6 months of age.

Metabolic abnormalities of the red cell such as deficiencies of the hexose monophosphate shunt (G6PD) lead to susceptibility to oxidative stresses, especially those generated by infection or certain chemicals. Most medications used in the neonatal period can be administered to children with defi-

ciency of G6PD without inducing hemolysis; there is no evidence that the usual dose of 1 mg of vitamin K-1 oxide is hazardous.

Glycolytic enzymopathies (e.g., pyruvate kinase, glucose phosphate isomerase, triose phosphate isomerase) cause small, spherical-appearing, "crenated" or "echinocytic" red cells shaped like sea urchins and may result in serious hemolytic anemia in the newborn period. It is especially important to recognize the latter deficiency since it is accompanied by severe neuromuscular deterioration in the first year of life that may lead to respiratory failure.

Galactosemia is frequently accompanied by hemolysis, and the child may develop additional problems with the institution of milk feeding.

Congenital erythropoietic porphyria is a very rare cause of severe hemolysis in the newborn and should be recognized promptly, since severe cutaneous blistering, necrosis, and scarring may result from exposure of these infants to phototherapy (and sunlight). The diagnosis may be made dramatically by exposing urine and stool to ultraviolet light (Woods Lamp), producing a brilliant orange fluorescence.

Routine pregnancy screening should include determination of maternal blood group (ABO) and Rh type, as well as a hemantigen screen. All Rh-negative mothers should be further studied for the presence of RH(D) antibodies. Regardless of maternal blood group and type, all cord bloods should be sent for ABO and Rh typing as well as for direct Coombs' testing. Positive Coombs' tests should be reported to the attending physician immediately and the nature of the antibody on the red cells determined. Hematocrit, reticulocyte, nucleated red cell, and platelet counts and blood smear should also be examined immediately in these cases. Total and direct serum bilirubin and albumin concentrations should also be determined. A similar workup is indicated in all cases of neonatal anemia, even when the Coombs' test is negative and there is no maternal-infant red cell immunoincompatibility.

If congenital infection is suspected, appropriate serum IgM and antibody titers should be obtained. Intrinsic red cell abnormalities can be diagnosed on cord blood and both heparinized and EDTA anticoagulated tubes should be stored for further study if necessary; many of these disorders can be diagnosed on blood retained for several weeks or longer. Peripheral smears of newborns are replete with unusually shaped red cells and red cell inclusions. However, after careful study of the peripheral smear, experienced observers can generally help guide diagnostic tests.

THERAPY

Although therapy for these disorders is based on experience accumulated over the last 30 years, many of the recommendations have not been carefully evaluated in well-designed trials; some aspects of management are necessarily controversial, especially in children who present with marginal hemolysis, anemia, and indirect bilirubinemia. The therapeutic options available include intrauterine transfusion, postnatal exchange transfusion, and phototherapy.

Intrauterine Transfusion. A discussion of intrauterine exchange transfusion is beyond the scope of this presentation. Mothers who appear to be at risk for Rh sensitization should be followed with serologic studies and, when appropriate, referred for amniocentesis to determine the rate of hemolysis in the fetus.

Resuscitation and Immediate Exchange Transfusion. The severely hydropic infant, with a cord blood hemacrit less than 5 to 8 gm/dl, whose condition is due to RH sensitization, may require intensive resuscitative measures in the delivery room and transfusion of plasma and red cells to correct shock and restore oxygen transport. The team may also have to support ventilation and correct acidemia. Immediately following stabilization of the infant, an exchange transfusion should be performed. Preparation for such catastrophic intervention improves the infant's chance for survival.

While some authorities have proposed a variety of additional bilirubin and hematologic parameters for exchange transfusion immediately following delivery, modern neonatal intensive care units are equipped to monitor biochemical, physiologic and hematologic parameters, and the stable, asymptomatic erthyroblastosis infant with moderate anemia and mild to moderate hyperbilirubinemia can be observed over the first few hours to determine whether the rate of rise of the serum bilirubin or the rate of fall in the hematocrit require intervention. The infant with falling hematocrit but only a modestly increasing serum bilirubin concentration may require only simple transfusion, at least initially. There is no evidence that performance of an exchange transfusion immediately after delivery reduces the need for subsequent exchange transfusions. In fact, exchange transfusions performed during this early period of life when major cardiovascular and pulmonary adjustments are occurring may well place the infant at undue risk.

Criteria for Therapy. Within the first 4 hours after delivery, the team should establish a maximum allowable serum bilirubin level. If it appears that the infant's bilirubin will exceed that level, efforts should then be made to use phenobarbital (see below), phototherapy, appropriate nutritional and general health management and, finally if these measures fail, exchange transfusion to prevent the serum bilirubin from exceeding that level. The total bilirubin rather than indirect bilirubin levels is generally used for these criteria. Only when the direct

bilirubin fraction exceeds 20% of the total bilirubin is it appropriate to subtract it from the total and use the net indirect-bilirubin concentration. It should also be recognized that laboratories differ on the accuracy of bilirubin determinations; neonatal bilirubin values should be subjected to regular quality control studies.

We recommend that phototherapy be instituted in *full-term* infants with hemolytic disease when the total serum bilirubin exceeds 10 mg/dl, in infants weighing *1500 to 2500 grams* (32 to 38 weeks) when the serum bilirubin exceeds 8 mg/dl, and in infants weighing less than 1500 grams as soon after birth as possible regardless of serum bilirubin concentration. Phototherapy units should be equipped with an equal mixture of "Special Blue" lamps and "Daylight" lamps to obtain optimal photodegradation of bilirubin and the energy output checked once daily. Energy levels fall dramatically after 2000 to 4000 hours of use.

Phototherapy should be continued until serum bilirubin levels have fallen to one half of the exchange transfusion indication level or stabilized at that level for a minimum of 12 hours. After stabilization of serum bilirubin levels, it is essential that they be monitored for an additional 48 hours, longer in some cases.

Should serum bilirubin levels rise despite phototherapy, exchange transfusion should be performed in a timely manner to prevent the bilirubin value from exceeding the predetermined maximum allowable level. This can best be predicted by graphing serum bilirubin concentrations. If the projected maximum allowable level will be reached within 4 hours of the last determination, the transfusion blood should be prepared and the exchange transfusion started without waiting for another bilirubin result. If laboratory data have been erratic, preparations for the exchange can be made while the serum bilirubin determination is repeated. If bilirubin values are still rising, the procedure can be initiated without further delay.

While there continues to be some controversy over maximum allowable levels and the use or nonuse of albumin-bilirubin binding data, it has been our policy to use the serum bilirubin criteria indicated in Table 2, based on birth weight and infant

Table 2. INDICATIONS FOR NEONATAL EXCHANGE TRANSFUSION (mg/dl)

	<1000	1000–1500	1500–2500	>2500
Healthy	10	14	18	20
High risk*	10	12	16	18

*Infants with hemolysis or asphyxia, hypoxia, acidosis, hypoalbuminemia, hypothermia, and septicemia.

condition. In our hands, this has resulted in a significant reduction in the incidence of autopsy-proven kernicterus.

In the past 10 years, with the use of phototherapy and prevention of Rh erythroblastosis with Rhogam, many pediatricians have become less experienced in the techniques of exchange transfusion. Since mortality due to exchange transfusion may be less than 0.5% in highly experienced hands and up to 10 times higher when performed by inexperienced physicians, the need for exchange transfusion should be anticipated and the infant transferred to an appropriate neonatal intensive care center with ample lead time.

Technique for Exchange Transfusion. The goal of exchange transfusion is to remove a substantial proportion of antibody coated or intrinsically abnormal red cells without subjecting the neonate to undue cardiovascular stress. Exchanges are less effective in removing circulating antibody or bilirubin than in removing red cells. CPD anticoagulated Rh negative red cells, preferably drawn less than 2 days before, are cross-matched against the mother's serum for infants with Rh erythroblastosis. The blood should match the infant's ABO type as well. For infants with ABO erythroblastosis, type O blood should be utilized. Type- and Rh-specific blood compatible with the infant should be utilized and cross-matched against maternal blood for all other hemolytic disorders. The cells should be sedimented and plasma removed to bring the hematocrit above 45%. In some centers, stored blood is supplemented with adenine to increase shelf life. There is a suggestion that blood donated by individuals with sickle trait or HbSC may compromise the hypoxic acidotic infant and, until more is known about this phenomenon, it is prudent to screen all donors with a test for sickling. Feedings are changed to clear liquids, and the blood is warmed, using a thermostatically controlled blood warmer. If none is available, allow blood to slowly warm to room temperature but never place the bag in hot water.

An umbilical venous catheter is passed through the ductus venosus into the inferior vena cava, avoiding, if possible, the portal circulation. Respiratory status, perfusion, and cardiovascular dynamics are closely monitored by electronic devices. Though early studies suggested that the hydropic infant was often volume overloaded, more recent studies indicate that this is unusual. The decision to decrease the infant's blood volume should be individualized and made only when there is evidence of cardiac overload as shown, for example, by a venous pressure exceeding 10 to 12 cm of water. In addition to obtaining necessary hematologic and bilirubin baseline studies, remaining portions of the first 10 to 20 ml exchange aliquot should be retained in anticoagulated tubes (heparin "green top" and ACD "yellow top") for additional studies should intrinsic causes of hemolysis be suspected. Using 5 to 10 ml aliquots for small infants, and 20 ml for larger infants, the blood is exchanged to a total of 160 to 180 ml/kg body weight. "Pushes" and "pulls" of blood should be slow and gentle, but intentional delays to allow "equilibration" are of little or no value and may prolong the procedure, increasing the risk of complications. The umbilical catheter should be removed at completion of the procedure. Phototherapy is instituted when the exchange is finished to help keep the bilirubin from rising. Antibiotic therapy is not indicated following exchange transfusion unless clinical or laboratory data suggest the presence of infection.

After exchange transfusion, glucose is continued through a separate peripheral intravenous line and bilirubin determinations and serum potassium and sodium levels repeated every 4 to 8 hours until stable. If bleeding and thrombocytopenia develop, 1 unit of platelets is given; thrombocytepenia without bleeding is not treated prophylactically unless the platelet count falls to less than 10,000 to 20,000/mm³. Serum ionized calcium can be monitored but supplementation is generally not necessary.

Whole blood, blood products, and even washed red cells contain considerable numbers of viable mononuclear cells. These cells are capable of immunologic reactivity and may carry viruses. Though there are currently no guidelines, further study of the use of frozen and/or irradiated cells may ultimately prove them to be safer; at the present time they are not recommended unless the infant is suspected of having congenital immunodeficiency.

Over a period of several days and occasionally over a period of several weeks, especially in infants with Rh erythroblastosis, the hemoglobin level may fall to values that require additional small, simple transfusions. Weekly hematocrit determinations are indicated for at least the first 6 weeks following birth, even when no exchange transfusion has been performed.

Phenobarbital. This antiepileptic sedative barbiturate also stimulates synthesis of microsomal drug metabolizing enzymes. The most important clinically is hepatic bilirubin glucuronosyl transferase, the major catalyst for bilirubin conjugation. Administration of this agent for at least 1 week prior to delivery will increase hepatic bilirubin conjugating capacity in near-term and term fetuses and neonates. This increased activity will persist if the drug is administered to the newborn. In this short-term situation, phenobarbital has little or no effect on prematures but can be useful in modestly reducing serum bilirubin levels and the frequency of exchange transfusions in full-term infants with hemolytic disease.

While we do not recommend the use of phenobarbital for general use in the prevention of physiologic jaundice because of its potential addicting effect, we start selected patients such as the mother carrying a fetus with proven Rh hemolytic disease with a daily dose of 60 mg per day at 34 weeks' gestation. The newborn should receive a dose of 5 mg per kg per day starting on the first day of life.

PREVENTION AND GENERAL MEASURES

It is now possible to dramatically reduce Rh sensitization in Rh-negative females by administering anti-Rh immunoglobulin following each exposure to Rh-positive red cells. Anti-Rh immunoglobulin should be given to all Rh-negative women as soon as possible and preferably within 72 hours after birth, abortion, amniocentesis, ruptured ectopic pregnancy, manual version, or transfusion or injection of blood products from an Rh positive donor. Women who have had very complicated deliveries with possible fetal to maternal bleeding should be studied for fetal red cell contamination by the Kleinhauer-Betke method. If significant fetal cells are seen, a double dose of anti-Rh immunoglobulin should be given to prevent sensitization.

Hyperviscosity Syndromes

VIRGINIA D. BLACK, M.D.

Infants with an elevated venous hematocrit may demonstrate a variety of symptoms that suggest a reduction in cardiac output. Cyanosis, peripheral pallor, and cardiopulmonary symptoms may be present. Less severely affected infants may be ruddy or have no obvious abnormalities.

The syndromes producing these disorders may be divided into two general categories: those associated with an elevated venous hematocrit and those associated with an elevated whole blood viscosity. The great majority of affected infants have both polycythemia and hyperviscosity. In most institutions, whole blood viscosity is not readily available, hence infants with a venous hematocrit of 70% or more can safely be regarded as having hyperviscosity. Infants with hematocrits as low as 55%, however, may also have an abnormal whole blood viscosity.

The treatment of these syndromes should be directed toward improving blood flow. This is best achieved by reducing the venous hematocrit and monitoring central venous pressure when indicated. An umbilical venous catheter should be inserted under sterile technique to a level just above the diaphragm. Central venous pressure can then be obtained and a partial plasma exchange transfusion can be carried out. Equal volumes of

blood are exchanged for either fresh frozen plasma or plasmanate. Electrolyte and water solutions should not be used. Our preference has been type-specific fresh frozen plasma because of its availability and the low risk of hepatitis.

The usual volume for exchange is determined by the following equation:

$$\frac{C\ Hct*-D\ Hct\dagger}{C\ Hct} \times weight\ (kg)\ (80\ ml/kg)$$

An arbitrary hematocrit of 50% is desired at the end of the exchange. This figure has been selected because it reduces the likelihood of continued hyperviscosity and yet should prevent later anemia. The procedure should be performed before 24 hours of age and preferably within 12 to 15 hours after birth. If an infant is not identified until after the first day of life the procedure should be performed only for serious symptoms.

The risks of partial plasma exchange are the same risks as an exchange transfusion: bleeding, vessel injury, infection, and clots occur in fewer than 1 in 100 patients. In addition, some institutions have had a high incidence of postexchange abdominal symptoms, including necrotizing enterocolitis. Infants with hyperviscosity already may have diminished flow to the gastrointestinal tract. The additional manipulation of blood flow during the exchange may further reduce flow to a compromised bowel.

Following the partial plasma exchange the infant's vital signs should be monitored for several hours. Feedings are held for 2 to 4 hours and then resumed. The hematocrit can be monitored immediately following the exchange and several hours later. It is uncommon for a second exchange to be needed if the volume exchanged is determined correctly. Although seizures and hyperbilirubinemia are frequently attributed to these syndromes, neither is common. Hypoglycemia is usually improved after the partial exchange.

A two year follow-up of infants randomized to either partial plasma exchange or symptomatic treatment has been completed. Data from this study suggest that partial plasma exchange will not prevent sequelae. Small but significant differences were seen in infants treated with exchange. Exchanged infants, however, had more immediate gastrontestinal symptoms, including necrotizing enterocolitis.

There is no good evidence that the sequelae of hyperviscosity persist into school age. Hence, it may be reasonable to observe or treat symptomatically the child who does not have symptoms. Before the decision to observe is made, a careful examination of the infant must reveal a thriving child. Par-

---

*C Hct = current hematocrit
†D Hct = desired hematocrit or 50%

ticular attention must be paid to the infant's alertness and tone. In the absence of hypotonia and without difficulty alerting, it may be safe to observe the infant further before treatment is initiated. If feedings are not tolerated or the infant's alertness changes, this decision must be re-evaluated. Frequent changes in sleep states and difficulty alerting are classically associated with this syndrome.

Long-term follow-up studies of infants with neonatal hyperviscosity suggest significant motor and neurologic sequelae. The sequelae have not been limited to symptomatic infants and are not eliminated by early partial plasma exchange transfusion. Infants with these syndromes should be followed closely for both fine and gross motor development as well as language. These sequelae are frequently subtle and often missed in the first year of life. The relationship between neonatal hyperviscosity and perceptual motor handicaps remains to be elucidated.

23

Special Problems in the Adolescent

Children Whose Parents Are Divorcing

DONALD P. ORR, M.D.

Divorce effects at least 1.2 million new children each year. It is estimated that approximately 18 million children under 17 years of age are living in homes headed by single parents. Since in some states, divorce and marriage rates are approximately equal, the pediatrician can expect a sizeable proportion of his patients will be affected. The role of the pediatrician can include 1) education and anticipatory guidance; 2) supportive treatment for parents to maximize their help to the child; 3) direct counseling of the children; 4) identification of vulnerable, at-risk groups in need of more intensive treatment or referral.

Divorce is traumatic for all involved; children of all ages are affected. However, the manifestations of the trauma and the extent and depth of the subsequent problems vary by age, level of development, previous psychological adjustment of the child and parents, amount and extent of continued parental bitterness, and quality of the subsequent contact with custodial and noncustodial parents. All must be considered by the physician in treatment these families.

Age Considerations. The immediate response for all age groups is one of pain, disbelief, bewilderment, sadness, and anxiety. As expected, the younger the child, the more likely it is that the response will be manifest behaviorally. The youngest preschool children regress, with loss of toilet training skills and temper tantrums. This is especially pronounced when there is no explanation given to the child about a parent's absence. One also sees

confusion, bewilderment, separation anxieties, sleep problems, and increased aggressive behavior. Pervasive neediness with clinging to strangers is a common, longer-term residual. Older preschool children are somewhat less disturbed,, but, again, one sees increased aggressive behavior, insecurity, confusion, and a significant amount of self-blame for the divorce, with expression of subsequent guilt. Decreased self-esteem is common, as are anxiety and sadness. Longer-term sequelae may include depression and interference with subsequent development. The oldest preschoolers are also upset by the divorce and manifest sadness and confusion, but they are better able to tolerate the divorce without breaking developmental stride. However, they still become anxious, display increased aggressive behavior, are irritable, and have separation problems. They are, fortunately, better able to verbalize the sadness and their concerns.

Nearly 50% of preschool children manifest psychological deterioration within a year following the divorce. Most vulnerable are those who remain depressed and regressed, and whose level of psychosexual development does not progress. The vulnerability seems to be related to the presence of maternal psychological problems and a poor quality of maternal-child relationship, which is *not* dependent on whether the mother works.

School-age children are sophisticated and better able to understand divorce and thus actively attempt to deal with it. They feel *less* responsible for it. Anger, however, appears at this age and may be directed at either or both parents. One sees temper tantrums and demandingness in addition to open verbal assaults. Since a child is fearful that he may be abandoned, the anger can be thinly disguised as stealing or aggressiveness toward others. Somatic symptoms, with headaches and stomachaches predominating, appear for the first time as common sequelae. Approximately one half of the children experience school difficulties in the period immediately following the divorce. Again, 50% of children whose parents divorce demonstrate diminished psychological functioning 1 year later. One sees depressive behavior, lowered self-esteem, and peer and school difficulties. A precocious interest and adolescent preoccupation with sexuality may also appear.

Adolescents, too, uniformly experience divorce as a painful experience; anger is a predominant effect. While they are angry at the parents for breaking up the family, they experience sadness and a sense of loss and betrayal. Included also is a sense of shame and embarassment about the divorce. At times, this impairs their ability to share the situation with others, and they may attempt to keep it a secret. They may find themselves caught in loyalty conflicts if they are asked to ally themselves with one parent at the expense of the other. However, adolescents are better able to deal with the trauma of divorce by psychologically and physically withdrawing from the family and by creating an emotional distance between their parents and themselves. The divorce forces them to relook at their parents, to rapidly deidealize them, and if dating resumes for the parent, to directly confront parental sexuality.

About one half of adolescents survive the divorce experience and develop into normal, well-adjusted young adults; however, even these are left with problems in heterosexual relationships. They fear intimacy and marriage, and may have doubts about their own sexuality. The other half of the adolescents experience more severe psychological conflicts and diminished school performance, deliquency, depression, and poor self-esteem. These children tend to enter into precipitous, clinging, multiple immature heterosexual relationships characterized by a high degree of sexual activity. The degree of vulnerability seems, to a large degree, to be related to parental responses—those parents who remain regressed, have a decreased ability to parent, and in whom overwhelming bitterness persists.

The goals of pediatric intervention are as follows: 1) to minimize pain and suffering of the child and parent; 2) to lessen the immediate psychological impact of the divorce; and, 3) to attempt to prevent subsequent, more serious psychological sequelae by supporting and strengthening the healthy coping responses of the parent and the child; by identifying the vulnerable group and intervening more agressively; and by referring those with more serious or longer lasting psychological responses.

Assessment and intervention are at several levels of complexity, and each clinician must identify his or her own capability. The pediatrician is at a particular advantage because frequently, he or she knows both parents. There is a danger, however, that the pediatrician will be seen as an ally of the mother at the expense of involvement with the father. One must look at the level of the previous psychological adjustment in evaluating the parent. Serious mental problems, especially psychosis and depression, leave the child at increased risk for subsequent problems. The pediatrician should estimate the strengths and vulnerabilities of the parent, judge how she or he is coping with the divorce and the extent of ongoing bitterness between the parents. It is helpful to support the parent either directly or by referral; self-help groups are especially valuable. This is a difficult time for parents who experience anger, anxiety, guilt, hurt, and a sense of shame, loss, and abandonment. However, the parent is still the single most important factor in helping the children.

One objective of this intervention is to educate the parent(s) about childrens' responses to divorce. By anticipating certain problems, they are better prepared to support their children through this difficult time. It must be stressed that although certain behaviors and reactions are common, children still require consistent limits. When rules change unpredictably, children become anxious and feel insecure, compounding problems. For children of all ages, the parent(s) must communicate that 1) although the parents are divorcing each other, they are not divorcing the children; 2) children are not responsible for the divorce; they need not feel guilt or shame; 3) the loyalty, affection, and commitment to the children will remain; 4) everyone is under stress; it will not be easy, but they must talk about it, especially their feelings.

Parents will be the most important helping person in most divorces and probably the sole helper for preschool children. In this age group, the quality of ongoing care taking is most important. In the many instances where the mother must work, this need not be detrimental to the child if a secure, stable provider can be identified. Because of the many regressive behaviors, including loss of toilet training skills, this may be a very trying time for all involved. Moreover, since these children remain exceedingly needy, clinging, and reaching out to strangers, they may be at particular risk of molestation from others and the parent must be particularly selective and protective.

Anger directed at the parent is very common with school-aged children and perhaps one of the most difficult aspects with which the parent must deal. However, because these children are increasingly verbal and actively seek to master the difficult situation, the custodial parent can take advantage. They must help to deal with the pain, the sense of loss, and not be allowed to maintain an unrealistic fantasy of reconciliation. The parent(s) must be vigilant for school problems. It is probably wise for the parent to contact a favorite teacher and alert him or her to the possibility of problems. Again, anticipation is important.

Adolescents must be given space—they need time to withdraw and distance to consolidate their feelings and thoughts. The parent can expect anger and expression of loss, grief, and sadness. When the parent resumes a heterosexual relationship, he or she must deal directly with the issues of dating and sexuality with the adolescent son or daughter. Discretion is the key.

The pediatrician may choose to see the school-aged child, particularly the adolescent, individually to assess the potential for subsequent problems and to counsel. The level of the predivorce psychosocial adjustment, including quality of peer relationships, degree of academic achievement, and whether or not behavior problems existed, is important. One can use this time, in addition, as anticipatory guidance with the parent. Sufficient time must be allowed for the result. It cannot be rushed. Younger children will have more need for play. This may be in the form of drawings or games. All ages should be permitted to proceed at their own pace. There is no correct way to begin or to counsel, and the pediatrician must call upon his or her previously acquired skills in interviewing and counseling.

Some suggestions: Although one begins slowly, the reason for the visit must be clearly stated at the beginning. Children may expect a physical examination or younger children fear an injection. The pediatrician must take the initiative. For example, "Your mother told me that she and your father have separated/divorced. I know that children have a lot of feelings about that. Sometimes they aren't sure about them or they aren't sure what these feelings mean. They don't know if they are OK or what to do with them." The child or adolescent will usually lead the way; however, again, direction and structuring of the interview without leading the patient is helpful. Long periods of silence are not helpful. Do not expect the patient to present feelings as if giving a book report. Important information will usually be interspersed with seemingly unrelated chatter. One may anticipate the typical areas of concern and suggest that *other* children have concerns about anger at parents, sense of responsibility for the divorce, shame or embarrassment. With adolescents, sexuality and their own future relationships and marriage need to be addressed at some time. This may only be relevant and useful to discuss months after the divorce.

Because of the high prevalence of persistent psychological problems following divorce, a subsequent visit should be routinely rescheduled in approximately 6 to 8 weeks. Persistent symptoms, particularly regression, depression, school problems, or poor coping responses of the parent indicate a further need for intervention. Unless the pediatrician is particularly skilled at counseling, these children should be referred to mental health colleagues.

Those vulnerable children at high-risk should be referred for preventive treatment at the time of initial evaluation when possible. However, because the parent may not see the need at that time, the pediatrician must be patient and persist in hopes of effecting a referral at a later time. Vulnerable situations include any of the following: 1) poor predivorce psychosocial adjustment of the child; 2) poor parent/child relationships before the divorce; 3) inadequate coping responses of the custodial parent; 4) poor parental communications; 5) lack of support network for the family; 6) ongoing depression and anger of the parent.

If the community is fortunate enough to have group programs for children of divorce, the pediatrician should make use of them. These are usually affordable and have the advantage of not labeling the patient as troubled or deviant but only as a child whose parents are undergoing a divorce. They are probably the single most effective preventive intervention.

Obesity

I. RONALD SHENKER, M.D.

The treatment of obesity in children and adolescents is not easy. It is time consuming, frustrating, and not infrequently unsuccessful. Obesity prevention and management remains an enigma for the physician. The basic tenets of therapy—reduced caloric intake and/or increased caloric utilization—are particularly difficult to achieve except in the most highly motivated patients. During childhood one must direct the bulk of attention to the parent while by the time of adolescence most management programs must deal in an intimate fashion with the patient.

Exogenous obesity is an eating disorder and as such therapy must be directed to reducing excessive intake. Psychological factors are undoubtedly important in the vast majority of patients, but dealing with these underlying factors alone will not control the symptomatology or outcome of the eating behavior. An active directive approach is needed.

Patient motivation is the key to success and must be assessed during the initial consultation. Although it has been demonstrated that self-image and self-assessment are more realistic in adolescent boys with obesity than in girls, the latter are often more motivated to reduce body fat and are more prone to follow a planned dietary and exercise regimen. Early adolescent boys are the least motivated

Table 1. 1000 CALORIE PER DAY SCHEDULE*

Breakfast Food	Serving	Cal.	Lunch Food	Serving	Cal.	Dinner Food	Serving	Cal.
Orange	1 whole	70	Chicken	3 oz.	170	Beef, lean	3 oz.	170
Tomato juice	1 cup	45	Turkey	3 oz.	190	Lamb, lean	3 oz.	170
Grapefruit	½ medium	55	Fish	3 oz.	160	Pork, lean	3 oz.	225
Grapefruit juice	¾ cup	75	Salmon (7¾ oz can, drained)	½ can	120	Veal, lean	3 oz.	185
Orange juice	¾ cup	80				Chicken	3 oz.	170
			Tuna (7 oz can drained)	½ can	170	Turkey	3 oz.	190
Bagel	½ whole	60				Fish	3 oz.	160
Bread	1 slice	60	Cottage cheese, low fat	¾ cup	145			
Cereal, cooked	½ cup	70				Bread	1 slice	60
Cereal, dry (sugar free)	¾ cup	70				Muffin	1 small	60
			Tossed green salad	1 cup	20	Toast, Melba	4 slices	60
			Carrot	1 small	20	Potato	1 small	70
Butter	1 tsp.	35	Pickle, dill	1 large	15	Beans, green lima	1/3 cup	60
Margarine	1 tsp.	35	Celery	2 stalks	10	Corn, whole kernel	1/3 cup	55
			Cauliflower	4–5 flowerets	15	Rice	1/3 cup	60
Nonfat milk	1 cup	90	Cabbage, shredded	½ cup	15	Mayonnaise	1 tbsp.	100
Buttermilk	1 cup	90	Pepper, green	1 whole	20	Margarine	1 tbsp.	100
Plain yogurt	1 cup	120	Radishes	9 medium	15	Oil	1 tbsp.	100
Coffee or Tea	—	—	Cantaloupe	¼ medium	30	Broccoli	3 spears	30
			Apple	½ medium	35	Brussels sprouts	4–5	30
			Blackberries, fresh or canned (drained)	½ cup	40	Asparagus	6 spears	20
						Beets	1/3 cup	20
			Orange	½ medium	35	Peas, green	1/3 cup	45
			Pear, fresh	½ medium	50	Beans, green	½ cup	20
			Grapefruit	½ medium	55	Cabbage, shredded	½ cup	15
						Carrots	½ cup	25
			Nonfat milk	1/3 cup	30	Tossed green salad	1 cup	20
			Buttermilk—nonfat	1/3 cup	30	Turnip	1 small	20
						Onions, green	5 med.	20
			Coffee or tea	—	—	Radishes	6 med.	10
						Lettuce Wedge	1/6 head	10
						Tomato	½ med.	15
						Peach	1 med.	35
						Honeydew	¼ med.	30
						Strawberries, fresh	½ cup	30
						Watermelon	½ cup	35
						Nonfat milk	1 cup	90
						Buttermilk	1 cup	90

Add (3) three times per week 1 egg—poached or boiled

Note: Substitute—2 ounces farmer cheese for one egg as desired.

*Select one food from each box for each meal.

or successful in adherence to a therapeutic plan.

The physician and patient must form an alliance for therapy. A transference undoubtedly occurs, but is less obvious than in conventional (psycho)therapy. Female adolescents may wish to please their (male) physicians. Although this is a poor long term motivation for weight reduction, any reasonable method of getting the patient on the right program for weight reduction should be utilized.

Preparation for new school entrance, such as high school or college, may be an important motivator. The physician should explore why the patient comes for treatment at a specific time, especially in the face of long term obesity. Motivation should be explored, exploited, and encouraged.

The goal of treatment is long term. An appropri-

ate assessment of ideal body weight based on standard growth charts is determined. An individual who is 20% over ideal weight for height is considered obese. In most instances, however, "eyeball" diagnosis of obesity is correct. Weight and skinfold measurements are useful in following therapeutic progress. For practical purposes, successful outcome is also easily "eyeballed."

The patient should be examined undressed at the initial visit. Naturally, causes for obesity other than overeating are to be excluded, such as genetic conditions, hypothalamic disorders, or endocrine causes. These are rare. However, the objectives of dietary control apply to all obesities.

The patient's body build should be noted and discussed with the patient. Realistic outcomes are

Table 2. 1400 CALORIE PER DAY SCHEDULE*

Breakfast Food	Serving	Cal.	Lunch Food	Serving	Cal.	Dinner Food	Serving	Cal.
Select one item			**Select one item**			**Select one item**		
Orange	1 whole	70	Chicken	3 oz.	170	Beef, lean	3 oz.	170
Tomato juice	1 cup	45	Turkey	3 oz.	190	Lamb, lean	3 oz.	170
Grapefruit	½ medium	55	Fish	3 oz.	160	Pork, lean	3 oz.	225
Grapefruit juice	¾ cup	75	Salmon (7¾ oz can, drained)	½ can	120	Veal, lean	3 oz.	185
Orange juice	¾ cup	80				Chicken	3 oz.	170
			Tuna (7 oz can drained)	½ can	170	Turkey	3 oz.	190
Select two items						Fish	3 oz.	160
Bagel	½ whole	60	Cottage cheese, low fat	¾ cup	145			
Bread	1 slice	60				**Select two items**		
Cereal, cooked	½ cup	70	**Select two items**			Bread	1 slice	60
Cereal, dry	¾ cup	70	Bagel	½ whole	60	Potato	1 small	70
Muffin (English)	½ whole	60	Bread	1 slice	60	Muffin	1 small	60
			Hamburger bun	½ whole	60	Corn, whole kernel	1/3 cup	55
Select one item						Rice	1/3 cup	60
Cream cheese	1 tbsp.	35	**Select one item**					
Margarine	1 tbsp.	35	Tossed green salad	1 cup	20	**Select one item**		
			Carrot	1 small	20	Broccoli	2 spears	30
Select one item			Pickle, dill	1 large	15	Brussels sprouts	4–5	30
Nonfat milk	1 cup	90	Celery	2 stalks	10	Asparagus	6 spears	20
Buttermilk	1 cup	90	Cauliflower	4–5 flowerets	15	Beets	1/3 cup	20
Plain yogurt	1 cup	120				Peas, green	1/3 cup	45
			Cabbage, shredded	½ cup	15	Beans, green	½ cup	20
As desired			Pepper, green	1 whole	20	Cabbage, shredded	½ cup	15
Coffee or Tea	—	—	Radishes	9 medium	15	Carrots	½ cup	25
			Select two items			**Select one item**		
Add (3) three times per week 1 egg—poached or boiled.			Cantaloupe	¼ medium	30	Tossed green salad	1 cup	20
			Apple	½ medium	35	Turnip	1 small	20
			Blackberries, fresh or canned (drained)	½ cup	40	Onions, green	5 med.	20
			Orange	½ medium	35	Tomato	½ med.	15
			Pear, fresh	½ medium	50	Lettuce wedge	1/6 head	10
			Grapefruit	½ medium	35	**Select one item**		
			Select one item			Mayonnaise	1 tbsp.	100
			Nonfat milk	1 cup	90	Oil	1 tbsp.	100
			Buttermilk	1 cup	90	Margarine	1 tbsp.	100
			Coffee or tea	—	—	**Select two items**		
						Peach	1 med.	35
						Tangerine	1 med.	40
						Honeydew	¼ med.	30
						Select one item		
						Nonfat milk	1 cup	90
						Buttermilk	1 cup	90

*Select food from each box for each meal.

to be agreed upon by patient, physician, and parent. "The apple doesn't fall far from the tree" is a worthwhile axiom to discuss with the patient and family. The role of genetic and environmental factors should be mentioned. An important goal of successful treatment is patient acceptance of self as he or she will be. Even if the ultimate weight loss is modest, the goal of self-acceptance is to be strived for.

Although many patients have short term motivation, no therapeutic program should have short term goals. Discuss the patient's goal in terms of 3, 6 or even 12 months from the initial visit. One pound of fat is equal to 3500 calories. Therefore, a program of caloric deprivation and exercise in which a deficit of 3500 calories per week is achieved results in weight loss of 1 pound per week or about 12 pounds in 3 months. This weight will not be reduced in an even manner. Typically weight loss is fastest in the first few weeks and then becomes more resitant. But an appreciation of a weight loss potential of 25 pounds in 6 months may be realistic and achievable for some adolescents with above average motivation.

The diet prescribed should be nutritionally sound and easy to follow. Examples are given in Tables 1 and 2 for nutritionally balanced 1000 and 1400 calories per day. Intake of calories only during mealtimes should be stressed. Dietary education should be occurring during weekly physician visits so that a newly learned eating behavior is maintained. Modification and individualization of the diet require time and detailed explanations. A nutritionist is particularly helpful in this regard. The pediatrician would be wise to seek out such a consultant. Being given a specific diet is an important tangible aid to the patient. Give duplicate copies to the patient and parent.

Frequent physician visits are essential to a successful weight reduction program. If follow-up visits are less than weekly for the first weeks, treatment is doomed to failure. Physician-patient rapport and trust occur during these visits, which always include a weight check under uniform conditions. Since enthusiasm is often high for both patient and physician at the outset, the first few weeks will often have a successful outcome, especially for the adolescent girl. Although intake of food is stressed in the earliest visits, weight maintenance with increased exercise and modestly increased calories if they have been severely restricted (i.e., 1000 or below) should be discussed in detail as follow-up proceeds beyond the first few weeks. Examples of 10 activities with caloric energy utilization as seen in Table 3 should be discussed.

Some patients will respond to specific behavior modification techniques utilized to reduce intake. The use of smaller plates, or prolonging the duration of the meals, or instructions to leave food on the plate, are specific techniques to be tried. Self-meditation may be useful in older adolescents. Parental rewards are a form of behavior modification and may be helpful in some children and adolescents.

The role of the family is often the key to outcome. Parents control the food coming into the home. Meals are usually not prepared by the patient. Ready access to high calorie foods or low calorie snacks are often parent dependent. If youngsters are in the center of family strife, they will be unable

to cooperate with a successful weight reduction program. The concept of the vulnerable child, a pathologic mechanism seen in the anorexic patient and in other psychosomatic conditions, is also applicable to the obese. Ancillary psychologic and psychiatric evaluation may be needed in some obese youngsters.

Dietary modification is frequently indicated for the entire family. A well balanced, calorically deficient diet may be beneficial to others in the family. Here again, the intact nonpathologic family can be of great support.

Since peer support and struggles for independence are so developmentally important for the adolescent, adjuncts to obesity therapy are group meetings, therapy, and counseling, which may be the primary appropriate treatment for some. Youngsters do best in peer groups. They generally should not become part of an adult obesity group. In the peer group, patients are able to see, identify with, and help themselves and others in the struggle to maintain an appropriate weight.

Drug treatment has no place in the treatment of childhood or adolescent obesity. However, some adolescents will respond to short term medication to "get started" on their diet. In some very resistant patients, it has been temporarily successful.

Finally, obesity prevention is obviously preferrable to obesity treatment. It should begin in infancy or in early childhood. However, the major therapeutic tool available, dietary restriction, cannot be prescribed without regard to nutritional needs and growth requirements. Allowing the child to "grow into his weight" is often indicated, as opposed to weight reduction. The results here are often less obvious and more frustrating to supervise. Natural periods of decreased intake after the rapid growth of the first 2 years of life should be appreciated. Parental guidance is essential to prevent obesity. Social and cultural factors must also be considered.

The final recommendation for the physician who treats the obese patient is to approach the patient with enthusiasm for potential success. An "upbeat" attitude may help patient motivation, which remains the single most important factor for a successful treatment outcome.

Table 3. BURNING OFF CALORIES BY THE HOUR

	Calories Utilized Per Hour If Body Weight Is:		
Activity	117 Pounds	152 Pounds	196 Pounds
Resting in bed or sleeping	55	72	93
Dancing, vigorous	264	344	444
Walking, 4 mph	307	400	518
Volleyball	265	345	445
Basketball, moderate	327	426	550
Bicycling, level 5.5 mph	233	304	392
Ping pong	180	235	302
Tennis, moderate	322	420	541
Bowling	310	404	520
Skiing downhill	449	585	755

Menstrual Disorders: Gynecologic Procedures and Problems

KAREN HEIN, M.D.

The most important principles in deciding to treat an adolescent with a menstrual disorder are that the condition poses sufficient threat to the health, well-being, or comfort of the teenager to warrant therapeutic intervention and that the benefits of treatment outweigh the risks of interfering with the normal maturation of the hypothalamic-pituitary-ovarian axis. Variation in the timing of menarche, frequency of menses, and amount and rate of menstrual flow are common in the teenage years.

AMENORRHEA

Since the average age of menarche varies among different populations, definition of primary amenorrhea must be specified for a given individual within her cultural context. In our experience, the average age of menarche in an inner city population was 12.4 years for whites, 11.9 years for blacks and 11.5 for Hispanic adolescents, whereas national data revealed a mean age of 13 years.

Primary Amenorrhea. Primary amenorrhea in the absence of pubertal delay or other nonendocrinologic dysfunction should be treated with reassurance and observation until approximately age 16 or 3 years after initial signs of puberty appear. Thereafter, evaluation is in order. Menstrual irregularities at time of stress or in the presence of weight changes should be viewed as alterations not requiring medical therapeutic intervention.

If amenorrhea is noted in the context of overall delayed puberty, the underlying cause must be sought and treated if possible. If the amenorrhea is due to a chronic disease, such as inflammatory bowel disease, renal or thyroid disease, or anorexia nervosa, effective treatment of the underlying disorder usually corrects the amenorrhea. In the rare instance when amenorrhea is caused by primary ovarian failure, such as in Turner's syndrome, or in testicular feminization syndrome or prolonged hypogonadotropic hypogonadism, replacement therapy with ovarian hormones is required. Estrogen therapy should be initiated at a chronologic age commensurate with the sexual development of normal peers. With recent evidence linking continuous long-term exogenous administration of estrogens to the development of endometrial carcinoma, it is currently recommended that periodic evaluation of the endrometrium be carried out and that therapy be discontinued for 1 week out of 4 once a maintenance schedule is instituted. Prolonged and unopposed estrogen therapy should be avoided.

Secondary Amenorrhea. Estrogen status can be determined through clinical or chemical means rather than a therapeutic trial of additional exogenous estrogen. In a normally estrogenized teenager, the addition of medroxyprogesterone acetate USP, 10 mg by mouth for 5 days, or a single dose of progesterone-in-oil, 25 to 100 mg IM, usually induces withdrawal bleeding. Although this may be reassuring to both physician and patient, it does not correct and may indeed worsen the underlying hormonal instability that produced the amenorrhea.

Teenagers with Stein-Leventhal syndrome should be treated in order to suppress excess endogenous hormone production. A combination estrogen-progestogen compound usually is employed and oral contraceptives are quite suitable. A combination of daily norethindrone, 1 mg, plus mestranol, 50 to 80 μg, or ethinyl estradiol, 35 to 50 μg, can be used for 21-day cycles, with 7 days of abstinence before the next cycle is begun.

Amenorrhea in Sexually Active Teenagers. Since more than half of the adolescent females in the U.S. have had first intercourse experience during adolescence, there are special considerations in treating amenorrhea in sexually active teenagers. Pregnancy status should be determined by appropriate blood and/or urine tests before any medications or radiologic studies are used to evaluate amenorrhea. In light of possible associations of congenital anomalies with progestins as well as synthetic estrogenic compounds, these hormones should not be administered to induce menses chemically until the possibility of pregnancy is excluded.

"Postpill" amenorrhea is more common among young adolescent females than older women when oral contraceptives are discontinued. Adolescents should not be given oral contraceptives until a pattern of ovulatory cycles is well established.

Inadequate residual endometrium with synechiae (Asherman's syndrome) may be suspected if amenorrhea following an abortion fails to respond to cycling with a conjugated estrogen, 1.25 mg daily by mouth for 3 weeks, or a combination of estrogen plus a progestogen. The diagnosis can then be confirmed by hysteroscopy.

Menstrual Irregularities with Weight Loss and Endurance Training. Rapid or profound weight loss, obesity, or endurance training are frequently accompanied by oligomenorrhea or amenorrhea. The long term effects of infrequent or absent menses in these patients are unknown. No medical therapeutic intervention is recommended if patients are otherwise in good health. Regulating or inducing menses by use of exogenous hormones is not recommended. When normal weight is regained or hours of training are reduced, menses usually resume normal patterns.

DYSFUNCTIONAL UTERINE BLEEDING

After menarche, the first several cycles are usually anovulatory, resulting in erratic menses that may be excessive in duration and amount of blood loss. Unless the patient becomes symptomatically anemic, the condition is best left alone, since it will be corrected once ovulation occurs more regularly. However, if the blood loss results in significant symptomatology, 3 modes of therapy are available. A progestogen such as norethinodrel, 5 mg by mouth daily, or medroxyprogesterone acetate, 10 mg by mouth daily, can be taken during the last 5 to 7 days of each cycle. Alternatively, a combination of high-dose estrogen plus progestin such as norethynodrel, 5 mg with mestranol, 75 μg, can be given by mouth in the following schedule: 5 tablets per day until the bleeding ceases (usually first day), then 4 tablets per day decreasing to 3, then 2, then 1 as long as bleeding does not recur. The single tablet should be continued for 21 days, at which time withdrawal bleeding will occur. If blood loss is so rapid or unrelenting that hospitalization is necessary, IV administration of conjugated estrogen for injection, USP 25 mg repeated after 4 hours (up to 6 times)*may be used. If medical therapy is unsuccessful, curettage might be indicated. Other causes of excessive or frequent bleeding (coagulopathy, aspirin sensitivity, or hypothyroidism) can be evaluated if the hypermenorrhea or polymenorrhea recurs.

DYSMENORRHEA

Dysmenorrhea is reported by approximately 60% of adolescent females and is the most common cause of short term recurrent school absenteeism. Recent developments in defining the role of prostaglandins in the production of menstrual cramps and the subsequent development of therapeutic agents to block the synthesis and action of prostaglandins have revolutionized the approach and treatment of dysmenorrhea. Aspirin, 650 mg 4 times per day, must be begun before menstrual flow commences to be effective. Newer, more effective agents, including fenamates and derivatives of arylpropionic acid, are now available. Pretreatment before onset of menstruation is not necessary. Prostaglandin production and release are maximal in the first 48 hours of menstrual flow; therefore, these preparations can be prescribed from onset through day two of menses. The following seem to offer comparable relief from dysmenorrhea:

Ibuprofen—400 mg 4 times daily not to exceed 2400 mg/day (loading dose 600–800 mg may be helpful).†

Naproxen—550 mg initially then 275 mg or 250 mg tablets not to exceed 1375 mg/day.†

Mefenamic Acid—250 to 500 mg three to four times per day.

Since these medications are used for only a few days per cycle, side effects are usually minimal and tolerable. Gastrointestinal symptoms (indigestion or change in stool frequency) are most common but tend to be mild. The long half-life of naproxen (10–17 hours) with corresponding need for infrequent dosages (often twice a day is sufficient) is an advantage of this preparation for teenagers.

Secondary dysmenorrhea is so common in intrauterine device wearers that routine use of prostaglandin synthetase inhibitors may be justifiable at the time of insertion, since their use will reduce cramping as well as the excessive blood loss that is experienced by many young women using an IUD.

Oral contraceptives are also effective in decreasing dysmenorrhea and should be considered for the adolescent also desiring contraceptive protection, or for the adolescent with a gastrointestinal ulcer for whom nonsteroidal anti-inflammatory agents are contraindicated.

Sexually Transmitted Diseases

JOHN W. KULIG, M.D.

Management of sexually transmitted infections in adolescents and children entails a search for coexisting infection, prescription of appropriate therapy, assurance of adequate follow-up, and provision of health education in hopes of preventing recurrence. Many sexually transmitted organisms produce asymptomatic infection; thus, in addition to the routine performance of gonococcal cultures and a serologic test for syphilis, consideration should be given to obtaining cultures for *Gardnerella vaginalis, Chlamydia trachomatis,* and herpes virus, as well as the examination of wet smears for *Trichomonas* and *Monilia*. In addition, a Papanicolaou smear should be obtained in all sexually active females, since the incidence of cervical dysplasia correlates with the onset of sexual activity, and cytologic changes may provide evidence of sexually transmitted infection including herpes genitalis and condylomata acuminata. Pregnancy should be excluded prior to use of either tetracycline or metronidazole in an adolescent female. Patients should be advised to abstain from intercourse during treatment. Partners must be treated to prevent recurrence, and condom use should be advocated. Diagnosis of sexually transmitted infection also provides an opportunity to discuss contraception. All patients should be scheduled for follow-up evaluation with cultures at an appropriate interval. Presence of a laboratory-confirmed sexually transmitted infection in a child should indicate the strong possibility of sexual abuse and lead to a sensitive but thorough investigation. Finally, many sexually transmitted infections must be reported by law to the appropriate local public health authority.

The following treatment recommendations are based on 1982 guidelines of the Venereal Disease Control Division of the Centers for Disease Control.

---

*This dosage may exceed that recommended by the manufacturer.

†Safety and efficacy in children have not been established.

Gonococcal Infections

Uncomplicated gonococcal urethritis or cervicitis may be treated with aqueous procaine penicillin G, 4.8 million units IM at two sites, with 1.0 gm of probenecid by mouth. Alternatives include amoxicillin, 3.0 gm, or ampicillin, 3.5 gm, either with 1.0 gm probenecid by mouth or tetracycline HC1, 500 mg by mouth, four times a day for 7 days. Tetracycline has the advantage of being effective against coexisting chlamydial infection but the disadvantages of requiring multiple doses and being contraindicated in pregnancy. Pharyngeal gonococcal infection should be treated with either aqueous procaine penicillin G or tetracycline as described above. Anorectal gonococcal infection should be treated with aqueous procaine penicillin G or spectinomycin,*2.0 gm IM in a single injection.

Children who weigh less than 45 kg with uncomplicated gonococcal vulvovaginitis, urethritis, pharyngitis, or proctitis can be treated with aqueous procaine penicillin G, 100,000 units/kg IM, plus probenecid, 25 mg/kg, by mouth (maximum 1.0 g). An alternative for vulvovaginitis or urethritis is amoxicillin, 50 mg/kg, plus probenecid, 25 mg/kg (maximum 1.0 g), both given orally. Children allergic to penicillins may be treated with spectinomycin, 40 mg/kg IM, and children older than 8 years may be treated with tetracycline, 40 mg/kg/day by mouth in four divided doses for 5 days.†Long-acting penicillins, such as benzathine penicillin G, are not effective in the treatment of gonococcal infections.

Treatment regimens for the gonococcal arthritis-dermatitis syndrome include 1) aqueous crystalline penicillin G, 10 million units IV per day until improvement occurs, followed by amoxicillin, 500 mg, or ampicillin, 500 mg, by mouth four times a day to complete at least 7 days of therapy; 2) amoxicillin, 3.0 gm or ampicillin, 3.5 gm by mouth, each with probenecid, 1.0 gm, followed by 7 days of therapy as above, 3) tetracycline HC1, 500 mg by mouth four times a day for at least 7 days, 4) either cefoxitin, 1.0 gm, or cefotaxime, 500 mg, given four times a day IV for at least 7 days, or 5) erythromycin, 500 mg by mouth 4 times a day for at least 7 days. Gonococcal meningitis and endocarditis require high dose IV penicillin therapy for 1 month.

Patients with penicillinase-producing *Neisseria gonorrhoeae* (PPNG) infection should receive spectinomycin, 2.0 gm IM in a single injection. Patients with positive cultures after spectinomycin therapy should be treated with cefoxitin, 2.0 gm IM in a single injection, plus probenecid, 1.0 gm by mouth, or cefotaxime, 1.0 gm IM in a single injection without probenecid. A daily single dose of 9 tablets of trimethoprim/sulfamethoxazole (80 mg/400 mg) for 5 days should be used to treat pharyngeal gonococcal infection due to PPNG.

An asymptomatic infant born to a mother with gonorrhea requires treatment with a single injection of aqueous crystalline penicillin G, 50,000 units, IM or IV, for full-term infants. Neonatal gonococcal ophthalmia requires hospitalization, isolation, and rapid initiation of treatment with aqueous crystalline penicillin G, 50,000 units/kg/day IV in two doses for 7 days. Eyes should be irrigated immediately and then at least hourly, as long as necessary to eliminate discharge. Neonates with arthritis and bacteremia should be hospitalized and treated with aqueous crystalline pencillin G, 75,000 to 100,000 units/kg/day IV in 4 divided doses for at least 7 days. Meningitis should be treated with aqueous crystalline penicillin G, 100,000 units/kg/day IV, divided in three or four doses and continued for at least 10 days. Parents of infants with gonococcal infection require treatment.

Chlamydia trachomatis Infections

Uncomplicated urethral, cervical, or rectal *Chlamydia* infections may be treated with tetracycline hydrochloride, 500 mg by mouth 4 times a day for at least 7 days, or doxycycline, 100 mg by mouth twice a day for at least 7 days. An alternative regimen for pregnant patients or those who do not tolerate tetracycline is erythromycin, 500 mg by mouth four times a day for at least 7 days, or 250 mg by mouth four times a day for at least 14 days if the higher dose is not tolerated. The regimens outlined above are also effective for nongonococcal urethritis, usually caused by *Chlamydia trachomatis* or *Ureaplasma urealyticum.*

Chlamydial conjunctivitis of the newborn is treated with oral erythromycin syrup, 50 mg/kg/day in four divided doses for at least 2 weeks. Topical antibiotic therapy is ineffective and provides no additional benefit. Chlamydial pneumonia of infancy is treated with oral erythromycin syrup, 50 mg/kg/day in four divided doses for at least 3 weeks. The optimal duration for most chlamydial therapy has not been well established.

Prevention of Ophthalmia Neonatorum

Neonatal prophylaxis should be directed against both gonococcal ophthalmia and chlamydial conjunctivitis. Effective preventive treatment against both diseases is provided by either erythromycin (0.5%) or tetracycline (1%) ophthalmic ointment given as a single application immediately postpartum with no rinsing of the eyes. Silver nitrate is effective prophylaxis for gonococcal ophthalmia, but will not prevent chlamydial conjunctivitis.

---

*Safety for use in infants and children has not been established.

†Manufacturer's Warning: Use of tetracycline during the period of tooth development may cause permanent discoloration and inadequate calcification of teeth.

Acute Pelvic Inflammatory Disease

Etiologic agents in acute pelvic inflammatory disease include *Neisseria gonorrhoeae, Chlamydia trachomatis,* anaerobic bacteria including *Bacteroides,* facultative gram-negative rods, *Actinomyces israelii,* and *Mycoplasma hominis.* Differentiating among agents is often impossible, thus antimicrobial therapy is directed against a broad range of pathogens.

Hospitalization should be strongly considered for all patients with PID, but certainly for those cases in which the diagnosis is uncertain, compliance or follow-up is questionable, systemic illness precludes outpatient management, pregnancy or pelvic abscess is suspected, or outpatient therapy has failed. Combined regimens with broad activity include cefoxitin, 2.0 gm IV four times a day, plus doxycycline, 100 mg IV twice a day, or clindamycin, 600 mg IV 4 times a day, plus gentamicin or tobramycin, 2.0 mg/kg IV, followed by 1.5 mg/kg IV three times a day in patients with normal renal function. Intravenous antibiotic therapy should be continued for at least 4 days and at least 48 hours after defervescence. Oral therapy may then be continued with either doxycycline, 100 mg by mouth twice a day, or clindamycin, 450 mg by mouth 4 times a day after discharge from the hospital to complete 10 to 14 days of therapy. A third alternative consists of doxycycline,*100 mg IV twice a day, plus metronidazole, 1.0 gm IV twice a day as above, followed by both drugs orally at the same dosage to complete 10 to 14 days of therapy. Outpatient regimens include 1) cefoxitin, 2.0 gm IM, 2) amoxicillin, 3.0 gm by mouth, 3) ampicillin, 3.5 gm by mouth, or 4) aqueous procaine penicillin G, 4.8 million units IM at two sites, each with probenecid, 1.0 gm by mouth, followed by doxycycline, 100 mg by mouth twice a day for 10 to 14 days.

Syphilis

Primary, secondary, or latent syphilis of less than 1 year's duration should be treated with benzathine penicillin G, 2.4 million units IM in a single injection. Patients who are allergic to penicillin should be treated with tetracycline HCl, 500 mg by mouth 4 times a day for 15 days. Penicillin-allergic patients who cannot tolerate tetracycline can be treated with erythromycin, 500 mg by mouth four times a day for 15 days. Syphilis of more than 1 year's duration, except neurosyphilis, should be treated with benzathine penicillin G, 2.4 million units IM once a week for three successive weeks (7.2 million units total). Alternatives include tetracycline HCl or erythromycin, 500 mg by mouth four times a day for 30 days.

Infants with congenital syphilis should have a cerebrospinal fluid (CSF) examination before treatment. Symptomatic infants or asymptomatic infants with abnormal CSF should be treated with aqueous crystalline penicillin G, 50,000 units/kg IM or IV daily in two divided doses for a minimum of 10 days or aqueous procaine penicillin G, 50,000 units/kg IM daily for a minimum of 10 days. Asymptomatic infants with normal CSF may be treated with benzathine penicillin G, 50,000 units/kg IM in a single injection. All patients with early syphilis and congenital syphilis should be scheduled to return for repeat quantitative nontreponemal tests at least 3, 6, and 12 months after treatment. Retreatment should be considered when clinical signs or symptoms of syphilis persist or recur, there is a fourfold increase in titer with a nontreponemal test, or a nontreponemal test showing a high titer initially fails to show a fourfold decrease within 1 year.

Gardnerella vaginalis Vaginitis

Gardnerella vaginalis (formally known as *Haemophilus vaginalis* or *Corynebacterium vaginale*) vaginitis is treated with metronidazole, 500 mg by mouth twice a day for 7 days. Ampicillin, 500 mg by mouth 4 times a day for 7 days, is less effective but costs much less than metronidazole and is very useful during pregnancy. Vaginal sulfa creams are ineffective.

Trichomoniasis

Trichomonas vaginitis is treated with metronidazole, 2.0 gm by mouth in a single dose, or metronidazole, 250 mg by mouth 3 times a day for 7 days. Ingestion of ethanol should be avoided for 48 hours after treatment owing to a possible disulfiram-like response associated with this medication. Metronidazole is contraindicated in pregnancy. Clotrimazole, 100 mg intravaginally, at bedtime for 7 days may provide symptomatic relief.

Herpes Genitalis

The first clinical episode of herpes genitalis may be treated with acyclovir ointment 5% applied in sufficient quantity to adequately cover all lesions every 3 hours, six times a day for 7 days. Acyclovir has been shown to reduce viral shedding and duration of symptoms in patients with primary infection who are treated within 6 days of onset. There is no effective therapy to prevent recurrence of genital herpes infection or to shorten the duration of symptoms. Symptomatic relief may be achieved with topical anesthetic ointments, povidone-iodine sitz baths, and oral analgesics.

Condylomata Acuminata

External genital and perianal warts may be treated with 10 to 25% podophyllin in compound tincture of benzoin applied carefully while avoiding normal tissue and washed off thoroughly within 4 hours. Podophyllin may be applied weekly for 4 weeks but should not be used during pregnancy. Alternative therapies include cryotherapy, electrosurgery, and surgical excision.

---

*Manufacturer's Warning: Use of drugs of the tetracycline class during tooth development (last half of pregnancy, infancy, and childhood to age 8 years) may cause permanent discoloration of the teeth.

Homosexual Behavior

RICHARD GREEN, M.D.

There is far more homosexual behavior during pre- and early adolescence than there are homosexually oriented adults. This has implications for both child and parent with regard to the enduring significance of such behaviors.

However, what of the minority of late pre- and early adolescents for whom a homosexual identity appears to be emerging? What are its phases of development? Are there differences for males and females?

While some adult homosexuals are aware of strong same-sex attractions during late childhood, most, particularly males, recall the onset during early adolescence. In the homosexually oriented male, there is an earlier emergence of erotic awareness than in the lesbian. Most male homosexuals become aware of the strong affective and erotic drive toward other males during early adolescence, while it is not until late adolescence, and in some cases adulthood, that many females with such an orientation become similarly aware.

The phases of evolving a homosexual identity have been enumerated in clinical studies. There is the phase of "feeling different" from others of the same-sex peer group, perhaps without a specific focus, or of having different interests, romantic and otherwise. "Crushes" on same-sex persons and idols of the same sex may emerge without a clear awareness of their erotic significance. Then, there is the beginning self-definition of oneself as homosexual. This may progress to the "coming out" phase when one defines oneself as having a homosexual orientation to self and to others. There may be a phase deemed "crashing out," in which a frenetic effort at public disclosure and experimentation, sometimes of a flamboyant nature, is made prior to settling into a modulated sexual lifestyle.

The meanings of homosexual behaviors differ for males and females. The meta meanings to males for being homosexual imply "femininity." Witness the terms "fairy," "girl," and "sissy" applied to men with a homosexual orientation, which strike at the core sexual identity of the male. The young man's psychosexual and psychosocial development is tethered—male, virile, and heterosexual. Being female, feminine, and heterosexual is less strongly linked in the female's development. For a female to have a same-sex erotic experience does not strike at her basic self-concept of being female or feminine. Thus, the conflict accompanying a homosexual orientation in adolescence differs for the male, both intrapsychically and as it evokes reaction from the environment.

Stigmatization of the male homosexual is clearly more powerful than that of the lesbian. Male-male relationships, particularly in adulthood, are viewed far more in sexual terms than are female-female relationships. Women may live together, publicly embrace, or kiss without stigma. And parents, prizing the male child, are more concerned with "imperfection" and are more troubled if they sense a "defect" in their son. Further, it is the heterosexually reproducing man who carries the family name.

Indeed, counseling with the parents of adolescents who may be "homosexual" is more problematic than counseling the adolescent. "Where did I go wrong?" is the oft-asked question. This is *not* a time for finger-pointing, but rather a time for reconciliation. No advantage is gained by blaming or responding directly to that question. Rather there is a need to maintain a family relating as harmoniously as possible. A significant sign of progress toward this goal has been the evolution in recent years of organizations of parents of gay adolescents. Here parents with similar feelings of guilt, shame, and embarrassment meet to share these feelings. The expectation is that they work them through so they may continue positive relationships with their children rather than experiencing the pain of parents who have "failed," or have been "betrayed."

What of dealing with the adolescent? First, find out what the adolescent *means* when he or she says, "I am homosexual" or "I think I'm homosexual." Does he or she mean that erotic fantasies involve both males and females? That homosexual fantasies exist along with heterosexual behaviors? That one's fantasies and behaviors are exclusively oriented to persons of the same sex? Or that one has had one or two "homosexual" experiments?

Adolescence is a time for keeping options open. Many primarily or exclusively homosexually oriented young adults recall a bisexual early adolescence. Sometimes, circumstances block off one of two paths. Other times, a premature decision is made to progress down one. With the vast majority of life ahead, more flexibility is available to the teenager.

But, how is flexibility to be maintained? One cannot always conjure up, with the rubbing of a magic ring, real life flesh and blood sexual partners. However, there is the readily available surrogate—fantasy. The flames of fantasy may be fanned by commercially available visual erotica. Pornography, in whatever form, whether it be a Sears Roebuck catalogue or a *Playboy* centerfold, is a readily available source for rehearsing and reinforcing erotic pleasures. This is done via masturbation.

Supportive options are open for the gay adolescent. Recent years have witnessed the advent of gay counseling centers and religious organizations committed to the compatibility of a homosexual orientation and maintenance of religious fidelity, such as the Metropolitan Community Church and Dignity, the latter being primarily for Catholics. Indeed there is a quiet (at times not so quiet) revolution going on within several churches with respect to accepting a homosexual orientation as compatible with the value systems considered important by these religious groups.

For the medical professional person, in addition to highlighting options there is also the responsibility of objectively balancing advantages versus disadvantages of a homosexual, heterosexual, or bisexual lifestyle. From what we know about the degree of stigma contemporaneously, historically, and in the future, other advantages and disadvantages associated with these lifestyles ought to be articulated in a nonjudgmental fashion. Caveat! Keep in mind that with the most highly motivated of patients and the best intentioned of therapists, two thirds of primarily or exclusively homosexual adults do not reorient to heterosexuality.

For the homosexually active adolescent, notably the young man, the clinician ought to be competent in those medical illnesses more likely to be associated with homosexual activities, including hepatitis, amebiasis, giardiasis, shigellosis, and AIDS.

A note about differential diagnosis. Consider homosexuality, transvestism, and transsexualism. The clinician is occasionally confronted by the anxious parent of a male adolescent who has been discovered secreting away or actually dressing in women's attire. Typically this is fetishistic (erotically arousing) behavior, properly termed "transvestism." Since the value system in our culture is such that parents are greatly concerned about homosexuality in their sons, it is usually reassuring for them to know that transvestites are typically heterosexual, marry, and father children. It is additionally reassuring that we have no idea how many adolescents experience a fetishistic cross-dressing phase in their psychosexual development that is transitory, fading by adulthood.

For the transsexual-appearing adolescent—the teenager who wishes hormones and sex reassignment procedures—the problems are more significant. Here we encounter the person with intrapsychic conflict of belonging to the "wrong sex," with accompanying social stigma and an anatomically same sex orientation. Management of these cases is detailed in the literature. By way of summary: do the reversible before the *ir*reversible. Enable the adolescent to continue school, perhaps "trying on" the new gender role through cross-dressing and a new school enrollment in the desired gender role. Adolescence, volatile as it is in most area, is especially volatile here. Some adolescents move away from transsexualism, perhaps settling into more comfortable lifestyles, including homosexuality. Deter self-destructive behavior, whether it be flamboyantly stealing wom-

ens' clothes as a "cry for help," dropping out of school, indiscriminate sexual behavior without understanding venereal disease symptoms, or cutting oneself off from a family social system that can be supportive during later years.

Finally, there is need for personal dignity, sexual privacy, and interpersonal responsibility to accompany sexual behavior by males and females, whether conducted by males with males or females, or by females with females or males. The quality, not the anatomy, of the relationship is central. The adolescent has the right to erect a sign on the bedroom door stating "Judgmentalists, Keep Out!"

Premarital Counseling

ELIZABETH R. McANARNEY, M.D.,
and DONALD E. GREYDANUS, M.D.

We shall define premarital counseling, or responsible sexuality, broadly and focus on the overall health education that occurs when the pediatrician actively teaches young patients about themselves. As developmentally oriented physicians, pediatricians are in an ideal position to work with children and their families to encourage responsible sexuality in their patients.

As children mature and services are directed toward them more than toward their parents, routine child and adolescent well visits should include discussions of normal growth and development, instruction about the differences between males and females, and breast and testicular self-examination.

Inclusion of Males and Females in Sexuality-Related Services. Pediatricians routinely examine the external genitalia of male infants, children, and adolescents, but, because of lack of visibility, may fail to include a routine inspection of the female genitals between infancy and adolescence. On the other hand, at adolescence we may focus pregnancy prevention services exclusively on females and fail to counsel male adolescents about their sexual responsibility. We suggest that pediatricians consider continuing an inspection of the female genitalia from infancy through adolescence and consider including males as well as females in their counseling about responsible sexuality. If the adolescent female is the pediatrician's patient and seeks pregnancy prevention services, then her male partner should be invited in to be included; conversely, if the male adolescent seeks preventive services, his female partner should be included.

Thus, by addressing sexuality-related concerns with parents initially and subsequently with their children and adolescents in the pediatrician's office, when the young person reaches adolescence there will be minimal discomfort on the pediatrician's and adolescent's part when specific sexuality-related services are required. By including males and females in sexuality-related services, there will be encouragement and an expectation of sexual responsibility by both males and females.

Normal Growth and Development. The pediatrician should ask prepubertal and pubertal young people about pubertal changes that they have observed. This history is best obtained in the absence of the parent. If the adolescent does not offer any personal observations about growth and development, questions can be addressed about the changes in the adolescent's height, weight, facial bones, breasts, and so on, which the pediatrician has documented on the physical examination. If, on physical examination, the pediatrician notices normal variants such as female breast asymmetry or gynecomastia, a discussion with the adolescent can be initiated: "Many young women's breasts are normally different sizes. (Pause) I notice yours are. (Pause) Have you noticed this? (Pause) This is normal." On examining a male adolescent with gynecomastia: "Some males have some breast enlargement, known as gynecomastia. I notice you have some gynecomastia, which may be embarrassing. (Pause) This is normal, but can make one feel uncomfortable." The pediatrician is encouraging the adolescent to be aware of his or her body and to become interested in normal bodily changes.

In addition to discussion about the adolescent's physical growth and development, the pediatrician should focus on the new sensations and feelings young people experience. Responsible sexuality discussions should include developing an understanding of other people's feelings and the fact that emotional relationships are an integral part of sexual relationships.

Instruction About Male and Female Differences. Sharing observations made during physical examination and actually teaching adolescents about male and female anatomy, menstruation, nocturnal emissions, erections, and responsibility in sexuality are important components of health education. Most young men and women are very interested in learning specific information about the opposite sex. Good reading materials and models of male and female anatomy are helpful in making the information more understandable to the adolescent.

Breast and Testicular Self-Examination. Patients often are the first to note changes in their bodies that may signify a pathologic process. Young women should be taught breast self-examination and young men, testicular self-examination. The breasts and male external genitalia during adolescence are charged with sexual feelings, which may make some adolescents uncomfortable about discussing such an examination and possibly even touching themselves. Since the incidence of breast carcinoma in adolescent women is low, the discovery of a malignant lesion during the adolescent years is minimal. Fibroadenomas may be identified by the adolescent. Testicular carcinoma may be initially noted in the late teens or early to mid 20s, so there is an immediate reason to teach testicular self-examination to adolescent males. A major reason for teaching breast and testicular self-examination is to develop a sense of responsibility for and comfort with one's body as one enters adulthood.

Adolescent Sexuality, Contraception, Abortion, and Pregnancy

ELIZABETH R. McANARNEY, M.D., *and* DONALD E. GREYDANUS, M.D.

PRIMARY PREVENTION OF ADOLESCENT PREGNANCY

Pregnancy during adolescence can be prevented by abstaining from coitus or, if the young person is sexually active,* by utilizing effective contraception. The pediatrician's role in these services will be emphasized.

Abstinence. Nearly 50% of unmarried women and 30% to 40% of males have not experienced coitus by 19 years of age. Many will at some time during adolescence question whether to delay or initiate coital activity. They may not be able to discuss their concerns about this with their parents, for whom the subject may be uncomfortable, and they may be unable to talk with peers for whom it appears that "everyone is doing it." Adolescents who are encouraged to discuss their feelings and concerns with their pediatricians may be relieved to find a nonparental, nonjudgmental professional with whom they can discuss their decision-making. Some may be seeking approval for their abstinence, while others may be seeking information from an adult about whether all their peers are sexually active. If they are considering initiating sexual activity, they may want to know what preventive services are available.

If sexuality-related concerns have been an integral part of the pediatrician's health care plan throughout the child's adolescent life, these issues can be addressed comfortably. Exploration of the adolescent's decision-making, of his or her future plans for family, and of future plans for education can be included in sexuality-related discussions. Instruction on the availability and accessibility of preventive services is also important.

Responsible Sexual Activity. Approximately

---

*Sexual activity is used interchangeably with coital activity.

50% of unmarried females and 60% to 70% of males have had coitus by the age of 19 years. Responsibility in sexual relationships becomes a critical theme in helping these young people prevent unwanted pregnancy. This theme can be initiated early in childhood and adolescence and should include responsibility in sexual matters as well as in other areas of life such as school, job, and family.

Well adolescent care should include specific questions about dating patterns and sexual activity, when appropriate. If the adolescent is group dating only, sexual activity is unlikely and, thus, specific questions about sexual activity can be eliminated. If the adolescent is sexually active, a thorough and honest discussion about whether he or she wants a pregnancy should follow. If pregnancy is not wanted, then a thorough discussion about contraceptive methods might be initiated.

Contraception during adolescence is a complex issue. The choice of a contraceptive method depends upon the cognitive development of the adolescent and the choice as to which method he or she prefers. Pediatricians should be knowledgeable about the adolescent's cognitive development, as, for example, a preformal operational young person would not be expected to take a diaphragm with her on her date and place it before coitus. The adolescent's choice of a method becomes particularly vital, as the effectiveness of the contraceptive method depends upon compliance, particularly with the birth control pill, diaphragm, condom, and foam.

It is imperative that the physician who discusses contraception needs with the adolescent patient also be fully prepared to perform a pelvic examination before prescribing specific methods. Indeed, a basic understanding of both adolescent sexuality and basic gynecology will allow the clinician to provide considerable primary and secondary care. The major gynecologic procedure pediatricians should learn is the pelvic examination.

There is considerable debate regarding the timing of a pelvic examination for non–sexually active asymptomatic adolescents, for whom we recommend examination between the ages of 15 and 18. A general physical examination, including careful evaluation of the breasts and abdomen, is usually done preceding pelvic evaluation. The girl who is sexually active needs a pelvic evaluation, regardless of her age.

The first procedure of the pelvic examination is inspection of the external genitalia, including visualization of the pubic hair, mons veneris, clitoris, labia, urethra, and hymenal ring. A reliable light source producing full illumination is critical. Visualization of the vagina and cervix is then undertaken. Although an otoscope, a vaginoscope, or a cystoscope are useful for examining a child, teenagers require the use of a speculum lubricated with warm water (not petroleum jelly or other sub-stances). The long, thin *Huffman speculum* is used for most adolescents, while the thicker *Pederson speculum* may be used for sexually active teenagers—if they can tolerate it. A *Graves type* can be utilized for multiparous youth.

Suggestions are as follows: 1) keep the instrument posterior to avoid irritating the urethra or clitoris. 2) place the speculum slowly, while you tell her what you are doing. Often, suggesting that the adolescent bear down as if she were having a bowel movement will facilitate insertion of the speculum. 3) Avoid long periods of silence and explain any sounds (such as the clicking of a speculum or the crackling of paper). 4) Stop and re-evaluate your procedure if pain or discomfort develops. Empathy is needed here, certainly *not* roughness or speed. 5) Carefully look for bleeding, discharge, tenderness, and abnormal vaginocervical pathology.

A common phenomenon is cervical erosion, in which the epithelium of the ectocervix is replaced by endocervical columnar epithelium. After the examination, carefully remove the speculum and perform a bimanual vaginal examination and a rectal examination, while observing for uterine-adnexal-rectal problems, such as pregnancy, ovarian cysts, salpingitis, proctitis, and others. After this procedure is completed, careful explanations are necessary to communicate your findings and to discuss therapeutic intervention and follow-up plans (to the patient and parents or guardians). Contraceptive advice can then be given. A discussion of the contraceptive methods now follows.

CONTRACEPTION

In view of the significant coital activity and resultant high pregnancy rate noted among today's adolescents, we recommend that health care professionals (including pediatricians) who care for sexually active adolescents also provide contraceptive information and/or contraception to them. The clinician who cannot provide contraception (or information) should refer them to appropriate sources.

Although most clinicians would recommend abstinence, it should be remembered that some sexually active young people will *not* accept this recommendation. Also, although some young people are *not* motivated to avoid pregnancy, many who are coitally active wish to avoid pregnancy by the use of specific contraceptive methods. Some of these methods are now reviewed.

Barrier Methods

The method of choice for sexually active adolescents is a barrier method, whether a diaphragm with vaginal cream (or foam) or condoms with or without vaginal contraceptives.

Diaphragm. This is a rubber cap with a metallic rim that is precoitally placed with contraceptive cream or jelly in the vagina. It is removed 6 hours or so after sexual activity. Coil-spring or flat-spring diaphragms are the types most commonly used, and the pediatrician can easily learn to fit the proper-size diaphragm (50 mm to 105 mm in diameter) for his or her patients. It is a safe and effective method if used properly with *each* coital act.

The side effects are few, including an occasional allergic reaction to the rubber or contraceptive agent and a foreign body vaginitis if the diaphragm is left in place for several days. Many adolescents, however, do not like either the normal genital intimacy or the constant need for sex preparation required for its use. Pediatricians should note that some adolescents are not ready to accept the diaphragm during adolescence but may later in their lives. Thus the diaphragm can always be offered, despite what the patient is or is not using.

Condom. This is another barrier method that can be used by many males as a very effective and safe contraceptive method whether used alone, with a diaphragm, or with various vaginal contraceptives. Lubricated types with a reservoir-tip are recommended, and there are many high-quality brands available today. Partial protection from sexually transmitted diseases is an added benefit. The use of the condom also allows the interested male to take an active and effective contraceptive role.

Vaginal Contraceptives. There are many types of vaginal contraceptives (topical spermicides) available, including creams, gels, foams, pastes, suppositories, and others. Foam appears to be the best agent, and cream the second best, because of greater intravaginal coverage. Most are effective as soon as applied, but suppositories need 10 to 15 minutes to melt. Vaginal contraceptives are placed in the vagina, usually near the cervix, prior to coitus. Repeated applications are needed with repeated coitus. In general, the topical spermicides should be used with other barrier methods and *not* be relied on as the *sole* contraceptive method. A new agent, the contraceptive collagen sponge (which is left in place for several days), is now being tested and may prove to be a better method than the basic vaginal contraceptive.

Oral Contraceptives

The most popular of the effective contraceptives is the combined birth control pill, which contains a fixed combination of an estrogen (ethinyl estradiol or mestranol) and a progestogen (norethynodrel, norethindrone, norethindrone acetate, ethynodiol diacetate, or norgestrel). If the young girl is having regular coitus and does not want a barrier method, the birth control pill is usually the best and safest method in the medically screened individual.

Absolute contraindications to use of the pill include a history of thromboembolism or thrombotic disease; active acute or chronic liver disease; undiagnosed uterine bleeding; pregnancy; breast cancer;

and other estrogen-dependent neoplasia. A 30 to 50 μg estrogen pill is currently recommended to reduce the risk of thromboembolism.

There are various conditions listed as *relative contraindications* for pill usage, in which the risks of pill-induced complications must be weighed against the pregnancy risks and in which the clinical judgment of a knowledgeable physician can help the adolescent female make appropriate decisions. In general, we recommend avoidance of the pill in those with hyperlipidemia, severe migraine headaches (especially with prolonged auras), hypertension, cyanotic heart disease, diabetes mellitus, uterine leiomyomata, lactation, coagulation disorders, major organ disease (such as renal, pulmonary, or hepatic), retinal disorders, porphyria, and chorea. Caution should be exercised in adolescents on regular medications. For example, failure of contraception (with subsequent pregnancy) has been reported in pill-taking women on antiepileptic drugs and also various antibiotics. If a specific medical problem is noted in the medical screening, the physician should understand current medical thinking about whether or not the pill is advisable.* However, the pill is not necessarily contraindicated just because a medical problem is noted.

Some issues are controversial and require clinical judgment. For example, the cause and effect relationship between pill use and depression is not clear, but women with severe depression are not usually given birth control pills. Nor is the pill usually prescribed for adolescents who experience irregular menstrual periods. The pill is usually prescribed for those who have been menstruating regularly for at least 6 months to a year. If the patient has irregular menses, she should be carefully evaluated for its reason. Oligomenorrhea, for example, may be due to various conditions. Before giving the pill, the physician should consult with a gynecologist. However, if the adolescent girl is at risk for pregnancy and a specific disorder is not found, the pill is usually warranted. Current studies do not support previous concerns that the pill causes oversuppression of the hypothalamic-pituitary axis and thus significant postpill amenorrhea.

Any young girl who is taking birth control pills should be carefully monitored for pill-induced side effects. We usually see the adolescent in 6 weeks for her first post-pill evaluation. A weight gain of 5 pounds with or without edema is common and is usually of little concern. A slight rise in blood pressure is also common. Acne vulgaris may develop or worsen and usually improves with current treatment modalities. Monilial vaginitis is not unusual and readily responds to intravaginal application of

---

*Greydanus, D.E.: Alternatives to adolescent pregnancy: A discussion of the contraceptive literature from 1960 to 1980. Semin. Perinatol. 5:53–90, 1981.

miconazole nitrate or clotrimazole cream for 7 nights. Intermenstrual spotting (breakthrough bleeding) may occur and frequently resolves over two to four cycles. Occasionally, 10–20 μg of ethinyl estradiol for 7 to 10 days is added to prevent recurrence. Intermenstrual bleeding that occurs after several months of pill use may be due to progestin deficiency, and may improve after switching to a brand with more progestin activity.

If any of the listed absolute contraindications develop, the pill is stopped immediately. If elective surgery is planned, the pill is stopped to reduce the incidence of postsurgical thrombosis. Heparin may be used for adolescents who must undergo emergency surgery. The development of relative contraindications may indicate the need to discontinue the pill. Other contraindications are melasma, erythema nodosum, angioedema, pseudotumor cerebri, cholelithiasis, mesenteric vascular disease, collagen vascular disease, inflammatory bowel disease, hypothalamic-pituitary dysfunction, and others. Another contraindication is the inability of some adolescents to take the pill each day or to return regularly for evaluations. After the first 6-week evaluation we recommend follow-ups every 3 to 6 months, depending on the situation. It is unwise to see teenage patients annually for contraceptive evaluation, since life circumstances can change so rapidly. Frequent monitoring for sexually transmitted diseases is important. We also recommend annual Papanicolaou smears for sexually active adolescents on oral contraceptives.

Most medically screened adolescents do well on the pill. Current studies do not support fears that long-term pill use causes post-pill amenorrhea, neoplasms, or thromboembolic disease in adolescents. Young girls may note improvement in such conditions as benign breast disease, cystic ovarian disease, dysmenorrhea, and/or dysfunctional uterine bleeding. Most major problems are found in adult women. However, we do not recommend long-term use in teenagers: an adolescent at high risk of pregnancy is placed on the pill, but she is changed to another method when she can accept such alternatives and is mature enough to use them safely. Pregnancy is prevented at a crucial time in the adolescent's life, and the risks of such an event far exceed any risk the pill may present. The mortality rate for women aged 15 to 19 is 1.2 deaths per 100,000 pill users (1.4 for those who smoke) versus 11.1 maternal deaths per 100,000 live births.

Finally, there are two other "pills" the clinician should consider. The "triphasic" pill has been introduced in Europe, and consists of three changes in concentrations of estrogen and progestogen during each monthly cycle. It seems to produce less breakthrough bleeding and less acne while remaining an effective contraceptive method. Also, the mini-pill, which is a progesterone-only type of pill,

has been available for many years. The mini-pill causes fewer vascular and metabolic effects than does the birth control pill. However, it produces less effective contraception and more abnormal menstrual irregularities. The mini-pill is an alternative when the combined birth control pill is contraindicated (as in diabetes mellitus, cyanotic heart disease, or sickle cell anemia). This pill is started on day 1 of the menstrual cycle, while the combined pill is usually started on day 5.

Intrauterine Devices (IUD)

The placement of a metallic or plastic device within the uterus for contraception remains a controversial issue. The most common IUDs used for teenagers are the copper 7 or T-types, in which copper wire is wrapped around the basic IUD stem. This IUD must be inserted (usually during menses) by a trained professional who is also capable of following the patient for the many possible side effects: menorrhagia, dysmenorrhea, uterine perforation (rare), ectopic pregnancy, pelvic infection, and others. The major problem associated with IUD's is the markedly increased incidence of pelvic inflammatory disease noted in wearers. Current literature indicates that there *is* a role for this effective contraceptive agent in teenagers, but potential IUD wearers must be carefully screened, must have a low risk for sexually transmitted disease, must accept no other effective method, and must allow for careful follow-up.

Postcoital Contraception

Diethylstilbestrol (DES)*has been used to prevent conception after coitus has taken place. It is given at an oral dose of 25 mg twice a day, for 5 days within 72 hours of coitus. Nausea and emesis are the main acute side effects. Pregnancy must be ruled out and a signed consent obtained prior to administration of the DES, in view of the genital abnormalities associated with some DES-offspring. Other postcoital methods that have been successfully used include other types of estrogen, synthetic progestogens, and even the IUD.

Injectable Contraceptives

Depo-medroxyprogesterone acetate (Depo-Provera)†can be given at an intramuscular dose of 150 mg every 3 months. It is as effective as the pill, and is recommended when the pill is difficult to administer or in situations where the pill is actually contraindicated. Depo-Provera has a specific role in mentally ill or mentally retarded adolescent females who are at high risk for pregnancy.

---

*FDA has concluded that the use of DES as a postcoital contraceptive is safe for use as emergency treatment only. Do not use as a routine method of birth control.

†This use of Depo-Provera is not listed by the manufacturer.

The major side effects include irregular menstrual bleeding, amenorrhea, abnormal glucose tolerance curves, nausea, emesis, headache, and weight gain. There has also been some concern by the Food and Drug Administration about a possible carcinogenic potential of Depo-Provera, but it should be noted that a direct association has not been proven, and it is approved in over 90 countries around the world as an effective contraceptive agent.

Miscellaneous Methods

Rhythm Methods. Avoidance of coitus around the estimated time of ovulation is a time-honored contraceptive method. Such estimation is based on various schemes, including observation of menstrual regularity, basal body temperature measurements, and changes in cervical mucus. The latter observation is called the Billings or ovulation method and relies on a "raw egg white appearance" of the cervical mucus (Spinnbarkeit) to identify the periovulatory period. Unfortunately, most adolescents are not motivated to use such methods of periodic abstinence, and it remains to be shown the real usefulness of these methods for the adolescent population. Methods of periodic abstinence may be considered for very motivated and trained teenagers.

Coitus Interruptus. Penile withdrawal prior to ejaculation is another common method that can be used by some teenage males. Considerable self-control is needed, however, and the possibility of sperm in the pre-ejaculatory fluid is a potential problem.

Noncoital Sex. Discussion with adolescents about their sexuality may lead to consideration of various aspects of noncoital sex, including kissing, fondling, oral-genital contact, masturbation and others. Clinicians, of course, have specific personal views in this area. It is important for clinicians to remember we are helping adolescents make *their own* judgments about sexual expression, not imposing *our* own. The value of noncoital sex in preventing coitus is variable, depending on the individual adolescent.

Douche. This is a common method among adolescents. Clinicians should discourage its use as a contraceptive method, since there is a very high failure rate ("pregnancy rate"), associated with its use. We can advise our patients of contraceptive methods that *may* work in selected cases (such as coitus interruptus or noncoital sex) and also those that simply do *not* work (such as postcoital douches). The douche, of course, can be part of normal perineal hygiene.

Lactation. The breastfeeding woman does delay her postpartum menstruation, but not indefinitely or predictably. Most will ovulate 7 to 9 months after birth despite lactation, and nearly all by 12 months.

Thus, lactation should not be relied on as the sole contraceptive method, especially 6 months or more after delivery.

Sterilization. Tubal ligation and vasectomy are certainly technically possible for any pubertal individual wishing permanent contraception. However, the moral and ethical overtones associated with the idea of sterilizing teenagers are such that it is not done, except in very unusual circumstances.

SECONDARY PREVENTION OF PREGNANCY

Once an adolescent is diagnosed as being pregnant, it is imperative that she and her partner decide about the disposition of the pregnancy. The pediatrician can initiate a discussion about this and should encourage inclusion of her partner or family, or both. They may choose to continue the pregnancy and keep or place the child for adoption or have an abortion. Whatever the decision, an early referral to obstetric or abortion services is imperative and maximizes outcome.

Obstetric services for those who choose to continue their pregnancies are delivered by obstetricians-gynecologists, certified nurse-midwives, or family physicians. Specialized adolescent maternity projects, such as the Rochester Adolescent Maternity Project (RAMP) in Rochester, New York, provide obstetric and psychosocial services to pregnant adolescents and their families and produce higher compliance with services and subsequently improved obstetric, neonatal, and psychosocial outcome than traditional services. Adolescents should have obstetric and neonatal outcome similar to that of adult women of similar backgrounds as long as they receive adequate prenatal services. Women less than 15 years of age have more premature babies than older adolescents and adult women, the exact reasons for which are unclear.

If the community does not have a specialized adolescent maternity project where obstetric and psychosocial services are delivered, and if the patient receives her prenatal care with an individual obstetric provider, the pediatrician may choose to provide psychosocial services and support to pregnant adolescents. This can be done by group work with pregnant adolescents in the office or through individual counseling. Subjects that warrant discussion include: the anatomy and physiology of pregnancy, labor and delivery, feelings about being pregnant, changing body structure, family response to the pregnancy, peers' responses to the pregnancy, responsibility for a child, and child care. Inclusion of the father of the baby as well as the families is often valued.

The adolescent who has an abortion will benefit from preabortion and postabortion discussion of her feelings. It is ideal to include the male partner as well, as he may need help about the way he feels about the abortion and may actually become depressed following the abortion. Specific discussions about the procedure, who will be present, what the procedure is like, what her family thinks, and if the family knows about the abortion are important.

The obstetrician-gynecologist has various abortion techniques available to him or her, including dilatation and currettage, dilatation and evacuation, vacuum curettage, intra-amniotic fluid injection (such as hypertonic saline, prostaglandins, or urea), hysterotomy and hysterectomy. The dilatation and curettage or suction abortion techniques are usually done in the first trimester (before the twelfth week), while the hypertonic injection method is used in the second trimester (usually not before the sixteenth week). Each method has its own risks and must be done by a very well-trained professional. Legal abortions are usually possible, in selected cases, up to the time of fetal viability (24–26 weeks).

The pediatrician can provide counseling to the adolescent contemplating abortion or refer the adolescent to a reputable agency or health care source where this counseling can be obtained. The individual who is postabortion should be provided with contraceptive information and, if requested, specific contraception. The current legal climate regarding abortion is quite dynamic, and the clinician should become aware of national and local laws and regulations regarding the availability of abortion to youth in his or her area.

Some adolescents who have either borne children or had abortions may need public health nurse referrals, which the pediatrician should utilize freely. The public health nurse can initiate open and thorough discussions of resolution of the initial pregnancy and prevention of subsequent pregnancies if the adolescents desire to remain nonpregnant.

Alcohol and Drug Abuse

MILTON WESTPHAL, M.D.

More than half of all American children will have experienced the effects of alcohol or an illicit psychoactive substance by the time they graduate from high school, and as many as 10% will have become regular alcohol or drug abusers. Although most abandon drug use before serious social or physiologic consequences occur, many experience acute effects of alcohol or drug use that demand medical intervention. These children are brought to doctors' offices and emergency rooms by friends, parents, or police, who frequently are unable to provide accurate information on the type or dose of the offending drug. Knowledge of the current street jargon is helpful, and drug screens of urine and blood help clarify diagnoses, but often treatment of

Table 1. DRUG CLASSIFICATION

Class	Examples
Cannabinols	Marijuana, hashish
Depressants	Barbiturates, diazepam, meprobamate, alcohol
Hallucinogens	LSD, mescaline, DOM, PCP
Opiates	Heroin, morphine, meperidine
Stimulants	Amphetamine, cocaine

acute reactions must be started with incomplete knowledge of drugs taken. Poison information centers and substance abuse programs are aware of the drugs currently popular in their areas. They can provide up-to-date information on diagnosis and treatment. See Table 1 for classifications of drugs.

ACUTE REACTIONS

There are six recognizable types of acute reaction to drug abuse. These can be classified as panic, flashback, pharmacologic response, psychotic behavior, overdose, and withdrawal.

Panic. Panic usually occurs in an inexperienced or first time user of marijuana, a hallucinogen, or a stimulant. Upon experiencing the effects of the drug the patient develops an acute anxiety state based on the belief that he has done himself serious physical harm, that he is losing control of himself, or that he is going insane. Physical manifestations are those of acute anxiety, tachycardia, mild hypertension, hyperreflexia, dilated pupils, and increased perspiration.

Treatment should be conservative. Once other causes of the symptoms have been reasonably well excluded, the patient should be kept in a quiet, nonthreatening environment with supportive friends or family around him. Repeated reassurance is important. The expected drug action and duration should be described and the patient should be frequently reoriented to time, space, and person, and given emotional support. Recovery usually will occur spontaneously as the drug effects wear off. Medication should be avoided if possible, but if absolutely necessary diazepam (Valium) orally or deep intramuscularly, 5 to 10 mg in children and 15 to 30 mg in the larger adolescents, may be used. The drug may be repeated in 1 to 3 hours, using a lower dose if possible.

Flashback. Flashbacks occur after prolonged use of cannabinols or the hallucinogens, and so are infrequent in preadolescents. History reveals prior experience but no recent drug exposure. In cannabinol users there is a sensation of slow thinking and mild disorientation in time, generally less intense than the experience of a marijuana high. The flashbacks last only 1 or 2 minutes. With hallucinogens lights or figures appear in the peripheral vision, and moving objects may be followed by a trail of light. The patients may feel euphoric, detached, may have feelings of depersonalization or have emotional reactions they had previously experienced immediately after taking the drug. Episodes often clear within minutes but may last for several hours. Exposure to marijuana may precipitate hallucinogen flashbacks, and the symptoms are generally milder than those that occur with drug use. Since the symptoms are self-limited, intervention should be restricted to reassurance and education about the nature of the episodes. Drug therapy should be avoided if possible. Patients should be told that flashbacks may occur for a month or more after the last exposure to a drug and should be warned that other medications such as stimulants, antihistamines, and particularly marijuana may precipitate flashbacks. Though the flashback itself is generally mild, the patient, believing that he suffered permanent brain damage or is becoming psychotic, may panic. If panic is severe, is not responsive to reassurance and comforting, and seems to be a threat to the patient, Valium, orally or deep intramuscularly at 5 to 10 mg in children and 15 to 30 mg in large adolescents, may be used. Repeated doses of 2 to 5 mg of diazepam may help when flashbacks are recurring.

Pharmacologic Response. The pharmacologic response to drug abuse varies with the drug used and the dose taken. The cannabinols, the stimulants, the opiates and analgesics, the depressants, and the hallucinogens each have distinct clinical manifestation that in the acute setting are self-limited. Once it has been determined that the symptoms are not a result of drug overdose and are not manifestations of trauma, psychosis, central nervous system injury or infection, hemorrhage, or other systemic disease, conservative management may be undertaken. The patient and parents should be reassured and an explanation of the timing and action of the suspected drug explained. State of consciousness and vital signs should be followed closely until symptoms are clearing so that the progressive manifestations of an overdose can be recognized and supportive therapy begun.

Relatively small doses of alcohol can produce severe hypoglycemia in children. The blood glucose may fall low enough to cause unconsciousness and seizures. The hypoglycemia responds to 2 ml/kg of 25% glucose IV but may recur over the next 12 hours and require retreatment.

Response to PCP is best treated by minimizing sensory input by dimming lights and reducing ambient noise or using ear plugs. Thirty gm of activated charcoal (Antichar) in 100 ml of magnesium citrate is given by mouth to children of 30 to 40 kg and repeated if vomited. The dose may be doubled for patients weighing over 40 kg. After allowing about 1 hour for gastric emptying of the charcoal and laxative, continuous gastric drainage is instituted, since the acidic gastric juice will contain a high concentration of PCP. The patient's vital signs, electrolytes, and urinary output must be carefully watched for signs of dehydration and electrolyte imbalance. Fluid and electrolyte losses, particularly potassium and chloride should be replaced intravenously. Gastric drainage is continued until the symptoms disappear. Then the patient is put on 1 to 2 grams of ascorbic acid and 100 to 200 ml of cranberry juice four times a day for 5 to 7 days to acidify the urine and speed urinary excretion of any remaining PCP.

Psychotic Behavior. Hallucinations, delusions, or paranoia with hostility and outbursts of violence may be seen after protracted use of the hallucinogens, PCP, atropine-like drugs, depressants, or stimulants and are occasionally seen after a single large dose of an amphetamine. In patients with no previous history of a psychiatric disorder, the psychotic reaction will usually clear spontaneously within a week and often clears within 24 hours. After excluding the possibility that a psychotic state preceded drug use, therapy should be directed at comforting and reassuring the patient while protecting him from injuring himself or others. Psychiatric hospitalization may be necessary until the reaction clears. Medication should be avoided if possible. Diazepam and other depressants may precipitate violence in a patient showing psychotic manifestations from amphetamines. Any use of psychoactive drugs in treating psychotic reactions should be guided by an expert in the field. Psychotic behavior from PCP may continue for as long as a month but will respond to acidification of urine as described in the section on pharmacologic response.

Overdose. Overdose occurs when the patient has taken enough drug to overwhelm his homeostatic mechanisms and threaten his survival. Overdose is most often seen when the patient has taken an opiate, alcohol, or other central nervous system depressant or one of the hallucinogens.

THE OPIATES. The opiates cause respiratory depression, hypoxia with cyanosis, cardiac arrhythmias, seizures, and shock. Immediate respiratory and circulatory support must be instituted and all of the parameters important to intensive care and life support must be monitored and managed. Naloxone (Narcan) is given intravenously in a dose of 0.01 mg/kg to a maximum of 0.4 mg. If improvement is not immediate, the dose may be repeated at 2 to 3 minute intervals for up to three doses. Supplemental intramuscular doses of naloxone may be required at 1 to 2 hour intervals until the opiate has been metabolized or excreted and its effects have disappeared. Naloxone is nontoxic and in the absence of opiates has negligible pharmacologic effects. In patients addicted to heroin or other opiates, naloxone may precipitate acute withdrawal symptoms that require management.

ALCOHOL AND OTHER CNS DEPRESSANTS. Overdose with alcohol and the CNS depressants causes cardiorespiratory depression and failure like that seen with the opiates, but the symptoms do not respond to naloxone. Management is based on the principles of life support and intensive care. Intubation, respiratory control, and cardiovascular support may be needed. If an overdose of barbiturates has been taken orally, repeated gastric lavage with activated charcoal (Antichar, each 30 grams suspended in 100 ml of water) may be useful as long as 24 hours after the ingestion. As large as possible a tube should be used. A cuffed endotracheal tube will protect against aspiration during lavage. 150 to 250 ml of the activated charcoal suspension should be left in the stomach. With alcohol overdose blood glucose must be followed closely since severe hypoglycemia often occurs. Prompt treatment with IV 25% glucose, 2 ml/kg, is important.

HALLUCINOGENS AND STIMULANTS. Hallucinogens and stimulants at very high doses cause respiratory depression, seizures, hyperthermia, and severe hypertension. The symptoms may require life support and intensive care. Seizures usually can be controlled with a slow intravenous injection of Valium in a dose of 5 to 20 mg. The hyperthermia may require use of a cooling blanket. Diazoxide* (Hyperstat) intravenously in a dose of 1 to 3 mg/kg (maximum 150 mg) is used to control dangerous degrees of hypertension. The dose may be repeated at intervals of 5 to 15 minutes until the blood pressure has returned to tolerable levels.

PCP overdose may cause muscle rigidity sufficient to require the use of muscle relaxants before intubation can be accomplished. When PCP has been taken orally, gastric lavage with a suspension of activated charcoal (Antichar, each 30 gram suspended in 50 to 100 ml of water) is used. Following lavage, 30 or 60 grams of activated charcoal suspended in 100 to 200 ml of magnesium citrate should be left in the stomach.

If the symptoms of overdose do not seem life-threatening, institute continuous gastric aspiration followed by urinary acidification as described in the section on pharmacologic reactions. If the overdose is severe with respiratory depression, unconsciousness or seizures, metabolic acidosis should be induced, since acidosis results in rapid clearing of PCP from the spinal fluid. Acidosis can be induced with ammonium chloride, 2.75 meq/kg q 6 hours by gastric tube or IV as a 1% solution in 0.25 normal saline. Blood pH, serum electrolytes, and molality must be monitored and managed very closely. The goal is to maintain blood pH between 7.2 and

7.3. Delay in lowering the urine pH suggests the presence of a potassium or chloride deficit, which should be corrected. When the urine pH falls to 5.0, furosemide (Lasix) 1 mg/kg (maximum 40 mg) IM q 8 hours is given to maintain diuresis. When the severe symptoms have cleared, gastric aspiration and the ammonium chloride and furosemide can be discontinued and urine acidification maintained with cranberry juice 100 to 200 ml and ascorbic acid 1 to 2 gm PO four times a day.

Withdrawal Syndromes. Withdrawal syndromes occur when the use of opiates, CNS depressants, or stimulants is abruptly discontinued. Withdrawal from the opiates, particularly heroin, has an acute phase which begins about 12 hours after the last dose with tearing, rhinorrhea, and diaphoresis and goes onto anorexia, back pain, tremor, insomnia, muscle spasm, abdominal pain, irritability, and a strong craving for the drug. The acute phase of withdrawal is usually much less intense by the fifth day and is over by 7 to 10 days. Vague discomfort and some mild autonomic dysfunction may last as long as a year. Treatment should be managed by a substance abuse program or a psychiatric service equipped to handle the legal, social, and medical problems of withdrawal therapy.

The withdrawal syndrome seen with the CNS depressants begins about 12 hours after the last dose with anorexia, nausea, vomiting, abdominal cramps, anxiety, and tremors plus some weakness and increased reflexes. Over the next 12 hours, the symptoms increase in severity and grand mal seizures and delirium may intervene. Beginning on the third day, the symptoms disappear, though abnormal autonomic responses and problems with sleep may last for as long as 6 months. A test dose of 3 mg/kg of pentobarbital up to a maximum of 200 mg should be administered PO or IM. If the patient falls asleep in 1 to 2 hours he is not addicted to a depressant drug. If at 2 hours severe symptoms of withdrawal remain, the dose may be doubled and then titrated at 2-hour intervals to determine the dose needed to control the symptoms. If the patient is normal at 2 hours, the initial dose may be repeated at 4 to 6 hours and then titrated to keep the patient symptom free. After 48 hours, the dose may be decreased by 1.5 mg/kg (maximum 100 mg) per day until the patient is off the drug. If significant symptoms of withdrawal appear on this schedule, the dose is being decreased too quickly. The patient should be given an extra 3 mg/kg (maximum 200 mg) IM, restabilized, and reduction begun again.

Alcohol withdrawal presupposes prolonged use and so is rare among adolescents. Its symptoms are like those of withdrawal from the other depressants. Hospitalization is usually needed. For a patient of adult size, Valium 10 mg PO, IM, or IV slowly, repeated three or four times during the first 24 hours will usually control the symptoms. Each subsequent day the dose may be reduced by one

---

*Safety in children has not been established.

third of the first day's dose if the patient remains symptom free. Thiamine, 100 mg, IM daily is needed for 3 days and then a daily multivitamin tablet should be given.

Long Term Management

The management of drug abuse in the older child and adolescent is a complex problem generally requiring the multidisciplinary approach available in substance abuse treatment centers. Many treatment centers currently try to maintain a satisfactory level of socioeconomic performance in their patients rather than to attain early complete abstinence. These centers stress that among chronic abusers the use of drugs serves as an important coping mechanism and more acceptable mechanisms must be found and substituted before the drug can be given up. Methodone therapy for her-

oin addiction is under strict legal control and should not be attempted outside of a substance abuse program. Success rates reported by experts are low, and even experienced therapists face frequent disappointment and risk involvement in the schemes and misrepresentations of their clients. Attempts at long term management by well meaning but inexperienced professionals lead almost invariably to disappointment and frequently to disaster.

Principles of management of chronic alcoholism in adolescence are poorly developed. Counseling, psychiatric treatment, support groups, modification of parental attitudes, and changes in environment have limited and irregular success. Sometimes adolescents, on their own or under pressure from concerned peers, will reduce or eliminate the use of alcohol.

24

Miscellaneous

Primary Immunodeficiency Disease

DIANE W. WARA, M.D.

DISORDERS OF ANTIBODY-MEDIATED IMMUNITY

Hypogammaglobulinemia

Four major groups of hypogammaglobulinemia exist: congenital, transient, acquired, and secondary. Gammaglobulin therapy provides adequate replacement of antibody to prevent life-threatening illness. Commercial gammaglobulin contains primarily IgG with only small amounts of IgA, IgM, IgD, and IgE. Human immune serum globulin (HISG) is prepared by alcohol fractionation of pooled human serum by Cohn's procedure (thus deriving its name of Cohn fraction 2). The fractionation procedure removes most other serum proteins and hepatitis viruses. HISG is approved for intramuscular use. Modified immune serum globulin (MISG) is now available for intravenous use. HISG may aggregate to form large molecular weight complexes, which are capable of spontaneously activating the complement system. These aggregates are probably responsible for the occasional systemic reaction to HISG. Although I consider gammaglobulin to be one of the safest biologic products available, rare anaphylactic reactions do occur following intramuscular injections. Immediate treatment with epinephrine and antihistamines is indicated in these instances.

I prefer to initiate therapy with 0.4 ml/kg of the commercially available 16.5 percent (165 mg/ml) HISG (given intramuscularly). Following this initial dose, I consider two factors in adjusting the amount of gammaglobulin administered: the quantity that the patient can tolerate and the quantity necessary to control infection. Initially, I

prescribe gammaglobulin once monthly. If the initial dose is not effective, I gradually increase the dose by 1 to 2 ml per injection each month, not to exceed 5 ml at any one site (10 ml in a large adult). The buttocks are the preferred site for injection, although the thighs may also be used.

I decrease the interval between doses from once monthly to once every 2 or 3 weeks if the patient continues to have infections or if a characteristic infection occurs immediately prior to the next injection (such as conjunctivitis, diarrhea, or arthralgia). Since no specific serum level of IgG has been correlated with control of infection, I do not obtain serial immunoglobulin levels.

If maximum amounts of intramuscular gammaglobulin given every 2 weeks do not adequately control infection, I utilize regular intravenous infusions of MISG. Intravenous MISG should be initiated at a dose of 100 mg/kg/month and may be increased to 400 mg/kg/month. The administration of MISG may be associated with anaphylactoid-like reactions, which can be controlled by decreasing the rate of infusion.

In addition to the routine use of gammaglobulin, selected antibiotics used on an intermittent or continuous basis may improve control of infection. Broad-spectrum antibiotics such as sulfa or ampicillin, both effective against *Hemophilus influenzae* and pneumococcus, are useful. In spite of adequate replacement therapy with gammaglobulin and appropriate use of antibiotics, chronic pulmonary disease may develop. Pulmonary physical therapy should be taught to parents and used intensively during acute respiratory infections. Chronic otitis media may be associated with hearing loss, and the appropriate use of polyethylene tubes may alter the course. Live viral immunizations (polio, mumps, measles, rubella) should not be given as these patients cannot form specific antibody and the attenuated virus may replicate, causing life-threatening disease.

Children with uncomplicated hypogammaglobulinemia may survive to adulthood without significant physical handicap. Chronic lung disease develops in some patients in spite of what appears to be adequate gammaglobulin therapy. The addition of antibiotic therapy may decrease the number of patients developing this complication, but prospective studies are not yet available. Patients with adult-acquired hypogammaglobulinemia may develop a thymoma and should have yearly chest radiographs as part of their regular evaluations.

Selected Immunoglobulin Deficiencies

Patients with selective IgA deficiency have less than 5 mg/dl of serum IgA and normal or increased levels of other immunoglobulins. The majority have absent secretory IgA. Cell-mediated immunity usually is intact. An increased incidence of allergy, sinopulmonary infection, gastrointestinal tract disease, and autoimmune disease occurs in these patients. The age at onset of symptoms varies. No specific replacement therapy is available. Patients with normal amounts of IgG may form antibodies against the immunoglobulin they lack if it is administered. Therefore, gammaglobulin therapy is contraindicated.

There appears to be a decrease in the number and severity of sino-pulmonary infections in some patients who are treated with broad-spectrum antibiotics at the onset of each respiratory illness, as viral infections often are followed by bacterial infections in these patients. Patients with selective IgA deficiency should be followed closely for the development of autoimmune disease. If patients require blood transfusions, packed washed red blood cells should be used. Some blood banks have available IgA-deficient donors who then can be utilized for cross-matching with IgA-deficient recipients; the possibility of an anaphylactic reaction following blood transfusion is decreased.

Too few patients with selective IgM deficiency have been identified to provide specific conclusions regarding treatment. I feel it is appropriate, in view of their particular susceptibility to certain bacteria to treat them with prophylactic ampicillin on a continuous basis. As these patients have the capacity to form specific antibody in immunoglobulin classes other than IgM, they should be immunized with Pneumovax (polyvalent pneumococcal polysaccharide vaccine) and *Hemophilus influenzae* and meningococcal vaccines, if available.

CELLULAR IMMUNODEFICIENCY DISORDERS

Severe Combined Immunodeficiency Disease

Severe combined immunodeficiency disease (SCID) is characterized by complete absence of antibody and cell-mediated immunity. Reconstitution of cellular immunity in infants with SCID appears more effective if infection is not present and the infant is well nourished. Alternatively, if the diagnosis of SCID is confirmed in an older infant already infected and malnourished, the infant should receive specific antimicrobials and hyperalimentation prior to efforts at reconstitution.

Bone marrow obtained from a compatible sibling donor as defined by nonreactivity in the mixed lymphocyte culture (MLC) reaction is the treatment of choice for severe combined immunodeficiency disease. If a compatible sibling donor is not available, a search of close relatives should be made. Rarely, an MLC-compatible nonsibling donor has been utilized. In spite of MLC identity and close matching at the histocompatibility loci, most patients experience a mild graft-versus-host reaction (GVHR) following transplantation. Successful bone marrow transplantation results in reconstitution both of cell-mediated and antibody-mediated immunity. The patient who received the first successful bone marrow transplant has now survived 14 years following the initial therapy, and more than 40 successful transplantations have been performed since that time.

In the absence of a compatible donor for bone marrow transplantation, there is no completely satisfactory approach to therapy. Transplantation of modified haplotype-identical bone marrow, obtained from a parent, is experimental. Mature T-cells capable of causing GVHR are removed by monoclonal antibody with complement-mediated lysis or by agglutination with soybean lectin. The residual cells appear capable of reconstituting cellular immunity.

Transplantation of fetal tissue has had limited success. Fetal thymus transplantation has resulted in T-cell reconstitution without evidence of B-cell reconstitution. The residual deficiency in antibody-mediated immunity can be managed by gammaglobulin injections. Depending on the extent of the cellular immunodeficiency disease, fetal thymus should be obtained from less than 14 weeks' gestational age fetuses to minimize the risk of GVHR.

Fetal liver, obtained at 9 weeks' gestation, may offer some benefit. Combined fetal liver and fetal thymus transplantation has been attempted by some investigators, although I have no experience with this approach to therapy.

Transplantation of thymus epithelium, obtained by cultured thymic fragments, has resulted in transient reconstitution of both B- and T-cell immunity. Survivors of thymic epithelial transplantation with malignancies have been reported. It is reported that thymic epithelial cultures do not contain viable lymphocytes and therefore transplantation does not induce GVHR. All patients are treated with gammaglobulin to provide passive antibody.

The therapies mentioned, other than bone marrow transplantation from a mixed lymphocyte culture identical sibling donor, have had varying results and are still considered experimental. The significant risk of fatal GVHR must be balanced with the possibility of reconstitution of cellular immunity.

Cellular Immunodeficiency with Abnormal Immunoglobulin Synthesis (Nezelof Syndrome)

Nezelof syndrome is a primary immunodeficiency disease characterized by varying degrees of cellular immunodeficiency and normal or nearly normal immunoglobulin levels, with absent specific antibody production.

Reconstitution of cell-mediated immunity has been attempted by various methods in these patients. Experience with histocompatible bone marrow transplantation in these patients is limited. Patients have been reconstituted successfully with fetal thymus transplants. Partial reconstitution of cell-mediated immunity in selected patients with this diagnosis has been achieved by repeated injections of thymic humoral factors, termed thymosin.

Combined Immunodeficiency Disease Associated with Adenosine Deaminase or Purine Nucleoside Phosphorylase Deficiency

Combined immunodeficiency disease associated with enzyme deficiency is characterized by an autosomal recessive inheritance and varying degrees of antibody and cellular immunodeficiency. Infants may have clinical and laboratory findings identical to those in patients with SCID or with a disease similar to the Nezelof syndrome.

Patients with immunodeficiency and associated enzyme deficiencies have been successfully treated utilizing bone marrow transplantation from histocompatible sibling donors. To date, this has been accomplished in patients with ADA deficiency, but not PNP deficiency. Following transplantation, enzyme levels in circulating red blood cells return to normal and there is a return of normal immunologic function.

In the absence of a matched bone marrow transplant donor, other forms of therapy have been utilized. Monthly transfusions of red cells as a source of ADA were utilized in a single patient and were associated with transient improvement of immunologic function following each transfusion. Red blood cells must be irradiated to prevent GVHR when this form of therapy is used. Although in theory biochemical treatment of patients with enzyme deficiency is possible, to date it has not been successful.

Thymic Hypoplasia with Hypocalcemia (DiGeorge Syndrome)

Children with thymic hypoplasia have congenital tetany, abnormal facies, congenital heart disease, and an increased susceptibility to infection. Treatment during the neonatal period is directed toward control of the hypoparathyroidism and surgical correction of the congential heart disease. If a cellular immune defect is documented, fetal thymus transplant is recommended. Reconstitution of cell-mediated immunity in patients with DiGeorge syndrome following fetal thymus transplant occurs rapidly and appears to be permanent. Alternative therapy to fetal thymus transplantation is injection of the thymic humoral factors contained within thymosin fraction V.

GENERAL CONSIDERATIONS IN MANAGEMENT OF PATIENTS WITH PRIMARY IMMUNODEFICIENCY DISEASE

Antibiotics

The use of broad-spectrum antibiotics such as sulfa or ampicillin may decrease the incidence of infections in some patients with immunodeficiency. I recommend the use of prophylactic antibiotics in patients with hypogammaglobulinemia and chronic lung disease, which develops or progresses in spite of the use of maximum replacement therapy with gammaglobulin. Trimethoprim-sulfamethoxazole is my choice of antibiotic. The adult dose is one half the therapeutic dose (1 tablet, 80 mg trimethoprim and 400 mg sulfamethoxazole), given twice daily. In children, 4 mg/kg of trimethoprim and 20 mg/kg of sulfamethoxazole each 24 hr, given in two divided doses, is adequate for prophylaxis. Trimethoprim-sulfamethoxazole is also given to all patients with significant cellular immunodeficiency disease as prophylaxis against *Pneumocystis carinii* infection.*

Pulmonary Assessment

Patients over age 6 with immunodeficiency disorders should have pulmonary function assessments performed at least annually. Their therapy should be changed if decreasing function is observed. Patients with chronic bronchitis and productive sputum should be placed on an aggressive pulmonary regimen similar to that used for patients with cystic fibrosis.

Pneumocystis carinii pneumonia is a frequent and serious complication of severe combined immunodeficiency disease. It should be suspected in a patient with cellular immunodeficiency disease and even mild respiratory distress. Mild perioral cya-

---

*The prophylactic use of trimethoprim-sulfamethoxazole is not listed in the manufacturer's directive.

nosis, associated with minimal tachypnea but a normal pulmonary examination and normal chest radiograph, may be found in an infant with diffuse *Pneumocystis carinii* pathologically on open lung biopsy. I recommend therapy with trimethoprim-sulfamethoxazole in addition to pentamidine for the treatment of *Pneumocystis carinii* pneumonia in patients with primary immunodeficiency disease. Although trimethoprim-sulfamethoxazole alone has been useful in treatment of *Pneumocystis carinii* pneumonia in patients with secondary immunodeficiency disease (malignancy), these results have not been achieved in children with primary immunodeficiency disease. Pentamidine is administered at 4 mg/kg daily for 10 to 14 days, intramuscularly.

Gastrointestinal Disease

Malabsorption and chronic diarrhea occur in patients with isolated defects in antibody-mediated immunity or combined immunodeficiency disease. Evaluation should include duodenal aspirates, which may reveal *Giardia lamblia*. The treatment of *Giardia* infestation is metronidazole[†] (Flagyl) in divided doses totaling 20 to 35 mg/kg/24 hr for 10 days. Stool cultures should be obtained from family members of diagnosed patients; if *Giardia lamblia* is isolated, these family members should be treated concurrently with the patient.

Immunizations

Patients with isolated B-cell deficiencies or combined immunodeficiency disease should not receive live virus vaccines. Fatal poliomyelitis has been reported in both patient groups. Control of varicella requires high-titer gammaglobulin prepared from individuals who have recently recovered either from the disease or from herpes zoster. It is available in limited supply from the National Red Cross Center (telephone (617) 881-4118), but must be given within 48 hours following exposure to varicella in order to be effective. Alternative but less effective therapy is the infusion of zoster-immune plasma, which is available from many local blood banks.

Blood Transfusions

All patients with cellular immunodeficiency are at risk for developing graft-versus-host disease (GVHD). Therefore, all blood products containing viable lymphocytes (plasma, whole blood,

---

†This use of metronidazole is not listed by the manufacturer.

packed red cells) should be irradiated with 3000 rad before transfusion. I recommend irradiating leukocytes with 1500 rad to preserve function and to decrease the risk of GVHD in neutropenic patients.

Sudden Infant Death Syndrome (SIDS) and Near-SIDS

DANIEL C. SHANNON, M.D.

Sudden infant death syndrome is death without sufficient pathology. Over the past 10 years, however, a pattern of subtle alterations in structure has emerged, suggesting that SIDS is related to recurrent or chronic hypoxia, perhaps caused by insufficient regulation of alveolar ventilation. The alterations include increased smooth muscle in the pulmonary circulation and astroglial proliferation in the brain stem. Unconfirmed alterations in the carotid body and cervical vagus nerve have been cited.

Infection appears to potentiate the risk of SIDS. Winter months and their attendant increased incidence of respiratory infections are associated with sudden infant deaths, both expected and unexpected. The full range of viruses is found. Other infections, such as botulism, may account for a small proportion of deaths. Host defense mechanisms have received little attention.

Altered plasma or liver composition of electrolytes or metal ions does not explain SIDS, and there is no evidence of altered glucose homeostasis. Altered thiamine and thyroid metabolism have been suggested but not proved. On the other hand, there are clear associations with maternal addiction to cigarettes and opiates, including methadone.

A variety of characteristics confirmed as different during pregnancy, labor, and delivery and in the home environment before and after birth all support the conclusion that the risk of altered physiology is seriously affected by the psychosocial milieu. As we will see, there are also subtle structural expressions of these alterations.

Although SIDS has occurred three and even four times in some families there is no evidence of genetic transmission in large studies. The risk of SIDS is increased in twins, especially those born second, but it is independent of zygosity. Some families have aggregation of SIDS, with a 2.1% risk in subsequent siblings of affected infants who were born singly and a 4.2% risk in survivors among twins. Nonmendelian factors or strong environmental influences during gestation or postnatal life may explain these observations. A number of twin pairs, both monozygous and dizygous, have died or have had near-SIDS events within hours of one another strengthening the argument for potent environmental factors.

Arrhythmias account for a small number of cases, and recent evidence from babies with near-SIDS suggests an alteration in control of the heart rate. Cardiovascular failure in SIDS may result either from exaggeration of a normal reflex response such as the laryngeal chemoreflex or from a qualitative defect in cardiovascular control.

Because sudden death without an obvious cause implies cessation of autonomic regulation of cardiovascular or respiratory activity, or both, it is important to understand how normal control mechanisms maintain ventilation and prevent or terminate apnea. It is even more pertinent because several investigators have identified abnormal breathing patterns or control mechanisms in infants in whom SIDS later occurred.

Episodes of prolonged apnea ($\geq$ 15 seconds) and excessive periodic and short apnea, sometimes with obstruction, characterize the breathing pattern of some infants in whom SIDS occurs. Abnormal ventilatory and arousal responses to both hypercapnia and hypoxia have been described. These observations point to a defect in the chemical regulation of respiratory muscles and their pattern of contraction.

The Child and Death of a Loved One

MORRIS A. WESSEL, M.D.

A child's personal physician has a unique opportunity to be helpful when a child suffers the loss through death of someone he or she loves. The manner in which adults care for a child at this tragic moment may determine to what extent the loss remains an overwhelming, unmasterable burden interfering seriously with a child's psychologic development and to what degree it is a stress that a child copes with and integrates as he grows and matures.

Adults—professionals, relatives, teachers, and friends—must realize that the loss of someone a child loves represents an incomparable stress for a child. Our task is to accept and respect children's feelings and anguish and to provide nurturing and comforting at this tragic moment. We cannot prevent their sadness, but we can support and comfort them as they grieve and mourn in their own unique ways. Even a very young child can be helped to succeed in this very difficult task, which may take many months or even years.

A child's preparation for coping with the death of a loved one begins prior to the event. Physicians and nurses providing comprehensive care during infancy and early childhood often suggest that parents try to help children develop understanding in the preschool years of the meaning of *being alive* and *being dead*. Children of 3 years of age—and some even younger—can understand what happens when a pet or other familiar animal dies. They realize that a dead goldfish no longer swims, and a bird lifeless on the ground can no longer sing or fly. These experiences can help a young child conceptualize the meaning of being alive and being dead.

Explanation of death as "no longer living," "not moving," "not eating," "just resting" is an appropriate way to help a child grasp the idea of what death is all about. Care must be taken to avoid suggesting that the deceased animal or person went to sleep, for this is likely to create undue fears that the child, too, might die while asleep.

Children feel deserted as members of a family anticipate the death of a loved one. They lose the attention of the person who is ill. Other family members, preoccupied with their own feelings, are also less and less available. Children may become angry with everyone around them. They feel abandoned at a time when they need more rather than less attention.

The solemnity and palpable gloom in a home as a family anticipates a death is frightening to a child. Explanations for the sadness and preoccupation are important. Adults should share the fact that "Uncle Joe is very sick; the doctors and nurses are doing everything they can to make him comfortable. He may die soon. That's why we're all so sad." A child may be unable to grasp fully, as are many adults, the reality of what is taking place. However, the conversation establishes an honest basis for later discussion, when one can say, "You remember I said Uncle Joe was very sick and might die? I'm very sad now to have to tell you that he did die."

When the primary caretaker, such as the mother, is the patient, a child wonders who will provide for his or her needs. It is wise to help a family designate one person who will assume the major care of the child. This may be a father, aunt, grandparent, close friend, older sibling, or housekeeper. Consistency of this person during a mother's illness and afterward is important. Whenever possible, it is helpful to maintain children in their own homes, where their familiar surroundings, their room, their toys, their own bed and furnishings serve as support during this stressful time.

Children experiencing the loss of a loved one wonder whether this could happen to other people who love and take care of them, or to themselves. Reassurance must be realistic, for who knows when any of us will die? It is best to say, "I don't think it will happen for a long, long time, and I'll be here to take care of you for many years." When it is a mother who dies, it is appropriate to approach the matter by saying, "We will miss Mommy very, very much. We will be sad for a long time as we miss her. I will see to it that someone will care for you and do the things Mommy used to do for you."

Although it is difficult for a grief-stricken relative to assume this approach, it is important to do so. It reassures children that their nurturing needs will be met; at the same time, it acknowledges their need to be sad. There is no way to protect children from being hurt when a loved one dies. It is a very real loss. They may, upon observing the adults crying, and their continued sadness, consider it as permission to release their own feelings of desolation. It helps them to initiate the process of grieving, which, for children as well as for adults, is appropriate and necessary when a loved one dies.

Parents often ask whether a child should attend the funeral of a loved one. I believe a child aged 4 years or older can make the decision. One should describe the service and mention that relatives and friends attending will be very sad. An appropriate way of presenting the opportunity is to say, "We're all very sad because we miss Nana so much. I will be sad, too. There will be music and prayers. Our minister (rabbi, priest) will talk about Nana. If you would like to come with us, I'll ask (a relative or a close friend) to join us. Or if you would rather stay home, that is all right, too. Someone you know will be here with you."

The gathering of relatives and friends and the ritual of the service can be supporting to children as it is to an adult. On the other hand, a child may decide that the experience is more than he or she can cope with, and choose wisely to remain at home. When a child does attend a funeral, it is important that someone be with him, preferably one who is not intensely grief-stricken. Nothing is sadder than the sight of a bewildered, grief-stricken child standing alone during a funeral service, ignored by adults who are preoccupied with their own anguish and feelings. An adult companion should be assigned the specific task of caring for the child and be ready to leave should the experience become overwhelming.

It is important to choose words carefully when explaining to a child what happens after death. The discussion should portray honestly the philosophic and religious beliefs of the family. The concept of life hereafter is, however, difficult for a young child to comprehend. A child may think of Heaven as a place far away, but accessible and a place from which people can return, or at least telephone or send a letter. It is not until the latter half of the first decade of life that a child begins to be able to grasp

meaningfully the concept of Heaven and a life hereafter. Nevertheless, if the family has this belief, it is wise to present the idea to a child of any age in forthright terms. One can say, "The body of a person who dies is placed in a special box in the cemetery. I'll show you where that is. The body rests there. I like to believe that part of the person, the spirit, the things we love that person for, rests in a place called Heaven, far far away, where there's no pain, or hunger, or suffering."

Every child is quick to sense dishonesty and insincerity. A disbelieving adult who presents a concept of life hereafter hoping that somehow this will aid a child only creates confusion and stimulates distrust. It is far better just to say, "I do not know exactly what I believe happens after death, but all I know is, Dad will no longer be with us."

A child who does not attend a funeral may request at a later date to visit the cemetery. It is wise to grant this wish. The sight of a fresh grave serves as a realistic documentation of the event; it often helps a child to begin the painful process of adapting to the reality of the loss.

Prolonged longing and wishing for the return of the deceased is normal in childhood, just as in adulthood. Knowing and understanding that a loved one has gone forever is only the initial phase of accepting reality and the permanence of the loss. A child, like an adult, must grapple for a long time to adapt to an important loss. Adults, finding the child's poignant struggle painful, often turn away to avoid dealing with a child's anguish. Physicians and nurses can be helpful by sharing with adults who care for a child how important it is to provide continuing support for a child grappling with the meaning of the loss of someone loved and from whom love was received.

Bereaved children become anxious when family members are away, fearing that they, too, might fail to return. It is important for adults who care for bereaved children to inform them where they are going and when they will return. They should keep in contact by phone if there is any unavoidable delay in returning home.

Children will often regress to behavior formerly abandoned during a period of bereavement. They may become anxious at bedtime and be fearful of leaving home. They may lose well-established urine and bowel control. They may be restless and out of sorts. Bodily complaints and a decrease in ability to meet educational challenges are common symptoms.

Bereaved children commonly dread illness, even of a minor sort. They imagine that they may be about to die, hence every call to a physician concerning a child's symptoms merits prompt response and careful consideration. This reassures both the child and the adult in a family. Also, one must bear in mind that illnesses do occur in bereaved children. Complaints during the stress of bereavement may reflect an early phase of significant gastrointestinal disease.

Bereaved children who present behavioral symptoms as they grapple with the loss may be far healthier than children who deny the loss and are unable to deal with it in any manner whatsoever.

Bereaved children benefit by knowing that their doctor cares about them. A phone call, a brief comment at the time of the first meeting after a death, or a letter is an important way of letting children know that their doctor understands and appreciates what they are experiencing in this sad moment. Parents and other caretakers need all the support we can give them as they continue to comfort and support a child at this tragic moment.

Child Abuse

NAHMAN H. GREENBERG, M.D.

Abuse and injury to young children by their parents or caretakers, that is, nonaccidental violence and neglect, is a major health and social problem. Starvation, neglect, violence, and exploitation contribute to damaged minds and bodies of infants and children. The increased interest in child abuse today can be attributed to a greater awareness of the problem rather than to an actual increase in the incidence of abuse. Health professionals have become more attentive to these problems in compliance with state laws that mandate reporting of child abuse and neglect to designated public child protective agencies.

Estimates of the number of children abused yearly in the United States are as high as 5,000,000. As many as 5% of all children have histories of sexual abuse. From 75,000 to 100,000 children are battered or otherwise severely attacked each year in the U.S., and neglect is reported for many times that number. Combinations of these maltreatments can be assumed in 30 to 40% of cases. The most seriously maltreated and injured children are the very young, below the age of 2 years.

MALTREATED INFANTS AND CHILDREN

Some Methodological Problems

It is difficult to make general statements about short-term and long-term consequences of infant and child abuse since, for the most part, we lack careful and long-range follow-up data that include careful and systematic assessments of infant and child rearing and care practices and family conditions in which abuse occurs. There are no consistent criteria and conditions determining whether a child is removed from the family or when, if removed, reunion will take place. There is no apparent control over the number and durations of placements to which a child might be subjected.

There are added problems of sampling. While studies can be done of the maltreated children who are brought to our attention, we cannot study those who avoid attention and detection, or the many who are lost to follow-up. We are unable also to explain the effects of abuse on overall personality development, on the development of behavioral disturbances, or on correlations with personality, psychoneurotic and psychotic disorders, and psychophysiologic dysfunctions.

The clinical study of abused children is a scientific nightmare. The amount of data collected is limited by lack of time, money, and expertise. The more impersonal the study, the less reliable are the results. Data interpretation is difficult; even mortality rates and reinjury rates can be misinterpreted. Mortality rates include death from reinjury, the long-term consequences of abuse, and deaths from unrelated causes. The severity and incidence of reinjury need to be evaluated; reinjury rates are easily misconstrued, especially when related to intervention and its consequences. A large proportion of children are lost to follow-up for various reasons.

Difficulties in assessing psychologic consequences, including possible harm, are also related to inadequate conceptualization in selecting measurements that can test for specific effects. The effects of earlier abuses on the child's current and future functioning depend on the interactions of a number of factors. The understanding of consequences requires an examination of interactions of major determinants of the child's psychologic development, including predispositional variables and the stage and characteristics of the developmental processes during which specific painful events and experiences occurred. The seriousness of the outcome is also linked with other factors, including the age and developmental phase of the child, the duration of the adverse relationship, the quality of care and experiences with parents in other matters, and inherent vulnerabilities. These factors also influence the nature of the traumatic experience, its content and intensity.

Clinical Evaluations and Observations of Abused Children

The infant or young child victimized by parental brutality causing obvious bodily injuries may also have experienced combinations of less brutal abuse, neglect, and deprivation. The consequences of any one may appear different in form and degree than the interactional effects of any two or more occurring in the history of the infant or child.

Factors that correlate with psychiatric symptoms are not only the type or severity of the physical assault but also environmental factors: emotional disturbance in parents, family instability, number of home changes, punitiveness and rejection by caretakers, and the child's perception of lack of permanence in the home setting. The assumption that trauma is typical or inevitable with abusive experiences implies consequent pathology or dysfunction whether of short or lengthy duration. The persistence of dysfunction may well depend on later developmental experiences, on conditions that promote health, and on the assimilation of the traumatic experience. This perspective on consequences of childhood abuse holds the view that no truly abusive event, experience, or relationship is ever wholly assimilated or neutralized; some increased vulnerability persists even when there are no obvious indications of untoward consequences. There is no one classic or typical personality profile for abused children. It is difficult to predict the conditions or events that will sensitize a child's mind. Whether a child has mastered an early experience or been made more vulnerable by it generally is not obvious until a later time, when predispositions can be tested.

Abused and neglected children exhibit low self-esteem and often behave in ways that invite rejection. They are not happy and seem unable to enjoy themselves in play or in social interactions in a manner appropriate to their ages. Untreated abused children in later childhood seem bitter, hostile, and suspicious of adults; depression is common, although on the surface the children may seem apathetic and shallow. Behavioral disorders and psychiatric illnesses are observed as abused children enter their teens.

The mental harm from overwhelmingly painful, traumatic experiences predisposes to a sense of devastation and to disorganized mental function. The abused child feels "damaged" and vulnerable, and fears repetition of these painful states. Evidence of trauma is found in anxiety dreams or nightmares and in the propensity for helplessness, fright, disorganized thought, psychosomatic symptoms, and dread. In later years, there tend to be disturbances that include an overall impairment of ego functioning associated with intellectual and cognitive defects; traumatic reactions with acute anxiety states; pathologic object relationships characterized by failure to develop basic trust; excessive use of "pathologic" defenses such as denial, projection, introjection, and splitting; impaired control of aggressive impulses, damaged self-concept accompanied by self-destructive behavior; and low frustration tolerance. Many have been enuretic and hyperactive; bizarre behavior or atypical habits, school learning problems, withdrawal, and oppositional behavior are common.

Phobias, avoidance responses, inhibitions, maladjustment reactions, behavioral problems (including delinquent behavior and aggressivity), depression, and disturbed relationships are frequent. There is a chronic sense of low self-esteem, with feelings of inadequacy and inferiority; their sense of self is of being small and unprotected, with a hostile self-rejection when longings for care are felt. They are very sensitive to separation and quickly feel rejected.

Aside from the pediatric or medical findings various clinical observations and studies have also shown language and general intellectual and development lag, atypical responses to maternal separation, and hypersensitivity of fear accompanied by avoidance responses. Data on speech and hearing development of abused children have shown them to have a much higher degree of language or speech delay. Children most affected are the younger ones who were seen during the critical periods of language development. Development in the older children seems to be less delayed. Many lack age-appropriate information such as knowing numbers and colors, and they also lack basic skills development. Children under 30 months may do well on motor skill items but perform less well in areas concerning object constancy, "means and end" relationships, and social relationships.

Where overt traumatic experiences are associated with an underlying fantasy, the imprint is probably more intense. For example, a neglected child left with intensified longings for nurturing care, touch, and affection will suffer physical punishment with even greater force and intensity and develop more enduring disturbing memories.

Attention must be given to the assessment of cognitive and attentional development to social responses, regulating functions, and stimulation tolerance. The breakdown of existing functions, the formation of unusual forms of behavior, the lag in development of or failure of emergence of functions are to be suspected as related to parental maltreatment. Neurologic studies are also indicated, particularly with evidence that children subjected to recurrent physical abuse during the first 2 years of life develop neurologic deficits in later years.

CHARACTERISTICS OF ABUSIVE PARENTS

It is important to separate abuse and neglect ascribed to cultural conditions from those due to the person responsible for child care or to interactions stimulated by the young child. If neglect is thought of in terms of deficiencies, restrictions, or the absence of specific environmental conditions, stimulations, and care needed for a child to thrive, then ignorance, famine, and poverty may result in child neglect. Faulty information combined with insufficient resources for educating an uninformed mother engaged in undesirable child care practices may also contribute to neglect. A withdrawn mother suffering from a serious mental disorder may neglect her child. Since experiences of the affected children in all three conditions may be similar, it is important to delineate cultural from subcultural or personal factors in planning treatment.

Parents who abuse their children have been characterized in many ways, even as "normal" if not healthy. Parents who beat their children often think of themselves as "disciplinarians"; some cite scripture to explain their use of physical pain. They think of corporal punishment as a desirable child-rearing practice, as a positive force for a child's well-being and instrumental in socialization. Unfortunately, these views are common and contribute to the avoidance of discovering personal and more significant motives in using physical punishment on young children.

The use of corporal punishment to modify behavior is widely accepted as both appropriate and a parental prerogative. Many people fail to see the connection between the cultural sanctioning of mild physical pain to discipline children and the occurrence of child abuse resulting in physical trauma or death. Corporal punishment is particularly inappropriate not only because of the strong emotions accompanying its use but also because of its side effect of teaching children aggression. A common description of abusive parents is that of emotional immaturity, low frustration tolerance resulting in aggression, rigidity in thought patterns and behaviors, and low self-esteem. They are assumed to have been abused as children and because they employ self-defeating defense mechanisms of regression, denial, and projection, they are prevented from realizing the consequences of their actions and in developing appropriate methods of expressing anger.

Our own studies indicate that most mothers of abused young children suffer from serious emotional disturbances. The majority qualified diagnostically as borderline, prepsychotic, severe character disordered, or psychotic. A predominance of their personalities were marked by a limited range of defenses: inflexibility, impaired judgment, and poor reality testing functions. Clinically, many seemed depressed, distant, apathetic, withdrawn, and emotionally impoverished. Little empathy and closeness was observed and gratifying relations with other adults were uncommon. Their fantasy life appeared sparse and most often consisted of primitive notions and fears, with hostility and violence a principal theme. Their world was commonly portrayed as a cruel place where people get stung, neglected, gobbled up, hurt, and taken advantage of even as they themselves sought for closeness and nurturance. Parents who abused young children were severely hostile, yet they seemed amazingly unaware of and unable to ac-

knowledge hostile feelings or urges where very young children had been most violently abused.

These parents experienced strong negative attitudes toward the earlier pregnancy, a significant unawareness of the child's needs, a lack of clarity about their role as parents, and especially the importance of affection as a necessary child care ingredient. The behavior of these mothers, observed in the presence of their children, revealed that they encouraged aggressive hostile acts between the children. They directed their child with strong, angry, verbal directives and abrupt harsh and painful hitting.

They never used gentle or simple physical restraint to alter the child's "objectionable" behavior. Impatience, unwarranted rejections, icy aloofness, and angry recriminations were often observed.

Parents who abuse their infants and children, including some who had committed infanticide, have been described as rigid, severely obsessive-compulsive, and "pseudoindependent," as well as demanding and aggressive toward the child, demanding strict compliance and obedience and physically punishing the child when frustrated by him. Low self-esteem and hypersensitivity to criticism, as well as a need for constant reassurance have also been attributed to the personality of observed abusive parents. Crises involving severe attacks on the child have been correlated with the taxing of circumstances that evoked such conditions, such as an excessively crying infant. The backgrounds of these parents have been described as lacking in care and impoverished of love and self-esteem, with a childhood history of pain and punishment.

TREATMENT

Some General Conditions

The service needs of these parents and children are many and consist of different combinations according to living conditions, service resources, treatment indications, and treatability. The abusive parent often experiences treatment as an intrusion. Therapists are perceived as unwelcome interlopers who exercise influence on the observed behavior of the family. A very punitive father who strongly considers beating children a necessary and legitimate right that serves the child well will strongly object to being informed that such practices not only are not acceptable but also are illegal.

It is not strange therefore that service plans include various emergency health and social services, individual and group therapies, parent groups, emergency and long-term foster homes, in-home services, and various health and child welfare agencies from the public and private sectors. It is important to not lose sight of the child and to always include indicated diagnostic and treatment child services. No significant family member should be allowed to remain outside the therapeutic plans.

The awareness that children are helpless and suffering often intensifies the response of service providers, who may not readily accept not being able to bring prompt relief and remediation; it is difficult to not feel helpless and incompetent. The pressure to provide services is especially felt when the problems are more complicated and in greater numbers than previously assumed and of moral and social consequence. These problems do not yield to easy answers.

Crisis intervention and collaboration with social agencies are required when protection of the child is necessary, when trying to bring a family together, and when trying to prevent additional cases. Experienced therapists are reluctant to take on these difficult and complicated, stormy, crisis ridden problems, which disrupt the professional's orderly life, and for which services tend to be limited.

The decision of what treatment approach to use is frequently made on the often inadequate basis of availability. Treatment services are usually provided by those with less formal training and experience, and usually with fewer treatment skills and less sensitivity and psychological understanding, who are less prepared to do psychotherapy and who are inadequately trained in diagnostic and insight oriented skills. How many cases of abuse do we know of that receive an adequate diagnostic evaluation?

The specialized treatments and living conditions needed for adults and children involved in maltreatment are not so difficult to determine even with our limited knowledge. Since treatment services cannot be postponed until sufficient knowledge is developed to guide the design and application of specific treatment plans, we must keep an open mind on the selection of treatment approaches, recognize preferences and biases, and realize that "service plans" often reflect local resources, biases, economics, political considerations, or priorities. Intervention programs have often developed without prior testing or regulation but based on hunches and assumptions that intuitive responses are better than inaction. We reward innovativeness in procedures in the absence of controls, test data, and a sound rationale.

Most identified abusive parents are amenable to psychotherapy. Group and individual psychotherapy as well as psychotherapy augmented by child management information have shown clinical usefulness. The use of multiple family therapy as a treatment modality in child abuse cases requires that the family's interaction be observed and treated with all members present; emphasis is on the inter-relationship of family members; and therapeutic interventions are geared toward changes within the family rather than in individuals. Psychoeducational programs teaching more effective pa-

rental practices, crisis nurseries, and family developmental centers have come into being as approaches to modifying if not preventing faulty parental behavior.

Initiating Child Protective Services

Awareness of a wide occurrence of child maltreatment has stimulated the development of legal and social service mechanisms designed to intervene on behalf of a child whose health was endangered and who required protection from further maltreatment. The ability to intervene, although not necessarily to provide ongoing services to such urgent condition, was enhanced through enactment of laws that gave child protective services legal authority to intervene into the lives of families to protect endangered children.

In the treatment of child abuse, there is a need to shift from the current reliance on placement to an emphasis on crisis intervention and comprehensive psychiatric and social services for the maltreated child and his or her family. The use of placement as a major intervention is recommended only as a last resort. Parents whose children have been placed or who were threatened with removal of their children respond with anger and frustration and question the genuineness of the offer of help. Sequelae of placement include depressive reactions in parents, the need to blame someone else, increased conflict with the spouse, and pregnancy within 1 year after placement.

Child protective services (CPS) responses to reported child abuse and neglect are a public promise of help through specialized social and mental health services. Intended to protect the "best interests of the child," they principally prevent further abuse by prompt intervention and introduction of services to assist the family in exercising responsibilities in the care and development of the children. Child protective services are in theory nonpunitive and noncondemning, and are an offer to help rehabilitate the family, to stabilize the home environment, and to treat the underlying factors causing child maltreatment. This depends on a study of presenting complaints, an adequate understanding of the persons and situational problems (i.e., a diagnostic work-up), a planning of the case's needs according to what requires changing and what services would bring that about, and finally, treatment proper, including arrangement and provision of services.

Services for abusive parents and abused children are founded on fundamental principles and practices of "helping relationships." The practices of professional social and mental health services are possible only insofar as certain conditions are met:
1. That clients or patients have the right to some degree of personal choice and decision on treatment.

2. That treatment be provided with respect; the patient is accepted as a worthy human being regardless of past actions, problems, and personal characteristics.
3. That the client has the right to have personal information treated with professional confidence.
4. That it is understood that the fundamental rights of patients cannot be violated by personal values or biases of the professional worker and there is an acceptance of the patient, so that evaluations are not influenced by personal opinions, differences, or personal values.
5. Time.

The severe increase in reports of abused and neglected children, causing caseloads that exceed the ability of professionals to provide adequate services, combined with the pressing into service of less well trained and experienced workers, decreases the amount and quality of services and promotes tougher management or administrative responses. Treatment skills and the influence of experience and professionalism are viewed as unaffordable luxuries, divorced from the realities of the situation. The situation encourages intercessions based on the power of coercion and threat, real and implied; changes are now to come about by demand and command. As the number of reported cases increases, as the child protective mandate is exercised in an increasingly narrow and legalistic way, the time for and expectation of understanding and use of skills essential to the development of working therapeutic relationships are reduced if not discarded. Initial interviews are no longer valued as crucial opportunities to assist families toward healthier futures; rather they become instruments to investigate without the commitment to bring about understanding and compassion.

With reduced options and increasing caseloads, immediate action is expected, and with less time for experience and education to develop and to improve skills. Protective custody and the placement of a young child in a foster home are the alternatives to professionalism and express the diversion into "removal of the problem" and the employment of an individualized form of "custodialism." This approach is relatively well oriented to management and narrow administrative ideas and to rigid and authoritarian individuals. Such legal devices reduce the demand and need for clinical skills and understanding to change behavior, to control and protect. They also reinforce the stereotype of the maltreating parent as someone who is inevitably dangerous and unpredictable, inferior and condemned; parents become vulnerable to attitudes and procedures of retribution and punishment. Psychotherapeutic and related clinical services become secondary if not tertiary in the hierarchy of methods to influence change.

The work of the therapist, the clinician, and the diagnostician involves an obligation to insure that no permanent physical or psychological harm will ensue from the procedures and that discomfort from such procedures or the loss of privacy will be remedied in an appropriate way during the course of treatment or at its completion.

The Initiation of Therapy and Collaboration in Child Abuse

The circumstances under which a person seeks treatment or is introduced to the need for treatment is very important to the initiation of psychotherapy and to the development of a treatment relationship. Likewise, the conditions under which a report is made of a child being abused and the characteristics of the response, usually by child protective service workers, can be powerful factors in the course of events and the quality of treatment services that follow. If we consider this phase of events a component of the initial phase of therapy, a phase concerned with the initiation of a treatment relationship leading to the establishment of a professional contractual involvement, then proper attention must be given to its difficulties, the technical skills required, the rationale underlying interventions, and a continuing attention to diagnosis. The initiation of child protective services and that of psychotherapeutic services differ even though the child protective services need to be employed to initiate treatment, fully recognizing that such interventions cannot always be performed with the neatness of a timed interpretation.

The nonvoluntary client or patient may or may not recognize the need for therapy or for change. The suggestion of a need for psychotherapeutic services based on a report of possible or actual child maltreatment is not a simple intervention to be carried out routinely without understanding the conditions and circumstances that will automatically influence the response to the suggestion and the possibility of bringing about a cooperative working relationship. The idea to seek treatment might originate in the patient or client, or it might be someone else's suggestion or wish; the idea to seek treatment might well have previously occurred in the nonvoluntary client.

Early contact with the social worker is essential for both diagnostic and treatment purposes, and in preparation for this, pediatricians and other specialists should maintain an honest relationship with the parents and keep them informed of the medical findings. An inquisitory or adversarial stature should be avoided. The earliest experiences in a psychotherapeutic relationship must be felt as helpful and as bringing about some lessening of distress, crises, and the sense of fear and anxiety. If an accusatory complaint, however valid, is made the abuser can be expected to experience greater initial fear and threat as a period of uncertainty, isolation, and loneliness is entered. In the encouragement of open discussion and in the urging of a renunciation of concealment by abusive parents of the injurious behavior towards one or more of their children, there is an understanding in psychotherapy that the discussion will not bring about punishment or rejection. The assurance of nonrejection and of a nonpunitive response is most difficult when being given by an agent of a legal agency not provided with the privilege of professional confidence or by a law enforcement officer serving as a child protective service worker.

Individuals respond to external conditions perceived as dangerous or threatening and to internal conditions or inner drives, emotions, or fantasies perceived as unacceptable with fears of retaliation, rejection, and social isolation. The responses are typically those that will avoid the discomfort or pain of the anxiety reflecting or signaling danger and threat, whether from external or internal sources. In psychotherapy, the therapist also represents change and symbolizes an advocacy for change. In that context, the therapist is also seen as an authority and as an "authoritarian," dominating, fearsome, and hostile. These "transference" responses are expected and are treated for their underlying determinants and thereby reduce resistances against further exploration and learning. The revelation of ideas, relationships, feelings, and activities recognized as forbidden and punishable, or as shameful and humiliating, is difficult even when the patient or client is safe from punitive consequences or their threat. To assume that this is any less difficult under punitive conditions or their threat or where ordered by an authority under coercive circumstances approaches the incredible. A therapeutic relationship involves the search for understanding without rebuff.

There are unfortunate misunderstandings about "treatment motivation" or treatment participation and continuity. The person who is reluctant to accept treatment is often inaccurately compared with individuals who request treatment and talk openly. The abusive parent who is reluctant to talk openly or freely is unfairly compared with the adult who has requested psychotherapy. In fact, the patient who talks freely is a rarity, and many months of work might be necessary to secure a halfway sufficient degree of honesty. The abusive parent who is unwilling to talk freely and honestly, who might angrily protest complaints or accusations, and who might insult and depreciate child protective service worker efforts might in fact be more honestly expositive than one who readily confesses or admits to physical and/or sexual abuse of a child. The abusive parent, like most clients or patients, is seldom accessible to treatment in the beginning, is reluctant to "open up," and certainly does not have

confidence in a total stranger, especially one initiating contact by means of a formal complaint even while offering services. A charge of maltreatment of a child cannot be expected to evoke initial responses of relief and calm in the parent so confronted.

The psychological treatment of members of a family with abusive relationships requires a dedication to interventions that initiate and aid in the development of a working relationship between the adult or child patient and the therapist. Genuine cooperation is vital during treatment sessions; the building of an effective treatment alliance is necessary if successful change is to be possible. A treatment alliance is not established immediately with first contacts and does not come about instantaneously. The alliance is, however, significantly facilitated or seriously obstructed by the quality of the earliest interactions during interviewing and other contacts. Abusive families are usually thought to be "hostile, concealing and rejecting the need of assistance." Participation in treatment also requires an understanding of the process and procedures of therapy, the expectations and purposes for some of the therapist's interventions. Confrontation, clarification, and the continuing encouragement of self-observation assisted by timed interpretations to facilitate the working alliance bring patients to a closer appreciation of why they resist assistance and change. Resistances cannot be ordered out of existence; they have developed for psychological reasons and they need to be treated.

The tendency in maltreatment is for chronic, however intermittent, patterns of abuse. Self-initiated treatment by abusive parents occurs and has been reported in the literature. The report of a family in which maltreatment of children is occurring probably involves persons who have not requested treatment, or at least not recently. Our experience with such families indicates a wide range of emotional disorders, including symptom neuroses and character neuroses, and such patients are well protected against insight, change, and intervention originating in the outer world.

Treatment of the Child

The dependency on parents is greater in abused children than in nontraumatized children, and the child's treatment itself is therefore dependent on the parents' attitudes toward treatment. A working alliance with parents is therefore essential not only to improve parent-child relationships but also to prevent the undermining of the child's therapy through failure of appointments or the child's perception of parental disinterest or disapproval and consequent fear of additional rejection and loss of care and hoped for affection.

The evaluation of children's emotional status or

mental health is facilitated by assessments of mastery of age-appropriate tasks. Evaluations and treatment need to be carried out under appropriate conditions, including provisions for play, drawing, and testing. Very young children may have difficulty in separating from a parent, and flexibility is needed to allow a parent to be present until a relationship is established permitting separation for the period of the session. Play and drawings and their interpretations are significant avenues for the child to express feelings and conflicts about self and parents, about their life situation and the emotional climate at home.

Interviewing older children is very similar to interviewing adults. History, early memories, attitudes, anxieties, mood, and other aspects of mental status can be assessed. Complaints by the child freely offered become crucial in facilitating a working relationship through the reduction of tension and awareness of "help" as symptoms are revealed and underlying pathology considered. Many young children with histories of abuse and neglect become highly dependent on their therapist, and the treatment of longings for intimate and nurturing gratification in children who were in fact deprived and brutalized requires great inner strength and resiliency in therapists.

The Psychotherapeutic Situation in the Treatment of Childhood Abuse

Like every medical endeavor, psychotherapies are concerned with symptoms and with the ways and means of removing them. Like any healing art, the first and foremost interest is not in how good or how bad a person the patient happens to be, but primarily in how sick a person the patient is, in how the patient became ill, regardless of the origins of the illness. Psychotherapeutic methods are from the outset a method of empirical, cool, objective investigation; the therapist is braced against any feelings of horror, disgust, shame, or anxiety that might occur when dealing with human aberrations. As human beings, psychotherapists are not devoid of these feelings, but they learn to proceed without swerving and without diffidence, regardless of the aberrations they are faced with: murder, falsehood, theft, incest, intrigue, chicanery, or child abuse. All are grist to the mill of psychological study.

Child abuse work is conducted under conditions structured by legal, political, and social considerations. These are set against treatment that must remain strictly scientific, that is, objective, cool, rational, unmoralistic, nonpolitical, and equally indifferent toward and curious about social passions and political trends. Clinicians need to concentrate on the psychological dynamics that are set into play when humans kill each other, including young children. As a person, the clinician, including the pediatrician is not at all immune to the torment of such inner queries but must maintain neutrality in his or her professional work and not get caught up in the decision-making and social action and experimentation that characterize the child protective system. Whether a person is allowed into treatment or whether the legal interventions are helpful are not the specific work of psychotherapy; however, the therapist cannot remain aloof from considerations about the conditions in which therapeutics are possible.

Fluid and Electrolyte Therapy

LEWIS A. BARNESS, M.D.

In health, fluid homeostasis is maintained by oral ingestion of fluids and foods that contain minerals, and fluid intake is regulated by thirst. Attention to fluid intake is necessary when the thirst mechanism is deranged, when fluid losses exceed intake, when the plasma volume is sub- or supranormal, or when the patient is unable to express his needs.

Water constitutes about 70% of lean body mass; 40 to 45% is intracellular, about 18% is interstitial, and 7% is intravascular. Intracellular cations are mainly potassium and magnesium; interstitial and intravascular mainly sodium (140–145 meq/l) and potassium (4–5 meq/l). Intracellular anions include phosphates, sulfates, bicarbonate, organic anions, and protein. Interstitial and intravascular cations are mainly chloride (95–105 meq/l) and bicarbonate (22–25 meq/l). Intravascular plasma also contains 6 to 7 gm of protein per dl (10 meq/l).

Maintenance water requirement, the volume required to replace insensible water loss (skin and respiratory tract) and water of urine formation in an afebrile patient at bed rest, is approximately 100 ml/100 kcal expended. Calculations for fluid requirements may be based on metabolic rate, surface area or weight (Table I).

Hydrogen ion homeostasis is maintained by plasma buffers, by control of P_{CO_2} by the lung and by renal excretion of acids or bases.

Maintenance Fluid Therapy. Maintenance fluids

Table 1. MAINTENANCE REQUIREMENTS

Weight (kg)	Surface Area (m²)	Water (ml/kg)	Cal/kg	Na⁺/kg (meq)	K⁺/kg (meq)
3	0.20	100	40–50	3–4	3–4
5	0.27	90	50–70	3–4	2–3
10	0.45	75	40–60	2–3	2–3
15	0.64	65	40–50	2–3	2–3
30	1.10	55	35–45	2–3	1–2
50	1.50	45	25–40	1–2	1–2
70	1.75	40	15–20	1–2	1–2

Requirements/m²: Water 1500 ml, Na⁺ 60 meq, K⁺ 50 meq.

are used in conditions when the child is in a normal state of hydration, such as in preoperative preparation. Such solutions should be made with sodium concentrations of 30 to 50 meq/l and potassium concentrations of 15 to 25 meq/l. Ordinarily, the anion can be entirely chloride, though basic anions (e.g., lactate, bicarbonate, acetate) may be used, up to one third of the total anions.

Dehydration. Assess the degree of dehydration. Volume depletion is estimated by weight loss as well as by blood pressure determination. Serum electrolytes and pH help determine status of individual ions. P_{CO_2} determination is useful in distinguishing pH abnormalities due to metabolic states in contrast to respiratory abnormalities. In respiratory acidosis the P_{CO_2} is high and in respiratory alkalosis it is low. These are reversed in metabolic acidosis and alkalosis.

Oral Rehydration. If the patient is alert, awake, and not in shock, first attempt to correct dehydration by oral fluids. Composition of three oral rehydration solutions are listed in Table 2.

Table 2. **COMPOSITION OF ORAL SOLUTIONS (mM/1)**

	Solution 1 (WHO)	Solution 2	Solution 3
Na+	90	50	30
K+	20	20	25
Cl-	80	40	30
HCO3-	30	30	—
Citrate	—	—	28
Glucose	111	111	278
Osmolality	331	251	391

The WHO solution (solution 1) has been successfully used worldwide for the treatment of diarrhea and dehydration, but is little used here because of fear of causing hyperelectrolytemia. This should be supplemented with water or breast milk to compensate for insensible water losses. Solution 2 provides sufficient electrolytes and water for many deficiency states and is usually well taken by ill children. Solution 3 is commercially available and convenient but does not provide as rapid correction, and may produce adverse osmotic effects.

For oral rehydration, give 50 ml/kg body weight within 4 hours for mild dehydration and 100 ml/kg over 6 hours for moderate dehydration. Amounts and rates should be increased if rehydration does not appear complete or if the patient continues to have excess losses, as with diarrhea. If the patient is nursing, these fluids should be supplemented with breastfeeding. In other patients, plain water should be offered after treatment has been given for 4 to 6 hours if solution 1 is used. Sufficient free water is available from solutions 2 and 3. In many

children with vomiting and diarrhea, vomiting will cease after 4 hours.

While diarrhea continues, an intake of 10 to 15 ml of electrolyte-containing solution per kg of body weight per hour is appropriate to compensate approximately for the stool losses. Maintenance therapy is added.

Parenteral Needs. Patients in shock, those with severe dehydration or with uncontrollable vomiting, those unable to drink for any reason including extreme fatigue or coma, and those with severe gastric distention require intravenous therapy.

Calculation of needs is similar to that above except that tolerance to intravenous fluids requires more frequent monitoring. Deficits of water and electrolytes can be estimated from Tables 3 and 4. Emergency management, especially if blood pressure is low, requires a central venous or pulmonary arterial catheter for more precise monitoring.

For severely dehydrated patients or those in shock, rapid intravenous administration of 20 to 40 ml/kg over 1 to 2 hours is given. Solution can be plasma, whole blood, human albumin, or other colloid. If these are not immediately available, start with a solution containing 75 meq/l of sodium and chloride in 5% to 10% glucose in water. A base such as lactate may be substituted for one third of the chloride. Next, the total volume of fluid to be administered over 24 hours is calculated. Half of this is given in the next 8 hours, and the remainder over the last 14 to 16 hours. This solution should

Table 3. **DEFICITS IN MODERATE DEHYDRATION**

	H2O (ml/kg)	Na+ (meq/kg)	K+ (meq/kg)	Cl- (meq/kg)
Fasting	100–120	5–7	1–2	4–6
Diarrhea				
Isotonic	100–120	8–10	8–10	8–10
Hypotonic	100–120	10–12	8–10	10–12
Hypertonic	100–120	2–4	0–4	–2 to –6
Pyloric stenosis	100–120	8–10	10–12	10–12
Diabetic				
ketoacidosis	100–120	8–10	5–7	6–8

Table 4. **ELECTROLYTE CONTENT OF BODY FLUIDS (meq/l)**

Source	Na+	K+	Cl-
Gastric	20–80	5–20	100–150
Small intestine, pancreas, bile	100–140	5–15	90–130
Ileostomy	45–135	3–15	20–115
Diarrhea	10–90	10–80	10–110
Sweat			
Normal	10–30	3–10	10–35
Cystic fibrosis	50–130	5–25	50–110
Burns	140–145	4–5	110

contain 40 to 75 meq/l NaCl in 5 to 10% glucose. Potassium, 20 to 30 meq/l, should be added as soon as the patient urinates.

For hypotonic or isotonic dehydration with adequate blood pressure, initial colloid can be eliminated but calculations are similar. For hypertonic dehydration, similar solutions are used but the rate of administration is decreased so that total fluids are given at a constant rate over 24 hours. Potassium concentration is 40 meq/l. Calcium gluconate, 10 ml of 10% solution, is added for each liter administered.

For acidosis with pH above 7.1, bicarbonate or other base is usually not necessary and, because H_2CO_3 traverses membranes including the CSF more rapidly than HCO_3^-, may be undesirable because the CSF pH will decrease while the blood pH is increasing. This is especially important when respiratory gas exchange is impaired. When the blood pH is 7.1 or less, bicarbonate, 15 to 25 meq/l, replaces an equal amount of chloride in the hydrating solution.

Diabetic Ketoacidosis. Elevations of blood sugar increase serum osmolality. Each 1000 mg/l has an osmolality of $1000 \div 180$ (the molecular weight) $= 5.6$ mosm. While each 100 mg glucose/dl would be expected to decrease serum sodium $5.6 \div 2 = 2.8$ meq, measurements have indicated that the true depression is about 1.6 meq/100 mg glucose. Serum sodium is decreased in hyperglycemic states. However, as the glucose is metabolized, water shifts out of the extracellular space and the serum sodium rises. Therefore, even in the presence of a low serum sodium with hyperglycemia, calculations are similar as in isotonic dehydration unless the serum sodium is depressed more than 1.6 meq/100 mg/dl of elevated glucose.

Premature Infants—Maintenance. Maintenance requirements are 80 to 100 ml/kg/day. However, Na^+ and K^+ are not needed on the first day. Na^+, 20 meq/l are added on the second and third day and increased to 40 meq/l on the fourth day. K^+, 2 meq/kg/day, is started on the second day. Fluids should be in 5 or 10% glucose with careful monitoring of blood sugar and electrolytes and appropriate modifications made.

Infants under radiant warmers or under phototherapy require 25 to 50% increase in maintenance fluids.

Anuria. Fluids are restricted to insensible water loss, approximately one fourth maintenance requirements, plus any urine output as 5 to 10% D/W. Hyperkalemia or hyponatremia may occur and require correction.

Inappropriate Secretion of Antidiuretic Hormone. This may occur with CNS disease or trauma, or postoperatively. Serum osmolality is low, while urine osmolality is inappropriately elevated. Treat with fluid restriction to one fourth to one half maintenance. In those with CNS disease without apparent fluid abnormalities, treat expectantly at two thirds to three fourths maintenance.

Cardiac Disease with Failure. Restrict fluids and Na^+ to two thirds maintenance. Diuretics may be needed. Serum electrolytes must be monitored, especially for the development of low serum sodium.

Parenteral Nutrition. Any child requiring prolonged intravenous therapy requires calories other than those provided by glucose in the electrolyte/glucose mixtures. Principles of administration are similar to those described on page 758. Caloric needs are those outlined in Table 1.

Malignant Hyperthermia

THOMAS P. KEON, M.D.

Temperature elevation accompanies a variety of physiologic processes and a broad spectrum of clinical diseases. Causes include vigorous exercise, ovulation, central nervous system dysfunction, infection by microorganisms, malignancy, collagen diseases, heat stroke, and malignant hyperthermia (MH).

Malignant hyperthermia is a muscular disorder in which rapid rises in body temperature to 43°C (109.4°F) or more have been recorded. This hereditary disorder is triggered by the administration of certain anesthetic agents or muscle relaxants used in anesthesia. On rare occasions a malignant hyperthermic crisis can be precipitated outside the operating room by high environmental temperatures, mild infections, extreme emotional excitement, muscle injury, or exercise. The incidence of MH is reported as 1:15,000 anesthetics in pediatric patients and 1:50,000 anesthetics in the adult population. The mortality rate has declined from a high of 70% in the 1960s to less than 30% in recent years. The decrease in mortality can be attributed to early recognition of a crisis, preoperative detection of susceptible individuals, and the recent use of dantrolene for pretreatment in susceptible individuals and in the management of acute MH crises.

Malignant hyperthermia is a disorder of muscle metabolism that results in a hypermetabolic state. The abnormality appears to be one of altered calcium dynamics, with a failure of uptake and storage of calcium by the sarcoplasmic reticulum inside the muscle cell. Relaxation is prevented by calcium, and there is increased glycogen utilization and heat production. Various pumping mechanisms of the cell membrane fail, with potassium, magnesium, and phosphate leaking out and sodium, water, and additional calcium leaking in. The potassium aggravates arrhythmias and water increases muscle edema. The increased metabolic rate results in excessive oxygen consumption, increased carbon dioxide production, and lactic acidosis. The effectiveness of dantrolene in this disorder is attributed to its attenuation of calcium release by the sarcoplasmic reticulum.

The earliest and most consistent sign of a developing malignant hyperthermic episode is tachycardia. Progression to multifocal ventricular dysrhythmia occurs with fulminant episodes. Blood pressure is unstable. Muscle stiffness and rigidity commonly occurs but is not a consistent sign. Profuse sweating accompanied by rapid and deep respirations may be observed. Fever may not be present initially but can rapidly rise to 45°C. Arterial blood gas analysis reveals acidemia with a mixed metabolic and respiratory acidosis. Hypoxemia occurs unless the inspired oxygen concentration is elevated. Serum potassium and calcium rise sharply. Creatinine phosphokinase (CPK) is grossly elevated. Myoglobinemia followed by myoglobinuria may induce acute renal failure. Disseminated intravascular coagulation (DIC) and heart failure occur with a severe crisis.

A written protocol in addition to appropriate equipment and drugs should be available in all surgical suites for the treatment of malignant hyperthermia.

1. Discontinue all triggering agents (potent inhalation anesthetics, succinylcholine).
2. Replace rubber hoses and soda lime or use a "clean" machine (anesthetic machine and breathing apparatus without prior exposure to triggering agents).
3. Hyperventilate with 100% oxygen and monitor with arterial line, Foley catheter, and central venous line.
4. Administer dantrolene,* 3 mg/kg as an initial bolus and increments of 1 mg/kg every 5 to 10 minutes until there is evidence that improvement is occurring. Up to 10 mg/kg may be required.
5. Initiate active cooling measures including a cooling blanket, ice bags or an iced bath, gastric, peritoneal, or thoracic lavage with cool saline (4°C), intravenous administration of iced normal saline solution. Cease cooling measures when temperature falls to 38°C.
6. Administer sodium bicarbonate, 1 meq/kg initially and in increments guided by arterial blood gas results.
7. Procainamide infusion, 1 mg/kg/min, is used for the treatment of ventricular arrhythmias.
8. Hyperkalemia may require treatment with glucose and insulin. (1 ml/kg of mixture containing 50 ml of 50% glucose and 10 units of regular insulin). Monitor blood glucose and potassium levels.
9. Maintain intravascular volume and urine output of 2 ml/kg/hr with normal saline. Mannitol,

0.25 gm/kg, and furosemide, 1 mg/kg, may be necessary to maintain urine output.
10. Continue dantrolene,* 1 mg/kg/6 hr for 3 days, to prevent recurrence. Ten percent of patients may have recurrence in the first 8 hours.
11. Supportive therapy with vigilant monitoring of arterial blood gases, serum electrolytes, osmolality, urine output, coagulation studies, and hemodynamic parameters is essential.

Malignant hyperthermia crisis may be prevented by the identification of susceptible individuals and the avoidance of known triggering agents. A family history of malignant hyperthermia or unexplained anesthetic death in a family member should alert the anesthesiologist and stimulate additional investigation. A muscle biopsy can be done and the caffeine-halothane contracture test performed to identify susceptible individuals. Anesthesia using nitrous oxide, diazepam, barbiturates, narcotics, and pancuronium has been administered without triggering a reaction in susceptible individuals. Agents to avoid include halogenated agents, depolarizing muscle relaxants, and amide type local anesthetics. Pretreatment of susceptible individuals using dantrolene, 1 mg/kg every 6 hours by mouth and 1 mg/kg intravenously, immediately prior to induction of anesthesia is recommended.

Infantile Colic

MAURICE A. KIBEL, D.C.H.

In Western countries the terms infantile, 3-month, and nocturnal colic have come to be associated with the regular occurrence of paroxysmal bouts of vigorous loud crying in infants between the ages of 2 weeks and 3 months. Attacks are commonest in the late afternoon or early evening. During the spells the infant cries persistently, cannot be placated, thrashes about, and draws up his legs or arches backward as though in pain. In all other respects the infant is healthy and thriving. There is no more spitting or vomiting than usual at this age, and the stools are normal. However, excessive wind may be passed per rectum during the paroxysm. The spells diminish after the age of 3 months and the infant shows no after effects.

Infantile colic is one of the commonest diagnoses made in pediatric office practice, yet there is still little agreement as to the nature of the infant's distress or the reasons for it. The confusion is exemplified by the range and ingenuity of treatments suggested by previous contributors to this section. These include gin, whiskey, making humming noises, and anal dilation! The measures we recommend are as likely as any to succeed in a condition that generally disappears spontaneously at around 3 months whatever the treatment.

---

*Safety of use of dantrolene in children under 5 years of age has not been established.

Crying is a normal and regular occurrence in young infants in response to a range of stimuli that are perceived as unpleasant. By crying the infant is signaling his need for help in the only way he knows and the commonest of these needs are for food, physical comfort, and close human contact. Nevertheless, even when these have been satisfied, a considerable portion of the waking hours are spent fretting or crying. As with infantile colic "normal" crying is most frequent between 6 P.M. and 10 P.M., at a time when the infant has accumulated a surfeit of stimuli from his new environment, hence the irritability. This pattern of behavior is universal, being seen in infants from all social strata and in both primitive and developed communities.

Infants with paroxysmal fretting or colic, often have a characteristic pattern of behavior. They appear to have a low threshold for discomfort and frustration. They gulp air during feeding, and this probably contributes to ongoing discomfort rather than being the primary cause. They often cry when a normal stool, or wind are passed per rectum. This behavior is as common in breast-fed infants as it is in bottle-fed infants.

Prolonged bouts of crying are unnerving and exhausting for parents, whose inability to console the infant leads to frustration, anxiety, and destroyed confidence. A vicious cycle then develops in which the crying infant is further stressed by the parents' tension and even more overstimulated by their futile efforts at rocking, burping, feeding, and pacifying.

Sometimes the difficulties in the mother-infant relationship may be primarily maternal. The infant is keenly sensitive of his mother's reactions, and lack of confidence and tension on her part may lead to excessive irritability in the infant. Less commonly, frank difficulties with bonding and post-partum depression are more serious causes that should always be borne in mind. Whether the infant or the mother is primarily at fault, it is not altogether surprising that in severe cases of "colic" the parent may be so exhausted from lack of sleep and frustration that severe family conflicts and even physical abuse of the infant may ensue.

MANAGEMENT

The diagnosis of infantile colic cannot be considered before an unhurried, comprehensive history has been taken and full physical and developmental examination carried out to exclude organic disease. The tympanic membranes should be inspected, as otitis media can cause persistent crying at night. One should ask about the strength of the urinary stream, and, if possible, micturition should be observed, since urinary obstruction may cause recurrent screaming spells in infants of both sexes. A urine culture and microscopy to exclude urinary tract infection are advisable in all cases of colic. The abdomen should be carefully examined for hernias and masses. The presence of persistent vomiting or spitting may point to esophagitis associated with gastroesophageal reflux. It is crucial to ensure that there is no developmental delay or neurologic abnormality in the unusually irritable or "colicky" infant. If screening for inherited metabolic disease is not routinely performed, this should be an essential test at this stage.

Having excluded organic disorders, the adequacy of feeding should be ascertained. Excessive crying is common in breast-fed infants who are underfed and the 6 P.M. feed is often the period when milk flow is at its lowest. A supplementary formula feed at this time is worth trying in these circumstances.

In most cases full explanation of the behavioral and benign nature of crying coupled with simple advice on handling will generally go a long way toward allaying fears, improving parents' confidence, and easing the situation. It must be emphasized to the parents that in responding to the crying by handling and loving the infant they are doing the normal thing and not spoiling him.

Attention to feeding technique and the mothers' method of bringing up wind may be fruitful. There are of course several ways of burping an infant after a feed, and experimentation may be necessary. Medications containing dill and bicarbonate of soda or preparations such as Telament drops also seem to help some infants. The hole in the teat should be checked, as one that is too large or too small may result in excessive air swallowing.

Attention to the infant's physical environment— a comfortable, warm room that is free of draughts along with firm wrapping to provide a feeling of being touched are other simple points that may be of value. Excessive stimulation by family and especially young siblings sometimes contributes to evening irritability.

A harness or sling to carry the infant on the mother's back or in front, allows close body contact and helps with the breaking of wind. The "infant seat" or chair is a further helpful measure and can be used from 1 month of age.

Sucking is a source of great comfort to babies. Parents often need to be reassured that pacifiers are useful and harmless, provided that reasonable hygiene is adhered to. Better still, finger or thumb sucking should be encouraged from an early age in these babies. Barry Zuckerman has described how this sort of anticipatory guidance to mothers immediately after birth may help in preventing problems later.*

I believe, therefore, that most so called colicky

---

*Behaviour Problems in Childhood: A Primary Care Approach. Gable, S(Ed), New York, Grune and Stratton, 1981.

infants simply represent the extreme end of a continuum of what is really normal behavior in young infants. Reassurance and attention to feeding and nursing technique are therapeutic in most cases. In only a minority is actual pain being experienced, presumably from smooth muscle spasm. In these infants a safe medication that undoubtedly helps is the antispasmodic dicyclamine hydrochloride (Bentyl) 5 ml of the syrup (containing 5 mg of active ingredient) are given in 10 ml of water 15 minutes before the evening feed or twice daily if necessary. However, mothers should never be fobbed off with medication before the steps mentioned above have been followed.

Many doctors and nurses readily turn to soya formulas in infants with colic, but I am convinced that in the majority of such infants changing the formula or discontinuing breast-feeding are totally unjustified. Nevertheless, in a few of these truly colicky infants, a specific item in the nursing mothers' diet may be responsible—spicy food or onions, for example—or true milk protein sensitivity may be present. Food intolerance should be suspected when there is a family history of atopy or when attacks are severe and persist past the age of 4 months. In the case of a breast-fed infant, a trial period in which cow milk is excluded from the mother's diet may be fruitful. If formula-fed, a change to soya milk (Prosobee, Isomil) is worth trying but clearly on a trial basis only. If the infant improves, the original formula should be reintroduced to see whether the symptoms can again be provoked and the trial repeated for confirmation of the intolerance.

Should all else fail sedation with phenobarbital, 2 mg/kg, or promethazine, 0.5 mg/kg, before the evening feed or twice daily may be required.

Genetic Diseases

BRUCE D. BLUMBERG, M.D.,
and DAVID L. RIMOIN, M.D., Ph.D.

Genetic diseases, although in most cases individually rare, are very common in aggregate. Population surveys reveal that 2 to 6% of all neonates exhibit some congenital malformation, and birth defects remain the third leading cause of mortality in the pediatric age group. Hospital surveys demonstrate that 20 to 50% of all pediatric inpatients suffer from disease processes with significant genetic components. In fact, many of the disorders discussed in this book are inherited or have important genetic aspects. Rather than recapitulating the specifics of these conditions, we will discuss the general approach to the management of patients with known or suspected genetic diseases.

Management of disease can involve prevention, therapy, or cure. In order to truly "cure" a genetic disorder, manipulations would be required at the gene level to repair or replace defective DNA sequences. To date, genetic "surgery" to reconstruct altered DNA has not been accomplished. However, recent experiments in mammals and humans have succeeded in altering gene expression and even in introducing functional "foreign" genes into an intact organism. To perfect these techniques as viable modes of therapy for any given genetic disorder, several sequential criteria must be met. First, it is necessary to identify the gene defect responsible for the disease. Then adequate quantities (numbers of copies) of the gene's normal human analog must be isolated or elaborated. Next, methods must be developed for the in vivo introduction of these copies into the cell nuclei of the patient. Finally, the gene must be incorporated into the recipient's genome in such a way that it is subject to normal mechanisms of regulated expression.

These sequential tasks for successful gene therapy have not been accomplished in their entirety even in experimental systems; preservation of normal gene regulation (tissue specific, developmentally sequenced, or feedback) almost certainly will continue to be the most difficult obstacle to gene therapy. Nevertheless, enormous recent advances suggest that therapy at the gene level may be a reality in the near future. It has been possible to introduce "foreign" growth hormone genes into intact mice (at the time of fertilization). Not only do these genes produce functional growth hormone in the recipient animals but these genes may then be transmitted to succeeding generations.

In the human, successful introduction and expression of foreign genes has not yet been achieved. However, it has been possible, in an experimental setting, to alter gene expression temporarily to compensate for a genetic defect. By administering 5-azocytidine to a patient suffering from β-thalassemia it has been possible to derepress the gene for the γ globin chain (presumably by interfering with the DNA methylation that is responsible for repression) and to thereby produce a transient increase in fetal hemoglobin synthesis. If techniques such as this become clinically applicable, it may become possible to artificially produce "persistence" of fetal hemoglobin and protect against the clinical consequences of β-thalassemia, sickle cell anemia, and other β-chain mutations.

While gene therapy remains a promise of the near future, effective therapy at other levels presently is available for many genetic disorders. Hereditary conditions frequently can be predicted, prevented, or managed to alleviate or avert clinical illness. Since the variety of surgical or medical treatments for genetic diseases is almost limitless, consideration will be given only to the general principles of management of hereditary disorders (Table 1). Of course, prior to embarking upon a

Table 1. MODES OF GENETIC THERAPY

Gene therapy
   e.g., i. β-thalassemia (experimental administration of 5-azocytidine to derepress hemoglobin F synthesis)

Replacement of missing (or defective) gene product
   e.g., i. Hemophilia A and B
        ii. Growth hormone deficiency
       iii. Agammaglobulinemia

Dietary elimination
   e.g., i. PKU and other disorders of amino acid metabolism
        ii. Galactosemia
       iii. Lactose or fructose intolerance
       iv. Urea cycle defects
        v. Organic acidemias

Avoidance of drugs and/or other environmental agents
   e.g., i. G6PD deficiency
        ii. Porphyrias
       iii. Mastocytosis
       iv. Malignant hyperthermia
        v. Pseudocholinesterase deficiency

End product supplementation (distal to an enzymatic block)
   e.g., i. Thyroid synthetic defects
        ii. Congenital adrenal hyperplasias
       iii. Glycogen storage diseases (frequent or continuous carbohydrate feedings)

Metabolic suppression (via feedback mechanisms)
   e.g., i. Congenital adrenal hyperplasias
        ii. Acute intermittent porphyria (hematin therapy)

Co-factor supplementation
   e.g., i. Methylmalonic acidemia (B_{12})
        ii. Proprionic acidemia or multiple carboxylase deficiency (biotin)
       iii. "Infantile convulsions" (pyridoxine)
       iv. Vitamin D dependent rickets

Enzyme induction
   e.g., i. Gilbert or Crigler-Najjar syndromes (induction of glucuronyl transferase with phenobarbital)
        ii. Methemoglobinemia (induction of NADPH dehydrogenase with methylene blue)

Metabolic inhibition
   e.g., i. Lesch-Nyhan syndrome (allopurinol)
        ii. Hyperlipoproteinemia, type III (clofibrate)
       iii. Nephrogenic diabetes insipidus (thiazide diuretics)

Detoxification (by depletion of substrate)
   e.g., i. Wilson disease or cystinuria (d-penicillamine)
        ii. Familial hypercholesterolemia (cholestyramine)
       iii. Hemochromatosis (desferoxamine)
       iv. Gout (uricosuric agents)
        v. Urea cycle defects (sodium benzoate)
       vi. Refsum disease (plasmapheresis)

Organ transplantation
   e.g., i. Immunodeficiency syndromes (marrow, fetal thymus, or fetal liver)
        ii. Osteopetrosis (bone marrow)
       iii. Polycystic kidneys (renal)
       iv. Mucopolysaccharidoses (fibroblasts questionably effective)

Prenatal therapy
   e.g., i. Erythroblastosis fetalis (intrauterine transfusion)
        ii. Methylmalonic acidemia (maternal B_{12} administration)
       iii. Multiple carboxylase deficiency (maternal biotin administration)
       iv. Hydrocephalus (transcutaneous ventriculoamniotic shunt placement)
        v. Urethral obstruction (transcutaneous vesicoamniotic shunt placement)
       vi. Fetal tachyarrhythmias (cardiac glycoside administration)

Surgery
   e.g., i. Complete androgen insensitivity (malignant prophylaxis)
        ii. Retinoblastoma (extirpation)
       iii. Cleft lip (cosmetic)
       iv. Multiple epiphyseal dysplasia (hip replacement)
        v. Hereditary spherocytosis (splenectomy)
       vi. Glycogen storage diseases (portacaval bypass)

Miscellaneous
   e.g., i. Arthrogryposis (physical therapy)
        ii. Huntington disease (psychological counseling)

particular course of treatment, a particular genetic defect must be identified as precisely as possible (at the molecular level, when feasible). Details of genetic differential diagnoses are beyond the scope of this summary, and the ensuing discussion will assume that an "exact" diagnosis has been ensured before considering therapy.

For some genetic diseases, symptoms are produced by an inability to synthesize an essential gene product. If the missing substance can be replaced exogenously, symptoms may be alleviated. In this manner, a transfusion of cryoprecipitate will temporarily correct the coagulopathy of the factor VIII deficient hemophiliac. In other instances, however, a single gene defect produces an enzyme deficiency, and enzyme replacement therapy is impractical for most diseases (owing to the difficulty of delivering the active enzyme to its intended site of action). In such cases, rather than supplying the absent gene product, therapeutic efforts must attempt to negate the effects of this deficiency. To this end, dietary elimination minimizes the accumulation of toxic metabolites, even in the face of a persisting enzymatic block (e.g., in phenylketonuria [PKU] or galactosemia). In other genetic disorders, symptoms are produced by an aberrant response to exogenous environmental agents. Avoidance of these agents, such as fava beans or offending medications in the G6PD deficient patient, may prevent clinical manifestation of the genetic defect.

Some other genetic diseases are characterized by the inability to synthesize a vital substance because of an enzymatic defect; this end product may be provided to the patient, thereby averting the consequences of the metabolic defect. Patients with iodine organification defects thus benefit from thyroid hormone supplementation even though the supplied substance is "distant" to the metabolic block. In the adrenogenital syndromes, treatment with corticosteroids or mineralocorticoids, or both, not only avoids the consequences of deficiency of these compounds, but also suppresses the overactive pathways that had been producing masculinizing or feminizing hormones.

In still other conditions, a metabolic block can be overdriven by the supplementation of pharmacologic doses of the appropriate vitamin cofactor (e.g., B_{12}-responsive methylmalonic aciduria). This strategy will be effective for conditions that involve decreased absorption of dietary cofactor, defective endogenous synthesis of active cofactor, or a decreased affinity of an abnormal enzyme for its normal cofactor. In yet other genetic disorders, resort must be made to detoxifying therapies. For example, the clinical abnormalities produced by copper in Wilson disease may be reversed by the administration of D-penicillamine, which chelates and forces excretion of excess stored copper.

For some genetic diseases for which it is not possible to enhance the activity of a deficient or defective enzyme, it may be possible to produce therapeutic benefit by manipulating other enzymes in the same or related pathways. In this fashion, phenobarbital may ameliorate the hyperbilirubemia of Gilbert or Crigler-Najjar syndromes by inducing glucuronyl transferase activity and stimulating conjugation. As another example, the inhibition of xanthine oxidase by allopurinol may avert the nephropathic consequences of the hyperuricemia seen in Lesch-Nyhan syndrome.

In recent years organ transplantation has assumed an expanding role in the therapy of genetic disorders. Of course, it is possible to replace organs that have been damaged or deformed as a result of a genetic defect; such is the case with renal transplantation in patients with adult polycystic kidney disease. Perhaps more significantly, organ transplantation in some diseases may provide a source of normal stem cells to replace their genetically abnormal counterparts, as is the case for some of the immunodeficiency syndromes. For still other disorders, transplanted tissue could potentially elaborate enzymes that the host had been genetically incapable of producing. This technique theoretically could benefit patients with Fabry's disease, mucopolysaccharidoses, or other conditions in which the missing enzyme is produced by transplantable tissues such as kidney or fibroblasts. However, the actual clinical benefit that has been derived from such transplants has thus far been limited.

The timing of therapy is of critical importance for many of the inborn metabolic errors. The pathologic consequences of a prolonged metabolic perturbation may be irreversible. The necessity of prompt diagnosis has stimulated the widespread institution of neonatal screening programs. Such testing is practical in diseases that can be inexpensively and accurately detected presymptomatically and for which early therapy is available and effective. Mandatory neonatal PKU screening is now performed in almost every state. The early recognition of this disorder and the prompt implementation of dietary restrictions allow the preservation of normal intellectual function in an individual who otherwise would be severely handicapped. Similar strategy has recently led to the expansion of neonatal screening in some states to include galactosemia, hypothyroidism, and other disorders of metabolism.

For some genetic diseases, even earlier recognition is required in order to minimize or avoid irreversible impairment. Although prenatal diagnosis has been available for some disorders for 10 to 15 years, it is much more recently that such diagnoses have provided opportunities for prenatal therapy. The best established antenatal therapeutic maneuver is the intrauterine transfusion of the fetus with erythroblastosis fetalis. Although still in a research stage, prenatal therapy has also been accomplished for some inborn errors of metabolism (i.e., maternal B_{12} administration in B_{12} responsive methylmalonic acidemia or maternal biotin administration in multiple carboxylase deficiency). Although results have not been uniformly encouraging thus far, procedures have been performed for the prenatal decompression of cranioventricular or urinary tract obstructions (i.e., by the transcutaneous, sonographically guided insertion of a one-way shunt to the amniotic cavity). Finally, in some instances, the antenatal recognition of a potentially life-threatening fetal anomaly (e.g., diaphragmatic hernia) has allowed life-saving surgery to be performed immediately after birth. It is likely that future advances will greatly broaden the spectrum of conditions amenable to similar forms of early intervention.

Prevention. One of the major facets of the management of genetic diseases is their prevention by genetic counseling, prenatal diagnosis, and screening programs. Genetic counseling has been defined as a communication process that deals with the human problems associated with the occurrence, or the risk of occurrence, of a genetic disorder in a family. This process involves an attempt by one or more appropriately trained persons to help the individual or family to 1) comprehend the medical facts, including the diagnosis, the probable course of the disorder, and the available management; 2) appreciate the way heredity contributes to the disorder, and the risk of recurrence in specified relatives; 3) understand the options for dealing with the risk of recurrence; 4) choose the course of action which seems appropriate to them in view of their risk and the family goals and act in accordance with that decision; and 5) make the best possible adjustment to the disorder in an affected family member and to the risk of recurrence of that disorder.

Several aspects of this definition merit elaboration. Genetic counseling, by its nature, is a family-oriented process. Even when a single individual is counseled, the familial implications of the discussed disease must be explored. Genetic counseling, like all counseling, is a communication process and thus requires a dialogue between the family and the health care provider. Genetic counseling ordinarily should be nondirective and focus upon the family's goals and values rather than reflect the counselor's subjective biases.

Genetic counseling is exceedingly time-consuming. A single new case, from initial data collection to completion, consumes almost 8 hours of professional time. The benefit of a team approach is an immediate corollary to the time-demanding nature of this process. Nurses, social workers, genetic associates, and psychiatric/psychologic professionals all may play indispensable roles.

A distinction should be made between "proband" and "nonproband" counseling. Usually genetic concerns are initiated by the presentation of a proband who has a specific inherited disease. Genetic medicine frequently departs from this disease-oriented model and instead focuses on health oriented medical activities. This preventive aspect of medical genetics attempts to minimize the incidence or impact of genetic diseases before they occur. Such efforts require the prospective identification of families at risk for the occurrence of a genetic illness. To implement this idea, several practical prerequisites must be met. A specific subpopulation at risk must be identifiable, an inexpensive screening test accurately predictive of risk must be available, and families at risk must be presented with options for dealing with this risk. This last requirement imposes the necessity of genetic counseling as a component of any screening program.

Several genetic diseases fulfill all these requirements. Heterozygote detection, for example, is available for sickle cell anemia in individuals of black African ancestry, for Tay-Sachs disease in Ashkenazi Jews, for β-thalassemia in individuals of Mediterranean ancestry, and for α-thalassemia in Orientals. It is likely that cystic fibrosis in Caucasians will join this list in the future when a noninvasive, reliable carrier test is developed. The beneficial effects of genetic screening are perhaps most evident in the case of Rh incompatibility. By prospectively identifying and treating women at risk for sensitization, the consequences of this genetic mismatch can be virtually eliminated.

As noted, genetic counseling must accompany screening if such testing is to achieve its intended goals. The challenges of this nonproband counseling are enormous. A couple prospectively discovered to be at genetic risk has had no personal experience with the disease in question in most cases. For example, Tay-Sachs disease is a completely abstract notion to the couple found to be at risk by carrier screening. It is difficult enough to illuminate the nature, course, and prognosis of a disease in proband-related counseling; these problems are magnified when the disease is predicted rather than experienced.

One of the most important goals of genetic counseling is the achievement of an understanding of the options available for dealing with risks of occurence or recurrence. A family may elect to accept their risk and continue with their prior reproductive plans, or they may alter their plans in a number of ways. A couple may decide to forego future reproduction, to adopt, or to employ donor insemination or a surrogate mother (in cases in which these methods circumvent the predicted genetic risk). It is not surprising that these options are unattractive to some couples. Fortunately, over the past decade, the development of prenatal diagnostic technologies has provided the additional option of selectively ensuring an unaffected offspring.

Midtrimester amniocentesis continues to be a widely employed prenatal diagnostic modality. Amniotic fluid obtained at 16 to 18 (menstrual) weeks of pregnancy contains cells that are thought to derive from the fetal skin and gastrointestinal, genitourinary, and/or respiratory tracts. These fibroblastoid and epithelioid cells may be placed in culture, thus establishing a viable fetal cell line. Within approximately 3 weeks, cell growth is usually adequate to allow cytogenetic or biochemical analysis. In this fashion, most chromosomal and many metabolic defects are detectable. Although at the present time, most of these diseases are not amenable to therapy, the family is at least afforded the option of selectively aborting an affected fetus (if such an action is consonant with their values).

In a smaller number of situations, direct analysis of the acellular amniotic fluid supernatant is of diagnostic value. In this manner, elevated alpha-fetoprotein may reflect an open neural tube defect, or an elevation of 17-hydroxyprogesterone may indicate the presence of 21-hydroxylase deficiency (since amniotic fluid is composed primarily of fetal urine). Recently, specialized techniques have been developed for the recognition of genetic defects that are not ordinarily expressed in amniotic fluid cells. Such methods may employ the known genetic linkage of an unmeasurable substance to an assayable marker (e.g., the linkage of 21-hydroxylase to the HLA locus). In other cases, it is actually possible to analyze cellular DNA to determine the presence or absence of a defect at the gene level (e.g., in α thalassemia or sickle cell anemia).

Ultrasonography is another broadly applicable technique of prenatal diagnosis. As an adjunct to amniocentesis, sonography aids in dating gestation, in localizing the placenta, and in detecting multiple gestations. As experience has accrued and technologic resolution has improved, many other fetal abnormalities have become amenable to sonographic diagnosis. An ultrasound examination can quantify amniotic fluid volume, assess fetal growth and well being (e.g., intrauterine growth retardation, ascites) and detect specific anomalies of the central nervous system (e.g., hydrocephalus, microcephaly), heart (valvular defects), gastrointestinal tract (obstructions), genitourinary system (e.g., cystic kidneys), and skeleton (e.g., abnormal limb length in some severe skeletal dysplasias).

Less frequently employed, but of value in specific situations, is fetal radiography, with or without the instillation of water-soluble (amniography) or lipid-soluble (fetography) contrast media into the amnionic sac. These methods may be useful, for example, in the assessment of bone mineralization in the fetus at risk for osteogenesis imperfecta. Since amniotic fluid is ordinarily swallowed, amniography may also allow evaluation of the fetal upper GI tract.

Also limited to specific situations are direct fetal visualization (fetoscopy) and fetal tissue sampling (e.g., blood drawing for the diagnosis of hemophilia or the hemoglobinopathies, skin biopsy for the diagnosis of lamellar ichthyosis, or liver biopsy for diagnosis of ornithine transcarbamylase deficiency). These latter techniques are accompanied by a much higher risk to pregnancy (3 to 5% spontaneous abortion) than is amniocentesis alone (total procedural risk $\leq 0.5\%$).

One of the more recent developments in prenatal diagnosis has been the emergence of methods to screen maternal blood for indicators of fetal disease. At the present time, maternal serum alpha-fetoprotein (AFP) determination represents the only screening test of this type (excepting routine antibody screening of all Rh negative women). By testing for elevated serum AFP in all pregnancies, it is possible to identify otherwise unsuspected women who are at an increased risk for fetal neural tube defect. It must be stressed that this is only a screening test, and persistently abnormal results must be followed by a more definitive examination (amniocentesis or ultrasonography, or both). It is likely that once the medical (e.g., quality control) and ethical (e.g., informed consent) questions surrounding this technique are resolved, maternal serum AFP screening, which is presently routine in Great Briatin and in some portions of the U.S., also will be adopted universally as a standard part of prenatal care.

Today, prenatal diagnosis is usually offered only to families known to be at increased risk for fetal disease. Advanced maternal age, with its concomitant increased risk for a chromosomally abnormal offspring, is by far the most common indication for prenatal studies. Couples known to be at risk for a detectable fetal condition by virtue of a previous affected child or positive family history compose a second group in which prenatal diagnosis may be performed. Other couples may be discovered to be at risk for a diagnosable fetal disease by virtue of the results of carrier or prenatal screening. Finally, prenatal diagnostic studies may be pertinent for undiagnosable conditions if test results are at least capable of refining the predicted risk of fetal disease. Amniocentesis in a Duchenne muscular dystrophy carrier serves as an example of this use of prenatal diagnosis; although this disorder cannot be diagnosed in utero, the a priori 25% risk of an affected offspring may be refined to a 50% risk, if the fetus is found to be male, or a near 0% risk in the instance of a female fetus.

In genetic disease, the broad connotation of "therapy" makes it difficult to maintain traditional distinctions between diagnosis and treatment. With the wide variety of genetic disorders confronting the clinician, accurate diagnosis is of paramount importance prior to a selection of therapeutic maneuvers. Many of these disorders require specific therapies, which follow the principles outlined above. Genetic counseling is one of the cornerstones of genetic therapy. Counseling serves to optimize the family's adjustment to a pre-existing disease and to present options for dealing with the understood risk for recurrence. Likewise, non-proband counseling performs a similar function by ac-

companying genetic screening in the absence of an index case. In many cases, prenatal diagnostic studies are an available response to a given risk of occurrence or recurrence.

With the current surge of interest in basic gene research, it is likely that future editions of this volume will detail many more techniques for the pre- and postnatal therapy of genetic diseases. Today's clinician may nevertheless derive satisfaction from the application of the many therapeutic modalities that are presently capable of markedly reducing the suffering associated with genetic disease.

Index

769